Georg E. Cold · Bent L. Dahl

Topics in Neuroanaesthesia and Neurointensive Care

Springer-Verlag Berlin Heidelberg GmbH

Georg E. Cold · Bent L. Dahl

Topics in Neuroanaesthesia and Neurointensive Care

Experimental and Clinical Studies upon Cerebral Circulation, Metabolism and Intracranial Pressure

Springer

Dr. Georg E. Cold
Department of Neuroanaesthesia
Århus University Hospital
8000 Århus, Denmark
(E-mail:gcold@aaa.dk)

Dr. Bent L. Dahl
Department of Neuroanaesthesia
Århus University Hospital
8000 Århus, Denmark

ISBN 978-3-642-07537-7 ISBN 978-3-662-04845-0 (eBook)
DOI 10.1007/978-3-662-04845-0

Library of Congress-Cataloging-in-Publication-Data
Cold, G. E. (Georg Emil), 1938- . Topics in neuroanaesthesia and neurointensive care: experimental and clinical studies upon cerebral circulation, metabolism, and intracranial pressure / Georg E. Cold and Bent L. Dahl. p.; cm.
Includes bibliographical references and index.
1. Cerebral circulation. 2. Anesthesiology. 3. Pharmacology. 4. Brain-Effect of drugs on. I. Dahl, Bent L., 1956- . II. Title.
[DNLM: 1. Brain-blood supply. 2. Anesthetics-pharmacology. 3. Brain-drug effects. 4. Brain-metabolism. 5. Intensive Care. 6. Intracranial Pressure. 7. Neurosurgical Procedures. WL 302 C688t 2002] RC388.5.C665 2002 616.8–dc21

http://www.springer.de

Originally published by Springer-Verlag Berlin Heidelberg New York in 2002.
Softcover reprint of the hardcover 1st edition 2002

Production: PRO EDIT GmbH, 69126 Heidelberg, Germany
Cover Design: E. Kirchner, 69121 Heidelberg, Germany
Typesetting: TBS, Sandhausen, Germany
Printed on acid-free paper SPIN: 10833918 21/3130Re - 5 4 3 2 1 0

Preface

The science of neuroanaesthesia and neurointensive care is fascinating, and the amounts of experimental and clinical studies are overwhelming. Surely, everyone can surf Medline and other database systems in order to get information. If you, however, ask for head injury, cerebral ischaemia or barbiturate, you will get hundreds, may be thousands of titles and even the same number of abstracts.

The aims of this book are to review important experimental and clinical data with emphasis on up-dated references. The text within each issue and sub-issue systematically covers experimental and clinical data separately, and details concerning cerebral blood flow, cerebral metabolism, intracranial pressure etc. are reviewed accordingly.

In our survey of the literature we did not use Medline or other database systems systematically. Rather, we used available medical journals which covered the topics of anaesthesia, neuroanaesthesia and neurointensive care. In this way we hope that relevant literature is presented. On the other hand, we cannot exclude that some important issues are omitted.

The book covers 12 topics. In three chapters methodology of CBF measurements, regulation of CBF, and intracranial pressure are described. In the next 6 chapters inhalation anaesthetics, hypnotic agents, analgesics, muscular relaxants, drugs used for control of blood pressure, and the sitting position are reviewed. The last three chapters cover head injury, subarachnoid haemorrhage and cerebral ischaemia.

We hope that the present book might offer some help in daily practice in neuroanaesthesia and in the care of neurointensive patients, when suddenly questions concerning therapy and management arise. Furthermore, we believe that the book might offer an assistance to researchers within the field of neuroanaesthesia, neurosurgery and neurointensive care in finding relevant up-dated references, and be an inspiration to people who want to perform even deeper exploration into the field of neuroscience.

Århus, Denmark, April 2001

Georg Emil Cold
Bent Lob Dahl

Contents

Chapter 1
Methods of cerebral blood flow measurement 1

Hydrogen clearance 1
Microsphere technique 1
The integral method of CBF measurement 2
Venous outflow technique 2
Autoradiographic method 2
The Kety and Schmidt method 3
The intraarterial approach 3
Inhalation and intravenous method 4
Arterio-venous oxygen difference and jugular saturation 4
Single-photon emission computed tomography 4
Positron emission tomography (PET) 5
Stable Xenon method 5
MR imaging methods 6
Doppler flowmetry 6
Laser flowmetry 7
References 7

Chapter 2
Regulation of cerebral blood flow (CBF) 13

Human studies of CBF 13
Human studies of cerebral metabolic rate oxygen (CMRO2) 13
Regulation of CBF (viscosity, haemodilution and cardiac output 16
Regulation by arterial oxygen tension (PaO2) 16
Metabolic regulation 17
Neurogenic regulation 19
Nitric oxide (NO) 20
The effects of different drugs upon CBF 21
Regulation by arterial carbon dioxide (PaCO2) 21
Cerebral autoregulation 26
References 30

Chapter 3
Intracranial pressure 43

Methodology 43
Patophysiology 44
Invasive or surgical approach to control of ICP-hypertension 47
Medical approach to control of ICP-hypertension 47
Control of cerebral blood volume 47

Cerebral arteriolar vasoconstriction . . . 50
Metabolic control of ICP . . . 56
Lidocaine . . . 59
Analgetics . . . 59
Muscular relaxation . . . 60
Osmotic agents and diuretics . . . 60
Kappa-opioid receptor agonists . . . 65
Corticosteroids . . . 65
Calcium blockers . . . 65
Inhibitors of excitatory amino acidss . . . 66
THAM . . . 66
Strategies in the control of ICP-hypertension . . . 66
References . . . 69

Chapter 4
Inhalation anaesthetics . . . 83

Effects of volatile anaesthetics on ion gates and cellular enzyme system . . . 83
Halothane (experimental studies) . . . 85
Haltohane (human studies) . . . 88
Enflurane (experimental studies) . . . 90
Enflurane (human studies) . . . 91
Isoflurane (experimental studies) . . . 92
Isoflurane (human studies) . . . 99
Sevoflurane (experimental studies . . . 102
Sevoflurane (human studies) . . . 103
Desflurane (experimental studies) . . . 104
Desflurane (human studies) . . . 105
Nitrous oxide (experimental studies) . . . 106
Nitrous oxide (human studies) . . . 107
Xenon . . . 108
General conclusion . . . 109
References . . . 110

Chapter 5
Hypnotic agents . . . 125

Receptor action . . . 125
Barbiturate (experimental studies) . . . 126
Barbiturate (human studies) . . . 130
Methohexitone (experimental studies) . . . 132
Methohexitone (human studies) . . . 132
Althesin (experimental studies . . . 132
Althesin (human studies) . . . 133
Etomidate (experimental studies . . . 133
Etomidate (human studies) . . . 134
Ketamin (experimental studies) . . . 135
Ketamin (human studies) . . . 136
Diazepam (experimental studies) . . . 137
Diazepam (human studies) . . . 138
Midazolam (experimental studies) . . . 138
Midazolam (human studies) . . . 139
Propofol (experimental studies) . . . 139
Propofol (human studies) . . . 141

Droperidol (experimental studies) 143
Droperidol (human studies) 144
GABA 144
Etanolone 145
References 145

Chapter 6
Analgesics 159

Action of receptors and transmitters 159
Morphine (experimental studies) 159
Morphine (human studies) 160
Pethidine 160
Phenoperidine 160
Fentanyl (experimental studies) 161
Fentanyl (human studies 162
Neurolept anaesthesia 163
Sufentanil (experimental studies) 163
Sufentanil (human studies) 164
Alfentanil (experimental studies 165
Alfentanil (human studies) 165
Remifentanil (experimental studies) 166
Remifentanil (human studies) 166
Comparative studies of central analgetics 167
Nalaxone (experimental studies) 168
Nalaxone (human studies) 168
References 168

Chapter 7
Neuromuscular blocking agents and local analgesics 173

Succinylcholine (experimental studies) 173
Succinylcholine (human studies) 173
D-tubocuranine (experimental studies) 174
D-tubocuranine (human studies) 174
Pancuronium 174
Atracurium (experimental studies) 174
Atracurium (human studies) 175
Cisatracurium 175
Vecuronium 175
Pipecuronium 175
Lidocaine (experimental studies) 175
Lidocaine (human studies) 177
Procaine 178
Tetracaine 178
Ropivacaine 178
References 178

Chapter 8
Drugs used for control of blood pressure 183

Sodium Nitroprusside (experimental studies) 184
Sodium Nitroprusside (human studies) 186

Nitroglycerin (experimental studies) 186
Nitroglycerin (human studies) 187
Trimethaphan (experimental studies) 187
Trimethaphan (human studies) 188
ATP and adenosine (experimental studies) 189
ATP and adenosine (human studies) 190
Theophylline 191
Dipyridamole 191
Isoflurane 191
α and β blocking agents 192
Ketanserin 193
Postoperative period 193
Calcium blockers 194
Central α_2-agonists 194
Angiotensin converting enzyme inhibitors 197
Prostaglandin E1 197
Clinical application 197
Hypertensive drugs 198
References 201

Chapter 9
The sitting position 211

Cardiovascular effects 211
Cerebrovascular and spinal cord dynamics 212
Air embolism 212
Treatment of air embolism 215
Clinical application 216
Reference 217

Chapter 10
Acute head injury 221

Experimental studies 221
Ischaemia 228
Cerebral oedema 229
Cellular integrity and biochemical disorders 231
Primary damage in human head injury 235
Secondary damage in human head injury 236
Prognostic indicators 239
Regulation of cerebral circulation and metabolism 241
Neurological assessment and monitoring 249
Biochemical studies and monitoring 251
Therapy in acute head injury 256
Guidelines for intensive care unit management 265
References 268

Chapter 11
Aneurysmal subarachnoid haemorrhage 291

Epidemiology 291
Experimental models 292
Intracranial pressure 293

Central and cerebral haemodynamics 294
Vasospasm 297
CSF biochemistry 302
Cardiac arrhythmia 303
Treatment 303
Monitoring 313
Perioperative management 316
References 321

Chapter 12
Ischaemia 337

Ischaemic thresholds 337
Spreading depression 340
Reperfusion after ischaemia 341
Brain oedema 344
Biochemical changes in the ischaemic cell 346
Gene expression 360
Cerebral acidosis and glucose 367
Temperature 369
Different receptors 370
Other drugs 374
References 376

Subject Index 405

Abbreviations

A	Adenosine
AMPA	Alpha-amino-3-hydroxy-5-methyl-4-isovasole proprionic acid
AVDO2	Arterio-venous oxygen content difference
AVS	N,N-propylenedinicotinamide
BBB	Blood-brain barrier
CA	Cerebral autoregulation
CBF	Cerebral blood flow
CBV	Cerebral blood volume
CMRO2	Cerebral metabolic rate of oxygen
CPP	Central venous pressure
CVR	Cerebral vascular resistance
CSF	Cerebrospinal fluid
CT	Computerized tomography
CT-Xe	Stable Xenon computerized tomography
DAI	Diffuse axonal injury
DHE	Dihydroergotamine
EAA	Excitatory amino acid
ECG	Electrocardiogram
EDRF	Endothelium-derived relaxing factor (NO)
EEG	Electroencephalogram
ET	Endothelin
GABA	γ-aminobutyric acid
HI	Head injury
HSP	Heat shock protein
ICAM-1	Intercellular adhesion molecule-1
ICP	Intracranial pressure
LOI	Lactate/oxygen index
IVP	Intraventricular pressure
MABP	Mean arterial blood pressure
MAC	Middle cerebral artery occlusion
MAC	Middle cerebral artery
MR	Magnetic resonance
MRI	Magnetic resonance imaging
MG	Nitroglycerin
NAME	NG-nitro-L-arginine methyl ester
NIRS	Near-infrared spectroscopy
NMDA	N-methyl-d-aspartate
NMMA	NG-monomethyl-L-arginine
OEF	Oxygen extraction fraction
PAF	Platelet-activating factor
PET	Positron emission tomography
PKC	Protein kinase C
PVI	Pressure volume index
Q10	The ratio of metabolic rates at two temperatures differing by 100C
SAH	Subarachnoid haemorrhage

SD	Spreading depression
SNP	Sodium nitroprusside
SOD	Superoxide dismutase
SPECT	Single photon emission computed tomography
TCD	Transcranial Doppler
THAM	Trishydroxy-methylaminomethan
TMP	Trimethaphan
VIP	Vasoactive intestinal polypeptide

Methods of cerebral blood flow measurements

Measurement of cerebral blood flow (CBF) is based on the use of freely diffusible indicators, which reach the brain tissue by the arterial system and give rise to a fast and complete equivalence in concentration between blood and tissue. The principle of calculation of CBF is based on the measurement of mean transit time. The technique has been developed during the last 40 years, and was originally introduced by Kety and Schmidt (1945) with the use of nitrous oxide as tracer. Later, the technique was elaborated to include diffusible indicators including ^{85}Kr and ^{133}Xe. The Kety and Schmidt and the intraarterial ^{133}Xe methods have been used in animal experiments and clinical studies. By surgical removal of soft tissue over the calvaria, and ^{133}Xe injection in the lingual artery it is possible to avoid extracerebral contamination in monkeys and rats (Harper and Jennett 1968, Hertz et al. 1977). During the last 25 years tomographic methods for regional CBF measurement have been developed. These methods include single-photon emission tomography (SPECT), stable Xenon method, positron emission tomography (PET) and technique based on magnetic resonance. Furthermore Doppler sonography and Laser Doppler flowmetry have been introduced.

Among techniques for CBF measurement the hydrogen clearance- , microsphere- venous outflow- , and autoradiographic methods are used in experimental studies. The Kety and Schmidt method, the intraarterial ^{133}Xe method, the arterio-venous oxygen difference method, SPECT, PET, stable Xenon method, magnetic resonance, Doppler flowmetry and Laser Doppler flowmetry are used for experimental as well as clinical studies.

Hydrogen clearance

The Hydrogen clearance technique introduced by Aukland et al. (1964) has some advantages in experimental studies, because of its ability to obtain multiple flow measurements over long periods of time (up to 10 hours), the ability to measure flow in a small tissue volume and the stability of the partition coefficient, especially in damaged tissue. The measurement of rCBF is based on a linear function between electrode current and tissue hydrogen concentration, provided that the thickness of the diffusion layer is constant. The limit of resolution is $5 \times 5 \times 5$ mm. Comparisons with other methodologies (venous outflow, ^{133}Xe, radioactive microspheres and ^{14}C antipyrine) have shown fairly good correlation's (Rowan et al. 1975, LaMorgese et al. 1975, Heiss and Traupe 1981). On the other hand, the technique is traumatic, giving rise to tissue injury due to electrode implantation resulting in loss of autoregulation, hyperaemia and oedema (Tuor and Farrar 1984). Moreover, zero baseline stability can be difficult to obtain. Arterial recirculation of hydrogen and inter-compartmental diffusion might be causes of error as well (For review see Farrar 1987).

Microsphere technique

Microsphere cerebral blood flow determination was introduced by Roth et al. (1970). A number of conditions must be fulfilled for the accurate reflection of CBF by microspheres. The microspheres must be well mixed at the injection site, the distribution in the blood stream must be proportional to the actual blood flow, the microspheres must be trapped completely on first passage and not disturb the regional or general circulation, and they must be stabely lodged until counted. Currently ten isotopes for labelling microspheres are available. Each isotope is characterised by specific gamma energy peak, thereby allowing detection by differential spectrometry. Organ blood flow in relative term is calculated as the percentage of spheres in an area of interest in relation to the total number of spheres injected. In absolute terms, blood flow can be calculated by measuring cardiac output by a separate technique (Nuetze et al. 1968, Mendell and Hollenberg 1971), or by determining a reference organ blood flow by withdrawing blood at a constant rate during the microsphere injection (Makowski et al. 1968, Domenech et al. 1969). Under normal physiological conditions good correlation between CBF determined by microsphere technique and CBF obtained with ^{133}Xe (Fan et al. 1979, Marcus et al. 1981), iodoantipyrine (Horton et al. 1980) and hydrogen clearance (Heiss and Traupe 1981) have been found. Under pathologic conditions a good correlation was found to the xenon technique at flow rates below 120 ml/100g/min, but not above this flow rate (Marcus et al. 1981). During middle cerebral artery occlusion, flow determined by the microsphere method consistently showed higher flow values than those obtained with the hydrogen clearance method (Heiss and Traupe 1981). In anaesthetized and awake animals the microsphere technique works well. Both regional and whole brain blood flow are easily obtained, and the calculation of flow is independent on the diffusion coefficient. Shunting of microspheres might occur especially under pathological conditions and during anaesthesia. It must be stressed that the use of microspheres in various pathologic models has not been fully evaluated. The limit of resolution is 8 x 8 x 8 mm.

The integral method of CBF measurement

In non-steady states, CBF measurement of shorter duration may be necessary. A method described by Gjedde et al. (1980) is based on an extension of the integral method of Landau et al. (1955). With this method a bolus injection of labelled butanol is given intravenously. Arterial blood is withdrawn into a syringe for 20 seconds. After 20 seconds the animal is decapitated, and the brain removed, dissected, and vials of brain tissue are analysed. The present method resembles the microsphere technique, but has the advantage that the indicator causes minimal circulatory derangement, and the microcirculation of the brain is not affected. Modification of this method has been used in rats (Gjedde et al. 1980), gerbil (van Uitert and Levy 1978) and monkeys (Raichle et al. 1976).

Venous outflow technique

Venous outflow from the confluence of the sagital and straight sinuses can be measured. If the lateral sinuses and the emissary veins are occluded, the venous outflow represents CBF. From the confluence of the sinuses the blood passes through a transducer probe or an electromagnetic flowmeter. This method was introduced by Rapela and Green (1964), and was further elaborated in the dog by Michenfelder et al. (1968) and Michenfelder and Theye (1968), who during normocapnia found a good correlation between flow determined by the venous outflow technique and CBF obtained by the ^{133}Xe method. In dogs, the obtained venous outflow represents drainage from 43% of the brain (Michenfelder et al. 1968). In rats continuous venous outflow can be measured after cannulation of the retroglenoid vein (Meldrum and Nilsson 1976, Nilsson and Siesjö 1983). This method has been investigated by Morii et al. (1986), who found minimal extracerebral contamination and a good correlation to flow obtained by the microsphere technique.

Autoradiographic methods

The autoradiographic method of measurement of CBF is based on Ketys study of the kinetics of exchange. The method was introduced by Landau et al. (1955) and Freygang and Sokoloff (1958) using J^{131}trifluoroiodomethane as a tracer. In 1969 Reivich and co-workers introduced antipyrine-14C, whilst Sukurada et al. (1978) introduced iodo-C^{14}antipyrine which has a greater blood-brain barrier permeability compared with C^{14}antipyrine. The calculation of local CBF is determined from the concentration of the tracer in the region of interest. Under the assumptions that the tracer is biologically inert, the tracer in the effluent veins of the tissue is in equilibrium with the brain, the CBF remains in a steady state during the period of measurement, and the value of the partition coefficient of the tracer can be determined, the values of CBF are correct. The limit of resolution is < 1 mm. It has been shown that autoradiographic strategy tends to underestimate flow, especially at increased flow rates (Eklöf et al. 1974) and under ischaemic conditions. Tomita and Gotoh (1981) have stressed that the method is inaccurate because of incomplete tracer mixing in ischaemic tissue and altered tracer permeability. However, if very short tracer infusion periods are used, local CBF can be measured by a modification of the indicator fractionation technique elaborated by Goldman and Sapirstein (1973). This technique has been used autoradiographically to estimate local CBF even in small animals (Pulsinelli et al. 1982).

After the development of the ^{14}C2-deoxyglucose method for measurement of regional cerebral glucose utilisation ($rCMR_{glucose}$) (Sokoloff et al. 1977), matched animal series for studies of rCBF and glucose utilisation have been possible. This double-tracer autoradiographic strategy has later on been developed (Lear et al. 1981, Ginsberg et al. 1986). Lear et al. (1984) have developed a generalised mathematic approach that allows two or more radionuclides with different half-lives to be used simultaneously to measure multiple aspects of cerebral function. In the method of Sokoloff for $rCMR_{glucose}$ determination, local 2-deoxyglucose accumulation is the basis for estimation of local glucose phosphorylation. However, only in normal tissue the rate of 2-deoxyglucose accumulation can be assumed to be a known fraction of glucose consumption. If the relationship between plasma and brain glucose has changed, a correction ratio of 2-deoxyglucose accumulation to glucose consumption (the lumped constant) might be determined separately by 3-O methylglucose autoradiography. Methods for this triple-tracer technique has been developed by Gjedde and Diemer (1983).

The Kety and Schmidt method

Measurement of CBF in humans was introduced by Kety and Schmidt with nitrous oxide as freely diffusible indicator (Kety 1945, Kety and Schmidt 1948). The method as originally described by Kety presumes catheterisation of the internal jugular vein, either by insertion of a catheter from the lateral or anterior approach of the neck. The tip of the catheter is directed cranially and placed at the base of the skull. Furthermore, a catheter in a peripheral artery is necessary. During a 15–30 min period of inhalation of the diffusible tracer, or during exhalation of the tracer after establishment of equilibrium between blood and brain tissue, samples of arterial and jugular venous blood are withdrawn at fixed intervals and the concentration of tracer determined. By the use of the height-over-area formula CBF is calculated globally in ml/100g/min. By simultaneous determination of arterial and venous blood oxygen content, the arterio-venous oxygen content difference ($AVDO_2$) is calculated in vol%, and by simple multiplication the cerebral metabolic rate of oxygen ($CMRO_2$) expressed as ml O_2/100g/min is calculated. In the adult the normal value of global CBF based on a 10 minutes saturation period and measured during normothermia and normocapnia is 50 ml/100g/min (Lassen and Munck 1955, Lassen 1959).

Insertion of a jugular venous catheter has been described by Oshima et al. (1991) and Jakobsen and Enevoldsen (1989). Other studies have shown that jugular bulb catheterisation does not increase intracranial pressure (Goetting and Preston 1991).

The method has been criticised because of contamination of extracranial venous blood (Lassen and Lane 1961), and central venous blood (Steinbach et al. 1976, Murray et al. 1978). Naturally, the method does not give information of regional distribution of CBF. The method is time consuming and requires a constant CBF and cerebral metabolism for at least 15 min. Moreover, the results of CBF calculation are not immediately available. On the other hand, the method gives a reliable estimate of global CBF and metabolism. Peroperatively, during intracranial surgery, the application of the method is fairly easy, and the operative procedure is not disturbed. Sapirstein and Ogden (1965) have argued, that erroneous results of CBF are obtained by this method, because the arterial and venous desaturation or saturation curves never reach each other during the period of investigation. This error results in an overestimation of CBF.

The intra-arterial approach

The Kety Schmidt method has been developed into an intra-arterial residue technique using ^{85}Kr, ^{133}Xe and nitrous oxide as a tracer (Lassen and Ingvar 1963, Høedt-Rasmussen et al. 1966). This modification presumes catheterisation of the internal carotid artery. Owing to neurological complications, due to microembolisation or spasms of the cerebral arteries, the method has been criticised (Ingvar and Lassen 1973). Using meticulous technique and heparinised catheters the neurological complications have been found to be negligible (Lassen 1986). The principles of calculation are identical with the original Kety Schmidt technique. Using externally placed scintillation detectors the technique has been sophisticated to include 254 regional detectors (Sveinsdottir et al. 1977). Together with compartmental analysis, the method gives information of flow in grey and white matter and the weight of these substances (Høedt-Rasmussen 1967). The method has been applied in clinical studies of cerebral diseases including cerebral tumours, stroke, aneurysm and head injury. Accordingly, important information concerning the regulation of CBF in relation to brain function and metabolic activity has been obtained (Ingvar and Lassen 1975).

By analysis of the first two minutes of the semilogarithmically displaced clearance curve, Olesen et al. (1971) stated that the initial slope correlates fairly well to the values obtained by the principles of mean transit time. The initial slope has been used extensively because it only requires 2 min of data collection. In studies of head injury (HI) an initial fast component referred to as tissue peak has been described (Kasoff et al. 1972, Enevoldsen et al. 1976, Cold et al. 1978). Tissue peaks are observed in regions with cerebral contusion and subdural hematoma, and are thought to develop secondarily to tissue ischaemia. It must be emphasised that compared with the compartmental analysis, the initial slope index underestimates grey matter flow by 20–30% (Lassen and Christensen 1976), and overestimates flow based on mean CBF. Consequently, the method does not give true values for calculation of $CMRO_2$. The normal value of CBF-initial in normothermic, normocapnic man is 65 ml/100g/min (Olesen et al. 1971).

Inhalation and intravenous methods

Inhalation or intravenous injection of ^{133}Xe have to some extent displaced the intra-arterial approach. These two methods have been developed by Mallett and Veall (1963) and Agnoli et al. (1969) respectively and have been elaborated by others (Obrist et al. 1967, Austin et al. 1972, Risberg et al. 1975, Wyper and Brooke 1977). In comparison with the intra-arterial approach both methods are atraumatic; consequently, these methods have gained some popularity. Via externally placed scintillation detectors often 10–32 in total, regional CBF (rCBF) is calculated. The calculation is complicated and cannot be done by visual analysis of the clearance curves. Corrections for flow in extracranial regions and remaining activity are necessary. However, the method has been accepted in clinical studies including repeated studies of CBF. It has been stated that flows determined by compartmental analysis are less stable than non-compartmental indices, especially when grey matter flow is less than 50 ml (Obrist and Wilkinson 1985). Accordingly, Risberg et al. (1975) have elaborated an initial slope index (ISI) based on the slope between 2 and 3 min. of the recirculation-corrected curve. With the inhalation technique the spatial resolution is fairly poor, the "cross-talk" from the opposite hemisphere being a constant phenomenon (Wyper and Brooke 1977), and it has been argued that reliable results in clinical studies of focal lesions of ischaemia or flow deprivation are not possible (Halsey 1981). Thus, it has been argued that regions with low perfusion will be "looked through" due to the high radiation from adjacent tissue areas (Donley et al. 1975), Risberg 1980, Ingvar and Lassen 1982). However, other studies including evaluation of sensitivity of the inhalation technique to ischaemic and probe-by-probe tests by use of ISI indices have shown that the inhalation technique is acceptable sensitive as regards ability to detect ischaemic flow (Ewing et al. 1981, Ewing et al. 1983). Another study in patients subjected to endarterectomy, indicates that the correlation between intra-carotid and intravenous method was excellent (Young et al. 1990). Stationary equipment with 32 channels has been used for several years. Mobile equipment with 10 to 16 detectors has the advantage that transport of the patient to the CBF equipment is avoided. Thus, bed-side studies in the intensive care unit are possible.

Arterio-venous oxygen difference ($AVDO_2$) and jugular venous saturation

From the formula $CBF \cdot AVDO_2 = CMRO_2$ it is obvious that $CBF = K/AVDO_2$. On the assumption that the physical dissolved oxygen content and the concentrations of haemoglobin in arterial and venous blood are identical $AVDO_2$ can be replaced by 100-SAT_{venous}. The inverse relationship between CBF and $AVDO_2$ can be used in longitudinal studies on the assumption that $CMRO_2$ is constant. Under circumstances where this assumption is fulfilled, repeated studies of $AVDO_2$ have been used in autoregulation studies to demonstrate the relationship between cerebral perfusion pressure and CBF and in studies of relative CO_2 reactivity.

Single-photon emission computed tomography (SPECT)

In comparison with PET, unpaired detectors are used during Single-photon emission computed tomography (SPECT). SPECT has been designed for regional studies using ^{133}Xe inhalation (Stokely et al. 1980. After xenon inhalation for 1-2 min. a series of tomogram is ready (Lassen et al. 1981). This method yields a resolution of 1.5 to 1.7 cm (Holm et al. 1985). With the introduction of iodine-, thallium- and technetium-labelled tracers SPECT has been shown to play an important role in the diagnosis and management of cerebral diseases (For review, see Holman and Hill 1987). Compared with CT scanning, SPECT is stated to have the following advantages: By reflecting changes in cerebral perfusion SPECT is more sensitive than CT scanning in demonstrating cerebral lesions, and SPECT demonstrates the lesions at an earlier stage compared with CT scanning (Abdel-Dayem et al. 1987).

Positron emission tomography (PET)

Positron emission tomography (PET) is based on positron emitting radionuclides, which after travelling few millimetres in the tissue interact with an electron, resulting in annihilation radiation with two gamma photons travelling in an opposite direction. Pairs of externally placed detectors are positioned on either side of the gamma source and connected by electronic coincidence circuits and only recording signals when two photons arrive within a very short time interval. In this way only photons arriving from positron annihilation are recorded (Phleps et al. 1975). A PET device consists of a large number of detector pairs. The information obtained from these detectors is combined to produce a two dimensional reconstruction of the regional radio-reactivity within the field (Ter-Pogossian 1977).

The radioisotopes used in PET to label compounds are ^{11}C, ^{13}N, $^{15}0$ and ^{18}F. Compounds for measurement of CBF include $^{15}0$-labeled H_2O, ^{15}C labelled CO_2, ^{18}F labelled CH_3F, [^{11}C] butanol and [^{18}F] fluoroethanol. For CBV [^{11}C]CO, [^{15}C]CO, [^{68}Ga] EDTA are used. For tissue pH [^{11}C] DMO and [^{11}C] CO_2, and for oxygen extraction and metabolism [^{15}O] O_2. Metabolism of glucose, amino acids, protein synthesis and free fatty acids can be studied with PET technique. Also neurotransmitters including dopamine, benzodiazepine, opiate, adrenergic- and cholinergic systems have been studied by PET. .

PET permits in vivo measurements of rCBF, regional blood volume, regional oxygen utilisation and regional values of lambda (blood brain partition coefficient) (Kanno and Lassen 1979, Phleps et al. 1982, Huang et al. 1982, Raichle 1983). The limit of resolution is 4 mm. rCBF is measured during inhalation of ^{15}O-labelled CO_2, which is transferred to ^{15}O-labelled H_2O in the pulmonary vascular bed. After 10 min. of inhalation a steady state is achieved where the amount of the tracer entering the brain equals the amount leaving by washout and radioactive decay. Another modification is based on iv bolus injection of tracer (PET-autoradiographic approach). In comparison with the inhalation-steady-state method a linear correlation between radioactivity and rCBF is obtained, and no amplification error is seen at higher flows. In cerebrovascular diseases PET studies can distinguish ischaemic from infarcted tissue by studying CBF and metabolism. In patients with stenosis of cerebral arteries, monitoring of rCBV with PET can indicate haemodynamically compromised regions of the brain. These patients are at a higher risk of infarction (Brooks 1991).

Clinical PET studies in healthy volunteers (Østergaard et al. 1998), cerebral arterial occlusion diseases (Yamauchi et al. 1996) and subarachnoid haemorrhage (Pichard et al. 2000) are available

Stable xenon method

Using Enhancement of CT scans during inhalation of 30-50% stable Xenon, an atraumatic tomographic approach to rCBF mapping is possible (Winkler et al. 1977, Drayer et al. 1978). Normal values of rCBF have been assessed by Yonas et al. (1991) who found mixed cortical flows averaging 51 ml/100g/min. This method has been developed by several groups and has been used in experimental studies of focal ischaemia (Yonas et al. 1988), in clinical studies of head injury (Yonas et al. 1984c, Wozney et al. 1985, Harrington et al. 1986, Darby et al. 1988), cerebral aneurysms (Yonas et al. 1984b), cerebral infarcts (Drayer et al. 1980, Yonas et al. 1984a) and multiple-vessel occlusion (Yonas et al. 1985). Available rCBF mapping 5 min after stable Xenon inhalation is possible, each voxel measuring 1 x 1 x 5 mm. The method has the interesting advantage, that it is possible to calculate both the regional distribution of rCBF and that of the partition coefficient (lambda) (Meyer et al. 1980, Dhawan et al. 1984). With this method important information on the occurrence of cerebral oedema and infarction is possible (Segawa et al. 1983, Yonas et al. 1984b).

Xenon, an anaesthetic gas, induces an increase in CBF (Junck et al. 1985, Gur et al. 1985, Obrist et al. 1985, Hartmann et al. 1991), an increase in the CO_2 reactivity and impairment of the cerebral autoregulation (Hartmann et al. 1987). Studies in primates subjected to freeze-injury indicate that stable Xenon does not increase ICP (Darby et al. 1991). However, in clinical studies of severe head injury stable Xenon inhalation sometimes increases ICP dangerously (Bergholt et al. 1994). Furthermore, stable Xenon inhalation gives rise to respiratory irregularities with bradypnea and bronchospasm and changes in the state of consciousness with risks of vomiting and aspiration (Yonas et al. 1987), and in awake normal volunteers the administration of stable xenon will be accompanied by hyperventilation suggesting that cautious interpretation is necessary in the assessment of rCBF with stable xenon (Hartmann et al. 1991).

In patients with impaired pulmonary function rCBF is underestimated when rCBF quantification is based on end-tidal xenon input curves and not arterial Xenon curves (von Oettingen et al. 2000). Stable Xenon CT studies in patients with acute head injury are published by Reinert et al. (2000).

MR imaging methods

Perfusion-weighted MR imaging

MR techniques to measure cerebral perfusion are devided into two main categories. MR CBF by non-diffusible tracers utilizes dynamical susceptibility contrast magnetic resonance imaging, tracking the passage of a rapidly injected MR contrast agent (paramagnetic Gd based chelate). The second catagory utilises diffusible tracers detectable by MR. The intrinsic water in blood is hence labeled by external radio excitation, and the inflow of labeled water into the tissue recorded. With this technique relative CBF values are obtained (Østergaard et al. 1996). In experimental studies of hypercapnia an approach was introduced to allow absolute quantification of CBF by introducing an empirical normalisation constant (Østergaard et al. 1998). With this technique comparison between PET-CBF and MR-CBF has been performed in healthy adults (Østergaard et al. 1998). Magnetic resonance technique has also been used for regional blood-brain barrier studies, and studies of regional cerebral blood volume (Østergaard et al. 1999).

By use of perfusion-weighted MR imaging a variety of markers including CBF, CBV, mean transit time, bolus-relaxivity, and bolus time-to-peak have been used for imaging (Warach et al. 1992, Sorensen et al. 1996, Tong et al. 1998, Neumann-Haefelin et al. 1999, Zaharchuk et al. 2000). In a recent study it was found that haemodynamic parameters, including CBF and CBV, were found to have significant discordant behaviour in the early ischaemic period. Thus care is required when interpreting perfusion-weighted imaging studies in humans that use different markers or combination of markers to assess ischaemic damage after human stroke (Zaharchuk et al. 2000).

Diffusion-weighted MR imaging

Diffusion-weighted MR imaging provides physiologic information about the self-diffusion of water, thereby detecting one of the first elements in the pathophysiological cascade leading to ischaemic injury (Baird and Warach 1998). The overall principle of diffusion measurement is that the spatial location of each water molecule over the time of observation results in a signal loss or darkening of the images. Because of restricted diffusion in biological tissue, self diffusion of water is referred to as apparent diffusion coefficient (ADC). The normal ADC in the brain is a weighted average of the diffusion constants in the extracellular and intracellular compartments (van Zijl et al. 1991, Benveniste et al. 1992). The values of ADC in grey matter range from 0.8 to 1.2 x 10^{-3} mm^2/sec, and in white matter from 0.3 to 1,2 10^{-3} mm^2/sec. In contrast ADC for CSF ranges from 2-3 10^{-3} mm^2/sec. Reduced ADC has been demonstrated as early as 105 min. after onset of ischaemic stroke (Warach et al. 1992a) On serial diffusion-weighted imaging the evolution and enlargement of acute stroke can be followed (Baird et al. 1997). By combining diffusion- and perfusion-weighted imaging it is possible to delineate the upper and lower boundaries of the volume of tissue at risk for eventual infarction (Sorensen et al. 1997), and define the ischaemic penumbra (Schlaug et al. 1997).

Clinical perfusion- and diffusion-weighted MR studies in stroke patients (Østergaard et al. 2000, Lansberg et al. 2000, Kluymans et al. 2000, Karonen et al. 2000, Karonen et al. 2001) are published recently. An experimental study in acute head injury is presented by Assaf et al. (1999), and a clinical study in acute head injury by Liu et al. (1999).

Blood oxygenation level-dependent (BOLD) contrast

The method is based on a change in the signal strength of the brain water protons produced by the paramagnetic effects of venous blood deoxyhemoglobin. BOLD has been used to image changes in brain haemodynamics produced by human mental operations. Several models suggest that BOLD contrast depends on tissue blood volume fraction, metabolic rate of oxygen, cerebral blood flow, hematocrit besides capillary and venous oxygenation state (Ogawa et al. 1993, Boxerman et al. 1995, Hathout et al. 1995, Buxton et al. 1998, van Zijl et al. 1998).

Doppler flowmetry

Using low frequency Doppler sonography transmitted through thin areas of the skull, e.g. the "temporal window" located above the zygomatic arch between the ear and orbit, direction-sensitive probes incorporating range gating can measure velocities in the cerebral arteries at selected depths within the skull.

This technique has the advantages of being non-invasive, accurate, reproducible and fast and ideal for continuous assessment of flow-velocity, especially in the middle cerebral arterial. Doppler measurement for velocity was developed by Aaslid et al. 1982). Like CBF, absolute velocities vary with age, haematocrit, $PaCO_2$, and cerebral metabolite activity (Caplan et al. 1990). Velocity is directly proportional to CBF and inversely proportional to the lumen of the vessel studied. This means that if spasm of the artery is present an increase in velocity is observed. The method has been used in clinical studies of vasospasm caused by subarachnoid haemorrhage (Lindegaard et al. 1989, Jakobsen et al. 1990) and traumatic brain lesion (Weber et al. 1990).The correlation between mean flow velocity and CBF measured by Xenon-CT has been analysed during acetazolamide administration and during hyperventilation. The correlation coefficient for relative changes in CBF and flow velocity for the overall population was r = 0.82. In subgroups of patients the correlation coefficient differed between 0.39 and 0.5, respectively, suggesting that the correlation between flow velocity and CBF varies with intracranial pathology (Brauer et al. 1998).

Laser Doppler flowmetry

The operating principles of laser Doppler flowmetry are similar to those of ultrasound Doppler. A low power laser beam is conducted to the cerebral tissue by an optical fibre. The shift in Doppler signal is proportional to the velocity of moving red cells. Blood flow is calculated by determining the product of blood volume and blood velocity, expressed in arbitrary units. In comatose patients a gradual increase in laser flow was correlated to clinical improvement (Meyerson et al. 1991). In patients with severe head injury changes in laser flow was found to be coupled to changes in cerebral perfusion pressure (Kirkpatrick et al. 1994). Lam et al. (1997) studied cerebral autoregulation in patients with severe head injury, and could identify patients with impaired and intact autoregulation. Likewise Smielewski et al. (1997) studied autoregulation by the hyperaemic response method using transcranial Doppler and laser flowmetry and found a significant correlation (r = 0.69) between the hyperaemic indices calculated by the two modalities.

References

Aaslid R, Markwalder TH, Nornes H. Noninvasive transcranial Doppler ultrasound recording of flow in basal cerebral arteries. J Neurosurg 1982: 57: 769–744

Abdel-Dayem HM, Sadek SA, et al. Changes in cerebral perfusion after acute head injury: comparison of CT with Tc-99m HM-PAO SPECT. Radiology 1987: 165: 221–226.

Agnoli A, Principe M, Priori AM, et al. Measurements of rCBF by intravenous injection of 113-Xe. In Cerebral Blood Flow. Brock M, Fieschi C, Ingvar DH, Lassen NA (eds). Springer Verlag, Berlin, Heidelberg, New York 1969: 31–34.

Assaf Y, Holokovsky A, Berman E, et al. Diffusion and perfusion magnetic resonance imaging following closed head injury in rats. J Neurotrauma 1999: 16: 1165–1176.

Aukland K, Bower BF, Berliner RW. Measurement of local blood flow with hydrogen gas. Circ Res 1964: 14: 164–187.

Austin G, Horn N, Rouhe S, Hayward W. Description and early results of an intravenous radioisotope technique for measuring regional cerebral blood flow in man. Europ Neurol 1972: 8: 43–51.

Baird AE, Warach S. Magnetic resonance imaging of acute stroke. J Cereb Blood Flow Metab 1998: 18: 583–609.

Benveniste H, Hedlund LW, Johnson GA. Mechanism of detection of acute cerebral ischemia in rats by diffusion-weighted magnetic resonance microscopy. Stroke 1992: 23: 746–754.

Baird AED, Benfield A, Schlaug G, et al. Enlargement of human cerebral ischemia lesion volumes measured by diffusion-weighted magnetic resonance imaging. Ann Neurol 1997: 41: 581–589.

Boxerman JL, Bandettini PA, Kwong KK, et al. The intravascular contribution to fMRI signal change: Monte Carlo modelling and diffusion weighted studies in vivo. Magn Reson Med 1995: 34: 4–10.

Brauer P, Kochs E, Werner C. et al. Correlation of transcranial Doppler sonography mean flow velocity with cerebral blood flow in patients with intracranial pathology. J Neurosurg Anesthesiol 1998: 10: 80–85.

Brooks DJ. The clinical role of PET in cerebrovascular disease. Neurosurg Rev 1991: 14: 91–96.

Buxton RB, Wong EC, Frank LR. Dynamics of blood flow and oxygenation changes during brain activation: the balloon model. Magn Reson Med 1998: 39: 855–864.

Caplan LR, Brass LM, DeWitt LD et al. Transcranial Doppler ultrasound: Present status. Neurology 1990: 40: 696–700

Cold GE, Jensen FT. Cerebral autoregulation in unconscious patients with brain injury. Acta Anaesth Scand 1978: 22: 270–280.

Darby JM, Yonas H, Marion DW, Latchaw RE. Local inverse steal induced by hyperventilation in head injury. Neurosurgery 1988: 23: 84–88.

Darby JM, Nemoto EM, Yonas H, Melick J. Stable Xenon does not increase intracranial pressure in primates with freeze-injury-induced intracranial hypertension. J Cereb Blood Flow Metab 1991: 11: 522–526.

Dhawan V, Haughton VM, Thaler HT, et al. Accuracy of stable Xenon/CT measurements of regional cerebral blood flow: Effect of extrapolated estimates of brain-blood partition coefficients. J Comput Assist Tomogr 1984: 8: 208–212.

Domenech RJ, Hoffman JIE, Noble MIN, et al. Total and regional coronary blood flow measured by radioactive mi-

crospheres in conscious and anesthetized dogs. Circ Res 1969: 25: 581–596.
Donley RF, Sundt TM, Anderson RE, Sharbrough FW. Blood flow measurements and the "look through" artifact in focal ischemia. Stroke 1975: 6: 121–131
Drayer BP, Wolfsen SK Jr, Reinmuth OM, et al. Xenon enhanced computed tomography for the analyses of cerebral integrity, perfusion and blood flow. Stroke 1978: 9: 123–212.
Drayer BP, Gur D, Yonas H, et al. Abnormalities of the Xenon brain-blood partition coefficient and blood flow in cerebral infarction. An in vivo assessment using transmission computed tomography. Radiology 1980: 135: 349–354.
Eklöf B, Lassen NA, Nilsson L, et al. Regional cerebral blood flow in the rat measured by tissue sampling technique; a critical evaluation using four indicators C14-antipyrine, C14-ethanol, H3-water, and 133-Xenon. Acta Physiol Scand: 1974: 91: 1–10.
Enevoldsen EM, Cold GE, Jensen FT, Malmros R. Dynamic changes in regional CBF, intraventricular pressure, CSF pH and lactate levels during the acute phase of head injury. J Neurosurg 1976: 44: 191–214.
Ewing JR, Keating EG, Sheehe PR, et al. Concordance of inhalation rCBFs with clinical evidence of cerebral ischaemia. Stroke 1981: 12: 188–195.
Ewing JR, Welch KMA, Robertson WM, et al. A probe-by probe identification of focal cerebral ischemia using the ^{133}Xe inhalation technique. J Cereb Blood Flow Metab 1983: 1: 586–587.
Fan FC, Chen RYZ, Schuessler GB, Chien S. Comparison between the ^{133}Xe clearance method and microsphere technique in cerebral blood flow determinations in the dog. Circ Res 1979: 44: 653–659.
Farrar JK, Hydrogen clearance technique. In Cerebral Blood Flow (ed) Wood JH. McGraw-Hill Company 1987: 275–287.
Freygang WH Jr, Sokoloff L. Quantitative measurement of regional circulation in the central nervous system by the use of radioactive inert gas. Adv Biol Med Physics 1958: 6: 263–279.
Ginsberg MD, Smith DW, Wachtel MS, et al. Simultaneous determination of local cerebral glucose utilization and blood flow by carbon-14, doulbe-label autoradiography: Method of procedure and validation studies in the rat. J Cereb Blood Flow Metab 1986: 6: 273–285.
Gjedde A, Hansen AJ, Siemkowicz E Rapid simultaneous determination of regional blood flow and blood-brain glucose in brain of rat. Acta Physiol Scand 1980: 108: 321–330
Gjedde A, Diemer NH. Autoradiographic determination of regional brain glucose content. J Cereb Blood Flow Metab 1983: 3: 303–310.
Goetting MG, Preston G. Jugular bulb catheterization does not increase intracranial pressure. Intensive Care Med 1991: 17: 195–198
Goldman H, Sapirstein LA. Brain blood flow in the conscious and anesthetized rat. Am J Physiol 1973: 224: 122–126
Gur D, Yonas H, Jackson DL, et al. Measurement of cerebral blood flow during Xenon inhalation as measured by the microspheres method. Stroke 1985: 16: 871–874.
Halsey J. Is there clinical value in measurement of rCBF? (Editorial). rCBF Bullitin 1981: 1: 5.
Harper AM, Jennett WB. Simultaneous measurement of beta and gamma clearance curves of radioactive inert gases from the monkey brain. In: Blood Flow through organs and tissues. Bin WH, Harper AM (eds), Livingstone Ltd, Edinburgh, London 1968: 214.
Harrington TR, Manwaring K, Hodak J. Local basal ganglia and brain stem blood flow in head injured patients using stable Xenon enhanced CT scanning. In: Intracranial Pressure VI, Miller JD, Teasdale GM, Rowan JO, Galbraith SL, Mendelow AD (eds). Springer Verlag, Berlin, Heidelberg 1986: 680–686.
Hartmann A, Wassman H, Czernicki Z, et al. Effect of stable Xenon in room air on regional cerebral blood flow and electroencephalogram in normal baboons. Stroke 1987: 18: 643–648.
Hartmann A, Dettmers C, Schuier FJ, et al. Effect of stable Xenon on regional cerebral blood flow and the electroencephalogram in normal volunteers. Stroke 1991: 22: 182–189
Hathout GM, Gambhir SS, Gopi RK, et al. A Quantitative physiologic model of blood oxygenation for functional magnetic resonance imaging. Invest Radiol 1995: 30: 669–682.
Heiss WD, Traube H. Comparison between hydrogen clearance and microsphere technique for rCBF measurement. Stroke 1981: 12: 161–167
Hertz MM, Hemmingsen R, Bolvig TG. Rapid and repetitive measurements of blood flow and oxygen consumption in the rat brain using intraarterial Xenon injection. Acta Physiol Scand 1977: 101: 501.
Holm S, Vorsted S, Lassen NA, Paulson OB. Physical factors affecting calculated cerebral blood flow values in hypoperfused areas in single photon emission computerized tomography. In: Hartman A, Hoyer S (eds) Cerebral Blood Flow and Metabolism, Springer Verlag, Heidelberg 1985: 234–237.
Holman BL, Hill TC. Perfusion imaging with single-photon-emission computed tomography. In: Wood JH (ed) Cerebral Blood Flow, Mc Graw-Hill Book Company 1987: 243–256.
Horton RW, Pedley TA, Meldrum BS, Chir B. Regional cerebral blood flow in the rat as determined by particle distribution and by diffusible tracer. Stroke 1980: 11: 39–44.
Huang S-C, Carson RE, Phleps ME. Measurement of local blood flow and distribution volume with short-lived isotopes. A general input technique. J Cereb Blood FLow Metab 1982: 2: 99–108.
Høedt-Rasmussen K, Sveinsdottir E, Lassen NA. Regional cerebral blood flow in man determined by intraarterial injection of radioactive inert gas. Circ Res 1966: 18: 237–247.
Høedt-Rasmussen K. Regional cerebral blood flow. The intraarterial injection method. Acta Neurol Scand 1967: 43 (suppl) 27: 1–81.
Ingvar DH, Lassen NA. Cerebral complications following measurements of regional cerebral blood flow (rCBF) with the intra-arterial 133-Xenon injection method. Stroke 1973: 4: 658–665.
Ingvar DH, Lassen NA. Atraumatic two-dimentional rCBF measurements using stationary detectors and inhalation of intravenous administration of 133-xenon. J Cereb Blood Flow Metab 1982: 2: 271–274
Jakobsen M, Enevoldsen E. Retrograde catherization of the right internal jugular vein for serial measurements of cerebral venous oxygen content J Cereb Blood Flow Metab 1989: 9: 717–720
Jakobsen M, Enevoldsen E, Dalager T. Spasm index in subarachnoid haemorrhage: Consequences of vasospam

upon cerebral blood flow and oxygen extraction. Acta Neurol Scand 1990: 82: 311–320
Junck L, Dhawan V, Thailer HT, Rottenberg DA. Effects of Xenon and Krypton on regional cerebral blood flow in the rat. J Cereb Blood Flow Metab 1985: 5: 126–132.
Kanno I, Lassen NA. Two methods for calculating regional cerebral blood flow from emission computed tomography of inert gas concentration. J Comput Assist Tomogr 1979: 3: 71–76.
Karonon JO, Liu Y, Vanninen RL, et al. Combined perfusion- and diffusion-weighted MR imaging in acute ischemic stroke during the 1st week: a longitudinal study. Radiology 2000: 217: 886–894.
Karonon JO, Partanen PL, Vanninen RL, et al. Evolution of MR contrast enhancement patterns during the first week after acute ischemic stroke. Am J Neuroradiol 2001: 22: 103–111.
Kasoff SS, Zingesser LH, Shulman K. Compartmental abnormalities of regional cerebral blood flow in children with head trauma. J Neurosurg 1972: 36: 463–470.
Kety SS, Schmidt CF. The determination of cerebral blood flow in man by the use of nitrous oxide in low concentrations. Am J Physiol 1945: 143: 53–66.
Kety SS, Schmidt CF. The nitrous oxide method for the quantitative determination of cerebral blood flow in man: Theory, procedure and normal values. J clin Invest 1948: 27: 476–483.
Kirkpatrick PJ, Smielewski P, Czosnyka M, Pickard JD. Continuous monitoring of cortical perfusion by laser Doppler flowmetry in ventilated patients with head injury. J Neurol Neurosurg Psychiatry 1994: 57: 1382–1388.
Kluymans M, van Everdingen KJ, Kappelle LJ, et al. Prognostic value of perfusion- and diffusion-weighted MR imaging in first 3 days of stroke. Eur Radiol 2000: 10: 1434–1441.
Lam JMK, Hsiang JNK, Poon WS. Monitoring of autoregulation using laser Doppler flowmetry in patients with head injury. J Neurosurg 1997: 86: 438–445.
LaMorgese J, Fein JM, Shulman K. Polarographic and microsphere analysis of ultraregional cerebral blood flow rates in the cat. In: Blood Flow and Metabolism in the Brain. Harper AM, Jennett WB, Miller JD, Rowan JO (eds), Churchill Livindstone, Edinburgh 1975: pp 7.3–7.8.
Landau WM, Freygang WH Jr, Roland LP, et al. The local circulation of the living brain; values in the unanesthetized and anesthetized cat. Trans Am Neurol Asic 1955: 80: 125–129.
Lansberg MG, Norbash AM, Marks MP, et al. Advantages of adding diffusion-weighted magnetic resonance imaging to conventional magnetic for evaluating acute stroke. Arch Neurol 2000: 57: 1311–1316.
Lassen NA, Munck O. The cerebral blood flow in man determined by the use of radioactive Krypton. Acta Physiol Scand 1955: 33: 30–49.
Lassen NA. Cerebral blood flow and oxygen consumption in man. Physiol rev 1959: 39: 183–238.
Lassen NA, Lane MH. Validity of internal jugular blood for study of cerebral blood flow and metabolism. J Appl Physiol 1961: 16: 313–320.
Lassen NA, Ingvar DH. Regional cerebral blood flow measurement in man. Arch Neurol 1963: 9: 615–622.
Lassen NA, Christensen MS. Physiology of cerebral blood flow. Br J Anesth 1976: 48: 719–735.
Lassen NA, Henriksen L, Paulson OB. Regional cerebral blood flow in stroke by 133-xenon inhalation using emission tomography. Stroke 1981: 12: 284–288.
Lassen NA. Cerebral and spinal cord blood flow. In Anaesthesia and Neurosurgery. Cottrell JE, Turndorff H (eds). Mosby Company, St Louis, Toronto 1986: 1–22.
Lear JL, Jones SC, Greenberg JH, et al. Use of 123-I and 14-C in a double radionuclide autoradiographic technique for simultaneous measurement of LCBF and LCMRgl: Theory and method. Stroke 1981: 12: 589–597.
Lear JL, Ackermann R, Kameyama M, et al. Multiple-radionuclide autoradiography in evaluation of cerebral function. J Cereb Blood Flow Metab 1984: 4: 264–269.
Liu AY, Maldjian JA, Bagley LJ, et al. Traumatic brain injury: diffusion-weighted MR imaging findings. Am J Neuroradiol 1999: 20: 1636–1641.
Lindegaard K-F, Nornes H, Bakke SJ, et al. Cerebral vasospasm diagnosis by means of angiography and blood velocity measurements. Acta Neurochir (Wien) 1989: 100: 12–24
Makowski EL, Meschia G, Droegenmueller W, Battaglia FC. Measurement of umbilical arterial blood flow to the sheep placenta and fetus in utero. Circ Res 1968: 23: 623–631.
Mallett BL, Veall N. Investigation of cerebral blood flow in hypertension, using radioactive-Xenon inhalation and extracranial recording. Lancet 1963: i: 1081–1082.
Marcus ML, Bischof CJ, Heistad DD. Comparison of microsphere and 133 Xenon clearance method in measuring skeletal muscle and cerebral blood flow. Circ Res 1981: 48: 748–761
Meldrum BS, Nilsson B. Cerebral blood flow and metabolic rate early and late in prolonged epileptic seizures induced in the rat by bicuculline. Brain 1976: 99: 523–543.
Mendell PL, Hollenberg NK. Cardiac output distribution in the rat. Comparison of rubidium and microsphere methods. Am J Physiol 1971: 221: 1617–1620.
Meyer JS, Hayman LH, Yamamoto M, et al. Local cerebral blood flow measured by CT after stable Xenon inhalation. Am J Radiol 1980: 135: 239–251.
Meyerson BA, Gunasekera L, Linderoth B, Gazelius B. Bedside monitoring of regional cortical blood flow in comatose patients using laser Doppler flowmetry. Neurosurgery 1991: 29: 750–755.
Michenfelder JD, Theye RA. Hypothermia: Effect on canine brain and whole-body metabolism. Anesthesiology 1968: 29: 1107–1112.
Michenfelder JD, Messick CM, Theye RA. Simultaneous cerebral blood flow measured by direct and indirect methods. J Surg Res 1968: 8: 475–481.
Morii S, Nagai AC, Ko KR, Winn HR. A venous outflow method for continuous monitoring cerebral blood flow in the rat. Am J Physiol 1986: 250: H304–H312.
Murray IPC, Hoschl R, Choy D. The jugular venous reflux. Clin Nucl Med 1978: 3: 56–57.
Neumann-Haefelin T, Wittsack HJ, Wenserski F, et al. Diffusion- and perfusion-weighted MRI. The DWI/PWI mismatch region in acute stroke. Stroke 1999: 30: 1591–1597.
Nilsson B, Siesjö BK. A venous outflow method for measurement of rapid change of cerebral blood flow and oxygen consumption in the rat. Stroke 1983: 14: 797–802.
Nuetze JM, Wyler F, Rudolph AM. Use of radioactive microspheres to assess distribution of cardial output in rabbits. Am J Physiol 1968: 215: 486–495.
Obrist WD, Thompson HK, King CH, Wang HS. Determination of regional cerebral blood flow by inhalation of 133-Xenon. Circ Res 1967: 20: 124–135.

Obrist WD, Jaggi JL, Harel D, Smith DS. Effect of stable Xenon inhalation of human CBF. J Cereb Blood Flow Metab 1985: 5: 557–558.

Obrist WD, Wilkinson WE. Stability and sensitivity of CBF indices in the noninvasive 133-Xe method. In: Cerebral Blood Flow and Metabolism Measurement; Hartmann A, Hoyer S (eds). Springer Verlag, Berlin 1985: 30–36.

Ogawa S, Menon RS, tank DW, et al. Functional brain imaging by blood oxygenation level-dependent contrast magnetic resonance imaging. A comparison of signal characteristics with a biophysical model. Biophys J 1993: 64: 803–812.

Olesen J, Paulson OB, Lassen NA. Regional cerebral blood flow in man determined by the initial slope of the clearance of the intra-arterially injected 133Xe. Stroke 1971: 2: 519–540.

Oshima E, Arai T, Urabe N. New anatomic landmarks for percutaneous catheterization of the internal jugular vein. Anesthesiology 1991: 74: 1164–1166

Phleps ME, Hoffman EJ, Mullani NA, Ter-Pogossian MM. Application of annihilation coincidence detection to transaxial reconstruction tomography. J Nucl Med 1975: 16: 210–223.

Phleps ME, Mazziotta JC, Huang SC. Study of cerebral function with positron computed tomography. J Cereb Blood Flow Metab 1982: 2: 113–162.

Pichard JD, Kirkpatrick PJ, Melsen T, et al. Potential role of NovoSeven in the prevention of rebleeding following aneurysmal subarachnoid haemorrhage. Blood Coagul Fibrolysis 2000: 11 (suppl 1): S117–120.

Pulsinelli WA, Bierley IB, Plum F. Temporal profile of neuronal damage in a model of transient forebrain ischaemia. Ann Neurol 1982: 11: 491–498.

Raichle ME, Eichling JO, Straatmann MG, et al. Blood-brain barrier permeability of 11-C-labeled alcohols and 15-0-labeled water. Am J Physiol 1976: 230: 532–552

Raichle ME. Positron emission tomography. Ann Rev Neurosci 1983: 6: 249–267.

Rapela CE, Green HD. Autoregulation of canine cerebral blood flow. Circ Res 1964: 15: 205–211.

Reinert M, Khaldi A, Zauner A, et al. High level of extracellular potassium and its correlates after severe head injury: relationship to high intracranial pressure. J Neurosurg 2000: 93: 800–807.

Reivich M, Jehle J, Sokoloff L, Kety SS. Measurement of regional cerebral blood flow with antipyrine-14C in awake cats. J Appl Physiol 1969: 27: 296–300.

Risberg J, Ali Z, Wilson EM, et al. Regional cerebral blood flow by 133-Xenon inhalation: Preliminary evaluation of an initial slope index in patients with unstable flow compartments. Stroke 1975: 6: 142–148.

Risberg J. Regional cerebral blood flow measurements by 133 xenon inhalation: methodology and application in neuropsychology and psychiatry. Brain Lang 1980: 9: 9–34

Roth JA, Greenfield AJ, Kaihara S, Wagner HN. Total and regional cerebral blood flow in unanesthetized dogs. Am J Physiol 1970: 219: 96–101.

Rowan JO, Reilly P, Farrar JK, Teasdale G. The Xenon-133 and hydrogen clearance methods-a comparative analysis. In Blood Flow and Metabolism in the Brain. Harper AM, Jennett WB, Miller JD, Rowan JO (eds). Churchill Livingstone, Edinburgh 1975: pp 7.9–7.10.

Sapirstein LA, Ogden E. Theoretic limitations of the nitrous oxide method for determination of regional blood flow. Circulation Research 1956: 4: 245–249.

Segawa H, Wakai S, Tamura A, et al. Computed tomographic measurement of local cerebral blood flow by Xenon enhancment. Stroke 1983: 14: 356–362.

Sakurada O, Kennedy C, Jehle J, et al. Measurement of local cerebral blood flow with iodo (14C) antipyrine. Am J Physiol 1978: 234: 59–66

Schlaug G, Benfield A, Siewert B, et al. The ischemic penumbra of human stroke: using functional MRI parameters to define tissue at risk for infarct progression. Neurology 1997: 48 (suppl 2): A204.

Smielewski P, Zcoskyka M, Kirkpatrick PJ, Pickard JD. Evaluation of the transient hyperemic response test in head-injured patients. J Neurosurg 1997: 86: 773–778.

Sokoloff L, Reivich M, Kennedy C, et al. The (14C) deoxyglucose method for measurement of local cerebral glucose utilization: Theory, procedure, and normal values in the conscious and anesthetized albino rat. J Neurochem 1977: 28: 897–916

Sorensen AG, Buonanno FS, Gonzales RG, et al. Hyperacute stroke: evaluation with combined multisection diffusion-weighted and hemodynamically weighted echo-planar MR imaging. Radiology 1996: 199: 391–401.

Steinbach JJ, Mattar AG, Mahin DT. Alteration of the cerebral blood flow study due to reflux in internal jugular veins. J Nucl Med 1976: 17: 61–64.

Stokely EM, Sveinsdottir E, Lassen NA, Rommer P. A single photon dynamic computer assisted tomography (DCAT) for imaging brain function in multiple cross sections. J Comput Assist Tomogr 1980: 4: 230–240.

Sveinsdottir E, Larsen B, Rommer P, Lassen NA. A multidetector scintillation camera with 254 channels. J Nucl Med 1977: 18. 168–174.

Ter-Pogossian MM. Basic principles of computed axial tomography. Semin Nucl Med 1977: 7: 109–127.

Tomita M, Gotoh F. Local cerebral blood flow values as estimated with diffusible tracers: validity of assumptions in normal and ischaemic tissue. J Cereb Blood Flow Metab 1981: 1: 403–411.

Tong DC, Yenari MA, Albers GW, et al. Correlation of perfusion- and diffusion-weighted MRI with NIHSS score in acute (6.5 hour) ischemic stroke. Neurology 1998: 50: 864–870.

Tuor UI, Farrar JK. Pial vessel caliber and cerebral blood flow during hemorrhage and hypercapnia in the rabbit. Am J Physiol 1984: 247: H40–51.

van Uitert RL, Levy DE. Regional brain blood flow in the conscious gerbil. Stroke 1978: 9: 67–72

van Zijl PCM, Moonen CTW, Faustino P, et al. Complete separation of intracellular and extracellular information in NMR spectra of perfused cells by diffusion-weighted spectroscopy. Proc Natl Acad Sci USA 1991: 88: 3228–3232.

van Zijl PC, Eleff SM, Ulatowski JA, et al. Quantitative assessment of blood flow, blood volume and blood oxygenation effects in functional magnetic resonance imaging. Nat Med 1998: 4: 159–167.

von Oettingen G, Bergholt B, Østergaard L, et al. Xenon CT cerebral blood flow in patients with head injury: influence of pulmonary trauma on the input function Neuroradiology 2000: 42: 168–173.

Warach S, Li W, Ronthal M, et al. Acute cerebral ischemia: evaluation with dynamic contrast-enhanced MR imaging and MR angiography. Radiology 1992: 182: 41–47.

Weber M, Grolimund P, Seiler RW. Evaluation of posttraumatic cerebral blood flow velocities by transcranial Doppler ultrasonography. Neurosurgery 1990: 27: 106–112

Winkler S, Sackett J, Holden J, et al. Xenon inhalation as a adjunct to computerized tomography of the brain: Preliminary study. Invest Radiol 1977: 12: 15–18.

Wozney P, Yonas H, Latchaw RE, et al. Central herniation revealed by focal decrease in blood flow without elevation of intracranial pressure.: A case report. Neurosurgery 1985: 17: 641–644.

Wyper DJ, Brooke MBD. Compensating for hemisphere crosstalk when measuring CBF. Acta Neurol Scand 1977: 56(suppl 64): 470–471.

Yamauchi H, Fukuyama H, Nagahama Y, et al. Evidence of misery perfusion and risk for recurrent stroke in major cerebral arterial occlusion diseases from PET. J Neurol Neurosurg Psychiatr 1996: 61: 18–25.

Yonas H, Wolfsen SK, Gur D, et al. Clinical experience with the use of Xenon-enhanced CT blood flow mapping in cerebral vascular disease. Stroke 1984a: 15: 443–450.

Yonas H, Good WF, Gur D, et al. Mapping cerebral blood flow by Xenon-enhanced computed tomography: Clinical experience. Radiology 1984b: 152: 425–442.

Yonas H, Snyder JV, Gur D, et al. Good BC. Local cerebral blood flow alterations (Xe-CT Method) in an accident victim. J Comput Assist Tomogr 1984c: 8: 990–991.

Yonas H, Gur D, Good BC, et al. Stable Xenon CT blood flow mapping in the evaluation of patients before and after extracranial/intracranial bypass surgery. J Neurosurg 1985: 62. 324–333.

Yonas H, Gur D, Latchaw RE, Wolfsen SK. Xenon computed tomographic blood mapping. In: Cerebral Blood Flow, Wood JH (ed) McGraw-Hill Book Company 1987: 220–242.

Yonas H, Gur D, Claassen D, et al. Stable Xenon enhanced computed tomography in the study of clinical and pathologic correlates of focal ischaemia in baboons. Stroke 1988: 19: 228–238.

Yonas H, Darby JM, Marks EC, et al. CBF measured by Xe-CT: Approach to analysis and normal values. J Cereb Blood Flow Metab 1991: 11: 716–725.

Young WL, Prohovnik I, Schroeder T, et al. Intraoperative 133Xe cerebral blood flow measurements by intravenous versus intracarotid methods. Anesthesiology 1990: 73: 637–643

Zaharchuk G, Yamada M, Sasamata M, et al. Is all perfusion-weighted magnetic resonance imaging for stroke equal? The temporal evolution of multiple hemodynamic parameters after focal ischemia in rats correlated with evidence of infarction. J Cereb Blood Flow Metab 2000: 20: 1241–1351.

Østergaard L, Weisskoff RM, Chester DA, et al. High resolution measurement of cerebral blood flow using intravascular tracer bolus passages. Part I: Mathematical approach and statistical analysis. Magn Reson Med 1996: 36: 715–725.

Østergaard L, Johanssen P, Høest-Poulsen P, et al. Cerebral blood flow measurements by magnetic resonance imaging bolus tracking: Comparison with $[^{15}O]H_2O$ positron emission tomography in humans. J Cereb Blood Flow Metab 1998: 18: 935–940.

Østergaard L, Hochberg FH, Rabinov JD, et al. Early changes measured by magnetic resonance imaging in cerebral blood flow, blood volume, and blood-brain barrier permeability following dexamethasone treatment in patients with brain tumors. J Neurosurg 1999: 90: 300–305.

Østergaard L, Sorensen G, Chesler DA, et al. Combined diffusion-weighted and perfusion-weighted flow heterogeneity magnetic resonance imaging in acute stroke. Stroke 2000: 31: 1097–1103.

Regulation of cerebral blood flow (CBF)

Human studies of CBF

Mean values

With the Kety and Schmidt technique the average values of CBF in awake normocapnic adult range from 45 to 67 ml/100g/min (Kety and Schmidt 1945, Schienberg and Stead 1949, Sokoloff et al. 1957, Lassen et al. 1960, Cohen et al. 1967). Generally, 50 ml/100g/min is used as reference (Lassen 1959). As incomplete tracer equilibrium influences the result, correction based on a computer-based simulation model indicates a global flow of 46 ml/100g/min (Lund Madsen et al. 1993). With the intraarterial approach, initial slope index as described by Olesen et al. (1971) averages 65 ml/100g/min. Using the same technique and compartment analysis CBF in the fast and slow compartments (grey and white matter) was 80 and 20 ml/100g/min respectively (Ingvar et al. 1965).

Ageing

Differences in anxiety, age and level of $PaCO_2$ might be the reason to the discrepancy in results. Studies with the inhalation technique and the initial slope index (ISI) calculated during the 2 to 3 min period (Risberg 1980) have shown CBF values averaging 58 ml/100g/min in young adults (mean age 24 years) against 48 ml/100g/min in subjects with mean age of 63 years (Ewing et al.1985).

With the stable Xenon method a significant decline in CBF with age has been found (Yonas et al. 1991). A preferential decline of CBF in the frontal cortex and a side-to-side asymmetry have also been found with advancing age (Waldemar et al. 1991).

Infants

In new-born infants global CBF ranges between 10 and 20 ml/100g/min and the glucose utilisation in the cerebral cortex is reduced. The relative few synaptic connections and thereby low neuronal activity are associated with a low cerebral oxygen uptake (Chugani and Phleps 1986, Greisen 1986, Altman et al. 1988, Pryds and Greisen 1990). According to the low CBF in neonates, the CO_2 reactivity is also reduced (Levene et al. 1988).

CT-Xe

Studies with the Xenon enhanced CT technique indicate that mixed cortical flow averaged 51 ml with highest and lowest flow rate of 84 and 20 ml/100g/min respectively. The highest flow rates were generally found in caudate, putamen and thalamus. Values within the high flow compartment demonstrated a decline with age. This was not found in low flow compartments (Yonas et al. 1991).

Human studies of cerebral metabolic rate of oxygen ($CMRO_2$)

Mean values

With the nitrous oxide method for the quantitative determination of $CMRO_2$, Kety and Schmidt (1948) found that cerebral oxygen uptake averaged 3.5 ml O_2/100g/min. Average values ranging from 3.0 to 3.8 have been found in other studies (Kety and Schmidt 1945, Schienberg and Stead 1949, Sokoloff et al. 1957, Lassen et al. 1960, Cohen et al. 1967). New studies with computer-based simulation models where correction for incomplete tracer equilibrium is performed indicate a mean value of 3.0 ml O_2 100 g/min (Madsen et al. 1993).

In PET studies $CMRO_2$ in grey and white structures has been calculated to be 6 and 2 ml O_2 /100g/min respectively (Frackowiac et al. 1980).

Active and basal metabolism

In his classical studies in anaesthetised dogs Michelfelder (1974,1975) showed that thiopental suppressed $CMRO_2$ only to the extend that EEG activity was silenced. This occurred when $CMRO_2$ was decreased 50%. The $CMRO_2$ associated with spontaneous EEG activity is functionally defined as "active". The basal $CMRO_2$ was assumed to represent the oxygen consumption necessary to maintain cell viability. In unanesthetised monkeys the active/basal distribution for $CMRO_2$ is 50/50 for CBF 40/60 and for glucose utilisation 60/40 (Nemoto et al. 1994).

Ageing

A decrease in $CMRO_2$ with ageing, and a higher level of $CMRO_2$ in children was described by Kennedy and Sokoloff (1957). A reappraisal of the original data , however, did not document a fall in $CMRO_2$ with chronological ageing (Dastur 1985). With PET glucose utilisation was found to be low in neonatal period. In infants 5 weeks of age PET studies of local glucose utilisation indicate that the metabolism was highest in the sensorimotor cortex, thalamus, midbrain-brainstem, and cerebellar vermis. By 3 months glucose metabolism had increased in the parietal, temporal, and occipital cortices, and basal ganglia, with subsequent increases in frontal and various association regions occurring by 8 months (Chugani and Phleps 1986). In the second and third year glucose utilisation exceeds adult values. By about 4 years, a plateau is reached until about 9 years. Later a gradual decline is found and adult values are obtained by the end of the second decade. The increase in glucose utilisation in children is most pronounced in neocortical regions, while phylogenetically older structures are similar to adult values (Chugani and Phleps 1986, Chugani et al. 1987).

In the kitten very low values of glucose utilisation are observed during the first 15 days of life. After 15 days many brain regions underwent sharp increase, to reach or exceed adult values by 60 days. This developmental period corresponds to the time of rapid synaptic proliferation. At 90 and 120 days, a slight decline in glucose utilisation, followed by a second peak at about 180 days, when sexual maturation occurs (Chugani et al. 1991).

Mental performance

In man global $CMRO_2$ is not influenced by mental and physical performance (Madsen et al. 1992). Where early studies indicated that sleep did not influence $CMRO_2$ significantly (Mangold et al. 1955). Studies indicate that $CMRO_2$ is suppressed during deep sleep and to a lesser degree during REM sleep. Thus, Madsen et al. (1991) found a 4% increase in CBF during REM sleep in the associative visual area, while a decrease by 9% was found in the inferior frontal cortex.

Starvation

PET studies during starvation indicate a 54% reduction in glucose utilisation (Redies et al. 1989). Instead ketone bodies account for about 50% of the energy supply (Owen et al. 1967). The human brain adapts to the changes in energy supply as early as 3 days following initiation of starvation, at which time ketone bodies account for approximately one-fourth of the cerebral energy requirements (Hasselbalch et al. 1994).

Stress

In animal studies stress, fear, hypotension, hypoglycaemia, hypoxia and ethanol withdrawal induce an increase in $CMRO_2$ as well as CBF. In studies of human volunteers with PET the results are more complex. For low anxiety subjects a linear increase in CBF with anxiety was found. For higher anxiety subjects, however, there was a linear decrease in CBF with increased anxiety and a linear decrease in cerebral metabolic rate with increased anxiety was also found (Gur et al. 1987). Beta-receptor stimulation with adrenaline and noradrenaline has the same effect (Bryan 1990).

CBF coupling

A coupling between metabolism and CBF has repeatedly been shown. Thus, Olesen (1971) found that CBF increased significantly in the part of the cerebral cortex representing the hand, during maximal physical efforts with the contralateral arm. Listening to speech and attention activates cortical areas in both hemispheres (Larsen et al. 1977, Larrue et al. 1994). During behavioural activation either by memory- or tactile somatosensory tasks an asymmetrical metabolic activation, which was opposite in direction within the cerebral and cerebellar hemispheres has been observed (Barker et al. 1991). Adenosine is involved in the regulation of pial vasodilation during cortical activation. Thus, dipyridamole, an adenosine uptake competitor, enhances the magnitude and duration of somatosensory cortical activation. In contrast theophyllamine, an adenosine receptor blocker, attenuates the response (Ko et al. 1990).

Epilepsy

Experimental studies have shown that epileptic seizure activity is associated with an increased flow and cerebral oxygen uptake, an increase in jugular venous oxygen tension and suspension of cerebral autoregulation (Plum and Posner 1968, Brodersen et al. 1973). Cerebral energy depletion (Collins et al. 1970) tissue acidosis occurring within 30 sec with postischaemic acidosis for 10–20 min (Yaksh and Andorson 1987) and an increase in the concentration of lactate in brain tissue have also been demonstrated (Beresford et al. 1969, Bolwig and Quistorff 1973). In rats CBF and cerebral oxygenation were studied by measuring relative changes in the oxidation/reduction level of cytochrome aa3. A relative hypoperfusion has been found during repeated seizures (Kreisman et al. 1991).

Diaschisis

A reduction in metabolism and CBF in the cerebellum contralateral to a lesioned cerebral hemisphere has been described as "crossed cerebellar diaschisis" (Baron et al. 1981, Lenzi et al. 1982, Martin and Raichle 1983, Pantano et al. 1986). The CO_2 reactivity is uniform across affected and unaffected cerebellar hemispheres (Ishii et al. 1994). In patients with crossed cerebellar diaschisis the cerebellar cortex contralateral to the stroke showed significant decrease in both oxygen consumption and glucose utilisation compared with the ipselateral cerebellar cortex. The decrease in oxygen consumption, however, was less than the decrease in glucose utilisation, resulting in a significant increase in the oxygen consumption/glucose utilisation ratio (Yamauchi et al. 1999). Studies in rats support that the mechanism underlying this phenomenon is interruption of the corticopontocerebellar tract (Serteser et al. 2001). Crossed cerebellocerebellar diaschisis has been described in patients with cerebellar stroke (Komaba et al. 2000).

Dementia

In patients suffering from organic and vascular dementia $CMRO_2$ is reduced (Lassen 1959, Gibbs et al. 1986). In demented patients with communicating hydrocephalus an increase in CBF and $CMRO_2$ has been observed after implantation of shunt (Greitz et al. 1969, Malmlund et al. 1972). In patients with normal pressure hydrocephalus shunt operation normalised or reduced the area of the subcortical low flow regions (Waldemar et al. 1993)

In Alzheimer's disease a CBF decrease in the parietal, frontal and temporal regions has been observed repeatedly (Komatani et al. 1988, Imran et al. 1999). In the same regions low values of $CMRO_2$ and $CMR_{glucose}$ have been revealed (Fukuyama et al. 1994). In another study by SPECT the flow pattern in Alzheimer was heterogeneous, predominantly with changes in frontal rCBF (Waldemar et al. 1994). In mild Alzheimer's disease decreased perfusion in the posterior cingulate has been demonstrated (Ishii et al. 1997). A close coupling between reduced rCBF and specific neurophysiological deficits has been demonstrated in patients with fronto-temporal dementia (Elfgren et al. 1996)

SPECT and PET data have been used to differentiate Alzheimer's disease from vascular dementia. The typical parieto-temporal pattern of hypoperfusion and hypometabolism with preserved vascular reactivity was observed in Alzheimer's disease, whereas the frontal lobe including the cingulate and superior frontal gyri, and vascular reactivity were predominantly affected in patients with vascular dementia (Komatani et al. 1988, Nagata et al. 2000).

Endotoxaemia

In volunteers a dose of Escheria Coli endotoxin sufficient to induce systemic vasodilation does not influence cerebral blood flow or the $CMRO_2$ (Pollard et al. 1997).

Head injury

In patients with severe head injury, a significant decrease in $CMRO_2$ parallels the deprivation of the consciousness (Obrist et al. 1984), and $CMRO_2$ as low as 0.4 ml O_2/100g/min has been found in the acute phase after head injury in patients who recover (Cold et al. 1978).

Subarachnoid haemorrhage

Likewise, a reduction of $CMRO_2$ has been found in patients with subarachnoid haemorrhage (SAH). The reduction in $CMRO_2$ correlates to the level of consciousness (Jakobsen et al. 1990), the Hunt and Hess graduation, degree of cerebral artery spasm (Voldby et al. 1985) and the amount of subarachnoid blood by CT scan (Jakobsen et al. 1991)

Regulation of CBF (viscosity, haemodilution and cardiac output)

Viscosity

Viscosity is determined by haematocrit, the deformability and aggregational properties of blood cells and plasma viscosity. Erythrocytes are deformed when passing through capillaries with vessel diameters of 4–6 μ. Brain haematocrit has been found to be about one-third lower than haematocrit in larger vessels (Blasberg et al.1983, Cremer and Seville 1983). Age of erythrocyte, pH and temperature and humoral factors may alter the erythrocyte internal viscosity. An increase in viscosity is followed by a decrease in microvascular circulation (Wood et al. 1983).

Haemodilution

Haemodilution increases CBF (Messmer et al. 1973, Thomas et al. 1977, Gottstein 1981). In rabbits subjected to profound haemodilution the maximum tolerable limit of anaemia was investigated. The haemoglobin concentration decreased from 142 g/L to 24 g/L. CBF increased from 37 to 66 ml/100g/min, brain tissue oxygen tension decreased from 27 to 12 mm Hg, brain tissue pH decreased from 7.22 to 7.12, $CMRO_2$ decreased from 4.3 to 1.9 ml O_2/100g/min, and loss of EEG amplitude was observed (Morimoto et al. 2001).

In volunteers the increase in CBF does not necessarily improve oxygen transport or tissue oxygenation. On the contrary tissue oxygen delivery is decreased (Hino et al. 1992).

Cardiac output

In the normal brains CBF does not change during expansion of the blood volume in spite of an increase in cardiac output. Volume expansion increases cerebral blood volume in proportion to CVP, suggesting passive venous distension (Todd et al. 1993).

In studies in monkeys subjected to MCAO local CBF was measured with the hydrogen technique during changes in cardiac output by exsanguination. The local CBF in non-ischaemic brain tissue was independent of cardiac output in contrast to ischaemic brain tissue where the local CBF varied directly with cardiac output (Tranmer et al. 1992).

Regulation of CBF by arterial oxygen tension

CBF

Generally CBF is unchanged until PO_2 has declined to about 50 mm Hg. At this point CBF will increase and at PO_2 30 mm Hg CBF will double (Kety and Schmidt 1948). At these levels of PO_2 an increase in ICP will occur, and somatosensory evoked potential is impaired (North et al. 1993). With 100% oxygen CBF decreases by 10% (Videen et al. 1987), and hyperbaric oxygen at 2 atm. reduces CBF 22% (Jacobsen et al. 1964). In rats the sensitivity of cerebrovascular receptors to moderate hypoxia are similar in young and aged animals but the maximum reactivity to severe hypoxia is attenuated in aged animals (Hoffman et al. 1984). Studies in ponies indicate that during severe hypoxia CBF increases within 45 sec and the change in CBF was completed after 90 sec. During very mild level of hypoxia (PaO_2 62 mm Hg) the increase in CBF occurred after 5 min of hypoxia (Wagerle et al. 1983). In volunteers hypoxic cerebral vasodilation occurs at peripheral oxygen saturation of 90% (Gupta et al. 1997).

With near infrared spectroscopy in healthy adult hypoxia results in a steady decrease of cerebral oxyhaemoglobin content and a decrease in oxidised cytochrome a1,a3 (Hampson et al. 1990).

Adenosine

An increase in adenosine concentration is supposed to be involved in hypoxic-mediated CBF increase (Hoffman et al. 1984). Thus, the adenosine uptake inhibitor dipyridamole and erythro-9-(2-hydroxy-3-nonyl) adenine (EHNA), an inhibitor of the enzyme adenosine deaminase, potentiates hypoxic vasodilation of pial arterioles while simultaneously increasing extracellular adenosine (Meno et al. 1993). Other studies indicate that basal adenosine levels are influenced to a greater extent by adenosine kinase than by adenosine deaminase, and strongly suggest a role for adenosine in CBF regulation (Sciotti and van Wylen 1993).

Nitric oxide

Also endothelium-derived relaxing factor, which has been identified as nitric oxide has been claimed to play a role (Kozniewska et al. 1992). The main action of nitric oxide is the stimulation of the soluble guanylate cyclase, which causes an increase in cGMP in vascular smooth muscle, leading to relaxation

(Moncada et al. 1989). On the other hand, glutamine metabolism is not involved (Hoop et al. 1990).

Sustained hypoxia

During sustained hypoxia for several days CBF and cerebral capillary pressure are elevated and brain water content increases without affection of ICP (Curran-Everett et al. 1991). These findings suggest that pressure gradients that would favour transcapillary fluid shift is created during hypoxia. Other studies have shown that cerebral venous pressure and haematocrit are increased during sustained hypoxia (Iwamoto et al. 1991). Vasogenic mechanisms including increased transcapillary filtration combined with arteriolar dilation and acute systemic episodes are supposed to be of importance for the development of high altitude cerebral oedema (Sutton and Lassen 1979) but cytotoxic oedema subsequent to hypoxia-mediated inhibition of the Na+ Ka+ adenosine triphosphatase has also been proposed (Klazo 1967).

Head injury

In severe head injury a PaO_2 above 80 mm Hg seems to correlate with a better outcome (Becker et al. 1977). On the other hand, experimental hyperoxygenation in these patients seems to be detrimental owing to the production of superoxide in the recirculation phase after ischaemia (Mickel et al. 1988). During craniotomy high oxygen tensions give a scattered oxygen tissue histogram (Eintrei and Lund 1986) which is supposed to indicate impaired tissue oxygenation (Lübbers 1977).

Metabolic regulation of CBF

Hypothermia

Q_{10}

Hypothermia decreases $CMRO_2$ and CBF proportionally (Rosomoff and Holaday 1954). In the temperature range 25–37 °C linear correlation between log $CMRO_2$ and body temperature has been found. Based on animal studies the constancy of the ratio delta log $CMRO_2$/delta temp Celsius ranges from 0.038 to 0.076, indicating a percentage change in $CMRO_2$ ranging from 9.1 to 19.1% per degree change in temperature (Feruglio et al. 1954, Adams et al. 1957, Bering 1961, Cohen et al. 1964, Michenfelder and Theye 1968, Tabaddor et al. 1972, Bering 1974, Hägerdal et al. 1975, Astrup et al. 1981). In dogs the temperature coefficient Q_{10} (defined as the ratio of metabolic rates at two temperatures differing by 10°C) was 2.2 at temperature between 37 and 27 °C. Below 27 °C the Q_{10} was doubled to 4.5, suggesting that the relationship of $CMRO_2$ to brain temperature is variable depending on the functional state of the brain. Below 27 °C progressive functional depression is supposed to account for the high Q_{10} value (Michenfelder and Milde 1991).

CO_2 reactivity and cerebral autoregulation

Pial arteriolar responses to hypercapnia and hypotension were studied in rats subjected to hypothermia. The response to hypercapnic vasodilation was intact, but vasodilation induced by hypotension was reduced (Irikura et al. 1998).

Coupling between regional oxygen consumption and rCBF

During hypothermic by-pass operation coupling between global $CMRO_2$ and CBF has been observed (Murkin et al. 1987, Stephan et al. 1992). One factor which could induce discrepancies between metabolism and CBF is anaesthesia (Maekawa et al. 1986). The relationship between local CBF and glucose utilisation during mild and moderate hypothermia has recently been studied in isoflurane (1 MAC) anaesthetised rats. Using *p*H-stat management a decrease in glucose utilisation at unchanged or increased rCBF was observed both during normo- and hypothermia. A strong linear correlation between rCBF and glucose metabolism was found suggesting an intact coupling that is reset to a higher blood flow/metabolism ratio (Frietsch et al. 2000).

Temperature differences

In neurosurgical patients the difference between rectal and cerebral temperature average 0.33 °C with the largest temperature difference being 2.30 °C (Mellergård and Nordström 1991).

Protection

Hypothermia exerts a protective effect on the brain in anoxia (Boyd and Connolly 1961) hypoxic hypoxia (Carlsson et al. 1976) global ischaemia (Chopp et al. 1989) incomplete ischaemia (Hoffman et al. 1991), transient MCAO (Chen et al. 1992) and in experimental head injury (Bouzarth et al. 1967, Clifton et al. 1991). It has been suggested that even a small decrease in temperature of 1–3 degree of Celsius might have a protective effect in global ischaemia (Marshall et al. 1956, Kramer et al. 1968, Michenfelder and Theye 1970, Kopf et al. 1975, Berntman et al. 1981, Young et al. 1983, Busto et al. 1987, Busto et al. 1989) and temporary focal ischaemia (Ridenour et al. 1992). Even when hypothermia is initiated during temporary focal ischaemia or during permanent focal ischaemia the infarct volume will be reduced without attenuating the reduction in cortical blood flow (Kader et al. 1992, Karibe et al. 1994). In another study an improvement of blood-brain barrier has been observed during hypothermia (Dietrich et al. 1989).

In rats, even small increments in temperature in ischaemic brain tissue seem to accentuate histopathological changes (Busto et al. 1987, Dietrich et al. 1990, Kitagawa et al. 1991).

ICP, head injury, ischaemia

The effects of hypothermia upon ICP are described in chapter 3. Furthermore, hypothermia is dealt within chapter 10 (acute head injury) and chapter 12 (cerebral ischaemia).

Barbiturate

A barbiturate in combination with hypothermia might effectively control intracranial hypertension in some patients with severe head injury (Shapiro et al. 1974). Likewise, the combination of barbiturate and hypothermia might accentuate the protective effect in brain ischaemia (Hägerdal et al. 1978, Lafferty et al. 1978, Nordström and Rehncrona 1978). However, animal experiments during anoxia indicate that although barbiturate and hypothermia might have potentially similar effects on $CMRO_2$, dissimilar mechanisms might be involved, because the rate of ATP depletion and lactate accumulation is considerably lower during hypothermia (Michenfelder and Theye 1970).

Mechanism

It has been suggested that the protective effect of more pronounced hypothermia is based on two mechanisms. 1) Since hypothermia shifts the oxygen haemoglobin-dissociation curve towards the left, and prevents or minimises a rightward shift due to acidosis, it maintains a high oxygen content in arterial blood. 2) By reducing $CMRO_2$ and consequently cellular energy requirement, hypothermia exerts a protective effect on cellular level (Carlsson et al. 1976b). However, experiments during hypoxia in rats indicate that the increased oxygen content in arterial blood produced by hypothermia is not a major determinant in hypothermic protection (Keykhah et al. 1980), and generally the protective effect is supposed to be caused by the decrease in $CMRO_2$.

Among the consequences of cerebral ischaemia known to be temperature sensitive are intracellular hydrogen ion homeostasis, calcium influx into neuronal structures, degradation of membrane lipids, and permeability of the blood-brain barrier (BBB) (Norwood and Norwood 1982, Krantis 1983, Rossi and Britt 1984, Lantos et al. 1986). Furthermore, hypothermia is supposed to inhibit various neurotransmitters (Vanhoutte et al. 1981, Boels et al. 1985, Haikala et al. 1986), whereas other studies suggest an accelerated metabolic turnover (Okuda et al. 1986). In many studies of mild hypothermia the cerebral metabolism as measured by cerebral metabolites was unchanged.

Other protective mechanisms have been proposed. It has been reported that mild hypothermia has an effect upon the arachidonic acid cascade during ischaemia in the gerbil (Dempsey et al. 1987). The lipoxygenase pathway is affected by mild hypothermia with decreased production of leucotriene B4. Thus, moderate hypothermia initiated after resuscitation after cardiac arrest in mongrel dogs, can inhibit the accumulation of lipid peroxidation products and the consumption of free radical scavengers in the brain tissue (Baiping et al. 1994).

Microtubule-associated protein 2 (MAP2), an important cross-linking component of the neuronal cytoskeleton, is decreased after traumatic brain injury. During hypothermia this decrease is not found, suggesting that attenuation of injury-induced MAP2 loss by hypothermia may contribute to the neuroprotective action of hypothermia (Taft et al. 1993).

Excitatory amino acids

A very important mechanism could be attenuation of the increase in excitatory neurotransmitters (Busto et al. 1989, Simpson et al. 1991, Baker et al. 1991). In transient global ischaemia in the rabbit, *in vivo* studies with microdialysis indicated that extracellular glutamate concentration increased by 11 uM in a group of 38 °C , while glutamate increased < 1 uM when the temperature was decreased to 32 °C (Illievich et al. 1994). Attenuation of the production of glycine which plays a role in the activation of NMDA-receptors has also been demonstrated (Baker et al. 1991, Simpson et al. 1991), and depletion of ubiquitin (Yamashita et al. 1991).

Hibernation

Natural tolerance to ischaemia has been studied during mammalian hibernation. Studies of ground squirrels during hibernation indicate a fall of CBF from 62 to 7 ml/100g/min (Frerichs et al. 1994). Hibernation appears to be actively regulated, and it is supposed that hormonal factors play a role (Swan and Schätte 1977).

Clinical studies

On the basis of the experimental studies hypothermia has been used in the intensive care of patients suffering from brain ischaemia (Connolly et al. 1962, Cohen 1981), during extracorporal circulation (du-Cailar et al. 1964), after circulatory arrest (White 1972), during neurosurgical operations (McKissock et al. 1960, Terry et al. 1962, Uihlein et al. 1962, Daw et al. 1964, Deligne and David 1966, Uihlein et al. 1966, White et al. 1967) and in the treatment of severe head injury (Sedzimir 1959, Shapiro et al. 1974). During the last decade, however, the once common use of hypothermia has been abandoned, and later experimental studies of hypothermia in the treatment of acute stroke did not prove any beneficial effect; on the contrary, a detrimental effect was observed in primates and cats (Michenfelder and Milde 1977, Steen et al. 1979). However, a study indicates that continuous circulation with aqueous solution after total exsanguination, can be accomplished at 1.7° C for several hours without neurological complications (Bailes et al. 1991). Mild hypothermia for brain protection has been suggested in clinical practice during temporary clipping of major cerebral arteries (Milde 1992). Schubert (1992), however, warns against this application as long as clinical controlled studies have not proved its effectiveness.

In acute head injury mild hypothermia has been used successfully. A decrease in ICP, CBF, $AVDO_2$ and $CMRO_2$ was found, and studies of outcome were promising (Shiozaki et al. 1993, Marion et al. 1993).

Neurogenic Regulation of CBF

A variety of nerves present on pial vessels has been described making nervous control of cerebral circulation a possibility (Duverger et al. 1987). Noradrenergic-containing nerve fibres in the wall of pial arteries arise from the superior cervical ganglion, and those along the intraparenchymal blood vessels arise mainly from the nucleus locus ceruleus (Hartman et al. 1972, Yokote et al. 1986). Concerning the effects of epinephrine and norepinephrine upon ceebral circulation, see chapter 8.

Locus ceruleus

Several studies have revealed a decrease in CBF following electrical stimulation of locus ceruleus (Raichle et al. 1975, De la Torré et al. 1977, Goadsby et al. 1982). During electrical stimulation of locus ceruleus volumetric estimate of cerebral blood volume by photoelectric method has shown a decrease in CBV in intraparenchymal vessels without any apparent effect on pial vessels (Otha et al. 1991).

Stimulation of the locus ceruleus also increases the blood-brain barrier permeability. Prior administration of phenoxybenzamine blocked this effect, while pindolol, a combined α-β-adrenoceptor antagonist, potentiated the effect (Sarmento et al. 1994).

Dorsal raphe nucleus

The dorsal raphe nucleus (DRN) provides serotonergic innervation of pial and intraparenchymal cerebral blood vessels (Moreno et al. 1991, Bonvento et al. 1991). Stimulation of DRN elicits changes in CBF in the rat (Bonvento et al. 1989, Cudennec et al. 1989). Sustained intermittent electrical stimulation of the DRN can evoke either increases or decreases of CBF depending on the anatomical localization. The DRN does not tonically maintain resting CBF, nor participate in the cerebrovascular response to change in PCO_2 (Underwood et al. 1992).

Trigeminal system

In primates, fibres pass directly from the trigeminal nerve to the internal carotid artery within the cavernous sinus (Ruskell and Simons 1987). The trigeminovascular nerves are predominantly unmyelinated C fibres, which form a network on the adventitial surface of cerebral vessels. In these nerves vesicles containing tachykinins, substance P, neurokinin A, calcitonin gene-related peptide (CGRP), galanin and cholecystokinin-8 are found. In animal experiments trigeminal ganglionectomy attenuates the increases in CBF accompanying acute severe hypertension (Sakas et al. 1989) and diminishes the extravasation of radiolabeled albumin resulting from disruption of the blood-brain barrier (Moskowitz et al. 1988). The caudal basilar artery and the vertebral arteries and their tributaries are innervated primarily by the upper cervical dorsal root ganglia (Nørregaard and Moskowitz 1985, Saito et al. 1989).

Sympathectomy

Chemical sympathectomy with six-hydroxy-dopamine leads to marked noradrenaline denervation in the nucleus ceruleus-innervated areas (Jonnson 1983) and to a decrease in noradrenaline levels measured in the cerebral cortex (Onesti et al. 1989).

Rats were subjected to chemical sympathectomy by stereotactic injection of 6-hydroxydopamine into the lateral ventricle. A hypertensive condition at a mean arterial pressure of about 160 mm Hg was maintained for 1 hour by intravenous phenylephedrine. Compared with a control group CBF increased, cerebral autoregulation was impaired and specific gravity of the cerebral tissue revealed cerebral oedema. It was suggested that depletion of brain noradrenaline levels causes a disturbance in cerebral microvasculatur tone and renders the cerebral blood vessels more vulnerable to hypertension (Kobayashi et al. 1991).

α-agonist

In dogs and goats (Ekström-Jodal et al. 1974, Oberdorster et al. 1973, Lluch et al. 1973), but not in rats (Drummond et al. 1989, Berntman et al. 1978, Tuor et al. 1986) α_1-agonists have a vasoconstrictor effect. In man intracarotid infusions of norepinephrine in doses that caused minimal change in blood pressure resulted in no change in CBF (Olesen 1972). If the blood-brain barrier is disrupted, norepinephrine and epinephrine, which both have a β-agonist activity, increase CBF and $CMRO_2$ (King et al. 1952, Berntman et al. 1978, MacKenzie et al. 1976, Artru et al. 1981).

Dopamine

D_2-like dopamine receptor density in the caudate nucleus is elevated in schizophrenia (Wong et al. 1997b). During normal aging the density of D_2-like dopamine receptors in the caudate nucleus declines 1% per year after the age of 18 years (Wong et al. 1997a).

The dopaminergic neural system has been proposed to play a role in the regulation of cerebrovascular tone (Edvinsson et al. 1978, Altura et al. 1980, Harik et al. 1986). A constrictor effect on pial arterioles is supposed to be activated through α-adrenoceptors (Edvinsson et al. 1978, Mc Culloch 1984) and not modified by endogenous prostanoids (Busija and Leffler 1988).

In dogs a triphasic effect has been observed with CBF reduction occurring at low (< 2 μg/kg/min) and high infusion rates (7–20 μg/kg/min), and an increase in CBF at infusion rates ranging from 2–6 μg/kg/min. No change in $CMRO_2$ was observed; the CBF reduction was blocked by phentolamine and the CBF decrease was blocked by dopamine receptor antagonists (haloperidol) (von Essen 1972, von Essen 1974, von Essen et al. 1980).

The effects of dopamine upon cerebral circulation is also mentioned in chapter 8.

Neuropeptides

There have been reports suggesting that GABA and neuropeptides (Onodera et al. 1987), such as neuropeptide Y (Edvinsson et al. 1987), substance P (Edvinsson et al. 1985), vasoactive intestinal peptides (Edvinsson et al. 1982, Kobayashi et al. 1983) and calcitonin-related gene peptide (Hanko et al. 1985, Edvinsson et al. 1987) play a role in the vasomotor regulation of cerebral circulation.

Vasopressin

Vasopressin and oxytocin are potent vasoconstrictors in a variety of vascular beds. *In vitro* and in situ studies have shown that vasopressin constricts cerebral arteries in human and several other species (Uchida et al. 1967, Lluch et al. 1984, Nakai 1987, de Aguilera et al. 1990). *In vivo* studies in dogs indicate that direct bolus injection of vasopressin in the vertebral artery produces a dose-dependent decrease in vertebral blood flow. With the same doses the mayor cerebral arteries dilate. Vasopressin is 10 times as potent as oxytocin (Suzuki et al. 1992).

Acetylcholine

Topical application of acetylcholine causes a massive increase in CSF prostanoid levels, and the cerebral constrictor effect caused by acetylcholine in piglets is abolished by treatment with indomethacin (Busija et al. 1988, Wagerle and Busija 1989).

Nitric oxide (NO)

The endothelium-derived relaxing factor is synthesised in endothelial cells and is supposed to be identical with NO derived from L-arginine (Fasehun et al. 1990, Palmer et al. 1990). L-arginine infusion increases basal but not activated CBF in humans (Reutens et al. 1997). Concerning NO and cerebral ischaemia see chapter 12.

NMMA

Formation of NO from L-arginine is inhibited by analogues of L-arginine such as L-NMMA (Gold et al. 1990, Johns et al. 1990). Under control conditions L-NMMA constricts cerebral blood vessels and this reaction is inhibited by L-arginine (Faraci 1990). Studies by the same author have shown that the constriction of small arteries (pial arterioles) is less than of greater arteries (basilar artery). The author suggests that the discrepancy is caused by a smaller basal production of NO in small arteries (Faraci 1991). Relaxation of systemic arteries to acetylcholine also depends on formation of NO. Tonic production of NO influences guanylate cyclase activity by which cyclic GMP is increased in smooth muscle.

CO_2

NO synthesis is critically involved in the CBF increase accompanying hypercapnia (Iadecola 1992, Wang et al. 1992, Pellegrino et al. 1993). Studies in rats suggest that pial arteriolar dilatory response to hypercapnia appears to involve NO. However, the source of the hypercapnic-induced NO production is apparently non endothelial (Wang et al. 1994).

Effects of different drugs upon CBF

Adenosine and eicosanoids influence tonus of the cerebral vasculature. Concerning adenosine and the effects upon CBF is mentioned in chapter 8 and 12. The effect of eicosanoids are mentioned in chapter 8 and 12.

Histamine and insulin

Histamine

Mast cells are localised in the meningeal investment of large cerebral arteries, resistance vessels, and veins (Edvinsson et al. 1977, Jarrott et al. 1979). Administrated intra-arterially, after blood-brain barrier disruption, histamine increases CBF and cerebrovascular transport of sucrose and aminoisobutyric acid (Gross et al. 1982), and it has been suggested that histamine may function as a neurotransmitter (Schwartz et al. 1980). Topical application of histamine induces cerebral vasodilation (Wahl and Kuschinsky 1979). This reaction is associated with increased CSF levels of prostanoids. The vascular response is eliminated after treatment with indomethacin (Mirro et al. 1988) and by the H_2 receptor antagonist cimitidine, but only incompletely by H_1 receptor blockers (Dacay and Bassett 1987).

Insulin

In diabetic man an increase in free insulin levels from 20 to 191 mU/L during euglycaemia did not alter total or regional glucose utilisation or CBF (Cranston et al. 1998).

Regulation by arterial carbon dioxide tension (P_aCO_2)

Hypercapnia

Hypercapnia has been used in the neurosurgical clinic in cases where an increase in CBF is intended, especially during carotid end-arterectomy. There is no doubt, however, that hypercapnia as a general rule is detrimental when intracranial compliance is exhausted. Release of tourniquets during orthopaedic operation increases ICP and CBF (Hirst et al. 1990).

During prolonged hypercapnia with 6% CO_2, (PaCO2 level 65 mm Hg), a 2,5-fold increase in CBF at 30 min. was observed in pigs. CBF decreased to basal values at three hrs. and gradually rose again at 6 and 8 hrs. This secondary CBF rise was associated with induction of endothelial NO synthase, mediated by prostaglandin E_2, which again was generated by a K(ATP) and Ca^{2+} channel-dependent process (Najarian et al. 2000).

In this review attention will be paid to hypocapnia which in experimental as well as clinical studies effectively reduces ICP.

Mechanism of hypocapnic vasoconstriction

The cerebrovascular resistance (CVR) is primarily regulated by changes in pH in the extracellular fluid surrounding cerebral vessels (Betz and Heuser 1967, Lassen 1968, Cotev and Severinghaus 1969, Plum and Siesjö 1975). The existence of a brain stem centre regulating hemispheric CBF during changes in $PaCO_2$ has been disproved by the fact that cortical CBF is not affected by change of $PaCO_2$ in the vertebral-basilar system (Skinhøj and Paulson 1969). Thus, an increase in pH constricts, and a decrease dilates cerebral resistance vessels. A decrease in CVR results in an increase in CBF and CBV, and an increase in CVR gives rise to an increase in flow and blood volume. As CO_2, in comparison with bicarbonate, is freely diffusible between arterial blood and brain tissue, changes in ventilation and consequently $PaCO_2$ are of utmost importance in the regulation of CBF.

Preliminary studies in rats suggest that endogenously released adenosine is involved in the increase in CBF response during hypercapnia (Phillis and De Long 1987).

Although indomethacin, a cyclo-oxygenase inhibitor, reduces the increase in CBF associated with hypercapnia (Dahlgren et al. 1981), recent studies do not indicate that prostaglandins are involved in the regulation of CBF during hypercapnia (Wei et al. 1980).

Nitric oxide

In experimental studies a pronounced diminution of hypercapnic response of CBF has been found after administration of NO synthase inhibitors (Iadacola 1992, Wang et al. 1992, Pelligrino et al. 1993). However, this effect was not demonstrated in other studies (Adachi et al. 1992, Sokoloff et al. 1992). In a study in rats L-NAME, a NO synthase inhibitor, inhibited the hypercapnic increase of both $CMRO_2$ and CBF (Horvath et al. 1994). This result suggests that at least part of the increase in CBF observed during hypercapnia is coupled to an increase in $CMRO_2$.

CO_2 reactivity

The absolute CO_2 reactivity is defined as delta CBF/delta $PaCO_2$ mm Hg). In the range of 4–6 kPa of $PaCO_2$ absolute CO_2 reactivity is 1–2 ml/mm Hg in dogs (Reivich 1964) and humans (McHenry et al. 1965). The relative CO_2 reactivity is defined as %change CBF/delta $PaCO_2$ mm Hg or delta ln CBF/delta $PaCO_2$ mm Hg. In normal subjects it averages 4%/mm Hg at $PaCO_2$ ranging from 5–6 kPa (Olesen et al. 1971). During hypocapnia, $PaCO_2$ ranging between 3–5 kPa, the relative CO_2 reactivity is 2%, and during hypercapnic level ($PaCO_2 > 6$ kPa) it is 6% (Tominaga et al. 1976). Comparative studies of regional CO_2 reactivity suggest that it is highest in the cerebrum, less pronounced in the cerebellum (x 0.6), and lowest in the spinal cord (x 0.5) (Sato et al. 1984).

Experimental studies

CBV and airway pressure

Rosomoff (1963) studied changes in CBV and CSF volume after 30 min of hypocapnia to $PaCO_2$ 20 mm Hg in dogs and found a fall in CBV, and an compensatory increase in CSF volume. With MRI technology the effect of hypocapnia to $PaCO_2$ 25 mm Hg was studied in the rat. CBV decreased 17% in the cerebellum, 15% in corpus striatum and 12% in neocortex (Payen et al. 2000). The changes in CVR and CBV during hypo- and hypercapnia are reflected in brain capillary diameter which is larger during hypercapnia (Duelli and Kuschinsky 1993).

During active hyperventilation cerebral venous drainage is not impaired, but during massive passive hyperventilation in dogs a high positive airway pressure impedes cerebral venous drainage, increases cerebral venous pressure, and consequently increases ICP (Kitahata et al. 1971).

Hypoxia

In dogs it has been shown that there is a hypoxic counteraction to hypocapnic vasoconstriction when the tissue oxygen tension in jugular venous blood has reached a critically low level. The venous oxygen tension, at which the hypoxic flow increases is initiated, does not indicate cerebral ischaemia, as ATP and phosphocreatine are not depleted (Granholm and Siesjö 1969). Following prolonged hyperventilation to $PaCO_2$ ranging from 1.3 to 1.6 kPa, however, a depletion of ATP and phosphocreatine have been observed in cats and dogs (Granholm and Siesjö 1969, Michenfelder et al. 1970), and a net intracellular acidosis has been observed during these circumstances (Nilsson and Busto 1973). Studies of brain tissue pH during respiratory alkalosis in dogs (Hilberman et al. 1984), and studies of cerebral tissue oxygen tension (Kennealy et al 1980) support the view that extreme hypocapnia might provoke cerebral ischaemia.

$CMRO_2$ and glucose utilisation

In a study by Samra et al. (1989) local glucose utilisation was increased heterogeneously throughout the brain in rats subjected to hypocapnia ($PaCO_2$ 25 mm Hg), with a significant increase in lateral and ventral thalamus, the inferior colliculus, lateral habenulla, medial geniculate body and auditory cortex.

In contrast, hypercapnia, which is tolerated well even for prolonged periods (Cohen et al. 1990), is associated with an increase in $CMRO_2$ (Berntman et al. 1979, Artru and Michenfelder 1980). This reaction is supposed to be caused by catecholamine, and the increase is inhibited by β-blocking agents.

Steal phenomenon

Experimental studies of focal ischaemia have shown a decrease in focal pial blood pressure during hypercapnia (Brawley et al. 1967, Symon 1970). This phenomenon is caused by a redistribution of blood flow from regions with a relatively high ICP and low CO_2 reactivity to regions with a high CO_2 reactivity and relatively low tissue pressure, referred to as a steal phenomenon.

Inverse steal phenomenon

Although studies in MACO indicate an increase in lactic-acidosis and a decrease in ATP in the focal region (Michenfelder and Sundt 1973), other studies indicate that hypocapnia might redistribute blood flow from regions with low tissue pressure and high CO_2 reactivity to regions with high pressures and relatively low CO_2 reactivity. This phenomenon is called inverse steal phenomenon.

Protection

The occurrence of inverse steal phenomenon is of considerably interest. Consequently, hypocapnia has been studied in experimental brain ischaemia. Studies in dogs and cats suggested that the size of an infarct was reduced when hypocapnia was applied prior to the insult (Soloway et al. 1968, Battistini et al. 1969). However, later experimental studies have not established this finding (Soloway et al. 1971). In a later investigation this item has been restudied. Dogs subjected to cardiac arrest were allocated to 8 hours resuscitation with or without hyperventilation. In hyperventilated dogs a significant histopathological amelioration was observed (Vanicky et al. 1992).

Impaired CO_2 reactivity

The CO_2 reactivity has been shown to be absent or impaired after ischaemia and traumatic brain injury. This abnormality has been associated with an increased activity of arachidonic acid metabolites and liberation of free oxygen radicals. In experimental studies inhibition of free oxygen radicals formation by indomethacin (inhibition of cyclooxygenase), superoxide dismutase and catalase (free oxygen radical scavengers) and n-acetylcysteine (free oxygen radical scavenger) normalise the CO_2 reactivity (Wei et al. 1981, Kontos et al. 1981, Ellis et al. 1991). In rats the CO2 reactivity was examined before, during and 4.5 hrs. after middle cerebral artery occlusion by perfusion MRI. The pre-ischaemic CO_2 reactivity averaging 3.5%/mm Hg decreased dramatically during occlusion in the ischaemic hemisphere. During reperfusion the CO_2 reactivity remained $< 1\%$/mm Hg in the region with end-ischaemic apparent diffusion coefficient $< 80\%$ of the preischaemic control value, but showed gradual recovery in the region with end-ischaemic apparent diffusion coefficient $>$ 80% of control. Although at the end of the experiment the CO_2 reactivity was higher in tissue with normal ATP levels than in tissue with decreased ATP levels, the CO_2 reactivity still remained far below the normal control value (Olah et al. 2000).

In dogs the CO_2 reactivity is sustained during drug-induced hypotension (Artru and Colley 1984) and in rats hypercapnic acidosis adversely affects energy metabolism during hypotension (Eklöf et al. 1972).

High dose barbiturate impairs the CO_2 reactivity. This finding has not been found with propofol or midazolam.

Adaptation (experimental studies)

Hypocapnia

In dogs and goats, adaptation to prolonged continuous hypocapnia occurs within 2–3 hours (Raichle et al. 1970, Albrecht et al. 1987). During prolonged respiratory alkalosis the greater fall in CSF-bicarbonate than in blood is supposed to be due to selective brain- and CSF-lactic acidosis (Wichser and Kazami 1975). Other studies in dogs subjected to sustained hypocapnia indicate that total and regional CBF correlates well with CSF-pH and a shift in the cerebrovascular sensitivity to CSF-pH was found (Warner et al. 1987).

Studies of pial arteriolar diameter by the cranial window technique in rabbits subjected to prolonged continuous hypocapnia indicate that hypocapnia is only effective in reducing pial vessel diameter for less than 24 hours. The authors argue that hyperventilation in clinical practice should only be used when ICP is elevated. If used preventively, its effect may have dissipated by the time ICP starts to rise (Muizelaar et al. 1988). The resetting phenomenon of CSF-pH has also been demonstrated by Fencl et al. 1965 and Severinghaus 1965).

Hypercapnia

Dogs subjected to normoxic hypercapnia initially show a dramatic increase in CBF accompanied by a decrease in CVR. The increase in CBF persists for three hours and is followed by a decrease in CBF and an increase in CVR. Regional variations occur. Areas with the highest initial CBF show a greater rate of decay in flow over time. CSF-pH, initially more acid during hypercapnia increases with time. This change is accompanied by an increase in CSF bicarbonate. In prolonged respiratory acidosis CSF-bicarbonate is formed in the choroid plexus and glia cells. The formation is catalysed by CO_2 anhydrase. Hansen et al.

(1986) in studies of piglets subjected to prolonged hypercapnia found an increase in CBF and $CMRO_2$ after 30 minutes.

CSF-formation

Prolonged hypocapnia decreases the rate of formation of CSF. After an initial decrease at 30 and 60 min formation of CSF returns to pre-hypocapnic values (Martins et al. 1976, Hochwald et al. 1976, Artru and Hornbein 1987).

In dogs with an intracranial mass-expanding lesion prolonged hypocapnia initially gives rise to a decrease in CBV. However, the CSF-pressure lowering effect is sustained by a reduction in CSF volume, despite reexpanding of CBV. In the same model brain water content did not contribute to changes in CSF pressure and volume (Artru 1987).

Human Studies

Cerebral blood volume (CBV)

The changes in CBV effected by hypo- and hypercapnia are correlated to changes in CBF. In normal brains CBV changes by about 0.04-0.05 ml/100g/mm Hg $PaCO_2$. In grey matter and white matter values of 0.053 and 0.043 ml/100g/mm Hg $PaCO_2$ have been found (Greenberg et al. 1975). For the total brain, this means an increase by 11 ml in CBV when $PaCO_2$ is increased from 4.0 to 6.7 kPa (Phleps et al. 1973, Grubb et al. 1974).

Hyperventilation and cerebral ischaemia

In awake, unsedated patients, active hyperventilation to $PaCO_2$ 2.7 kPa induces changes in EEG compatible with cerebral hypoxia (Morgan and Ward 1970). These changes disappeared when hyperbaric oxygenation was provided (Reivich et al. 1966). During hypocapnia EEG slowing is observed when jugular venous oxygen tension is about 22 mm Hg (Gotoh et al. 1965). Accordingly, during prolonged hyperventilation in comatose patients an improvement of consciousness has been observed when $PaCO_2$ became normal (Froman 1968).

On the basis of theoretical considerations proposed by Sørensen (1978), hypoxemia to 4.0 kPa, a level at which consciousness is altered and eventually lost, equals hyperventilation to $PaCO_2$ 3.5 kPa at a $CMRO_2$ value of 3.0 ml O_2/100g/min, as regards the decrease in jugular oxygen tension, which under these conditions should average 3.0 kPa. At this level signs of cerebral hypoxaemia are evident (Allen and Morris 1962, Wollman and Orkim 1968).

The threshold at which deterioration in consciousness occurs and EEG signs compatible with cerebral hypoxaemia are observed is a jugular venous oxygen tension of about 2.5–3.0 kPa. These low tensions occur at PaO_2 ranging between 3.5 and 4.0 kPa and at a $PaCO_2$ level of 2.5 - 3.0 kPa. In humans subjected to extreme hypocapnia, a moderate increase in $CMR_{glucose}$ has been found, indicating anaerobic cerebral metabolism (Alexander et al. 1968). This change occurs at CBF levels ranging from 10 to 20 ml/100g/min, and at jugular venous oxygen tensions of 2.7 kPa (Gotoh et al. 1965).

Bohr effect

The decrease in oxygen delivery capacity effected by hypocapnia is partly caused by the decrease in CBF (part 75%) and partly by a shift of the dissociation curve of oxyhaemoglobin (part 25%) (Cain 1963, Gotoh t 1965, Harp and Wollman 1973).

CO2 reactivity

In several studies of severe head injury the CO_2 reactivity has been shown to be low in the acute phase and that a low hemispheric CO_2 reactivity is correlated to a poor outcome (Fieschi et al. 1974, Overgaard and Tweed 1974, Cold et al. 1977a, Messeter et al. 1986).

ICP

In patients with intracranial hypertension, hypocapnia effectively reduces ICP and CBF. It is accepted that the fall in ICP is caused by vasoconstriction of cerebral vessels and a decrease in CBV. Although the decrease in CBV is small in comparison with the total brain volume, hypocapnia can be life-saving in patients with a mass-expanding cerebral lesion, and acute hyperventilation is, therefore, an important tool in the management of acute intracranial hypertension (Lundberg et al. 1959, Slocum et al. 1961, Bozza et al. 1961).

Diaschisis

In diaschisis regions with low CBF hypocapnia only reduces CBF little, while hypercapnia gives rise to a pronounced CBF increase (Takano et al. 1988).

Steal phenomenon

In patients with apoplexy and cerebral tumours, hypercapnia might provoke a steal phenomenon by promoting a decrease in CBF in the focal region (Palvölgyi 1969, Paulson et al. 1970).

Inverse steal phenomenon

In severe head injury, apoplexy, and brain tumours, an inverse steal phenomenon or Robin Hood phenomenon has been observed during hypocapnia (Palvölgyi 1969, Paulson et al. 1970, Pistolese et al. HI1972, Fieschi et al. 1974, Cold et al. 1977b, Obrist et al. 1984). Regions with inverse reactions are shattered over the cerebral hemisphere and sparsely localised to abnormal radiological findings (Cold et al. 1977b).

Darby et al.(1988), in a study with enhanced Xenon CT scanning, demonstrated that hypocapnia might provoke a pronounced CBF increase resulting in cerebral oedema.

Regional studies of CO_2 reactivity

In patients with severe head injury the CO_2 reactivity ranged from 1.3 to 8.5%/mm Hg $PaCO_2$. Lobar, cerebellar, basal ganglia and brain-stem CO_2 reactivities frequently varied from the mean global value by more than 25%. The greatest variability occurred in patients with acute subdural haematoma and patients with diffuse injuries (Marion and Bouma 1991).

Carotid surgery apoplexy and head injury

A beneficial effect of hypocapnic inverse steal has been postulated during carotid end-arterectomy (Fourcade et al. 1970). In another study inverse steal was observed very rarely (Artru and Merriman 1989). In studies of carotid end-arterectomy routinely use of hypocapnia is not advocated, and hypocapnia in comparison with hypercapnia decreases carotid stump pressure (Boysen et al. 1971).

In the majority of patients with carotid occlusion the CO_2 reactivity is impaired. These patients have an increased risk of developing a stroke during the follow-up period (Kuroda et al. 1993, Yonas et al. 1993, Powers 1991, Kleiser and Widder 1992). In many patients an initially impaired CO_2 reactivity improves with time (Widder et al. 1994).

The occurrence of inverse steal reaction is of considerable interest. Studies of cerebral autoregulation during hypocapnia indicate a normalisation of autoregulation during hypocapnia in patients with apoplexy and cerebral tumours (Paulson et al. 1972). Studies of hypocapnia as a therapeutic tool in the control of intracranial hypertension have suggested prolonged artificial hyperventilation as a rational treatment in patients suffering from brain ischaemia. However, controlled studies of the effect of artificial hyperventilation in cerebral apoplexy have been discouraging, no improvements in recovery or outcome being demonstrated (Christensen 1976).

In patients with severe traumatic head injury an uncontrolled study of artificial hyperventilation suggests improvement of outcome (Gordon 1979). This finding was opposed by Jennett et al. (1980) who in an uncontrolled multicentre study found that patients undergoing mechanical ventilation had outcomes which were worse than expected.

In a clinical outcome study by Muizelaar et al. (1991) patients with head injury were randomized to respiratory treatment during normocapnia, hypocapnia ($PaCO_2$ level 25 mm Hg) and a third group with hypocapnia and in addition treatment with THAM. At 3 and 6 months after injury the number of patients with favourable outcome was lower in the hyperventilation group than in the control- and the THAM group. However, this occurred only in patients with an initial motor score of 4–5, and at 12 months posttrauma this difference was not found.

Adaptation (human studies)

The adaptation to prolonged hypocapnia has been investigated in patients with apoplexy. The half-life of the adaptation mechanism of CSF-pH and CSF bicarbonate averages 6 hours, and adaptation was found to be complete within 24–30 hours (Christensen et al. 1974). Studies in healthy adults support these findings (Rehde et al. 1977). Recently, studies using non-invasive Doppler ultrasound technique and calculation of the instantaneous mean blood velocity during hypocapnia in normal subjects indicated that blood velocity showed adaptation within 10 min after induction of hypocapnia (Ellingsen et al. 1987). However, in patients with severe head injury an uncontrolled study did not reveal signs of CSF-pH adaptation within periods of 6–24 hours, and it is suggested that the mechanism of adaptation is impaired in severe generalised cerebral lesions with lactic-acidosis or ischaemia (Cold et al. 1977a). When hyperventilation is used for several days to reduce ICP in the presence of brain oedema, withdrawal of hypocapnia should be cautious as ICP-hypertension very often reappears (Havill 1984).

Clinical use of prolonged continuous hyperventilation. Pro et contra

Some arguments for and against the use of prolonged artificial hyperventilation have already been advanced. Other arguments against this therapeutic measure are as follows: 1) Inhibition of oxygen delivery from oxyhaemoglobin to the tissue, because of a left shift of the saturation curve of haemoglobin (Bohr effect). Besides impairment of the oxygen delivery to the brain this effect includes impairment of oxygen supply to the myocardium (Neill and Hattenhauer 1975). 2) Decrease in cardiac output and blood pressure caused by a reduction in the central venous blood flow and diastolic filling. These effects are mediated via an increase in mean airway pressure. An increase in airway pressure combined with a decrease in blood pressure also induces a decrease in renal function and an associated retention of water and sodium. 3) Hypocapnia increases whole body CO_2 production (Cain 1970, Khambatta and Sullivan 1974) and in experimental studies an increase in $CMRO_2$ has been observed (Hassan and Kazemi 1976). 4) Prolonged hypocapnia provokes disruption of the blood-brain barrier (Rengachery et al. 1967). 5) Hypocapnia decreases collateral perfusion in ischaemic regions (Brock et al. 1969). 6) The risk of barotrauma might be stressed as a function of increased airway pressure.

Acetazolamide

pH

Acetazolamide, a potent carbonic anhydrase inhibitor, is a potent cerebral vasodilator. After intravenous administration a rapid decrease of pH in brain tissue and extracellular fluid, despite a constant cerebral tissue PCO_2 occur (Severinghaus and Cotev 1968). The CBF increase after acetazolamide is dose dependent (Posner and Plum 1960), and the effect is maximal after 10 minutes (Gotoh et al. 1966, Friis et al. 1980). $CMRO_2$ is unchanged after acetazolamide (Posner and Plum 1960).

In patients with carotid stenosis or occlusion acetazolamide has been used for measuring of vasoreactivity reserve capacity (Vorstrup et al. 1988, Brown et al. 1986, Russell et al. 1990, Dahl et al. 1994). It has been demonstrated that an increased risk of ischaemic episodes in the ipsilateral hemisphere to the occluded artery is present when the cerebrovascular reactivity is reduced (Kleister and Widder, 1992, Yonas et al. 1993).

Cerebral autoregulation (CA)

Cerebral autoregulation refers to the ability in the brain to maintain a constant CBF despite changes in cerebral perfusion. Evaluation of CA is performed under steady state conditions where a measurement of CBF is obtained first at a constant baseline MABP, followed by another steady-state measurement of CBF at a higher or lower MABP. This method is referred to as static autoregulation test. If the CBF changes with either an increase or a decrease in MABP, CA is impaired or lost. If CBF is maintained at the baseline level, despite changes in MABP, CA is intact.

Static and dynamic studies of CA

A non-invasive method of dynamic approach to evaluate cerebral autoregulation was introduced by Aaslid et al. (1989). This so called leg-cuff approach uses the rapid drops in blood pressure caused by release of tight blood pressure cuffs as an autoregulatory stimulus, and compares MABP and CBF velocity by transcranial Doppler sonography. At least three iterations of the test procedure should be performed and averaged to obtain valuable results (Mahony et al. 2000). Good correlation between results of static and dynamic studies of CA has been documented (Larsen et al. 1994, Tiecks et al. 1995).

During the transient hyperaemic response test a brief compression of the ipselateral carotid artery is performed during continuos recording of flow velocity in the middle cerebral artery. If cerebral autoregulation is present, the reduction in middle cerebral artery pressure during carotid artery compression should cause vasodilatation in the arterioles distal to the middle cerebral artery. Consequently, a release of the compression results in a transient increase in CBF and flow velocity (Giller 1991, Czosnyka et al. 1992). The ratio of blood flow velocity immediately after release of compression to baseline flow velocity is a valid index of cerebral autoregulation, and has the same sensitivity as the leg-cuff method (Smielewski et al. 1996). In a recent study it was concluded that experimental factors such as duration of carotid artery compression and magnitude of the decrease in blood flow velocity during carotid compression significantly influence the transient hyperaemic response (Cavill et al. 1998).

Using transcranial Doppler the correlation between slow waves in arterial blood pressure and blood flow velocity has been analysed (Steinmeier et al. 1996, Zhang et al. 1998, Czosnyka et al. 1996). This method is less laborious and may be used in a wider range of patients. With this method a good prediction of outcome in patients with severe head injury has been obtained, and an optimal CPP in sedated, paralysed patients is easily defined (Czosnyka et al. 1996, Czosnyka et al. 1997). The method is potential useful in situations in which a change in cerebral autoregulation in response to change of ventilation pattern, osmotherapy, or hypertension/hypervolaemia therapy, is to be monitored (Piechnik et al. 1999).

Experimental studies of cerebral autoregulation

Evidence of an intrinsic regulation of CBF designed to maintain a constant cerebral perfusion during changes in blood pressure was first presented by Fog (1934), and later confirmed by others (Forbes et al. 1937, Lassen 1959).

Cranial window technique

Studies in cats with the cranial window technique for direct observation of the pial microcirculation indicate that the adjustments in calibre within the autoregulatory range occur in vessels larger than 200 μ in diameter, whilst small arterioles less than 100 μ in diameter only dilate at pressures equal or less than 90 mm Hg (Kontos et al. 1978). However, adjustments also occur in large arteries. 20–45% of the change in CVR during adjustments occurs in large resistance arteries (Heisand et al. 1978)

Flow velocity studies

Studies with transcranial Doppler technique in rabbits indicate that below the lower limit of CA pulsative amplitude varies with the CPP. Above the break point pulsative amplitude varies inversely with CPP. Thus, lower limit of CA can be estimated by this technique (Nelson et al. 1992).

Lower limit of cerebral autoregulation

The lower limit of CA differs for different species. Below this level CBF decreases and becomes pressure dependent. At pressure decreases below the lower limit of CA maximal distension of the cerebral vessels does not occur. Thus, Häggendal and Johanssom (1965) in dogs demonstrated that hypercapnia increases CBF further. By a stepwise increase in ICP a shift of the lower limit of CA towards lower levels of CPP has been demonstrated in rats (Hauerberg et al. 1994).

Upper limit of cerebral autoregulation

In dogs an upper limit of CA has been defined (Ekström-Jodal et al. 1972). This limit is dependent on species, and is increased in experimental renovascular hypertension in baboons (Strandgaard et al. 1975b). In rats subjected to stepwise intracranial hypertension the upper limit of autoregulation is shifter to lower levels of CPP, and a narrowing of the autoregulated interval has been demonstrated (Hauerberg et al. 1998).

Energy metabolism

In cats subjected to mock installation and examined by MR spectroscopy, lactate rises at an average CPP of 49 mm Hg, and an increase in phosphocreatine was observed at an average CPP of 29 mm Hg. However, in cats considerable variation was found in the CPP at which failure of brain energy metabolism occurred, suggesting differences in CA curves in this animal (Sutton et al. 1987).

Different factors

In dogs the lower limit of CA is unaltered during hypocapnia (Artru et al. 1989). In experimental studies (Jarden et al. 1984) as well as human studies (Waldemar et al. 1989) the lower limit of CA is decreased by the angiotensin converting enzyme, captopril. Other studies by Stone and Raichle (1974) demonstrate that the lower limit of CA is dose-dependently increased during hypercapnia. Studies in MCAO indicate that in the focal region of ischaemia, CA is lost when CBF is decreased to values of 20–30% of control (Symon et al. 1976, Dirnagl and Pulsinelli 1990).

In rats a shift of the lower limit of CA towards lower CPP was observed during severe intracranial hypertension effected by infusion of mock-CSF. Thus, the lower limit of CA was 73 mm Hg in control studies, but 59 and 51 mm Hg during moderately and pronounced increased ICP. These results indicate that an acute elevation of ICP activates a reserve capacity of cerebral resistance vessels (Hauerberg and Juhler 1994). In another study by the same group it was found that intracranial hypertension by mock-CSF infusion is followed by a shift of the upper limit of CA towards lower CPP values (Hauerberg et al. 1998).

Time

In baboons CA regulation starts within 5–8 seconds of change in MABP, and is largely completed within 20 seconds (Symon et al. 1973). In dogs the regulation is completed within 45 seconds (Ekström-Jodal 1970).

Rate of change in blood pressure

The function of CA also depends upon the rate of change in MABP, even within the autoregulatory range. Moreover, the autoregulatory limit defined as the change in CBF in response to the rate of change in MABP differs in normotensive and spontaneously hypertension animals (Barzo et al. 1993).

CPP and CVR

From the equation CBF = CPP/CVR, complete cerebral autoregulation means that changes in CPP and CVR are in concert. In this equation CPP is defined as MABP ICP. If cerebral autoregulation, however, is absent, and MABP and/or ICP are changed in parallel so that CPP remains unchanged, CBF increases with MABP (Miller et al. 1971).

CPP or MABP

Studies in cats indicate that at CPP of 40 mm Hg, where cerebral autoregulation is impaired or absent, CBF depends more on arterial driving pressure than upon CPP. In the same study it was demonstrated that non-autoregulating blood vessels had an increased CBF for a given MABP or CPP (Chan et al. 1992)

The CA is lost during hypoxaemia (Häggendal and Johansson 1965, Kogure et al. 1970), during hypercapnia (Ekström-Jodal et al. 1970), and during hyperthermia (Katsumura et al. 1993).

Blood-brain barrier (BBB)

Above the upper limit of CA, disruption of the blood-brain barrier occurs. Studies with Evans blue indicate, that cerebral oedema and focal haemorrhage supervene (Johansson et al. 1970), Häggendal and Johansson 1992). Acute hypertension to this level of blood pressure is associated with endothelial lesions and abnormalities of the vascular smooth muscle in pial arterioles. These changes are inhibited by pre-treatment with indomethacin, or topical application on the brain surface with the free oxygen radical scavenger, superoxide dismutase (Kontos et al. 1981).

Hypertension above the upper limit of CA for about one hour is associated with long-lasting disruption of the blood-brain barrier and development of cerebral oedema (Ekström-Jodal et al. 1975). In contrast, hypertension of short duration (< 3 min) results in reversible blood-brain barrier dysfunction, which is normalised within 10 min (Johansson and Linder 1978). The disruption of the BBB primarily occurs in the venules, and the dysfunction is supposed to be due to an increase in venous pressure (Auer 1978, Mayhan et al. 1986a).

Brain acidosis does not influence BBB (Olesen and Chrone 1986), and in total energy depleted animals the BBB has been found to be intact (Greenwood et al. 1989).

Regional differences in CA

Studies in cats suggest that the derangement of CA is heterogeneous within the brain, with relatively resistance of the cerebellum (Sato et al. 1984). In contrast, acute hypertension in rats indicates that hyperperfusion is most prominent in the cerebellum, parietal grey, thalamus, striatum and pons. These anatomical regions are recognised sites of hypertensive haemorrhage in human (Burke et al. 1987). Other studies in rats suggest that the CA is more effective in the brain stem than in the cerebrum (MacKenzie et al. 1976, Suzuki et al. 1984, Baumbach and Heistad 1985, Murphy and Johanson 1985, Mayhan et al. 1986). Moreover, distribution of blood flow occurs with relatively high flow in favour of thalamus, hypothalamus, pons and medulla oblongata (Chen et al. 1984). Regional derangement of CA seems to be influenced by stress, e.g. insulin-induced hypoglycaemia. The presence of disturbed CA is related to the occurrence of neuropathological findings (Siesjö et al. 1983).

Ischaemia

Studies in rats subjected to unilateral cerebral embolization by microspheres (Hardebo and Beley 1984), and studies in dogs with multifocal cerebral ischaemia induced by air embolism (Dutka et al. 1987) indicate that arterial hypertension during the ischaemic period increases the leakage through the BBB, resulting in haemorrhage in the infarcted brain region. Furthermore, acute hypertension induces delayed deterioration of brain function as evaluated by evoked responses, and worsens CBF. Other studies in gerbils subjected to carotid artery ligation have unveiled that hypertension after blood flow restoration, following ischaemia, induces an accelerated BBB damage (Ito et al. 1980).

Cerebral vasoconstrictors

The CA has been studied extensively with the aid of norepinephrine and angiotensin II. These drugs were assumed to have no action on cerebral vessels (King et al. 1952, Agnoli et al. 1965, Greenfield and Tindall 1968, Olesen 1972) except when the MABP exceeded the upper limit of CA, resulting in disruption of the BBB (MacKenzie et al. 1976, Edvinsson et al. 1978). Later studies, however, indicate that these drugs have a direct constrictive effect upon cerebral vessels (Sercombe et al. 1985, Speth and Harik 1985). In large doses angiotensin II produces cerebral vasodilation, particularly of pial vessels. Prostaglandin synthesis does not seem to be involved in this action (Tamaki et al. 1992). Kuschensky et al. (1982) found a reduced cerebral glucose utilisation, and an increase in CBF during norepinephrine infusion. Furthermore, Reynier-Rebuffet et al. (1987) in studies in rabbits observed non-uniformity of CBF during norepinephrine or angiotensin II-induced hypertension, suggesting that the cerebrovascular regulatory mechanisms in hypertension are more complex, and cannot be explained by a simple myogenic theory as proposed by Symon et al. (1972).

Autoregulatory mechanism

It is generally believed that myogenic reactions of smooth muscle in the arterial walls are responsible for the CA regulation. *In vivo* studies of isolated arteries support this view (Vinaull and Simeone 1981). Experimental studies, however, suggest that adenosine also plays an important role as chemical mediator during induced hypotension (Winn et al. 1980, Winn et al. 1981). Released adenosine predominantly appears to remain inside the cerebral cells (McIlwain and Poll 1986), and contrary to the study of Winn et al. (1980). Other studies indicate that interstitial fluid adenosine concentration failed to increase during autoregulation stress in the rat (Van Wylen et al. 1987, Park et al. 1988).

Sympathetic innervation

Activation of perivascular sympathetic nerves modifies the CA thresholds of lower and upper limits of CA by a shift towards higher levels (Papela et al. 1967, Eklöff et al. 1971, Waltz et al. 1971). Other studies suggest that neurogenic activity influences the CA under stress (Salanga and Waltz 1973, Fitch et al. 1975, Bill and Linder 1976, MacKenzie et al. 1979, Edvinsson et al. 1983). The vascular responses are brought about by nervous, and not by purely muscular mechanisms (Mchedlischvili et al. 1975). Thus, acute sympathectomy and α-blockade decrease lower limit of CA (Fitch et al. 1975, MacKenzle et al. 1979). On the other hand, an increase in upper limit of CA has been demonstrated during sympathetic stimulation (Bill and Linder 1976) and during β-blockade (Sadoshima et al. 1989). The same limit is decreased during sympathetic denervation (Sadoshima et al. 1986). Moreover, studies in rats have shown that increased sympathetic activity during acute hypertension seems to blunt the vulnerability of the BBB (Johansson and Auer 1983). The CA is easily abolished when vasodilation of cerebral vessels is induced by papaverine (Johansson 1974), during hypercapnia (Häggedal and Johansson 1975, and during hypoxia (Häggendal and Johansson 1965).

Human studies of cerebral autoregulation

Limits of autoregulation

In humans the lower limit of CA lies between 50 and 80 mm Hg (Shenkin et al. 1950, McKrell et al. 1955, Kleinerman et al. 1958). Through many years a level of 60 mm Hg has been supposed to be the lower limit of CA. However, studies in healthy volunteers indicate that the lower limit of CA is about 85 mm Hg in normotensive and 113 in hypertensive subjects (Schmidt et al. 1990). An upper limit of CA has been demonstrated in normotensive subjects (Strandgaard et al. 1975a), and is thought to be about 150–170 mm Hg of MABP (Lassen 1974). Dynamic cerebral autoregulation, as assessed by flow velocity responses to transient and induced blood pressure stimuli, is unaffected by ageing (Carey et al. 2000).

Time related changes

In humans the CA regulation starts within 5–8 seconds and it is completed within 20 seconds (Greenfield et al. 1984). In chronic hypertension the lower and upper limit of CA are shifted to the right (Strandgaard et al. 1973a). After 2–3 weeks of antihypertensive therapy, however, a shift to the left has been observed (Strandgaard 1976). For review Strandgaard and Paulson (1984).

Hypertensive encephalopathy

The human equivalent to disrupted BBB is acute hypertensive encephalopathy (Skinhøj and Strandgaard 1973).

The influence of drugs etc.

Drugs with vasodilatatory capacity on cerebral vessels, like papaverine and inhalation agents (halothane, enflurane, isoflurane and sevoflurane) impair the CA. Impairment of CA has also been demonstrated during hyperthermia (Allen et al. 1986). On the other hand, a normalisation of $PaCO_2$ and the use of hypnotic drugs, which induce a suppression of cerebral oxygen uptake, restore the CA. Studies in humans with cerebral tumours and apoplexy have shown that induced hypocapnia restores CA, which otherwise was abolished during normocapnia (Paulson et al. 1972, Hadjidimos et al. 1975). The upper limit of CA is shifted to the left after pre-treatment with captopril (Paulson et al. 1989, Waldemar et al. 1989)

Dissociation between CO_2 reactivity and cerebral autoregulation

In the acute phase of head injury CA generally is abolished. This impairment might be focal, localised to one hemisphere or global. Several studies of CA in the acute phase of head injury, however, indicate that CA is un-impaired during the acute phase (first day of trauma), abolished later on, and might normalise during recovery of the patient (Fieschi et al. 1974, Enevoldsen and Jensen 1979, Cold and Jensen 1978). Enevoldsen and Jensen (1979) found that in comatose patients with severe head impaired CO_2 reactivity was accompanied by intact" cerebral autoregulation. This dissociation between CO_2 reactivity and CA was also demonstrated in another study indicating that acute hypocapnia changes regions with unimpaired CA and abolished CO_2 reactivity, to regions with impaired CA (Cold et al. 1981). As CA in experimental studies is very easily disturbed, the initial unimpaired CA may be a "false" phenomenon. The presence of "false" CA has been debated, and it is thought that CA tests by angiotensin-induced blood pressure increase, might provoke an increase in cerebral tissue pressure due to extravasation of water and electrolytes, which secondary obstructs the cerebral vessels, leaving CPP unchanged. Clinical studies, however, do not support this view, since angiotensin-induced hypertension in patients with "false" CA is not always followed by an increase in ICP. Therefore, either other mechanisms are responsible for "false" CA, or with available technique it is not possible accurately to detect changes in tissue pressure.

References

Aaslid R, Lindegaard KF, Sorteberg W, Nornes H. Cerebral autoregulation dynamics in human. Stroke 1989: 20: 45-52.

Adams JE, Elliot H, Sutherland VC, et al. Cerebral metabolic studies of hypothermia in the human. Surg Forum 1957: 7: 535–539.

Agnoli A, Battistini N, Bozza L, Fieschi C. Drug action on regional cerebral blood flow in cases of acute cerebrovascular involvment. Acta Neurol Scand 1965: suppl 14: 142–144.

Albrecht RF, Ruttle M. Central effect of extended hyperventilation in unanaeshtetizewd goats. Stroke 1987: 18: 649–655.

Alexander SC, Smith TC, Strobel G, et al. Cerebral carbohydrate metabolism of man during respiratory and metabolic alkalosis. J Appl Physiol 1968: 24: 66–72.

Allen GC, Morris LE. Central nervous system effects of hyperventilation during anaesthesia. Br J Anaesth 1962: 24: 296–306.

Allen SJ, Giezentanner A, Cronau LH, et al. Whole body hyperthermia increases cerebral blood flow and impairs cerebral autoregulation. Anesthesiology 1986: 65: A321.

Altman DI, Powers WJ, Perlman JM, et al. Cerebral blood flow requirement for brain viability in newborn infants is lower than adults. Ann Neurol 1988: 24: 218–226.

Altura BM, Gebrewold A, Lassoff S. Biphasic reponsiveness of rat pial arterioles to dopamine. Direct observation of the microvasculature. Br J Pharmacol 1980: 69: 543–544.

Artru AA, Michenfelder JD. Effects of hypercapnia on canine cerebral metabolism and blood flow with simultaneous direct and indirect measurement of blood flow. Anesthesiology 1980: 52: 466–469.

Artru AA, Nugent M, Michenfelder JD. Anesthetics affect the cerebral metabolic reponse to circulatory chatecholamines. J Neurochem 1981: 36: 1941.

Artru AA; Coley PS. Cerebral blood flow responses to hypocapnia during hypotension. Stroke 1984: 15: 878–883.

Artru AA, Reduction of cerebrospinal fluid pressure by hypocapnia. J Cereb Blood Flow Metab 1987: 7: 471–479.

Artru AA, Hornbein TF. Prolonged hypocapnia does not alter the rate of CSF production during halothane anaesthesia or sedation with nitrous oxide. Anesthesiology 1987: 67: 66–71.

Artru AA, Katz RA, Coley PS, Autoregulation of cerebral blood flow during normocapnia and hypocapnia in dogs. Anesthesiology 1989: 70: 288–292.

Artru AA, Merriman HG. Hypocapnia added to hypertension to reserve EEG changes during carotid end-arterectomy. Anesthesiology 1989: 70: 1016–1018.

Astrup J, Møller Sørensen P, Sørensen HR. Inhibition of cerebral oxygen and glucose consumption in the dog by hypothermia, pentobarbital, and lidocaine. Anesthesiology 1981: 55: 263–268.

Auer L. Origin and localization of Evans blue extravasation in acutely-induced hypertension in cats. Europ Neurol 1979: 17: 211–215.

Bailes JE, Leavitt ML, Teeple E, et al. Ultraprofound hypothermia with complete blood substitution in a canine model. J Neurosurg 1991: 74: 781–788.

Baker AJ, Zornow MH, Grafe MR, et al. Hypothermia prevents ischemia-induced increases in hippocampal glycine concentrations in rabbits. Stroke 1991: 22: 666–673.

Barker WW, Ysohii F, Loewenstein DA, et al. Cerebrocerebellar relationship during behavioral activation. J Cereb Blood Flow Metab 1991: 11: 48–54.

Baron JC, Bousser MG, Comar D, et al. Noninvasive tomographic study of cerebral blood flow and oxygen metabolism in vivo. Potentials, limitations, and clinical applications in cerebral ischemic disorders. Eur Neurol 1981: 20: 273–284.

Battistini N, Casacchia M, Bartolini A, et al. Effects of hyperventilation on focal brain damage following middle cerebral artery occlusion. In: Cerebral blood flow, clinical and experimental results. Brock M et al. (eds) Springer Verlag, Berlin, 1969: 249–253.

Baumbach GL, Heistad DD. Heterogeneity of brain flow and permeability during acute hypertension. Am J Physiol 1985: 249: 629–637.

Becker DP, Miller JD, Greenberg RP, et al. The outcome from severe head injury with early diagnosis and intensive management. J Neurosurg 1977: 47: 491–502.

Beresford HR, Posner JB, Plum F. Changes in brain lactate during induced cerebral seizures. Arch Neurol 1969: 20: 243–248.
Bering EA. Effects of profound hypothermia and circulatory arrest on cerebral oxygen metabolism and cerebrospinal fluid electrolyte composition in dogs. J Neurosurg 1974: 39: 199–205.
Berntman L, Dahlgren N, Siesjö BK. Influence of intravenously administered catecholamines on cerebral oxygen consumption and blood flow in the rat. Acta Physiol Scand 1978: 104: 101.
Berntman L, Dahlgren N, Siesjö BK. Cerebral blood flow and oxygen consumption in the rat brain during hypercapnia. Anesthesiology 1979: 50: 299–305.
Berntman L, Welch FA, Harp JR. Cerebral protective effect of low-grade hypothermia. Anesthesiology 1981: 55: 495–498.
Betz E, Heuser D. Cerebral cortical blood flow during changes of acid-base equilibrium of the brain. J Appl Physiol 1967: 23: 726–733.
Bill A, Linder J, Sympathetic effect on cerebral blood vessels in acute hypertension. Acta Physiol Scand 1976: 96: 114–121.
Blasberg RG, Fenstermacher JD, Patlak SC. Transport of alpha-aminoisobutyric acid across brain capillary and cellular membranes. J Cereb Blood Flow Metab 1983: 3: 8–32.
Boels PJ, Verbeuren TJ, Vanhoutte PM. Moderate cooling depresses the accumulation and the release of newly synthetized catecholamines in isolated canine saphenous veins. Experientia 1985: 41: 1374–1377.
Bolwig TG, Qistorff B. In vivo concentration of lactate in the brain of conscious rats before and during seizures: A new ultra-rapid technique for freeze-sampling of brain tissue. J Neurochem 1973: 21: 1345–1348.
Bouzarth WF, Kazi KH, Bubelis I, Shenkin HA. Effect of temperature upon craniocerebral trauma. Am Med Ass 1967: 199: 567–569.
Boyd RJ, Connolly JE. Tolerance of anoxia of dogs brain at various temperature. Surg Forum 1961: 12: 408–410.
Boysen G, Ladegaard-Pedersen HJ, Henriksen H, et al. The effect of $PaCO_2$ on regional cerebral blood flow and internal carotid arterial pressure during carotid clamping. Anesthesiology 1971: 35: 286–300.
Bozza MM, Maspes PE, Rossanda M. The control of brain volume and tension during intracranial operations. Br J Anaesth 1961: 33: 132–147.
Brawley BW, Strandness DE, Kelly WA. The phsyiologic response to therapy in experimental cerebral ischemia. Arch Neurol 1967: 17. 180–½87.
Brock M, Furuse M, Weber R, et al. Brain tissue pressure gradients. In: Intracranial Pressure II. Lundberg N, et al. (eds). Springer Verlag, Brilin. 1975: 215–220.
Brodersen P, Paulson OB, Bolwig TG, et al. Cerebral hyperaemia in electrically induced epileptic seizures. Arch Neurol 1973: 28: 334–338.
Bryan RM, Cerebral blood flow and energy metabolism during stress. Am J Physiol 1990: 259- 269–280.
Burke AM, Greenberg JH, Sladky J, Reivich M. Regional variation in cerebral perfusion during acute hypertension. Neurology 1987: 37: 94–99.
Busija DW, Wagerle LC, et al. Acetylcholine dramatically increases prostanoids synthesis in piglet parietal cortex. Brain Res. 1988: 439: 122–126.
Busto R, Dietrich D, Globus MY et al. Small differences in intra-ischemic brain temperature critically determine the extent of ischaemic neuronal injury. J Cereb Blood Flow Metab 1987: 7: 729–738.
Busto R, Globus MY, Dietrich WD, et al. Effect of mild hypothermia on ischemia-induced release of neurotransmitters and free fatty acids in rat brain. Stroke 1989: 20: 904–910.
Cain SM. An attemp to demonstrate cerebral anoxia during hyperventilation of anaesthetized dogs. J Appl Physiol 1963: 204: 323–326.
Cain SM. Increased oxygen uptake with passive hyperventilation of dogs. J Appl Physiol 1070: 28: 4–7
Carey BJ, Eames PJ, Blake MJ, et al. Dynamic cerebral autoregulation is unaffected by aging. Stroke 2000: 31: 2895–2900.
Carlsson C; Häggendal M, Siesjö BK. Protective effect of hypothermia in cerebral oxygen deficiency caused by arterial hypoxia. Anesthesiology 1976a: 44: 27–34.
Carlsson C, Hägerdal M, Sisjö BK. The effects of hyperthermia upon oxygen consumption and upon organic phosphate, glycolytic metabolites, citric acid cycle intermediates, and associated aminoacids in rat cerebral cortex. J Neurochem 1976b: 26: 1001–1006.
Cavill G, Simpson EJ, Mahajan RP. Factors affecting assessment of cerebral autoregulation using the transient hyperaemic response test. Br J Anaesth 1998: 81: 317–321.
Chan KH, Miller JD, Piper IR. Cerebral blood flow at constant cerebral perfusion pressure but changing arterial and intracranial pressure. Relationship to autoregulation. J Neurosurg Anesthesiol 1992: 4: 188–193.
Chen H, Chopp M, Zhang ZG, et al. The effect of hypothermia on transient middle cerebral artery occlusion in the rat. J Cereb Blood Flow Metab 1992: 12: 621–628.
Chen RYZ, Fan FC, Schuessler GB, et al. Regional cerebral blood flow and oxygen consumption of the canine brain during hemorrhagic hypotension. Stroke 1984: 15: 343–350.
Chopp M, Knight R, Tidwell CD, et al. The metabolic effects of mild hypothermia on global cerebral ischemia and recirculation in the cat. J Cereb Blood Flow Metab 1989: 9: 141–148
Christensen MS. Acid-base changes in cerebrospinal fluid and blood, and blood volume changes following prolonged hyperventilation in man. Br J Anaesth 1974: 46: 348–357.
Christensen MS. Prolonged artificial hyperventilation in cerebral apoplexy. Acta Anaesthesiol Scand 1976: suppl 62: 1–24.
Chugani HT, Phleps ME. Maturational changes in cerebral function in infants determined by 18FDG positron emission tomography. Science 1986: 231: 840–843.
Chugani HT, Hovda DA, Villablance JR, et al. Metabolic maturation of the brain: A study of local cerebral glucose utilization in the developing cat. J Cereb Blood Flow Metab. 1991: 11: 35–47.
Clifton GL, Jiang JY, Lyeth BG. et al. Marked protection by moderate hypothermia after experimental traumatic brain injury. J Cereb Blood Flow Metab 1991: 11: 114–121.
Cohen PJ, Wollman H, Alexander SC, et al. Cerebral carbohydrate metabolism in man during halothane anaesthesia. Effects of $PaCO_2$ on some aspects of carbohydrate utilization. Anesthesiology 1964: 25: 185–191.
Cohen PJ. To dream the impossible dream (editorial view). Anesthesiology 1981: 55. 491–493.
Cohen Y, Chang LH, Litt L, et al. Stability of brain intercellular lactate and 31P-metabolite levels at reduced intracellular

pH during prolonged hypercapnia in rats. J Cereb Blood Flow Metab 1990: 10: 277–284.
Cold GE Jensen FT, Malmros R. The cerebrovascular CO_2 reactivity during the acute phase of brain injury. Acta Anaesthesiol Scand 1977a: 21: 222–231.
Cold GE, Jensen FT, Malmros R. The effects of $PaCO_2$ reduction on regional cerebral blood flow in the acute phase of brain injury. Acta Anaesthesiol Scand 1977b: 21: 359–367.
Cold GE, Jensen FT. Cerebral autoregulation in unconscious patients with brain injury. Acta Anaesthesiol Scand 1978: 22: 270–280.
Cold GE. Cerebral metabolic rate of oxygen ($CMRO_2$) in the acute phase of brain injury. Acta Anaesthesiol Scand 1978: 22: 249–256.
Cold GE, Christensen MS, Schmidt K. Effect of two levels of induced hypocapnia on cerebral autoregulation in the acute phase of head injury coma. Acta Anaesthesiol Scand 1981: 25: 397–401.
Collins RC, Posner JB, Plum F. Cerebral energy metabolism during electroshock seizures in mice. Am J Physiol 1970: 218: 943–950.
Connolly JE, Boyd RJ, Calvin JW. The protective effect of hypothermia in cerebral ischaemia. Experimental and clinical application by selective brain cooling in the human. Surgery 1962: 52: 15–24.
Cotev S. Severinghaus JW. Role of cerebrospinal fluid pH in management of respiratory problems. Anesth Analg 1969: 48: 42–47.
Cranston I, Marsden P, Matyka K, et al. Regional differences in cerebral blood flow and glucose utilization in diabetic man: the effect of insulin. J Cereb blood Flow Metab 1998: 18: 130–140.
Cremer JE, Seville MP. Regional brain blood flow, blood volume and haematocrit values in the adult rat. J Cereb Blood Flow Metab 1983: 3: 254–256.
Curran-Everett DC, Iwamoto J, Meredith MP, Krasney JA. Intracranial pressures and O_2 extraction in conscious sheep during 72 h of hypoxia. Am J Physiol 1991: 261: 103–109.
Czosnyka M, Picard J, Whitehouse H, Piechnik S. The hyperaemic response to transient reduction in cerebral perfusion pressure. Acta Neurochir 1992: 115-90-97.
Czosnyka M, Smielewski P, Kirkpatrick P, et al. Monitoring of cerebral autoregulation in head-injured patients. Stroke 1996: 27: 829–834.
Czosnyka M, Smielewski P, Kirkpatrick P, et al. Continuous assessment of cerebral vasomotor reactivity in head injury. Neurosurgery 1997: 41: 11–19.
Dacey RG, Basett JE. Histaminergic vasodilation of intracerebral arterioles in the rat. J Cereb Blood Flow Metab 1987: 7: 327–331.
Dahlgren N, Nilsson B, Sakabe T, Siesjö BK. The effect of indomethacin on cerebral blood flow and oxygen consumption in the rat at normal and increased carbon dioxide tensions. Acta Physiol Scand 1981: 111: 475–485.
Dastur DK. Cerebral blood flow and metabolism in normal human aging, pathological aging and senile dementia. J Cereb Blood Flow Metab 1985: 5: 1-9.
Daw EF, Moffitt EA, Michenfelder JD, Terry HR. Prrofound hypothermia. Can Anesth Soc J 1964: 11: 382–393.
Darby JM, Yonas H, Marion DW, Latchaw RE. Local inverse steal induced by hyperventilation in head injury. Neurosurgery 1988: 23: 84–88.
DeAguilera ME, Vila JM, Irurzun A, et al. Endothelium-independent contractions of human cerebral arteries in response to vasopressin. Stroke 1990: 21: 1687–1793.
De la Torré JC, Surgeon JW, Walker RH. Effects of locus coeruleus stimulation on cerebral blood flow in selected brain regions. Acta Neurol Scand, suppl 64: 104–105.
Deligne P, David M. Hibernation artificielle en neuro-chirugie. Evolution de nos techniques. Ann Anesth Franc 1966: 7: 117–129.
Dempsey RJ, Combs DJ, Maley ME, et al. Moderate hypothermia reduces postischemic edema development and leucotriene production. Neurosurgery 1987: 21: 177–181.
Dietrich WD, Busto R, Valdes I, Loor Y. Effects of normothermic versus mild hyperthermic forebrain ischemia in rats. Stroke 1990: 21: 1318–1325.
Dirnagl U, Pulsinelli W. Autoregulation of cerebral blood flow in experimental focal brain ischemia. J Cereb Blood Flow Metab 1990: 10: 327–336.
Drummond JC, Oh YS, Cole DJ, et al. Phenylephedrine-induced hypertension decreases the area of ischemia following middle cerebral artery occlusion in the rat. Stroke 1989: 20: 1538.
DuCailar J, Rioux J, Groleau D, Villard F. Hypothermie au dessous de 25 par refrigeration externe et sans circulation extra-corporelle. Ann Anesth Franc 1964: 4: 781–800.
Duelli R, Kuschinsky W. Changes in brain capillary diameter during hypocapnia and hypercapnia. J Cereb Blood Flow Metab 1993: 13: 1025–1028.
Dutka AJ, Hallenbech JM, Kochanek P. A brief episode of severe arterial hypertension induces delayed deterioration of brain function and worsens blood flow after transient multifocal cerebral ischaemia. Stroke 1987: 18: 386–395.
Duverger D, Edvinsson L, MacKenzie ET, et al. Concentrations of putative neurovascular transmitters in major cerebral arteries and small pial vessels of various species. J Cereb Blood Flow Metab 1987: 7: 497–501.
Edvinsson L, Cervos-Navarro J, Larsson LI, et al. Regional distribution of mast cells containing histamine, dopamine, or 5-hydroxytryptamine in the mammalian brain. Neurology 1977: 27: 878–883.
Edvinsson L, Hardelia JE, MCCulloch J, Owman C. Vasomotor response of the cerebral blood vessels to dopamine and dopaminergic agonists. Adv Neurol 1978: 20: 85–96.
Edvinsson L, Hardebo JE, MacKenzie ET, Owman C. Effects of exogeneous noradrenaline on local cerebral blood flow after osmotic opening of the blood-brain barrier in the rat. J Physiol (Lond) 1978: 274: 149–156.
Edvinsson L, McCulloch J, Rossell S. Uddman R. Antagonism by (D-pro 2, D-Trp 7,9)-substance P on the cerebrovascular dilatation induced by substance P. Acta Physiol Scand 1982: 116-411-423.
Edvinsson L, Dequerce A, Duverger D, et al. Central serotonergic nerves project to the pial vessels of the brain. Nature 1983: 306: 55–58.
Edvinsson L, Jansen I, Uddman R. Substance P and cerebral blood vessels. In: Hakanson R, Sundler F (eds). Nerve fibre supply and characterization of postsynaptic receptors in tachykinin antagonists. Amsterdam, Elsevier, 1985: 57–64.
Edvinsson L, Copeland JR, Emson PC, et al. Nerve fibers containing neuropeptide Y in the cerebrovascular bed: Immunocytochemistry, radioimmunoassays, and vasomotor effects. J Cereb Blood Flow Metab 1987: 7: 45.

Edvinsson L, Ekman R, Jansen I, et al. Calcitonin gene-related peptide and cerebral blood vessels: Distribution and vasomotor effects. J Cereb Blood Flow Metab 1987: 7: 720–728.

Eintrei C, Lund N, Effects of increases in inspired oxygen fraction on brain surface pressure fields in pig and man. Acta Anaesthesiol Scand 1986: 30: 194–198.

Eklöff B, Ingvar DH, Kågström E, Olin T. Persistance of cerebral blood flow autoregulation following chronic bilateral cervical sympathetomy in the monkey. Acta Physiol Scand 1971: 82: 172–176.

Ekström-Jodal B, Häggendal E, Nilsson NJ. On the relation between blood pressure and blood flow in the cerebral cortex of dogs. Acta Physiol Scand 1970: (suppl) 350: 29–42.

Ekström-Jodal B, Häggendal Em Linder LE, et al. Cerebral blood flow autoregulation at high arterial pressures and different levels of carbondioxide tension in dogs. Europ Neurol 1972: 6: 6–10.

Ekström-Jodal V, von Essen C, Häggendal E. Effects of noradrenaline on the cerebral blood flow in the dog. Acta Neurol Scand 1974: 50: 11.

Ekström-Jodal B, Häggendal E, Johansson B, et al. Acute arterial hypertension and the blood-brain barrier. In Langfitt TW, et al. (eds) Cerebral Circulation and Metabolism, Springer Verlag, New York, 1975: 7–9.

Elfgren CI, Ryding E, Passant U. Performance on neuropsychological tests related to single photon emission computerised tomography findings in frontotemporal dementia. Br J Psychiatry 1996: 169: 416–422.

Ellingsen I, Hauge A, Nicolaysen G, et al. Changes in human cerebral blood flow due to step changes in PaO_2 and $PaCO_2$. Acta Physiol Scand 1987: 129: 157–163.

Ellis EF, Dodson LY, Police RJ. Restoration of cerebrovascular responsiveness to hyperventilation by oxygen radical scavenger n-acetylcysteine following experimental traumatic brain injury. J Neurosurg 1991: 75: 774–779.

Enevoldsen EM, Jensen FT. Autoregulation and CO_2 responses of cerebral blood flow in patients with severe head injury. J Neurosurg 1978: 48: 689–703.

Ewing JR, Robertson WM, Brown GG. et al. ^{133}Xenon inhalation: Accuracy in detection of ischaemic cerebral regions and angiographic lesions. In Wood JH (ed). Cerebral Blood Flow Physiology and Clinical Aspects, McGraw-Hill Book Company 1985: 202–219.

Faraci FM. Role of nitric oxide in regulation of basilar artery tone in vivo. Am J Physiol 1990: 259: 1216–1221.

Faraci FM. Role of endothelium-derived relaxing factor in cerebral circulation: Large arteries vs. microcirculation. Am J Physiol 1991: 261: 1038–1042.

Fasehun OA, Gross SS, Rubin LE, et al. L-arginine but not N-benzoyl-L-arginine ethyl ester is a precursor of endothelium-derived relaxing factor. J Pharmacol Exp Ther 1990: 255: 1348–1353.

Feruglio FS, Ruiu P, Ruiu L. La protata circulatoria, il consumo di O_2 e la resistanza vascolare cerebrale delluomo nello stato di ibernazione artificiale con ipotermia. Minerva Med 1954: 45: 1655–1660.

Fieschi C, Battistini N, Beduchi A, et al. Regional cerebral blood flow and intraventricular pressure in acute head injuries: J Neurol Neurosurg Psychiat 1974: 37: 1378–1388.

Fitch W, MacKenzie ET, Harper AM. Effects of decreasing arterial blood pressure on cerebral blood flow in the baboon. Circulation Res 1975: 37: 550–557.

Fog M. Om piaarteriernes vasomotoriske reaktion. Leven (ed), Munksgaard, Copenhagen 1934.

Forbes HS, Nason GI, Wortman RC. Cerebral circulation. Arch Neurol Psychiat 1937: 37: 334–360.

Fourcade HE, Larson P, Ehrenfeld WK, et al. The effect of CO_2 and systemic hypertension on cerebral perfusion pressure during carotid endarterectomy. Anesthesiology 1970: 33: 383–391.

Frackowiak RSJ, Lenzi GL, Jones T, Heather JD. Quantitative measurement of regional cerebral blood flow and oxygen metabolism in man using ^{15}O and positron emission tomography. Theory, procedure, and normal values. J Comput Assist Tomogr 1980: 4: 727–736.

Frerichs KU, Kennedy C, Sokoloff L, Hallenbeck JM. Local cerebral blood flow during hibernation, a model of natural tolerance to "cerebral ischemia. J Cereb Blood Flow Metab 1994: 14: 193–205.

Frietsch T, Krafft P, Piepgras A. et al. Relationship between local cerebral blood flow and metabolism during mild and moderate hypothermia in rats. Anesthesiology 2000: 92: 754–763.

Fromann C. Adverse effects of low carbon dioxide tensions during mechanical over-ventilation of patienst with combined head and chest injuries. Br J Anaesth 1968: 40: 383–386.

Fukuyama H, Ogawa M, Yamauchi H, et al. Altered cerebral energy metabolism in Alzheimer's disease: a PET study. J Nucl Med 1994: 35: 1–6.

Gibbs JM, Frackowiak RS, Legg NJ. Regional cerebral blood flow and oxygen metabolism in dementia due to vascular disease. Gerontology 1986: 32 (suppl 1): 84–88.

Giller CA. A bedside test for cerebral autoregulation using transcranial Doppler ultrasound. Acta Neurochir 1991: 108: 7–14.

Goadsby PJ, Lambert GA, Lance JW. Differential effects on the internal and external carotid circulation of the monkey evoked by locus coeruleus stimulation. Brain Research 1982: 249: 247–254.

Gold ME, Wood KS, Byrns RE, et al. N-methyl-L-arginine causes endothelium-dependent contraction and inhibition of cyclic GMP formation in artery and vein. Proc Natl Acad Sci USA 1990: 87: 4430–4434.

Gordon E. Nonoperative treatment of acute head injuries (The Karolinska Experience) Intern Anaesth Clin 1979: 17: 181–199.

Gotoh F, Meyer JS, Takagi Y. Cerebral effects of hyperventilation in man. Arch Neurol 1965: 12: 410–423.

Granholm L, Siesjö BK. The effect of hypercapnia and hypocapnia upon the cerebrospinal fluid lactate and pyruvate concentrations and upon the lactate, pyruvate, ATP, ADP, phosphocreatine and creatine concentrations of the cat brain. Acta Phyiol Scand 1969: 75: 257–266.

Greisen G. Cerebral blood flow in preterm infants during the first week of life. Acta Paediatr Scand 1986: 75: 43–51.

Grote J, Zimmer K, Schubert R. Effects of severe arterial hypocapnia on regional cerebral blood flow regulation, tissue PO_2 and metabolism in the brain cortex of cats. Phlügers Arch 1981: 391: 195–199.

Greenberg JH, Alavi A, Reivich M, et al. Local cerebral blood volume response to carbon dioxide in man. Circ Res 1975: 43: 324–331.

Greenfield JC, Tindall GT. Effect of norepinephrine, epinephrine and angiotensin on blood flow in the internal carotid artery of man. J Clin Invest 1968: 47: 1672–1684.

Greenfield JC, Rembert JC, Tindall GT. Transient changes in cerebral vascular resistance during the Valsalva maneuver in man. Stroke 1984: 15: 76–79.
Greenwood J, Hazell AS, Luthert PJ. The effect of low pH saline perfusate upon the integrity of the energy-depleted rat blood-brain barrier. J Cereb Blood Flow Metab 1989: 9: 234–242.
Greitz TV, Grepe AO, Kalmer MS, Lopez J. Pre- and postoperative evaluation of cerebral blood flow in low-pressure hydrocephalus. J Neurosurg 1969: 31: 644–651.
Gross PM, Teasdale GM, Graham DI, et al. Intra-arterial histamine increases blood-brain barrier transport in rats. Am J Physiol 1982: 243: 307–317.
Grupp RL, Raichle ME, Eichling JO, Ter-Pogossian MM. The effects of changes in $PaCO_2$ on cerebral blood volume, blood flow, and vascular mean transit time. Stroke 1974: 5: 630–638.
Gupta AK, Menon DK, Czosnyka M, et al. Thresholds for hypoxic cerebral vasodilation in volunteers. Anesth Analg 1997: 85: 817–820.
Gur RC, Gur RE, Resnick SM, et al. The effect of anxiety on cortical cerebral blood flow and metabolism. J Cereb Blood Flow Metab 1987: 7: 173–177.
Hägerdal M, Harp JR, Siesjö BK. Influence of changes in arterial $PaCO_2$ on cerebral blood flow and cerebral energy state during hypothermia in the rat. Acta Anaesthesiol Scand 1975: suppl 57: 25–33.
Hägerdal M, Welch FA, Keykhah MM, et al. Protective effects of combinations of hypothermia and barbiturate in cerebral hypoxia in the rat. Anesthesiology 1978: 49: 165–169.
Häggendal E, Johansson B. Effects of arterial carbon dioxide tension and oxygen saturation on cerebral blood flow autoregulation in dogs. Acta Physiol Scand 1965: suppl 258: 27–53.
Häggendal E, Johansson B. On the pathophysiology of the increased cerebrovascular permeability in acute arterial hypertension in cats. Acta Neurol Scand 1972: 48: 265–270.
Haikala H, Karmalathi T, Ahtee L. The nicotine-induced changes in striated dopamine metabolism of mice depend on body temperature. Brain Res 1986: 375: 313–319.
Hampson NB, Camporesi EM, Stolp BW, et al. Cerebral oxygen availability by NIR spectroscopy during transient hypoxia in humans. J Appl Physiol 1990: 69: 907–913.
Hanko J, Hardebo JE, Kahrström J, et al. Calcitonin gene-related peptide is present in mammalian cerebrovascular nerve fibers and dilates pial and peripheral arteries. Neurosci Lett 1985: 57: 91–95.
Hansen NB, Nowicki PT, Miller RR, et al. Alterations in cerebral blood flow and oxygen consumption during prolonged hypocapnia. Pediatr Res 1986: 20: 147–150.
Hardebo JE, Beley A. Influence of blood pressure on blood-brain barrier function in brain ischaemia. Acta Neurol Scand 1984: 70: 356–359.
Harik SI, Yoshida S, Busto R, Ginsberg MD. Monoamine neurotransmitters in diffuse reversible forebrain ischemia and early recirculation: Increased dopaminergic activity. Neurology 1986: 36: 971–976.
Harp JR, Wollman H. Cerebral metabolic effects of hyperventilation and deliberate hypotension. Br J Anaesth 1973; 45: 256–262.
Hartman BK, Zide D, Udenfriend S. The use of dopamine-beta-hydroxylase as a marker for the central noradrenergic nervous system in the rat brain. Proc Natl Acad Sci USA 1972: 69: 2722–2726.
Hassan FM, Kazemi H, Dual contribution theory of regulation of CSF HCO_3^- in respiratory acidosis. J Appl Physiol 1976: 40: 559–567.
Havill JH. Prolonged hyperventilation and intracranial pressure. Critical Care Medicin 1984: 12: 72–74
Hauerberg J, Juhler M. Cerebral blood flow autoregulation in acute intracranial hypertension. J Cereb Blood Flow Metab 1994: 14: 519–525.
Hauerberg J, Xiaodong M, Willumsen L, et al. The upper limit of cerebral blood flow autoregulation in acute intracranial hypertension. J Neurosurg Anesthesiol 1998: 10: 106–112.
Heistad DD, Marcus ML, Abboud FM. Role of large arteries in regulation of cerebral blood flow in dogs. J Clin Invest 1978: 62: 761–768.
Hilberman M, Nioka S. Subramanian H, et al. Brain pH during respiratory acidoses and alkalosis, a ^{31}P NMR study. Anesthesiology 1984: 61: A317.
Hino A, Ueda S, Mizukawa N, et al. Effect of hemodilution on cerebral hemodynamics and oxygen metabolism. Stroke 1992: 23: 423–426.
Hirst RP, Slee TA, Lam AM. Changes in cerebral blood flow velocity after release of intraoperative tournequets in humans: A transcranial Doppler study. Anesth Analg 1990: 71: 503–510
Hochwald GM, Wald A, Malhan C. The sink action of cerebrospinal fluid volume flow. Arch Neurol 1976: 33: 339–344.
Hofmann WE, Albrecht RF, Miletich DJ. The role of adenosine in CBF increases during hypoxia in young vs. aged rats. Stroke 1984: 15: 124.
Hoffman WE, Albrecht RD, Miletich DJ. Cerebrovascular response to hypoxia in young vs. aged rats. Stroke 1984: 15: 129.
Hoffman WE, Werner C, Baughman VL, et al. Postischemic treatment with hypothermia improves outcome from incomplete cerebral ischemia in rats. J Neurosurg Anesthesiol 1991: 3: 34–38.
Hoop B, Masjedi M-R, Shih VE, Kazemi H. Brain glutamate metabolism during hypoxia and peripheral chemodenervation. Am J Physiol 1990: 69: 147–154
Horvath I, Sandor NT, Ruttner Z, McLaughlin AC. Role of nitric oxide in regulating cerebrocortical oxygen consumption and blood flow during hypercapnia. J Cereb Blood Flow Metab 1994: 14: 503–509.
Iadecola C. Does nitric oxide mediate the increase in cerebral blood flow elicited by hypercapnia? Proc Natl Acad Sci USA. 1992: 89: 3913–3916.
Illievich UM, Zoenow MH, Choi KT, et al. Effects of hypothermic metabolic suppression on hippocampal glutamate concentrations after transient global cerebral ischemia. Anesth Analg 1994: 78: 905–911.
Imran MB, Kawashima R, Awata S, et al. Tc-99m HMPAO SPECT in the evaluation of Alzheimer's disease: correlation between neuropsychiatric evaluation and CBF images. J Neurol Neurosurg Psychiatry 1999: 66: 228–232.
Ingvar DH, Cronquist S, Ekberg R, et al. Normal values of regional cerebral blood flow in man, including flow and weight estimates of gray and white matter. A preliminary summary. Acta Neurol Scand 1965: 41 [suppl 14]: 72–78
Irikura K, Miyasaka Y, Nagai S, et al. Moderate hypothermia reduces hypotensive, but not hypercapnic vasodilation of pial arterioles in rats. J Cereb Blood Flow Metab 1998: 18: 1294–1297.
Ishii K, Kanno I, Uemura K, et al. Comparison of carbon dioxide responsiveness of cerebellar blood flow between af-

fected and unaffected sides with crossed cerebellar diaschisis. Stroke 1994: 25: 826–830.
Ishii K, Sasaki M, Yamaji S, et al. Demonstration of decreased posterior cingulate perfusion in mild Alzheimer's disease by means of $H_2{}^{15}O$ positron emission tomography. Eur J Nucl Med 1997: 24: 670–673.
Ito U, Ohno K, Yamaguchi T, Takei H, et al. Effect of hypertension on blood-brain barrier change after restoration of blood flow in post-ischaemic gerbil brains. Stroke 1980: 11: 606–611.
Iwamoto J, Curran-Everett DC, Krasney E, Krasney JA. Cerebral metabolic and pressure-flow responses during sustained hypoxia in awake sheep. J Appl Physiol 1991: 71: 1447–1453
Jacobsen I, Harper MB, McDowall DG. The effect of O_2 at 1 and 2 atmospheres on the blood flow and oxygen uptake of the cerebral cortex. Surg Gynecol Obstet 1964: 119: 737–742
Jakobsen M, Enevoldsen EM, Bjerre P. Cerebral blood flow and metabolism following subarachnoid hemorrhage: Cerebral oxygen uptake and global blood flow during the acute period in patients with SAH. Acta Neurol Scand 1990: 82: 174–182.
Jakobsen M, Skjødt T, Enevoldsen EM. Cerebral blood flow and metabolism following subarachnoid hemorrhage: Effect of subarachnoid blood. Acta Neurol Scand 1991: 83: 226–233.
Jarden JO, Barry DI, Juhler M, et al. Cerebrovascular aspects of converting-enzyme inhibition: II. Blood-brain barrier permeability and effect of intracerebroventricular administration of captopril. J Hypertension 1984: 2: 599–604
Jarrott B, Hjelle JT, Spector S. Association of histamine with cerebral microvessels in regions of bovine brain. Brain Res 1979: 168: 323–330.
Jennett B, Teasdale G, Fry J, et al. Treatment for severe head injury. J Neurol Neurosurg Psychiat 1980: 43: 289–295
Johansson BB, Li C, Olsson Y, Klatzo I. The effect of acute arterial hypertension on the blood-brain barrier to protein tracers. Acta Neuropath 1970: 16: 117–124.
Johansson BB. Blood brain barrier dysfunction in acute arterial hypertension after papaverine-induced vasodilatation. Acta Neurol Scand 1974: 50: 573–580.
Johansson BB, Linder LE. Reversibility of the blood-brain barrier dysfunction induced by acute hypertension. Acta Neurol Scandinav 1978: 57: 345–348.
Johansson BB, Auer LM. Neurogenic modification of the vulnerability of the blood-brain barrier during acute hypertension in conscous rats. Acta Physiol Scand 1983: 117: 507–511.
Johns RA, Peach MJ, Linden J, Tichotsky A. N-monomethyl-L-arginine inhibits endothelium-derived relaxing factor-stimulated cyclic GMP accumulation in cocultures of endothelial and vascular smooth muscle cells by an action specific to the endothelial cell. Circ Res 1990: 67: 979–985
Jonsson G. Chemical lesioning techniques; monoamine neurotoxins. In Björklund A, Hökfelt T (eds) Handbook of Chemical Neuroanatomy, Amsterdam, Elsevier 1983: 1: 463–507
Kader A, Brisman MH, Maraire N, et al. The effect of mild hypothermia on permanent focal ischemia in the rat. Neurosurgery 1992: 31: 1056–1061.
Karibe H, Chen J, Zarow GJ, et al. Delayed induction of mild hypothermia to reduce infarct volume after temporary middle cerebral artery occlusion in rats. J Neurosurg 1994: 80: 112–119.
Katsumura H, Hosotani K, Kabuto M, et al. Influences of total body hyperthermia by extracorporal circulation on intracranial hemodynamics in dogs. In Intracranial Pressure VIII. Avezaat CJJ, van Eijndhoven JHM, Maas IAR, Tans JThJ (eds). Springer Verlag 1993: 203–206.
Kennealy JA, McLennan JE, Loudon G, McLaurin RL. Hyperventilation-induced cerebral hypoxia. Am Rev Resp Dis 1980: 122: 407–412.
Kennedy C, Sokoloff L. An Adaptation of the nitrous oxide method to the study of the cerebral circulation in children; normal values for cerebral blood flow and cerebral metabolic rate in children. J Clin Invest 1957: 36: 1130–1137.
Kety SS, Schmidt CF. The determination of cerebral blood flow in man by the use of nitrous oxide in low concentrations. Am J Physiol 1945: 143: 53–66.
Kety SS, Schmidt CF. The nitrous oxide method for the quantitative determination of cerebral blood flow in man: Theory, procedure and normal values. J clin Invest 1948: 27: 476–483.
Kety SS; Schmidt CF. Effects of altered arterial tensions of carbon dioxide and oxygen on cerebral blood flow and cerebral oxygen consumption of normal young men. J Clin Invest 1948: 27: 484–492
Keykhah MM, Hagerdal M, Welsh FA, et al. Effect of high vs. low arterial blood oxygen content on cerebral energy metabolite levels during hypoxia with normothermia and hypothermia in the rat. Anesthesiology 1980: 52: 492–495.
King BD, Sokoloff L, Wechsler L. The effects of l-epinephrine and l-norepinephrine upon cerebral circulation and metabolism in man. J clin Invest 1952: 31: 273–279.
Kitagawa K, Matsumoto M, Tagaya M, et al. Hyperthermia-induced neuronal protection against ischaemic injury in gerbils. J Cereb Blood Flow Metab 1991: 11: 449–452
Kitahata LM, Galicich JM, Sato I. The effect of passive hyperventilation on intracranial pressure. J Neurosurg 1971: 34: 185–193.
Khambatta HJ, Sullivan SF. Carbon dioxide production and washout during passive hyperventilation alkalosis. J Appl Physiol 1974: 37: 665–669
Klazo I. Presidential address - Neuropathological aspects of brain edema. J Neuropathol Exp Neurol 1967: 26: 1–14
Kleinerman J, Sencetta SM, Hackel DB. Effects og high spinal anaesthesia on cerebral circulation and metabolism in man. J clin Invest 1958: 37: 285–293.
Kleiser B, Widder B. Course of carotid artery occlusion with impaired cerebrovascular reactivity. Stroke 1992: 23: 171–174.
Ko KR, Ngai AC, Winn HR. Role of adenosine in regulation of regional cerebral blood flow in sensory cortex. Am J Physiol 1990: 259: H1703–H1708
Kobayashi S, Kyoshima K, Olschsowka JA, Jacobowitz DM. Vasoactive intestinal polypeptide immunoreactive and cholinergic nerves in the whole mount preparation of the major cerebral arteries. Histochemistry 1983: 79: 377–381
Kobayashi H, Hayashi M, Kuwana H, et al. Effect of chemical sympathectomy on cerebral blood flow in rats. J Neurosurg 1991: 75: 906–910
Kogure K, Schieberg P, Fujishima M, et al. Effects of hypoxia on cerebral autoregulation. Am J Physiol 1970: 219: 1393–1396

Komaba Y, Osono E, Kitamura S, Katayama Y. Crossed cerebellocerebral diaschisis in patients with cerebellar stroke. Acta Neurol Scand 2000: 101: 8–12.

Komatani A, Yamaguchi K, Sugai Y, et al. Assessment of demented patients by dynamic SPECT of inhaled xenon-133. J Nucl Med 1988: 29: 1621–1626.

Kontos HA, Wei EP, Navari RM, et al. Responses of cerebral arteries and arterioles to acute hypotension and hypertension. Am J Physiol 1978: 234: H371–383.

Kontos HA, Wei EP, Dietrich WD, et al. Mechanism of cerebral arteriolar abnormalities after acute hypertension. Am J Physiol 1981: 240: H511–527.

Kopf GS, Mirvis DM, Myers RE. Central nervous system tolerance to cardiac arrest during profound hypothermia. J Surg Res 1975: 18: 29–34.

Kozniewska E, Oseka M, Stys T. Effects of endothelium-derived nitric oxide on cerebral circulation during normooxia and hypoxia in the rat. J Cereb Blood Flow Metab 1992: 12: 311–317.

Kramer RS, Sanders AP, Lesage AM et al. The effect of profound hypothermia on preservation of cerebral ATP content during circulatory arrest. J Thorac Cardiov Surg 1968: 56: 699–709.

Krantis A. Hypothermia-induced reductions in the permeation of the radiolabelled tracer substances across the blood-brain barrier. Acta Neuropathol 1983: 60: 61–69.

Kreisman NR, Magee JC, Brizzee BL. Relative hypoperfusion in rat cerebral cortex during recurrent seizures. J Cereb Blood Flow Metab 1991: 11: 77–87

Kuroda S, Kamiyama H, Abe H et al. Acetazolamide test in detecting reduced cerebral perfusion reserve and predicting long-term prognosis in patients with internal carotid artery occlusion. Neurosurgery 1993: 32: 912–918.

Kuschinsky W, Suda S, Bunger R, Sokoloff L. The influence of L-norepinephrine on the local coupling between brain metabolism and blood flow. In: Cerebral Blood Flow: Effects of Nerves and Neurrotransmitters, Heistad DD, Marcus ML (eds). New York: Elsevier/North-Holland 1982: 169–176.

Lafferty JJ, Keykhah MM, Shapiro HM, et al. Cerebral hypometabolism obtained with deep pentobarbital anesthesia and hypothermia (30° C). Anesthesiology 1978: 49: 159–164.

Lantos J, Temes G, Torok B. Changes during ischaemia in extracellular potassium ion concentration of the brain under nitrous oxide or hexobarbital-sodium anesthesia and moderate hypothermia. Acta Physiol Scand 1986: 67: 141–153.

Larsen B, Skinhøj E, Soh K, Endo H, Lassen NA. The pattern of cortical activity provoked by listening and speech revealed by rCBF measurements. Acta Neurol Scnad 1977: 56 (suppl 64): 268–269.

Larsen FS, Olsen KS, Hansen BA, et al. Transcranial Doppler is valid for determination of the lower limit of cerebral blood flow autoregulation. Stroke 1994: 25: 1985–1988.

Larrue V, Celsis P, Bès A, Marc-Vergnes JP. The functional anatomy of attention in humans: Cerebral blood flow changes induced by reading, naming, and the Stroop effect. J Cereb Blood Flow Metab. 1994: 14: 958–962.

Lassen NA. Cerebral blood flow and oxygen consumption in man. Physiol Rev 1959: 39: 183–238.

Lassen NA, Feinberg I, Lane MH. Bilateral studies of cerebral oxygen uptake in young and aged normal subjects and in patients with organic dementia. J clin Invest 1960: 39: 491–500.

Lassen NA. Brain extracellular pH: The main factor controlling cerebral blood flow (editorial). Scand J clin Lab Invest. 1968: 22: 247–249

Lassen NA. Control of cerebral circulation in health and disease. Circ Res 1974: 34: 749–760.

Lenzi GL, Frackowiak RSJ, Jones T. Cerebral oxygen metabolism and blood flow in human cerebral ischaemic infarction. J Cereb Blood Flow Metab 1982: 2: 321–335

Levene MI, Shortland D, Gibson N, Evans DH. Carbon dioxide reactivity of the cerebral circulation in extremely premature infants: Effects of postnatal age and indomethacin. Pediatr Res 1988: 24: 175–179

Lluch S, Reimann C, Glick G. Evidence for a direct effect of adrenergic drugs on the cerebral vascular bed of the unanesthetized goat. Stroke 1973: 4: 50–56.

Lluch S, Conde MV, Diéguez G et al. Evidence for the direct effect of vasopressin on human and goat cerebral arteries. J Pharmacol Exp Ther 1984: 228: 749–755

Lundberg N, Kjällquist A, Bien C. Reduction of increased intracranial pressure by hyperventilation. Acta Psychiat neurol Scand 1959: 34 (suppl 139).

Lübbers DW. Quantitative measurement and describtion of oxygen supply to the tissue. In: Jöbsis FF (ed) Oxygen and Physiological Function. Dallas: Professional Information Library, 1977: pp 254–276

MacKenzie ET, McCulloch J, O'Keane M et al. Cerebral circulation and norepinephrine: Relevance of the blood-brain barrier. Am J Physiol 1976: 231: 483-

MacKenzie ET, McGeorge AD, Graham DT et al. Effects of increasing arterial pressure on cerebral blood flow in the baboon, influence of the sympathetic nervous system. Phlügers Arch Eur J Physiol 1979: 378: 189–195.

Madsen PL, Holm S, Vorstrup S, et al. Human regional cerebral blood flow during rapid-eye-movement sleep. J Cereb Blood Flow Metab 1991: 11: 502–507

Madsen PL, Schmidt JF, Holm S, et al. Mental stress and cognitive mental performance do not increase the overall level of cerebral O_2 uptake in humans. J Appl Physiol 1992: 73: 420–426.

Madsen PL, Holm S, Herning M, Lassen NA. Average blood flow and oxygen uptake in the human brain during resting wakefulness: a critical appraisal of the Kety-Schmidt technique. J Cereb Blood Flow Metab 1993: 13: 646–655.

Maekawa T, Tommasono C, Shapiro HM et al. Local cerebral blood flow and glucose utilization during isoflurane anaesthesia in the rat. Anesthesiology 1986: 65: 144–151.

Mahony PJ, Panerai RB, Deverson ST et al. Assessment of the thigh cuff technique for measurement of dynamic cerebral autoregulation. Stroke 2000: 31: 476–480.

Martin WRW, Raichle ME. Cerebral blood flow and metabolism in cerebral hemisphere infarction. Ann Neurol 1983: 14: 168–176

McHenry LC, Slocum HC, Bivens HE, et al. Hyperventilation in awake and anesthetized man. Arch Neurol 1965: 12: 270–277

McIlWain H, Poll JD. Adenosine in cerebral homeostatic role: appraisal through actions of homocysteine, colchicine and dipyridamole. J Neurobiol 1986: 17: 39–49.

Malmlund HO, LyingTunell U, Bohmer G. The effect of ventricular-atrial shunting on cerebral oxygen consumption in patients with dementia. Europ Neurol 1972: 6: 340–345.

Mangold R, Sokoloff L, Conner E, et al. The effects of sleep and lack of sleep on the cerebral circulation and metabolism of normal young men. J clin Invest 1955: 34: 1092–1100.

Marion DW, Bouma GJ. The use of stable xenon-enhanced computed tomographic studies of cerebral blood flow to define changes in cerebral carbon dioxide vasoresponsivity caused by a severe head injury. Neurosurgery 1991: 29: 869–873

Marshall SB, Owens JC, Swan H. Temporary circulatory occlusion to the brain of the hypothermic dog. Arch Surg 1956: 72: 98–106.

Martins AN, Doyle TF, Newby N. PCO_2 and rate of formation of of cerebrospinal fluid in the monkey. Am J Physiol 1976: 231: 127–131.

Mayhan WG, Heistad DD. Role of veins and cerebral venous pressure in disruption of the blood-brain barrier. Circ Res 1986a: 59: 216-220.

Mayhan WG, Faraci FM, Heistad DD. Disruption of the blood-brain barrier in cerebrum and brain stem during acute hypertension. Am J Physiol 1986b: 251: H1171–1175.

Mc Culloch J. Role of dopamine in interactions among cerebral function, metabolism, and blood flow. In: Neurotransmitters and the Cerebral Circulation, MacKenzie ET, Seylas J, Bès A (eds), New York, Raven Press, L.E.R.S. monograph series; 1984: vol 2, pp 137–155

McKissock W, Paine KWE, Walsh LS. The value of hypothermia in the surgical treatment of ruptured intracranial aneurysms. J Neurosurg 1960: 17: 700–707.

McKrell TN, Stone HH, Wechsler RL. Effect of drug induced hypotension on cerebral circulation in man. Surg Forum 1955: 5: 730–736.

Mchedlishvili GI, Mitagcaria NP, Ormotsadze LG. Vascular mechanisms controlling a constant blood supply to the brain ("autoregulation"). Stroke 1973. 4: 742–750

Mellergård P, Nordström C-H. Intracerebral temperature in neurosurgical patients. Neurosurgery 1991: 28: 709–713

Meno JR, Ngai AC, Winn HR. Changes in pial arteriolar diameter and CSF adenosine concentrations during hypoxia. J Cereb Blood Flow Metab 1993: 13: 214–220.

Messeter K, Nordström C-H, Sundbärg G, et al. Cerebral hemodynamics in patients with severe head trauma. J Neurosurg 1986: 64: 231–237.

Messmer K, Gornandt L, Jesch F, et al. Oxygen transport and tissue oxygenation during hemodilution with dextran. Adv Exp Med Biol 1973: 37: 669–680.

Michenfelder JD, Theye RA. Hypothermia: Effect on canine brain and whole-body metabolism. Anesthesiology 1968: 29: 1107–1112.

Michenfelder JD, VanDyke RA, Theye RA. The effects of anesthetic agents and techniques on canine cerebral ATP and lactate levels. Anesthesiology 1970: 33: 315–321.

Michenfelder JD, Theye RA. The effects of anaesthesia and hypothermia on canine cerebral ATP and lactate during anoxia produced by decapitation. Anesthesiology 1970: 33: 430–439.

Michenfelder JD, Sundt TM. The effect of $paCO_2$ on the metabolism of ischaemic brain in squirrel monkeys. Anesthesiology 1973: 38: 445–453

Michenfelder JD. The interdependency of cerebral functional and metabolic effects following massive doses of thiopental in the dog. Anesthesiology 1974: 41: 231–236.

Michenfelder JD. The in vivo effect of massive concentrations of anesthetics on canine cerebral metabolism. In: Fink BR, (ed), Molecular mechanisms of anesthesia, progress in anesthesiology. Raven Press, New York, 1975: 1: 537–543.

Michenfelder JD, Milde JH. Failure of prolonged hypocapnia, hypothermia or hypertension to favourably alter acute stroke in primates. Stroke 1977: 8: 87–91.

Michenfelder JD, Milde JH. The relationship among canine brain temperature, metabolism, and function during hypocapnia. Anesthesiology 1991: 75: 130–136

Mickel HS, Vaishnav YN, Kempski O, et al. Breathing 100% oxygen after global brain ischemia in Mongolian Gerbils results in increased lipid peroxidation and increased mortality. Stroke 1987: 18: 426–430.

Milde LN. Points of view - Clinical use of mild hypothermia for brain protection: A dream revisited. J Neurosurg Anesthesiol 1992: 4: 211–215.

Miller JD, Stanek AE, Langfitt TW. Concepts of cerebral perfusion pressure and vascular compression during intracranial hypertension. In: Meyer JS, Schade JD (eds). Progress in Brain Research. Amsterdam: Elsevier, 1971: 411–432

Mirro R, Busija DW, Armstead WM, Leffler CW. Histamine dilates the pial arterioles of newborn pigs through prostanoid production. Am J Physiol 1988: 23: H1023–H1026

Moncada S, Palmer RMJ, Higgs EA. The discovery of nitric oxide as endogenous nitrovasodilator. Hypertension 1988: 12: 365–372

Moreno MJ, Conde MV, De la Luz Fraile M, et al. Lesion of the dorsal raphe nucleus induces supersensitivity to serotonin in isolated cat middle cerebral artery. Brain Res 1991: 538: 324–328.

Morgan P, Ward B. Hyperventilation and changes in the electroencephalogram and electroretinogram. Neurology 1970: 20: 1009–1014.

Morimoto Y, Mathru M, Martinez-Tica J, Zornow MH. Effects of profound anemia on brain tissue oxygen tension, carbon dioxide tension, and pH in rabbits. J Neurosurg Anesthesiol 2001: 13: 33–39.

Moskowitz MA, Wei EP, Saito K et al. Trigeminalectomy modifies pial arteriolar reponses to hypertension or norepinephrine. Am J Physiol 1988: 255: H1–H6

Muizelaar JP, van Der Poel HG, Li Z, et al. Pial arteriolar vessel diameter and CO_2 reactivity during prolonged hyperventilation in the rabbit. J Neurosurg 1988: 69: 923–927.

Muizelaar JP, Marmarou A, Ward JD, et al. Adverse effects of prolonged hyperventilation in patients with severe head injury: a randomized clinical trial. J Neurosurg 1991: 75: 731–739

Murkin JM, Farrar JK, Tweed A, et al. Cerebral autoregulation and flow/metabolism coupling during cardio-pulmonary bypass: The influence of $PaCO_2$. Anesth Analg 1987: 66: 825–832.

Murphy VA, Johanson CE. Adrenergic-induced enhancement of brain barrier system permeability to small nonelectrolytes: choroid plexus versus cerebral capillaries. J Cereb Blood Flow Metab 1985: 5: 401–412.

Nagata K, Maruya H, Yuya H, et al. Can PET data differentiate Alzheimer's disease from vascular dementia? Ann N Y Acad Sci 2000: 903: 252–261.

Najarian T, Marrache AM, Dumont I, et al. Proponged hypercapnia-evoked cerebral hyperemia via K(+) channel- and prostaglandin E (2)-dependent endothelial nitric oxide synathase induction. Circ Res 2000: 87: 1149–1156.

Nakai M. Contractile effects of perivascularly applied vasopressin on the pial artery of the cat brain. J Physiol (Lond) 1987: 387: 441–452

Neill WA, Hattenhauer M. Impairment of myocardial O_2 supply due to hyperventilation. Circulation 1975: 52: 854–858.

Nelson RJ, Czosnyka M, Pickard JD, et al. Experimental aspects of cerebrospinal hemodynamics: The relationship between blood flow velocity waveform and cerebral autoregulation. Neurosurgery 1992: 31: 705–710.

Nemoto EM, Yao L, Yonas H, Darby JM. Compartmentation of whole brain blood flow and oxygen and glucose metabolism in monkeys. J Neurosurg Anesthesiol 1994: 6: 170–174.

Nilsson L, Busto R. Controlled hyperventilation and its effect on brain energy and acid-base parameters. Acta Anesthesiol Scand 1973: 17: 243–252

Nordström C-H, Rehncrona S. Reduction of cerebral blood flow and oxygen consumption with a combination of barbiturate anesthesia and induced hypothermia in the rat. Acta Anaesthesiol Scand 1979: 22: 7–12.

North JB, Reilly PL, Gorman D, et al. The effect of hypoxia on intracranial pressure and cerebral blood flow. In Intracranial Pressure VIII. Avezaat CJJ, van Eijndhoven JHM, Maas IAR, Tans JThJ (eds). Springer Verlag 1993: 238–243.

Norwood WE, Norwood CR. Influence of hypothermia on intracellular pH during anoxia. Am J Physiol 1982: 243: 62–65.

Nørregaard TV, Moskowitz MA. Substance P and the sensory innervation of intracranial and extracranial feline cephalic arteries. Implications for vascular pain mechanisms in man. Brain 1985: 108: 517–533

Oberdorster G, Lang R, Zimmer R. Direct effect of alpha- and betasympathomimetic amines on cerebral circulation of the dog. Pflügers Arch 1973: 340: 145–160.

Obrist WD, Langfitt TW, Jaggi JL, et al. Cerebral blood flow and metabolism in comatose patients with acute head injury. Relationship to intracranial hypertension. J Neurosurg 1984: 61: 241–253.

Okuda C, Saito A, Miyazaki M, Kuriyama K. Alteration of the turnover of dopamine and 5-hydroxtryptamine in rat brain associated with hypothermia. Pharmacol Biochem Behav 1986: 25: 79–83.

Olah L, Franke C, Schwindt W, Hoehn M. CO_2 reactivity measured by perfusion MRI during transient focal cerebral ischemia in rats. Stroke 2000: 1: 2236–2244.

Olesen J. Contralateral focal increase of cerebral blood flow in man during arm work. Brain 1971: 94: 635-646.

Olesen J, Paulson OB, Lassen NA. Regional cerebral blood flow in man determined by the initial slope of the clearance of the intra-arterially injected ^{133}Xe. Stroke 1971: 2: 519–540.

Olesen J. The effect of intracarotid epinephrine, norepinephrine and angiotensin on regional cerebral blood flow in man. Neurology (Minneap.) 1972: 22: 978–987.

Olesen S–R, Chrone C. Rapid increase in blood–brain barrier permeability during severe conductance of cerebral microvascular walls. Acta Physiol Scand 1986: 127: 233–241

Onadera H, Sata G, Kogure K. GABA and benzodiazepine receptors in the gerbil brain after transient ischemia: demonstration by quantitative-receptor antoradiography. J Cereb Blood Flow Metab 1987: 7: 82–88

Onesti ST, Strauss RC, Mayol B, et al. The effects of norepinephrine depletion on cerebral blood flow in the rat. Brain Res 1989: 477: 378–381

Otha K, Gotoh F, Shimazu K, et al. Locus coeruleus stimulation exerts different influences on the dynamic changes of cerebral pial and intraparenchymal vessels. Neurol Res 1991: 13: 164–167

Overgaard J and Tweed WA. Cerebral circulation after head injury. Part I: Cerebral blood flow and its regulation after closed head injury with emphasis on clinical correlations. J Neurosurg 1974: 41: 531–541.

Owen OE, Morgan AP, Kemp HG, et al. Brain metabolism during fasting. J Clin Invest 1967: 46: 1589–1595.

Palmer RMJ, Ashton DS, Moncada S. Vascular endothelial cells synthetize nitric oxide from L-arginine. Nature 1988: 333: 664–666

Palvölgyi R. Regional cerebral blood flow in patients with intracranial tumors. J Neurosurg 1969: 31: 149–163.

Pantano P, Baron JC, Samson Y, et al. Crossed cerebellar diaschisis: Further studies. Brain 1986: 109: 677–694

Park TS, van Wylen DGL, Rubio R, Berne RM. Brain interstitial adenosine and sagital sinus blood flow during systemic hypotension in piglet. J Cereb Blood Flow Metab 1988: 8: 822–828

Paulson OB. Regional cerebral blood flow in apoplexy due to occlusion of the middle cerebral artery. Neurology 1970: 20: 63–77.

Paulson OB, Olesen J, Christensen MS. Restoration of autoregulation of cerebral blood flow by hypocapnia. Neurology (Minneap.) 1972: 22: 286–293.

Paulson OB, Strandgaard S, Edvinsson L. Cerebral Autoregulation. Cerebrovascular and Brain Metabolism Reviews 1990: 2: 161–192.

Payen JF, Briot E, Tropres I, et al. Regional cerebral blood volume response to hypocapnia using susceptibility constrast MRI. NMR Bioned 2000: 13: 384–391.

Pelligrino DA; Koenig HM, Albrecht RF. Nitric oxide synthesis and regional cerebral blood flow responses to hypercapnia and hypoxia in the rat. J Cereb Blood Flow Metab 1993: 13: 80–87.

Phillis JW, De Long RE. An involvement of adenosine in cerebral blood flow regulation during hypercapnia. Gen Pharmac 1987: 18: 133–139.

Phleps ME, Grubb RL, Ter-Pogosian MM. Correlation between $PaCO_2$ and regional cerebral blood volume by x-ray fluorescence. J Appl Physiol 1973: 35: 274–280

Piechnik SK, Xang X, Czosnyka M, et al. The continuous assessment of cerebrovascular reactivity: a validation of the method in healthy volunteers. Anesth Analg 1999: 89: 944–949.

Pistolese GR, Faraglia V, Agnoli A, et al. Cerebral hemispheric "counter-steal" phenomenon during hyperventilation in cerebrovascular diseases. Stroke 1972: 3: 456–461.

Plum F, Siesjö BK. Recent advances in CSF physiology. Anesthesiology 1975: 42: 708–730.

Pollard V, Prough DS, Deyo DJ, et al. Cerebral blood flow during experimental endotoxemia in volunteers. Crit Care Med 1997: 25: 1700–1706.

Posner JB, Plum F. The toxic effect of carbon dioxide and acetazolamide in hepatic encephalopathy. J Clin Invest 1960: 39: 1246–1258.

Powers WJ. Cerebral hemodynamics in ischaemic cerebrovascular disease. Ann Neurol 1991: 29: 231–240.

Proctor HJ, Carins C, Fillipo D, et al. Brain metabolism during increased intracranial pressure as assessed by niroscopy. Surgery 1984: 96: 273–278

Pryds O, Greisen G. Preservation of single flash visual evoked potentials at very low cerebral oxygen delivery in sick newborn, preterm infants. Pediatr Neurol 1990: 6: 151–158

Raichle ME, Posner JB, Plum F. Cerebral blood flow during and after hyperventilation. Arch Neurol 1970: 23: 394–403

Raichle ME, Plum F. Hyperventilation and cerebral blood flow. Stroke 1972: 3: 566–575.

Raichle ME, Hartman BK, Eichking JO, Sharpe LG. Central noradrenergic regulation of cerebral blood flow and vascular permeability. Proc Nat Acad Sci USA 1975: 72: 3726–3730

Rapela CE, Green HD, Denison AB. Baroreceptor reflexes and autoregulation of cerebral blood flow in the dog. Circ Res 1967: 21: 559–568.

Redies C, Hoffer LJ, Beil C, et al. Generalized decrease in brain glucose metabolism during fasting in human studied by PET. Am J Physiol 1989: 256: E805–E810.

Reivich M. Arterial PCO_2 and cerebral hemodynamics. Am J Physiol 1964: 206: 25–35

Reivich M, Cohen PJ, Greenbaum L. Alterations in the electroencephalogram of awake man produced by hyperventilation: Effects of 100% oxygen at 3 atmospheres (absolute) pressure. Neurology 1966: 16: 304.

Rengachery SS, Roth DA, Andrew NW, Mark VH. Alteration of the blood-brain barrier with hyperventilation. 1967: 614–617

Reutens DC, McHugh MD, Toussaint P-J, et al. L-arginine infusion increases basal but not activated cerebral blood flow in humans. J Cereb Blood Flow Metab 1997: 17: 309–315.

Reynier-Rebuffel A, Aubineau P, Issertial O, Seylaz J. Nonuniformity of CBF response to NE- or ANG II-induced hypertension in rabbits. Am J Physiol 1987: 253: H47–H57.

Ridenour TR, Warner DS, Todd MM, McAllister AC. Mild hypothermia reduces infarct size resulting from temporary but not permanent focal ischemia in rats. Stroke 1992: 23: 733–738

Risberg J. Regional cerebral blood flow measurements by ^{133}Xenon inhalation: Methodology and applications in neuropsychology and psychiatry. Brain and Language 1980: 9: 9–34

Rosner MJ. Cerebral perfusion pressure: Link between intracranial pressure and systemic circulation. In: Wood JH (ed) Cerebral Blood Flow, Physiological and Clinical Aspects 1987: 425–448.

Rosomoff HL, Holaday DA. Cerebral blood flow and cerebral oxygen consumption during hypothermia. Am J Physiol 1954: 179: 85–88.

Rossi GT, Britt RH. Effects of hypothermia on the cat brainstem auditory evoked response. Electroencephalogr Clin Neurophysiol 1984: 57: 143–155.

Ruskell GL, Simons T. Trigeminal nerve pathways to the cerebral arteries in monkeys. J Anat 1987: 155: 23–37

Russell D, Dybevold S, Kjartansson O, et al. Cerebral vasoreactivity and blood flow before and 3 months after carotid endarterectomy. Stroke 1990: 21: 1029–1032.

Sadoshima S, Fujii K, Yao H, et al. Regional cerebral blood flow autoregulation in normotensive and spontaneously hypertensive rats - effects of sympathetic denervation. Stroke 1986: 17: 981–984.

Saito DE, Moskowitz MA. Contributions from the upper cervical dorsal roots and trigeminal ganglia to the feline circle of Willis. Stroke 1989: 20: 524–526

Sakas DE, Moskowitz MA, Wei EP, et al. Trigeminovascular fibers increase blood flow in cortical gray matter by axon reflex-like mechanisms during acute severe hypertension or seizures. Proc Natl Acad Sci USA 1989: 86: 1401–1405

Salanga VD, Waltz AG. Regional cerebral blood flow during stimulation of seventh cranial nerve. Stroke 1973: 4: 213–217.

Samento A, Borges N, Lima D. Influence of electrical stimulation of locus coeruleus on the rat blood-brain barrier permeability to sodium fluorescein. Acta Neurochir (Wien) 1994: 127: 215–219.

Samra SK, Turk P, Arens JF. Effect of hypocapnia on local cerebral glucose utilization in rats. Anesthesiology 1989: 70: 523–526.

Sato M, Pawlik G, Heiss WD. Comparative studies of regional CNS blood flow autoregulation and responses to CO_2 in the cat. Effects of altering arterial blood pressure and $PaCO_2$ on rCBF of cerebrum, cerebellum, and the spinal cord. Stroke 1984: 15: 91–97.

Schienberg P, Stead EA. The cerebral blood flow in male subjects as measured by the nitrous oxide technique: Normal values for blood flow, oxygen utilization, glucose utilization, and peripheral resistance with observations on the effect of tilting and anxiety. J Clin Invest 1949: 28: 1163.

Schmidt JF, Waldemar G, Vorstrup S, et al. Computerized analysis of cerebral blood flow autoregulation in humans: validation of a method for pharmacologic studies. J Cardiovasc Pharmacol 1990: 15: 983-988

Schubert A. Points of view - Should mild hypothermia be routinely used in human cerebral protection? The flip side. J Neurosurg Anesthesiology 1992: 4: 216–220

Schwartz JL, Pollard H, Quach TT. Histamine as a neurotransmitter in mammilian brain: neurochemical evidence. J Neurochem 1980: 35: 26–33.

Sciotti VM, van Wylen DGL. Increases in interstitial adenosine and cerebral blood flow with inhibition of adenoisne kinase and adenosine deaminase. J Cereb Blood Flow Metab 1993: 13: 201-207.

Sedzimir CB. Therapeutic hypothermia in cases of head injury. J Neurosurg 1959: 16: 407–414.

Sercombe R, Verrechia C, Oudart N, et al. Pial artery response to norepinephrine potentiated by endothelium removal. J Cereb Blood Flow Metab 1985: 5: 312–317.

Serteser M, Ozben T, Gumuslu S, et al. Biochemical evidence of crossed cerebellar diaschisis in terms of nitric oxide indicators and lipid peroxidation products in rats during focal cerebral ischemia. Acta Neurol Scand 2001: 103: 43–48.

Severinghaus JW, Cotev S. Carbonic acidosis and cerebral vasodilation after diamox. Scand J Clin Lab Invest (suppl) 1968:102: VII: I:E.

Shapiro HM, Wyte SR, Loeser J. Barbiturate augmented hypothermia for reduction of persistant intracranial hypertension J Neurosurg 1974: 40: 90–100.

Shenkin HA, Hafkenschiel JH, Kety SS. Effects of sympathectomy on the cerebral circulation of hypertensive patients. Arch Surg 1950: 61: 319–324.

Siesjö BK, Ingvar M, Pelligrino D. Regional differences in vascular autoregulation in the rat brain in severe insulin-induced hypoglycemia. J Cereb Blood Flow Metab 1983: 3: 478–485.

Skinhøj E, Paulson OB. Carbon dioxide and cerebral circulatory control. Arch Neurol 1969: 20: 249–252

Skinhøj E, Strandgaard S. Pathogenesis of hypertensive encephalopathy. Lancet 1973: i: 461–462.

Slocum HC, Hayes HJ, Laezman BL. Ventilator technique of anaesthesia for neurosurgery. Anesthesiology 1961: 22: 143–145.

Smielewski P, Czosnyka M, Kirkpatrick P, et al. Assessment of cerebral autoregulation using carotid artery compression. Stroke 1996: 27: 2197–2203.

Sokoloff L, Perland S, Konetsky C, Kety SS. The effect of D-lysergic acid diethylamide on cerebral circulation and overall metabolism. Ann NY Acad Sci 1957: 66: 468–477

Sokoloff L, Kennedy C, Adachi K, et al. Effects of inhibition of nitric oxide synthase on resting local cerebral blood flow and on changes induced by hypercapnia or local functional activity. In: Pharmacology of Cerebral Ischemia. Kriegstein J, Oberpichler-Schwenk H (eds). Stuttgart, Wissenschaftliche Verlagsgesellschaft 1992, pp 371–381.

Soloway M, Nadel W, Albin MS, White RJ. The effect of hyperventilation on subsequent cerebral infarction. Anesthesiology 1968: 29: 975–980.

Soloway M, Moriarty G, Fraser JG, White RJ. Effect of delayed hyperventilation on experimental cerebral infarction. Neurology 1971: 21: 479–485.

Speth RC, Harik SI. Angiotensin II receptor binding sites in brain microvessels. Proc Natl Sci 1985: 82: 6340–6343.

Steen PA, Milde JH, Michenfelder JD. No barbiturate protection in a dog model of complete cerebral ischaemia Ann Neurol 1979: 5: 343–349.

Steinmeier R, Bauhof C, Hubner U, et al. Slow rhytmic oscillations of blood pressure, intracranial pressure, microcirculation, and cerebral oxygenation: dynamic interaction and time course in humans. Stroke 1996: 27: 2236–2243.

Stephan H, Weyland A, Kazmaier S, et al. Acid-base management during hypothermic cardiopulmonary bypass does not affect cerebral metabolism but does affect blood flow and neurological outcome. Br J Anaesth 1992: 69: 51–57.

Strandgaard S, Olesen J, Skinhøj E, Lassen NA. Autoregulation of brain circulation in severe hypertension. Br Med J 1973: 1: 507–510.

Strandgaard S, McKenzie ET, Jones JV, Harper AM. Studies on cerebral blood flow following breakthrough of autoregulation. Blood flow and metabolism in the brain, Harper M, Jennett B, Miller D. Rowan J (eds). Churchill Livingstone, Edinburgh, London, New York 1975a: 5.15.

Strandgaard S, Jones JV, MacKenzie ET, Harper AM. Upper-limit of cerebral blood flow autoregulation in experimental renovascular hypertension in the baboon. Circ Res 1975b: 37: 164–167.

Strandgaard S. Autoregulation of cerebral blood flow in hypertensive patients. The modifying influence of profound antihypertensive treatment on the tolerance to acute, drug-induced hypotension. Circulation 1976: 53: 720–727.

Strandgaard S, Paulson OB. Cerebral autoregulation. Stroke 1984: 15: 413–416.

Swan H, Schätte C. Antimetabolic extract from the brain of the hibernating ground squirrel Citellus tridecemlineatus. Science 1977: 195: 84–85.

Sutton JR, Lassen N. Pathophysiology of acute mountain sickness and high altitude pulmonary edema: an hypothesis. Bull Eur Physiopathol Respir 1979: 15: 1045–1052

Sutton LN, McLaughlin AC, Kemp W, et al. Effects of increased ICP on brain phosphocreatine and lactate determined by simultaneous 1H and 31P NMR spectroscopy. J Neurosurg 1987: 67: 381–386.

Suzuki R, Nitsch C, Fujiwara K, Klatzo I. Regional changes in cerebral blood flow and blood-brain barrier permeability during epileptiform seizures and in acute hypertension in rabbits. J Cereb Blood Flow Metab 1984: 4: 96–102.

Suzuki Y, Satoh S-I, Kimura M, et al. Effects of vasopressin and oxytocin on canine cerebral circulation in vivo. J Neurosurg 1992: 77: 424–431

Symon L. Regional cerebrovascular responses to acute ischaemia in normocapnia and hypercapnia. J Neurol Neurosurg Psychiat 1970: 33: 756–762

Symon L, Held K, Dorsch MWC. On the myogenic nature of the autoregulatory mechanism in the cerebral circulation. Europ Neurol 1972: 6: 11–18.

Symon L, Held K, Dorsch NWC. A study of regional autoregulation in the cerebral circulation to increased perfusion pressure in normocapnia and hypercapnia. Stroke 1973: 4: 139–147.

Symon L, Branston NM, Strong J. Autoregulation in acute focal ischemia. An experimental study. Stroke 1976: 7: 547–554

Sørensen SC. Theoretical considerations on the potential hazards of hyperventilation during anesthesia. Acta Anaestheiol Scand 1978: suppl 67: 106–110.

Tabaddor K, Gardner TJ, Walker AE. Cerebral circulation and metabolism at deep hypothermia. Neurology (Minneap.) 1972: 22: 1065–1070.

Taft WC, Yang K, Dixon CE, et al. Hypothermia attenuates the loss of hippocampal microtubule-associated protein 2 (MAP2) following traumatic brain injury. J Cereb Blood Flow Metab 1993. 13: 796–802.

Takano T, Nagatsuka K, Ohnishi Y, et al. Vascular response to carbon dioxide in areas with and without diaschisis in patients with small, deep hemispheric infarction. Stroke 1988: 19: 840–845

Terry HR, Daw EF, Michenfelder JD. Hypothermia by extracorporeal circulation for neurosurgery: an anesthetic technique. Anesth Analg 1962: 41: 241–248.

Thomas DJ, du Boulay GH, Marshall J, et al. Effect of hematocrit on cerebral blood flow in man. Lancet 1977: 2: 941–943.

Tiecks FP, Lam AM, Aaslid R, Newell DW. Comparison of static and dynamic cerebral autoregulation measurements. Stroke 1995: 26: 1014–1019.

Todd MM, Weeks JB, Warner DS. The influence of intravascular volume expansion on cerebral blood flow and blood volume in normal rats. Anesthesiology 1994: 78: 945–953.

Tominaga S, Strandgaard S, Eumera K, et al. Cerebrovascular CO_2 reactivity in normotensive and hypertensive man. Stroke 1976: 7: 507–510.

Tamaki K, Saku Y, Ogata J. Effects of angiotensin and atrial natriuretic peptide on the cerebral circulation. J Cereb Blood Flow Metab 1992: 12: 318–325

Tranmer BI, Keller TS, Kindt GW, Archer D. Loss of cerebral regulation during cardiac output variations in focal cerebral ischemia. J Neurosurg 1992: 77: 253–259

Tuor UI, Edvinsson L, McCulloch J. Catecholamines and the relationship between cerebral blood flow and glucose use. Am Physiol Soc 1986: 251: H824–833.

Uchida E, Bohr DF, Hoobler SW. A method for studying isolated resistance vessels from rabbit mesentery and brain and their responses to drugs. Circ Res 1967: 21: 525–536

Uihlein A, Terry HR, Payne WS, Kirklin JW. Operations on intracranial aneurysms with induced hypothermia below 15 C and total circulatory arrest. J Neurosurg 1962: 19: 237–239.

Uihlein A, MacCarty CS, Michenfelder JD, et al. Deep hypothermia and surgical treatment of intracranial aneurysms. Am Med Ass 1966: 195: 639–641.

Underwood MD, Bakalian MJ, Arango V, et al. Regulation of cortical blood flow by the dorsal raphe nucleus: Topographic organization of cerebrovascular regulatory regions. J Cereb Blood Flow Metab 1992: 12: 664–673.

Vanhoutte PM, Verbeuren TJ, Webb RC. Local modulation of the adrenergic neuroeffector interaction in the blood vessel wall. Physiol Rev 1981: 61: 151–247.

Vanicky I, Marsala M, Murár J, Marsala J. Prolonged postischemic hyperventilation reduces acute neuronal damage after 15 min of cardiac arrest in the dog. Neuroscience Lett 1992: 135: 167–170.

Van Wylen DGL, Park TS, Rubio R et al. Brain dialysate adenosine concentration during cerebral autoregulation in the adult rat. Fed Proc 1987: 46: 354.

Videen TO, Perlmutter JS, Herscovitch P, Raichle ME. Brain blood volume flow, and oxygen utilization with ^{15}O radiotracers and positron emission tomography: Revised metabolic computations. J Cereb Blood Flow Metab 1987: 7: 513–516

Vinall PE, Simeone FA. Cerebral autoregulation: An in vitro study. Stroke 1981: 12: 640–642.

Voldby B, Enevoldsen EM, Jensen FT. Regional CBF, intraventricular pressure, and cerebral metabolism in patients with ruptured intracranial aneurysms. J Neurosurg 1985: 62: 48–58.

von Essen C, Zervas NT, Brown DR, et al. Local cerebral blood flow in the dog during intravenous infusion of dopamine. Surg Neurol 1980: 13: 181–188.

von Essen C. Effects of dopamine on cerebral blood flow in the dog. Acta Neurol Scand 1974: 50: 39–52.

von Essen C. Effects of dopamine, noradrenaline and 5-hydroxytryptamine on cerebral blood flow in the dog. J Pharm Pharmacol 1972: 24: G68

Vorstrup S. Tomographic cerebral blood flow measurements in patients with ischaemic cerebrovascular disease and evaluation of the vasodilatory capacity by the acetazolamide test. Acta Neurol Scand 1988: 114: 77: 1–48.

Wagerle LC, Orr JA, Shirer HW, et al. Cerebrovascular response to acute decreases in arterial PO_2. J Cereb Blood Flow Metab 1983: 3: 507–515

Wagerle LC, Busija DW. Cholinergic mechanisms in the cerebral circulation of the newborn piglet: effect of inhibitors of arachidonic acid metabolism. Circ Res 1989: 64: 1030–1036.

Wahl M, Kuschinsky W. The dilating effect of histamine on pial arteries of cats and its mediation of H_2 receptors. Circ Res 1979: 44: 161–165.

Waldemar G, Schmidt JF, Andersen AR, et al. Angiotensin converting enzyme inhibition and cerebral blood flow autoregulation in normotensive and hypertensive man. J Hypertension 1989: 7: 229–235

Waldemar G, Hasselbalch SG, Andersen AR, et al. 99m-Tc-d,l-HMPAO and SPECT of the brain in normal aging. J Cereb Blood Flow Metab 1991: 11: 508–521

Waldemar G, Schmidt JF, Delecluse F, et al. High resolution SPECT with (99mTc)-d,l-HMPAO in normal pressure hydrocephalus before and after shunt operation. J Neurol Neurosurg Psychiatry 1993: 56: 655–664.

Waldemar G, Bruhn P, Kristensen M, et al. Heterogeneity of neocortical cerebral blood flow deficits in dementia of the Alzheimer type: a (99mTc)-d.1-HMPAO SPECT study. J Neurol Neurosurg Psychiatry 1994: 57: 285–295.

Waltz AG, Yamaguchi T, Regli F. Regulatory responses of cerebral vasculatur after sympathetic denervation. Am J Physiol 1971: 221: 298–302

Wang Q, Paulson OB, Lassen NA. Effect of nitric oxide blockade by NG-nitro-L-arginine on cerebral blood flow response to changes in carbon dioixide tension. J Cereb Blood Flow Metab 1992: 12: 947–953.

Wang Q, Pelligrino DA, Koenig HM, Albrecht RF. The role of endothelium and nitric oxide in rat pial arteriolar dilatory responses to CO_2 in vivo. J Cereb Blood Flow Metab 1994: 14: 944–951.

Warner DS, Turner DM, Kassell NF. Time-dependent effects of prolonged hypercapnia on cerebrovascular parameters in dogs: Acid-base chemistry. Stroke 1987: 18: 142-149.

Wei EP, Ellis EF, Kontos HA. Role of prostagladins in pial arteriolar response to CO_2 and hypoxia. Am J Physiol 1980: 238: H226-230

Wei EP, Kontos HA, Dietrich WD et al. Inhibition by free radical scavengers and by cyclooxygenase inhibitors of pial arteriolar abnormalities from concussive brain injury in cats. Circ Res 1981: 48: 95-103

Wichser J, Kazemi H. CSF bicarbonate regulation in respiratory acidosis and alkalosis. J Appl Physiol 1975: 38: 504–512

Widder B, Kleiser B, Krapf H. Course of cerebrovascular reactivity in patients with carotid artery occlusions. Stroke 1994: 25: 1963–1967.

White RJ, Albin MS, Verdura J, Locke GE. Differential extracorporal hypothermic perfusion of and circulatory arrest to the human brain. Med Res Engineering 1967: 6: 18–24.

White RJ. Preservation of cerebral function during circulatory arrest and resuscitation: Hypothermic protective considerations. Resuscitation 1972: 1: 107–115.

Winn HR, Welsh JE, Rubio R, Berne RM. Brain adenosine production in the rat during sustained alteration in systemic blood pressure. Am J Physiol 1980: 239: H 636–641.

Winn HR, Rubio R, Berne RM. The role of adenosine in the regulation of cerebral blood flow. J Cereb Blood Flow Metab 1981: 1: 239–244.

Winsö I. Cerebral blood flow at hyperventilation. The interrelation between oxygen and carbon dioxide tensions in the cerebrovascular response to hyperventilation in dogs. Elanders Boktruckeri aktiebolag, 1971: Göteborg

Wollman SB, Orkim LR. Postoperative human reaction time and hypocapnia during anesthesia. Br J Anaesth 1968: 40: 920–927.

Wong DF, Young D, Wilson PD, et al. Quantification of neuroreceptors in the living human brain. D_2-like dopamine receptors: theory, validation, and changes during normal aging. J Cereb Blood Flow Metab 1997a: 17: 316–330.

Wong DF, Young D, Wilson PD. Quantification of neuroreceptors in the living human brain: IV. Effect of aging and elevations of D_2-like receptors in schizophrenia and bipolar illness. J Cereb Blood Flow Metab 1997b: 17: 331–342.

Wood JH, Simeone FA, Fink EA, Golden MA. Hypervolemic hemodilution in experimental focal cerebral ischemia: Evaluations of cardiac output, regional cerebral blood flow, and ICP after intravascular volume expansion with low molecular weight dextran. J Neurosurg 1983: 59: 500–509

Yakch TL, Anderson RE. In vivo studies on intracellular pH, focal flow, and vessel diameter in the cat cerebral cortex: Effects of altered CO_2 and electrical stimulation. J Cereb Blood Flow Metab 1987: 7: 332–341

Yamashita K, Eguchi Y, Kajiwara K, et al.: Mild hypothermia ameliorates ubiquitin synthesis and prevents delayed neuronal death in the gerbil hippocampus. Stroke 1991: 22: 1574–1581.

Yamauchi H, Fukuyama H, Nagahama Y, et al. Uncoupling of oxygen and glucose metabolism in persistent crossed cerebellar diaschisis. Stroke 1999: 30: 1424–1428.

Yano M, Ikeda Y, Kobayshi S, et al. The outcome with barbiturate therapy in severe head injuries. In: Intracranial Pressure VI, Miller JD, Teasdale GM, Rowan JO, Galvraith SL, Mendelow AD (eds), Springer Verlag, Berlin, Heidelberg 1986: 769–773.

Yokote H, Itakura T, Nakai K, et al. A role of the central catecholamine neuron in cerebral circulation. J Neurosurg 1986: 65: 370–375

Yonas H, Darby JM, Marks EC, et al. CBF measured by Xe-CT: Approach to analysis and normal values. J Cereb Blood Flow Metab 1991: 11: 716–725

Yonas H, Smith HA, Durham SR, et al. Increased stroke risk predicted by compromized cerebral blood flow reactivity. J Neurosurg 1993: 79: 483–489.

Young RS, Olenginski TP, Yagel SK, Towfighi J. The effect of graded hypothermia on hypoxic-ischaemic brain damage: a neuropathologic study in the neonate rat. Stroke 1983: 14: 929–934.

Zhang R, Zuckerman JH, Giller CA, Levine BD. Transfer function analysis of the dynamic cerebral autoregulation in human. Am J Physiol 1998: 274: H233–241.

Intracranial pressure

In this chapter methodology, indication for ICP measurement, critical levels of ICP and regional differences in ICP are described. Medical approaches to ICP control, including body position, hyperventilation, hypothermia, barbiturate, are considered. The effects upon ICP of inhalationanaesthetics, hypnotic drugs, analgetics, muscular relaxant and drugs used for control of blood pressure are described in chapter 4–8. ICP measurement in patients with severe head injury, and patients with subarachnoid haemorrhage is reviewed in chapter 10 and 11 respectively.

Methodology

Lundberg (1960) introduced continuous intraventricular pressure (IVP) monitoring in the neurointensive clinic. This method, based on an intraventricular catheter connected to a pressure transducer, has remained the gold standard method, with which other methods are compared. A standard practice is to zero the ICP at the external auditory meatus, and to correct for differences between heart level when calculating cerebral perfusion pressure (CPP). Owing to the traumatic nature of the method, difficulties concerning the surgical procedure, especially when the cerebral ventricles are compressed, and the relatively high infection rate, other methods have been introduced.

Besides the standard gold technique of Intraventricular pressure monitoring the following approaches have been used: Epidural transducer; subdural bolt via a burr hole; subdural catheter; peroperative placement of subdural needle; intraparenchymal transducer, lumbar spinal fluid pressure, and lumbar epidural pressure.

The subdural bolt, screwed through the bone, and placed into contact with the dura was introduced by Vries et al. (1973). Advantages of the bolt-method are that it does not require brain tissue penetration or anatomical knowledge of the position of the ventricular system. A subdural catheter can be placed below the dura in connection with craniotomy (Sugiura et al. 1985, Rosenwasser et al. 1989) eventually introduced via a Tuohy needle (Yano et al. 1988). This method has been used in traumatic head injury and during the postoperative period after tumour surgery (Constantini et al. 1988). Perioperative ICP measurement can be obtained with a thin needle placed subdurally during the operation (Cold et al. 1996). Epidural transducer based upon an external transducer coupled to a pressure sensitive switch was described by Crutchfield et al. (1990). Similarly, Gaeltec subdural catheter tip pressure transducer has been introduced. Its advantage is that both zero and catheter checks can be carried out after insertion (Roberts et al. 1983). Also intracranial transducers are available, but some of them are fraught with technical problems related to calibration and system stability.

In neonates and infants monitoring of the anterior fontanelle pressure has been practiced (Wayenberg et al. 1993). Using the Rotterdam teletransducer Wayenberg (1998) concludes that it is technically possible and clinically helpful to obtain accurate information about ICP and changes in cerebral compliance in a wide range of clinical conditions with this technique.

New methods for ICP recording are based on the algorithms for realtime calculation of ICP from continuously monitored blood flow velocity and arterial blood pressure (Zabolotny et al. (2000). An MR-based noninvasive method for ICP measurements has been developed. Early results show sensitivity sufficient to differentiate between normal and elevated ICP (Alperin et al. 2000).

Comparison among methods

In a series of 378 recordings of ICP ventricular catheter, the Richmond screw, and subdural catheter were compared. The Richmond screw became blocked more often (16%) than the subdural catheter (2,7%) or the ventricular catheter (2,5%). Complications of infection, and intracerebral haemorrhage were observed mostly in patients with ventricular catheter (North and Redally 1986). In a recent study, based on 739 own studies and 14500 literature cases, a cumulative infection risk of 6,7% in ventricular measurements, 0,7% in brain tissue, and 0% in epidural registrations were found (Aschoff et al. 2000). In another study subarachnoid catheter and subarachnoid bolt were compared with intraventricular catheter. The subarachnoid bolt was shown to be relatively inaccurate, while the subarachnoid catheter was demonstrated to be an accurate, reliable, and safe method and an acceptable alternative to ventriculostomy (Mollman et al. 1988). Case reports (Miller et al. 1986), and other comparison of subarachnoid bolts and intraventricular pressure demonstrate the same conclusion (Mendelow et al. 1983). In another study the Gaeltec subdural method and subdural catheter technique were compared with the IVP method. Only 44% of the fluid filled catheter readings corresponded with the IVP recordings in series of 10 mm Hg ranges, while 53% of readings were lower than the IVP recordings. This tendency was even more marked at higher pressures. With the Gaeltec catheter 72% of the readings corresponded with IVP. Thus, the subdural catheter appeared less reliable compared with the Gaeltec monitor (Barrow et al. 1985). Sundberg et al. (1986) compared intra-parenchymal transducer with IVP at IVP levels ranging from zero to 80 mm Hg. Difference between the pressures did not exceed 5 mm Hg. In another study it was emphasized that drift of the intraparenchymal tip catheter occurs. This tendency is potentiated by inability to recalibrate the transducer (Ghajar 1995). Comparison between the plastimed extradural sensor and the Camino fiberoptic system unveiled that extradural pressure was higher than the Camino-pressure (bias 9 mm Hg). The lack of agreement between the two methods was supposed to be the unreliability of extradural pressure monitoring (Bruder et al. 1995).

Lumbar spinal and epidural pressure have been compared experimentally during cisternal infusion. The degree of pressure rises and the time course was identically. Calculated compliance, however, differed between the two methods (Kinuta et al. 1987). Lumbar CSF-pressure has been used for studies of anesthetic action, and for studies of the influence of head position upon pressure (Macrocordatos et al. 2000).

Normal values

CSF pressure data of spinal origin are numerous. Normal pressure is generally defined as pressures below 200 cm H_2O, corresponding to 15 mm Hg. In subjects without cerebral disorders intracranial pressure measured in the supine position averages 11 mm Hg (SD: 2 mm Hg, range 7–15 mm Hg) (Albeck et al. 1991).

Pathophysiology

The tolerance to intracranial hypertension depends on the pathophysiology. Thus, high ICP-levels are tolerated fairly well as regards neurological status and consciousness, if the pressure-increase is developed over months or years and the high pressure is not accompanied by major shifts of the intracranial content. This is observed in obstructive hydrocephalus and slow-growing tumours. On the other hand, if ICP-hypertension is caused by haematomas or cytotoxic oedema, secondary to ischaemia, and accompanied by major shift of the intracranial compartments, it is tolerated badly.

Pressure waves

Waves occur syncroneously with the cardiac cycle and respiration. Waves syncronised with pressure ventilation are supposed to be caused by an increase in intrathorasic pressure. Cyclic variation of cerebral pial arteriolar diameter also occurs. The amplitude of these variations are greater during normal arteriolar tone than during vasodilation caused by hypercapnia (Daley et al. 2000).

Lundberg (1960) described plateau or A-waves, B-waves and C-waves. A-waves are characterized as large plateau-like formations recurring at intervals of varying length with duration of 5 to 20 min, and pressure increase of maximally 100 mm Hg. A-waves occur in space-occupying lesions. They are associated with an increase in cerebral blood volume (Risberg et al. 1969), which again may be a caused by changes in cerebral perfusion pressure in patients with intact autoregulation (Rosner and Becker 1984). Experimentally, spontaneous activity of the locus coeruleus complex is suppressed during plateau waves, while the activity of neurons from the cholinoceptive pontine area is increased (Maeda et al. 1989). Other studies indicate that lesion in the ventral noradrenergic system evoked ICP changes resembling plateau-waves while activation of the same system by glutamate microinjection produced a decrease in ICP (Maeda et al. 1993). Thus, activity within the cholinergic basal forebrain, as well as the central noradrenergic system, contributes to ICP changes resembling plateau-waves (Maeda and Miyazaki 1998).

B-waves are defined as rhythmic oscillations occurring more or less regularly at a frequency of 1–2 per minute often occuring synchroneously with respiration (Lundberg 1960). B-waves are provoked by a decrease in cerebral perfusion pressure (Rosner and Coley 1986).

C-waves are defined as rhythmic iscillations , occurring with a frequency of 4–8 per minute with an amplitude from discernibility to 20 mm Hg. C-waves are related to rhythmic variations of systemic arterial pressure described as Traube-Hering waves.

Critical levels

Experimental studies

In baboons ischaemic oedema (cytotoxic oedema) is a threshold phenomenon which develops when CBF is reduced below 20 ml/100g/min (Symon et al. 1979). However, oedema formation is also dependent on the duration of the ischaemic period and whether ischaemia is complete or incomplete (Ito et al. 1979, Schuier et al. 1980, Todd et al. 1986). With this in mind drugs which prevent cerebral ischaemia also are supposed to prevent the formation and/or propagation of cerebral oedema.

Studies in dogs of brain tissue- and CSF oxygen tension indicate that CPP below 80 mm Hg is critical. Below this level brain tissue oxygen tension decreases. In the CPP range of 40–60 mm Hg a sharp decline in oxygen tensions was found indicating development of cerebral ischaemia (Maas et al. 1993).

In rabbits the critical level at which ICP rises in response to hypoxia is PaO_2 level of 50 mm Hg. Below this level ICP rises steeply (North et al. 1993).

In cats subjected to epidural balloon insufflation CBF increases when ICP began to rise. At ICP levels of 20–30 mm Hg CBF and CBV started to decrease. Decompression of the balloon led to an abrupt decrease in ICP and a transient increase in CBF and CBV, after which both CBF and CBV recovered to control values (Kojima et al. 1993).

In cats posttraumatic hypoventilation exacerbates the ICP increase and reduces the pressure-volume index (PVI). It is supposed that these events accelerate neuronal damage and produce more extensive brain oedema (Shima and Marmarou 1993).

Human studies

During craniotomy the critical level of ICP for cerebral swelling after opening of dura is 10 mm Hg. This threshold has been demonstrated in supratentorial (Bundgaard et al. 1998) and infratentorial tumours (Jørgensen et al. 1999).

Studies of ICP in patients with severe head injury indicate that pressure levels above 30–40 mm Hg for several hours are associated with a poor outcome (Troupp 1967, Vapalahti et al. 1969, Cold et al. 1975, Changaris et al. 1987). In a study of 160 patients with severe head injury Miller et al. (1977) found intracranial hypertension (ICP 10 mm Hg) in 82% of the patients and in 97% of the patients with a mass lesion. Although ICP 40 mm Hg was only observed in 10% of the patients, intracranial hypertension was found to be a primary reason for death in 50% of the patients.

The relationships between ICP, the pulse wave amplitude, and CPP indicate a gradual increase in amplitude with CPP decreasing from 75 to 30 mm Hg. For CPP below 30 mm Hg there is a sharp decrease in amplitude. This change indicates critical disturbance in cerebral circulation (Czosnyka et al. 1994).

In the American Guidelines (2000) the following recommendations are proposed: There are insufficient data to support a treatment standard for this topic". As option the American Guidelines propose that "intracranial pressure (ICP) treatment should be initiated at an upper threshold of 20–25 mm Hg". "Interpretation and treatment of ICP based on any threshold should be corroborated by frequent clinical examination and cerebral perfusion pressure data".

Regional difference in ICP

Experimental studies

It is generally believed that ICP is the same throughout the cerebrospinal fluid spaces within the cranial cavity. In an experimental study of monkeys subjected to inflation of a balloon it was found that pressure forces were not uniformly transmitted from an expanding mass. Even pressure decreases were observed in some brain regions (Kuchiwaki et al. 1992). In a porcine model subjected to a frontal mass lesion, intraparenchymal ICP monitors were placed in the right and left hemispheres. During expansion of the mass, a pressure difference that increased as the size of the mass increased, developed between intracranial regions. The regional pressures were found to vary in a consistent fashion.Right and left frontal pressures were equal. The pressure gradients through the brain were as follows: Frontal pressures temporal pressures midbrain pressures cerebellar pressures (Wolfla et al. 1996).

Clinical studies

Pressure differentials have not been demonstrated in clinical studies of head injury with bilateral frontal placement of transducers (Yano et al. 1987). Significant and lasting ICP gradients (10 mm Hg) between bilateral frontal hemispheres were found in all patients with an acute subdural haematoma (Chambers et al. 1998). In clinical studies of head injury interhemispheric supratentorial pressure gradients have been demonstrated. Mindermann and Gratzl (1998) argue that simultaneous bilateral ICP measurement may be warranted in the initial posttraumatic phase. Transient gradients that disappear with time are frequently observed, and may indicate an increase in the size of the lesion (Sahuquillo et al. 1999).

During craniotomy pressure gradients between supra- and infratentorial compartments have been demonstrated (Cold et al. 1996). Likewise pressure gradients related to the underlying tumour and/or gravity have been found in patients with cerebral tumours (Bundgaard et al. 2000).

Monitoring technology

In the American Guidelines (2000) the following recommendations are proposed: in the current state of technology, the ventricular catheter connected to an external strain gauge is the most accurate, low cost, and reliable method of monitoring intracranial pressure (ICP). It also allows therapeutic CSF drainage. ICP transduction via fiberoptic or strain gauge devices placed in the ventricular catheters, provides similar benefits, but at higher cost. Parenchymal ICP monitoring with fiberoptic or strain gauge catheter tip transduction is similar to ventricular ICP monitoring, but has the potential for measurement drift. Subarachnoid, subdural, and epidural monitors (fluid coupled or pneumatic) currently are less accurate". These arguments are in agreement with a study where the reliability of epidural transducers was not improved. Using epidural transducers, one must be aware of the possibility of overestimating ICP by more than 10 mm Hg, and the possibility of significant drifting over time (Raabe et al. 1998).

Pressure volume relationship

Complaince is defined as the pressure reaction to a change in intracranial volume ($\Delta V/\Delta P$). The exponential nature of the pressure volume curve indicates that a similar volume increment at different points of the curve results in a different pressure response. The slope of the pressure volume curve is dependent on factors contributing to compensatory mechanisms. Thus, compensatory changes in ventricular fluid volume and cerebral blood volume influence the pressure increase obtained during volume expansion. Furthermore, the steepness of the pressure volume curve varies under different pathological circumstances, and is also influenced by therapy with mannitol and steroid.

The pressure volume index is defined as the volume necessary to raise the ICP by a factor of 10. By plotting the pressure on a logarithmic axis against volume, the otherwise exponential curve becomes linear. The slope of this curve is the pressure volume index.

Recently the Spiegelberg intracranial pressure and intracranial compliance monitor system have been tested. Good correlation of compliance was found with the CSF-bolus injection technique in experimental (Yau et al. 2000) and clinical studies (Piper et al. 1999). In a recent study of patients with severe head injury it was found that at high ICP (ICP 20 mm Hg) compliance was linearly correlated to CPP suggesting failure of autoregulatory mechanism (Protella et al. 2000). In another study of patients with closed head injury it was found that at similar values of ICP intracranial compliance depends on the age of the patients (Kiening et al. 2000).

Indications to ICP monitoring

In the American Guidelines for the Management of Severe Traumatic Brain Injury (2000), the authors summarize: ICP monitoring per se has never been subjected to a prospective, randomized clinical trial (PRCT), to establish its efficacy (or lack there of) in improving outcome from severe head injury. Hence there are insufficient data to support the use as a standard. However, there is a large body of published clinical experience that indicates, that ICP monitoring (1) helps in the earlier detection of intracranial mass lesions, (2) can limit the indiscriminate use of therapies to control ICP which themselves can be potentially harmful, (3) can reduce ICP by CSF drainage, and thus improve cerebral perfusion (4) helps in determining prognosis, and (5) may improve outcome. ICP monitoring is therefore used by most head injury experts in the United States, and it is accepted as a relatively low-risk high yield, modest-cost intervention. Comatose head injury patients (GCS 3-8) with abnormal CT scans should undergo ICP monitoring. Comatose patients with normal CT scans have much lower incidence of intracranial hypertension, unless they have two or more of the following features at admission: Age over 40 years, unilateral or bilateral motor posturing, or a systolic blood pressure of less than 90 mm Hg. ICP monitoring in patients with normal CT scans with two of these risk factors is suggested as a guideline. Routine ICP monitoring is not indicated in patients with mild or moderate head injury. However, it may be undertaken in certain conscious patients with traumatic mass lesions at the discretion of the treating physician".

Invasive or surgical approach to control of ICP-hypertension

Hydrocephalus

In the neurosurgical clinic intracranial hypertension may develop as a consequence of increased volume of ventricular fluid, blood volume or the volume of the brain tissue components. In hydrocephalus the volume of ventricular fluid is increased. The rational therapy under this circumstance is drainage or surgical shunt operation.

Mass lesion and decompression craniectomy

The amount of intracranial content might be increased owing to tumour, contusion, haematoma and cerebral oedema. The rational therapy is surgical with removal of the space occupying process.

Decompression craniectomy has recently gained increasing interest. Bardt et al. (2000) performed decompression craniectomy in 70 patients with uncontrolled ICP-hypertension and found a decrease in ICP from 39 to 10 mm Hg one hour after decompression. The six month mortality rate was 33.3%. Similar results were found in patients subjected to bilateral decompression (Yoo et al. 2000).

Ventricular drainage

Ventricular drainage is used in the neurointensive clinic in patients with subarachnoid haemorrhage, severe head injury, intraventricular haemorrhage and hydrocephalus. Drainage can be continuous or intermittent. With the drainage system connected to a pressure transducer, the system both gives continuous ICP recording and opportunities for biochemical analysis of the CSF (lactate, pyruvate etc). Risks include infection, overdrainage of the ventricular system with collapse of the ventricular system.

Spinal CSF drainage

Since the publication by Vourc'h (1963), describing the use of plastic catheter inserted percutaneously for the drainage of CSF, spinal drainage has been rarely used. Controlled studies of spinal pressure and ICP, however, are not available. The technique is useful in lowering ICP and achieving brain relaxation during intracranial surgery (cerebral aneurysm and basal tumours), and as prevention and/or treatment of intracranial and spinal fistulas (Basouri et al. 1999).

Medical approach to control of ICP-hypertension

Operative approach to surgical correction of intracranial hypertension may be restricted, because the main reason for cerebral swelling is brain oedema or increased cerebral blood volume. The control of intracranial hypertension under such circumstances is based on the control of intracranial blood volume either via control of cerebral venous distension (central venous pressure, neck compression, dihydroergotamine) or control by neurophysiological mechanisms including the chemical (P_aCO_2,PO_2, indomethacin, theophyllamine), neurogenic or hormonal (catecholamine), metabolic (hypnotics, analgetics, hypothermia) and autoregulatory control of cerebral circulation. At last, control of cerebral tissue water content can be effected by osmotic acting drugs like mannitol, diuretics and hypertonic saline.

In this review, non-surgical principles of control of intracranial pressure will be reviewed. New principles of prevention of ischaemic damage of the brain will shortly be commented, as regards their influence on intracranial pressure and/or the pressure/volume relationship.

Control of cerebral blood volume (CBV)

In adults the intracranial blood volume is about 60–80 ml with 2/3 in the capillary and venous bed and 1/3 in the arterial vessels. With an average global CBF of 50 ml/100g/min, about 700–1000 ml blood (20% of cardiac output) is perfused through the cerebrum per minute. As cerebral blood flow, under normal situations, is precisely adjusted to metabolic demand, adjustment of cerebral blood volume by changes in the cerebral vascular resistance (hypocapnia, indomethacin, theophyllamine) may be potentially detrimental. On the other hand, a decrease in the cerebral venous blood volume does not influence oxygen delivery. As the blood content in venous vessels is the double of the arterial bed, the potentials of manipulation of the venous blood volume theoretically should have a greater impact upon intracranial pressure.

Central venous pressure and head position

Experimental studies

An increase of central venous pressure (CVP), whatever the reason, may contribute to ICP-hypertension and changes in PVI. Experimental studies indicate that reduction in brain compliance can occur secondary to elevation of CVP following resuscitation from haemorrhagic shock (Hariri et al. 1993). Thus, fluid volume replacement in patients with head injury should be done with careful attention to CVP.

In pigs a significant and linear increase in ICP with increased intraabdominal pressure has been demonstrated. This tendency is augmented during head-down position (Josephs et al. 1994, Rosenthal et al. 1997), but is ameliorated when apneumic retractors are applied (Este-McDonald et al. 1995).

Human studies

Acutely increased intra-abdominal pressure causes significant increase in ICP and a decrease in cerebral perfusion pressure. Increased intra-abdominal pressure appears to produce this effect by augmenting pleural and other intrathoracic pressures, and causing a functional obstruction to the cerebral venous outflow via the jugular venous system (Bloomfield et al. 1997).

Head and body position

Changes in head position, including maximal flexion and lateral rotation will give rise to an increase in intracranial pressure, and elevation of the head give rises to a fall in ICP (Hulme and Cooper 1976, Nornes and Magnäs 1971, Kenning et al. 1981, Yoshida et al. 1991, Urlesberger et al. 1991, Williams and Coyne 1993, Meixensberger et al. 1997, Hung et al. 2000). The ICP increase during head rotation is reduced by concomitant head elevation (Hung et al. 2000). The most alarming increase in ICP, however, is observed during head-down position (Hulme and Cooper 1976, Lee 1989, Feldman et al. 1992, Schneider et al. 1993, Yoshida et al. 1993, Mavrocordatos et al. 2000). The mechanisms are intracranial venous distension and an increase in cerebral blood volume (Mcedlishvili 1988). During bilateral radical neck dissection measurement of ICP indicates a marked increase in ICP immediately after internal jugular vein ligation with a maximum peak at 30 minutes. Pressure levels of 40 mm Hg were observed as well as systemic arterial hypertension in response to the elevated ICP (Weiss et al. 1993).

Some studies indicate that moderate flexion of the head 15–30 degree, is associated with a decrease in ICP owing to the improved venous drainage (Kanter et al. 1991). In another study tilting of the head at a steep angle from neutral position (head-tilt position) was compared with the “sniffing position”. The sniffing position was found to be superior to the head-tilt position as regards ICP and CPP (Yoshida et al. 1993).

Head position and CPP

In one study the decrease in ICP is smaller than the decline in blood pressure, and a decrease in cerebral perfusion pressure is therefore observed. Under these circumstances elevation of the head might precipitate ICP waves of the B-type (Rosner and Coley 1986). In another study head elevation was not accompanied by a change in cerebral perfusion pressure because the decrease in ICP corresponded to that of blood pressure (Feldman et al. 1992).

CSF formation

The changes in ICP and sagital sinus pressure do not impair CSF absorption in cats, because the differences between ventricular pressure and sagital sinus pressure are unchanged during change in body position (Kotani et al. 1993).

Pressure volume index (PVI)

During head-down position PVI is higher than during horizontal position indicating an increase in pressure-buffering ability (Kotani et al. 1993). The same group studied PVI and cranial cavity compliance in cats, and found that the values of PVI and compliance were significantly greater in the head-down tilt in spite of an increase in ICP. During craniospinal blockade by epidural ligation of spinal cord at C2 level the PVI and compliance were also higher in the head-down position. This result indicates that the pressure buffering capacity is increased with head-down tilt with respect to intracranial volume loading. The buffering mechanism does not depend on movement of the cerebrospinal fluid, but on the increased cerebral venous vascular bed with communication between extracranial and intracranial compartments (Adachi and Kotani 1990). In contrast, Raabe et al. (1999) found that variation in body position did not change intracranial compliance. A change in hydrostatic offset pressure causes a shifting of the volume-pressure curve along the pressure axis without its shape being affected.

PEEP and CPAP

Coughing, Valsalva maneuver, application of PEEP and CPAP, and neck compression are supposed to increase ICP. The mechanisms should be an increase in cerebral venous pressure. Even appplication of a cervical collar for immobilisation might increase ICP (Raphael and Chotai 1994).

Experimental studies

In rabbits subjected to elevation of ICP by an epidural balloon, it was demonstrated that the volume needed to reach the deflection point of the volume/pressure course was lower, when PEEP at 10 cm H_2O was applied, compared to the values at PEEP zero. The study suggested that PEEP decreased intracranial compliance (Feldman et al. 1997).

Human studies

The effect of CPAP upon cerebral flow velocity is conflicting. Haring et al. (1994) in volunteers found that 12 cm H_2O CPAP caused a significant increase in middle cerebral artery velocity. In contrast Bowie et al. (2001) did not find any significant change in velocity during application of 5 and 10 cm H_2O CPAP.

The effects of PEEP upon ICP in the clinical setting are conflicting. When patients are maintained in the 30 degree head-up position, PEEP improves arterial oxygenation without increasing ICP (Frost et al. 1977). In another study, including patients with head injury, SAH and hydrocephalus, PEEP at 5 cm H_2O did not alter ICP, and the clinical relevance of ICP increase at PEEP levels of 10 and 15 cm H_2O was questionable, because CPP did not change and remained 60 mm Hg. Furthermore, in patients with increased ICP higher levels of PEEP did not change ICP or CPP (McGuire et al. 1997). In a recent study application of PEEP at 10 and 15 cm produced an increase in ICP without significant effect on CPP (Videtta et al. 2000). Generally, PEEP is considered as a valuable form of therapy for the comatose patient with pulmonary disorders such as pneumonia or pulmonary oedema (Frost 1977). In another study, however, the effects of PEEP were studied in patients with severe head injury and acute lung injury. PEEP did not induce any change in CPP and CBF, but ICP was correlated to static elastance of the respiratory system due to alveolar overdistension (Mascia et al. 2000). These findings are in agreement with a study by Kolbitsch et al. (2000). They found that application of CPAP breathing at 6 cm H_2O, which does not exceed the physiological PEEP, had no influence on cerebral compliance. In contrast, CPAP at 12 cm H_2O increased cerebrospinal fluid peak velocity measured by phase-contrast MR imaging. Increased cerebral blood volume which impairs systolic craniocaudal CSF displacement was considered the most likely underlying mechanism.

Warnings against PEEP are also based upon a study in volunteers indicating that CPAP of 12 cm increased CSF pressure from 7 to 11 mm Hg (Hörmann et al. 1994). In the sitting position the combination of head flexion and rotation with institution of PEEP might cause a dangerous increase in ICP (Lodrini et al. 1989).

Suction and other procedures

All procedures in the upper airway, including suction, intubation, coughing, vomiting, and Valsalva maneuver provoke an increase in ICP. During coughing ICP raises instantaneously to a high level, but normally the basal level is reached within a few seconds. If intracranial compliance, however, is deranged, upper airway procedures might result in permanent ICP increase. Relaxants, lidocaine, central analgesics, and hypnotics prevent the ICP increase.

Dihydroergotamine (DHE)

Peripheral vascular resistance

Dihydroergotamine (DHE) increases peripheral vascular resistance (PVR), mainly by constriction of the venous capacitance vessels (Mellander and Nordenfelt 1970, Müller-Schweinitzer and Rosenthaler 1987).

Experimental studies

In a porcine model of ICP-hypertension DHE administrated for 60 min caused a lasting decrease in ICP probably achieved by a decrease in cerebral blood volume due to constriction of both arterial and venous capacitance vessels (Nilsson et al. 1995).

Human studies

DHE is a potent constrictor of human basilar arteries *in vitro*. In normal adult DHE does not influence CBF (Andersen et al. 1987). Neither does hydergine, a mixture of three ergotoxines, alter CBF even after intraarterial carotid injection (McHenry et al. 1971, Olesen and Skinhøj 1972).

In a preliminary study Grände (1989) reported that DHE 0.25 mg intravenously decreased ICP in head injured patients. The duration of this effect was about one hour and after this period ICP was stabilised at a lower level. Further studies from the same group and others concluded that the decrease in ICP was accompanied by a 30% increase in CBF, a decrease in $AVDO_2$, an increase in CPP, and a 6% decrease in cerebral blood volume (Ryding et al. 1990, Gopinath et al. 1994). In severe HI the effect of DHE upon ICP is not correlated to CO_2 reactivity. Thus, a decrease in ICP was obtained by DHE in patients with or without impaired CO_2 reactivity (Asgeirsson et al. 1995)

DHE was used in dose of 0.25 mg during craniotomy for cerebral tumours subjected to isoflurane/nitrous oxide anesthesia. In accordance to the study in head injury patients a significant increase in MABP was observed. ICP, however, increased significantly as well. In several patients the increase in MABP was associated with an increase in CBF, and a fall in $AVDO_2$, suggesting that these patients had impaired cerebral autoregulation. Thus, the increase in ICP was associated with an increase in both CBF and MABP (Bundgaard et al. 2000).

The Lund model

DHE combined with metoprolol, clonidine, and prostaglandin has been introduced in the treatment of severe head injury. Metoprolol and clonidine elicit only minor effect upon cerebral haemodynamics in severely injured patients (Asgeirsson et al. 1995). The main concept is that opening of the BBB upsets the normal regulation of brain volume and aggravates oedema formation.

The patients are subjected to moderate hyperventilation (30–33 mm Hg), and thiopental sedation (0.5–3.0 mg/kg/h). Both metoprolol and clonidine are supposed to decrease hydrostatic capillary pressure, and reduce fluid filtration across the damaged blood-brain barrier. DHE in doses declining from 0.8 ug/kg/h to 0.1 ug/kg/h are administered to reduce ICP by precapillary and venous vasoconstriction. Low dose prostaglandin infusion 0,5–0.8 Ng/kg/min is given to improve microcirculation around contusion, and to heal the disrupted blood-brain barrier (Grände et al. 1977).

Although clinical controlled studies have not been performed, preliminary results with this regime seem promising (Asgeirsson et al. 1994, Asgeirsson et al. 1995).

Cerebral arteriolar vasoconstriction

Blood pressure control and cerebral autoregulation

Traditionally, the lower limit of cerebral autoregulation (CA) lies between 50 and 80 mm Hg in normotensive adults. Recently Schmidt et al. (1990), with computerized analysis found that the limit averaged 85 mm Hg. The corresponding upper limit of CA is between 130 and 170 mm Hg (Lassen 1974). In chronic hypertension the lower and upper limits are shifter to the right (Strandgaard et al. 1973).

Head injury

In the acute phase of severe head injury (HI) the CA is generally impaired or lost. The abolished CA can be focal, localized to one hemisphere or global (Fieschi et al. 1974, Enevoldsen and Jensen 1978, Cold and Jensen 1978).

In patients with severe head injury the combination of abolished CO_2 reactivity and "preserved" cerebral autoregulation occurs. In some patients the increase in MABP is accociated with an increase in ICP, the result being an unchanged CPP. "False" CA has been reported by several authors, and regional change from "false" to abolished CA is a common phenomenon (Review Cold 1990).

Subarachnoid hemorrhage, apoplexy and tumour

In experimental (Mendelow et al. 1981) and human subarachnoid hemorrhage (Heilbrun et al. 1972) the CA is generally impaired. This impairment is especially observed in patients with severe spasms (Ishii 1979, Voldby et al. 1985). In apoplexy (Paulson et al. 1970), cerebral tumors (Palvölgyi 1969) and transient focal cerebral ischaemia (Skinhøj et al. 1970) CA likewise is impaired or abolished.

Vasoparalysis

Complete vasoparalysis, a condition where the CO_2 reactivity as well as the CA are lost, has been described in the above mentioned diseases. In acute severe head injury with haemorrhagic hypovolemia restoration of blood pressure with transfusion is often followed by a simultaneous increase in ICP, leaving the cerebral perfusion pressure unchanged and critical low. On the other hand, Rosner (1987) in acute severe head injury found that a deliberate increase in blood pressure, generally releases a fall in ICP. This reaction, called vasoreactive cascade, implies that the CA predominantly is preserved. Accordingly, the author recommends a cerebral perfusion pressure about 85 mm Hg in patients with severe head injury.

Guidelines

In the America Guidelines for the Management of Severe Traumatic Brain Injury (2000) resuscitation of blood pressure and oxygenation is discussed..“A. *Standards:* There are insufficient data to support a treatment standard. B. *Guidelines:* Hypotension (systolic blood pressure < 90 mm Hg) or hypoxia (apnea, cyanosis or an O2 saturation < 90 in the field or PaO2 < 60 mmHg) must be monitored and scrupulously avoided, if possible, or corrected immediately in severe TBI patients. C. *Options:* The mean arterial blood pressures should be maintained above 90 mmHg through the infusion of fluids throughout the patients course to attempt to maintain Cerebral Perfusion Pressure (CPP) > 70 mmHg.

Guidelines for Cerebral Perfusion Pressure have the following recommendations (2000). A *Standards:* There are insufficient data to support treatment standards. B. *Guidelines:* There are insufficient data to support treatment guidelines. C. *Options:* Cerebral perfusion pressure should be maintained at a minimum of 70 mm Hg.

The European Guideline does not discuss a specific threshold over which CPP should be maintained. Volume expansion and inotropes, or vasopressors are indicated when arterial blood pressure is insufficient to maintain CPP in a normovolemic patient (Maas et al. 1997).

Hyperventilation (HV)

Hypercapnia has been used in the neurosurgical clinic in cases where an increase in CBF is desired, especially during carotid endarterectomy. There is no doubt, however, that hypercapnia as a general rule is detrimental when intracranial compliance is exhausted. Instead attention will be paid to hypocapnia, which in experimental as well as clinical studies effectively reduces ICP.

Experimental studies of hyperventilation

CBV

Rosomoff (1963) studied changes in CBV and CSF volume after 30 min of hypocapnia to $PaCO_2$ 20 mmHg in dogs and found a fall in CBV, and a compensatory increase in CSF volume. The changes in CBV effected by hypo- and hypercapnia are correlated to changes in CBF. In normal brains CBV changes by about 0.04–0.05 ml/100g/mm Hg $PaCO_2$. In grey- and white matter values of 0.053 and 0.043 ml/100g/mm Hg $PaCO_2$ have been found (Greenberg et al. 1975). For the total brain, this means an increase by 11 ml in CBV, when $PaCO_2$ is increased from 4.0 to 6.7 kPa (Phleps et al. 1973, Grubb et al. 1974).

Active and passive hyperventilation

During active hyperventilation cerebral venous drainage is not impaired. During massive passive hyperventilation in dogs a high positive airway pressure impedes cerebral venous drainage, increases cerebral venous pressure, and consequently might increase ICP (Kitahata et al. 1971).

Steal phenomenon

Studies of focal ischaemia indicate a decrease in focal pial blood pressure during hypercapnia (Brawley et al. 1967, Symon 1970). This phenomenon is caused by a redistribution of blood flow from regions with a relatively high ICP and low CO_2 reactivity to regions with a high CO_2 reactivity and relatively low tissue pressure, referred to as a steal phenomenon.

Inverse steal phenomenon

Although studies in MCAO indicate an increase in lactic-acidosis and a decrease in ATP in the focal region (Michenfelder and Sundt 1973), other experimental studies indicate that hypocapnia might redistribute blood flow from rather healthy regions with low tissue pressure and high CO_2 reactivity to more injured regions with high pressures and relatively low CO_2 reactivity. This reaction is called inverse steal phenomenon. The occurrence of inverse steal phenomenon is of considerably interest and has focused the attention on hypocapnia as a therapeutic tool in experimental brain ischaemia. Preliminary studies in dogs and cats suggested that the size of an infarct was reduced if hypocapnia was applied prior to the insult (Soloway et al. 1968, Battistini et al. 1969). However, later experimental studies have not corroborated this finding (Soloway et al. 1971).

Human studies of hyperventilation

Ischaemia

In awake, unsedated patients, active hyperventilation to $PaCO_2$ 2.7 kPa induces changes in EEG compatible with cerebral ischaemia (Morgan and Ward 1970). These changes disappeared when hyperbaric oxygenation was provided (Reivich et al. 1966). During hypocapnia EEG slowing is observed when jugular venous oxygen tension is about 22 mm Hg (Gotoh et al. 1965). The threshold at which deterioration in consciousness occurs and EEG signs compatible with cerebral hypoxemia are observed, is a jugular venous oxygen tension of about 2.5–3.0 kPa. These low tensions occur at PaO_2 ranging between 3.5 and 4.0 kPa and at a $PaCO_2$ level of 2.5–3.0 kPa. In humans subjected to extreme hypocapnia, a moderate increase in $CMR_{glucose}$ has been found, indicating anaerobic cerebral metabolism (Alexander et al. 1968). This change occurs at CBF levels ranging from 10 to 20 ml/100g/min, and at jugular venous oxygen tensions of 2.7 kPa (Gotoh et al. 1965).

Bohr effect

The decrease in oxygen delivery capacity effected by hypocapnia is partly caused by the decrease in CBF (part 75%) and partly by a shift of the dissociation curve of oxyhemoglobin (part 25%) (Cain 1963, Gotoh et al 1965, Harp and Wollman 1973).

CO_2 reactivity

In studies of acute head injury the CO_2 reactivity is low during the acute phase. A low hemispheric CO_2 reactivity is correlated to a poor outcome (Fieschi et al. 1974, Overgaard and Tweed 1974, Cold et al. 1977a, Messeter et al. 1986).

Using enhanced Xe-CT technique it was found that hemispheric CO_2 reactivity ranged between 1,3 and 8.5%/mm Hg $PaCO_2$. Lobar, cerebellar, basal ganglia, and brain-stem CO_2 reactivities frequently varied from the mean global value by more than 25%. The greatest variability occurred in patients with acute subdural hematoma and patients with diffuse injuries (Marion and Bouma 1991).

Hyperventilation as a life saving procedure

In patients with intracranial hypertension, hypocapnia effectively reduces ICP and CBF. It is accepted that the fall in ICP is caused by vasoconstriction of cerebral arterioles and a secondary decrease in CBV. Although the decrease in CBV is small in comparison with the total brain volume, hypocapnia can be life-saving in patients with a mass-expanding cerebral lesion. Acute hyperventilation is, therefore, an important tool in the management of acute intracranial hypertension (Lundberg et al. 1959, Slocum et al. 1961, Bozza et al. 1961). On the other hand, hyperventilation must be used cautiously, because it might provoke a dangerous decrease in CBF especially in regions with low CBF (Cold 1989a). Ideally the use of prolonged artificial hyperventilation should be guided by measurement of rCBF, $AVDO_2$, venous saturation or tissue oygen tension.

Risk of ischaemia in adults

This issue has been debated vigorously during the last decade. The monitored data include rCBF, jugular venous saturation, $AVDO_2$, and brain tissue oxygen tension. The definition of hyperemia where CBF outstrips the metabolic demand of the tissue is used by Obrist et al. (1984) and Bruce et al. (1979). Their studies were primarily based upon the $CMRO_2$/CBF relationship ($AVDO_2$) and jugular venous saturation. Real CBF data was used by Cold (1989) in adult victims, and Skippen et al. (1997) in pediatric head injury patents. Data based upon jugular venous saturation are problematic. The two jugular veins have been shown to drain asymmetric parts of the brain, and a significant difference in oxygen saturation in the same patient has been described (Stocchetti et al. 1994). In addition, jugular bulb saturation, per definition, is unable to detect regional areas of ischaemia.

Cerebral oligaemia is observed in regions with low CBF and preserved CO_2 reactivity (Cold et al. 1989, Meixensberger et al. 1993). In these regions hyperventilation decreases rCBF below ischaemic threshold of 18–20 ml/100g/min. Studies of brain tissue oxygen tension indicate that hyperventilation may reduce oxygen tensions to very low values (Dings et al. 1996). Likewise, manual bagging causes cerebral oligaemia, and precipitates compensatory hypoperfusion with fall in cerebral venous saturation (Procaccio et al. 1993).

Hyperventilation in pediatric patients

In pediatric patients with severe head injury diffuse brain swelling occurs with high frequency (Bruce et al. 1979, Aldrich et al. 1992). Increase in blood volume attributed to partial or complete impairment of cerebral autoregulation and dysfunction of the blood-brain barrier allowing pathologic vasodilation have been proposed (Bruce et al. 1979). Evidence for this assumption has never emerged. Nevertheless, vasoconstrictory therapy to decrease CBV has been suggested as particularly appropriate in pediatric patients with head injury. Hyperventilation to a $PaCO_2$ level below 25 mm Hg has been standard therapy in many pediatric units. In a study by Skippen et al. (1997) 23 pediatric head injury patients were followed with Xe-CT scanning, jugular bulb saturation, and ICP monitoring. They found that there is a very little evidence of absolute" hyperaemia in their patients. Furthermore, they found CBF values < 18 ml/100g/min even in normocapnic patients. The percentage of areas with oligaemic flow increased during hypocapnia.

Steal phenomenon

In patients with apoplexy and cerebral tumours, hypercapnia might provoke a steal phenomenon by promoting a decrease in CBF in the focal region of incomplete ischaemia (Palvölgyi 1969, Paulson 1970).

Inverse steal phenomenon

On the other hand, in patients with severe head injury, apoplexy, and brain tumours, an inverse steal phenomenon or Robin Hood phenomenon has been observed during hypocapnia (Palvölgyi 1969, Paulson 1970, Pistolese et al. 1972, Fieschi et al. 1974, Cold et al. 1977b, Obrist et al. 1984). However, regions with inverse reactions are scattered over the cerebral hemisphere and sparsely localized to abnormal radiological findings (Cold et al. 1977b). Darby et al.(1988), in a study with enhanced Xenon scanning, demonstrated that hypocapnia might provoke a pronounced CBF increase probably resulting in cerebral oedema.

Recently Dings et al. (1996) introduced measurement of brain tissue oxygen tension in patients with severe head injury. In many cases hypocapnia was associated with an increase in tissue oxygen tension during the first day after trauma.

Cerebral autoregulation

Studies of CA during hypocapnia show a normalization of the CA during hypocapnia in patients with apoplexy and cerebral tumours Paulson et al. 1972).

Outcome

Prolonged artificial hyperventilation with hypocapnia has been suggested as an effective tool in the control of ICP-hypertension. However, controlled studies of the effect of artificial hyperventilation in cerebral apoplexy have been discouraging, no improvements in recovery or outcome being demonstrated (Christensen 1976). In patients with severe traumatic head injury an uncontrolled study of artificial hyperventilation suggested improvement of outcome (Gordon 1979). This finding was opposed by Jennett et al. (1980) who in an uncontrolled multicenter study found that patients undergoing mechanical ventilation had outcomes which were worse than expected. In a clinical outcome study by Muizelaar et al. (1991) patients with head injury were randomised to respiratory treatment during normocapnia, hypocapnia ($PaCO_2$ level 25 mm Hg), and a third group where hypocapnia was supplemented with treatment with THAM. At 3 and 6 months after injury the number of patients with favourable outcome was lower in the hyperventilation group than in the control- and the THAM group. However, this occurred only in patients with an initial motor score of 4–5, and at 12 months post-trauma this difference was not found.

Guidelines and strategies

In the American Guidelines for the Management of Severe Traumatic Brain Injury (2000) the use of hyperventilation in the acute management is discussed. The following guidelines are proposed. A. *Standards:* In the absence of increased ICP chronic prolonged hyperventilation therapy ($PaCO_2$ of 25 mm Hg or less) should be avoided. B. *Guidelines:* The use of prophylactic hyperventilation ($PaCO_2$ < 35 mm Hg) during the first 24 h. after severe TBI should be avoided, because it can compromise cerebral perfusion when CBF is reduced. C. *Options:* Hyperventilation therapy may be necessary for brief periods when there is an acute neurologic deterioration, or for longer periods if intracranial hypertension, refractory to sedation, paralysis, CSF-drainage and osmotic diuretics is present. Jugular venous saturation (SjO2), $AVDO_2$, brain tissue oxygen monitoring and CBF monitoring may help to identify cerebral ischaemia, if hyperventilation resulting in $PaCO_2$ values less than 30 mm Hg is necessary.

In the 1997 European guidelines for management of severe head injury, a basal $PaCO_2$ level of 4.0–4.5 kPa is recommended. Accepted methods for ICP management include: A. Sedation, analgesia, and mild hyperventilation ($PaCO_2$ 4.0–4.5 kPa). B. Volume expansion and inotropes or vasopressors when arterial blood pressure is insufficient to maintain CPP in a normovolemic patient. C. Osmotic therapy with mannitol, given repeatedly, or administrated in accordance with ICP level. Serum osmolality should be maintained < 315. Other agents, such as glycerol or sorbitol are not advocated. If osmotherapy has insufficient effect, furosemide can be given additionally. D. CSF-drainage. E. If these methods fail to reduce ICP, more intensive hyperventilation ($PaCO_2$ <

30 mm Hg), preferably with monitoring of cerebral oxygenation to detect cerebral ischaemia, for instance by jugular venous saturation, should be used. Alternatively the use of barbiturate in high doses may be considered (Maas et al. 1997).

Whether hyperventilation is detrimental, and provokes cerebral ischaemia has been discussed vigorously. Cold (1990) and Miller et al,. (1992) have summarised their approach to the management of ICP-hypertension. In patients with cerebral hyperaemia, and elevated ICP, cerebral autoregulation presumably is lost, $AVDO_2$ is low, and the CO_2 reactivity is preserved. Hyperventilation to a $PaCO_2$ level of 20–25 mm Hg is expected to produce a beneficial effect, and normalises venous saturation and $AVDO_2$. On the other hand, in patients with compromised CPP and relatively high $AVDO_2$, hyperventilation may produce cerebral oligaemia.

Cruz (1998) in a prospective study compared outcome of 178 patients with severe head injury undergoing continuous monitoring of cerebral extraction of oxygen ($SAT_{arterial}$ - SAT_{venous}) and CPP with a group of 175 patients undergoing monitoring of CPP only. They found that in patients with ICP-hypertension associated with compromised CSF space, monitoring with cerebral extraction in conjunction with CPP resulted in a better outcome (12% vegetative survivals or death) compared with 32% when CPP is monitored alone. The strategies as presented by Cruz et al. (1998) have been criticized by Chestnut (1998), who argues that the CPP management group was not identical with the CPP regime proposed by Rosner (1995), and stress that the jugular venous saturation values must be interpreted with caution.

Adaptation to prolonged hyperventilation

Experimental studies

In studies in dogs and goats, adaptation to prolonged continuous hypocapnia occurs within 2–3 hours (Raichle et al. 1970, Albrecht and Ruttle 1987). Prolonged hypocapnia decreases the rate of formation of CSF. After an initial decrease at 30 and 60 min, however, formation of CSF returns to prehypocapnic values (Martins et al. 1976, Hochwald et al. 1976, Artru and Hornbein 1987). In dogs with an intracranial mass-expanding lesion prolonged hypocapnia initially gives rise to a decrease in CBV. However, the CSF-pressure lowering effect is sustained by a reduction in CSF volume, despite reexpanding of CBV. In the same model brain water content did not contribute to changes in CSF pressure and volume (Artru 1987).

Human studies

Half-life of adaptation. The adaptation to prolonged hypocapnia has been investigated in patients with apoplexy. The half-life of the adaptation mechanism of CSF-pH and CSF bicarbonate average 6 hours, and adaptation is said to be complete within 24–30 hours (Christensen et al. 1974). Studies using non-invasive Doppler ultrasound technique and calculation of the instantaneous mean blood velocity during hypocapnia in normal subjects indicate that blood velocity showed adaptation within 10 min after induction of hypocapnia (Ellingsen et al. 1987).

*Impaired adaptation.*In an uncontrolled study of patients with severe head injury no signs of CSF-pH adaptation within periods of 6–24 hours were disclosed. It was suggested that ischaemia prevented the CSF-pH adaptation (Cold et al. 1977a). When hyperventilation is used for several days to reduce ICP in the presence of brain oedema, withdrawal of hypocapnia should be cautious as ICP-hypertension very often reappears (Havill 1984). Mechanism of adaptation is supposed to play a role in this rebound ICP-hypertension.

The use of prolonged continuous hyperventilation. Pro et contra

Some arguments for and against the use of prolonged artificial hyperventilation have already been discussed. Other arguments against this therapeutic measure are as follows: 1) inhibition of oxygen delivery from oxyhaemoglobin to the tissue, because of a left shift of the saturation curve of haemoglobin (Bohr effect). Besides impairment of the oxygen delivery to the brain this effect includes impairment of oxygen supply to the myocardium (Neill and Hattenhauer 1975). 2) decrease in cardiac output and blood pressure caused by a reduction in the central venous blood flow and diastolic filling. These effects are mediated via an increase in mean airway pressure causing an increase in CVP, cerebral venous pressure and to a decrease in CPP. An increase in airway pressure and CVP, combined with a decrease in blood pressure also induces a decrease in renal function and an associated retention of water and sodium. 3) Hypocapnia increases whole body CO_2 production (Cain 1970, Khambatta and Sullivan 1974). 4) In experimental studies an increase in $CMRO_2$ has been observed (Hassan and Kazemi 1976). 5) Prolonged hypocapnia provokes disruption of the blood-brain barrier (Rengachery et al. 1967). 6) Hypocapnia decreases collateral perfusion in ischaemic regions (Brock et al. 1969). 7) The risk of barotrauma is increased as a function of increased airway pressure.

The beneficial and detrimental effects of prolonged hyperventilation are summarised as follows:

Beneficial effects

1. Decrease in ICP (control of ICP hypertension).
2. Respiratory alkalosis, neutralising metabolic acidosis in extracellular tissue.
3. Normalisation of cerebral autoregulation.
4. Inverse steal phenomenon (Robin Hood reaction).
5. Normalisation of regional cerebral blood flow pattern (disappearance of tissue peaks) (Cold and Jensen 1978).
6. Prolonged hyperventilation reduces energy consumption and exhausting respiratory work.
7. Reduction of CSF formation.

Detrimental effects

1. Cerebral oligaemia or ischaemia in focal regions and water-shed areas (Michenfelder and Sundt 1973, Proctor et al. 1984)
2. Decrease in diastolic filling and cardiac output.
3. Decrease in MABP and CPP.
4. Increase in CVP, and cerebral venous pressure.
5. Water and salt retention.
6. Inhibition of oxygen delivery to the tissues (Bohr effect).
7. Barotrauma.
8. Increase in whole body oxygen consumption and CO_2 production
9. Hypocapnia decreases collateral perfusion (Brock et al. 1969)
10. Prolonged hypocapnia provokes BBB disruption (Rengachery et al. 1967)
11. Rebound hyperaemia after prolonged artificial hyperventilation is accompanied by ICP-hypertension

Indomethacin (experimental studies)

CBF $CMRO_2$

Indomethacin is a blocker of cyclooxygenase and thereby prostaglandin synthesis. Indomethacin acts as a cerebral vasoconstrictor and reduces CBF while $CMRO_2$ remains unchanged (Pichard and MacKenzie 1973, Sakabe and Siesjö 1979, Dahlgren et al. 1981, Wennmalm et al. 1981).

Cerebral oedema

Studies of canine basilar arteries indicate that prostaglandin mediates cerebral oedema (Shohami et al. 1987). In cats subjected to focal ischaemia (Dempsey et al. 1985) and rats subjected to freezing lesions (Yen and Lee 1987) indomethacin reduces cerebral oedema. Also the rapid accumulation of eusanoids during reperfusion is blocked by indomethacin (Gaudet et al. 1980). In other experimental studies of focal ischaemia (Harris et al. 1982; Awad et al. 1983, Sutherland et al. 1988, Suzuka et al. 1989) and traumatic head injury (Shapira et al. 1988), indomethacin administration was not followed by a decrease in cerebral oedema.

Protection

Indomethacin reduces cerebral infarct size in focal ischaemia (Sasaki et al. 1988), enhances post-ischaemic re-perfusion after MCAO (Shigeno et al. 1985) and reduces cerebral fluid compression injury (Hallenbeck and Furlow 1979). Furthermore, in rats subjected to fluid percussion trauma pre-treatment with indomethacin improves recovery (Kim et al. 1989).

Other experimental studies suggest that the infarct size in focal cerebral ischaemia was not influenced by indomethacin (Harris et al. 1982, Koide et al. 1986).

Indomethacin, human studies

In healthy volunteers the decrease in CBF after a bolus dose of indomethacin followed by continuous infusion is sustained. During hypoxia and during hypercapnia CBF increases indicating normal regulation of CBF (Jensen et al. 1993). In healthy volunteers 0.1, 0.2 and 0.3 mg/kg/h indomethacin decreased CBF to about 45 ml/100g/min (Jensen et al. 1996).

Head injury

The vasoconstrictor effect of indomethacin has been used in the treatment of ICP-hypertension in patients with head injury. In a preliminary study, indomethacin 30 mg was followed by an immediately decrease in ICP of about one hour duration. The fall in ICP was accompanied by a decrease in CBF, an increase in $AVDO_2$ and AVD-lactate, whilst $CMRO_2$ was unchanged (Jensen et al. 1991). In another study the effect of a bolus dose (30 mg) of indomethacin on ICP was comparable with the effect of a 1.5 kPa decrease in $PaCO_2$ (Dahl et al. 1991). Considerable rCBF decrease has been observed after iv. indomethacin in patients with head injury, also in focal regions where CBF is decreased (Plougman et al. 1992). However, only transient increase in AVD-lactate has been observed (Jensen et al. 1991, Dahl et al. 1992).

Cerebral tumours

In patients subjected to craniotomy for cerebral tumours indomethacin immediately and within seconds after iv. administration, decreased ICP accompanied by a decrease in CBF (Bundgaard et al. 1996).

Adenosine receptor blockers (Theophyllamine)

CBF

In human studies (Wechsler et al. 1954, Gottstein and Paulson 1972) the adenosine receptor blocker theophyllamine, reduces CBF. The CBF decrease is dose-dependent (Magnussen and Høedt-Rasmussen 1977, Skinhøj and Paulson 1970). The decrease in CBF is accompanied by a decrease in ICP (Rich et al. 1953).

Inverse steal phenomenon

The occurrence of "inverse cerebral steal" in focal regions suggests that this reciprocal flow increase is favourable in some patients with apoplexy (Skinhøj and Paulson 1970).

Ischaemia

In gerbils subjected to moderate forebrain ischaemia, theophylline-pretreatment moderately aggravates neurological outcome and enhances the ischaemic cell damage (Rudolphi et al. 1987). Local application of theophyllamine has no effect on the hypoxic dilatation of pial arteries, suggesting that adenosine may not be the main causative factor for the development of hypoxic hyperaemia (Haller and Kuschinsky 1987).

Apoplexy

In apoplectic patients a striking improvement in neurological status has been reported after theophyllamine administration (Smith-Voigt 1951, Mainzer 1953, Olivarius 1957). In a controlled study intravenous theophyllamine was used in patients with cerebral infarction. After aminophylline an improvement in neurological performance was observed in 35 versus 15% in the control group. However, after three weeks there was no difference in neurological status and residual disability between the two groups (Geismar et al. 1976). Theophyllamine has not been used in the treatment of ICP-hypertension in head injury or subarachnoid haemorrhage.

Metabolic control of ICP

Metabolic control of intracranial pressure is based on the concept that cerebral blood flow is adjusted to metabolic demand of the brain tissue. If the metabolic demand of the tissue decreases, cerebral blood flow and volume will decrease, and the intracranial pressure will decline. Metabolic regulation of intracranial pressure is effected by hypothermia and drugs, which reduce the metabolic rate of oxygen in the brain (hypnotics, analgesics). As hypnotic and analgesic treatment depress the respiration, patients subjected to these treatments are intubated and respiration is supported with a respirator. As this treatment is often supplemented with treatment with muscle relaxants, the effect of muscle relaxants upon intracranial pressure will also be discussed.

Hypothermia, experimental studies

CBF, $CMRO_2$ and Q_{10}

Hypothermia decreases $CMRO_2$ and CBF proportionally. In dogs the temperature coefficient Q_{10} (defined as the ratio of metabolic rates at two temperatures differing by 10°C) was 2.2 at temperatures between 37° and 27° C. Below 27° C the Q_{10} was doubled to 4.5 suggesting that the relationship of $CMRO_2$ to brain temperature is variable depending on the functional state of the brain; below 27° C progressive functional depression is supposed to account for the high Q_{10} value (Michenfelder and Milde 1991).

Protection

Hypothermia exerts a protective effect on the brain in hypoxic hypoxia (Carlsson et al. 1976), global ischaemia (Chopp et al. 1989), incomplete ischemia (Hoffman et al. 1991), and in experimental head injury (Clifton et al. 1991). It has been suggested that even a small decrease in temperature of 1–3 degrees of Celsius has a protective effect in experimental brain ischemia (Busto et al. 1989) and an improvement of blood-brain barrier has been observed (Dietrich et al. 1989).

On the other hand, in rats, even small increments in temperature in ischaemic brain tissue seem to accentuate histopathologic damage (Kitagawa et al. 1991).

Hypothermia, clinical studies

A barbiturate in combination with hypothermia might effectively control intracranial hypertension in some patients with severe head injury (Shapiro et al. 1974). Likewise, the combination of barbiturate and hypothermia might accentuate the protective effect in brain ischaemia (Nordström and Rehncrona 1978).

On the basis of the experimental studies the use of hypothermia has been discussed and suggested in the intensive care of patients suffering from brain ischaemia (Cohen 1981).

Hypothermia has been used in the treatment of cerebral ischaemia in humans (Connolly et al. 1962), during extracorporal circulation (duCailar et al. 1964), after circulatory arrest (White 1972), during neurosurgical operations (Uihlein et al. 1966, White et al. 1967) and in the treatment of severe head injury (Sedzimir 1959, Shapiro et al. 1974). Later on, the once common use of hypothermia was abandoned, because studies of hypothermia in the treatment of acute stroke did not prove any beneficial effect. On the contrary, a detrimental effect was observed in primates and dogs (Michenfelder and Milde 1977, Steen et al. 1979).

Mild hypothermia, however, has again been introduced in the treatment of ICP hypertension in severe head injury. A decrease in ICP accompanied by a decrease in CBF, $AVDO_2$ and $CMRO_2$ have been found (Shiozaki et al. 1993, Marion et al. 1993), and a decrease in $CMR_{lactate}$ has been found (Metz et al. 1996). These changes are accompanied by a moderate decrease in cardiac index, fall in platelet count, and an increased level of serum lipase with signs of pancreatitis (Metz et al.1996). In a small allocated study hypothermia was found to improve outcome (Clifton et al. 1993). In a recent randomised study Marion et al. (1997) found that patients kept at 33°C for 24 hours after the injury did not show improved outcome in comparison with normothermic patients.

Hypnotic agents

CBF, $CMRO_2$ and ICP

In experimental as well as human studies it has been documented that hypnotic agents, including barbiturate, benzodiazepines, etomidate and propofol, increase cerebrovascular resistance and reduce CBF and ICP (Pierce et al. 1951, Michenfelder 1974, Stullken et al. 1977, Larsen et al. 1981, Cold et al. 1986, Stephan et al. 1987). These effects are effected through a metabolic suppression of $CMRO_2$. The metabolic suppression is dose-dependent until the EEG is isoelectric. Beyond this level no further suppression of $CMRO_2$ or CBF occurs (Michenfelder 1974, Kassell et al. 1980, Milde and Milde 1985). Hypnotics have been used in the control of ICP-hypertension (Gordon 1970, Hunter 1972, Shapiro et al. 1973).

CPP

More or less, hypnotics also decrease blood pressure, either by a cardiac depression or by peripheral dilatation. The peripheral dilatation effected by propofol is well known. Cerebral perfusion pressure (CPP) changes accordingly. CPP increases if the decrease in ICP is more pronounced as compared with the decrease in mean arterial blood pressure. CPP is unchanged or decreases if the fall in blood pressure either levels the decrease in ICP or is more pronounced. Generally, a bolus dose of these drugs, corresponding to induction dose during anaesthesia, gives rise to a pronounced ICP decrease. However, owing to the intracranial pressure/volume relationship the decrease in ICP is dependent on the pressure before administration and the intracranial compliance.

Sedation

Chronic administration of barbiturate has been used in the intensive care management of apoplexy, severe head injury and cerebral aneurysm. As a consequence of respiratory obstruction/failure, risk of aspiration and failure of reflexes combined with unconsciousness these patients are often intubated and eventually hyperventilated. This regime is supported by sedation with hypnotics/analgetics in order to prevent coughing, stress and anxiety. For sedation pentobarbitone or thiopental are administered with hours interval. Alternatively, continuous infusion thiopental, propofol or midazolam are used. Etomidate is not used for continuous sedation because of its inhibitory effect upon adrenal steroidogenesis.

Propofol sedation was compared with morphine combined with midazolam sedation in patients with severe head injury. Propofol led to a fall in $AVDO_2$ from 6 to 3 ml O_2 /100 ml. However, there was no effect on MABP, ICP or CPP, and outcome was similar in the 2 groups (Stewart et al. 1994). In a study of head injury patients bolus doses of propofol 1.5 mg/kg were compared with thiopental 3 mg/kg. The ICP reducing effects were comparable. However, the MABP reducing effect was more pronounced and lasted a longer period, when propofol was used (Merlo et al. 1993). Hypnotic drugs for sedation or ICP reduction therapy, whether thiopental, propofol or midazolam, should be administered by continuous infusion, and continuous monitoring of CPP and cerebral venous saturation are recommended (Andrews et al. 1993).

ICP-hypertension

On the basis of the regulatory effect of hypnotic agents upon acute ICP-hypertension (Shapiro et al. 1974, Sidi et al. 1983) and the abundance of documentation of a protective effect in acute focal and incomplete ischaemia, prolonged hypnotic sedation has been used prophylactically in severe head injury. In several uncontrolled studies barbiturate-coma-treatment has been claimed to prevent or attenuate ICP-hypertension and improve outcome (Rockoff et al. 1979, Saul and Ducker 1982, Eisenberg et al. 1988). In other uncontrolled studies these findings are not supported (Yano et al. 1986).

Ward et al. (1985), however, did not find any improvement of outcome in a controlled study where barbiturate was administrated in doses sufficient to suppress the EEG to burst suppression level for several days. In the barbiturate-treated group the incidence of arterial hypotension and septicaemia were higher than in the control group. Likewise, Abramson et al. (1983) did not find any beneficial effects of barbiturate in a controlled study of thiopentone administrated to patients after cardiac arrest.

Guidelines

In the American Guidelines for the Management of Severe Traumatic Brain Injury (2000) the use of barbiturate in the control of ICP-hypertension has been discussed. A. *Standards:* There are insufficient data to support standards for the use of barbiturate. B. *Guidelines:* High dose barbiturate therapy may be considered in haemodynamically stable salvageable patients with ICP-hypertension, refractory to maximal medical and surgical intracranial pressure lowering therapy.

In the European guidelines sedation and analgesics in combination with moderate hyperventilation are recommended. The use of specific high-dose barbiturate, however, is not discussed (Maas et al. 1997).

EEG

The question why hypnotic agents are not effective in promoting a good outcome is supposed to be multifactorial. As pointed out by Astrup (1982) the effect of hypnotic agents upon cerebral ischaemia is only to be expected in focal ischaemia, hypoxia and in incomplete ischaemia where maximal functional suppression is not to be expected, and some EEG activity is preserved. In these pathological situations hypnotic agents might suppress oxygen uptake to some degree and thus induce some degree of cerebral protection. In complete cerebral ischaemia the EEG is isoelectric and CMRO2 is decreased accordingly. Under this circumstance a protective effect of barbiturate is not to be expected.

$CMRO_2$

In severe head injury (Bruce et al. 1973, Cold 1978, Obrist et al. 1979) and comatose patients with subarachnoid hemorrhage (Grubb et al. 1977, Voldby et al. 1985), CMRO2 is decreased severely, often to values averaging 50% of the values obtained in awake adults. Accordingly, the effect of barbiturate upon CBF and $CMRO_2$ is decreased or absent (Messeter et al. 1986, Cold 1989). Thus, in the acute phase of head injury the barbiturate reactivity, as measured by the decrease in $CMRO_2$ after a bolus dose of 5 mg/kg seems to be dependent on the $CMRO_2$ level before thiopental injection (Cold 1989), and in comatose patients with a 50% decrease in $CMRO_2$ the barbiturate reactivity averaged zero (Dahl et al. 1992).

Tolerance

Other reasons to diminished effect of barbiturate during chronic treatment is development of tolerance (Sawada et al. 1982).

Vasodilation

A direct vasodilatory effect of barbiturate has been found on cerebral vessels (Altura et Altura 1975, Edvinsson and Mc Culloch 1981, Marin et al. 1981). Thus, Edvinsson and Mc Culloch (1981) in feline middle cerebral arteries found that maximum contractions effected by potassium, noradrenaline, and prostaglandin F_2 were reduced in the presence of pentobarbital. Gross and Abel (1985) in a rabbit basilar artery model found that concentrations of 3×10^{-5} thiopental caused relaxation of norepinephrine-induced contraction. In the monkey Tsuji and Chiba (1986, 1987) demonstrated a biphasic vascular response, with an initial vasoconstriction followed by a vasodilation in a dose-dependent manner. It is supposed that this effect modifies the ICP-lowering effect of barbiturate when $CMRO_2$ and electrical and functional capacity are low.

Lidocaine

Experimental studies

Protection

In rabbits lidocaine (0.05 mg/kg/min) accelerates the time course of neuroelectrical recovery after global ischaemia (Sustch and Rubinstein 1991). In dogs subjected to deep barbiturate anaesthesia or hypothermia, leading to isoelectric EEG, the addition of lidocaine (160 mg/kg) caused an additional cerebral metabolic inhibition of 15–20% (Astrup et al. 1981b). In the same studies lidocaine caused reduction in the potassium efflux rate of about 50%, probably by reducing membrane ion permeability in accordance with its local anaesthetic action (Astrup et al. 1981a). These results indicate that lidocaine might have some protective effects against cerebral ischaemia.

In cats subjected to spinal cord injury a certain protective effect has indeed been observed (Kobrine et al. 1984, Chang et al. 1986).

A protective effect, however, has not been observed in studies of cats subjected to spinal injury and monitored with spinal evoked responses (Haghighi et al. 1987), in rats subjected to near complete global ischaemia (Warner et al. 1988), and in cats subjected to MCAO (Shokunbi et al. 1986, Gelb et al. 1988). However, in a recent study cats were subjected to MCAO. Lidocaine (5 mg/kg) followed by continuous infusion induced better preservation of evoked potentials. Smaller infarct size and higher CBF in the peripheral region of the infarct were also demonstrated (Shokunbi et al. 1987).

In studies in cats, subjected to cerebral ischaemia induced by air embolism, lidocaine stabilises blood pressure (Evans et al. 1984), and pre-treatment with lidocaine attenuates the intracranial hypertension caused by the air embolism (Evans et al. 1989). Furthermore, lidocaine given after the air embolus was also effective in reducing ICP hypertension (Evans and Kobrine 1987).

Clinical studies

During endotracheal intubation (Bedford et al. 1980b, Hamill et al. 1981), scalp incision (Bedford et al. 1980a) and suction procedures in neurointensive patients (Donegan et al. 1980, White et al. 1982, Yano et al. 1986), intravenous lidocaine in doses of 1.5 mg/kg inhibits or attenuates the ICP increase. However, in patients subjected to repeated tracheal suction lidocaine toxicity is to be expected.

Analgetics

Spontaneous ventilation

Morphine and analogue drugs should be administered with extreme caution in the spontaneous breathing patient with exhausted intracranial compliance. On the other hand, these drugs are used in subarachnoid haemorrhage and in the postoperative course after craniotomy. Careful monitoring of conscious state, respiration, blood pressure, and eventually gas analysis (PaO_2 $PaCO_2$) or capnometry/oximetry is mandatory. Even a small dose of morphine (3 mg iv) might provoke a decrease in $AVDO_2$ suggesting a state of hyperaemia (Cold and Felding 1992).

Controlled ventilation

In the ventilator-treated patient morphine and fentanyl do not increase CBF or ICP. On the contrary, a decrease in ICP is repeatedly observed. This is caused by the sedative effect giving rise to a decrease in CO_2 production, and a decreased level of circulating catecholamines, which otherwise increases cerebral oxygen uptake and CBF when the blood-brain barrier is disrupted (MacKenzie et al. 1976, Berntman et al. 1978, Artru et al. 1981). An additive effect of hypnotic and analgesics on cerebral oxygen uptake may also play a role.

Sufentanil, alfentanil

Sufentanil and alfentanil should be used with reservation because animal experiments indicate that sufentanil provokes a prolonged period of CBF and CBV increase (Milde et al. 1990). Comparative studies of fentanyl, alfentanil and sufentanil in patients subjected to craniotomy indicate, that the use of the two latter drugs was accompanied by a decrease in CPP and an increase in CSF-pressure (Marx et al. 1989). Cerebral autoregulation may play a role, because correction of blood pressure normalised ICP. Both sufentanil and alfentanil elicit a decrease in blood pressure. As a consequence, a decrease in CVR and an increase in CBV may occur. Under these circumstances an increase in ICP is observed.

Muscular Relaxation

Suxamethonium

In experimental (Cottrell et al. 1983, Lanier 1986) as well as human studies (March et al. 1980) succinylcholine increases ICP. The rise in ICP is caused by activation from peripheral impulses from the muscles (Lanier et al. 1989).

Non-depolarization agents

Pancuronium, atracurium and vecuronium do not increase ICP (Lanier et al. 1985, Giffin et al. 1986, Rosa et al. 1986).

Risk of aspiration

Choice of muscle relaxants during acute intubation depends on a rational analysis where risk of aspiration is weighed against the risk of enhancing ICP hypertension. In patients with limited intracranial compliance aspiration of the ventricle before intubation may provoke dangerous ICP-hypertension. An association between delayed gastric emptying and intracranial hypertension has been described repeatedly (Norton et al. 1988, Garrick et al. 1988, Ott et al. 1991); the mechanism is supposed to be increased release of corticotropin-releasing factor from cerebrum (Taché et al. 1987). Furthermore, reduced lower oesophageal sphincter pressure has been found after acute and chronic brain injury (Vane et al. 1982). If the risk of aspiration is supposed to be greater than the risk of dangerous ICP-hypertension, cross-induction technique with succinylcholine is justified. In other situation where intracranial compliance is exhausted, non-depolarisating relaxants are to be preferred.

Long term use of neuromuscular blocking agents in patients with head injury to manage ICP- hypertension, does not improve overall mortality, and may actually be detrimental because of the prolongation of their ICU stay. Thus, neuromuscular blockade should be reserved for patients with ICP-hypertension alone, who require escalation of treatment intensity (Hsiang et al. 1994).

Controlled outcome studies, elucidating the effect of non-depolarisating relaxants are not available.

Osmotic acting drugs and diuretics

Electrolytes and proteins and the blood-brain barrier (BBB)

Cerebral tissue is protected by the blood-brain barrier, which allows the passive diffusion of non-electrolytes inclusive water. The extracellular space in cerebral tissue is negligible under normal circumstances. The electrophysical balance between intra- and extracellular milieu is adjusted with a high intracellular potassium concentration and a high extracellular sodium concentration.

Na^+

Low Pl-sodium concentration is accompanied by an increase in cerebral tissue water content. During extreme hyponatriaemia brain oedema may develop. If the blood-brain barrier is disrupted an increase in extracellular space with filtration of plasma proteins also occurs.

Crystalloid

Patients with severe HI might have impaired peripheral circulation, even when normotensive. Volume infusion with crystalloid improves oxygen transport without increasing ICP (Scale et al. 1994).

Protein

Changes in protein concentration do not influence the volume of the extracellular space whether the blood-brain barrier is disrupted or not, because the architecture of the extracellular space does not allow any expansion.

Mannitol

Osmotic gradient

In patients with intracranial hypertension, early studies of intravenous infusion of mannitol showed that this drug effectively reduces ICP (Wise and Chater 1962). After fast intravenous infusion of 0.5–1 g/kg ICP is reduced after 2–5 min. The ICP reducing effect is of hours` duration, dependent on the dose and the infusion rate (James 1980).

The osmotic effect of mannitol is dependent on the osmotic gradient in blood (Shenkin et al. 1962). The faster the mannitol concentration difference between plasma and extracellular fluid developes, the stronger and the longer the reduction in ICP (Takagi et al. 1993). A difference in osmotic gradient exceeding 10 mOs always gives rise to a reduction in ICP (Marshall et al. 1978). The decrease in ICP is correlated to the decrease in the water content in brain tissue (Nath and Galgraith 1986).

Mannitol, experimental studies

Pial vessels

Following mannitol infusion in cats, blood viscosity decreases immediately. The greatest decrease occurs at 10 min. At 75 min a rebound increase in viscosity occurs. The pial vessel diameter decreased simultaneously, the largest decrease being at 10 min. The changes in pial vessels were interpreted as an autoregulatory process (Muizelaar et al. 1983). Further studies indicate that if cerebral autoregulation is impaired, mannitol infusion is followed by a decrease in ICP, while ICP is unchanged in studies where the autoregulation is intact (Muizelaar et al. 1984). The authors hypothesized that changes in blood viscosity might give rise to compensatory changes in the degree of constriction in cerebral vessels. In studies of vessel diameters with the cranial window technique in cats, it was concluded that mannitol in clinically relevant doses does not exert significant constriction on cerebral vessels. Mannitol therefore exerts its effect on ICP through its osmotic effect, rather than by a direct effect on cerebral blood volume (Auer and Haselsberger 1987).

CBF and $CMRO_2$

Studies of mannitol infusion at normal intracranial pressure in baboons (Johnstone and Harper 1973) and dogs (Kassell et al. 1982) have shown an increase in CBF, while CBF is unchanged in animals subjected to intracranial hypertension by an epidural balloon (Johnstone and Harper 1973). In the same study mannitol infusion was followed by an increase in $CMRO_2$.

Oedema

Studies of cryogenic oedema in the cat indicate that a single dose of mannitol decreases cerebral oedema. However, repeated dose of mannitol leads to an increased water content in oedematous regions (Kaufmann and Cardoso 1993).

Ischaemia

Mannitol has a beneficial effect in experimental cerebral ischaemia (Little 1978, Watanabe et al. 1979). In studies of experimental cytotoxic oedema mannitol induces a normalisation of EEG (James et al. 1978). Studies in rabbits subjected to MCAO have shown that mannitol administration improves CBF in regions of ischaemia, and that a gradual decline in intercellular pH is prevented (Meyer et al. 1987). Shirane and Weinstein (1992) found that mannitol intensified reperfusion hyperaemia after 30 minutes temporary ischaemia in rats. In cats mannitol improves postischaemic recovery of blood flow (Tanaka and Tomonaga 1987), and in rats subjected to forebrain ischaemia mannitol considerably ameliorated the ischaemic injury (Sutherland et al. 1988). In a swine model of retractor brain ischaemia, mannitol plus nimodipine is superior to either agent alone in maintaining both CBF and evoked potential (Andrews and Muto 1992).

Other experimental studies of cerebral ischaemia have failed to demonstrate any enhancement of CBF by mannitol (Seki et al. 1981, Pena et al. 1982).

Mannitol, human studies

Central haemodynamic, Na^+ and K^+

Studies of central haemodynamic (CH) in patients undergoing craniotomy have shown that mannitol infusion is followed by an increase in blood volume, CVP, pulmonary artery wedge pressure and cardiac output and a decrease in the concentration of haemoglobin, plasma-sodium and the peripheral resistance (Rudehill et al. 1983, Brown et al. 1986). The concentration of plasma-potassium decreases after mannitol 1 g/kg and increases after 2 g/kg (Manninen et al. 1987).

CBV, CBF and $CMRO_2$

An increase in CBV a few minutes after mannitol infusion has been demonstrated (Ravussin et al. 1986a). Following mannitol infusion blood viscosity decreases for at least two hours, suggesting an enhancement of cerebral microcirculation (Burke et al. 1981). Accordingly, studies of cerebral circulation indicate an increase in CBF occurring after 10–20 min and lasting for up to 24 hours, and a variable increase in $CMRO_2$ (Jafar et al. 1986).

ICP

The effect of mannitol upon ICP has been studied in patients with cerebral tumours and aneurysms. In patients with normal ICP a transient but significant increase in ICP followed by a steady decrease towards values below control were found. In contrast, patients with intracranial hypertension showed no increase in ICP, which decreased immediately after mannitol infusion (Ravussin et al. 1986b).

CPP

Other studies suggest that the effect of mannitol is at least partly dependent upon other haemodynamic mechanisms. Thus, patients with CPP > 70 mm Hg responded relatively poorly to mannitol, while ICP decreased in patients with CPP < 70 mm Hg, suggesting that at CPP > 70 mm Hg the vasoconstriction is already nearly at maximum. Under this circumstance mannitol is unable to increase resistance further (Rosner and Coley 1987). In general, administration of large doses of mannitol is safe in the presence of ICP-hypertension (Abou-Madi et al. 1993).

PVI

In neurointensive patients the volume pressure relationship improves after mannitol, often without change in ICP (Miller et al. 1975).

Guidelines

In the Guidelines for the Management of Severe Traumatic Brain Injury (2000), the following recommendations are suggested. A. *Standards:* There are insufficient data to support a treatment standard. B. *Guidelines:* Mannitol is effective for control of raised ICP after severe HI. (Limited data suggest that intermittent boluses may be more effective than continuous infusion). Effective doses range from 0.25 to 1g/kg. C. *Options:* The indications for use of mannitol prior to ICP monitoring are signs of transtentorial herniation or progressive neurological deterioration not attributable to systemic pathology. Hypovolaemia, however, should be avoided by fluid replacement. Serum osmolality should be kept below 320 mOsm because of concern for renal failure. Euvolaemia should be maintained by adequate fluid replacement. A Foley catheter is essential in these patients. Intermittent boluses may be more effective than continous infusion.

In the European guideline osmotic therapy, preferably mannitol given as repeated infusion, is advocated. Serum osmolality should be maintained < 315. Other agents, such as glycerol or sorbitol are not advocated. If osmotherapy has insufficient effect, furosemide can be given additionally (Maas et al. 1997).

In a Cochrane database review Schierhout and Roberts (2000) conclude that there are insufficient data to recommend one form of mannitol infusion over other. Mannitol therapy for raised ICP may have a beneficial effect on mortality when compared to pentobarbital treatment. ICP–directed treatment shows a small beneficial effect compared to treatment directed by neurological signs and physiological indicators. There are insufficient data on the effectiveness of pre-hospital administration of mannitol to preclude either a harmful or a beneficial effect on mortality.

Mannitol and Blood-Brian Barrier

Tight junction

Osmotic opening of the brain-blood barrier by infusion of hyperosmolar solutions like mannitol has repeatedly been demonstrated. In patients with cerebral tumours hyperosmolar blood-brain barrier disruption with mannitol is used to overcome the relatively inaccessibility of inflitrating glioma cells to chemotherapy. It has been argued that opening of tight-junctions is the dominant mode of leakage in hyperosmolar opening. The opening of the barrier is independent of energy-producing metabolism. It is supposed that osmotic barrier opening is the result of passive shrinkage of endothelial cells and the surrounding tissue (Greenwood et al. 1988). As a result of the impaired barrier function mannitol diffuses into the cells. In this respect it is of interest that hydroxyethyl starch macromolecyles protect against blood-brain barrier disruption due to intracarotid injection of mannitol in rats (Chi et al. 1996).

Rebound phenomenon

Brain cells are able to create osmotic active particles. These particles reduce the transcellular osmotic gradient (Jennett and Teasdale 1981).

After discontinuing the mannitol infusion the osmotic gradient is reversed because mannitol is excreted through the urine, decreasing the concentration in the plasma. Consequently, the concentration of mannitol is found to be higher in the extracellular and intracellular compartments as compared with the concentration in the blood. This rebound phenomenon gives rise to water influx into brain cells, and an increase in ICP (McQueen and Jeanes 1964).

Glycerol

Glycerol is an alternative to mannitol in the treatment of ICP-hypertension. Glycerol is effective by the oral and iv. route. Haemolysis can be provoked but is avoided by reducing the concentration and infusion rate (Quandt and Reyes 1984). In one study equipotent doses of mannitol and glycerol were used in children with ICP-hypertension. Mannitol was found to be superior to glycerol (MacDonald and Uden 1982). In a study of adult patients with ICP-hypertension a greater and longer lasting pressure reduction was found when glycerol was used (Smedema et al. 1993). In another study by Biestro et al. (1997) glycerol and mannitol were compared in patients with head injury. At one and two hours after infusion both agents induced an effective decrease on ICP and increase in CPP. The results suggested that mannitol would be most indicated as a bolus to control sudden rises in ICP, whereas glycerol would be most indicated as a basal treatment.

Hypertonic saline (HS), experimental studies

Central haemodynamic

Pigs subjected to haemorrhagic hypotension were resuscitated with hypertonic saline or Ringers solution. Normalisation of blood pressure and oxygen delivery were faster with hypertonic saline (Schmoker et al. 1991). An improved cardiac performance has likewise been observed (Kien et al. 1990).

In dogs subjected to haemorrhagic hypotension, resuscitation with either 7.2% saline or 20% hydroxyethyl starch was used. Both fluids restored MABP and cardiac output equally. At 60 min after resuscitation, however, cardiac output decreased in the hypertonic resuscitated group. ICP, CPP and CBF were similar in both groups (Whitney et al. 1991).

The effect of hypertonic saline on the heart function has been documented. In the isolated blood-perfused heart of rabbits hypertonic saline induces an increase in contractility, relaxation of the myocardium, combined with coronary dilation. The improvement of cardiac performance is inhibited by amiloride, a Na^{+}/Ca^{2+} exchange blocker, suggesting that calcium influx through the sarcolemma is a mayor mechanism by which hypertonic saline improves cardiac performance (Mauren et al. 1995). In contrast, studies of isolated hearts indicate that hypertonic saline exerts myocardial depression, both in the ischaemic and non-ischaemic heart (Waagstein et al. 1995).

In a blinded, randomised study in swine hypertonic saline/dextran caused an immediate, transient acidaemia, which primarily was due to hyperchloraemic, hypokalemic metabolic acidosis with normal anion gab. The acidaemia was transient because of the off-setting alkalotic effects of decreasing serum protein, normalisation of electrolytes, and the transient nature of an increase CO_2 tension (Moon and Kramer 1995).

ICP, CBF and blood-brain barrier

During resuscitation of acute haemorrhage the ICP level is lower in animals treated with hypertonic saline (Prough et al. 1985, Ducey et al. 1990, Schmoker et al. 1991, Prough et al. 1991). Under this circumstance hypertonic saline also reduces water content in cerebral tissue (Todd et al. 1985), but not in the injured part of the brain (Wisner et al. 1990). CBF improves (Todd et al. 1985, Whitley et al. 1988, Schmoker et al. 1991, Prough et al,. 1991, Schürer et al. 1992), and brain tissue oxygen tension normalises (Schürer et al. 1992).

In cats subjected to fluid percussion injury, and mild haemorrhage hypotension, rCBF does not increase sufficiently to restore cerebral oxygen delivery or normalise EEG activity (DeWitt et al. 1996). Studies of rCBF and regional glucose utilisation in rats indicate a perfect coupling after resuscitation, although the ratio glucose utilisation/rCBF was reset to a higher level (1,5 ml/mol in the control group, contra 2.7 ml/mol in the hypertonic saline group)(Waschke et al.1996).

It is supposed that the improvement of CBF and the decrease in ICP are caused by a reduction in the cellular volume of uninjured brain parenchyma, endothelial cells, and erythrocytes (Shackford et al. 1992). However, hypertonic saline disrupts the blood-brain barrier (Durwald et al. 1983), and rapid infusion of hypertonic saline might cause acute hypotension by a decrease in total peripheral resistance (Kien et al. 1991).

Comparative studies

In a canine model of intracranial haemorrhage the effect of 3 and 23.4% hypertonic saline was compared with mannitol (1g/kg). Hypertonic saline, in both concentrations, is as effective as mannitol in the treatment of intracranial hypertension. Hypertonic saline has a longer duration of action, particularly when used in 3% solution (Qureshi et al. 1999). In rats subjected to cortical cryogenic lesion hypertonic saline was more effective in reducing ICP than equi-osmolar mannitol, and in mannitol treated animals rebound ICP-hypertnesion was observed (Mirski et al. 2000). In rabbits subjected to cryogenic lesion infusion of HS induces a decrease in ICP (Härtl et al. 1993). Berger et al. (1995) studied the effect of 7.2% saline/dextran or 20% mannitol in rabbits subjected to focal lesion of vasogenic edema. They found that hypertonic saline/dextran was as effective as mannitol in reducing ICP.

Hypertonic saline, human studies

Prehospital resuscitation

In a double-blind randomised trial Vassar et al. (1993) used Ringer solution, 7.5% saline, 7.5% saline combined with dextran 70, and 7.5% saline combined with 12% dextran. Patients with systolic pressure < 90 mm Hg were included. They found that hypertonic saline was associated with an increase in blood pressure, and an increase in survival at hospital discharge. Patients with low baseline GCS seemed to benefit most from 7.5% NaCl. Hypertonic NaCl without added dextran 70 was as effective as solution that contained dextran 70.

Cardiac performance

In patients without cardiovascular disease hypertonic saline improves cardiac performance. The improvement of left ventricular function is caused mainly by a combined effect of increased left ventricular preload and reduced afterload. In these patients hypertonic NaCl reduced blood pressure significantly (Goertz et al. 1995).

Repeated administration of hypertonic saline as bolus during neurosurgery suggests that repetitive amounts of hypertonic NaCl cause no serious overload when 30 min. intervals are kept. Osmolality, however, should be checked before each bolus (Henchen et al. 1991).

Cerebral dynamics

Although experimental studies indicate that hypertonic saline is not superior to mannitol in its ability to reduce ICP in cryogenic brain oedema (Scheller et al. 1991), hypertonic saline has been used successfully in children with head injury (Fisher et al. 1992, Khenna et al. 2000), in patients with intractable intracranial hypertension (Worthley et al. 1988), and in patients with brain-stem trauma (Gemma et al. 1996).

Points of view

Zornow (1996) in an editorial concludes that hypertonic saline reduces ICP and brain volume, and can be used safely in humans with minimal potential for morbidity. On the other hand, Schell et al. (1996) summarise that further studies are needed to measure the functional outcome rather than early parameters of CNS function. In addition hypertonic NaCl has a defined risk including the potential detrimental effects of hypernatraemia (lethargy, seizure and coma), tearing of bridging veins, development of subdural haematoma, central myelinose, cardiac failure and arrhythmia.

Furosemide, experimental studies

CSF formation and cerebral oedema

Furosemide induces an inhibition of CSF production and a concurrent reduction of ICP. These changes are thought to enhance the clearance of vasogenic oedema (Reulen et al. 1977).

In cats subjected to cold injury furosemide effectively reduces the amount of brain oedema (Long et al. 1976). In dogs subjected to cold injury furosemide decreases brain water content in normal dogs, but not in nephrectomized dogs, indicating that the effect of furosemide is mediated by diuresis (Marshall et al. 1982).

Administration with mannitol

In dogs mannitol and furosemide, when used together produce a greater and more sustained fall in ICP than mannitol alone (Pollay et al. 1983, Roberts et al. 1987).

Furosemide, clinical studies

ICP

Furosemide does not provoke an initial increase in ICP and does not change serum osmolality or electrolytes to the same degree as does mannitol (Cottrell et al. 1977). Furosemide decreases CSF formation rate and increases CSF absorption capacity (Sklar et al. 1980).

Administration of mannitol

In patients, with brain tumour or cerebral aneurysm, subjected to a rapid infusion of mannitol (1.4 g/kg) or the same dose combined with furosemide (0.3 mg/kg), brain shrinkage was greater and more consistent with mannitol plus furosemide than with mannitol alone. Rapid electrolyte depletion of sodium was observed with the combination of the two drugs and must be corrected (Schettini et al. 1982).

High dose

In patients with intracranial hypertension, the combination of Ringer's solution and furosemide 250 mg resulted in a definite improvement in general condition occurring after 24 hours. Forced diuresis with high doses of furosemide is suggested as treatment of choice for acute cerebral oedema (Thilmann and Zeumer 1974).

Kappa-opioid receptor agonists

It has been demonstrated that kappa-opioid receptor agonists inhibit antidiuretic hormone secretion and promote water excretion in animals and humans. Receptor-binding studies have demonstrated the presence of kappa opioid receptors in the supraoptic and paraventricular nuclei of the hypothalamus and neurohypophysis. Niravoline, a kappa opioid agonist, has marked diuretic activity and low analgesic potency. It induces a dose-dependent increase in urine output and decreases urine osmolality and free water reabsorption without changing urinary electrolyte excretion. Niravoline and other kappa agonists have been reported to reduce ischaemic brain oedema in mice and rats (Silvia et al. 1987, Gueniau et al. 1995), and in experimental studies in cats it effectively reduces ICP and improves CPP without significant changes in serum osmolality (Bemana et al. 1998, Nagao et al. 2000).

Corticosteroids

Experimental studies

Glucocorticoids are useful in the resolution of altered vascular permeability in experimental brain oedema (Maxwell et al. 1971). Steroids reduce CSF-production (Weiss and Nulsen 1970), attenuate free radical production, and have other beneficial effects in experimental models (Bracken et al. 1985, Bracken et al. 1990, Hall et al. 1988, Pappius and McCain 1969).

Human studies

In patients with brain tumours steroids result in a marked clinical improvement, also in the perioperative period to patients undergoing craniotomy (French and Galicich 1964, Renaudin et al. 1973).

In patients with severe head injury Gobiet et al. (1976) compared low-dose and high-dose decadron therapy, and documented a beneficial effect in patients on high-dose therapy. A beneficial effect was also found by Faupel et al. (1976) in a double-blind trial. Subsequently, six major studies were performed. None of these revealed substantial benefits of steroid therapy (Braakman et al. 1983, Cooper et al. 1979, Dearden et al. 1986, Gobiet et al. 1976, Gudeman et al. 1979, Saul et al. 1981).

In the American Guidelines for the Management of Severe Traumatic Brain Injury (2000) and the European EBIC-guidelines (Maas AIR et al. 1997) glucocorticoids are not recommended in the treatment of severe head injury.

Calcium blockers

Acute head injury

Clinical studies concerning the effect of Calcium-blockers upon outcome in patients with acute head injury have been inconclusive (Koston et al. 1985, Teasdale et al. 1989, Compton et al. 1990, Bailey et al. 1991, European study group 1994). In contrast Harders et al. (1996) in a controlled study found that nimodipine-treated patients had a better outcome. In the same study ICP was measured in 33% of the patients. ICP values in excess of 20 mm Hg were observed more frequently in the placebo group. In a Cochrane Review Langham et al (2000) concluded that there is still considerable uncertainty over the effect on Nimodipine on brain injury patients.

Subarachnoid hemorrhage

Early studies indicated that Nimodipine improves neurological recovery after subarachnoid hemorrhage (Allen et al. 1983, Petruk et al. 1988, Pichard et al. 1989). Other studies indicate that nimodipine treatment is associated with a reduction of cerebral infracts (Ôhman et al. 19991a), low incidence of delayed neurological dysfunction (Gilsbach et al. 1990), and a low incidence of death caused by delayed cerebral ischaemia (Ôhman and Heiskanen 1988, Ôhman et al. 1991b). In a metaanalysis it was demonstrated that nimodipine improved outcome (Barker and Ogilvy 1996). ICP recordings during controlled studies of nimodipine are not available.

Cardiac arrest

Preliminary studies of nimodipine in cardiac arrest have shown an improvement of postischemic hypoperfusion and an enhancement of recovery rate. There were no evidence of seriously increased cerebrospinal fluid pressure in either groups the first 48 hours (Forsman et al. 1989).

Inhibitors of excitatory amino acids

ICP

In experimental studies of subdural hematoma NMDA antagonists attenuate the ICP increase otherwise found (Kurudo et al. 1991).

THAM

Experimental studies

Studies in cats demonstrate that THAM (trihydroxymethylaminomethan) decreases the production of brain lactate and brain oedema and promotes the recovery of cerebral energy dysfunction. The same study indicated that THAM ameliorates the deleterious effects of hyperventilation by minimising energy disturbances and that it also decreases the formation of brain oedema (Yoshida and Marmarou 1991).

Human studies

Intrathecal administration of THAM in patients with severe cerebral acidosis causes an alkaline shift of CSF pH, and secondary efflux of lactate resulting in a decrease of CSF elastance and a reduction of the risk of ICP elevation (Kuklane et al. 1993).

Clinical controlled studies in patients with severe HI indicate that intravenous treatment with THAM effectively controls ICP-hypertension (Pfenninger et al. 1989a). When used prophylactically another controlled study revealed lower levels of CSF-lactate and probably improved recovery (Rosner et al. 1989). In a randomised prospective clinical study treatment with THAM versus conventional treatment were compared. The THAM group had fewer episodes of ICP elevation than those in the control group, and the rate of patients needing hyperventilation for control of ICP was higher in the control group (Wolf et al. 1993).

Strategies in the control of ICP-hypertension

Surgical intervention

Strategies of treatment in acute intracranial hypertension are dependent upon the pathogenesis of the intracranial disease. Surgical evacuation or decompression of a mass lesion, whether it is caused by tumour, abscess or hematoma is the primary goal. If hydrocephalus, as evaluated by CT-scanning is an element, ventricular drainage eventually followed by shunt surgery is the treatment of choice.

Ventricular drainage

Ventricular drainage is common practice in patients with subarachnoid haemorrhage and in patients with intracerebral hematoma with penetration to the ventricular system. Ventricular drainage is used in severe traumatic head injury, and drainage is included in guidelines for the management of severe head injury. Owing to compression of the ventricular system, with difficulties in insertion of a ventricular catheter, risk of infection and not least the popularity of other less traumatic methods including subarachnoid bolt and epidural transducers, ventricular drainage is used rarely in acute traumatic head injury. On the other hand, in patients with subarachnoid haemorrhage and intraventricular haematoma ventricular drainage is routinely used.

Ischaemia

When an intracranial space-occupying process is present it might be accompanied by focal or global cerebral ischaemia. The degree of ischaemia is dependent on the size of the intracranial space-occupying lesion and the tissue pressure it exerts focally and globally. The pressure of the mass upon the surrounding cerebral tissue gives rise to an increase in tissue pressure, reduced cerebral perfusion pressure and impaired cerebral perfusion. Under these circumstances the oxygen demand of cerebral tissue might exceed the oxygen delivery capacity. In the ischaemic brain tissue cytotoxic brain oedema develops. Blood-brain barrier dysfunction and impairment of cerebral autoregulation are present, and vasogenic brain oedema very easily develops. These events are aggravated if accompanied by hypoxia, hypercapnia and arterial hypertension/hypotension.

Primary and secondary damage

Traditionally, discrimination between primarily irreversible and secondary potentially reversible ischaemic damages is discussed: The aim of intensive care being prevention of the secondary ischaemic damage. Early surgical removal of space-occupying lesions, prevention of hypotension, hypoxaemia, hypercapnia and hyperthermia are cornerstones in avoiding secondary brain ischaemia.

Protection

Measures which antagonise, prevent or abolish secondary ischaemic damage (hypothermia, hypnotics, Calcium blockers (nimodipine), antagonists to excitatory amino acids, lazaroids and methylprednisolone in spinal injury theoretically also prevent the development of cytotoxic oedema secondary to ischaemia.

Ventilation

In the treatment of cerebral ischaemia and intracranial hypertension adequate ventilation and a sufficient central circulation are of importance. Ventilatory support and support of the circulation are essential principles in treatment.

Monitoring

Monitoring of arterial gas analysis, oximetry and capnometry is mandatory in prevention and management of ICP-hypertension. Central circulation must be optimised by continuous monitoring of intraarterial blood pressure, central venous pressure, diuresis, peripheral and central temperature and eventually wedge pressure and cardiac output with the Swan Ganz technique.

If pre-hospital blood pressure level is known blood pressure level should be adjusted accordingly. However, stipulation of blood pressure level can be difficult in intracranial hypertension, where an element of Cushing response might be present. In these cases measurement of ICP and the result of CT scanning are instructive.

Drug-induced reduction of blood pressure should be done with caution in order to prevent a dangerous fall in cerebral perfusion pressure with development of ischemia. On the other hand, elevation of blood pressure beyond the upper level of autoregulation might provoke cerebral oedema and haemorrhage.

Cerebral autoregulation

Cerebral autoregulation is abolished or impaired focally or globally in the comatose neurosurgical patient. In traumatic head injury combined with severe haemorrhagic hypotension total vasoparalysis of the cerebral arterioles is often found. Restoration of blood pressure by transfusion is accompanied by an increase in ICP and under this circumstance CPP is never restored.

Dopamine

Even in unconscious patients with ICP-hypertension regions with intact cerebral autoregulation might exist. At the assumption that cerebral autoregulation predominantly is intact, it has been shown that careful, drug-induced (dopamine) increase in blood pressure might be accompanied by a decrease in ICP and an increase in CPP.

CVP, PEEP, CPAP

Measurement of central venous pressure may predict the intracranial venous pressure. Compression of the jugular veins is prevented by using a neutral position of the head, eventually combined with 30 degree elevation of the head which facilitates emptying of the cerebral venous vessels. PEEP and CPAP should be used with caution as both procedures might increase cerebral venous pressure.

Water and electrolyte balance

Careful evaluation and correction of water and electrolyte balance disturbances should be performed repeatedly, eventually with intervals of few hours. Especially hyponatraemia, owing to the decrease in osmolality, may aggravate cerebral oedema. The dehydration therapy, previously used in the neurointensive care, is now abandoned and replaced with a neutral fluid balance. If respiratory support with a ventilator is indicated or cardiac performance is reduced, a positive fluid balance, not exceeding 500-1000 ml, may optimise cardiac filling pressure, eventually supplemented with inotropic drugs like dopamine. Depletion of potassium during prolonged osmotic or diuretic therapy, and during prolonged hyperventilation should be replaced.

ICP monitoring

Indication for continuous intracranial pressure monitoring should be critically evaluated. In traumatic head injury CT scanning predicts ICP-hypertension fairly good if a mass lesion (subdural, intracerebral and subdural haemorrhage), compression of the basal cisterns or diffuse cerebral contusion are present. In diffuse axonal injury and localised cerebral contusion monitoring of ICP can be omitted, unless deterioration in consciousness and/or repeated neurological examinations suggest development of intracranial mass-expanding lesion or oedema. In such cases CT scanning is repeated, and the indication of continuous ICP monitoring is re-evaluated.

ICP hypertension

In the treatment of ICP-hypertension it is of importance to distinguish between acute catastrophes indicating immediate neuroradiological examination, and the more prolonged chronic intracranial hypertension so often observed during the intensive care of neurosurgical patients.

Acute ICP-hypertension

In patients with acute intracranial hypertension the consciousness of the patient deteriorates abruptly. Neurological examination may unveil abnormal peripheral reflexes and brain-stem reflexes. In this situation any therapeutic measure which decreases ICP should be used, including oxygen therapy, artificial hyperventilation, eventually intubation, sedation with hypnotics/analgetics and osmotic acting drugs like mannitol. Blood pressure should be maintained at normal pressure during drug administration, and hypertensive crisis should be treated cautiously, because it may be a part of a Cushing response.

Sustained ICP-hypertension

Sustained intracranial hypertension developing over hours or days may be secondary to ischaemic cytotoxic oedema, development and propagation of intracranial haematoma, and eventually hydrocephalus. Again, acute neurological examination (CT-scanning) is indicated to confirm or exclude surgical intervention.

Prophylactic hyperventilation and barbiturate treatment

Although clinical controlled studies indicate that prophylactic use of artificial hyperventilation, and the use of barbiturate coma sedation do not improve the clinical outcome, clinical practice convincingly has demonstrated that acute ICP-hypertension can be treated effectively. When clinical studies do not show any beneficial effect it might be caused by impairment of the effect on cerebral vasculature (abolished CO_2 - or barbiturate reactivity), development of ischaemia elicited by hyperventilation, hypoxaemia and reduction of blood pressure, and extracranial complications (pulmonary infection, decreased immune response, barotrauma, abdominal distension). However, analysis of the cerebral circulation and its regulation are supposed to be instructive and helpful as a guide to therapy.

CBF and $AVDO_2$ and tissue oxygen tension

Measurement of cerebral blood flow, arterio-venous oxygen content difference ($AVDO_2$), $CMRO_2$ and CO_2 reactivity together with ICP have been used as indicators for decision as regards therapy. If the CBF is high, relative to the $CMRO_2$ ($AVDO_2$ is low), a relative luxury perfusion exists (oxygen supply > oxygen demand). Under this circumstance the effect of hyperventilation can be estimated by measurement of the CO_2 reactivity, either globally ($\%AVDO_2/\Delta PaCO_2$ kPa) or regionally ($\%rCBF/\Delta PaCO_2$ kPa). On this basis the effect of hyperventilation upon acute change (decrease) in ICP and acute change in CBF (ischaemia) can be balanced. However, a risk of regional ischaemia still exists as this monitoring only reflects global perfusion. Measurement of tissue oxygen tensions might reveal focal ischemia.

$CMRO_2$

As regards barbiturate sedation, a relatively high $CMRO_2$, as calculated from the product of CBF and $AVDO_2$, indicates a preserved barbiturate reactivity, which otherwise is to be calculated as the difference in $CMRO_2$ before and after a thiopental loading dose of thiopental 5 mg /kg. Continuous EEG monitoring before and after a barbiturate dose, as regards the appearance of burst suppression level, can also guide the therapy.

Degree of hypocapnia

If artificial hyperventilation is decided, the initial fall in $PaCO_2$ should be 1–1.5 kPa and the resulting ICP decrease should be evaluated over 1–2 hours. A further decrease in $PaCO_2$ can be decided if the ICP level still is too high (> 25 mm Hg for hours).

Adaptation

As adaptation to acute hypocapnia occurs within 6-8 hrs. evaluation of the treatment should be repeated with intervals of 8–12 hrs. In order to prevent reactive hyperaemia weaning of hyperventilation must occur gradually over 6–12 hours. Otherwise, a rebound increase in cerebral perfusion and ICP might occur.

Mannitol

Mannitol should be used if intracranial hypertension is sustained, or if the result of clinical CBF measurement contraindicates the use of hyperventilation or hypnotics. Under these circumstances repeated dosages of mannitol (0.25–0.5 g/kg) are administered with intervals of 6–8 hours for several days without the formation of rebound edema otherwise observed during prolonged continuous mannitol treatment.

Steroids

In the American and the European guidelines (2000, Maas et al. 1997) steroids are not recommended in the treatment of severe head injury.

Dihydroergotamine, indomethacin and hypertonic saline

In intractable ICP-hypertension other non-surgical measures can be life-saving. Preliminary clinical studies of indomethacin, dihydroergotamine and hypertonic saline suggest prolonged amelioration of the intracranial pressure profile.The indication for these therapeutic interventions is still debated.

References

Abramson NS, Safar P, Detre K et al. Results of a randomized clinical trial of brain resuscitation with thiopental. Anesthesiology 1983: 59: A101.

Abou-Madi M, Trop D, Ravussin P. The early role of mannitol-induced hemodynamic changes in the control of intracranial hypertension. In Intracranial Pressure VIII. Eds.: Avezaat CJJ, van Eijndhoven JHM, Maas AIR, Tans J ThJ. Springer Verlag 1993: 601–604.

Adachi R, Kotani J. Changes in the intracranial pressure dynamics with head-down tilt in cats. Masui 1990: 39: 1343–1350.

Albech MJ, Børgesen SE, Gjerris F, et al. Intracranial pressure and cerebrospinal fluid outflow conductance in healthy subjects. J Neurosurg 1991: 74: 597–600.

Albrecht RF, Ruttle M. Cerebral effect of extended hyperventilation in unanesthetized goats. Stroke 1987: 18: 649–655

Alexander SC, Smith TC, Strobel G, et al. Cerebral carbohydrate metabolism of man during respiratory and metabolic alkalosis. J Appl Physiol 1968: 24: 66–72.

Allen GS, Ahn HS, Preziosi TJ, et al. Cerebral arterial spasms – a controlled trial of nimodipine in patients with subarachnoid hemorrhage. N Eng J Med 1983: 308: 619–624

Altura BT, Altura BM. Pentobarbital and contraction of vascular smotth muscle. Am J Physiol 1975: 229: 1635–1640

Alperin N, Lee SB, Raksin BP, et al. Noninvasive ICP measurements using magnetic resonance imaging. Proceeding XI ICP symposium 2000, 02-6, page 37.

Andersen AR, Tfeft-Hansen P, Lassen NA. The effect of ergotamine and dihydroergotamine on cerebral blood flow in man. Stroke 1987: 18: 120–123

Andrews PJD, Dearden NM, Miller JD. Comparison of thiopentone and propofol at two rates of intravenous administration in severily head injured patients. In Intracranial Pressure VIII. Avezaat CJJ, van Eijndhoven JHM, Maas AIR, Tans J ThJ. (eds) Springer Verlag 1993: 623–628.

Andrews RJ, Muto RP. Retraction brain ischaemia: mannitol plus nimodipine preserves both cerebral blood flow and evoked potentials during normoventilation and hyperventilation. Neurol Res 1992: 14: 19–25.

Artru AA, Nugent M, Michenfelder JD. Anesthetics affects the cerebral metabolic response to circulatory catecholamines. J Neurochem 1981: 36: 1941–1946.

Artru AA. Reduction of cerebrospinal fluid pressure by hypocapnia: Changes in cerebral blood volume, cerebrospinal fluid volume, and brain tissue water and electrolytes. J Cereb Blood Flow Metab 1987: 7: 471–479.

Artru AA, Hornbein TF. Prolonged hypocapnia does not alter the rate of CSF production in dogs during halothane anesthesia or sedation with nitrous oxide. Anesthesiology 1987: 67: 66–71.

Aschoff A, Muenkel K, Hashemi B, et al. Risk of ICP-monitoring. 739 own and 14500 literature cases. Proceeding XI ICP Symposium, Cambridge 2000, 02–1, page 32.

Asgeirsson B, Grände PO, Nordström C-H. A new therapy of posttrauma brain edema based on haemodynamic principles for brain volume regulation. Intensive Care Medicine 1994: 20: 260–267.

Asgeirsson B, Grände PO, Nordström C-H, et al. Cerebral haemodynamic effects of dihydroergotamine in patients with severe traumatic brain lesions. Acta Anesthesiol Scand 1995: 39: 922–930.

Astrup J, Skovsted P, Gjerris F, Sørensen HR. Increase in extracellular potassium in the brain during circulatory arrest: Effects of hypothermia, lidocaine, and thiopental. Anesthesiology 1981a: 55: 256–262.

Astrup J, Møller Sørensen P, Sørensen HR, Inhibition of cerebral oxygen and glucose consumption in the dog by hypothermia, pentobarbital, and lidocaine. Anesthesiology 1981b: 55: 263–268.

Astrup J. Energy-requiring cell functions in the ischemic brain. Their critical supply and possible inhibition in protective therapy. J Neurosurg 1982: 56: 482–497.

Auer LM, Haselsberger K. Effect of intravenous mannitol on cat pial arteries and veins during normal and elevated intracranial pressure. Neurosurgery 1987: 21: 142–146.

Awad I, Little JR, Lucas F, et al. Modification of focal cerebral ischemia by prostacyclin and indomethacin. J Neurosurg 58: 714–719, 1983

Bailey I, Bell A, Gray J et al. A trial of the effect on nimodipine on outcome after head injury. Acta Neurochir 1991: 110: 97–105.

Bardt T, Schneider GH, Lanksch WR, Unterberg A. Decompressive craniectomy following traumatic brain injury: ICP, CPP and neurological outcome. Proceeding XI ICP Symposium. 2000, 09–5, page 79.

Barker FG, Ogilvy C. Efficacy of prophylactic nimodipine for delayed ischaemic deficit after subarachnoid haemorrhage: A metaanalysis. J Neurosurg 1996: 84: 405–414.

Barlow P, Mendelow D, Lawrance A, et al. Clinical evaluation of two methods of subdural pressure monitoring. J Neurosurg 1985: 63: 578–582.

Bassauri LT, Concha-Julio E, Selman JM, et al. Cerebrospinal fluid spinal lumbar drainage: Indications, technical tips, and pitfalls. Crit Rev Neurosurg 1999: 9: 21–27.

Battistini N, Casacchia M, Bartolini A, et al. Effects of hyperventilation on focal brain damage following middle cerebral artery occlusion. In Cerebral blood flow, clinical and experimental results. Brock M, Fieschi C, Ingvar DH, Lassen NA, Schurmann K (eds). Springer-Verlag, Berlin, Heidelberg, New York, 1969: 249–253.

Bedford RF, Persing JA, Pobereskin L, Butler A. Lidocaine or thiopental for rapid control of intracranial hypertension? Anesth Analg 1980a: 59: 435–437.

Bedford RF, Winn HR, Tyson G, Park TS, Jane JA. Lidocaine prevents increased ICP after endotracheal intubation. In: Shulman K, Marmarou A, Miller JD, Becker DP, Hochwald GM, Brock M (eds); Intracranial Pressure IV, Springer Verlag, Berlin Heidelberg, New York 1980b: 595–598.

Bemana I, Nagao S. Effects of niravoline (RU 51599), a selective kappa-opiod receptor agonist on intracranial pressure in gradually expanding extradural mass lesion. J Neurotrauma 1998: 15: 117–124.

Berger S, Schürer L, Härtl R, et al. Reduction of posttraumatic intracranial hypertension by hypertonic/hyperoncotic saline/dextran and hypertonic mannitol. Neurosurgery 1995: 37: 98–108.

Berntman L, Dahlgren N, Siesjö BK. Influence of intravenously administered catecholamines on cerebral oxygen consumption and blood flow in the rat. Acta Physiol Scand 1978: 104: 101–108.

Biestro A, Alberti R, Galli R, et al. Osmotherapy for increased intracranial pressure: Comparison between mannitol and glycerol. Acta Neurochir 1997: 139: 725–733.

Bloomfield GL, Ridings PC, Blockers CR. Et al. A proposed relationship between increased intraabdominal, intrathoracic, and intracranial pressure. Crit Care Med 1997: 25: 496–503.

Bowie RA, O´Conner PJ, Hardman JG, Mahajan RP. The effect of continuous positive airway pressure on cerebral blood flow velocity in awake volunteers. Anesth Analg 2001: 92: 415–417.

Bozza MM, Maspes PE, Rossanda M. The control of brain volume and tension during intracranial operations. Br J Anaesth 1961: 33: 132–147.

Braakman R, Schouten HJA, et al. Megadose steroids in severe head injury. J Neurosurg 1983: 58: 326–330.

Bracken MB, Shepard MJ, Collins WF, et al. A randomized, controlled trial of methylprednisolone or naloxone in the treatment of acute spinal-cord injury. Results of the national Acute Spinal Cord Injury Study. J Neurosurg 1985: 63: 704–713.

Bracken MB, Shepard MJ, Collins WF, et al. A randomized, controlled trial of methylprednisolone or naloxone in the treatment of acute spinal cord injury. N Engl J Med 1990: 322: 1405–1411.

Brawley BW, Strandness DE, Kelly WA. The physiologic response to therapy in experimental cerebral ischaemia. Arch Neurol 1967: 17: 180–187.

Brock M, Hadjidimos AA, Schürmann K (1969) Possible adverse effects of hyperventilation on rCBF during the acute phase of total proximal occlusion of a main cerebral artery. In Cerebral Blood Flow. Brock M, Fieschi C, Ingvar DH, Lassen NA, Schürmann K (eds). Springer Verlag Berlin Heidelberg New York, 1969: 254–257.

Brown SC, Lam AM, Manninen PH. Haemodynamic effects of high-dose mannitol in man. Can Anaesth Soc J 1986: 33: S92–S93.

Bruce DA, Langfitt TW, Miller JD, et al. Regional cerebral blood flow, intracranial pressure, and brain metabolism in comatose patients. J Neurosurg 1973: 38: 131–145.

Bruce DA, Raphaely RC, Goldberg AI, et al. Pathophysiology, treatment and outcome following severe head injury in children. Childs Brain 1979: 5: 174–191.

Bruce DA, Schut L, Bruno LA, et al. Outcome following severe head injuries in children. J Neurosurg 1978: 48: 679–688.

Bruder N, N'Zoghe P, Graziani N, et al. A Comparison of extradural and intraparenchymatous intracranial pressures in head injured patients. Intensive Care Med 1995: 21: 850–852.

Bundgaard H, Landsfeldt U, Cold GE. Subdural monitoring of ICP during craniotomy: Thresholds of cerebral swelling/herniation. Acta Neurchir 1998 (suppl) 71: 276–278.

Bundgaard H, Cold GE. Studies of regional subdural pressure gradients during craniotomy. Br J Neurosurg 2000: 14: 229–234.

Bundgaard H, von Oettingen G, Jørgensen H, et al. The effects of dihydroergotamine on intracranial pressure, cerebral blood flow and cerebral metabolism in patients subjected to craniotomy for brain tumors. J Neurosurg Anesthesiol 2000, (in press)

Burke AM, Quest DO, Chien S, Cerri C. The effects of mannitol on blood viscosity. J Neurosurg 1981: 55: 550–553.

Busto R, Globus MYT, Dietrich WD, et al. Effect of mild hypotehrmia on ischemic-induced release of neurotransmitters and free fatty acids in rat brain. Stroke 1989: 20. 904–910

Cain SM. An attemp to demonstrate cerebral anoxia during hyperventilation of anaesthetized dogs. Am J Physiol 1963: 204: 323–326.
Cain SM (1970) Increased oxygen uptake with passive hyperventilation of dogs. J Appl Physiol 28: 4–7
Cardoso ER, Piatek D. Intracranial and venous pressures Part I: Intracranial pulse wave changes during hemodynamic maneuvers in humans. In Intracranial Pressure VII. Hoff JT, Betz AL (eds) 1989, 203–205.
Carlsson C, Hägerdal M, Siesjö BK. Protective effect of hypothermia in cerebral oxygen deficiency caused by arterial hypoxia. Anesthesiology 1976: 44: 27–34.
Chang JL, Chang GL, Nemoto EM, Hung TK, Nemmer JP. Protective effect of i.v. lidocaine in acute experimental spinal cord injury. Anesthesiology 1986: 65: A319.
Chambers IR, Kane PJ, Signorini DF, et al. Bilateral ICP monitoring: Its importance in detecting the severity of secondary insults. Acta Neurochir 1998 (suppl) 71: 42–43.
Changaris DG, McGraw CP, Richardson JD, et al. Correlation of cerebral perfusion pressure and Glasgow coma scale to outcome. J Trauma 1987: 27: 1007–1012
Chestnut RM. Hyperventilation versus cerebral perfusion pressure management. Time to change the question. Crit Care Med 1998: 26: 210–212.
Chi OZ, Lu X, Wei HM, et al. Hydroxyethyl starch solution attenuates blood-brain barrier disruption caused by intracarotid injection of hyperosmolar mannitol in rats. Anesth Analg 1996: 83: 226–341.
Chopp M, Knight R, Tidwell CD, et al. The metabolic effects of mild hypothermia on global cerebral ischemia and recirculation in the cat: Comparison to normothermia and hyperthermia. J Cereb Blood Flow Metab 1989: 9: 141–148
Christensen MS. Acid-base changes in cerebrospinal fluid and blood, and blood volume changes following prolonged hyperventilation in man. Br J Anaesth 1974: 46: 348–357.
Christensen MS. Prolonged arteficial hyperventilation in cerebral apoplexy. Acta Anaesthesiol Scand 1976: suppl 62: 1–24.
Clifton GL, Jiang JY, Lyeth BG, et al. Marked protection by moderate hypothermia after experimental traumatic brain injury. J Cereb Blood Flow Metab 1991: 11: 114–121
Clifton GL, Allen S, Barrodale P, et al. A phase II study of moderate hypothermia in severe brain injury. J Neurotrauma 1993: 10: 263–271.
Cohen PJ. To dream the impossible dream. (editorial view). Anesthesiology 1981: 55: 491–493.
Cold GE, Enevoldsen EM, Malmros R. The prognostic value of continuous intraventricular pressure recording in unconscious brain-injured patients under controlled ventilation. In: Intracranial Pressure II, Lundberg N, Pontén U, Brock M (eds). Springer Verlag, Berlin, Heidelberg, New York 1975: 517–521
Cold GE, Jensen FT, Malmros R. The cerebrovascular CO_2 reactivity during the acute phase of brain injury. Acta Anaesthesiol Scand 1977a: 21: 222–231.
Cold GE, Jensen FT, Malmros R. The effects of $PaCO_2$ reduction on regional cerebral blood flow in the acute phase of brain injury. Acta Anaesth Scand 1977b: 21: 359–367.
Cold GE, Jensen FT. Cerebral autoregulation in unconscious patients with brain injury. Acta Anaesthesiol Scand 1978: 22: 270–280
Cold GE. Cerebral metabolic rate of oxygen ($CMRO_2$) in the acute phase of brain injury. Acta Anaesthesiol Scand 1978: 22: 249–256
Cold GE, Christensen MS, Schmidt K. Effect of two levels of induced hypocapnia on cerebral autoregulation in the acute phase of head injury coma. Acta Anaesthesiol Scand 1981: 25: 397–401.
Cold GE, Eskesen V, Eriksen H, Blatt Lyon B. Changes in $CMRO_2$, EEG and concentration of etomidate in serum and brain tissue during craniotomy with continuous etomidate supplemented with N_2O and fentanyl. Acta Anaesthesiol Scand 1986: 30: 159–163.
Cold GE. Does acute hyperventilation provoke cerebral oligaemia in comatose patients after acute head injury?. Acta Neurochir (Wien) 1989: 96: 100–106
Cold GE. Measurement of CO_2 reactivity and barbiturate reactivity in patients with severe head injury. Acta Neurochir (Wien) 1989: 98: 153–163
Cold GE. Cerebral blood flow in acute head injury. Acta Neurochir (Wien) [suppl 49]: 1990: 1–64.
Cold GE, Tange M, Jensen TM, Ottesen S. Subdural pressure measurement during craniotomy. Correlation with tactile estimation of dural tension and brain herniation after opening of dura. Br J. Neurosurg 1996: 10: 69–75.
Collins RC, Posner JB, Plum F. Cerebral energy metabolism during electroshock seizures in mice. Am J Physiol 1970: 218: 943–950.
Compton JS, Lee T, Jones NR, et al. A double-blind placebo controlled trial in the calcium entry blocking drug, nicardipine, in the treatment of vasospasm following severe head injury. Br J Neurosurg 1990: 4: 8–15.
Connolly JE, Boyd RJ, Calvin JW. The protective effect of hypothermia in cerebral ischaemia. Experimental and clinical application by selective brain cooling in the human. Surgery 1962: 52: 15–24.
Constantini S, Cotev S, Rappaport H, Pomeranz S, Shalit MN. Intracranial pressure monitoring after elective intracranial surgery. J Neurosurg 1988: 69: 540–544.
Cooper PR, Moody S; Clark WK, et al. Dexamethasone and severe head injury. A Prospective double-blind study. J Neurosurg 1979: 51: 307–316.
Cottrell JE, Robustelli A, Post K, Turndorf H. Furosemide- and mannitol-induced changes in intracranial pressure and serum osmolality and electrolytes. Anesthesiology 1977: 47: 28–30.
Cottrell JE, Hartung J, Giffin JP, Shwirly B. Intracranial and hemodynamic changes after succinylcholine administration in cats. Anesth Analg 1983: 62: 10006–1009
Crotchfield JS, Narayan RK, Robertson CS, et al. Evaulation of fiberoptic intracranial pressure monitor. J Neurosurg 1990: 72: 482.
Cruz J. The first decade of continuous monitoring of jugular bulb oxyhemoglobin saturation. Management strategies and clinical outcome. Crit Care Med. 1998: 26: 344–351.
Czosnyka M, Price DJ, Williamson M. Monitoring of cerebrospinal dynamics using continuous analysis of intracranial pressure and cerebral perfusion pressure in head injury. Acta Neurochir (Wien) 1994: 126: 113–119.
Dahl B, Bergholt B, Kjærgaard JO, et al. The correlation between CO_2 - and indomethacin reactivity in severe head injury. Acta Neurochir 1996: 138: 265–273.
Dahlgren N, Nilsson B, Sakabe T, Siesjö BK. The effect of indomethacin on cerebral blood flow and oxygen consumption in the rat at normal and increased carbon dioxide tensions. Acta Physiol Scand 1981: 111: 475–485
Daley ML, Han S, Leffler C. Cyclic variation of cerebral pial arteriolar diameter synchronized with positive pressure

inhalation. Proceeding XI ICP Symposium, Cambridge 2000, P5-1, page 167.
Darby JM, Yonas H, Marion DW, Latchaw RE. Local inverse steal induced by hyperventilation in head injury. Neurosurgery 1988: 23: 84–88.
Dempsey RJ, Roy MW, Meyer KL, Donaldson DL. Indomethacin-mediated improvement following middle cerebral artery occlusion in cats. Effects of anesthesia. J Neurosurg 1985: 62: 874–881.
Dearden NM, Gibson SJ, McDowall DG, et al. Effect of high-dose dexamethasone on outcome from severe head injury. J Neurosurg 1986: 64: 81–88.
DeWitt DS, Prough DS, Deal DD, et al. Hypertonic saline does not improve cerebral oxygen dilivery after head injury and mild hemorrhage in cats. Crit Care Med 1996: 24: 109–117.
Dietrich WD, Busto R, Valdes I, Loor Y. Effects of normothermic versus mild hyperthermic forebrain ischemia in rats. Stroke 1990: 21: 1318–1325
Dings J Meixenberger J, Amschler J, et al. Brain tissue pO_2 in relation to cerebral perfusion pressure, TCD findings and CO_2 reactivity after severe head injury. Acta Neurochir 1996: 138: 425–434.
Donegan MF, Bedford RF. Intravenously administered lidocaine prevents intracranial hypertension during endotracheal suctioning. Anesthesiology 1980: 52: 516–518.
DuCailar J, Rioux J, Groleau D, Villard F. Hypothermie au dessous de 25 par refrigeration externe et sans circulation extra-corporelle. Ann Anesth Franc 1964: 4: 781–800.
Ducey JP, Lamiell JM, Gueller GE. Cerebral electrophysiologic effects of resuscitation with hypertonic saline-dextran after hemorrhage. Critical Care Medicine 1990: 18: 744–749
Durwald QJ, Del Maestro RF, Amacher AL, Farrar JK. The influence of systemic arterial pressure and intracranial pressure on the development of cerebral vasogenic edema. J Neurosurg 1983: 59: 803–809
Edvinsson L, Mc Culloch J. Effects of pentobarbital on contractile responses of feline cerebral arteries. J Cereb Blood Flow Metab 1981: 1: 437–440
Eisenberg HM, Frankowski RF, Contant CF, et al. High-dose barbiturate control of elevated intracranial pressure in patients with severe head injury. J Neurosurg 1988: 69: 15–23.
Ellingsen I, Hauge A, Nicolaysen G, et al. Changes in human cerebral blood flow due to step changes in PAO_2 and $PACO_2$. Acta Physiol Scand 1987: 129: 157–163.
Enevoldsen EM, Jensen F, Autoregulation and CO_2 responses of cerebral blood flow in patients with actute severe head injury. J Neurosurg 1978:48: 689–703
Este-McDonald JR, Josephs LG, Birkett DH, et al. Changes in intracranial pressure associated with apneumic retractors. Arch Surg 1995: 130: 362–365.
European Study Group on Nimodipine in Severe Head Injury. A multicenter trial of the efficacy of nimodipine on outcome after severe head injury. J Neurosurg 1994: 80: 797–804.
Evans DE, Kobrine AI, Legrys DC, Bradley ME. Protective effect of lidocaine in acute cerebral ischaemia induced by air embolism. J Neurosurg 1984: 60: 257–263.
Evans DE, Kobrine AI. Reduction of experimental intracranial hypertension by lidocaine. Neurosurgery 1987: 20: 542–547.
Evans DE, Catron PW, McDermott JJ, et al. Effect of lidocaine after experimental cerebral ischaemia induced by air embolism. J Neurosurg 1989: 70: 97–102.
Faupel G, Reulen HJ, Muller D, et al. Double-.blind study on the effects of steroids on severe closed head injury. In: Dynamics of Brain Edema. Pappius HM, Feindal W (eds), Springer Verlag 1976: 337–343.
Feldman Z, Kanter MJ, Robertson CS, et al. Effect of head elevation on intracranial pressure, cerebral perfusion pressure, and cerebral blood flow in head-injured patients. J Neurosurg 1992: 76: 207–211.
Feldman Z, Roberson CS, Contant CSF, et al. Positive end-expiratory pressure reduces intracranial compliance in the rabbit. J Neurosurg Anesthesiol 1997: 9: 175–179.
Ficher B, Thomas D, Peterson B. Hypertonic saline lowers raised intracranial pressure in children after head trauma. J Neurosurg Anesthesiol 1992: 4: 4–10
Fieschi C, Battistini N, Beduschi A, et al. Regional cerebral blood flow and intraventricular pressure in acute head injuries. J Neurol Neurosurg Psychiat 1974: 37: 1378–1388.
Forsman M, Aarseth HP, Nordby HK, et al. Effects of nimodipine on cerebral blood flow and cerebrospinal fluid pressure after cardiac arrest: Correlation with neurologic outcome. Anesth Analg 1989: 68: 436–443
French LA, Galicich JH. The use of steroids for control of cerebral edema. Clin Neurosurg 1964: 10: 212–223.
Frost EA. Effects of positive end-expiratory pressure on intracranial pressure and compliance in brain-injured patients. J Neurosurg 1977: 47: 195–200.
Garrick T, Mulvihill S, Buack S, et al. Intracerebroventricular pressure inhibits gastric antral and duodenal contractility but not acid secretion in conscious rabbits. Gastroenterology 1988: 95: 26–31
Gaudet RJ, Alam I, Levine L. Accumulation of cyclooxygenase products of arachidonic acid metabolism in gerbil brain during reperfusion after bilateral common carotid artery occlusion. J Neurochem 1980: 35: 653–658
Geismar P, Marquardsen J, Sylvest J. Controlled trial of intravenous aminophylline in acute cerebral infarction. Acta Neurol Scand 1976: 54: 173–180
Gelb AW, Steinberg GK, Lam AM, et al. The effects of a bolus of lidocaine in focal cerebral ischaemia. Can J Anaesth 1988: 35: 489–493.
Gemma M, Cozzi S, Piccoli S, et al. Hypertonic saline fluid therapy following brain stem trauma. J Neurosurg Anesthesiology 1996: 8: 137–141.
Ghajar J. Intracranial pressure monitoring techniques. New Horiz 1995: 3: 395–359.
Giannotta SL, Weiss MH, Apuzzo MLJ, et al. High-dose glucocorticoids in the management of severe head injury. Neurosurg 1984: 15: 497–501.
Giffin JP, Hartung J, Cottrell JE, et al. Effect of vecuronium on intracranial pressure, mean arterial pressure and heart rate in cats. Br J Anaesth 1986: 58: 441–443
Gilsbach JM, Reulen HJ, Ljunggren B, et al. Early aneurysm surgery and prevention therapy with intravenously administrered nimodipine: A multicenter, double-blind, dose-comparison study. Neurosurgery 1990: 26: 458–464.
Gobiet W, Bock WJ, Liesgang J, et al. Treatment of acute cerebral edema with high dose of dexamethasone. In: Intracranial Pressure III. Beks JWF, et al. (eds), Springer Verlag 1976: 231–235.
Goertz AW, Mehl T, Lindler KH, et al. Effect of 7.2% hypertonic saline/6% hetastarch on left ventricular contractility in anaesthetized humans. Anesthesiology 1995: 82: 1389–1395.

Goldberg RN, Jonshi A, Moscoso P, Castillo T. The effect of head position on intracranial pressure in the neonate. Crit Care Med 1983: 11: 428–430.

Gopinath SP, Robertson CS, Narayan RK. Cerebrovascular effects of dihydroergotamine in head injury. Critical Care Medicine 1994 [abstract] A204.

Gordon E. The action of drugs on intracranial contents. In: Boulton TB, Bryce-Smith R et al. (eds); Progress in Anaesthesiology, Excerpta Medica, Amsterdam 1970: 60.

Gordon E. Nonoperative treatment of acute head injuries (The Karoliska Experience). Intern Anaesth Clin 1979: 17: 181–199.

Gotoh F, Meyer JS, Takagi Y. Cerebral effects of hyperventilation in man. Arch Neurol 1965: 12: 410–423.

Gottstein U, Paulson OB. The effect of intracarotid aminophylline infusion on the cerebral circulation. Stroke 1972: 3: 560–565

Grände P-O. The effects of dihydroergotamine in patients with head injury and raised intracranial pressure. Intensive Care Med 1989: 15: 523–527

Grände P-O, Asgeirsson B, Nordström CH. Physiologic principles for volume regulation of the tissue enclosed in a rigid shell with application to the injured brain. J Trauma 1997: 42: S23–S31.

Greenberg JH, Alavi A, Reivich M, et al. Local cerebral blood volume response to carbon dioxide in man. Circ Res 1975: 43: 324–331

Greenwood J, Luthert PJ, Pratt OE, Lantos PL. Hyperosmolar opening of the blood-brain barrier in energy-depleted rat brain. Part I. Permeability studies. J Cereb Blood Flow Metab 1988: 8: 9–15.

Gross CE, Abel PW. Contraction and relaxation of rabbit basilar artery by thiopental. Neurosurgery 1985: 17: 433–435

Grubb RL, Raichle ME, Eichling JO, Ter-Pogossian MM. The effects of changes in $PaCO_2$ on cerebral blood volume, blood flow, and vascular mean transit time. Stroke 1974: 5: 630–638.

Grubb RL, Raichle ME, Eichling JO, Gado MH. Effects of subarachnoid hemorrhage on cerebral blood volume, blood flow and oxygen utilization in humans. J Neurosurg 1977: 46: 446–453

Gudeman SK, Miller JD, Becker DP, Failure of high-dose steroid therapy to influence intracranial pressure in patients with severe head injury. J Neurosurg 1979: 51: 301–306.

Gueniau C, Berteleau L, Oberlander C. Protection from ischemic focal cerebral oedema in mice by two kappa opioid receptor agonists, Niravoline and U 50488. J Cereb Blood Flow Metab 1995: suppl1, S383.

Guidelines for the Management of Severe Traumatic Brain Injury (2000). Indications for intracranial pressure monitoring. J Neurotrauma 2000: 17: 667–679.

Guidelines for the Management of Severe Traumatic Brain Injury. Intracranial pressure treatment thresholds J Neurotrauma 2000: 17: 681–683.

Guidelines for the Management of Severe Traumatic Brain Injury. The use of hyperventilation in the acute management of severe traumatic brain injury. J Neurotrauma 2000: 17: 699–705.

Guidelines for the Management of Severe Traumatic Brain Injury. The use of mannitol in severe head injury J Neurotrauma 2000: 17: 705–709.

Guidelines for the Management of Severe Traumatic Brain Injury. The use of barbiturate in the control of intracranial hypertension. J Neurotrauma 2000: 17: 711–714.

Guidelines for the Management of Severe Traumatic Brain Injury. Guidelines for cerebral perfusion pressure. J Neurotrauma 2000: 17: 693–699.

Guidelines for the Management of Severe Traumatic Brain Injury. Resuscitation of blood pressure and oxygenation J Neurotrauma 2000: 17: 661–667.

Guidelines for the Management of Severe Traumatic Brain Injury. Recommandations for intracranial pressure monitoring technology. J Neurotrauma 2000: 17: 685–692.

Hallenbeck JM, Furlow TW. Prostaglandin I_2 and indomethacin prevent impairment of post-ischemic brain reperfusion in the dog. Stroke 1979: 10: 629–637

Haller C, Kuschinsky W. Moderate hypoxia: reactivity of pial arteries and local effect of theophylline J Appl Physiol 1987: 63: 2208–2215.

Harders A, Kakarieka A, Braakman R et al. Traumatic subarachnoid hemorrhage and its treatment with nimodipine. J Neurosurg 1996: 85: 82–89.

Haring HP, Hormann C, Schalow S, Benzer A. Continuous positive airway pressure breathing increases cerebral blood flow volocity in humans. Anesth Analg 1994: 79: 883–885.

Hariri RJ, Firlich AD, Shepard SR, et al. Traumatic brain injury, hemorrhagic shock, and fluid resuscitation: Effects on intracranial pressure and brain compliance. J Neurosurg 1993: 79: 421–427.

Harp JR, Wollman H. Cerebral metabolic effects of hyperventilation and deliberate hypotension. Br J Anaesth 1973: 45: 256–262.

Harris RJ, Bayhan M, Branston NM, et al. Modulation of the pathophysiology of primate focal cerebral ischaemia by indomethacin. Stroke 1982: 13: 17–24

Hassan FM, Kazemi H. Dual contribution theory of regulation of CSF HCO_3^- in respiratroy acidosis. J Appl Physiol 1976: 40: 559–567

Havill JH. Prolonged hyperventilation and intracranial pressure. Critical Care Medicin 1984: 12: 72–74

Härtl R, Schürer L, Dautermann C, et al. Effect of hypertonic-hyperoncotic solutions (HHS) on increased intracranial pressure after a focal brain lesion and inflation of an epidural balloon. In Intracranial Pressure VIII. Avezaat CJJ, van Eijndhoven JHM, Maas AIR, Tans J ThJ (eds). Springer Verlag 1993: 612–614.

Heilbrun MP, Olesen J, Lassen NA. Regional cerebral blood flow studies in subarachnoid hemorrage. J Neurosurg 37: 36–44

Henschen S, Busse MW, Zisowsky S, et al. Short term volume effects of a hypertonic saline bolus during neurosurgery. Neurchirurgica 1991: 34: 163–165.

Hochwald GM, Wald A, Malhan C. The sink action of cerebrospinal fluid volume flow. Arch Neurol 1976: 33: 339–344.

Hoffman WE, Werner C, Baughman VL, Thomas C, Miletich DJ, Albrecht RF. Postischemic treatment with hypothermia improves outcome from incomplete cerebral ischemia in rats. J Neurosurg Anesthesiol 1991: 3: 34–38.

Hörmann C, Mohsenipour I, Gottardis M, Benzer A. Response of cerebrospinal fluid pressure to continuous positive airway pressure in volunteers. Anesth Analg 1994: 78: 54–57.

Hsiang JK, Chestnut RM, Crisp CB, et al. Early routine paralysis for intracranial pressure control in severe head injury: Is it necessary? Crit Care Med 1994: 22: 1471–1476.

Hulme A. Cooper R. The Effects of head position and jugular vein compression on intracranial pressure. A clinical study. Intracranial Pressure III. Beks JWF, Bosch DA, Brock M

(eds). Springer-Verlag, Berlin, Heidelberg, New York 1976, 259–263
Hung OR, Hare GM, Brien S. Head elevation reduces head-rotation associated increased ICP in patients with intracranial tumours. Can J Anaesth 2000: 47: 415–420.
Hunter AR. Thiopentone supplemented anaesthesia for neurosurgery. Br J Anaesth 1972: 44: 506–510.
Ishii R. Regional cerebral blood flow in patients with ruptured intracranial aneurysm. J Neurosurg 1979: 50: 587–594
Ito U, Ohno K, Nakamura R, et al. Brain edema during ischemia after restoration of blood flow. Measurement of water, sodium, potassium content and plasma protein permeability. Stroke 1979: 10: 542–547
Jafar JJ, Johns LM, Mullan SF. The effect of mannitol on cerebral blood flow. J Neurosurg 1986: 64: 754–759.
James HE, Cytotoxic edema produced by 6-Aminonicotinamide and its response to therapy. Neurosurgery 1978: 3: 196–200.
James HE. Methodology for the control of intracranial pressure with hypertonic mannitol. Acta Neurochir (Wien) 1980: 51: 161–172
Jennett B, Teasdale G, Fry J, et al. Treatment for severe head injury. J Neurol Neurosurg Psychiat 1980: 43: 289–295
Jennett WB, Teasdale C. Management of head injuries in the acute state. Philadelphia: FA Davis Company 1981: 240–241.
Jensen K, Öhrström J, Cold GE, Astrup J. The effects of indomethacin on intracranial pressure, cerebral blood flow, and cerebral metabolism in patients with severe head injury and intracranial hypertension. Acta Neurochir (Wien) 1991: 108: 116–121
Jensen K, Freundlich M, Bünemann L, et al. The effect of indomethacin upon cerebral blood flow in healthy volunteers. The influence of moderate hypoia and hypercapnia. Acta Neurochir (Wien) 1993: 124: 114–119.
Johnstone IH, Harper AM. The effect of mannitol on cerebral blood flow. An experimental study. J Neurosurg 1973: 38: 461–471.
Josephs LG, Este-McDonald E, Birkett DH, Hirsch EF, Diagnostic laparoscopy increases intracranial pressure. J Trauma 1994: 36: 815–818.
Jørgensen HA, Bundgaard H, Cold GE. Subdural pressure measurement during fossa posterior surgery. Br J Neurosurg 1999: 13: 449–453.
Kanter MJ, Robertson CS, Sheinberg MA, et al. Changes in cerebral hemodynamics with head elevated vs. head falt. Intracranial Pressure 8, 1991, abstract 079.
Kassell NF, Hitchon PW, Gerk MK, et al. Alterations in cerebral blood flow, oxygen metabolism, and electrical activity produced by high dose sodium thiopental. Neurosurgery 1980: 7: 598–603.
Kassell NF, Baumann KW, Hitchon PW, et al. The effects of high dose mannitol on cerebral blood flow in dogs with normal intracranial pressure. Stroke 1982: 13: 59–61.
Kaufmann AM, Cardoso ER. Effects of mannitol treatment on cerebral water content. In Intracranial Pressure VIII. Avezaat CJJ, van Eijndhoven JHM, Maas AIR, Tans J ThJ (eds). Springer Verlag 1993: 592–595.
Kenning JA, Toutant SM, Saunders RL. Upright patient positioning in the management of intracranial hypertension. Surg Neurol 1981: 15: 148–152.
Khambatta HJ, Sullivan SF. Carbon dioxide production and washout during passive hyperventilation alkalosis. J Appl Physiol 1974: 37: 665–669
Khanna S, Davis D, Peterson B, et al. Use of hypertonic saline in the treatment of severe refractory posttraumatic intracranial hypertension in pediatric traumatic brain injury. Crit Care Med 2000: 28: 4: 1144–1151
Kien ND, Kramer GC, White DA. Acute hypotension caused by rapid hypertonic saline infusion in anesthetized dogs. Anesth Analg 1991: 73: 597–602.
Kim HJ, Levasseur JE, Patterson JL, et al. Effect of indomethacin prestreatment on acute mortality in experimental brain injury. J Neurosurg 1989: 71: 565–572
Kinuta Y, Ishikawa M, Hirai O, et al. Clinical validity of lumbar subarachnoid pressure measurement No To Shinkei 1987: 39: 673–678.
Kitagawa K, Matsumoto M, Tagaya M, et al. Hyperthermia-induced neuronal protection against ischemic injury in gerbils. J Cereb Blood Flow Metab 1991: 11: 449–452
Kitahata LM, Galicich JM, Sato I. The effect of passive hyperventilation on intracranial pressure. J Neurosurg 1971: 34: 185–193.
Kiening KL, Schoening WN, Unterberg AW, Lanksch WR. Intracranial compliance as bed-side monitoring technique in severely head-injured patients. Proceeding XI ICP Symposium, Cambridge 2000: 01–5, page 30.
Kinuta Y, Ishikawa M, Hirai M, et al. Clinical calidity of lumbar subarachnoid pressure measurement. No To Shinkei 1987: 39: 673–678.
Kluklane M, Eelmäe J, Roose M, Kaasik AE. Correction of CSF acidosis and craniospinal system viscoelastic parameters with intrathecal THAM. In Intracranial Pressure VIII. Azezaat CJJ, van Eijdnhoven JHM, Maas AIR, Tans JThJ (eds). Springer Verlag 1993: 620–622.
Kobrine AI, Evans DE, LeGrys DC, et al. Effects of intravenous lidocaine on experimental spinal cord injury. J Neurosurg 1984: 60: 595–601.
Koide T, Wieloch TW, Siesjö BK. Chronic dexamethasone pretreatment aggravates ischaemic neuronal necrosis. J Cereb Blood Flow Metab 1986: 6: 395–404
Kojima T, Iwat K, Tamai K. Change of cerebral electrophysiological activity, regional cerebral blood flow and regional cerebral blood volume in acute intracranial hypertension. In Intracranial Pressure VIII. Avezaat CJJ, van Eijndhoven JHM, Maas AIR, Tans J ThJ (eds). Springer Verlag 1993: 249–252.
Kolbitsch C, Lorenz IH, Hoermann C, et al. The influence of increased intrathoracic pressure on cerebral compliance in humans. Proceeding XI ICP symposium, Cambridge 2000, P17–8, page 286.
Koston H, Rumpf E, Stampfl G, et al. Treatment of cerebral vasospasm following severe head injury with the calcium influx blocker nimodipine. Neurochirgica 1985: 28: 103–109.
Kotani J, Adachi R, Fujita N, et al. Effect of cerebral venous congestion on the pressure-volume index in the evaluation of intracranial pressure dynamics. J Neurosurg Anesthesiol 1993: 5: 121–126.
Kotani J, Momota Y, Sugioka S, Umemura A, Ueda Y. Effect of head-down tilt on intracranial pressure and sagital sinus pressure during general anesthesia in cats. Anesth Prog 1993: 39: 209–211.
Kuchiwaki H, Misu N, Takada S, et al. Measurement of local directional pressures in the brain with mass. Neurosurgery 1992: 31: 731–738.

Langham J, Goldfrad C, Teasdale G, et al. Calcium channel blockers for acute traumatic brain injury. Cocrane Database Syst Rev 2000: CD000565
Lanier WL, Milde JH, Michenfelder JD. The cerebral effects of pancuronium and atrachurium in halothane-anesthetized dogs. Anesthesiology 1985: 63: 589–597
Larsen R, Hilfiker O, Radle J Sonntag H. Midazolam: Wirkung auf allgemeine Hämodynamik, Hirndurchblutung und Cerebralen Sauerstoffverbrauch bei Neurochirurgischen Patienten. Anaesthesist 1981: 30: 18–21.
Lassen NA. Control of cerebral circulation in health and disease. Circ Res 1974: 34: 749–760
Lee ST. Intracranial pressure changes during positioning of patients with severe head injury. Heart Lung 1989: 18: 411–414.
Little JR. Modification of acute focal ischaemia by treatment with mannitol. Stroke 1978: 9: 4-9.
Lodrini S, Montolivo M, Pluchino F, Borroni V. Positive end-expiratory pressure in supine and sitting positions: its effects on intrathoracic and intracranial pressures. Neurosurgery 1989: 24: 873–877.
Long DM, Maxwell R, Choi KS. A new therapy regimen for brain edema. In: Pappius HM, Feidal W (eds). Dynamics of brain edema, Springer Verlag, Berlin, Heidelberg, New York 1976: 293–300.
Lundberg N, Kjällquist A, Bien C. Reduction of increased intracranial pressure by hyperventilation. Acta Psychiat neurol Scand 1959: 34 (suppl 139).
Lundberg N. Continuous recording and control of ventricular fluid pressure in neurosurgical practice. Acta Psychiat Scand 1960: (suppl 149): 36: 1–193.
Maas AIR, Flecken stein W, deJong DA, Wolf M. Effect of increased ICP and decreased cerebral perfusion pressure on brain tissue and cerebrospinal fluid oxygen tension. In Intracranial Pressure VIII. Avezaat CJJ, van Eijndhoven JHM, Maas AIR, Tans J ThJ (eds). Springer Verlag 1993: 233–237.
Maas AIR, Dearden M, Teasdale GM, et al. EBIC-guidelines for management of severe head injury in adults. Acta Neurochir 1997: 139: 286–294.
MacDonald JT, Uden DL. Intravenous glycerol and mannitol therapy in children with intracranial hypertension. Neurology 1982: 32: 437–440.
MacKenzie ET, McCullock J, O'Keane M et al. Cerebral circulation and norepinephrine: relevance of the blood-brain barrier. Am J Physiol 1976: 231: 483–408.
Maeda M, Miyazaki M, Ishii S. The role of the mutual interaction between the locus coeruleus complex and the cholinoceptive pontine area in the plateau wave. In: Hoff JT, Betz AL (eds). Intracranial Pressure VII. Springer Verlag, Berlin Heidelberg New York Tokyo 1989: 228–231.
Maeda M, Miyazaki M, Ishii S. Control of ICP by the medullary reticular formation. In: Intracranial Pressure VIII. Avezaat CJJ, van Eijndhoven JHM, Maas AIR, Tans JThJ (eds). Springer Verlag, Berlin Heidelberg, New York Tokyo 1993: 207–213.
Maeda M, Miyazaki M. Control of ICP and cerebrovascular bed by the cholinergic basal forebrain. Acta Neurochir 1998 (suppl) 71: 293–296.
Magnussen I, Høedt-Rasmussen K. The effect of intraarterial administered aminophylline on cerebral hemodynamics in man. Acta Neurol Scand 1977: 55: 131–136
Mainzer F. Treatment of incipient apoplexy with intravenous aminophylline, Acta Med Scandinav 1953: 146: 362–374
Manninen PH, Lam AM, Gelb AW, Brown SC. The effect of high-dose mannitol on serum and urine electrolytes and osmolality in neurosurgical patients. Can J Anaesth 1987: 34: 442–446.
March ML, Dunlop BJ, Shapiro HM, et al. Succinylcholine-intracranial pressure effects in neurosurgical patients. Anesth Analg 1980: 59: 550–551
Marx W, Shah N, Long C, et al. Sufentanil, alfentanil, and fentanyl: Inpact on cerebrospinal fluid pressure in patients with brain tumours. J Neurosurg Anesthesiol 1989: 1: 3–7
Marin J, Lobato RD, Rico ML, et al. Effect of pentobarbital on the reactivity of isolated human cerebral arteries. J Neurosurg 1981: 54: 521–524
Marion DW, Bouma GJ. The use of stable xenon-enhanced computed tomographic studies of cerebral blood flow to define changes in cerebral carbon dioxide vasoresponsivity caused by a severe head injury. Neurosurgery 1991: 29: 869–873
Marion DW, Obrist WD, Carlien PM, et al. The use of moderate therapeutic hypothermia for patients with severe head injuries: A preliminary report. J Neurosurg 1993: 79: 354-362.
Marion DW, Penrod LE, Kelsey SF, et al. Treatment of traumatic brain injury with moderate hypothermia. New Eng J Med 1997: 336: 540–545.
Marshall LF, Smith RW, Rauscher LA, Shapiro HM. Mannitol dose requirements in brain-injured patients. J Neurosurg 1978: 48: 169–172
Marshall WK, Page RB, Milchak MA. Furosemide reduces brain water in cerebral injury in dogs. Anesthesiology 1982: 57: A308.
Martins AN, Doyle TF, Newby N. PCO_2 and rate of formation of of cerebrospinal fluid in the monkey. Am J Physiol 1976: 231: 127–131.
Mascia L, Grasso S, Puntillo F, et al. The effects of positive end expiratory pressure on cerebral hemodynamics in severe brain injured patients with acute lung injury. Proceeding XI ICP symposium, Cambridge 2000, P12–9, page 245.
Mavrocordatos P, Bissonnette P, Ravussion P. Effects of neck position and head elevation on intracranial pressure in anaesthetized neurosurgical patients: preliminary results. J Neurosurg Anesthesiol 2000: 12: 10–14.
Maxwell WK, Page RB, Milchak MA. Furosemide reduces brain water in cerebral injury in dogs. Anesthesiology 1982: 57: A308.
Mchedlishvili G. Pathogenetic role of circulatory factors in brain edema development. Neursurg Rev. 1988: 11: 7–13.
McGuire G, Crossley D, Richards J, Wong D. Effects of varying levels of positive end-expiratory pressure on intracranial pressure and cerebral perfusion pressure. Crit Care Med 1997: 25: 1059–1062.
McHenry LC Jr, Jaffe ME, West JW, et al. Regional cerebral blood flow and cardiovascular effects of hexobendine in stroke patients. Neurology (Minneap.) 1972: 22: 217–223
McQueen JD, Jeanes LD. Dehydration and rehydration of the brain with hypertonic urea and mannitol. J Neurosurg 1964: 11: 118–128.
Meixensberger J, Brawanski A, Danhauser-Leistner I, et al. Is there a risk to induce ischemia by hyperventilation therapy? In Intracranial Pressure VIII. Avezaat CJJ, van Eijndhoven JHM, Maas AIR, Tans J ThJ (eds). Springer Verlag 1993: 589–591.
Meixensberger J, Baunach S, Amschler J, et al. Influence of body position on tissue-pO_2, cerebral perfusion pressure

and intracranial pressure in patients with acute brain injury. Neurol Res 1997: 19: 249-253.
Mellander S, Nordenfelt I. Comparative effects of dihydroergotamine and noradrenaline on resistance exchange and capacipance functions in the peripheral circulation. Clin Sci 1970: 39: 183-201
Mendelow AD, McCalden TA, Hattingh J, et al. Cerebrovascular reactivity and metabolism after subarachnoid hemorrhage in baboons. Stroke 1981: 12: 58-65
Mendelow AD, Rowan JO, Murray L, Kerr AE. A clinical comparison of subarachnoid screw pressure measurements with ventricular pressure. J Neurosurg 1983: 58: 45-50.
Merlo F, Demo P, Moreth T, et al. Propofol vs. thiopental for the control of elevated ICP in head injured patients. In Intracranial Pressure VIII. Avezaat CJJ, van Eijndhoven JHM, Maas AIR, Tans J ThJ (eds). Springer Verlag 1993: 629-631.
Messeter K, Nordström C-H, Sundbärg G, et al. Cerebral hemodynamics in patients with severe head trauma. J Neurosurg 1986: 64: 231-237.
Metz C, Holzschuh M, Bein T, et al. Moderate hypothermia in patients with severe head injury: Cerebral and extracerebral effects. J Neurosurg 1996: 85: 533-541.
Meyer FB, Anderson RE, Sundt TM, Yakch TL. Treatment of experimental focal cerebral ischaemia with mannitol J Neurosurg 1987: 66: 109-115.
Michenfelder JD, Sundt TM. The effect of $PaCO_2$ on the metabolism of ischemic brain in squirrel monkeys. Anesthesiology 1973: 38: 445-453
Michenfelder JD. The interdependency of cerebral functional and metabolic effects following massive doses of thiopental in the dog. Anesthesiology 1974: 41: 231-236.
Michenfelder JD, Milde JH. Failure of prolonged hypocapnia, hypothermia or hypertension to favourably alter acute stroke in primates. Stroke 1977: 8: 87-91.
Michenfelder JD, Milde JH. The relationship among canine brain temperature, metabolism, and function during hypocapnia. Anesthesiology 1991: 75: 130-136
Milde LN, Milde JH, Michenfelder JD. Cerebral functional, metabolic, and hemodynamic effects of etomidate in dogs. Anesthesiology 1985: 63: 371-377.
Milde LN, Milde JH Gallagher W. Effects of sufentanil on cerebral circulation and metabolism in dogs. Anesth Analg 1990: 70: 138-146
Miller JD, Leech P. Effects of mannitol and steroid therapy on intracranial volume-pressure relationships in patients. J Neurosurg 1975: 42: 274-281.
Miller JD, Becker DP, Ward JD, et al. Significance of intracranial hypertension in severe head injury. J Neurosurg 1977: 47: 503-513
Miller JD, Bobo H, Kapp JP. Inaccurate pressure reading for subarachnoid bolts. Neurosurgery 1986: 19: 253-155.
Mindermann T, Gratzl O. Interhemispheric pressure gradients in severe head trauma in humans. Acta Neurochir 1998 (suppl) 71: 56-58.
Mirski AM, Denchev ID, Schnitzer SM, Hanley FD. Comparison between hypertonic saline and mannitol in the reduction of elevated intracranial pressure in a rodent model of acute cerebral injury. J Neurosurg Anesthesiol 2000: 12: 334-344.
Mollman HD, Rockswold GL, Ford SE. A clinical comparison of subarachnoid catheters to ventriculostomy and subarachnoid bolts: a prospective study. J Neurosurg 1988: 68: 737-741.
Morgan P, Ward B. Hyperventilation and changes in the electroencephalogram and electroretinogram. Neurology 1970: 20: 1009-1014.
Moon PF, Kramer GC. Hypertonic saline/dextran resuscitation from hemorrhagic shock induces transient acidosis. Crit Care Med 1995: 23: 323-331.
Mouren S, Delayance S, Mion G, et al. Mechanisms of increased myocardial contractility with hypertonic saline solutions in isolated blood-perfused rabbit hearts. Anesth Analg 1995: 81: 777-782.
Muizelaar JP, Wei EP, Kontos HA, Becker DP. Mannitol causes compensatory cerebral vasoconstriction and vasodilatation in response to blood viscosity changes J Neurosurg 1983: 59: 822-828.
Muizelaar JP, Lutz HA, Becker DP. Effect of mannitol on ICP and CBF and correlation with pressure autoregulation in severely head-injured patients. J Neurosurg 1984: 61: 700-706.
Muizelaar JP, Marmarou A, Ward JD, et al. Adverse effects of prolonged hyperventilation in patients with severe head injury: a randomized clinical trial. J Neurosurg 1991: 75: 731-739
Müller-Schweinitzer E, Rosenthaler J. Dihydroergotamine: Pharmacodynamics, and mechanism of venoconstrictor action in beagle dogs. J Cardiovasc Pharmacol 1987: 9: 686-693
Nagao S, Bemana I, Kuratani H, et al. Niravoline, a selective kappa-opioid receptor antagonist effectively reduces elevated intracranial pressure. Exp Brain Res 2000:130: 338-344
Nath F, Galbraith S. The effect of mannitol on cerebral white matter water content. J Neurosurg 1986: 65: 41-43.
Neill WA, Hattenhauer M. Impairment of myocardial O_2 supply due to hyperventilation. Circulation 1975: 52: 854-858.
Nilsson F, Messeter K, Grände PO, et al. Effects of dihydroergotamine on cerebral circulation during experimental intracranial hypertension. Acta Anaesthesiol Scand 1995: 39: 916-921.
Nordström C-H, Rehncrona S. Reduction of cerebral blood flow and oxygen consumption with a combination of barbiturate anesthesia and induced hypothermia in the rat. Acta Anaesthesiol Scand 1979: 22: 7-12.
Nornes H, Magnäs B. Supratentorial epidural pressure recording during posterior fossa surgery. J Neurosurg 1971: 35: 541-549.
North JB, Reilly PL, Gorman D, et al. The effect of hypoxia on intracranial pressure and cerebral blood flow. In Intracranial Pressure VIII. Avezaat CJJ, van Eijndhoven JHM, Maas AIR, Tans J ThJ (eds). Springer Verlag 1993: 238-243.
North JB, Reilly PI. Comparison among three methods of intracranial pressure recording. Neurosurgery 1986: 18: 730-732.
Norton JA, Ott LG, McClain C, Adams L, et al. Intolerance to enteral feeding in the brain-injured patients. J Neurosurg 1988: 68: 62-66.
Obrist WD, Gennarelli TA, Segewa H, et al. Relation of cerebral blood flow to neurological status and outcome in head-injured patients. J Neurosurg 1979: 51: 292-300
Obrist WD, Langfitt TW, Jaggi JL, et al. Cerebral blood flow and metabolism in comatose patients with acute head injury. Relationship to intracranial hypertension. J Neurosurg 1984: 61: 241-253.

Öhman J, Heiskanen O. Effect of nimodipine on the outcome of patients after aneurysmal subarachnoid hemorrhage and surgery. J Neurosurg 1988: 69: 683–686.
Ohman J, Servo AM, Heirkanen O. Risks factors for cerebral infarction in good-grade patients after aneurysmal subarachnoid hemorrhage and surgery: A prospective study. J Neurosurg 1991a: 74: 14–20.
Ohman J, Servo A, Heiskanen O. Long-term effects of nimodipine on cerebral infarcts and outcome after aneurysmal subarachnoid hemorrhage and surgery. J Neurosurg 1991b: 74: 8–13.
Olesen J, Skinhøj E. Effects of ergot ankaloids (Hydergine) on cerebral haemodynamics in man. Acta Pharmacol 1972: 31: 75–85
Olivarius B deFine. Theophyllamin behandling af udvalgte tilfælde af apoplexia cerebri thrombotica. Ugeskr f Læger 1957: 119: 623–625
Ott L, Young B, Phillipts R, et al. Altered gastric enptying in the head-injured patient: relationship to feeding intolerance. J Neurosurg 1991: 74: 738–742
Overgaard J and Tweed WA. Cerebral circulation after head injury. Part I: Cerebral blood flow and its regulation after closed head injury with emphasis on clinical correlations. J Neurosurg 1974: 41: 531–541.
Ozyurt E, Graham DI, Woodruff GN, McCulloch J. Protective effect of the glutamate antagonist, MK-801 in focal cerebral ischemia in the cat. J Cereb Blood Flow Metab 1988: 8: 138–143
Palvölgyi R. Regional cerebral blood flow in patients with intracranial tumors. J Neurosurg 1969: 31: 149–163.
Pappius HM, McCann WP. Effects of steroids on cerebral edema in cats. Arch Neurol 1969: 20: 207–216.
Paulson OB, Lassen NA, Skinhøj E. Regional cerebral blood flow in apoplexy without arterial occlusion. Neurology (Minneap.) 1970: 20: 125–138
Paulson OB. Regional cerebral blood flow in apoplexy due to occlusion of the middle cerebral artery. Neurology 1970: 20: 63–77.
Paulson OB, Olesen J, Christensen MS. Restoration of autoregulation of cerebral blood flow by hypocapnia. Neurology (Minneap.) 1972: 22: 286–293.
Petruk KC, West M, Mohr G, et al. Nimodipine treatment in poor-grade aneurysm patients. J Neurosurg 1988: 68: 505–517.
Pena H, Gaines C, Suess D, et al. Effect of mannitol on experimental focal ischaemia in awake monkeys. Neurosurgery 1982: 11: 477–481.
Pfenninger E, Lindner KH, Ahnefeld FW. Die Infusion von THAM (trishydroxymethyl- aminomethan) als Therapie zur Senkung des erhöhten intrakraniellen Druckes beim akuten Schädel-Hirn-Trauma. Anesthesist 1989: 38: 189–192.
Phleps ME, Grubb RL, Ter-Pogosian MM. Correlation between $PaCO_2$ and regional cerebral blood volume by x-ray fluorescence. J Appl Physiol 1973: 35: 274–280
Pichard JD, MacKenzie ET. Inhibition of prostaglandin synthesis and the response of baboon cerebral circulation to carbon dioxide. Nature New Biol 1973: 245: 187–188
Pichard JD, Murray GD, Illingworth R, et al. Effect of oral nimodipine on cerebral infarction and outcome after subarachnoid hemorrhage.: British aneurysm nimodipine trial. Br Med J 1989: 298: 636–642
Pierce EC, Lambertsen CJ, Deutsch S, et al. Cerebral circulation and metabolism during thiopental anesthesia and hyperventilation in man. J Clin Invest 1962: 41: 1664–1671.
Piper I, Spiegelberg A, Whittle I et al. A comparative study of the Spiegelberg compliance devices with a manual volume-injection method: a clinical evaluation in patients with hydrocephalus. Br J Neurosurg 1999: 13: 581–586.
Pistolese GR, Faraglia V, Agnoli A, et al. Cerebral hemispheric "counter-steal" phenomenon during hyperventilation in cerebrovascular diseases. Stroke 1972: 3: 456–461.
Pollay M, Fullenwider C, Roberts A, Stevens FA. Effect of mannitol and furosemide on blood-brain osmotic gradient and intracranial pressure. J Neurosurg 1983: 59: 945–950.
Portella G, Cormio M, Cierio G. Continuous cerebral compliance monitoring in severe head injury. Relationship with intracranial pressure and cerebral perfusion pressure. Proceeding XI ICP Symposium, Cambridge 2000: 01–3, page 28
Procaccio F, Menasce G, Sacchi L, et al. Ischemic insult due to manual ventilation in head injured pateints with intracranial hypertension. In Intracranial Pressure VIII. Avezaat CJJ, van Eijndhoven JHM, Maas AIR, Tans J ThJ (eds). Springer Verlag 1993: 583–588.
Proctor HJ, Carins C, Fillipo D, et al. Brain metabolism during increased intracranial pressure as assessed by niroscopy. Surgery 1984: 96: 273–278
Prough DS, Johnson JC, Poole GV, et al. Effects on intracranial pressure of resuscitation from hemorrhagic shock with hypertonic saline versus lactated Ringer's solution. Crit Care Med 1985: 13: 407–410.
Prough DS, Withney JM, Taylor CL, et al. Regional cerebral blood flow following resuscitation from hemorrhagic shock with hypertonic saline: Anesthesiology 1991: 75: 319–327.
Quandt CM, Reyes RA de los. Pharmacologic management of acute intracranial hypertension. Drug Intelligence and Clin Pharmac 1984: 18: 105–112.
Qureshi AI, Wilson DA, Traystman RJ. Treatment of elevated intracranial pressure in experimental intracerebral hemorrhage: Comparison between mannitol and hypertonic saline. Neurosurgery 1999: 44: 1055–1064.
Raabe A, Totzauer R, Meyer O, et al. Reliability of epidural pressure measurement in clinical practice: Behavior of three modern sensors during simultaneous ipselateral intraventricular or intraparenchymal pressure measurement. Neurosurgery 1998: 43: 306–311.
Raabe A, Czosnyka M, Piper I, Seifert V. Monitoring of intracranial compliance: correlation for a change in body position. Acta Neurochir 1999: 141: 31–36.
Raichle ME, Posner JB, Plum F. Cerebral blood flow during and after hyperventilation. Arch Neurol 1970: 23: 394–403
Raphael JH, Chotai R. Effects of cervical collar on cerebrospinal fluid pressure. Anaesthesia 1994: 49: 437–439.
Ravussin P, Archer DP, Tyler JL, et al. Effects of rapid mannitol infusion on cerebral blood volume. J Neurosurg 1986a: 64: 104–113.
Ravussin P, Chiolero R, Buchser E, deTribolet N, Freeman J. CSF pressure changes following mannitol in patients undergoing craniotomy. Anesthesiology 1986b: 65: A303.
Reivich M, Cohen PJ, Greenbaum L. Alterations in the electroencephalogram of awake man produced by hyperventilation: Effects of 100% oxygen at 3 atmospheres (absolute) pressure. Neurology 1966: 16: 304.

Rengachery SS, Roth DA, Andrew NW, Mark VH. Alteration of the blood-brain barrier with hyperventilation. J Neurosurg 1967: 614–618.

Renaudin J, Fewer D, Wilson CB, et al. Dose dependency of decadron in patients with partially excised brain tumors. J Neurosurg 1973: 39: 302–305.

Reulen HJ, Graham R, Spatz M, Klatzo I. Role of pressure gradients and bulk flow in dynamics of vasogenic edema. J Neurosurg 1977: 46: 24–35.

Risberg J, Lundberg N, Ingvar D. Regional cerebral blood volume during acute transient rises of the intracranial pressure (plateau waves). J Neurosurg 1969: 31: 303–310.

Roberts PA, Pollay M, Engles C, et al. Effect on intracranial pressure of furosemide combined with varying doses and administration rates of mannitol. J Neurosurg 1987: 66: 440–446.

Rockoff MA, Marchall LF, Shapiro HM. High-dose barbiturate therapy in humans: A clinical review of 60 patients. Ann Neurol 1979: 6: 194–199.

Ropper MJ, Coley IB. Cerebral perfusion pressure, intracranial pressure, and compliance. Neurology 1982: 32: 1288-1291.

Rosa G, Orfie P, Sanfilippo M, et al. The effects of atrachurium besylate (Tracrium) on intracranial pressure and cerebral perfusion pressure. Anesth Analg 1986: 65: 381–384

Rosenthal RJ, Hiatt JR, Phillips EH, et al. Intracranial pressure. Effect of pneumoperitoneum in a large-animal model. Surg Endosc 1997: 11: 376–380.

Rosenwasser RH, Kleiner LI, Krzeminski JP, Buchheit WA. Intracranial pressure monitoring in the posterior fossa: A preliminary report. J Neurosurg 1989: 71: 503–505.

Rosner MJ, Becker DP. Origin and evolution of plateau waves, experimental observations and a theoretical model. J Neurosurg 1984: 60: 312–324.

Rosner MJ, Coley IB. Cerebral perfusion pressure, intracranial pressure, and head elevation. J Neurosurg 1986: 65: 636–641.

Rosner MJ, Coley I. Cerebral perfusion pressure: A hemodynamic mechanism of mannitol and postmannitol hemogram. Neurosurgery 1987: 21: 147–156.

Rosner MJ. Cerebral perfusion pressure: Link between intracranial pressure and systemic circulation. In: Wood JH (ed) Cerebral Blood Flow, Physiology and Clinical Aspects. McGraw-Hill Book Company, 1987: 425–448

Rosner MJ, Elias KG, Coley I. Prospective, randomized trial of THAM therapy in severe brain injury: Preliminary results. In: Intracranial Pressure VII. Hoff JT, Betz AL (eds). Springer Verlag 1989: 611–615.

Rosomoff HL, Holaday DA. Cerebral blood flow and cerebral oxygen consumption during hypothermia. Am J Physiol 1954: 179: 85–88.

Rosomoff HL. Distribution of intracranial contents with controlled hyperventilation: Implications of neuroanesthesia. Anesthesiology 1963: 24: 640–645

Rudehill A, Lagerkranser M, Lindquist C, Gordon E. Effects of mannitol on blood volume and central hemodynamics in patients undergoing cerebral aneurysm surgery. Anesth Analg 1983: 62: 875–880.

Ryding E, Asgeirsson B, Bertman L, et al. Dihydroergotamine treatment of increased ICP following severe head injury. 5 th Nordic CBF symposium, Lund 1990, abstract

Rudolphi KA, Keil M, Hinze H-J. Effect of theophylline on ischemically induced hippocamapal damage in Mongolian gerbils: a behavioral and histopathological study. J Cereb Blood Flow Metab 1987: 7: 74–81.

Sahuquillo J, Poca M-A, Arribas M, et al. Interhemispheric supratentorial intracranial pressure gradients in head-injured patients: Are they clinically important. J Neurosurg 1999: 90: 16–26.

Sakabe T, Siesjö BK. The effect of indomethacin on blood flow-metabolism couple in the brain under normal, hypercapnic and hypoxic conditions. Acta Physiol Scand 1979: 107: 283–284

Sasaki T, Nakagomi T, Kirino T, et al. Indomethacin ameliorates ischemic neuronal damage in the gerbil hippocampal CA1 sector. Stroke 1988: 19: 1399–1403

Saul TG, Ducker TB. Effect of intracranial pressure monitoring and aggressive treatment on mortality in severe head injury. J Neurosurg 1982: 56: 498–503.

Sawada Y, Sugimoto H, Kobayashi H, et al. Acute tolerance to high-dose barbiturate treatment in patients with severe head injuries. Anesthesiology 1982: 56: 53–54

Scalea TM, Meltz S, Yelon J, et al. Resuscitation of multiple trauma and head injury: Role of crystalloid fluids and inotropes. Crit Care Med 1994: 22: 1610–1615.

Schackford SR, Zhuang J, Schmoker J. Intravenous fluid tonicity: Effect on intracranial pressure, cerebral blood flow, and cerebral oxygen delivery in focal brain injury. J Neurosurg 1992: 76: 91–98

Schell RM, Applegate RL, Cole DJ, Salt, strach and water on the brain. Points of view. J Neurosurg Anesthesiol 1996: 8: 178–182.

Scheller MS, Zornow MH Oh YS. A comparison of the cerebral and hemodynamic effects of mannitol and hypertonic saline in a rabbit model of acute cryogenic brain injury. J Neurosurg Anesthesiol 1991: 3: 291–296

Schettini A, Stahurski B, Young HF. Osmotic and osmotic-loop diuresis in brain surgery. Effects on plasma and CSF electrolytes and ion excretion. J Neurosurg 1982: 56: 679–684.

Schierhout G, Robert I. Mannitol for acute traumatic brain injury. Cochrane Database Syst Rev 2000: 2: CD001049.

Schmidt JF, Waldemar G, Vorstrup S, et al. Computerized analysis of cerebral blood flow autoregulation in humans; Validation of a method for pharmacologic studies. J Cardiovascular Pharmacol 1990: 15: 983–988

Schmidt-Voigt J. Fortschrittliche Frühbehandlung des Schlaganfalles. Med Welt 1951: 20: 1090–1095

Schmoker JD, Zhuang J, Shackford SR. Hypertonic fluid resuscitation improves cerebral oxygen delivery and reduces intracranial pressure after hemorrhagic shock. J Trauma 1991: 31: 1607–1613.

Schneider GH, von H, Franke R, Lanksch WR, Unterberg A. Influence of body position and cerebral perfusion pressure. Acta Neurochir 1993: 59: 107–112.

Schuier FJ, Hossmann KA. Experimental brain infarct in cats II: Ischemic brain edema. Stroke 1980: 11: 593–601.

Schürer L, Dautermann C, Härtl R. et al. Treatment of hemorrhagic hypotension with hypertonic/hyperoncotic solutions: Effects on regional cerebral blood flow and brain surface oxygen tension. Europ Surg Res 1992: 24: 1–12.

Sedzimir CB. Therapeutic hypothermia in cases of head injury. J Neurosurg 1959: 16: 407–414.

Seki H, Ogawa A, Yoshimoto T, Suzuki J. Effect of mannitol on rCBF in canine thalamic ischemia. An experimental study. Brain Nerve (Tokyo) 1981: 33: 1101–1105.

Shapira Y, Davidson E, Weidenfeld Y, et al. Dexamethasone and indomethacin do not affect brain edema following head injury in rats. J Cereb Blood Flow Metab 1988: 8: 395–402

Shapiro HM, Galindo A, Wyte SR, Harris AB. Rapid intraoperative reduction of intracranial pressure with thiopental. Br J Anaesth 1973: 45: 1057–1061.

Shapiro HM, Wyte SR, Loeser J. Barbiturate augmented hypothermia for reduction of persistant intracranial hypertension. J Neurosurg 1974: 40: 90–100.

Shenkin HA, Goluboff B, Haft H. The use of mannitol for the reduction of intracranial pressure in intracranial surgery. J Neurosurg 1962: 19: 897–901.

Shigeno S, Fritschka E, Shigeno T, Brock M Effects of indomethacin on rCBF during and after focal cerebral ischemia in the cat. Stroke 1985: 16: 235–242.

Shima K, Marmarou A. Effect of posttraumatic hypoventilation. In: Intracranial Pressure VIII. Avezaat CJJ, van Eijndhoven JHM, Maas AIR, Tans J ThJ (eds). Springer Verlag 1993: 476–478.

Shirane R, Weinstein PR. Effect of mannitol on local cerebral blood flow after temporary complete cerebral ischemia in rats. J Neurosurg 1992: 76: 486–492.

Shiozaki T, Sugimoto H, Taneda M. et al. Effect of mild hypothermia on uncontrollable intracranial hypertension after severe head injury. J Neurosurg 1993: 79: 363–368.

Shohami E, Shapira Y, Sidi A, Cotev S. Head injury induces increased prostaglandin synthesis in rat brain. J Cereb Blood Flow Metab 1987: 7: 58–63

Shokunbi MT, Gelb AW, Peerless SJ, et al. An evaluation of the effect of lidocaine in experimental focal cerebral ischemia Stroke 1986: 17: 962–966.

Shokunbi MT, Gelb AW, Miller DJ, Wu XM. A continuous infusion of lidocaine protects in temporary focal cerebral ischemia. Anesthesiology 1987: 67: A580.

Sidi A, Cotev S, Hadani M, et al. Long-term barbiturate infusion to reduce intracranial pressure. Critical Care Medicin 1983: 11: 478–481.

Silvia RC, Slizgi GR, Ludens JH, Tang AH. Protection from ischemic-induced cerebral edema in the rat by U-50488H, a kappa opioid receptor agonist. Brain Res 1987: 403: 52–57.

Skinhøj E, Paulson OB. The mechanism of action of aminophylline upon vascular disorders. Acta Neurol Scand 1970: 46: 129–140

Skinhøj E, Høedt-Rasmussen K, Paulson OB, Lassen NA. Regional cerebral blood flow and its regulation in patients with transient focal cerebral ischemia. Neurology (Minneap.) 1970: 20: 485–493

Skippen P, Sear M, Poskitt K, et al. Effect of hyperventilation on regional cerebral blood flow in head-injured children. Crit Care Med 1997: 25: 1402–1409.

Sklar FH, Beyer CW, Ramanathan M, Clark WK. The effects of furosemide on CSF dynamics in patients with pseudotumor cerebri. In: Intracranial Pressure IV. Shulman K, Marmarou A, Miller JD, Becker DP, Hochwald GM, Brock M (eds); Springer Verlag, Berlin, Heidelberg, New York 1980: 660–663.

Slocum HC, Hayes GW, Laezman BL. Ventilator technique of anesthesia for neuroanesthesia. Anesthesiology 1961: 22: 143–145

Smedena RJ, Gaab MR, Hesiler HE. A conparison study between mannitol and glycerol therapy in reducing intracranial pressure. In Intracranial Pressure VIII. Avezaat CJJ, van Eijndhoven JHM, Maas AIR, Tans J ThJ (eds). Springer Verlag 1993: 605–608.

Soloway M, Nadel W, Albin MS, White RJ. The effect of hyperventilation on subsequent cerebral infarction. Anesthesiology 1968: 29: 975–980.

Soloway M, Moriarty G, Fraser JG, White RJ. Effect of delayed hyperventilation on experimental cerebral infarction. Neurology 1971: 21: 479–485.

Steen PA, Milde JH, Michenfelder JD. No barbiturate protection in a dog model of complete cerebral ischaemia Ann Neurol 1979: 5: 343–349.

Stephan H, Sonntag H, Schenk HD, Kohlhausen S. Einfluss von disoprivan (Propofol) auf die Durchblutung und Sauerstoffverbrauch des Gehirns and die CO_2 Reaktivität der Hirngefässe beim Menschen. Anaesthetist 1987: 36: 60–65.

Stewart L, Bullock R, Rafferty C, et al. Propofol sedation in severe head injury fails to control high ICP but reduces brain metabolism. Acta Neurochir 1994 [suppl] 60: 544–546.

Stocchetti N, Paparella A, Bridelli F, et al. Cerebral venous oxygen saturation studied with bilateral samples in the internal jugular veins. Neurosurgery 1994: 34: 38–43.

Strandgaard S, Olesen J, Skinhøj E, Lassen NA. Autoregulation of brain circulation in severe arterial hypertension. Br Med J 1973: 1: 507–510

Stullken AH, Milde JH, Michenfelder JD, Tinker JH. The nonlinear responses of cerebral metabolism to low concentrations of halothane, enflurane, isoflurane and thiopental. Anesthesiology 1977: 46: 28–34.

Sugiara K, Hayama N, Tachisawa T, et al. Intracranial pressure monitoring by a subdurally placed silicone catheter. Technical note. Neurosurgery 1985: 16: 241–244.

Sundberg G, Messeter K, Nordström CH, Söderström S. Intracerebral versus intraventricular pressure recording. In: Intracranial Pressure VI. Miller JD, Teasdale GM, Rowan JO, et al. (eds), Springer Verlag 1986: 187–192.

Sustch G, Rubinstein EH. Lidocaine accelerates recovery of brain electrical activity after 3 minutes of complete ischaemia in the rabbit. J Neurosurg Anesthesiol 1991: 3: 124–131.

Sutherland G, Lesiuk H, Bose R, Sima AAF. Effect of mannitol, nimodipine, and indomethacin singly or in combination on cerebral ischaemia in rats. Stroke 1988: 19: 571–578.

Suzuka T, Mabe H, Nagai H. Role of arachidonic acid metabolites on development of ischemic cerebral edema in rat middle cerebral artery occlusion. J Cereb Blood Flow Metab 1989: 9: suppl 1, S 89

Symon L. Regional cerebrovascular responses to acute ischaemia in normocapnia and hypercapnia. J Neurol Neurosurg Psychiat 1970: 33: 756–762

Symon L, Branston NM, Chikovani O. Ischemic brain edema following middle cerebral artery occlusion in baboons: relationship between regional cerebral water concent and blood flow at 1 and 2 hours. Stroke 1979: 10: 184–191

Taché Y, Maeda-Hagiwara M, Turkelson CM Central nervous system action of corticotropin-releasing factor to inhibit gastric emptying in rats. Am J Physiol 1987: 253: G241–G245

Takagi H, Tanaka M, Ohwada T, Tomonaga F. Pharmacokinetic analysis of mannitol in relation to the decrease of ICP. In Intracranial Pressure VIII. Avezaat CJJ, van Eijndhoven JHM, Maas AIR, Tans J ThJ (Eds). Springer Verlag 1993: 596–600.

Tanaka A, Tomonaga M. Effect of mannitol on cerebral blood flow and microcirculation during experimental middle cerebral artery occlusion. Surg Neurol 1987: 28: 189–195.

Thilmann J, Zeumer H. Untersuchungen zur Behandlung des Hirnödems mit hohen Dosen Furosemid. Dtsch med Wschr 1974: 99: 932–935.

Todd MM, Tommasino C, Moore S. Cerebral effects of isovolemic hemodilution with a hypertonic solution. J Neurosurg 1985: 63: 944–948
Todd NV, Picozzi P, Crockard A, Russell RR Reperfusion after cerebral ischemia: Influence of duration of ischemia. Stroke 1986: 17: 460–466
Troupp H. Intraventricular pressure in patients with severe brain injuries. J Trauma 1967: 7: 875–883
Tsuji T, Chiba S. Responses of isolated canine and simian basilar arteries to thiopentone by a newly designed pharmacological method for measuring vascular responsiveness. Acta Neurochir 1986: 80: 57–61
Tsuji T, Chiba S. Mechanism of vascular responsiveness to barbiturates in isolated and perfused canine basilar arteries. Neurosurgery 1987: 21: 161–166
Uihlein A, MacCarty CS, Michenfelder JD, et al. Deep hypothermia and surgical treatment of intracranial aneurysms. Am Med Ass 1966: 195: 639–641.
Urlesberger B, Muller W, Ritschi E, Reiterer F. The influence of head position on the intracranial pressure in preterm infants with posthemorrhagic hydrocephalus. Childs Nerv Syst 1991: 7: 85–87.
Vane DW, Shiffer M, Grosfeld JL, Hall P Reduced lower esophageal sphincter (LES) pressure after acute and chronic brain injury. J Pediatr Surgery 1982: 17: 960–964.
Vapalahti M, Troupp H, Heiskanen O. Extremely severe brain injuries treated with hyperventilation and ventricular drainage. In: Cerebral Blood Flow. Brock M, Fieschi C, Ingvar DH, Lassen NA, Schurmann K (eds). Springer Verlag, Berlin, Heidelberg, New York 1969: 266-267
Vassar MJ, Fischer RP, OBrien PE. A multicenter trial for resuscitation of injured patients with 7.5% sodium chloride. Arch Surg 1993: 128: 1003–1013.
Videtta W, Villarejo F, Cohen M, et al. Effects of PEEP on ICP and cerebral perfusion pressure. Proceeding XI ICP Symposium, Cambridge 2000, O15–1, page 114.
Voldby B, Enevoldsen EM, Jensen FT. Regional cerebral blood flow, intraventricular pressure, and cerebral metabolism in patients with ruptured intracranial aneurysms. J Neurosurg 1985: 62: 48–58
Voldby B, Enevoldsen EM, Jensen FT. Cerebrovascular reactivity in patients with ruptured intracranial aneurysms. J Neurosurg 1985: 62: 59–67
Vourc'h G. Continuous cerebrospinal fluid drainage by indwelling spinal catheter. Br J Anaesth 1963: 35: 118–120.
Vries JK, Becker DP, Young HF. A subdural screw for monitoring intracranial pressure. J Neurosurg 1973: 39: 416.
Waagstein L, Haljamäe H, Ricksten SE, Sahlman L. Effect of hypertonic saline on myocardial function and metabolism in nonischemic and ischemic isolated owrking hearts. Crit Care Med 1995: 23: 1890–1897.
Ward JD, Becker DP, Miller JD, et al. Failure of prophylactic barbiturate coma in the treatment of severe head injury. J Neurosurg 1985: 62: 383–388.
Warner DS, Godersky JC, Smith M-L. Failure of pre-ischaemic lidocaine administration to ameliorate global ischaemic brain damage in the rat. Anesthesiology 1988: 68: 73–78.
Waschke KF, Albrecht DM, van Ackern K, Kuschinsky W. Coupling between local cerebral blood flow and metabolism after hypertonic/hyperoncotic fluid resuscitation from hemorrhage in conscious rats. Analg Anesth 1996: 82: 52–60.
Watanaba T, Yoshimoto T, Ogawa A, et al. The effect of mannitol in preserving the development of cerebral infarction. An electron microscopic investigation. Neurol Surg (Tokyo) 1979: 7: 859–866.
Wayenberg JL, Raftopoulos C, Vermeylen D, Pardou A. Non-invasive measurement of ICP in the newborn and the infant: The Rotterdam Teletransducer. Arch Dis Child 1993: 69: 493–497.
Wayenberg JL. Non-invasive measurement of intracranial pressure in neonates and infants: Experience with the Rotterdam teletransducer. Acta Neurochir 1998 (suppl) 71: 70–73.
Wechsler RE, Kleiss LM, Kety SS. The effect of intravenous administrated aminophylline on cerebral circulation and metabolism in man. J Clin Invest 1954: 29: 28–30
Weiss KL, Wax MK, Haydon RC, et al. Intracranial pressure changes during bilateral radical neck dissections. Head Neck 1993: 15: 546–552.
Weiss MH, Nulsen FE. The effect of glucocorticoids on CSF flow in dogs. J Neurosurg 1970: 32: 452–458.
Wennmalm Å, Eriksson S, Wahren J. Effect of indomethacin on basal and carbon dioxide stimulated cerebral blood flow in man. Clin Phys 1981:1: 227–234
White PF, Schlobohm RM, Pitts LH, Lindauer JM. A randomized study of drugs for preventing increases in intracranial pressure during endotracheal suctioning. Anesthesiology 1982: 57: 242–244.
White RJ, Albin MS, Verdura J, Locke GE. Differential extracorporal hypothermic perfusion of and circulatory arrest to the human brain. Med Res Engineering 1967: 6: 18–24.
White RJ. Preservation of cerebral function during circulatory arrest and resuscitation: Hypothermic protective considerations. Resuscitation 1972: 1: 107–115.
Whitley JM, Prough DS, Lamb AK, et al. Regional cerebral blood flow following resuscitation from hemorrhagic shock in dogs with a subdural mass. Anesthesiology 1988: 69 [suppl] A 539
Whitley JM. Prough DS, Taylor CL, et al. Cerebrovascular effects of small volume resuscitation from hemorrhagic shock: Comparison of hypertonic saline and concentrated hydroxyethyl starch in dgos. J Neurosurg Anesthesiol 1991: 3: 47–55.
Williams A, Coyne SM. Effects of neck position on intracranial pressure. Am J Crit Care 1993: 2: 68–71.
Wise BL, Chater N. The value of hypertonic mannitol solution in decreasing brain mass and lowering cerebrospinal-fluid pressure. J Neurosurg 1962: 19: 1038–1043.
Wisner DH, Schuster L, Quinn C. Hypertonic saline resuscitation of head injury: Effects on cerebral water content. J Trauma 1990: 30: 75–78.
Wolf AL, Levi L, Marmarou A, et al. A prospective randomized clinical trial of tromethamine (THAM) and its effect upon outcome in severe head injury. In Intracranial Pressure VIII. Avezaat CJJ, van Eijndhoven JHM, Maas AIR, Tans J ThJ (eds). Springer Verlag 1993: 615–619.
Wolfla C, Luerssen TG, Bowman RM, Putty TK. Brain tissue pressure gradients created by expanding frontal epidural mass lesion. J Neurosurg 1996: 84: 642–647.
Worthley IGL, Cooper DJ, Jones N. Treatment of resistant intracranial hypertension with hypertonic saline. J Neurosurg 1988: 68: 478–481
Yano M, Nishiyama H, Yokota H, et al. Effect of lidocaine on ICP response to endotracheal suctioning. Anesthesiology 1986: 64: 651–653.
Yano M, Ikeda Y, Kobayashi S, Otsuka T. Intracranial pressure in head-injured patients with various intracranial lesions

is identical throughout the supratentorial intracranial compartment. Neurosurgery 1987: 21: 688–692.

Yano M, Kobayashi S, Otsuka T. Useful ICP monitoring with subarachnoid catheter method in severe head injuries. J Trauma 1988: 28: 476–480.

Yau YH, Piper IR, Clutton RE, Whittle IR. Experimental evaluation of the Spiegelberg intracranial pressure and intracranial compliance monitor. Technical note. J Neurosurg 2000: 93: 1072–1077.

Yen MH, Lee SH. Effects of cyclooxygenase and lipoxygenase inhibitors on cerebral edema induced by freezing lesions in rats. Europ J Pharmacol 1987: 144: 369–373.

Yoo DS, Kim DS, Park CK, et al. Ventricular pressure monitoring during the decompressive craniectomy. Proceeding ICP XI Symposium, Cambridge, 2000, P11–5, page 230.

Yoshida A, Shima T, Okada Y, Yamada T. Effects of postural changes on epidural pressure in patients with serious intracranial lesions. Intracranial Pressure VIII, Avezaat CJJ, van Eijndhoven JHM, Maas AIR, Tans JTJ (eds) 1991: 433–436.

Yoshida A, Shima T, Okada Y, Yamada T, Kurino H. Effects of postural changes on epidural pressure and cerebral perfusion pressure in patients with serious intracranial lesions. In Intracranial Pressure VIII. Avezaat CJJ, van Eijndhoven JHM, Maas AIR, Tans J ThJ (eds). Springer Verlag 1993: 4336436.

Yoshida K, Marmarou A. Effects of tromethamine and hyperventilation on brain injury in the cat. J Neurosurg 1991: 74: 87–96.

Zabolotny WM, Zaworski W, Czosnyka M, et al. Method for real time estimation of intracranial pressure from blood flow velocity and arterial blood pressure. Proceeding XI ICP symposium, Cambridge 2000, 02–5, page 36.

Zornow MH. Hypertonic saline as a safe and efficacious treatment of intracranial hypertension. J Neurosurg Anesthesiology 1996: 8: 175–177.

Inhalation anaesthetics

During the last fifty years the attitude concerning the use of inhalation agents in neuroanaesthesia has changed dramatically. Before experimental and human studies of ICP and CBF were available, volatile anaesthetics, including ether, cyclopropane and trichlorethylene were used routinely, and these agents were praised for the stability of cerebral haemodynamics. With the introduction of halothane in the fifties a new era was introduced, where halothane was used for all intracranial surgical procedures. However, the impact of experimental and human studies in the sixties showing that halothane increased ICP and CBF, together with studies of neurolept anaesthesia and intravenous hypnotics (barbiturate, althesin, etomidate, propofol) indicating a stabilised ICP, and a fall in CBF and $CMRO_2$ resulted in warning against and omission of halothane. During these years neuroanaesthesia was predominantly performed with intravenous hypnotics supplemented with central analgesics and nitrous oxide. In the seventies, the introduction of isoflurane changed the neuroanaesthetic practice. Isoflurane, in comparison with halothane, increases ICP and CBF much lesser, whereas the suppression of $CMRO_2$ was much more pronounced. During the last twenty years, nitrous oxide has been studied extensively, and warnings have been raised because of its cerebral stimulating effects. Total intravenous anaesthesia with propofol or midazolam, supplemented with central analgesics has been introduced. Simultaneously, the new inhalation agents, sevoflurane and desflurane have been studied experimentally and clinically. Both drugs act more or less like isoflurane as regard cerebral circulation and metabolism. The advantages of these drugs include the fast induction of anaesthesia and shortened emergency. During the years to come further clinical studies will answer the question whether these agents have a place in neurosurgical anaesthesia.

Another issue concerning inhalation agents is their ability to induce brain protection. This issue was first analysed in the mouse hypoxia model, and later in experimental studies of focal and global ischaemia. Although inhalation agents potential brain protective effect has been clarified experimentally, clinical studies until now have not proved any effect.

Whether the effects of anaesthetics upon cerebral circulation, metabolism, brain protection and anaesthetic action are discussed, the principle biomolecular effect is thought to be mediated through ion gate and cellular enzyme systems. As a consequence, the effect of volatile anaesthetics upon ion gates and cellular enzyme systems is described.

Effects of volatile anaesthetics on ion gates and cellular enzyme systems

According to Lynch and Pacrazio (1994) volatile anaesthetics appear to elicit two neurobiologic actions independently generated by (1) an stereoselective activation of GABA-gated chloride receptor channels (Quinlan et al. 1995) and (2) inhibition of presynaptic Ca^{2+} influx. *In vivo* studies of guinea pig synaptosomes indicate that volatile anaesthetics decrease $[Ca^{2+}]_i$ in a manner consistent with inhibition of Ca^{2+} entry, possibly by specific voltage-gated neuronal calcium channels (Miao et al. 1995), and inhibit multiple voltage-gated (type T,L and N) calcium currents in hippocampal pyramidal neurones (Study 1994). Contrary to this concept other studies indicate that volatile anaesthetics increase $[Ca^{2+}]_i$. Thus, it has been proven that 1 MAC isoflurane increases $[Ca^{2+}]_i$ in cortical neurones (Bickler et al. 1994). The same finding has been demonstrated during halothane, isoflurane and xenon in mouse cortical neurones (Franks et al. 1998) Studies of rat cortical brain slices furthermore indicate that isoflurane and halothane reversibly increase $[Ca^{2+}]_i$ in isolated neurones, and that this increase is caused primarily by release from intracellular stores (Kindler et al. 1999).

Other mechanisms include voltage-dependent sodium channels Rehberg et al. 1996). One or more of these mechanisms are supposed to generate anaesthetic effect. On hypothetical basis other mechanisms, however, have been proposed. G-protein provides receptor-effector coupling at the membrane surface for several intercellular transmitters including opioids and α_2-adrenergic agents. The protein kinase C enzyme family modulates functions on both GABA receptors (Kellenberger et al. 1992) and Ca^{2+} channels (Slater et al. 1993); and protein kinase C inhibition lowers anaesthetic requirements (Firestone et al. 1993). Isoflurane and halothane alter the Ca^{2+} binding properties of calmodulin. However this interaction is complex. A biphasic effect was observed both for halothane and for isoflurane, Calmodulin undergoes a conformational shift when binding Ca^{2+}, exposing several hydrophobic residues (Levin and Blanck 1995).

$GABA_A$ receptor inhibition

Electrophysiological studies have demonstrated that inhalation anaesthetics enhance the duration of GABA-induced chloride currents in cultured hippocampus neurones (Jones et al. 1992), and that these agents prolong the decay phase of inhibitory postsynaptic currents in pyramidal neurones in brain slices (Lukatch and MacIver 1997, Banks and Pearce 1999). In other studies it has been shown that volatile anaesthetics differential enhance $GABA_A$ receptor-mediated synaptic inhibition, suggesting that hippocampal interneurones circuits are depressed by volatile anaesthetics (Nishikawa and MacIver 2001).

Excitatory amino acids

Glutamate is the most ubiquitous excitatory neurotransmitter in the central nervous system. Glutamate, that is released from the presynapnic terminals as a transmitter, should be scavenged to terminate synaptic transmission. The presynaptic terminals themselves can uptake a part of the glutamate from the synaptic cleft. However, a large part of glutamate is removed by astrocytes. Astrocytes play an important role for termination of excitatory glutamatergic neurotransmission. In the presence of halothane 0–4% cultured astrocytes increase the glutamate uptake, and potentially attenuate excitatory synaptic transmission in the central nervous system (Miyazaki et al. 1997).

Nitric oxide mechanisms

The vascular endothelium synthesises and releases nitric oxide (NO), which stimulates cytosolic guanyl cyclase to increase GMP (cGMP) concentrations within vascular smooth muscle cells, resulting in vasorelaxation. Inhibition of nitric oxide synthase (NOS) has been reported to be antinociceptive, and to reduce the threshold of general anaesthesia. Volatile anaesthetics, including halothane and isoflurane, attenuate agonist-stimulated, endothelium-dependent NO-cGMP pathways (Stone and Johns 1989, Toda et al. 1992, Nakamura et al. 1994). Inhibition of NOS and soluble guanylate cyclase dose-dependently decrease the MAC values of halothane and isoflurane (Johns et al. 1992, Pajewski et al. 1996, Pajewski et al. 1998). An acute selective inhibition of neuronal NOS also decreases sevoflurane MAC and cerebellar cGMP concentrations in mice. However, during long-term neuronal NOS inhibition there was a dissociation between the decrease in sevoflurane MAC concentration and the cerebellar cGMP concentration, suggesting that cGMP-independent compensatory mechanisms may occur when NOS in chronically inhibited (Ichinose et al. 1998).

Cyclic GMP dependent protein kinases also serve as major effectors for cGMP in the vascular and nervous system. Thus, cyclic GMP-dependent protein kinase Iα inhibitor markedly reduces MAC for isoflurane, but also completely blocks the NO-induced increase in isoflurane MAC, which suggests that cyclic GMP-dependent protein kinase Iα may mediate the action for the NO-cGMP pathway in anaesthetic mechanisms at the spinal cord level (Tao et al. 2000).

Noradrenergic noncholinergic nerves play a role in the regulation of vascular tone in cerebral arteries via the nitric oxide-cGMP pathway. It has been demonstrated, however, that in the isolated canine cerebral arteries, halothane and isoflurane inhibit the relaxation caused by nonadrenergic noncholinergic nerve stimulation (Yamamoto et al. 1998). The volatile anaesthetics influence nitric oxide production differently. It has been demonstrated that nitric oxide production in rat cerebellar slices is enhanced by isoflurane, but not by halothane (Rengasamy et al. 1997). These findings have been restated by microdialysis study (Loeb et al. 1998).

Effects upon plasma membrane Ca^{2+}-ATPase

In vitro studies indicate that halothane, isoflurane, xenon and nitrous oxide at clinically relevant partial pressure diminished plasma membrane Ca^{2+}-ATPase activity in cerebral synaptic plasma membranes (Horn et al. 1992, Franks et al. 1995a). *In vivo* study with halothane confirms this observation (Franks et al. 1995b).

Effect upon K^+ channels

One of the potential mechanisms for arterial vasodilation is enhanced K^+ efflux resulting in an increased opening frequency of membrane K^+ channels. Halothane and isoflurane, however, suppress the activity of K^+ channels in canine cerebral arterial cells (Eskinder et al. 1995). Another study in pentobarbital-anaesthetised dogs indicate that the vasodilation of cerebral pial vessels induced by isoflurane and sevoflurane appears to be mediated, at least in part, via activation of ADP-sensitive K^+ channels (Iida et al. 1998).

Halothane, experimental studies

CVR, CBF and $CMRO_2$

In animal experiments halothane induces a decrease in CVR (Harp et al. 1976, Todd and Drummond 1984b), an increase in CBF (McDowall et al. 1963, Theye and Michenfelder 1968a, Smith and Wollman 1972, Smith 1973, Harp et al. 1976, Stullken et al. 1977, Todd and Drummond 1984b, Scheller et al. 1984), and a decrease in $CMRO_2$ (McDowall et al. 1963, Theye and Michenfelder 1968a, Smith 1973, Harp et al. 1976, Stullken et al. 1977, Todd and Drummond 1984b). The changes in CVR and CBF give rise to an increase in CBV and ICP (Fitch and McDowall 1971, DiGiovanni et al. 1974, Drummond et al. 1983a, Todd and Age Drummond 1984b).). The increase in CBF occurs few minutes after induction, and is recorded before any change in CMRO2 (Albrecht et al. 1977).

The increase in CBF is dependent on the age. Thus, the increase in CBF is more pronounced in young animals (Hoffman et al. 1982a).

Nitric oxide (NO)

In vitro studies of cerebral arteries suggest that the halothane-induced vasodilation is partly mediated through a rise in tissue NO by stimulation of guanylate cyclase catalyzing the formation of cyclic guanosine 3.5-monophosphate (cGMP) (Eskinder et al. 1992). This effect is related to the capacity for cGMP to reduce intracellular Ca^{2+} levels (Lincoln et al. 1988). At clinically relevant concentrations, halothane dilates intracerebral arterioles. Dilation is mediated, in part, by neuronally derived nitric oxide, whereas endothelial NO synthase does not play a major role in halothane-induced dilation of hippocampal microvessels (Staunton et al. 2000). Using the closed window technique, a recent study indicated that release of NO produced from L-arginine by NO synthase is an intermittent step in the halothane-induced vasodilation (Koenig et al. 1993), and McHerson et al. (1994) found that NO synthase inhibition prevents the increase in CBF by halothane. Others have found that halothane seems to modify the NO half-life or its activated redox form (Blaise et al. 1994). This observation is in accordance with findings that halothane has an inhibitory effect on cGMP production (Kant et al.1980) and NO production in the brain (Tobin et al. 1994). That volatile anaesthetics cause reversible inhibition of NO production in rat thoracic aorta (Uggeri et al. 1992, Muldoon et al. 1988) and that halothane greatly diminished or eliminated all systemic and regional haemodynamic responses to L-NAME (Sigmon et al. 1995). Discrepancies in results concerning the effect of inhalation agents upon NO pathways are evident. Further work is needed to elucidate this issue.

CBF changes related to time

During halothane administration over several hours a normalisation of CBF occurs, and at the same time a moderate increase in CVR and $CMRO_2$ is observed (Albrecht et al. 1983). According to Warner et al. (1985), this cerebrovascular adaptation to prolonged halothane administration is not related to changes in CSF-pH, which is unchanged. Simultaneous administration of nitrous oxide gives rise to an increase in CBF, and a decrease in CVR

Regional CBF

Halothane induces regional changes in CBF. Related to cardiac output a relative increase in rCBF has been observed in hypothalamus and in the brainstem (Chen et al. 1982). It has been suggested that these regional differences in perfusion play an important role in the regulation of the general circulation during halothane anaesthesia. Other studies using an autoradiographic technique have unveiled regional differences in cerebral glucose utilisation as well. Thus, CMR-glucose decreases relatively more in the occipital lobe, the brain-stem, cerebellar cortex and the anterior commissure (Shapiro et al. 1978). According to Harkin et al. (1997) studies of rat brain slices indicate that both superficially localised pial arterioles and intraparenchymal arterioles are dilated by halothane.

CBF/$CMRO_2$

The dissociation between CBF and $CMRO_2$ which occurs after halothane administration is dose dependent. Thus, an increase in the ratio CBF/$CMRO_2$, indicating a luxury perfusion has repeatedly been observed, and the same observation has been made during enflurane and isoflurane anaesthesia (Smith and Wollman 1972). However, the increase in this ratio during iso-MAC administration of the three anaesthetic agents is most pronounced during halothane anaesthesia (Drummond and Todd 1985).

CPP

Halothane has a negative inotropic effect on the myocardium. This effect together with a decrease in peripheral systemic resistance, are responsible for the decrease in blood pressure. The net result is a decrease in CPP, partly caused by a decrease in MABP and partly owing to the increase in ICP (Jennett et al. 1967). The changes in CBF during halothane induction are dependent on CPP. Thus, during gradual suppression of MABP, an associated decrease in CBF and $CMRO_2$ has been observed (McDowall et al. 1963), and during halothane induced hypotension to MABP 30 mm Hg a 50% decrease in CBF and $CMRO_2$ has been found. These changes are followed by a decrease in saturation of cerebral venous blood (Okuda et al. 1976, Militich et al. 1976), but not by CSF-acidosis. Normalisation of MABP after reduction of the inspiratory concentration of halothane induces an increase in CBF above control level. In this phase the cerebral autoregulation is impaired.

Cerebral autoregulation (CA) and blood-brain barrier (BBB)

Generally, the cerebral autoregulation is impaired or lost, dose dependently, during halothane anaesthesia (Okuda et al. 1976, Miletich et al. 1976, Morita et al. 1977, Albrecht et al. 1983). This impairment is more pronounced during normo- and hypercapnia, but partly or completely normalised during hypocapnia (Miletich et al. 1976). Halothane induced impairment of the cerebral autoregulation is accompanied by a defect blood-brain barrier, and extravasation of protein and water in the extracellular fluid (Forster et al. 1978).

Brain oedema

In animals subjected to cryogenic lesion, halothane in comparison with barbiturates and neurolept anaesthesia induces an increase in the water content in cerebral tissue close to the lesion (Smith and Marque 1976). However, in recent studies with magnetic resonance scanning no difference in the water content has been disclosed (Fuller et al. 1980). In a recent study of cryogenic brain oedema in the rabbit it was found that isoflurane anaesthesia attenuates cerebral oedema compared to fentanyl, thiopental or alpha-chlorose (Murr et al. 1995).

CO_2-reactivity

During halothane anaesthesia, at normal CPP, the CO_2 reactivity is generally preserved (Drummond and Todd 1985). During 1% halothane administration the CO_2 reactivity averages 2 ml/100g/min/mm Hg $PaCO_2$ (Young et al. 1991a). In the same study it was found that halothane is a selective cortical vasodilator compared with isoflurane, but at iso-MAC administration both anaesthetics have similar effect on global CO_2 reactivity. The CO_2 reactivity can be impaired during halothane induced hypotension (Okuda et al. 1976). In rats the intensity of halothane- and hypercapnia-induced cerebral hyperaemia is strain-dependent (Takahashi et al. 1996).

Energy metabolism

At high concentrations of halothane (5–10% inspiratory), a pronounced reduction of $CMRO_2$ has been found. At these high concentrations an increase in lactate, the lactate/pyruvate ratio and a decrease in ATP and phosphocreatine in cerebral tissue occur (Michenfelder et al. 1970, Michenfelder and Theye 1975). Halothane induces an increase in the electrical impedance of the brain, a result which is supposed to be caused by a reversible intracellular translocation of electrically, inactive ions from the extracellular space, possibly caused by an increased binding of cations to proteins (Schettini and Moreshead 1978).

ICP

Halothane gives rise to an increase in ICP (Fitch and McDowall 1971, DiGiovanni et al. 1974, Todd and Drummond 1984b). The increase in ICP is generally accompanied by a fall in CPP, and together these changes impede cerebral circulation, and augment the risks of cerebral ischaemia (Fitch and McDowall 1971). Experimentally, an increase in intracranial pressure gradients between supra- and infratentorial compartments has been observed. These pressure gradients can increase considerably up to 50–60 mm Hg, and are followed by increased impaction at the tentorium and pupillary dilatation (Fitch and McDowall 1971).

Cerebral protection

In the dog the infarct size resulting from MCAO is greatest in animals anaesthetised with halothane compared with dogs undergoing insult while awake or when anaesthetised with pentobarbital (Smith et al. 1974). Studies in primates confirmed this finding (Michenfelder and Milde 1975). Later studies, however, indicate that when brain temperature was maintained normothermic throughout the focal ischaemic insult, a neurological and histological protective effect was observed (Warner et al. 1995). In a later study the same group, however, found that long-term (5 hours) halothane administration after an ischaemic insult did not ameliorate damage from focal cerebral ischaemia (Sarraf-Yadzi et al. 1999). It has been shown that halothane protects against spinal cord injury in the rat. This effect of halothane was equal to that observed with fentanyl, nitrous oxide anaesthesia or spinal lidocaine (Cole et al 1989). In another study, in gerbils, it was demonstrated that halothane causes substantial protection of the CA1 sector of hippocampus after brief episodes of ischaemia, provided that the anaesthesia was continued for at least 45 min into the recirculation period. This effect was found to be equal to that of barbiturates, suggesting that both anaesthetics interfere with the same biochemical or functional events that lead to post-ischaemic neuronal injury (Kuroiwa et al 1989).

In the cat halothane strongly inhibits potassium-evoked spreading depression (SD) (Saito et al. 1995. Focal ischaemia induces SD-like depolarisations in border zones of the ischaemic focus (Nedergaard and Astrup 1986). This ischaemic transient depolarisation is associated with a stepwise deterioration of regional tissue PO_2 probably resulting from lack of compensatory CBF enhancement (Back et al. 1994). In a final stage, it may turn into terminal depolarisation (Graf et al. 1995). Intercellular communication through gap junction is blocked by halothane (Mantz et al. 1993). Compared with α-choralose anaesthetised cats, halothane decreased the number of transient depolarisations and reduced infarct volume in MCAO-induced severe ischaemia (Saito et al. 1997).

GABA

In the brain cells, halothane inhibits GABA (gamma-aminobutyric acid), resulting in an increase in the concentration of GABA in the synapses and inhibition of their function (Cheng et al. 1981). In connection with halothane anaesthesia, the concentration of GABA particularly increases in the pons (Fontenot et al. 1984). In mouse brain halothane at 1% increases the aminosynthesis of neuroactive amino acids including GABA, aspartate, glutamate. In another study, however, 2% halothane decreased the synthesis (Watanabe et al. 1993). Halothane affects the inhibitory GABA-mediated transmitter system in various sites. Firstly, in cortical slices, it reduces the breakdown of GABA, thus potentially increasing its concentration in the synaptic cleft. Secondly, it prolongs the time constant of decay of spontaneous GABA receptor-mediated postsynaptic currents in hippocampal slices through release of intracellular calcium.

Excitatory amino acids

N-methyl-D aspartate (NMDA) receptor antagonists induce heterogeneous changes in glucose utilisation in conscious rats (Nehls et al. 1988). This effect has been found to be markedly modified by halothane anaesthesia (Kurumaji and Mc Culloch 1989). Studies of mouse hippocampal slice indicate that halothane depresses glutamate receptor-mediated excitatory postsynaptic currents, most likely by inhibition of glutamate release (Perouansky et al. 1995).

It has been demonstrated that antagonists of glutamatergic neurotransmission decrease the MAC value for volatile anaesthetic agents (Scheller et al. 1989, McFarlane et al. 1992, Mantz et al. 1992, Koruda et al. 1993). During forebrain ischaemia, which is known to perturb glutamatergic neurotransmission, the MAC value of halothane is not affected. However, anatomical foci for motor responses elicited during MAC determination could be localised at levels caudal to the forebrain (McFarlane et al. 1994).

Dopamine

Several lines of evidence suggest that halothane like isoflurane anaesthesia is associated with changes in extracellular dopamine concentrations in the striatum *in vivo*. An inverse correlation has been reported between the striatal dopamine content and halothane anaesthesia requirements in mice (Segal et al. 1990). In addition, the striatal levels of dopamine or its metabolites measured *in vivo* by microdialysis were increased by clinical halothane and isoflurane concentrations (Stahle et al. 1990, Miyano et al. 1993, Opacka-Juffry et al. 1991). This might be explained in part by blockade of the dopamine carrier by these agents (El-Maghrabi and Eckenhoff 1993). In the rat halothane and isoflurane decrease the NMDA-evoked dopamine release by acting directly at dopamine terminals in striatal slices. This finding supports the involvement of both depression of presynaptic NMDA receptor-mediated responses and enhancement of GABA receptor-mediated responses (Keita et al. 1999).

Cerebrospinal fluid

Considering the increase in ICP effected by halothane, studies by Artru (1983) have shown that resistance to CSF resorption is increased, but CSF production is normal or decreased. The increased resistance to outflow is supposed to be a factor mediating sustained ICP increase after halothane anaesthesia (Artru 1983).

Dose requirement

Studies in rats indicate that neurologic status following head trauma can influence anaesthetic requirement. Thus, the anaesthetic requirement of halothane is reduced in severely injured animals (Shapira et al. 1992).

Halothane, human studies

CBF, CVR and $CMRO_2$

Studies in human support the findings in animal experiments. Thus, a decrease in CVR, a dose-related increase in CBF, and a decrease in $CMRO_2$ have repeatedly been observed (Alexander et al. 1964, Wollman et al. 1964, McHenry et al. 1964, Christensen et al. 1967). In the study by Christensen et al.(1967), 1% halothane in oxygen during normocapnia and maintained MABP increased CBF by 27% and decreased $CMRO_2$ by 26%. However, during normocapnic hypotension a 18% decrease in CBF was observed. These changes are supposed to be caused by impaired cerebral autoregulation as MABP support induced a considerable increase in CBF. In comparison Iso-MAC studies of halothane, enflurane and isoflurane during normocapnia and MABP support have shown a dose related increase in CBF with all three anaesthetics. However, the increase in CBF during halothane already occurs during 0.6 MAC halothane, while the increase in CBF by enflurane and isoflurane is only registered with 1.6 MAC enflurane or isoflurane (Murphy et al. 1974). Studies during craniotomy using topical application of 133-Xe on the cerebral cortex close to cerebral tumours have supported these findings (Eintrei et al. 1985).

ICP and CPP

The increase in CBF might induce critical intracranial hypertension, and a decrease in CPP (S¢ndergård 1961, Marx et al. 1962, Jennett et al. 1967, Jennett et al. 1969, Shapiro et al. 1972a, Adams et al. 1972). These dangerous changes in ICP and CPP are frequently observed during induction of anaesthesia with halothane, especially during normo- and hypercapnia. In contrast, the increase in ICP to some extent can be prevented if hypocapnia is applied before administration of halothane (Adams et al. 1972). The attenuating effect of hypocapnia on ICP hypertension is most pronounced if hypocapnia is applied about 5 min before halothane administration (Misfeldt et al. 1974).

Studies with Doppler technique

With transcranial Doppler sonography it has been demonstrated that halothane causes an increase in vessel diameter measured in the middle cerebral artery (Schregel et al. 1992) and in the large basal cerebral arteries (Schregel et al. 1991).

Infants

In preterm neonates without neurological diseases and subjected to halothane, isoflurane, fentanyl or ketamine anaesthesia ICP decreases slightly (Friesen et al. 1987). The authors suggest that the difference between these results and those concerning studies of ICP in adults is due to compliance of the neonate's open-sutured cranium.

CBF/$CMRO_2$ and $AVDO_2$

In studies of the arterio-venous oxygen content difference during anaesthesia with neurolept anaesthesia or an anaesthetic procedure with halothane 0.45–0.9% supplemented with nitrous oxide as described by Madsen et al. (1987), it has been shown that these two procedures generally provoke a decrease in $AVDO_2$ (Engberg et al. 1989). Clinically controlled studies with subcutaneous application of plain bupivacaine in the scalp indicate, that the increase in MABP, and the decrease in AVDO2 can be prevented by regional analgesia of the scalp before incision (Engberg et al. 1990).

CO_2-reactivity

The CO_2 reactivity is preserved during halothane anaesthesia (Alexander et al. 1964), also when space-occupying lesions are present (Eintrei et al. 1985, Madsen et al. 1987a). In healthy children subjected to halothane 1 MAC anaesthesia the CO_2 -reactivity is intact (Leon and Bissonnette 1991). During carotid endarterectomy the CO_2 reactivity during isoflurane or halothane administration was found to average 4.8 and 5.2%/mm Hg $PaCO_2$ respectively (Young et al. 1991b).

Cerebral autoregulation (CA)

The cerebral autoregulation is generally impaired in patients with space-occupying lesion (brain tumours, severe head injury etc). During craniotomy the autoregulation is especially challenged during incision and after extubation, where blood pressure increases occur.

Craniotomy

During craniotomy for cerebral tumours in pentobarbitone induction, and maintenance of anaesthesia with fentanyl, nitrous oxide 67%, halothane 0.5% and moderate hypocapnia, an associated decrease in CBF and $CMRO_2$ has been observed (Astrup et al. 1984). The same associated decrease has been observed after thiopentone induction, supplemented with nitrous oxide 67% and halothane 0.45% when hypocapnia has been applied. During these conditions only minimal increase in CBF was found when the halothane concentration was increased from 0.45% to 0.9% (Madsen et al. 1987a). Considering the values of CBF and $CMRO_2$ obtained during the two investigations, they are identical to those obtained during neurolept anaesthesia (Cold et al. 1988). However, comparative studies of the arterio-venous oxygen content difference ($AVDO_2$) during halothane and neurolept anaesthesia with the same degree of hypocapnia, have shown that the $AVDO_2$ is maintained at lower levels during halothane anaesthesia. As $AVDO_2$ indicates the ratio CBF/$CMRO_2$, these dynamic studies are indirect evidence of the presence of a relative luxury perfusion elicited during halothane anaesthesia (Engberg et al. 1989).

As indicated before, animal experiments supported by human investigations have attenuated the reputation of halothane in neurosurgical practice, especially in patients with space-occupying lesions (Jennett et al. 1969, Gordon 1970, Fitch and McDowall 1971). However, clinical studies of MABP, CPP, ICP, CBF and $CMRO_2$ during halothane anaesthesia show that halothane, like isoflurane, under controlled circumstances and during the application of hypocapnia, can be used during neurosurgical intervention for small space-occupying processes (Astrup et al. 1984, Madsen et al. 1987a). As the CO_2 reactivity and the metabolic effect of thiopental in doses of 4–5 mg/kg under these circumstances are preserved, perioperative complications such as brain prolapse or oedema can to some extent be controlled by intensifying the hypocapnia, or by intravenous injection of small doses of barbiturates (Astrup et al. 1984, Madsen et al. 1987a). Furthermore, clinical practice indicates that mannitol in doses of 0.5–1 gr./kg or furosemide will produce shrinkage of the brain before or after opening of the dura

Hyperventilation

Hyperventilation is generally advocated to patients subjected to neurosurgical procedures for space-occupying lesions. In clinical practice the lower limit of hypocapnia is supposed to be 2.7–3.3 kPa (20–25 mm Hg)(Gordon 1974). Below this level jugular venous saturation is low, and risk of cerebral ischaemia must be considered. Animal experiments have shown that $PaCO_2$ below this limit does not reduce ICP further. On the contrary, the CPP might be reduced, and ICP increases if these limits are exceeded owing to an increase in CVP and a decrease in venous blood flow to the heart (Kitahata et al. 1971). In clinical practice moderate hypocapnia to $PaCO_2$ ranging from 3.6–4.0 is advocated (Frost 1984).

Barbiturate

Injection of thiopentone as a bolus doses during halothane anaesthesia, induces a further decrease in $CMRO_2$. Thus, thiopentone in doses of 4–6 mg/kg will reduce $CMRO_2$ to values of 1.7 ml O_2/100g/min, which is close to the maximal suppression of $CMRO_2$ obtained by barbiturates alone (Astrup et al. 1984). As experimental studies indicate that barbiturates have a brain-protective effect, thiopentone supplemented general anaesthesia with halothane has been used in surgery for cerebral aneurysms. Barbiturate given in doses of 10–20 mg/kg during craniotomy for aneurysms results in delayed postoperative recovery and postoperative respiratory insufficiency, which make postoperative artificial ventilation necessary (Bendtsen et al. 1984, Belapavlovic et al. 1985). Controlled studies, however, concerning the beneficial effects of barbiturates have not been performed.

Clinical application

Animal experiments and clinical research concerning the effect of halothane on cerebral circulation and ICP, have to some extent resulted in avoidance of halothane in neuroanaesthesiological practice, especially in patients with space-occupying cerebral diseases (Jennett et al. 1969, Fitch and McDowall 1971, Gordon 1970). Other studies support this view, especially comparative studies of halothane, enflurane and isoflurane have shown that during Iso-MAC concentrations of these anaesthetics, the increase in ICP is dose-dependent and most pronounced during halothane (Todd and Drummond 1984b). The same study indicates that the increase in ICP is related to the increase in CBF. Furthermore, experimental studies in cats have shown that the tendency to brain prolapse during craniotomy is considerably higher during Iso-MAC halothane anaesthesia (Drummond et al. 1983a).

Repeated experimental as well as human studies have shown that halothane elicits a dose-related increase in CBV, CBF and ICP, and a decrease in CVR,

$CMRO_2$, CMR-glucose and CPP. These results, combined with studies indicating an impairment of cerebral autoregulation, and the brain-blood barrier with risks of a development of cerebral oedema, have discredited the use of halothane in surgery for space-occupying intracranial diseases.

The risks of intracranial hypertension and decrease in CPP are related to the concentration of halothane used, the age of the patient and the haemodynamic stability. The changes in cerebral circulation, are to some extent modified by the application of hypocapnia, barbiturate induction and a sufficient doses of analgesic. Thus, clinical studies in selected patients subjected to craniotomy for small space-occupying lesions like tumours, have shown that halothane in the concentration of 0.5–0.9%, combined with nitrous oxide and fentanyl safely can be used, and peroperative complications such as brain prolapse or oedema can be controlled by the use of intensified hyperventilation, intravenous bolus doses of thiopentone, and infusion of mannitol and furosemide. Nevertheless, presently halothane is hardly used in neuroanaesthesia, and has been replaced by the newer inhalation anaesthetics, isoflurane, sevoflurane and desflurane.

Enflurane, experimental studies

CBF and $CMRO_2$

In animal experiments enflurane induces a dosage dependent increase in CBF (Michenfelder and Cucchiara 1974, Takasaki 1974). However, if arterial pressure is not maintained, a fall in CBF has been observed (Sakabe 1975). $CMRO_2$ is decreased dose-dependently by enflurane (Stullken et al. 1977). At concentrations of enflurane above 2.2% in dogs a 34% decrease in $CMRO_2$ occurred. At higher concentrations of enflurane, however, no further decrease in $CMRO_2$ was observed (Michenfelder and Cucchiara 1974).

Combined with nitrous oxide

In rats subjected to 1.2 MAC combination of nitrous oxide and enflurane a biphasic metabolic response was observed. Local cerebral glucose utilisation was activated in sensory input structures and components of the limbic system, when nitrous oxide was increased from 0 to 30%, with a relative depression in metabolism when nitrous oxide was further increased from 30 to 60%. At all spinal cord levels a homogeneous increase in metabolism was observed when enflurane was replaced by 0–30% nitrous oxide, with a return to control when nitrous oxide was further increased from 30–60% (Cole and Shapiro 1989).

ICP

At normal ICP in dogs enflurane only increases ICP slightly if at all (Boop and Knight 1978, Hans et al. 1980). However, a significant increase in ICP was observed in animals with intracranial hypertension (Boop and Knight 1978), but the increase in ICP was smaller compared with halothane (Hans et al. 1980).

CSF formation

In cats the degree of brain protrusion found during craniotomy was more pronounced during halothane, compared to enflurane and isoflurane anaesthesia (Drummond et al. 1983a). After discontinuing the administration of enflurane a significant increase in ICP without correlation to changes in CBV has been observed (Artru 1983). These changes are supposed to be caused by an increase in resistance to CSF reabsorption and in the production rate of CSF during enflurane anaesthesia (Mann et al. 1980, Artru 1984c).

EEG and energy metabolism

During the first experimental studies with enflurane, twitching of the extremities and face were observed (Virtue et al. 1966, Botty et al. 1968). Later on, de Jong and Heavner (1971), found that the twitching was synchronous with spike discharge activity obtained by EEG. Joas et al. (1971) studying dogs subjected to hypocapnic enflurane anaesthesia, observed seizure-like EEG tracings and focal twitching in response to hand clapping, and disappearance of spike activity when $PaCO_2$ was increased. In cats, there is a prolonged period of abnormal EEG activity up to 16 days following enflurane anaesthesia (Julien and Kavan 1972). In the same animal, diazepam, thiopentone, methohexitone and ketamine all attenuated established EEG seizure activity (Darimont and Jenkins 1977). Studies in cats indicate that the involvement of the sensorimotor cortex is essential for the development of enflurane-induced seizure (Kurata et al. 1994).In dogs the seizure activity associated with enflurane anaesthesia is accompanied by a 48% increase in $CMRO_2$ (Michenfelder and Cucchiara 1974). The hyperexcitability appears to originate in the limbic system, with subsequent spread to all other areas (Darimont and Jenkins 1977). Myers and Shapiro (1979) have suggested that the enflurane induced epileptogenic foci are located in the hippocampus and related structures, and from the same group a significant decrease in the ratio rCBF/CMR-glucose in the hippocampus was observed, suggesting that substrate demand could potentially outstrip supply within the hippocampus (Ray et al. 1979). In another study enflurane-induced release of excitatory amino acid, glutamate, was found in mouse brain synaptosomes (Hiroso et al. 1992). However, other studies in rats have shown that the cerebral cortical energy state is not depleted during enflurane induced seizure activity (Seo et al. 1984), and neuropathological studies in rats, subjected to long-time enflurane EEG spiking activity have not shown any signs of irreversible neuronal damage (Lin et al. 1986). However, in rats subjected to haemorrhage to blood pressure of 35 mm Hg, brain tissue oxygenation is better maintained during isoflurane and ketamine than during enflurane anaesthesia (Longnecker et al. 1986).

Enflurane, human studies

CBF

In patients without neurological diseases enflurane has no effect on global CBF (Wollman et al. 1969, van Aken et al. 1977), but a significant decrease in regional CBF in the frontal and occipital regions at 2% enflurane has been observed (Rolly and van Aken 1979). In patients with subacute or chronic brain lesions, enflurane causes a decrease in CBF (Reinhold et al. 1974, Reinhold and DeRood 1976), and in patients with head injury where blood pressure was maintained with phenylephedrine, 1% enflurane had no effect on global CBF (De Rood et al. 1980). However, in many of these studies the patients were premedicated, and anaesthesia was maintained with nitrous oxide. Consequently, Sakabe et al. (1983) compared pure enflurane anaesthesia at two concentrations with values obtained at awake state, and found that enflurane at 2 and 3.5% is a cerebral vasodilator causing a 15 and 32% increase in CBF respectively. In comparative clinical studies of enflurane, halothane and isoflurane isoMAC concentrations of isoflurane and enflurane give rise to an increase in CBF, which is much smaller than the increase obtained with halothane (Murphy et al. 1974, Entree et al. 1985).

$CMRO_2$

Enflurane gives rise to a decrease in $CMRO_2$ (Wollman et al. 1969, Sakabe et al. 1983). In patients with supratentorial cerebral tumours, subjected to craniotomy with thiopentone induction and maintenance of anaesthesia with nitrous oxide 67%, fentanyl and enflurane 1 or 2% during hypocapnia, an associated decrease in CBF and $CMRO_2$, and a dose related decrease in $CMRO_2$ were observed (Madsen et al. 1986) Compared to iso-MAC concentrations of isoflurane and halothane, the suppression of $CMRO_2$ was more pronounced, and the effect on global CBF identical (Madsen and Cold 1987).

ICP and CPP

Induction of anaesthesia with 3% enflurane in patients with intracranial lesions gives rise to a marked increase in ICP (Tambuniello et al. 1978). In contrast, enflurane 1% during induction in high-risk neurosurgical patients does not change ICP (McLeskey et al. 1974), and in patients with cerebral tumours, enflurane 2% has very little effect on ICP, but decreases blood pressure and CPP significantly (Moss et al. 1983). In patients with intracranial lesions and high ICP level, enflurane 1–2% increases ICP by up to 9–15 mm Hg (Zattoni et al. 1974)., and in patients with severe head injury, having an initial ICP above 20 mm Hg, enflurane 1.5% induces a considerable increase in ICP, similar to nitrous oxide and halothane (Schulte am Esch et al. 1979). However, in other studies the ICP increase elicited by enflurane was smaller than that obtained with halothane (Cunitz et al. 1976).

In many of these studies, enflurane decreased CPP significantly (Zattoni et al. 1974, Cunitz et al. 1976, Schulte am Esch et al.1979, Moss et al. 1983) often to values less than 50 mm Hg, which is at the lower end of the range of CA. Thus, changes in CA capacity, and the fact that most studies were performed in patients with impaired or lost CA, might influence the changes in ICP. It is supposed that the increase in ICP during enflurane anaesthesia might be even more pronounced if blood pressure is maintained.

EEG

Human studies have confirmed that epileptic activity might be elicited by enflurane. The incidence of muscle twitching in patients receiving enflurane has been reported to be 7% (Lebowitz et al. 1972). In children enflurane consistently produced spike waves on EEG even at concentrations as low as 1% (Neundörfer and Klose 1975). Increasing depth of enflurane anaesthesia is characterised by the appearance of high-voltage spikes (Stockard and Bickford 1975), but with elevation of $PaCO_2$, signs of cerebral irritability appear to be reduced. In the same study, the addition of nitrous oxide did not alter the EEG pattern (Neigh et al. 1971). The EEG changes can persist for several days (Burchiel et al. 1977, Kruczek et al. 1980), and epileptic seizures have been observed days after enflurane administration (Ohm et al. 1975, Grant 1986). However, in a retrospective analysis of patients undergoing intracranial surgery 14% of isoflurane against 8% of enflurane anaesthetised patients had one or more convulsions (Christys et al. 1989). In a study of 14 patients subjected to craniotomy for small cerebral tumours, the combined use of hypocapnia and enflurane in concentrations of 1–2% did not elicit epileptic seizure activity (Madsen et al. 1986).

Evoked potential

Enflurane increases the latency of brain-stem auditory evoked potential response in humans (Dubois et al. 1982, Thornton et al. 1983). Inter-peak latencies are also affected, and the abnormalities are suggestive of a maximal effect of enflurane on midbrain reticular formation. These observations seem to confirm the hypothesis of the rostral brain-stem playing a role in the mechanism of generalised seizure activity (Mirsky et al. 1979).

Clinical application

Experimental as well as human studies have shown that enflurane is a cerebral vasodilator which gives rise to an increase in CBF and ICP, and a decrease in CVR. Simultaneously enflurane induces a marked decrease in $CMRO_2$. Owing to the phenomena of epileptic seizure activity observed during enflurane anaesthesia, especially provoked by hypocapnia, this inhalation agent is generally avoided in the neurosurgical clinic. Provided EEG monitoring can be practised during craniotomy clinical studies, however, suggest that enflurane might be an alternative to halothane (Madsen et al. 1986).

Isoflurane, experimental studies

CBF, CVR and $CMRO_2$

In animal experiments, isoflurane induces an increase in CBF and a decrease in CVR and $CMRO_2$ (Cucchiara et al. 1974, Stullken et al. 1977, Newberg et al. 1983, Todd and Drummond 1984b, Gelman et al. 1984). In dogs, the benzodiazepine antagonist, flumazenil, partially antagonises the suppression of $CMRO_2$, and EEG is changed from sleep to awake pattern (Roald et al. 1988). The changes in CBF and $CMRO_2$ give rise to an increase in the ratio $CBF/CMRO_2$ (Smith and Wollman 1972).

With Laser-Doppler flowmetry isoflurane causes a dose-related increase in flow. Cerebral autoregulation is present but attenuated at low concentrations of isoflurane. The same study suggested that isoflurane is superior in maintaining the oxygen supply in the cerebrocortical microcirculation than halothane (Lee et al. 1994).

CBV

In dogs isoflurane, even during hypocapnia, increases CBV (Archer et al. 1987). However in rats subjected to 1 MAC isoflurane or halothane there was no difference in CBV (Katz et al. 1988). In the study by Archer and co-workers CBF and CBV were not measured concomitantly. The same group therefore has repeated the study with measurement of rCBF and rCBV with PET in hypocapnic baboons, and found that the addition of 1.3% isoflurane did not change rCBF or rCBV (Archer et al. 1990). In a study by Weeks et al. (1989), CBV changes during halothane and isoflurane anaesthesia were identical and the responsiveness of CBF to changing $PaCO_2$ was preserved during the administration of both volatile anaesthetic. Todd and Weeks (1996) made a comparative study of the effects of propofol, pentobarbital, and isoflurane on CBF and CBV. They found that CBF in isoflurane anaesthetised animals was 2.0–2.6 times greater than with propofol or pentobarbital. Nevertheless, although CBV was greater in the isoflurane group than in the propofol and pentobarbital groups, the magnitudes of the inter-group differences were much smaller (about 20%).

Regional CBF

The increase in CBF occurs faster and more pronounced in the deep structures of colliculus superior and inferior, the limbic system and the cerebellum, as compared with the cerebral cortex (Maekawa et al. 1986, Manohar and Parks 1984, Mutch and Ringaert 1987). Comparative experimental studies in cats and dogs indicate that isoflurane possesses cerebrovascular properties that are different from halothane. Thus, the increase in CBF and decrease in CVR elicited by isoflurane are much smaller (Todd and Drummond 1984b), and rCBF to cortical and subcortical areas, including diencephalon and the brain stem, was lower during isoflurane than during halothane anaesthesia (Chen et al. 1984). Studies of CBF by hydrogen clearance in rabbits subjected to hypo-, normo- and hypercapnia support these findings. Thus, CBF during 1 MAC isoflurane decreased during hypocapnia, was unchanged during normocapnia and increased regionally during hypercapnia. In comparison, during 1 MAC halothane CBF increased during all three conditions (Scheller et al. 1986). In another study discrepancies also exist as regards the degree of vasodilatation effected by the two agents. Recently, Hansen et al. (1989b) studied CBF autoradiographically in rats, and found that cortical CBF was greater during halothane anaesthesia, while subcortical CBF was greater during isoflurane anaesthesia. The reason for these anatomically selective CBF effects by the two agents is unknown. It is supposed to be related to their different cortical electrophysiological effects. On the other hand, the overall effect of the two drugs in other studies in the same animal was identical. Isoflurane differentially produces dose-dependent dilation of intraparenchyman cerebral microvessels (Farber et al. 1997).

Changes related to time

During prolonged isoflurane anaesthesia in dogs, CBF declines over a period of hours despite constant CPP (Brian et al. 1988). In the same animal McPherson et al. (1989b) found that CBF declines over time during continued isoflurane anaesthesia despite constant CPP and $PaCO_2$. The same authors found that stabilisation of MABP with angiotensin II to support haemorrhage-induced hypotension produced a prolonged cerebral hyperaemia, whereas support of MABP with phenylephedrine did not provoke hyperaemia (Brian et al. 1990). Changes in CBF during prolonged isoflurane anaesthesia are still unclear because Roald et al. (1989) in the same animal found that CBF as well as $CMRO_2$ remained unchanged. The blood pressure in these animals was not supported during the experiment. That blood pressure support with angiotensin II affects CBF differently from phenylephedrine has been demonstrated by Patel and Mutch (1990), who concluded that either phenylephedrine results in indirect cerebral vasodilation or angiotensin II has intrinsic cerebral vasoconstricting effects. The same group found that during isoflurane anaesthesia phenylephedrine, infused to support MABP following haemorrhagic hypotension, effectively restores rCBF (Mutch et al. 1989).

Cerebral arteries

The effects of halothane, isoflurane, sevoflurane and pentobarbital on hypocapnia- and bicarbonate-induced constriction of isolated canine middle cerebral arteries have been investigated *in vitro*. Constriction was attenuated more potently by halothane than by isoflurane, sevoflurane and pentobarbital at clinically relevant concentrations, supporting the view that decreased CBF induced by both respiratory and metabolic alkalosis may be reversed during halothane anaesthesia, but is largely unaffected by isoflurane, sevoflurane and pentobarbital (Ogawa et al. 2000).

Pial vessels

In experimental studies of isolated human pial arteries halothane and isoflurane act as direct dose dependent vasodilators. During hypocapnia the dilation effected by halothane is diminished, and isoflurane acts as a vasoconstrictor under this condition (Reinstrup et al. 1994).

Nitric oxide

It has been suggested that isoflurane and halothane exert their vasodilating properties by NO liberation (McPherson et al. 1993, McPherson et al. 1994, Todd et al. 1994). With the cranial window technique isoflurane causes cerebral microvessel dilation. Both NO synthesis and an intact endothelium are essential for this response (Koenig et al. 1994). Cholinergic-induced cerebral hyperaemia is observed in isoflurane- but not in pentobarbital-anaesthetised dogs. This difference is caused by stimulation of NO synthase by isoflurane (Sturaitis et al. 1994). Several laboratories, however, provide strong evidence that anaesthetics are not able to stimulate NO release (Flynn et al. 1992). Thus, both halothane and isoflurane appear to be potent inhibitors of NO-release (Muldoon et al. 1988, Stone and Johns 1989, Uggeri et al. 1992, Toda et al. 1992). Johns et al. (1995) studied cultured vascular smooth muscle and endothelial cell-vascular smooth muscle. The effects of inhalation agents on cyclic GMP content in NO stimulated and non-NO stimulated cells were investigated. Under these circumstances volatile agents do not stimulate or inhibit basal cyclic GMP production, suggesting that volatile anaesthetics do not activate soluble of particulate guanyl cyclase and do not activate NO synthase. In the brain, under normal physiologic conditions, NO is produced by two constitutive isoforms of NO-synthase (NOS), endothelial NOS (eNOS), and neuronal NOS (nNOS). In nNOS knockout mice, the cerebral hyperaemic response to isoflurane is preserved by compensatory mechanisms that is NO-independent at 2.4 vol%, although it may involve eNOS at 1.2 and 1.8 vol% (Okamoto et al. 1997).

Other studies in pentobarbital anaesthetised dogs indicate that the vasodilation of pial vessels induced by isoflurane and sevoflurane is mediated, at least in part, via activation of ATP-sensitive K^+ channels (Iida et al. 1998).

Vasodilation

In studying the direct cerebral vasodilating potencies of halothane and isoflurane in rabbits Drummond et al. (1986) found that the relative effect of halothane and isoflurane on CBF is dependent on the $CMRO_2$ present prior to their administration. When the pre-existing $CMRO_2$ is not markedly depressed, isoflurane decreases $CMRO_2$ and causes less cerebral vasodilatation than halothane. However, if the initial $CMRO_2$ is depressed by a high dose of pentobarbitone, which caused a 43% decrease in $CMRO_2$, halothane and isoflurane have similar vasodilating potencies. Other studies in the same animal indicate that pentobarbitone given in a bolus dose during isoflurane anaesthesia until burst suppression on EEG, will increase CBF (Scheller et al. 1987a). The reason might be that barbiturate under these circumstances of severe metabolic depression has a vasodilatory effect on vascular smooth muscles in cerebral arteries (Altura et Altura 1975, Edvinsson and Mc Culloch 1981, Marin et al 1881).

Glucose metabolism

The effect of isoflurane anaesthesia on local cerebral glucose utilisation has been studied in rats. A significant decrease was observed in all cortical areas and in the primary sensory relay nuclei of the central visual and auditory pathways. Furthermore, the utilisation of glucose was decreased in the cerebellum, red nucleus, the ventral thalamus, in the CA1 field and dentate gyrus in the hippocampus. However, the utilisation was increased in the substantia nigra pars compacta and in the medial habenulo-interpenducular system and the CA3 field of the hippocampus (Ori et al. 1986, Maekawa et al 1986). During isoflurane anaesthesia in rats, hypocapnia to $PaCO_2$ 20 mm Hg at normotension does not change glucose utilisation. rCBF becomes homogeneously reduced by 40%. On the other hand, hypocapnia combined with isoflurane-induced hypotension to MABP 50 mm Hg causes a heterogeneous response with CMR-glucose decreased in the frontal-, the parietal cortex and the thalamus. Unaltered utilisation was observed in the mesencephalon and the medulla oblongata, and increased utilisation in the hippocampus and the cerebellum (Waaben et al. 1989). In comparative studies in rats, during 1 MAC isoflurane or halothane, a strong correlation between glucose utilisation and CBF within individual anatomic regions was found. At a given value for glucose utilisation CBF during isoflurane was higher than with halothane, suggesting that CBF and oxygen consumption remain coupled, and that at a given level of glucose utilisation, isoflurane possesses greater cerebral vasodilating capabilities than halothane (Hansen et al. 1989).

Cerebral autoregulation (CA) and blood-brain barrier (BBB)

Comparative studies of CA during isoflurane and halothane anaesthesia indicate an impairment of CA during halothane, while CA is partly preserved during isoflurane anaesthesia (Todd and Drummond 1984b). During isoflurane-induced hypotension in baboons, the CA is totally abolished. After normalisation of blood pressure, secondary to the reduction of the isoflurane concentration, a short lasting increase in CBF was observed, indicating a hyperaemic phase (Van Aken et al. 1986). Studies in dogs by McPherson and Traystman (1987) indicate that during decrease in MABP or increase in CSF pressure the CA is preserved at 1 MAC isoflurane, but absent at 2 MAC. In another study in dogs it was demonstrated that early during the administration of 1 MAC isoflurane the CA was abolished. However, after 3 h CBF was maintained constant despite changes in CPP by haemorrhage or inflation of an aortic balloon (Mc Pherson et al. 1990). In rats isoflurane decreased the transport of small hydrophilic molecules across the blood-brain barrier. The mechanism and importance of this decreased transport are not clear (Chi et al. 1992).

CO_2-reactivity

In animals without cerebral lesions, and blood pressure within a normal range of CA, the CO_2-reactivity is preserved (Cucchiara et al. 1974). The reactivity is higher with 1 MAC isoflurane compared with 1 MAC halothane (Drummond and Todd 1985). In baboons subjected to isoflurane-induced hypotension the CO_2 reactivity was found to be intact at base-line blood pressure; however, at 20 and 50% decrease in blood pressure the CO_2 reactivity was found to be impaired and absent respectively (Van Aken et al. 1986). Other studies in dogs subjected to 1.4% isoflurane indicate preserved CO_2 reactivity to hypo- as well as hypercapnia; however with 2.8% isoflurane vasoconstriction to hypocapnia is retained, but vasodilation to hypercapnia is abolished (McPherson et al. 1989). In dogs subjected to 1.4% isoflurane during normocapnia, CBF and CO_2 reactivity decreased over time. These changes were not caused by changes in brain metabolism. Studies with laser-Doppler measurement of the effects of halothane and isoflurane on the CO_2 reactivity suggest that hypercapnia increases cerebrocortical red cell flow more with isoflurane than with halothane, at least at moderate anaesthetic concentrations (Lee et al. 1995).

ICP and CSF formation

In studies in cats and dogs, isoflurane only increases ICP minimally if at all (Todd and Drummond 1984b). The same results were found in dogs with intracranial hypertension caused by inflation of an epidural balloon and subjected to 1 MAC isoflurane. If nitrous oxide was supplemented to isoflurane, an increase in ICP was observed (Albin et al. 1986). It is supposed that species differences might exist, because Scheller et al. (1987) in rabbits subjected to cryogenic brain lesion observed an increase in ICP independent of the level of $PaCO_2$ and a similar ICP increasing effect with both halothane and isoflurane. In cats subjected to craniotomy, brain surface protrusion during enflurane and isoflurane anaesthesia is much less than during halothane anaesthesia, and when anaesthetic-induced differences in blood pressure were eliminated by arterial pressure support, the protrusion caused by halothane compared with that caused by enflurane or isoflurane was exaggerated (Drummond et al. 1983a). In other studies the increase in ICP during isoflurane administration seems to follow changes in CBV, which is increased by 10%. The increase in ICP is only of 30 min duration as opposed to more than three hours duration with halothane and enflurane (Artru 1984a). In dogs, isoflurane in comparison with enflurane does not change the rate of CSF production (Artru 1984b).

EEG

Isoflurane causes progressive changes in the EEG. At concentrations less than 0.5 MAC an increase in alpha frequency from 8–12 Hz to more than 15 Hz occurs; voltage increases concomitantly. When isoflurane concentration is increased above 0.4 MAC, the regions with high voltages shift from the posterior to the anterior part of the brain. At 1 MAC, frequency decreases and voltage increases further. At 1.5 MAC, burst suppression appears, and the voltage begins to diminish. At 2 MAC, the EEG becomes isoelectric (Stullken et al. 1977, Tinker et al. 1977, Newberg et al. 1983).

At sub-MAC isoflurane concentrations, noxious stimulation activates cortical and subcortical structures (midbrain reticular formation, thalamus). At concentrations exceeding MAC, however, isoflurane abolishes these responses (Antognini and Carstens 1999).

Brain protection

Studies in mice subjected to hypoxia have shown that isoflurane has a brain-protective effect (Newberg and Michenfelder 1983). In dogs isoflurane-induced hypotension to MABP 40 to 50 mm Hg produced a 40% decrease in $CMRO_2$, accompanied by a 60% decrease in CBF. The cerebral energy state indicated by the concentrations of ATP, ADP, AMP, phosphocreatine and lactate were unchanged (Newberg et al. 1984).

During exposure to isoflurane in concentrations of 5–6%, an increase in the concentrations of lactate and lactate/pyruvate ratio, but an unchanged concentration of ATP and phosphocreatine in cerebral tissue was found (Newberg et al. 1983). The brain protective effect of isoflurane has been evaluated in several studies. In one study isoflurane 2% showed significantly better protection than the protection found during nitrous oxide anaesthesia. The outcomes of the animals subjected to either isoflurane or methohexital were comparable (Baughman et al. 1990a). In another study of incomplete forebrain ischaemia in rats, the animals were subjected to either halothane or isoflurane anaesthesia. Studies of rCBF and glucose utilisation indicated that the ratio flow/metabolism was highest in the isoflurane group and lowest during nitrous oxide 70%. These results relate to reappearing time of EEG in the reperfusion period and suggest indirectly a brain protective effect of isoflurane (Maekawa et al. 1989). *In vitro* data indicate that isoflurane can reduce α-amino-*d*-hydroxy-4-isoxazole-propionate (AMPA) receptor-mediated toxicity (Carla and Moroni 1992). In a recent *in vivo* study in the rat cerebral cortex isoflurane reduced AMPA-induced cortical injury in a dose-dependent manner. The simultaneous injection of NBQX, an antagonist of AMPA receptor, inhibited the development of this lesion (Kimbro et al. 2000). Studies of MCAO, in which a nylon filament is advanced into the middle cerebral artery via the carotid artery, indicated that isoflurane anaesthetised rats developed smaller infarct compared with awake and fentanyl/nitrous oxide anaesthetised animals (Soonthon-Brant et al. 1999). Another study of global cerebral ischaemia indicates that isoflurane reduced damage to selective vulnerable cerebral structures compared with rats anaesthetised with fentanyl/nitrous oxide (Miura et al. 1998). In a recent study it was found that isoflurane, in comparison with fentanyl, improves long-term neurological outcome after traumatic brain injury in rats (Statler et al. 2000).

Unfortunately, other experimental results have been negative. Thus, Warner et al. (1986) studied the effect of isoflurane on neuronal necrosis following near-complete forebrain ischaemia in the rat (bilateral carotid occlusion and hypotension to 50 mm Hg). They found morbidity and pathophysiological changes unaffected by isoflurane. Studies in rats subjected to MCAO during controlled hypotension with either sodium nitroprusside, isoflurane or controlled hypovolaemia did not disclose any difference in zero flow areas as evaluated by the 14C-antipyrine technique (Cole et al. 1987). Studies in monkeys subjected to MCAO during thiopentone or isoflurane induced EEG suppression until burst suppression level, and where MABP was maintained with support of blood pressure indicate that isoflurane does not offer advantages compared with thiopentone as regards cerebral protection (Nehls et al. 1987, Milde et al. 1988). In a recent study in rabbits the effects of pentobarbital and isoflurane on conditioned learning after transient global cerebral ischaemia were investigated. During this condition it was demonstrated that a brief episode of cerebral ischaemia results in impairment of associative learning. Hypothermia and burst-suppressive doses of pentobarbital but not isoflurane were able to improve neurobehavioral outcome as measured by ability to acquire a trace conditioned response (Young Kwon et al. 2000). In a study by Warner et al. (1991), MCAO was applied in hypertensive rats subjected to either halothane, isoflurane or methoxyhexitone anaesthesia. Isoflurane and methoxyhexitone were administrated in dosages sufficient to produce the same level of EEG burst-suppression. Under these circumstances the infarct volume was less during methoxyhexitone than during isoflurane, although rCBF in the damaged hemisphere was higher during isoflurane. Kawaguchi et al. (2000) recently studied rats subjected to filament MCAO while awake or anaesthetised with isoflurane. The animals were allowed to survive 2 days or 2 weeks. The isoflurane group had major protection at 2 days. At 2 weeks, however, both the awake and isoflurane anaesthetised animals had large and similar-sized infarcts. These results are supported by *in vitro* studies of evoked population spikes recorded from brain hippocampus slices, where isoflurane compared with thiopentone did not elicit any brain protective effect (Bendo et al. 1987), and studies with Laser flowmetry indicating that the CBF threshold for cortical depolarisation did not differ between halothane and isoflurane (Verhaegen et al. 1994).

Altogether, it has not been proved that isoflurane offers any brain protective effects in regional ischaemia, and if so, whether isoflurane and thiopentone during strictly comparative circumstances offer the same degree of protection (Michenfelder 1987). Based on the studies by Warner et al. (1991) and Sano et al. (1992) it has been argued that interventions that reduce cerebral metabolic rate of oxygen not "per se" are to be viewed as protective. Todd and Warner (1992) in an editorial have discussed this issue, and called attention to the fact that the protective effect of anaesthetics and hypothermia cannot be explained by metabolic depression alone. The role of excitatory amino acids, which result in postsynaptic depolarisation and calcium entry into the cell may be influenced by hypothermia (Busto et al. 1989). Other authors stress that we do not know how anaesthetics influence the release of excitatory amino acids or free radicals. Recently, Warner (2000) in an editorial summarised that we still are in an era of uncertainty regarding isoflurane neuroprotection.

On the other hand, anaesthetics probably have some protective properties. Thus, Verhaegen et al. (1992) observed a 1,5 min. delay in time to depolarisation between iso-MAC concentrations of isoflurane/nitrous oxide, versus halothane/nitrous oxide. The delay in time to depolarisation correlated with the depression of cerebral glucose- and oxygen metabolism. In a similar study Nellgård et al. (2000) provided evidence that cerebral metabolic rate reduction has an advantageous effect on outcome from severe ischaemia, but that such benefit is likely to be small.

Glucose

The discrepancies in results concerning the brain-protective effect of isoflurane in focal ischaemia might be influenced by the brain glucose concentration, as a high brain concentration of glucose during incomplete ischaemia might worsen the outcome. That this factor might play a role in studies of isoflurane-induced brain protection, has indirectly been shown by Kofke et al. (1986). They found that brain concentration of glucose during isoflurane anaesthesia was higher than during halothane, suggesting that cerebral lactic-acidosis might be increased if isoflurane is given.

Exitatory amino acids

Recent *in vitro* studies indicate that isoflurane inhibits glutamate receptors and delays cellular injury induced by simulated ischaemia (Bickler et al. 1994). The same group studied brain slice models of cerebral anoxia. They found that isoflurane decreased glutamate release to a similar extent as hypothermia (28°C) does. However, the increased glutamate release with hyperthermia (39°C) was not prevented by isoflurane (Eilers and Bickler 1996). The relative neuroprotective effects of dizocilpine, a glutamate receptor antagonist, and isoflurane during focal cerebral ischaemia in the rat have been studied during ridig maintenance of brain temperature. Dizocilpine was effective in reducing cerebral infarction size. In contrast, isoflurane administration at 0.7% did not reduce infarction size (Sarraf-Yazdi et al. 1998). *In vivo* studies of guinea pig synaptosomes indicate that volatile anaesthetic including isoflurane decrease $[Ca^{2+}]_i$ in a manner consistent with inhibition of Ca^{2+} entry, possibly through specific voltage-gated neuronal calcium channels (Miao et al. 1995). Another *in vivo* study in the rat indicates that isoflurane can reduce N-methyl-D-aspartate-mediated cortical injury in a dose-dependent manner (Harada et al. 1999). In contrast to these studies animals subjected to complete global ischaemia in pentobarbital or isoflurane a prolongation of the time to terminal depolarisation was observed. Anaesthesia, however, did not influence the rate at which the extracellular concentrations of glutamate, aspartate, or glycine increased. By contrast hypothermia reduced the release of all excitatory amino acids (Nakashima and Todd 1996).

The effects of volatile anaesthetic agents on NMDA receptor mediated excitatory synaptic transmission have not been completely characterised. Field excitatory postsynaptic potentials in the CA1 area were recorded with extracellular electrodes after electrical stimulation of Schaffer-collateral-commissural fiber inputs. The findings suggest that field excitatory postsynaptic potentials mediated by postsynaptic NMDA receptors are more sensitive to clinically relevant concentrations of isoflurane than non-NMDA receptor-mediated responses are. This selective effect was not observed for halothane. Both agents appeared to depress release of glutamate from nerve terminals via presynaptic actions (Nichikawa et al. 2000).

Brain temperature

Other factors also might influence the discrepancies in results found in comparative studies of isoflurane- and halothane-induced cerebral protection. It is supposed that a large portion of variability in histopathologic damage is attributed to the difference in brain temperature during and after ischaemia. Busto et al. (1987) found that during ischaemia brain temperature rapidly decreased unless actively maintained. Sano et al. (1992) studied incomplete ischaemia in rats subjected to either 1.3 MAC isoflurane or halothane at normothermia and compared with 1.3 MAC halothane at mild hypothermia. They found that isoflurane with this model did not confer cerebral protection relative to halothane anaesthetised animals, but that mild hypothermia by only 3 degree Celsius was markedly protective. This study confirms the result obtained by Baughman et al. (1989b), that outcome with halothane was not different from isoflurane despite difference in metabolic suppression effected by the two anaesthetics.

Brain tissue oxygen tension

Studies in dogs indicate that increased oxygen ventilation will increase brain tissue PO_2 90% during 3% isoflurane compared to baseline, if MABP is supported. This hyperoxygenated state appears to be due to abolition of normal constrictor regulatory mechanisms by high dose isoflurane, combined with maintenance of adequate cerebral perfusion pressure (Hoffman and Edelman 2000b). Another study from the same group indicates that brain oxygen reactivity, defined as the increase in brain tissue oxygen tension divided by the increase in PaO_2, is increased during 3% isoflurane compared with 1.5% isoflurane and propofol anaesthetised dogs (Hoffman and Edelman 2000c).

Spreading depression

One mechanism by which volatile anaesthetics can reduce injury is by reducing the frequency of spreading depression-like depolarisations in the penumbra during focal ischaemia. The occurrence of spreading depression during focal ischaemia has been demonstrated by several investigators. These ischaemic depolarisations increase calcium influx into the penumbra neurones. Because of their constrained energy supply, these neurones might not be able to re-establish ionic homeostasis, and consequently they may undergo ischaemic death (Hossmann 1994). Both isoflurane and pentobarbital reduce the frequency of ischaemic depolarisation. This effect might, in part, mediate some of the documented neuroprotective effect found with these drugs (Patel et al. 1998).

Combined with nitrous oxide

Theoretically, nitrous oxide (an agent with cerebral stimulatory effect), might attenuate the cerebral protective effect of isoflurane. Mortality studies in rats suggest that isoflurane provides better cerebral protection alone, than nitrous oxide, but does not indicate that nitrous oxide combined with isoflurane worsens the outcome (Baughman et al. 1988). In a later study the same group found that during moderate ischaemia 0.5 and 1 MAC isoflurane produced better neurologic outcome and less histopathologic damage from ischaemia than did nitrous oxide 70% alone. Addition of nitrous oxide to 0.5 MAC isoflurane attenuated the improvement in neurologic outcome and produced more histopathologic damage compared with the damage produced during isoflurane alone. However, the addition of nitrous oxide to 1 MAC isoflurane did not significantly change outcome or histopathologic score (Baughman et al. 1989b).

Oedema and cryogenic ischaemic injury

In rabbits subjected to cryogenic brain lesion it was found that 1 MAC halothane anaesthesia resulted in less oedema formation compared to animals subjected to pentobarbitone or isoflurane anaesthesia (Kaieda et al. 1989). In the same animal it was found that a cryogenic injury attenuates the normal CBF response to isoflurane both in the damaged hemisphere as well as in the apparently uninjured regions distant from the injury focus. The CO_2 reactivity in the injured hemisphere was abolished, but present in the contralateral hemisphere and the cerebellum (Ramani et al.1991).

This study has been followed up by Murr et al.(1993) who measured rCBF and formation of brain oedema in the presence of a cold injury in rabbits, and compared the effects of isoflurane, fentanyl and thiopentone anaesthesia. In their report they demonstrated a marked cerebral hyperaemia during isoflurane anaesthesia, although MABP was even lower than in the other experimental group. They found no evidence of an anaesthetic dependent enhancement or attenuation of brain oedema, suggesting that modification of the hyperaemic blood flow response in the focal ischaemic region by anaesthetic does not influence formation of perifocal oedema. In a study of cryogenic brain oedema in the rabbit it was found that isoflurane anaesthesia attenuates cerebral oedema compared to fentanyl, thiopental or alpha-chlorose (Murr et al. 1995).

Controlled hypotension

In comparative studies in dogs of controlled hypotension to MABP 40 mm Hg with trimethaphan, nitroprusside, halothane or isoflurane, the energy charge in cerebral tissue was found to be unchanged during isoflurane-induced hypotension. In the same study CBF and $CMRO_2$ were significantly decreased during isoflurane-induced hypotension (Newberg et al. 1984). Comparative studies of pO_2 in cerebral tissue during isoflurane and 2-chloroadenosine induced hypotension indicate higher pO_2 levels during isoflurane-induced hypotension (Seyde and Longnecker 1986). Furthermore, studies in dogs subjected to isoflurane-induced hypotension to 40 mm Hg of MABP and hypocapnia ($PaCO_2$ 20 mm Hg) suggest no adverse effects on cerebral metabolism or function (Artru 1986a). The responses of CBF, $CMRO_2$, and ICP during varying rates of isoflurane-induced hypotension have recently been studied in dogs. On the one hand, slow induction of hypotension to MABP 45 mm Hg within 6–10 min, in comparison with fast induction within 1–5 min, resulted in a transient increase in ICP, and a more prolonged ICP increase after reestablishment of normotension. The authors conclude that the increase in ICP might be deleterious when intracranial compliance is already jeopardised (Hickey et al. 1986b). On the other hand, rapid induction of hypotension in comparison with slow induction results in a transient reduction of CBF that is not accompanied by a similar reduction in $CMRO_2$, suggesting that isoflurane-induced hypotension should be initiated gradually to permit initiation of homeostatic mechanisms that result in the least alteration in CBF (Hickey et al. 1986a). The comparative studies combined with experimental evidence of a cerebral protective effect of isoflurane have focused attention on isoflurane as an agent used in clinical practice for controlled hypotension. Recently, the effect of isoflurane-induced hypotension on cerebral autoregulation has been studied with angiotensin II in anaesthetised pigs. CA was tested at two levels of MABP representing a 32 and 59% decrease of control. 1.7 and 2.7% isoflurane was used. At both levels of hypotension isoflurane produced a dose dependent impairment of the autoregulatory response to angiotensin as well as a decrease in MABP caused by caval block. After hypotension the autoregulatory response to increased blood pressure was restored within 15–25 min and to decreased blood pressure within 25–50 min (Stånge et al. 1990).

Elimination

Studies concerning the elimination of isoflurane from the brain are conflicting. In studies by Wyrwicz et al. (1983), a 43% decrease of the 19-F NMR signal was still observed 5 hours after a 90 min isoflurane anaesthesia. This result suggested a very slow elimination of isoflurane disagrees with invasive results with end-tidal gas chromatography (Cohen et al. 1972, Carpenter et al. 1986). Recently NMR studies in which signals from extracerebral compartments were eliminated have shown a half-life of isoflurane elimination of 36 min (Mills et al. 1987).

Isoflurane, human studies

CBF and $CMRO_2$

Comparative clinical studies in patients without cerebral lesions (Murphy et al. 1974, Algotsson et al. 1988, Olsen et al. 1994), and in patients with mass-expanding cerebral lesions (Entree et al. 1985, Madsen and Cold 1987b) have shown that the increase in CBF, if present at all, is less with iso-MAC isoflurane and enflurane than with halothane, and that the increase in CBF is dose-dependent. Simultaneously, isoflurane induces a decrease in $CMRO_2$ (Murkin et al. 1986, Madsen et al. 1987b, Algotsson et al. 1988, Olsen et al. 1994).

Infants

In pre-term neonates anterior fontanel pressure recorded with the Ladd AFP monitor, decreases by 11% during administration of 0.75% isoflurane (Friesen et al. 1987). In children without cerebral diseases, aged one to eight years, cerebral blood flow velocity did not change when the initial isoflurane MAC concentration of either 0.5, 1.0 or 1.5 MAC was varied. No change in velocity when isoflurane was administered over time was observed (Bisonnette and Leon 1992).

Regional studies of CBF and metabolism

The pattern of rCBF differs between halothane and isoflurane with higher subcortical flows during isoflurane than during halothane anaesthesia at 1 MAC. Despite this redistribution, isoflurane anaesthesia results in a lower mean CBF value than anaesthesia with halothane (Reinstrup 1994). In adults without cerebral disorders isoflurane (0.5% end-expiratory) is associated with a global, fairly uniform, reduction of glucose utilisation by 46% (Alkire et al. 1997).

CO_2 reactivity

During isoflurane/nitrous oxide anaesthesia for supratentorial cerebral tumours the CO_2 reactivity is preserved, averaging 4.4%/mm Hg $PaCO_2$ (Madsen et al. 1987b).

In healthy subjects the rate at which cerebral blood flow responds to changes in PaCO2 was faster during 1–1.5 MAC isoflurane compared with halothane in iso-MAC concentrations (Chong et al 2000).

Cerebral autoregulation

In patients without cerebral disorders CBF autoregulation is disrupted at 2 MAC isoflurane, but not during 1 MAC isoflurane anaesthesia (Olsen et al. 1994). Another study, analysed with transcranial Doppler, indicates that dynamic autoregulation was better preserved during 1.5 MAC sevoflurane than during isoflurane (Summors et al. 1999).

Combined with nitrous oxide

Regional CBF measured with SPECT is greater with combined nitrous oxide and isoflurane than with iso-MAC concentration of isoflurane alone. The relative flow distribution, however, was similar (Reinstrup et al. 1997).

Craniotomy

In studies of patients subjected to craniotomy for small supratentorial tumours with thiopentone induction, and maintenance of anaesthesia with isoflurane 0.75%, nitrous oxide 67%, fentanyl and moderate hypocapnia, CBF was decreased by 27%, and $CMRO_2$ by 29% in comparison with the values obtained in the awake state. Under these circumstances, an increase in isoflurane concentration to 1.5% does not change CBF, while CVR and $CMRO_2$ decreased significantly. In the same study the relative CO_2 reactivity was found to be intact (Madsen et al. 1987b). Other studies indicate that the CO_2 reactivity in oedematous brain tissue might be absent during isoflurane anaesthesia, but preserved during fentanyl anaesthesia (Shah et al. 1988). In a recent study including patients with brain tumours, rCBF was measured during two levels of $PaCO_2$ with Doppler Laser flowmetry. The probe was placed over oedematous cerebral cortical tissue. The patients were anaesthetised with either isoflurane/nitrous oxide or fentanyl/nitrous oxide. During isoflurane anaesthesia a wide variety of responses to hypocapnia was observed. In some patients CBF increased markedly (inverse reaction). These patterns were not observed during fentanyl, nitrous oxide anaesthesia (Shah et al. 1990).

Jugular venous bulb saturation

Jugular venous bulb oxygen tension was measured in patients undergoing normothermic cardiopulmonary by-pass. The patients received a standardised anaesthesia consisting of fentanyl and midazolam and were randomly allocated to receive either isoflurane, sevoflurane or propofol. Jugular bulb saturation values were significantly higher during by-pass in the isoflurane group and significantly lower six hours after by-pass in the sevoflurane group when compared with the propofol group (Nandate et al. 2000).

In a randomized study patients undergoing craniotomy for supratentorial cerebral tumours, were randomized to propofol, isoflurane or sevoflurane. $AVDO_2$ was significantly higher and jugular venous bulb saturation was significantly lower in the propofol group compared with the isoflurane- and sevoflurane group (Petersen et al. 2000).

Comparative studies of ICP during craniotomy

Todd and Weeks (1996) compared ICP during propofol/fentanyl, isoflurane/nitrous oxide and fentanyl/nitrous oxide for elective supratentorial craniotomies. They found that epidural ICP measured through first burr hole did not differ between the three groups. In the isoflurane group, however, more patients had a relatively high ICP. In a non-randomized study of patients with cerebral tumours, however, ICP was lowest during propofol/fentanyl anaesthesia, compared with isoflurane/nitrous oxide and sevoflurane. In the same study it was found that the number of patients with an ICP above 10 mm Hg, which represents threshold of cerebral swelling, was significantly lower in propofol/fentanyl anaesthetised patients (Bundgaard and Cold 1997a, Bundgaard and Cold 1997b). These findings recently have been confirmed in a randomized controlled study (Petersen et al. 2000).

Coronary by-pass

In patients without intracranial diseases undergoing a coronary by-pass operation, 1 MAC isoflurane or enflurane at normothermia produced a 35 and 39% fall in CBF respectively. $CMRO_2$ was decreased by 50% with either agents. The cerebral autoregulation was impaired with both agents, and the CO_2 reactivity in both adults and children was maintained at 1 MAC (Larsen et al. 1988, Leon and Bissonnette 1991). During cardiopulmonary by-pass for closed heart surgery, the combination of hypothermia to about 26 C°, and isoflurane until burst suppression level of EEG reduced CBF to levels of 10 ml/100g/min, and $CMRO_2$ to about 0.3 ml O_2 /100g/min. Thiopentone infusion used to obtain the same level of EEG suppression reduces $CMRO_2$ to the same level, but reduces CBF even further until the level of 8 ml/100g/min (Woodcock et al. 1987).

Blood pressure, ICP and CPP

Generally isoflurane elicits a decrease in MABP. Studies of the central haemodynamics have shown that the decrease in MABP primarily is caused by peripheral vasodilatation and not a fall in cardiac output (Stevens et al. 1971, Shimosato et al. 1982). In clinical studies isoflurane increases ICP and decreases MABP and CPP during normocapnia. The increase in ICP and the decrease in CPP can be diminished if hyperventilation or barbiturate injections are applied prior to or simultaneously with the administration of isoflurane (Adams et al. 1981, Campkin 1984, Saintz et al. 1988, Campkin and Flinn 1989). During neuroleptic anaesthesia for tumour and aneurysm surgery, isoflurane 1% increases ICP and reduces MABP and CPP, but controlled hyperventilation partially restores the ICP and CPP values (Gordon et al. 1988). In other studies where the patients were premedicated with droperidol and fentanyl, isoflurane 1% during normocapnia did not increase ICP, while 1% isoflurane during hypocapnia was associated with a decrease in ICP (Mazzarella et al. 1986). It is supposed that the discrepancy in results between this study and the study by Adams and co-workers, where ICP increased during normocapnic isoflurane administration, is due to differences in the regime of premedication. In other studies of patients with space-occupying cerebral lesions, an increase in ICP has also been observed (Grosslight et al. 1985, Belopavlovic and Buchthal 1986, Pfeifer et al. 1987). Caution in using isoflurane in patients with limited intracranial compliance has consequently been advanced.

EEG

In clinical studies, isoflurane administration is followed by suppression of the EEG activity just like the suppression obtained in experimental studies (Eger et al. 1971, Homi et al. 1972, Clark et al. 1973). At concentrations of 2–3% isoflurane, the EEG is isoelectric. Similar changes are not observed during halothane anaesthesia (Stockard and Bickford 1975). In comparison with enflurane, epileptic seizure activity cannot be provoked by stimulation or hypocapnia (Eger et al. 1971). Accordingly isoflurane has been used successfully in patients with status epilepticus where halothane did not eliminate the seizure activity (Ropper et al. 1986). Prolonged low-flow isoflurane anaesthesia has been used successfully for the control and treatment for status epilepticus (Kofke et al. 1985, Sasaki et al. 1992). Although perioperative seizure activity has been associated with the administration of isoflurane (Hymes 1985, Harrison 1986), isoflurane as the offending agent has been questioned (Keats 1985). During recovery from isoflurane anaesthesia an EEG arousal phenomenon occurring immediately before awakening has been observed. This phenomenon does not occur during enflurane and is rarely observed during halothane anaesthesia (Erdmann and Brandt 1986). Supplementation with nitrous oxide during 1 MAC isoflurane, enflurane and halothane anaesthesia also induces marked EEG changes. Generally, a shift to lower frequencies was accompanied by a pronounced reduction of amplitude resulting in a decrease of total EEG power (Brandt et al. 1985). In elderly patients isoflurane induces EEG changes with a greater proportion of total electrical silence, and a greater number of isoelectric periods suggesting a discrete alteration with age in the central nervous system sensitivity to isoflurane (Schwartz et al. 1989).

Changes in EEG do not predict depth of anaesthesia as defined by the response to surgical incision, the response to verbal command or the development of memory (Dwyer et al. 1994). On the other hand, studies with topographic EEG indicate that surgical stimulation induces a graded arousal phenomenon, most dominant in frontal regions (Kochs et al. 1994). The changes in EEG always precede the change in flow velocity by 5–7 s. These observations suggest that some flow/metabolism coupling is preserved during isoflurane anesthesia (Lam et al. 1995)

Evoked potential

During isoflurane anaesthesia, a dose dependent increase in evoked potential latencies, a decrease in amplitudes and a prolongation of central conduction time have been observed (Peterson et al. 1984, Sebel et al. 1986, Heneghan et al. 1987).

Cerebral protection

In patients undergoing isoflurane anaesthesia for carotid endarterectomy, critical CBF, defined as flow below which the majority of patients developed ipsilateral EEG changes of ischaemia within 3 min of carotid occlusion, was found to be 8–10 ml/100g/min (Messick et al. 1987). This value is considerably lower compared with the values obtained during halothane anaesthesia (Sharbrough et al. 1973. In a retrospective study from the same group patients were subjected to carotid endarterectomy in either halothane, enflurane or isoflurane anaesthesia. The values for the ischaemic threshold for isoflurane and halothane were confirmed, and for enflurane the ischaemic threshold was found to be 15 ml. The incidence of ischaemic EEG changes was significantly less during isoflurane anaesthesia (18%), than during enflurane (26%) or halothane (25%) (Michenfelder et al. 1987). In another study isoflurane, in comparison with halothane anaesthesia, prevented EEG amplitude depression during trimethaphan-induced hypotension to MABP 40 mm Hg (Lloyd-Thomas et al. 1990). In clinical studies a neuroprotective effect of isoflurane has never been proved. Nevertheless, neuroanaesthesia with isoflurane has been practised, and is recommended during aneurysm surgery (Meyer and Muzzi 1992).

Controlled hypotension

Clinical studies indicate that isoflurane is a safe and effective agent for the induction of hypotension in neurosurgical patients (Campkin and Flinn 1986). Another point of view has been stressed by Young et al. (1989b). These authors compared CBF and $CMRO_2$ in patients subjected to carotid endarterectomy during either isoflurane, halothane or fentanyl anaesthesia supplemented with nitrous oxide, and found that the metabolic suppression, evaluated as decrease in $CMRO_2$,was equally affected. They concluded that choice of anaesthetic agents for cerebrovascular surgery should not be made on the basis of metabolic suppression. During relatively light anaesthesia, vasoactive properties of anaesthetics were suggested to be more important. An increase in adenylate kinase activity in CSF (a marker of brain cell injury) was observed after prolonged isoflurane-induced hypotension for correction of dento-facial deformities. During anaesthesia MABP was reduced to 50 mm Hg during several hours. (Enlund et al. 1989).

Aneurysm surgery

During surgery for cerebral aneurysm in isoflurane-induced hypotension to MABP 50–60 mm Hg, cardiac output is unchanged (Lam and Gelb 1983), and the pulmonary shunt fraction is unaffected (Nicholas and Lam 1984). Three studies of CBF and metabolism during isoflurane-induced hypotension in patients subjected to craniotomy for cerebral aneurysm have been published (Newman et al. 1986, Roth et al. 1986, Madsen et al. 1987c). In all three studies, CBF was unchanged during isoflurane-induced hypotension, while $CMRO_2$ was reduced by 9–58%, and CBF was considerably higher, compared with the threshold values of cerebral ischaemia of 10 ml/100g/min obtained during carotid endarterectomy (Messick et al. 1987). In the study by Madsen et al. (1987c) a significant increase in CBF during the post-hypotensive period was observed. This increase was not associated with changes in $PaCO_2$ or MABP. It was suggested that increased isoflurane concentration was still present in cerebral tissue at the time of investigation, but hyperaemia, secondary to regional cerebral ischaemia cannot be excluded, although global CBF was far above ischaemic threshold.

The effects of fast and slow increase in isoflurane concentration on cerebral haemodynamic have recently been studied during isoflurane-induced hypotension to MABP 60 mm Hg by repeated determination of AVDO2 in patients undergoing cerebral aneurysm surgery. The results indicate that rapid induction, in comparison with slow induction, is accompanied by an early and more prolonged decrease in AVDO2, suggesting a state of relative luxury-perfusion (Haraldsted et al. 1991).

Moyamoya disease

Regional cortical blood flow was measured by Laser-Doppler flowmeter in patients with Moyamoya disease. During isoflurane administration cortical blood flow decreased in some regions. The jugular venous bulb saturation increased in most patients, while the frontal near infra-red spectroscopy indicated a decrease. The results suggesting the occurrence of intracerebral steal (Sato et al. 1999).

Sevoflurane, experimental studies

Sevoflurane has a very low blood/gas solubility ratio compared to isoflurane (0.59 versus 1.41), suggesting that it may offer some advantages over isoflurane in neuroanaesthesia (Wallin et al. 1975). Emergency time for prolonged anaesthesia indicates conflicting results. In a comparison of isoflurane and sevoflurane it was found that emergency times increased with increasing duration for isoflurane but not for sevoflurane (Ebert et al. 1998). On the other hand, Eger et al. (1998) found that with increasing duration of administration (up to 8 hours) decrease in alveolar concentration of sevoflurane was increasingly delayed, and this was correlated to slower recovery times.

CSF formation and resistance to reabsorption

In rabbits sevoflurane did not influence CSF formation and resistance to reabsorption of CSF (Artru and Momota 2000).

CBF, $CMRO_2$ and EEG

In rabbits the effects of sevoflurane on CBF, ICP, $CMRO_2$ and the EEG are similar to those of isoflurane (Scheller et al. 1988). However, the study was performed during morphine, nitrous oxide anaesthesia and the blood pressure was maintained with angiotensin, all factors which might influence the results. The same group in non-paralysed dogs studied the effects of only sevoflurane or isoflurane as anaesthetic agents. The results indicate that sevoflurane, in common with isoflurane, had minimal effects on CBF at concentration of 0.5, 1.5 and 2.15 MAC, and significantly reduced $CMRO_2$ at end-tidal concentrations sufficient to produce a burst suppression pattern (Scheller et al. 1990). Another study indicates that compared with isoflurane the CBF increase is lesser during iso-MAC concentration of sevoflurane (Conzen et al. 1992). According to studies in pentobarbital-anaesthetised dogs the vasodilation of cerebral pial vessels induced by isoflurane and sevoflurane appears to be mediated, at least in part, via activation of ATP-sensitive K^+ channels (Iida et al. 1998).

ICP

In cats sevoflurane increases ICP and intracranial elastance (Kotani et al. 1992). However, sevoflurane does not increase ICP in hyperventilated dogs (Takahashi et al. 1993). The effect of cryogenic brain injury upon ICP was studied in sevoflurane and halothane anaesthetised rabbits. After cryogenic injury the concentration of inhaled anaesthetic drugs was increased to achieve a blood pressure of 35 mm Hg. Neo-synephrine was infused to raise the blood pressure to 100 mm Hg, During this procedure ICP increased from 11 to 44 mm Hg in the sevoflurane anaesthetised animals, against 9 to 32 mm Hg during halothane. The study indicates that neo-synephrine-induced increases in blood pressure in animals receiving sevoflurane are associated with a higher level of intracranial hypertension than in comparable halothane-anaesthetised animals (Kim et al. 1994). In another study in cats halothane and sevoflurane were compared as regard brain energy metabolism. It was found that hyperventilation and fluctuating blood pressure contributed to the occurrence of abnormal brain energy metabolism during both anaesthetic agents. The metabolic disturbances, however, were most pronounced during halothane administration (Fujibayashi et al. 1993).

Autoregulation

In rats cerebral autoregulation is intact with 1 MAC sevoflurane, but impaired with 2 MAC (Lu et al. 1998).

EEG activity

In cats spontaneous EEG spike activity and somatic stimulation-induced seizures during sevoflurane anaesthesia were reported (Osawa et al. 1994).

Sevoflurane, human studies

Central haemodynamic

Sevoflurane appears to offer a more stable heart rate profile than either isoflurane or desflurane (Malan et al. 1995, Ebert et al. 1995). In the guinea pig ventricular papillary muscle model the direct myocardial depressant effects of sevoflurane are similar to those described by isoflurane. The contractile depression is partly related to the attenuation of Ca^{2+} influx through the cardiac membrane. Another effect seems to be a depression of the delayed outward K^+ current, which appears to underlie the increased action potential duration (Park et al. 1996).

Nephrotoxicity

At low ventilatory flow rate sevoflurane compromises renal function. Under this circumstance sevoflurane is degraded by CO_2 absorbents to compound A (Gonsowski et al. 1994). The production of compound A is directly related to the temperature of the carbon dioxide absorbent, increasing as gas flow decreases (Bito and Ikeda 1994). In clinical studies of short duration, where gas flow of 1–2 l/min was used, serum creatinine and BUN were unchanged. However, after 8 hours 1.2 MAC sevoflurane administration renal toxicity, as indicated by high albumine excretion was found (Eger et al. 1997). In recent studies, where specific analysis to detect renal tubule cytotoxicity was applied, nephrotoxicity was not detected (Kharasch et al. 1997, Bito et al. 1997). Until the question of sevoflurane´s nephrotoxicity is solved, low-flow sevoflurane should not be administrated (flow < 2 l/min), and < 3l/min for daylong surgery. Sevoflurane should not be used in patients with impaired kidney function (Mazze and Jamison 1995, 97).

CBF and $CMRO_2$

In patients with supratentorial cerebral tumours sevoflurane increased CBF and decreased CVR dose-dependently. $CMRO_2$, was unchanged (Bundgaard et al. 1998). In cardiac patients CBF and $CMRO_2$ are coupled with a reduction of flow and metabolism averaging 38% and 47% respectively during one MAC sevoflurane (Mielck et al. 1999). Artru et al. (1997) found that sevoflurane and isoflurane at 0.5, 1.0 and 1.5 MAC decreased flow velocity in the middle cerebral artery, and an increase jugular venous oxygen saturation was observed. ICP was not significantly altered by either anaesthetics. In another study of patients without cerebral diseases flow velocity was reduced during sevoflurane anaesthesia compared with the awake condition. The addition of nitrous oxide caused flow velocity to increase towards the values obtained in the awake state (Cho et al. 1996). In children flow velocity studies indicate that sevoflurane and halothane combined with nitrous oxide decrease blood pressure and increase cerebral blood flow velocity, suggesting that sevoflurane produces cerebrovascular effects similar to those of halothane during anaesthetic induction (Berkowitz et al. 1996). During baseline propofol anaesthesia in patients with cerebral tumours 1% sevoflurane did not change flow velocity or jugular venous saturation. In contrast 3% sevoflurane reduced $AVDO_2$ by 25%, but flow velocity was still unchanged. The authors conclude that sevoflurane might provide a certain degree of luxury perfusion (Heath et al. 1997). In another study by Kuroda et al. (1996) sevoflurane increased the CBF/$CMRO_2$ ratio dose-dependently. At 1.5 MAC the increase of the ratio was maintained with minimal fluctuation for three hours. In a follow up study transcranial flow velocity was monitored during prolonged 1.5 MAC sevoflurane anaesthesia. No decay in flow velocity over time during a three hour period was observed (Kuroda et al. 1997). During surgical incision sevoflurane and isoflurane elicit similar impairment of $AVDO_2$ (Inada et al. 1996). In a recent review Duffy and Matta (2000) summarise that sevoflurane compares favourable to halothane and causes less disturbance of cerebral haemodynamic. The effects of sevoflurane on the central nervous system are not markedly dissimilar to isoflurane. Sevofluranes insolubility confers rapid onset, intraoperative titratability and rapid offset, which should facilitate early postoperative evaluation in the neurosurgical setting. However, it appears that with prolonged administration recovery times may be delayed.

Regional CBF

In studies of volunteers with MR technology 0.4 MAC of sevoflurane causes regional cerebral vasodilation as regional cerebrovascular resistance decreases and rCBF increases. Regional mean transit time showed that rCBF increased relatively more than regional cerebral blood volume, thereby indicating that the observed increase in rCBF during inhalation of sevoflurane cannot be explained by vasodilation alone (Kolbitsch et al. 2000).

EEG

In healthy volunteers EEG studies during sevoflurane anaesthesia have reported no evidence of neuroexcitation (Holaday and Smith 1981). Yet, several case reports have noted seizure-like movements, as well as EEG-recorded seizures during induction of sevoflurane anaesthesia (Adachi et al. 1992, Komatsu et al. 1994). In patients with refractory epilepsy the effects of sevoflurane and isoflurane on interictal spike activity were studied. It was found that under identical conditions, both sevoflurane and isoflurane provoke interictal spike activity at near burst-suppression dosages. This property, however, was more prominent with sevoflurane than with isoflurane (Watts et al. 1999). EEG studies have been performed in children. In comparison with halothane sevoflurane induction was accompanied by sharp slow waves, while slow waves and fast rhythms (spindles) were observed during halothane induction. Sevoflurane induction elicits a marked inhibition of parasympathetic control of heart rate (Constant et al. 1999). In adult women sevoflurane induction provokes epileptiform EEG activity with spikes or polyspikes. These changes are associated with an increase in heart rate (Yli-Hankala et al. 1999). Nevertheless, agitation observed during sevoflurane induction is never associated with seizure activity.

In patients undergoing elective carotid endarterectomy during 0.6–1.2% sevoflurane in 50% nitrous oxide, CBF was measured before and during carotid occlusion. Ischaemic EEG occurred at rCBF values of 7,8,11,11 and 13 ml. The $rCBF_{50}$,defined as the rCBF value at which 50% of patients will not demonstrate EEG evidence of cerebral ischaemia, was 11.5 ml/100g/min (Grady et al. 1998).

ICP

In patients undergoing transphenoidal hypophysectomy without evidence of mass effect sevoflurane at 0.5 and 1 MAC increases lumbar CSF pressure (Talke et al. 1999). The changes produced by 1 MAC sevoflurane did not differ from those found by the same authors during 1 MAC isoflurane or desflurane (Talke et al. 1996).

A relatively high ICP averaging 11 mm Hg was found during sevoflurane anaesthesia for patients with supratentorial cerebral tumours. An increase in ICP was not observed when sevoflurane concentration was increased (Bundgaard et al. 1998). In a non-randomized comparative study in patients with cerebral tumours ICP during sevoflurane and isoflurane anaesthesia were comparable, but significantly higher compared with propofol/fentanyl anaesthetised patients (Bundgaard and Cold 1997). These findings have been confirmed in an open randomized study including patients subjected to craniotomy for small supratentorial tumours. During near normocapnic CO_2 level ICP was significantly lower in patients subjected to propofol anaesthesia compared with isoflurane- and sevoflurane-anaesthetised patients. After hyperventilation propofol anaesthetised patients still had a lower ICP compared with isoflurane and sevoflurane, but the differences in ICP were much smaller (Petersen et al. 2000).

Cerebral autoregulation

In patients without cerebral diseases autoregulation is intact during 1.2 MAC sevoflurane (Cho et al. 1996). In a study of hypotensive anaesthesia induced by prostaglandin E_1 autoregulation was intact as well (Kitaguchi et al. 1992). In another study, in patients subjected to extra-intracranial by-pass anastomosis, cerebral autoregulation was intact (Kitaguchi et al. 1993). Studies of dynamic cerebral autoregulation with transcranial Doppler indicate that during 1.5 MAC sevoflurane dynamic autoregulation was better preserved during sevoflurane than with isoflurane anaesthesia (Summors et al. 1999).

CO_2-reactivity

In patients without cerebral diseases (Cho et al. 1996), cardiac patients (Mielck et al. 1999), patients with cerebral tumours (Inada et al. 1996), and patients subjected to extra-intracranial by-pass anastomosis (Kitaguchi et al. 1993) the CO_2 reactivity was intact. CO_2-reactivity in young adults, ranging 20 to 40 years, is greater than in adults in the 50 to 70 years of age (Nishiyama et al. 1997). In patients subjected to craniotomy for supratentorial cerebral tumours, the CO_2 reactivity was higher for sevoflurane and isoflurane, compared with propofol anaesthetised patients (Petersen et al. 2000). In another study adults undergoing surgery without cerebral or cardiovascular system disease, transcranial Doppler was monitored during stepwise change in end-tidal CO_2. The patients were randomly assigned to either sevoflurane or isoflurane anaesthesia. Flow velocity was smaller in the isoflurane group at end-tidal CO_2 ranging from 20 to 40 mm Hg. The rate of change in flow velocity with change in CO_2, however, was larger in the isoflurane compared with the sevoflurane group (Nishiyama et al. 1999).

Desflurane, experimental studies

Haemodynamic effect

At equi-anaesthetic concentrations, desflurane and isoflurane produced similar haemodynamic effects. However, in the absence of drugs that inhibited autonomic reflexes, desflurane had less negative inotropic activity and produced less decrease in arterial pressure. The coronary vasodilator actions of desflurane and isoflurane within the limitations of the actual model were not similar. When the increase in heart rate and rate-pressure product produced by desflurane were prevented with autonomic nervous blockade, desflurane produced no change in coronary blood flow velocity (Pagel et al. 1991).

CBF, $CMRO_2$ and ICP

In dogs desflurane produces a dose-related decrease in CVR and an increase in CBF. These changes are followed by a decrease in $CMRO_2$ and suppression of EEG. Maintenance of blood pressure with phenylephedrin increases CBF even more. ICP increased during desflurane anaesthesia as well (Lutz et al. 1990). In comparison with halothane, enflurane and isoflurane hypocapnia do not decrease ICP during 0.5–1 MAC desflurane (Lutz et al. 1991). In other studies the ICP increase is not completely prevented by hypocapnia.

Compared with isoflurane desflurane is not associated with major differences in the effects on cerebral glucose utilisation, CBF, and the coupling between local CBF and local glucose utilisation (Lenz et al. 1999).

CSF formation

The formation rate of CSF is increased during desflurane anaesthesia (Artru 1993). Desflurane, like isoflurane decreases intracranial compliance at normal CSF pressure. This effect was independent of anaesthetic concentration or $PaCO_2$ (Artru 1994).

EEG

Similar to isoflurane, the EEG is progressively suppressed. At 2 MAC desflurane elicits a burst suppression pattern, interrupted by periodic polyspiking activity. In swine no EEG evidence of tolerance to desflurane was observed (Rampil et al. 1991a). The effect of higher concentrations of Desflurane on EEG activity is attenuated with time (Lutz et al. 1990).

Evoked potential

Somato-sensory evoked potentials are depressed at concentrations > 1.5 MAC (Black et al. 1990).

CO_2 reactivity

During desflurane anaesthesia the CO_2 reactivity at all concentrations of desflurane ranging from 0.5 to 1.5 MAC remained intact (Lutz et al. 1991).

Protection

Studies in dogs indicate that during desflurane-induced hypotension CBF, though decreased, was able to provide adequate cerebral perfusion to meet cerebral demand of oxygen uptake, even during profound hypotension of MABP 40 mm Hg with 2.4% MAC desflurane (Milde and Milde 1991).

Brain tissue oxygen tension

Studies during prolonged MCAO occlusion indicate that brain tissue oxygen tension is better maintained during desflurane compared with etomidate anaesthetised animals (Hoffman et al. 1998b).

Recovery

Studies with MR technique indicate that anaesthesia residues in the brain is of shorter duration with desflurane than with isoflurane and halothane, suggesting that recovery from anaesthesia should be more rapid (Lockhart et al.1991). In a recent study Tsai et al. (1992) found that desflurane anaesthesia was superior to isoflurane anaesthesia in the recovery of cognitive function.

Desflurane, human studies

Induction and emergency.

In randomized studies the emergency from desflurane anaesthesia is more rapid than from isoflurane (Smiley et al. 1991).

Studies of transcranial Doppler

Healthy adult patients for non-neurological surgery in propofol anaesthesia were recruited to either desflurane 7.2% or sevoflurane 2.2% respectively. The concentration of the two anaesthetic gases were increased to 10.8% and 3.3% or desflurane two minutes later. The patients receiving desflurane had greater middle cerebral artery velocities and blood pressure than those receiving sevoflurane (Bedforth et al. 2000).

Brain tissue oxygen tension

In patients subjected to craniotomy for cerebral aneurysm brain tissue oxygen tension was monitored during either desflurane alone or desflurane supplemented with thiopental until the same burst suppression level. Temporary arterial clipping in thiopental-treated patients decreased brain tissue PO_2 by 30%, whereas desflurane increased brain tissue PO_2 by 70% (Hoffman et al. 1998a). The same group studied patients subjected to cerebral aneurysm surgery. Desflurane increases brain tissue oxygen tension and brain tissue pH, when desflurane concentration is increased form 4 to 9% end-tidal (Hoffman et al. 2000a).

ICP

In patients with supratentorial mass lesions, ICP increases progressively during 45 min of hypocapnia and 1 MAC desflurane. Under the same conditions this is not observed with isoflurane (Muzzi et al. 1992).

Combined with nitrous oxide

In a study of patients with supratentorial mass lesions tight brain after opening of dura occurred with higher frequency during 1 MAC isoflurane or desflurane compared with 0.5MAC of either isoflurane or desflurane plus 50% nitrous oxide. Spinal-fluid pressure was measured, but did not correlate to the occurrence of tight brain (Turner et al. 1996).

EEG

Desflurane produces EEG changes comparable to those observed with equipotent levels of isoflurane (Rampil et al. 1991b, Hoffman and Edelman 1995). The onset of silence of EEG is associated with a sudden reduction of blood flow velocity in the middle cerebral artery. The changes in EEG always precede the change in flow velocity by 5–7 s. These observations suggest that some flow/metabolism coupling is preserved during desflurane anaesthesia (Lam et al. 1995)

Clinical application

Recently con and pro regarding desflurane and sevoflurane have been discussed. On the one hand, the titratability of these inhalation agents has previously been unavailable. This creates a potential for tight haemodynamic control during the rapidly changing levels of stimulation in neurosurgery (Baker 1997). On the other hand, other neuroanaesthesiologists argue that intravenous anaesthetics are a better choice for neuroanaesthesia when considering their effects upon cerebral metabolism, protection against ischaemia, and toxicity (Tempelhoff 1997).

Nitrous oxide, experimental studies

Anaesthetic action

Nitrous oxide-induced analgesia is partially reversed by naloxone in humans (Yang et al. 1980, Chapman and Benedetti 1979) and mice (Berkowitz et al. 1976, Smith and Rees 1981). Nitrous oxide-induced analgesia is attenuated in mice by opioid receptor antagonists (Finck et al. 1988). During long exposure to nitrous oxide opioid receptor density in the brain stem decreased, indicating a down regulation of opioid receptors (Ngai and Finck 1982). In chronically cannulated canine inhalation of nitrous oxide causes a marked increase in enkephalin, suggesting a selective involvement of opioid neuropeptides in the mediation of nitrous oxide-induced analgesia (Finck et al. 1995). In microcultures of rat hippocampal neurones, nitrous oxide acts as non-competitive NMDA-receptor antagonist (Mennerick et al. 1998).

CBF and $CMRO_2$

Repeated studies in mice and rats indicate that CBF and $CMRO_2$ are unchanged during N_2O administration (Carlsson et al. 1976b, Harp et al. 1976, Ratcheson et al. 1977, Dahlgren et al. 1981, Ingvar and Siesjö 1982). However, in dogs an increase in both blood flow and oxygen uptake has been found (Theye and Michenfelder 1968a, Sakabe et al. 1978, Oshita et al. 1979, Gibson and Duffy 1981, Fitzpatrick and Gilboe 1982). In the same animal CBF increases during normocapnic nitrous oxide administration, but not during hypocapnia. Nitrous oxide increases ICP both during normo- and hypocapnia. This effect is observed in animals with normal ICP as well as animals subjected to ICP hypertension by inflation of an epidural balloon (Albin et al. 1986).

Regional CBF and glucose metabolism

In rats glucose utilisation was increased by 15–25% in subcortical structures (red nucleus, thalamus, geniculate bodies and superior colliculus), but decreased in nucleus accumbens and sensorimotor cortex by comparable amounts (Ingvar and Siesjö 1982, Pelligrino et al. 1984). *In vitro* studies of cerebral cortex mitochondria from the goat show that the increased oxygen consumption accompanying nitrous oxide anaesthesia, cannot be attributed to a direct effect of nitrous oxide on mitochondrial respiration (Becker et al. 1986). In dogs, the concentration of ATP and lactate is unchanged during N_2O anaesthesia (Michenfelder et al. 1970).

Dopaminergic activation

In rats nitrous oxide activates dopaminergic neuronal activity in the mesocortical projection and the medullary network. It is supposed that the emetic and euphoric properties of nitrous oxide may be caused by this activation. The activation of dopaminergic activity was, however, attenuated after four hours of exposure indicating development of acute tolerance (Murakawa et al. 1994).

Protection

In mice subjected to hypoxia nitrous oxide reduces survival and reverses thiopental-induced prolongation of survival time (Hartung and Cottrell 1987). Another study from the same group indicates that nitrous oxide impairs electrophysiologic recovery after severe hypoxia in rat hippocampal slices (Amorim et al. 1997). On the other hand, Milde (1988) found that nitrous oxide had no effect on survival time. As stated by Artru (1988b) methodological errors including ambient temperature and the inspiratory concentration of oxygen might be responsible for the discrepancy in results.

Stress and nitrous oxide sedation

Nitrous oxide only influences cerebral circulation and metabolism minimally, but a certain degree of activation may occur if stress factors are not eliminated (Carlsson et al. 1976b). These considerations are interesting because nitrous oxide in experimental studies as well as human investigations is used for sedation. It has been observed that CBF and $CMRO_2$ in paralysed animals increase considerably when nitrous oxide is exchanged with nitrogen. This increase is not observed in rats subjected to adrenectomy and rats undergoing treatment with β-blocking agents (Carlsson et al. 1975a). In unrestrained rats 70% nitrous oxide produces cerebral vasodilatation with 100% increase in cortical flow while $CMRO_2$ is unchanged. CBF remained increased even after 60 min nitrous oxide exposure (Baughman et al. 1990b).

Supplement to other anaesthetics

In cats where halothane or isoflurane were used as basis anaesthetic, nitrous oxide induces a significant increase in CBF (Drummed and Todd 1985, Hansen et al. 1988c). The increase in CBF elicited by nitrous oxide is highest at high end-tidal concentrations of halothane or isoflurane (Drummed et al. 1987). Studies in rats have demonstrated that the addition of nitrous oxide to background halothane anaesthesia was associated with dilatation of cerebral vasculature and an increase in ICP (Seyde et al. 1986). In rabbits the increase in CBF and ICP are accompanied by an increase in EEG frequency and decrease in amplitude. These changes as well as the increase in CBF and ICP were also observed during hypocapnia (Todd 1987, Kaieda et al. 1989a). Even during 1.4–3.5% isoflurane anaesthesia, giving rise to isoelectric EEG, nitrous oxide increases CBF, but has no effect on $CMRO_2$ (Roald et al. 1991). Hansen et al. (1989b) studied equipotent doses of isoflurane or halothane with or without nitrous oxide in rats. It was found that the addition of 0.5 MAC nitrous oxide to 0.5 MAC halothane resulted in flow similar to those produced by 1 MAC halothane alone. In contrast, the addition of nitrous oxide to 0.5 MAC isoflurane resulted in flow values significantly greater than those measured during 1.0 MAC isoflurane alone. It was concluded that the use of nitrous oxide as opposed to increased dose of volatile halogenated agents has no advantage in respect of minimising anaesthetic-induced increases in CBF (Hansen et al. 1989). Similar studies have been performed in pigs subjected to isoflurane-induced hypotension with or without nitrous oxide. It was found that nitrous oxide has no significant effect on CBF, flow velocity or ICP compared with isoflurane alone (Tsai et al. 1994). In rats it has been demonstrated that 70% nitrous oxide does not alter glucose utilisation when administrated with 0.5 MAC isoflurane. These data suggest that the effect of nitrous oxide on CBF when administrated with volatile agents is direct and mediated by factors other than change in cerebral metabolic rate (Reasoner et al 1990). Contrary to these observations, nitrous oxide combined with diazepam in rats elicits an associated and pronounced decrease in CBF and CMRO2 (Carlsson et al. 1976b, Carlsson and Chapman 1981). The effects of combinations of nitrous oxide with enflurane or isoflurane on blood flow, metabolism and outcome in experimental ischaemia are described in the sections of enflurane and isoflurane.

Nitrous oxide, human studies

CBF and rCBF

In humans, CBF is unchanged or increased during nitrous oxide administration, while $CMRO_2$ is decreased by 10–20% (Wollman et al. 1965, Alexander et al. 1968, Smith et al. 1970). Studies in adult volunteers indicate a dose-dependant increase in CBF especially in the frontal regions, while a decrease in the posterior cortical regions was observed (Deutsch and Samra 1990, Reinstrup et al. 1994). Administered together with halothane, nitrous oxide gives rise to an increase in jugular venous oxygen tension, suggesting cerebral vasodilatation (Sakabe et al. 1976).

PET studies indicate that nitrous oxide inhalation is associated with activation in the anterior cingulate cortex, a limbic area known to mediate psychomotor and cognitive processes. Deactivation was found in the posterior cingulate, hippocampus, parahippocampus gyrus, and visual association cortices in both hemispheres (Gyulai et al. 1996).

ICP

During induction of anaesthesia in patients with space-occupying lesions, nitrous oxide induces an increase in ICP (Henriksen and Balslev-J¢rgensen 1973, Misfeldt et al. 1974, Moss and McDowall 1979), and an increase in CBF and jugular venous oxygen tension (Sakabe et al. 1976). The increase in ICP disappears when nitrous oxide is withdrawn, and during hypocapnia (Misfeldt et al. 1974, Balslev-J¢rgensen and Misfeldt 1975). It is suggested that the increase in ICP during nitrous oxide induction, partly is caused by an increase in $PaCO_2$, provoked by a decrease in pulmonary minute ventilation owing to absorption of nitrous oxide in the lungs (Cold 1975). In adults without intracranial diseases isoflurane was compared with isoflurane supplemented with nitrous oxide. Under these comparable iso-MAC conditions nitrous oxide administration caused a 43% increase in CBF during normocapnia but not during hypocapnia. $CMRO_2$ was unaltered by nitrous oxide, but EEG demonstrated an activated pattern (Algotsson et al. 1992). Studies with transcranial Doppler indicate that nitrous oxide, when added to an isoflurane, is a potent cerebral vasodilator. The vasodilating effect of nitrous oxide, however, is not uniform; it progressively increased with an increasing isoflurane concentration (Strebel et al. 1995). In another study of patients without neurologic disease it was found that nitrous oxide is a more potent vasodilator than an equipotent dose of isoflurane (Lam et al. 1994).

The incidence of pneumocephalus after supratentorial craniotomy has been reported to be 100% (Domino et al. 1992, Reasoner et al. 1994). Tension pneumocephalus after neurosurgery in the supine position occurs very rarely (Satapathy and Dash 2000). After fossa posterior surgery tension pneumocephalus is common (Kitahata and Katz 1976, Lunsford et al. 1979, Friedman et al. 1981, Toung et al. 1983, Dash et al. 1990), and nitrous oxide has been claimed to increase ICP when air is entrapped. In the sitting and the steep head-up position nitrous oxide should immediately be withdrawn if clinical signs of air-embolism occur, and the use of nitrous oxide should be avoided during pneumoencephalography or when pneumoencephalocele is present. The effects of nitrous oxide on ICP after dural closure have been studied in patients undergoing craniotomy. It was found that continuation of nitrous oxide after dural closure did not affect ICP during this period, suggesting that it is not necessary to discontinue nitrous oxide prior to dural closure for reasons of avoiding expansion of intracranial air and increasing ICP (Domino et al. 1992).

Evoked potential.

In humans subjected to painful tooth pulp electrical shocks under nitrous oxide analgesia, evoked potential latencies and amplitudes are restored after naloxone administration (Chapman and Benedetti 1979).

EEG

The EEG changes described during nitrous oxide administration include acceleration of the volatile anaesthetic-induced fast activity, activation of beta range frequencies (Yamamura et al. 1981), along with a shifting temporal pattern which may represent acute tolerance (Avramow et al. 1990). Bispectral EEG studies during 50% nitrous oxide inhalation did not differ significantly from baseline values. Abrupt decreases from high to low concentration frequently evoked a profound, transient slowing of the EEG activity (Rampil et al. 1998).

Clinical application

The use of nitrous oxide in neuroanaesthesiological practice has been discussed, and it has been argued that the use of iv. infusion of hypnotic and analgesic agents can suitably be an alternative to techniques of anaesthesia with nitrous oxide (Barker 1987).

Xenon

Xenon, an inactive gas, has anaesthetic properties. 1 MAC Xenon is achieved with 71% suggesting that Xenon is more potent that nitrous oxide (Cullen et al. 1969). With transcranial Doppler sonography no adverse effects on myocardial function were detected (Luttropp et al. 1993). Xenon is used during stable Xenon enhanced CT-scanning in patients with intracranial disorders.

Receptor action

In a recent study the actions of isoflurane and Xenon on GABAergic and glutamatergic synapses were investigated using voltage-clamp techniques on cultures of the rat hippocampal neurones. In comparison with isoflurane, Xenon had no measurable effect upon GABAergic inhibitory postsynaptic currents or on currents evoked by exogenous application of GABA, but it inhibits total charge transfer through the excitatory postsynaptic current. Xenon selectively inhibits NMDA receptor-mediated component of the current, but has little effect on the AMPA/kainate receptor-mediated component (de Sousa et al. 2000).

CBF and ICP

During 30–40% Xenon inhalation an increase in CBF has been observed (Gur et al. 1985, Obrist et al. 1985, Hartmann et al. 1987). This finding has also been recorded with transcranial Doppler (Broich et al. 1992, Giller et al. 1990, Marks et al. 1992, Bergholt et al. 1996). In pigs studied with the sagital sinus outflow technique, however, xenon inhalation had no effect upon rCBF and cerebral autoregulation (Fink et al. 2000). In a recent study the effects of xenon inhalation on mean and local CBF and local glucose utilisation were studied in rats. Compared with conscious control inhalation with 30 and 70% xenon did not result in changes of lCBF or mean CBF. Two minutes after xenon inhalation, however, CBF increased by 48%. During steady state inhalation the correlation between CBF and glucose utilisation was maintained (Frietsch et al. 2001).

Studies of ICP are conflicting. Harrington et al. (1986) demonstrated an increase in ICP. This has been confirmed by Plougmann et al. (1994). In contrast other studies indicate no significant increase in ICP during xenon administration (Darby et al. 1989, Marion and Crosby 1991).

During xenon inhalation a specific deactivation in the anterior cingulate has been disclosed (Cold et al. 1998).

General Conclusion

Nitrous oxide, used for many years in neuroanaesthetic practice, has been criticised, because of its stimulating effects upon cerebral metabolism, and because it increases ICP. The results of several experimental as well as clinical studies suggest that nitrous oxide should be omitted. The epileptogenic character of enflurane makes this anaesthetic a bad choice for neurosurgical anaesthesia.

Isoflurane, in comparison with halothane and enflurane, possesses interesting qualities which make it an inhalation agent to be considered in neuroanaesthetic practice. Experimental and clinical studies indicate that isoflurane induces a moderate dose-dependent increase in CBF, CBV and ICP, and a decrease in CVR and $CMRO_2$. The CO_2 reactivity generally is preserved, and the changes in CBF, CBV and ICP can be attenuated by controlled hyperventilation. The pronounced suppression of $CMRO_2$ suggests a moderate brain protective effect, and compared to halothane the cerebral autoregulation is only partly impaired. However, a protective effect of isoflurane compared with halothane has never been proved. In comparison with halothane isoflurane suppresses the EEG dose-dependently, and at concentrations of 2–3% the EEG is isoelectric. The effect of isoflurane on the peripheral resistance can be used therapeutically when controlled hypotension is decided. However, isoflurane administration might result in uncontrolled decrease in MABP and CPP, especially during hypovolaemia and in patients with reduced cardiac reserves. These effects necessitate reduction in inspiratory concentration or infusion of considerable amounts of plasma expanders or crystalloid.

The effects on cerebral circulation and metabolism of sevoflurane and desflurane, are comparable to isoflurane. The benefits including rapid induction, emergence, and adjustments of anaesthetic depth make these anaesthetics a valuable tool in neurosurgical anaesthesia (Koenig 1994).

Measurement of CBF during neuroanaesthesia, as practised by Madsen and Cold (1991), was supposed to correlate to ICP. In an experimental comparative study of CBF and CBV it was found that CBF alone did not adequately describe the cerebrovascular effects of anaesthetics, at least with respect to predicting the magnitude of the likely effect on ICP (Todd and Weeks 1996). Comparative studies of ICP during isoflurane, nitrous oxide anaesthesia, and intravenous anaesthesia with propofol/fentanyl, did not disclose any difference in short-time outcome in patients subjected to supratentorial craniotomy. ICP level measured with epidural transducer through first burr hole were identical (Todd et al. 1993). Nevertheless, the opinion that total intravenous anaesthesia represents the best anaesthetic technique for neurological surgery has recently been advanced (Ravussin et al. 1994). Using a subdural approach described recently (Cold et al 1996) threshold of cerebral swelling during craniotomy has been defined. At ICP levels 10 mm Hg cerebral swelling occurs with high probability (Bundgaard et al. 1998). With this technique it was found, in a retrospective study, that ICP is lower during propofol/fentanyl anaesthesia compared with sevoflurane and isoflurane/nitrous oxide. The same study indicates that the number of patients with ICP above the threshold level of cerebral swelling (ICP >10 mm Hg) was significantly lower in patients undergoing anaesthesia with propofol/fentanyl (Bundgaard and Cold 1997a, Bundgaard and Cold 1997b). In a recent prospective study these findings have been confirmed (Petersen et al. 2000).

References

Adachi M, Ikemoto Y, Kubo K, Takuma C. Seizure-like movements during induction of anaesthesia with sevoflurane. Br J Anaesth 1992: 68: 214–215.

Adams RW, Gronert GA, Sundt TM, Michenfelder JD. Halothane, hypocapnia, and cerebrospinal fluid pressure in neurosurgery. Anesthesiology 1972: 37: 510–517.

Adams RW, Cucchiara RF, Gronert GA, et al. Isoflurane and cerebrospinal fluid pressure in neurosurgical patients. Anesthesiology 1981: 54: 97–99.

Antognini JF, Carstens E. Isoflurane blunts electroencephalographic and thalamic-reticular formation responses to noxious stimulation in goats. Anesthesiology 1999: 91: 1770–1779.

Albin MS, Bunegin L, Gelineau J. ICP and CBF reactivity to isoflurane and nitrous oxide during normocapnia, hypocapnia and intracranial hypertension. In: Miller JD, Teasdale GM, Rowan JO; Galbraith SL, Mendelow AD (Eds) Intracranial Pressure VI. Springer Verlag, Berlin, Heidelberg 1986: 719–724.

Albrecht RF, Miletich DJ, Rosenberg R, Zahed B. Cerebral blood flow and metabolic changes from induction to onset of anesthesia with halothane or pentobarbital. Anesthesiology 1977: 47: 252–256.

Albrecht RF, Miletich DJ, Madala LR. Normalization of cerebral blood flow during prolonged halothane anaesthesia. Anesthesiology 1983: 58: 26–31.

Alexander SC, Wollman H, Cohen PJ, et al. Cerebrovascular response to $PaCO_2$ during halothane anaesthesia in man. J Appl Physiol 1964: 19: 561–565.

Algotsson L, Messeter K, Nordstrom CH, Ryding E. Cerebral blood flow and oxygen consumption during isoflurane and halothane anaesthesia in man. Acta Anaestheiol Scand 1988: 32: 15–20.

Algotsson L, Messeter K, Rosén I, Holmin T. Effects of nitrous oxide on cerebral haemodynamics and metabolism during isoflurane anaesthesia in man. Acta Anaesthesiol Scand 1992: 36: 46–52.

Alkire MT, Haier RJ, Shah NK, Anderson CT. Positron emission tomography study of regional cerebral metabolism in humans during isoflurane anesthesia. Anesthesiology 1997: 86: 549–557.

Amorim P, Chanbers G, Cottrell J, Kass IS. Nitrous oxide impairs electrophysiologic recovery after severe hypoxia in rat hippocampal slices. Anesthesiology 1997: 87: 642–651.

Archer DP, Labrecque P, Tylor JL, et al. Cerebral blood volume is increased in dogs during administration of nitrous oxide or isoflurane. Anesthesiology 1987: 67: 642–648.

Archer DP, Lebrecque P, Tylor JL, et al. Measurement of cerebral blood flow and volume with positron emission tomograpy during isoflurane administration in the hypocapnic baboon. Anesthesiology 1990: 72: 1031–1037.

Artru AA, Steen PA, Michenfender JD. Cerebral metabolic effects of nalaxone administered with anaesthetic and subanaesthetic concentrations of halothane in the dog. Anesthesiology 1980: 52: 217–220.

Artru AA. Relationship between cerebral blood volume and CSF pressure during anesthesia with halothane or enflurane in dogs. Anesthesiology 1983: 58: 533–539.

Artru AA. Effects of enflurane and isoflurane on resistance to reabsorption of cerebrospinal fluid in dogs. Anesthesiology 1984c: 61: 529–533.

Artru AA. Effects of halothane and fentanyl anesthesia on resistance to reabsorption of CSF. J Neurosurg 1984d: 60: 252–256.

Artru AA. Isoflurane does not increase the rate of CSF production in the dog. Anesthesiology 1984a: 60: 193–197.

Artru AA. Relationship between cerebral blood volume and CSF pressure during anesthesia with isoflurane or fentanyl in dogs. Anesthesiology 1984b: 60: 575–579.

Artru AA. Cerebral metabolism and EEG during combination of hypocapnia and isoflurane-induced hypotension in dogs. Anesthesiology 1986a: 65: 602–608.

Artru AA. Survival time during hypoxia: Effects of nitrous oxide, thiopental, and hypothermia (Editorial) Anesth Analg 1988b: 67: 913–916.

Artru AA. rate of cerebrospinal fluid formation, resistance to reabsorption of cerebrospinal fluid, brain tissue water content, and electroencephalogram during desflurane anesthesia in dogs. Journal of Neurosurgical Anesthesiology 1993: 5: 178–186.

Artru AA. Intracranial volume/pressure relationsship during desflurane anesthesia in dogs: Comparison with isoflurane and thiopental/halothane. Anesth Analg 1994: 79: 751–760.

Artru AA, Lam AM, Johnson JO, Sperry RJ. Intracranial pressure, middle cerebral artery flow velocity, and plasma inorganic cencentrations in neurosurgical patients receiving sovoflurane or isoflurane. Anesth Analg 1997: 85: 587–592.

Artru AA, Momota Y. Rate of CSF formation and resitance to reabsorption of CSF during sevoflurane or remifentanil in rabbits. J Neurosurg Anesthesiol 2000: 12: 37–43.

Astrup J, Rosen¢rn J, Cold GE, et al. Minimum cerebral blood flow and metabolism during craniotomy. Effect of thipental loading. Acta Anaesthesiol Scand 1984: 28: 478–481.

Avramov MN, Shingu K, Morris K. Pregressive changes in electroencephalographic responses to nitrous oxide in humans. A possible acute drug tolerance. Anesth Analg 1990: 70: 369–374.

Back T, Kohno K, Hossmann KA. Cortical negative DC deflections following middle cerebral artery occlusion and KCl-induced spreading depression: effect on blood flow, tissue oxygenation, and electroencephalogram. J Cereb Blood Flow Metab 1994: 14: 12–19.

Baker KZ. Desflurane and sevoflurane are valuable additions to the practice of neuroanesthesiology: pro. J Neurosurg Anesthesiol 1997: 9: 66–68.

Balslev-J¢rgensen B, Misfeldt BB. Intracranial pressure during recovery from nitrous oxide and halothane anesthesia in neurosurgical patients. Br J Anaesth 1975: 47: 977–981.

Banks MI, Pearce RA. Dual actions of volatile anesthetics on $GABA_A$ IPCs: Dissociation of blocking and prolonging effects. Anesthesiology 1999: 90: 120–134.

Barker J. Nitrous oxide in neurosurgical anaesthesia (editorial). Br J Anaesth 1987: 59: 146–147.

Baughman VL, Hoffman WE, Miletich DJ, et al. Neurologic outcome in rats following incomplete cerebral ischaemia during halothane, isoflurane, or N_2O. Anesthesiology 1988: 69: 192–198.

Baughman VL, Hoffman WE, Miletich DJ, Albrecht RF. Isoflurane vs. methohexital during incomplete cerebral ischaemia in the rat. Anesth Analg 1989a: 68: S19.

Baughman VL, Hoffman WE, Thomas C, et al. The interaction of nitrous oxide and isoflurane with incomplete cerebral ischemia in the rat. Anesthesiology 1989b: 70: 767–774.

Baughman VL, Hoffman WE, Thomas C, et al. Comparison of methohexital and isoflurane on neurologic outcome and histopathology following incomplete ischemia in rats. Anesthesiology 1990a: 72: 85–94.

Baughman VL, Hoffman WE, Thomas C, et al. Cerebrovascular and cerebral metabolic effects of N_2O in unrestrained rats. Anesthesiology 1990b: 73: 269–272.

Becker GL, Pelligrino DA, Miletich DJ, Albrecht RF. The effect of nitrous oxide on oxygen consumption by isolated cerebral cortex mitochondria. Anesth Analg 1986: 65: 355–359.

Bedforth N, Hardman JG, Nathanson MH. Cerebral hemodynamics response to the introduction of desflurane: A comparison with sevoflurane. Anesth Analg 2000: 91: 152–155.

Belapavlovic M, Buchthal A, Beks JWF. Barbiturates for cerebral aneurysm surgery. Acta Neurochir 1985: 76: 73–81.

Belapavlovic M, Buchthal A. Effect of isoflurane on intracranial pressure in patients with intracranial mass lesions. In: Miller JD, Teasdale GM, Rowan JO, Galbraith SL, Mendelow AD (eds); Intracranial Pressure VI, Springer Verlag, berlin, Heidelberg 1986: 725–731.

Bendo AA, Kaas IS, Cottrell JE. Anesthetic protection against anoxic damage in the rat hippocampal slice. Brain Research 1987: 403: 136–141.

Bendtsen AO, Cold GE, Astrup J, Rosen¢rn J. Thiopental loading during controlled hypotension for intracranial aneurysm surgery Acta Anaesthesiol Scand 1984: 28: 473–477.

Bergholt B, Plougmann B, Astrup J, et al. Blood flow velocities in middle cererbal artery during inhalation of 30% stable xenon. Acta Neurol Scand 1996: (suppl) 166: 46–49.

Berkowitz RA, Ngai SH, Finck AD. Nitrous oxide analgesia: resenblance to opiate action. Science 1976: 194: 967–968.

Berkowitz RA, Hoffman WE, Cunnigham F, McDonald T. Changes in cerebral blood velocity in children during sevoflurane and halothane anesthesia. J Neurosurg Anesthesiol 1996: 8: 194–198.

Bickler PE, Buck LT, Hansen BM. Effects of isoflurane and hypothermia on glutamate receptor-mediated calcium influx in brain slices. Anesthesiology 1994: 81: 1461–1469.

Bito H, Ikeda K. Plasma-inorganic fluoride and intracircuit degradation product concentrations in long-duration, low-flow sevoflurane anesthesia. Anesth Analg 1994: 79: 946–951.

Bito H, Ikeuchi Y, Ikeda K. Effects of low-flow sevoflurane anesthesia on renal function: comparison with high-flow sevoflurane anesthesia and low-flow isoflurane asneshtesia. Anesthesiology 1997: 86: 1231–1237.

Bisonnette B, Leon JE Cerebrovascular stability during isoflurane anaesthesia in children. Can J Anaesth 1992: 39: 128–134.

Black S, Konstadt S, Sami H, Roa T. Effect of I-653 (desflurane) on somatosensory evoked potentials [abstract]. Anesthesiology 1990: 73: A181.

Blaise G, To Q, Parent M, et al. Does halothane interfere with the release, action, or stability of endothelium-derived relaxing factor/Nitric oxide? Anesthesiology 1994: 80: 417–426.

Boop WC, Knight R. Enflurane anesthesia and changes of intracranial pressure. J Neurosurg 1978: 48: 228–231.

Botty C, Brown B, Stanley V, et al. Clinical experiences with the compound 347, a halogenated anesthetic compound. Anest Analg 1968: 47: 499–505.

Brandt L, Dick W, Erdmann K. Nitrous oxide influences EEG changes induced by halothane, enflurane and isoflurane. Anesthesiology 1985: 63: A409.

Brian JE, McPherson RW, Traystman RJ. Evolution of cerebral blood flow with time during 1.4 and 2.8% isoflurane in dog. Anesthesiology 1988: 69: A532.

Brian JE, Traystman RJ, McPherson RW. Changes in cerebral blood flow over time during isoflurane anesthesia in dogs. J Neurosurg Anesthesiol 1990: 2: 122–130.

Broich H, Bülau P, Hartmann A. et al. The effect of stable xenon inhalation on cerebral blood flow velocities and topographic electroencephalography in normal volunteers. In Yonas H (ed): Cerebral blood flow measurement with stable xenon enhanced computed tomography. New York; Raven Press 1992: 292–295.

Bundgaard H, Jensen K, Cold GE, et al. Effects of perioperative indomethacin on intracranial pressure, cerebral blood flow, and cerebral metabolism in patients subjected to craniotomy for cerebral tumors. J Neurosurg Anesthesiol 1966: 8: 273–279.

Bundgaard H, Cold GE. A prospective comparative study of ICP during three anesthetics for elective craniotomy. Acta Anaestheiol Scand 1997: 41: (suppl10): 166.

Bundgaard H, Cold GE. A prospective study of ICP during two anesthetics for elective craniotomy. Acta Anaesthesiol Scand 1997: 41: (suppl 110): 195.

Bundgaard H, Landsfeldt U, Cold GE. Subdural monitoring of ICP during craniotomy.Acta Neurochir 1998: (suppl 71): 276–278.

Bundgaard H, von Oettingen G, Larsen KM, et al. Effects of sevoflurane on intracranial pressure, cerebral blood flow, and cerebral metabolism. A dose-response study in patients subjected to craniotomy for cerebral tumours. Acta Anaesthesiol Scand 1998: 42: 621–627.

Burchiel KJ, Stockard JJ, Calverley RK, Smith NT. Relationship of pre and postanaesthetic EEG abnormalities to enflurane-induced seizure activity. Anesth Analg 1977: 56: 509–514.

Busto R, Dietrich W, Globus M, et al. Small differences in intraischemic brain temperature critically determine the extent of neuronal injury. J Cereb Blood Flow Metab 1987: 7: 729–738.

Busto R, Globus M-T, Dietrich W, et al. Effect of mild hypothermia on ischemic-induced release of neurotransmitters and free fatty acids in rat brain. Stroke 1989: 20: 904–910.

Campkin TV. Isoflurane and cranial extradural pressure, A study in neurosurgical patients. Br J Anaesth 1984: 56: 1083–1087.

Campkin TV, Flinn RM. Isoflurane: Its use to induce hypotension in neurosurgical patients. Europ J Anesthesiology 1986: 3: 395–401.

Campkin TV, Flinn RM. Isoflurane and cerebrospinal fluid pressure. A study in neurosurgical patients undergoing intracranial shunt procedures. Anaesthesia 1989: 44: 50–54.

Carlsson C, Hagerdal M, Siesjo BK. Increase in cerebral oxygen uptake and blood flow in immobilization stress. Acta Physiol Scand 1975a: 95: 206–208.

Carlsson C, Hagerdal M, Siesjo BK. The effect of nitrous oxide on oxygen consumption and blood flow in the cerebral cortex of the rat. Acta Anaesth Scand 1976a: 20: 91–95.

Carlsson C, Hagerdal M, Kaasik AE, Siesjo BK. The effects of diazepam on cerebral blood flow and oxygen consumption in rats and its synergistic interaction with nitrous oxide. Anesthesiology 1976b: 45: 319–325.

Carlsson C, Chapman AG. The effects of diazepam on the cerebral metabolic state in rats and its interaction with nitrous oxide. Anesthesiology 1981: 54: 488–495.

Carpenter RL, Eger EI II, Johnson BH, et al. Pharmacokinetics of inhaled anaesthetics in humans: Measurements during and after the simultaneous administration of enflurane, halothane, isoflurane, methoxyplurane and nitrous oxide. Anesth Analg 1986: 65: 575–582.

Chapman CR, Benedetti C. Nitrous oxide effects on cerebral evoked potential to pain: partial reversal with a narcotic antagonist. Anesthesiology 1979: 51: 135–138.

Chen RYZ, Fan FC, Schuessler GB, Chien S. Distribution of cerebral blood flow (CBF) during halothane anesthesia. Anesthesiology 1982: 57: A37.

Chen RYZ, Fan FC, Carlin RD, et al. Comparison of regional cerebral blood flow during isoflurane and halothane induced hypotension. Anesthesiology 1984: 61: A21.

Cheng S-C, Brunner Ea. Inhibition of GABA metabolism in rat brain slices by halothane. Anesthesiology 1981: 55: 26–33.

Chi OZ, Anwar M, Sinha AK, et al. Effects of isoflurane on transport across the blood-brain barrier. Anesthesiology 1992: 76: 426–431.

Cho S, Fujigaki T, Uchiyama Y, et al. Effects of sevoflurane with and without nitrous oxide on human cerebral circulation. Anesthesiology 1996: 85: 755–760.

Chong KY, Craen RA, Murkin JM, et al. Rate of change of cerebral blood flow velocity with hyperventilation during anaesthesia in humans. Can J Anesth 2000: 47: 125–130.

Christensen MS, H¢edt-Rasmussen K, Lassen NA. Cerebral vasodilatation by halothane anaesthesia in man and its potentiation by hypotension and hypercapnia. Br J Anaesth 1967: 927–934.

Christys AR, Moss E, Powell D. Retrospective study of early postoperative convulsions after intracranial surgery with isoflurane or enflurane anaesthesia. Br. J Anaesth 1989: 62: 624–627.

Clark DL, Hosick EC, Adams N, et al. Neural effects of isoflurane (Forane) in man Anesthesiology 1973: 39: 261–270.

Cohen EN, Chow KL, Mathers L. Autoradiographic distribution of volatile anaesthetics within the brain. Anesthesiology 1972: 37: 324–331.

Cold GE. Nitrous oxide and intracranial pressure. Br J Anaesth 1975: 47: 1119.

Cold GE, Christensen KJS, Nordentoft J, et al. Cerebral blood flow, cerebral metabolic rate of oxygen and relative CO_2 reactivity during neurolept anesthesia in patients subjected to craniotomy for supratentorial cerebral tumors. Acta Anaesthesiol Scand 1988. 32: 310–315.

Cold GE, Tange M, Jensen TM, Ottesen S. Subdural pressure measurement during craniotomy. Correlation with tactile estimation of dural tension and brain herniation after opening of dura. Br J Neurosurg 1996: 10: 69–75.

Cold GE, Bergholt B, von Oettingen G, et al. Is focal decline of blood flow to anterior cingulate during inhalation of 33% stable Xenon a key to anaesthesia. Acta Anaesthesiol Scand 1999 (suppl 114): 43: 113.

Cole DJ, Drummond JC, Shapiro HM. A comparison of the extent of ischaemia following middle cerebral artery occlusion during three induced hypotensive techniques. Anesthesiology 1987: 67: A571.

Cole DJ, Shapiro HM. Different 1.2 MAC combinations of nitrous oxide-enflurane cause unique cerebral and spinal cord metabolic responses in the rat. Anesthesiology 1989: 70: 787–792.

Constant I, Dubois M-C, Piat V et al. Changes in electroencephalogram and autonomic cardiovascular activity during induction of anesthesia with sevoflurane compared with halothane in children. Anesthesiology 1999: 91: 1604–1615.

Conzen PF, Vollmar B et al. Systemic and regional hemodynamics of isoflurane and sevoflurane in rats. Analg Anesth 1992: 74: 79–88.

Cucchiara RF, Theye RA, Michenfelder JD. The effects of isoflurane on canine cerebral metabolism and blood flow. Anesthesiology 1974: 40: 571–574.

Cullen SC, Eger EI II, Cullen BF, Gregory P. Observations on the anesthetic effect of combination of xenon and halothane. Anesthesiology 1969: 31: 305–309.

Cunitz G, Danhauser I, Gruss P. Die Wirkung con Enflurane (Etrane) im Vergleich zu Halothan auf den intracranielle Druck. Anaesthesist 1976: 25: 323–330.

Dahlgren N, Ingvar M, Yokoyama H, Siesjo BK. Effect of indomethacin on local cerebral blood flow in awake, minimally restrained rats. J Cereb Blood Flow Metab 1981: 1: 233–236.

Darimont PC, Jenkins LC. The influence of intravenous anaesthetics on enflurane-induced central nervous system seizure activity. Can Anesth Soc J 1977: 24: 42–56.

Darby JM, Yonas H, Pentheny S. et al. Intracranial pressure response to stable xenon inhalation in patients with head injury. Surg Neurol 1989: 32: 343–345.

Dash hh, Bithal PK, Muley S, et al. Tension pneumocephalus following posterior fossa surgery in sitting position. J Anaesth Clin Pharmacol 1990: 6: 207–212.

De Jong RH, Heavner JE. Correlation of the Ethrane Electroencephalogram with motor activity in cats. Anesthesiology 1971: 35: 474–481.

DeRood M, Deloof T, Berre J, et al. Effect of 1% enflurane anesthesia on cerebral blood flow and metabolism in neurosurgical patients during normo- and hyperventilation. Acta Anaesthesiol Belg 1980: 31 (suppl): 3–19.

DeSousa SLM, Dickinson R, Lieb WR, Franks NP. Contrasting synaptic actions of the inhalational general anesthetics isoflurane and Xenon. Anesthesiology 2000: 92: 1055–1066.

Deutsch G, Samra SK. Effects of ntrous oxide on global and regional cortical blood flow. Stroke 1990: 21: 1293–1298.

Dewitt DS, Fatouros PP, Wist AO, et al. Stable xenon versus radiolabeled microsphere cerebral blood flow measurements in baboons. Stroke 1989: 20: 1716–1723.

DiGiovanni AJ, Goodrick J, Neigh JL, et al.. The effect of halothane anaesthesia on intracranial pressure in the presence of intracranial hypertension. Anesth Analg 1974: 53: 823–828.

Domino KB, Hemstad JR, Lam AM, et al. Effect of nitrous oxide in intracranial pressure after cranial-dural closure in patients undergoing craniotomy. Anesthesiology 1992: 77: 421–425.

Drummond JC, Todd MM, Toutant SM, Shapiro HM. Brain surface protrusion during enflurane, halothane and isoflurane anesthesia in cats. Anesthesiology 1983a: 59: 288–293.

Drummond JC, Todd MM. Shapiro HM. Cerebral blood flow autoregulation in the cat during anesthesia with halothane and isoflurane. Anesthesiology 1983b: 55: A305.

Drummond JC, Todd MM. The response of feline cerebral circulation to $PaCO_2$ during anesthesia with isoflurane and halothane and during sedation with nitrous oxide. Anesthesiology 1985: 62: 268–273.

Drummond JC, Todd MM, Scheller MS, Shapiro HM. A comparison of the direct cerebral vasodilating potencies of halothane and isoflurane in the New Zealand White Rabbit. Anesthesiology 1986: 65: 462–467.

Drummond JC, Scheller MS, Todd MM. The effect of nitrous oxide on cortical blood flow during anaesthesia with halothane and isoflurane, with and without morphine, in the rabbit. Anesth Analg 1987: 66: 1083–1089.

Dwyer RC, Rampil IJ, EgerII EI. Bennett HL. The electroencephalogram does not predict depth of isoflurane anesthesia. Anesthesiology 1994: 81: 403–409.

Dubois MY, Sato S, Chassy J, Macnamara TE. Effects of enflurane on brainstem auditory evoked responses in humans. Anesth Analg 1982: 61: 898–902.

Duffy C, Matta BF. Sevoflurane and anaesthesia for neurosurgery. J Neurosurg Anesthesiol 2000: 12: 128–140.

Ebert TJ, Harkin CP, Muzzi M. Cardiovascular responses to sevoflurane: a review. Anesth Analg 1995: 81: S11–22.

Ebert TJ, Robinson BJ, Uhrich TD, et al. Recovery from sevoflurane anaesthesia: a comparison to isoflurane and propofol anaesthesia. Anesthesiology 1998: 89: 1524–1531.

Eger EI, Stevens WC, Cromwell TH. The electroencephalogram in man anesthetized with forene. Anesthesiology 1971: 35: 504–508.

Eger EI II, Koblin DD, Bowland T, et al. Nephrotoxicity of sevoflurane versus desflurane anesthesia in volunteers. Anesth Analg 1997: 84: 160–168.

Eger EI II, Gong D, Koblin DD, et al. The effect of aneshtetic duration on kinetic and recovery characteristic of desflurane versus sevoflurane, and on the kinetic charactiristic of compound A in volunteers. Anesth Analg 1998: 86: 414–421.

Eilers H, Bickler PE. Hypothermia and isoflurane similarly inhibit glutamate release evoked by chemical anoxia in rat cortical brain slices. Anesthesiology 1996: 85: 600–607.

Eintrei C, Leszniewski W, Carlsson C. Local application of 133-Xenon for measurement of regional cerebral blood flow (rCBF) during halothane, enflurane and isoflurane anaeshesia in humans. Anesthesiology 1985: 63: 391–394.

Engberg M, Öberg B, Christensen KS, et al. The arterio-venous oxygen content differences ($AVDO_2$) during halothane and neuroleptanaesthesia in patients subjected to craniotomy. Acta Anaesthiol Scand 1989: 33: 642–646.

Engberg M, Melsen NC, Herlevsen P, et al. Changes of blood pressure and cerebral arterio-venous oxygen content differences ($AVDO_2$) with and without bupivacain scalp infiltration during craniotomy. Acta Anaesthiol Scand 1990: 34: 346–349.

Erdmann K, Brandt L. Paradoxical EEG arousal phenomenon following anesthesia with isoflurane. Anesthesiology 1986: 65: A347.

Eskinder H, Hillard CJ, Flynn N, et al. Halothane-induced vasodilation of canine cerebral arteries may be mediated through cyclic GMP formation. Anesth Analg 1992: 74: S91.

Eskinder H, Gebremedhin D, Lee JG, et al. Halothane and isoflurane decrease the open state probability of K+ channels in dog cerebral arterial muscle cells. Anesthesiology 1995: 82: 479–490.

Farber NE, Harkin CP, Niedfeldt J, et al. Regional-specific and agent-specific dilation of intracerebral microvessels by volatile anesthetics in rat brain slices. Anesthesiology 1997: 87: 1191–1198.

Finck AD, Samaniego E. Ngai SH. Irreversible opoid receptor blockade decreases the analgetic effects of ketamine and nitrous oxide in mice. Anesthesiology 1988: 69: A604.

Finck DA, Samaniego E, Ngai SH. Nitrous oxide selectively releases Met^5-Enkephalin and Met^5-enkephalin-Arg^6-Phe^7 into canine third ventricular cerebrospinal fluid. Anesth Analg 1995: 80: 664–670.

Fink H, Blobner M, Bogdanski R, et al. Effects of xenon on cerebral blood flow and autoregulation: an experimental study in pigs. Br J Anaesth 2000: 84: 221–225.

Firestone S, Firestone LL, Ferguson C, Blanck D. Staurosporine a protein kinase C inhibitor, decreases the general anesthetic requirement in Rana Pipiens tadpoles. Anesth Analg 1993: 77: 1026–1030.

Fitch W, McDowall DG. Effect of halothane on intracranial pressure gradients in the presence of intracranial space-occupying lesions. Br J Anaesth 1971: 43: 904–911.

Fitzpatrick JH, Gilboe DD. Effects of nitrous oxide on the cerebrovascular tone, oxygen metabolism, and electroencephalogram of the isolated perfused canine brain. Anesthesiology 1982: 57: 480–484.

Flynn NM, Buljubasic N, Bosnjak ZJ, Kampine JP. Isoflurane produces endothelium-independent relaxation in canine middle cerebral arteries. Anesthesiology 1992: 76: 461–467.

Fontenot HJ, Wilson RD, Norris JC, Ho IK. The GABA system: New evidence of neurotransmitter involvement in the mechanism of anesthesia. Anesthesiology 1984: 61: A327.

Forster A, VanHorn K, Marshall LF, Shapiro HM. Anesthetic effects on blood-brain barrier function during acute arterial hypertension. Anesthesiology 1978: 49: 26–30.

Franks JJ, Horn J-L, Janicki PK, Singh G. Halothane, isoflurane, xenon, and nitrous oxide inhibit calcium ATPase activity in rat brain synaptic plasma membranes. Anesthesiology 1995a: 82: 108–117.

Franks JJ, Horn J-L, Janicki PK, Singh G. Stable inhibition of brain synaptic plasma membrane calcium ATPase in rats anesthetized with halothane. Anesthesiology 1995b: 82: 118–128.

Franks JJ, Wamil AW, Janicki PK, et al. Anesthetic-induced alteration of Ca^{2+} homeostasis in neural cells: A temperature-sensitive process that is enhanced by blockade of plasma memebrane Ca^{2+}-ATPase isoforms. Anesthesiology 1998: 89: 149–164.

Friedman GA, Norfleet EA, Bedford RF. Discontinuation of nitrous oxide does not prevent pneumocephalus. Anesth Analg 1981: 60: 57–58.

Friesen RH, Thieme RE, Honda AT, Morrison JE. Changes in anterior fontanel pressure in preterm neonates receiving isoflurane, halothane, fentanyl or ketamine. Anesth Analg 1987: 66: 431–434.

Frietsch T, Bogdanski R, Blobner M, et al. Effects of Xenon on cerebral blood flow and cerebral glucose utilization in rats. Anesthesiology 2001: 94: 290–297.

Fujibayashi T, Sugiura Y, Yanagimoto M, et al. Brain energy metabolism and blood flow during sevoflurane and halothane anesthesia: effects of hypocapnia and blood pressure fluctations. Acta Anaesthesiol Scand 1993: 37: 806–810.

Fuller J, Gelb AW, Karlik S. The influence of halothane and innovar on brain oedema formation. Can Anesth Soc J 1980: S110.

Gelman S, Fowler KC, Smith LR. Regional blood flow during isoflurane and halothane anaesthesia. Anesth Analg 1984: 63: 557–565.

Gibson GE, Duffy TE. Impaired synthesis of acetylcholine by mild hypoxia or nitrous oxide. J Neurochem 1981: 36: 28–33.

Giller CA, Purdy P, Lindstrøm WW. Effects of inhaled stable xenon on cerebr of the Ethrane Electroencephalogram with motor activity in cats. Anesthesiology 1971: 35: 474–481.

Giller CA, Purdy P, Lindstrøm WW. Effects of inhaled stable xenon on cerebral blood flow velocity. AJNR 1990: 11: 177–182.

Gonsowski CT, Laster MJ, Eger II EI, et al. Toxocoty of compound A in rats. Effect of a 3-hour administration. Anesthesiology 1994: 80: 556–565.

Gordon E. The action of drugs on intracranial contents. In: Boulton TB, Bryce-Smith R et al. (eds); Progress in Anaesthesiology, Excerpta Medica, Amsterdam 1970: 60.

Gordon E. Anaesthesia for neurosurgery. In Emeric Gordon (ed) A basis and practice of neuroanaesthesia. Excerpta Medica 1974:173–198.

Gordon E, Lagerkranser M, Rudehill A, von Host H. The effect of isoflurane on cerebrospinal fluid pressure in patients undergoing neurosurgery. Acta Anaesthesiol Scand 1988: 32: 108–112.

Grady RE, Weglinsky MR, Sharbrough FW, Perkins WJ. Correlation of regional cerebral blood flow with ischemic electroencephalographic changes during sevoflurane- nitrous oxide anesthesia for carotid endarterectomy. Anesthesiology 1998: 88: 892–897.

Graf R, Saito K, Hübel K. et al. Spreading depression-like DC-negativations turn into terminal depolarization after prolonged focal ischemia in cats. J Cereb Blood Flow Metab 1995: (suppl) 15: S15.

Grant IS. Delayed convulsions following enflurane anaesthesia. Anaesthesia 1986: 41: 1024–1025.

Grosslight K, Foster R, Colohan AR, Bedford RF. Isoflurane for neuroanesthesia: Risk factors for increases in intracranial pressure. Anesthesiology 1985: 63: 533–536.

Gur D, Yonas H, Jackson DL, Wolfson SK, et al. Measurement of cerebral blood flow during xenon inhalation as measured by the microsphere method. Stroke 1985: 16: 871–874.

Gyulai FE, Firestone LL, Mintun MA. Winter PM. In vivo imaging of human limbic responses to nitrous oxide inhalation. Anesth Analg 1996: 83: 291–298.

Hans P, Dethier JC, Godin D, Stevenaert A. Compared effects of enflurane and of halothane on the intracranial pressure and the cerebral perfusion pressure in dog. Acta Anaestheiol Belg 1980: 31 (suppl): 49–59.

Hansen TD, Warner DS, Todd MM, et al. Distribution of cerebral blood flow during halothane versus isoflurane anesthesia in rats. Anesthesiology 1988a: 69: 332–337.

Hansen TD, Warner DS, Todd MM. Nitrous oxide is a more potent cerebral vasodilator than either halothane or isoflurane. Anesthesiology 1988b: 69: A537.

Hansen TD, Warner DS, Todd MM, Vust LJ. The role of cerebral metabolism in determining the local cerebral blood flow effects of voliatile anesthetics: Evidence for persistent flow-metabolsm coupling. J Cereb Blood Flow Metab 1989a: 9: 323–328.

Hansen TD, Warner DS, Todd MM, Vust LJ. Effects of nitrous oxide and volatile anaesthetics on cerebral blood flow. Br J Anaesth 1989b: 63: 290–295.

Harada H, Kelly PJ, Cole DJ, et al. Isoflurane reduces N-methyl-D-aspartate toxicity in vivo in the rat cerebral cortex. Anesth Analg 1999: 89: 1442–1447.

Haraldsted V, Asmussen J, Herlevsen P, Cold GE. Cerebral arteriovenous difference of oxygen during gradual and sudden increase of the concentration of isoflurane for induction of deliberate hypotension. Acta Anaesthesiol Scand 1992: 33: 142–144.

Harkin CP, Hudetz AG, Schmeling WT, et al. Halothane-induced tation of intraparenchymal arterioles in rat brain slices: a conparison to sodium nitroprusside. Anesthesiology 1997: 86: 885–894.

Harp JR, Nilsson L, Siesjö BK. The effect of halothane upon cerebral oxygen consumption in the rat. Acta Anaesth Scand 1976: 20: 83–90.

Harrington TR, Manwaring K, Hodak J. Local basal ganglia and brain stem blood flow in the head.injured patient using stable xenon-enhanced CT scanning. In Miller JD, Teasdale GM, Rowan JO et al. (eds) Intracranial Pressure VI, Berlin, Springer Verlag 1986: 680–686.

Harrison JL. Postoperative seizures after isoflurane anesthesia. Anesth Analg 1986: 65: 1235–1236.

Hartmann A, Wassman H, Czernicki Z, et al. Effect of stable xenon in room air on regional cerebral blood flow and electroencephalogram in normal baboons. Stroke 1987: 18: 643–648.

Hartung J and Cottrell JE. Nitrous oxide reduces thiopental-induced prolongation of survival in hypoxic and anoxic mice. Anesth Analg 1987: 66: 47–52.

Heath KJ, Gupta S, Matta BF. The effects of sevoflurane on cerebral hemodynamics during propofol anesthesia. Anesth Analg 1997: 85: 1284–1287.

Heneghan CPH, Thornton C, Navaratnarajah M, Jones JG. Effect of isoflurane on auditory evoked response in man. Br J Anaesth 1987: 59: 277–282.

Henriksen HT, Balslev J¢rgensen P. The effect of nitrous oxide on intracranial pressure in patients with intracranial disorders. Br J Anaesth 1973: 45: 486–492.

Hickey R, Bunegin L, Albin MS, et al. Cerebral blood flow responses during varying rates of isoflurane induced hypotension. Anesthesiology 1986: 65: A580.

Hickey R, Albin MS, Bunegin L, et al. Intracranial pressure dynamics during and subsequent to induced hypotension with isoflurane. Anesthesiology 1986: 65: A460.

Hiroso T, Inoue M, Uchida M et al. Enflurane-induced release of an excitatory amino acid, glutamate, from mouse brain synaptpsomes. Anesthesiology 1992: 77: 109–113.

Hoffman WE, Miletich DJ, Albrecht RF. Cardiovascular and regional blood flow changes during halothane anesthesia in the aged rat. Anesthesiology 1982a: 56: 444–448.

Hoffman WE, Edelman. Comparison of isoflurane and desflurane anesthetic depth using burst suppression of the elec-

troencephalogram in neurosurgical patients. Anesth Analg 1995: 81: 811–816.
Hoffman WE, Charbel FT, Edelman G, Ausman JI. Thiopental and desflurane treatment for brain protection. Neurosurgery 1998a: 43: 1050–1053.
Hoffman WE, Charbel FT, Edelman G, et al. Comparison of etomidate and desflurane on brain gases and pH during prolonged middle cerebral artery occlusion. Anesthesiology 1998b: 88: 1188–1194.
Hoffman WE, Wheeler P, Edelman G, et al. Hypoxic brain tissue following subarachnoid hemorrhage. Aneshtesiology 2000a: 92: 442–446.
Hoffman WE, Edelman G. Enhancement of brain tissue oxygenation during high dose isoflurane anaesthesia in the dog. J Neurosurg Anesthesiol 2000b: 12: 95–98.
Hoffman WE, Edelman G. Isoflurane increase brain oxygen reactivity in dogs. Anesth Analg 2000c: 91: 637–641.
Holadya DA, Smith FR. Clinical characteristics and biotransformation of sevoflruane in healthy human volunteers. Anesthesiology 1981: 54: 100–106.
Homi J, Konchigeri HN, Exkenhoff JE, Linde HW. A new anesthetic agent-Forane. Preliminary observations in man. Anesth Analg 1972: 51: 439–477.
Horn J-L, Franks JJ, Sastry BVR, Singh G. Xenon reduces Ca^{2+} adenosine triphosphatase pump activity in synaptic plasma membranes from the rat (abstract). Anesthesiology 1992: (suppl): A417.
Hossmann KA. Glutamate-mediated injury in focal cerebral ischemia: the excitotoxin hypothesis revised. Brain Pathol 1994: 4: 22–36.
Hymes JA. Seizure activity during isoflurane anesthesia. Anesth Analg 1985: 64: 367–368.
Ichinose F, Mi W-D, Miyazaki M, et al. Lack of correlation between the reduction of sevoflurane MAC and the cerebellar cyclic GMP concentrations in mice treated with 7-nitroindazole. Anesthesiology 1998: 89: 143–148.
Iida H, Ohata H, Iida M, et al. Isoflurane and sevoflurane induce vasodilation of cerebral vessels via ATP-sensitive channel activation. Anesthesiology 1998: 89: 954–960.
Inada T, Shingu K, Uchida M, et al. Changes in the cerebral arteriovenous oxygen content difference by surgical incision are similar during sevoflurane and isoflurane anaesthesia. Can. J Anaesth 1996: 43: 1019–1024.
Ingvar M, Siesjo BK. Effect of nitrous oxide on local cerebral glucose utilization in rats. J Cereb Blood Flow Metab 1982: 2: 481–486.
Jennett WB, McDowall DG, Barker J. The effect of halothane on intracranial pressure in cerebral tumors. J Neurosurg 1967: 26: 270–274.
Jennett WB, Barker J, Fitch W, McDowall DG. Effect of anesthesia on intracranial pressure in patients with space-occupying lesions. Lancet 1969: i: 61–64.
Joas TA, Stevens WC, Eger II EI. Electroencephalographic seizure activity in dogs during anesthesia. Br J Anaesth 1971: 43: 739–745.
Johns RA, Mosciki JC, DiFazio CA. Nitric oxide sunthase inhibitor dose-dependently and reversibly reduces the threshold for halothane anaesthesia. Anesthesiology 1992: 77: 779–784.
Johns RA, Tichotsky A, Muro M. et al. Halothane and isoflurane inhibit endothelium-derived relaxing factor-dependent cyclic guanosine monophsphate accumulation in endothelial cell-vascular smooth muscle Co-cultures independent of an effect on guanylyl cyclase activation. Anesthesiology 1995: 83: 823–834.
Jones MV, Brooks PA, Harrison NL. Enhancement of gamma-aminobutyric acid-activated Cl^- currents in cultured rat hippocampal neurones by three volatile anaesthetics. J Physiol (Lond) 1992: 449: 279–293.
Julien RM, Kavan EM. Electrographic studies of a new volatile anaesthetic agent: Enflurane (Ethrane). J Pharmacol and Exper Therapeut 1972: 183: 393–403.
Junck L, Dhawan V, Thaler HT et al. Effects of xenon and krypton on regional cerebral blood flow in the rat. J Cereb Blood Flow Metab 1985: 126–132.
Kaieda R, Todd MM, Cook LN, Warner DS. The effects of anesthetics and $PaCO_2$ on the cerebrovascular, metabolic, and electroencephalographic responses to nitrous oxide in the rabbit. Anesth Analg 1989a: 68: 135–143.
Kaieda R, Todd MM, Weeks JB, Warner DS. A comparison of the effects of halothane, isoflurane, and pentobarbital anesthesia on intracranial pressure and cerebral edema formation following brain injury in rabbits. Anesthesiology 1989c: 71: 571–579.
Kant GJ, Muller TW, Lenox RH, Meyerhoff JL. In vivo effects of pentoparbitla and halothane anesthesia on levels of adenosine 3.5-monophosphate and guanosine 3,5-monophosphate in rat brain regions and pituitary. Biochem Pharmacol 1980: 29: 1891–1896.
Katz JJ, Todd MM, Warner DS. Quantitative comparison of cerebral blood volume in rats receiving halothane or isoflurane. Anesthesiology 1988: 69: A534.
Kawaguchi M, Kimbro JR, Drummond JC, et al. Isoflurane delays but does not prevent cerebral infarction in rats subjected to focal ischaemia. Anesthesiology 2000: 92: 1335–1342.
Keats AS. Seizures from isoflurane. Anesth Analg 1985: 64: 1225–1226.
Keita H, Henzel-Rouellé D, Dupont H, et al. Halothane and isoflurane increase spontaneous but reduce the N-methyl-D-aspartate-evoked dopamine release in rat striatal slices. Anesthesiology 1999: 91: 1788–1797.
Kellenberger S. Malherbe P, Spiegel E. Function of the $\alpha 1\beta 2\gamma 2S\gamma$-aminobutyric acid type A receptor is modulated by protein kinase C via multiple phsophorylation sites. J Biol Chem 1992: 267: 25660–25663.
Kharasch ED, Frink Jr EJ, Zager R. et al. Assessment of low-flow sevoflurane and isoflurane effects on renal function using sensitive markers of tubular toxociti. Anesthesiology 1997: 86: 1238–1254.
Kim HK, Zornow MH, Illievich UM, et al. Sevofulrane versus halothane anesthesia after acute cryogenic brain injury in rabbits: relationship between arterial and intracranial pressure. J Neurosurg Anesthesiol 1994: 6: 260–264.
Kimbro JR, Kelly PJ, Drummond JC, et al. Isoflurane and pentobarbital reduce AMPA toxicity in vivo in the rat cerebral cortex. Anesthesiology 2000: 92: 806–812.
Kindler CH, Eilers H, Donohoe P, et al. Volatile anesthetics increases intracellular calcium in cerebrocortical and hippocampal neurons. Anesthesiology 1999: 90: 1137–1145.
Kitaguchi K, Nakajia T et al. The change in cerebral blood flow during hypotensive anesthesia induced by prostaglandin E1. Masui 1992: 41: 766–771.
Kitaguchi K, Ohsumi H et al. Effects of sevoflurane on cerebral circulation and metabolism in patients with ischemic disease. Anesthesiology 1993. 79: 704–709.

Kitahata LM, Galicich JM, Sato I. The effect of passive hyperventilation on intracranial pressure. J Neurosurg 1971: 34: 185–193.

Kitahata LM, Katz JD. Tension pneumocephalus after posterior fossa craniotomy, a complication of the sitting position. Anesthesiology 1976: 44: 448–450.

Kochs E, Bischoff P, Pichlmeier U, Schulte am Esch J. Surgical stimulation induces changes in brain electrical activity during isoflurane/nitrous oxide anesthesia. Anesthesiology 1994: 80: 1026–1034.

Koenig HM, Pelligrino DA, Albrecht RF. Halothane vasodilation and nitric oxide in rat pial vessels. J Neurosurg Anesthesiol 1993: 5. 264–271.

Koenig HM What's up with the new volatile anesthetics, desflurane and sevoflurane, for neurosurgical patients?. Editorial. J Neurosurg Anesthesiol 1994. 6: 229–232.

Koenig HM, Pelligrino DA, Wang Q, Albrecht RF. Role of nitric oxide and endothelium in rat pial vessel dilation response to isoflurane. Anesth Analg 1994: 79: 886–891.

Kofke WA, Snider MT, Young RSK, Ramer JC. Prolonged low flow isoflurane anesthesia for status epilepticus. Anesthesiology 1985: 62: 653–656.

Kofke WA, Hawkins RA, Davis DW, Biebuyck JF. Increased brain glucose during isoflurane anesthesia. Anesthesiology 1986: 65: A582.

Kolbitsch C, Lorenz IH, Hörmann C, et al. A subanesthetic concentration of sevoflurane increases regional cerebral blood flow and regional cerebral blood volume and decreases regional mean transit time and regional cerebrovascular resistance in volunteers. Anesth Analg 2000: 91: 156–162.

Komatsu H, Taie S, Endo S, et al. Electrical seizures during sevoflruane anesthesia in two pediatric patients with epilepsy. Anesthesiology 1994: 81: 1535–1537.

Kotani J, Sugioka S, Momota Y, Ueda Y. Effect of sevoflurane on intracranial pressure, sagittal sinus pressure, and the intracranial volume-pressure relation in cats. J Neurosurg Anesthesiol 1992: 4: 194–198.

Kruczek M, Albin MS, Wolf S, Bertoni JM. Postoperative seizure activity following enflurane anesthesia. Anesthesiology 1980: 53: 175–176.

Kurata J, Nakao S-i, Murakawa M, et al. The cerebral cortex origin of enfluran-induced generalized seizures in cats. Anesth Analg 1994: 79: 713–718.

Kuroda Y, Strebel S, Rafferty C, Bullock R. Neuropretective doses of N-methyl-D-aspartate receptor antagonists profoundly reduce the minimum alveolar anesthetic concentration (MAC) for isoflurane in rats. Anesth Analg 1993: 77: 795–800.

Kuroda Y, Murakami M, Tsuruta J, et al. Preservation of the ratio of cerebral blood flow/metabolic rate for oxygen during prolonged anesthesia with isoflurane, sevoflurane, and halothane in humans. Anesthesiology 1996: 84: 555-561. .

Kuroda Y, Murakami M, Tsuruta J, Murakawa T. Blood flow velocity of middle cerebral artery during prolonged anesthesia with halothane, isoflurane, and sevoflurane in humans. Anesthesiology 1997: 87: 527–532.

Kuroiwa T, Bonnekoh P, Hossmann K-A. Post-ischemic halothane anesthesia prevents delayed neuronal death of CA1 neurons in gerbils. J Cereb Blood Flow Metab. 1989: (suppl 1): S756.

Kurumaji A, Mc Culloch J. Halothane anaesthesia modifies the changes in local cerebral glucose use induced by NMDA receptor blockade. J Cereb Blood Flow Metab. 1989: (suppl 1): S753.

Lam AM, Gelb AW. Cardiovascular effects of isoflurane-induced hypotension for cerebral aneurysm surgery. Anesth Analg 1983: 62: 742–748.

Lam AM, Mayberg TS, Eng CC, et al. Nitrous oxide-isoflurane anesthesia causes more cerebral vasodilation than an equipotent dose of isoflurane in humans. Anesth Analg 1994: 78: 462–468.

Lam AM, Matta BF, Mayberg TS, Strebel S. Changes in cerebral blood flow velocity with onset of EEG silence during inhalation anaesthesia in humans: Evidence of flow-metabolism coupling? J Cereb Blood Flow Metab 1995: 15: 14–17.

Larsen R, Maurer I, Khambatta H. Wirkungen von Isofluran und Enfluran auf die zerebrale Hämodynamik und den zerebralen Sauerstoffverbrauch des Menschen. Anesthesist 1988: 37: 173–181.

Lebowitz MH, Blitt CD, Dillon JB. Enflurane-induced central nervous system excitation and its relation to carbon dioxide tension. Anesth Analg 1972: 51: 355–363.

Lee JG, Hudetz AG, Smith JJ, et al. The effect of halothane and isoflurane on cerebrocortical microcirculation and autoregulation as assessed by Laser-Doppler flowmetry. Anesth Analg 1994: 79: 58–65.

Lee JG, Smith JJ, Hudetz AG, et al. Laser-Doppler measurement of the effect of halothane and isoflurane on the cerebrovascular CO_2 response in the art. Anesth Analg 1995: 80: 696–702.

Lenz C, Frietsch T, Fütterer C, et al. Local coupling of cerebral blood flow to cerebral glucose metabolisme during inhalation anesthesia in rats. Anesthesiology 1999: 91: 1720–1723.

Leon JE, Bissonnette B. Cerebrovascular responses to carbon dioxide in children anaesthetized with halothane and isoflurane. Can J Anaesth 1991: 38: 817–825.

Levin A, Blanck TJJ. Halothane and isoflurane alter the Ca^{2+} binding properties of calmodulin. Anesthesiology 1995: 83: 120–126.

Lin DM, Powell HC, Shapiro HM. Absence of longterm neuropathology after sustained enflurane epileptiform activity. Anesthesiology 1986: 65: A348.

Lloyd-Thomas AR, Cole PV, Prior PF, Isoflurane prevents EEG depression during trimetaphan-induced hypotension in man. Br J Anaesth 1990: 65: 313–318.

Lockhart SH, Cohen Y, Yasuda N, et al. Cerebral uptake and elimination of desflurane, isoflurane, and halothane from rabbit brain: An In Vivo NMR study. Anesthesiology 1991: 74: 575–580.

Loeb AL, Raj NR, Longnecker DE. Cerebellar nitric oxide is increased during isoflurane anesthesia compared to halothane anesthesia. A microdialysis study in rats. Anesthesiology 1998: 89: 723–730.

Longnecker DE, Shuptrine JR, Seyde WC, Walker MS. Hemorrhage and cerebral tissue oxygenation: A comparison of ketamine, isoflurane and enflurane. Anesthesiology 1986: 65: A324.

Lu H, Werner C, Engehard K, Scholz M, Kochs E. The effect of sevoflurane on cerebral blood flow autoregulation in rats. Anesth Analg 1998: 87: 854–858.

Lukatch HS, MacIver MB. Voltage-clamp analysis of halothane effects on GABA (A fast) and GABA (A slow) inhibitory currents. Brain Res 1997: 765: 108–112.

Lunsford LD, Maroon JC, Sheptak PE, Albin MS. Subdural tension pneumocephalus: report of two cases. J Neurosurg 1979: 50: 525–527.

Luttropp HH, Rommer B, Perhag L, et al. Left ventricular performance and cerebral haemodynamics during xenon anaesthesia. Anaesthesia 1993: 48: 1045–1049. .

Lutz LJ, Milde JH, Milde LN. The cerebral function, metabolic, and hemodynamic effects of desflurane in dogs. Anesthesiology 1990: 73: 125–131.

Lutz LJ, Milde JH, Milde LN. The response of the canine cerebral circulation to hyperventilation during anesthesia with desflurane. Anesthesiology 1991: 74: 504–507.

Lynch C, Pancrazio JJ. Snails, spiders and streospecificity-Is there a role for calcium channels in anesthtic mechanisms. Anesthesiology 1994: 81: 1–5 .

Madsen JB, Cold GE, Eriksen HO, et al. CBF and $CMRO_2$ during craniotomy for small supratentorial cerebral tumous in enflurane anaesthesia. A dose-response study. Acta Anaesthesiol Scand 1986: 30: 633–636.

Madsen JB, Cold GE, Hansen ES, Bardrum B.Cerebral blood flow, cerebral metabolic rate of oxygen and relative CO_2 reactivity during craniotomy for supratentorial cerebral tumours in halothane anaesthesia. A dose-response study. Acta Anaesthesiol Scand 1987a: 31: 454–457.

Madsen JB, Cold GE, Hansen ES, Bardrum B. The effect of isoflurane on cerebral blood flow and metabolism in humans during craniotomy for small supratentorial cerebral tumors. Anesthesiology 1987b: 66: 332–336.

Madsen JB, Cold GE, Hansen ES, et al. Cerebral blood flow and metabolism during isoflurane-induced hypotension in patients subjected to surgery for cerebral aneurysms. Br J Anaesth 1987c: 59: 1204–1207.

Madsen JB, Cold GE. Cerebral blood flow and oxygen uptake during anesthesia with halothane, enflurane or isoflurane. J Cereb Blood Flow Metab 1987: 7 (suppl 1): S628.

Maekawa T, Tommasino C, Shapiro HM, et al. Local cerebral blood flow and glucose utilization during isoflurane anesthesia in the rat. Anesthesiology 1986: 65: 144–151.

Maekawa T, Ishikawa T, Nakakimura K, et al. Effects of volatile anesthetics on local cerebral blood flow and glucose utilization in brain ischemia. J Cereb Blood Flow Metab 1989: (suppl 1): S289.

Malan TP, DiNardo JA, Isner RJ. et al. Cardiovascular effects of sevoflurane compared with those of isoflurane in volunteers. Anesthesiology 1995: 83: 918–928.

Mann JD, Cookson SL, Mann ES. Differential effects of pentobarbital, ketamine hydrochoride, and enflurane anaesthesia on CSF formation rate and outflow resistance in the rat. In Shulman K, Marmarou A, Miller JD, Becker DP, Hochwald GM, Brock M (eds); Intracranial Pressure IV. Springer Verlag, Berlin, Heidelberg 1980: 466–471.

Manohar M, Parks C. Regional distribution of brain and myocardial perfusion in swine while awake and during 1.0 and 1.5 MAC isoflurane anesthesia produced without and with 50% nitrous oxide. Cardiovasc Res 1984: 18: 344–353.

Mantz J, Cheramy A, Thierry A-M, et al. Anesthetic properties of riluzole (54272 RP), a new inhibitor of glutamate neurotransmission. Anesthesiology 1992: 76: 844–848.

Marion DW, Crosby K. The effect of stable xenon on ICP. J Cereb Blood Flow Metab 1991: 11: 347–350.

Marks EC, Yonas H, Sanders HM, et al. Effects of xenon and CO_2 inhalation on flow velocity measured with transcranial Doppler. In Yonas H (ed) Cerebral Blood Flow Measurement with Stable Xenon Enhanced Computed Tomography. New York, Raven Press. 1992: 286–291. .

Marx GF, Andrews IC, Orkin LR. Cerebrospinal fluid pressures during halothane anesthesia. Can Anaesth Soc J 1962: 9: 239–245.

Mazzarella B, Mastronardi P, Cafiero T, et al. Isoflurane and intracranial pressure. In: Miller JD, Teasdale GM, Rowan JO, Galbraith SL, Mendelow AD (eds); Intracranial Pressure VI, Springer Verlag, Berlin, Heidelberg 1986: 732–735.

Mazze RI, Jamison R. Renal effect of sevoflurane. Anesthesiology 1995: 83: 443–445.

Mazze RI, Jamison R. Low-flow (1l/min) sevoflurane. Is it safe. Anesthesiology 1997: 86: 1225–1227.

McDowall DG, Harper AM, Jacobsen I. Cerebral blood flow during halothane anesthesia. Br J Anaesth 1963: 35: 394–402.

McFarlane C, Warner D, Todd M, Nordholm L. AMPA-receptor competitive antagonism reduces halothane MAC in rats. Anesthesiology 1992: 77: 1165–1170.

McFarlane C, Warner DS, Dexter F, Ludwig PA. Minimum alveolar concentration for halotahne in the rat is resistant to effects of forebrain ischemia and reperfusion. Anesthesiology 1994: 81: 1206–1211.

McHenry LC. Quantitative cerebral blood flow determination. Application of a krypton 85 desaturation technique in man. Neurology (Minneap.) 1964: 14: 785–793.

McLeskey CH, Cullen BF, Kennery RD, Galindo A. Control of cerebral perfusion pressure during induction of anesthesia in high-risk neurosurgical patients. Anesth Analg 1974: 53: 985–992.

McPherson RW, Traystman RJ. Effects of isoflurane on cerebral autoregulation. Anesthesiology 1987: 67: A 576.

McPherson RW, Brian JE, Traystman RJ. Cerebrovascular responsiveness to carbon dioxide in dogs with 1.4% and 2.8% isoflurane. Anesthesiology 1989a: 70: 843–850.

McPherson RW, Brian JE, Traystman RJ. Evaluation of cerebral blood flow with time during isoflurane anesthesia. J Cereb Blood Flow Metab 1989b: 9: (suppl 1): S472.

McPherson RW, Derrer SA, Traystman RJ. The effect of 1 MAC isoflurane on cerebrovascular response to increased or decreased cerebral perfusion pressure. Anesthesiology 1990: 73; No 3A, A1219.

McPherson RW, Derrer SA, Traystman RJ. Changes in cerebral CO_2 responsivity over time during isoflurane anesthesia in the dog. J Neurosurg Anesthesiol 1991: 3: 12–19.

McPherson RW, Kirsch JR, Moore LE, Trystman RJ. N-Nitro-L-arginine methyl ester prevents cerebral hyperemia by inhaled anesthetics in dogs. Anesth Analg 1993: 77: 891–897.

McPherson RW, Kirsch JR, Tobin JR, et al. Cerebral blood flow in primates is increased by isoflurane over time and is decreased by nitric oxide synthase inhibition. Anesthesiology 1994: 80: 1320–1327.

Mennerick S, Jevtovic-Todorovic V, Todorovic SM, et al. Effect of nitrous oxide on excitatory and inhibitory synaptic transmission in hippocampal cultures. J Neurosci 1998: 18: 9716–9726.

Messick JM, Casement B, Sharbrough FW, et al. Correlation of regional cerebral blood flow (rCBF) with EEG changes during isoflurane anesthesia for carotid endarterectomy: Critical rCBF. Anesthesiology 1987: 66: 344–349.

Meyer FB, Muzzi DA. Cerebral protection during aneurysm surgery with isoflurane anaesthesia. J Neurosurg 1992: 76: 541–543.

Michenfelder JD, VanDyke RA, Theye RA. The effect of anesthetic agents and techniques on canine cerebral ATP and lactate levels. Anesthesiology 1970: 33: 315–321.

Michenfelder JD, Cucchiara RF. Canine cerebral oxygen consumption during enflurane anesthesia and its modification during induced seizures. Anesthesiology 1974: 40: 575–580.

Michenfelder JD, Theye RA. In vivo toxic effects of halothane on canine cerebral metabolic pathways. Am J Physiol 1975: 229: 1050–1055.

Michenfelder J. Milde J. Influence of anesthetics on metabolic functional, and pathological responses to regional cerebral ischemia. Stroke 1975: 6: 405–410.

Michenfelder JD, Theye RA. Canine systemic and cerebral effects of hypotension induced by hemorrhage, trimethaphan, halothane or nitroprusside. Anesthesiology 1977: 46: 188–195.

Michenfelder JD. Does isoflurane aggravate regional cerebral ischaemia? (Editorial). Anesthesiology 1987: 66: 451–452.

Michenfelder JD, Sundt TM, Fode N, Sharbrough FW. Isoflurane when compared to enflurane and halothane decreases the frequency of cerebral ischaemia during carotid endarterectomy. Anesthesiology 1987: 67: 336–340.

Michenfelder JD, Milde JH. The interaction of sodium nitroprusside, hypotension, and isoflurane in determining cerebral vasculature effects. Anesthesiology 1988: 69: 870–875.

Mielck F, Stephan H, Weyland A, Sonntag H. Effect of one minimum alveolar anesthesic concentration sevoflurane on cerebral metabolisme, blood flow, and CO_2 reactivity in cardiac patients. Anesth Analg 1999: 89: 364–369.

Milde LN, Milde JH, Lanier WL, Michenfelder JD. Comparison of the effects of isoflurane and thiopental on neurologic outcome and neuropathology after temporary focal cerebral ischemia in primates. Anesthesiology 1988: 69: 905–913.

Milde LN. The hypoxic mouse model for screening cerebral protective agents: A re-examination. Anesth Analg 1988: 67: 917–922.

Milde LN, Milde JH. The cerebral and systemic hemodynamic and metabolic effects of desflurane-induced hypotension in dogs. Anesthesiology 1991: 74: 513–518.

Miletich DJ, Ivankovich AD, Albrecht RF, et al. Absence of autoregulation of cerebral blood flow during halothane and enflurane anesthesia. Anesth Analg 1976: 55: 100–109.

Mills P, Sessler DI, Moseley M, et al. An in vivo 19-F nuclear magnetic resonance study of isoflurane elimination from the rabbit brain. Anesthesiology 1987: 67: 169–173.

Mirsky AF, Stockard JJ, Skoff BF, Jones TA. Brainstem auditory evoked potential alterations during induced and spontaneous generalized spike-wave activity in animals and humans Neuroscience 1979: 5: 196.

Misfeldt BB, Balslev J¢rgensen P, Rish¢j M. The effect of nitrous oxide and halothane upon the intracranial pressure in hypocapnic patients with intracranial disorders. Br J Anaesth 1974: 46: 853–858.

Miura Y, Grocott H, Bart RD, et al. Differential effects of anesthetic agents on outcome from near-complete but not incomplete global ischaemia in the rat. Anesthesiology 1998: 89: 391–400.

Miyazaki H, Nakamura Y, Arai T, Kataoka K. Increase of glutamate uptake in astrocytes A possible mechanism of action of volatile anesthetics. Anesthesiology 1997: 86: 1359–1366.

Miyono K, Tanifiji Y, Eger El. The effect of halothane dose on striatal dopamine: An in vivo microdialysis study. Brain Res 1993: 605: 342–344.

Morita H, Nemoto EM, Bleyaert AL, Stezoski SW. Brain blood flow autoregulation and metabolism during halothane anesthesia in monkeys. Am J Physiol 1977: 233: H670–676.

Moss E, McDowall DG. ICP increases with 50% nitrous oxide in oxygen in severe head injuries during controlled ventilation. Br J Anaesth 1979: 51: 757–760.

Moss E, Dearden NM, McDowall DG. Effects of 2% enflurane on intracranial pressure and cerebral perfusion pressure. Br J Anaesth 1983: 55: 1083–1087.

Muldoon SM, Hart JL, Bowen KA, Freas W. Attenuation of endothelium-mediated vasodilation by halothane. Anesthesiology 1988: 68: 31–37.

Murakawa M, Adachi T, Nakao S, et al. Activation of the cortical and medullary dopaminergic systems by nitrous oxide in rats: A possible neurochemical basis for psychotropic effects of postanesthetic nausea and vomiting. Anesth Analg 1994: 78: 376–381.

Murkin JM, Farrar JK, Tweed WA, Guiraudon G. Cerebral blood flow, oxygen consumption and EEG during isoflurane anesthesia. Anest Analg 1986: 65: S107.

Murphy FL, Kennell EM, Johnstone RE, et al. The effects of enflurane, isoflurane and halothane on cerebral blood flow and metabolism in man. Abstracts and scientific papers. Annual meeting of the American Sos Anaesth 1974: 61–62.

Murr R, Schürer L, Berger S. et al. Effects of isoflurane, fentanyl, or thiopental anesthesia on regional cerebral blood flow in rabbits. Anesth Analg 1993: 77: 898–907.

Murr R, Berger S, Schürer L, et al. Influence of isoflurane, fentanyl, thiopental, and α-chloralose on formation of brain edema resulting from focal cryogenic lesion. Anesth Analg 1995: 80: 1108–1115.

Mutch WAC, Ringaert KRA. Effects of haemorrhage and phenylephedrine on cerebral blood flow in rats during isoflurane anaesthesia. Can J Anaesth 1987: S106–Sl07.

Mutch WAC, Malo LA, Ringaert KRA. Phenylephedrine increases regional cerebral blood flow following hemorrhage during isoflurane-oxygen anesthesia. Anesthesiology 1989: 70: 276–279.

Muzzi DA, Losasso TJ, Dietz NN et al. The effect of desflurane and isoflurane on cerebrospinal fluid pressure in humans with supratentorial mass lesions. Anesthesiology 1992: 76: 720–724.

Myers RR, Shapiro HM. Local cerebral metabolism during enflurane anesthesia:identification of epileptigenic foci. Electroenceph Clin Neurophysiol 1979: 47: 153–162.

Nakamura K, Terasako K, Toda H, et al. Mechanisms of endothelium-dependent relaxation by halothane, isoflurane, and sevoflurane. Can J Anesth 1994: 41: 340–346.

Nakashima K, Todd MM. Effects of hypothermia, pentobarbital, and isoflurane on postdepolarization amino acid release during complete global cerebral ischemia. Anesthesiology 1996: 85: 161–168.

Nandate K, Vuylsteke A, Ratsep I, et al. Effects of isoflurane, sevoflurane and propofol anaesthesia on jugular venous oxygen saturation in patients undergoing coronary artery bypass surgery. Br J Anaesth 2000: 84: 631–633.

Nedergaard M, Astrup J, Infarct rim: effect of hyperglycemia on direct current potential and [^{14}C]2-deoxyglucose phosphorylation. J Cereb Blood Flow Metab 1986: 6: 607–615. .

Nehls DG, Todd MM, Spetzler RF, et al. A comparison of the cerebral protective effects of isoflurane and barbiturates during temporary focal ischaemia in primates. Anesthesiology 1987: 66: 453–464.

Neigh JL, Garman JK, Harp JR. The electroencephalographic pattern during anesthesia with ethrane: Effects of depth of anesthesia, $PaCO_2$ and nitrous oxide. Anesthesiology 1971: 35: 482–487.

Nellgård B, Mackensen GB, Pineda J, et al. Anesthetic effects on cerebral metabolic rate predict histologic outcome from near-complete forebrain ischemia in the rat. Anesthesiology 2000: 93: 431–436.

Neundorfer B, Klose R. EEG-veränderungen bei kindern während enflurane-anästhesie. Prakt Anesth 1975: 10: 271–284.

Newberg LA, Michenfelder JD. Cerebral protection by isoflurane during hypoxemia or ischemia. Anesthesiology 1983: 59: 29–35.

Newberg LA, Milde JH, Michenfelder JD. The cerebral metabolic effects of isoflurane at and above concentrations that suppress cortical electrical activity. Anesthesiology 1983: 59: 23–28.

Newberg LA, Milde JH, Michenfelder JD. Systemic and cerebral effects of isoflurane-induced hypotension in dogs. Anesthesiology 1984: 60: 541–546.

Newman B, Gelb AW, Lam AM. The effect of isoflurane-induced hypotension on cerebral blood flow and cerebral metabolic rate for oxygen in humans. Anesthesiology 1986: 64: 307–310.

Ngai SH, Finck AD. Prolonged exposure to nitrous oxide decreases opiate receptor density in rat brainstem. Anesthesiology 1982: 57: 26–30.

Nicholas JF, Lam AM. Isoflurane-induced hypotension does not cause inpairment in pulmonary gas exchange. Can Anesth Soc J 1984: 31: 352–358.

Nichikawa K-I and MacIver MB. Excitatory synaptic transmission mediated by NMDA receptors is more sensitive to isoflurane than are non-NMDA receptor-mediated responses. Anesthesiology 2000: 92: 228–236.

Nischikawa K, MacIver M. Agent-selective effects of volatile anesthetics on $GABA_A$ receptor-mediated synaptic inhibition in hippocampal interneurons. Anesthesiology 2001: 94: 340–347.

Nishiyama T, Sugai N, Hanaoka K. Cerebrovascular CO_2 reactivity in elderly and younger adlut patients during sevoflurane anaesthesia. Can J Anaesth 1997: 44: 160–164.

Nishiyama T, Matsukawa T, Yokoyama T, Hanaoka K. Cerebrovascular carbon dioxide reactivity during general anaesthesia: A comparison between sevoflurane and isoflurane. Anesth Analg 1999: 89: 1437–1441.

Obrist WD, Jaggi JL, Harel D, Smith DS. Effect of stable xenon inhalation on human CBF. J Cereb Blood Flow Metab 1985: 5 (suppl 1): 557–558,.

Ohm WW, Cullen BF, Amory DW, Kennedy RD. Delayed seizure activity following enflurane anesthesia. Anesthesiology 1975: 42: 367–368.

Okamoto H, Meng W, Ma J, et al. Isoflurane-induced cerebral hyperemia in neuronal nitric oxide synthase gene deficient mice. Anesthesiology 1997: 86: 875–884.

Ogawa K, Yamada S, Mizumoto K, et al. Inhibitory effects of halothane, isoflurane, sevoflurane, and pentobarbital on the constriction induced by hypocapnia and bicarbonate in isolated canine cerebral arteries. J Neurosurg Anesthesiol 2000: 12: 99–106.

Okuda Y, McDowall DG, Ali MM, Lane JR. Changes in CO_2 responsiveness and in autoregulation of the cerebral circulation during and after halothane-induced hypotension. J Neurol Neurosurg Psychiat 1976: 39: 221–230.

Olsen KS, Henriksen L, Owen-Falkenberg A, et al. Effect of 1 or 2 MAC isoflurane with or without ketanserin on cerebral blood flow autoregulation in man. Br J Anaesth 1994: 72: 66–71.

Opacka-Juffry J, Ahier RG, Cremer JE. Nomifensine-induced increase in extracellular striatal dopamine is enhanced by isoflurane anesthesia. Synapse 1991: 7: 169–171.

Ori C, Dam M, Pizzolato G, et al. Effects of isoflurane anesthesia on local cerebral glucose utilization in the rat. Anesthesiology 1986: 65: 152–156.

Osawa M, Shingu K, Murakawa M, et al. Effects of sevoflurane on central nervous system electrical activity in cats. Anesth Analg 1994: 79: 52–57.

Oshita S, Ishikawa T, Tokutsu Y, Takeshita H. Cerebral circulatory and metabolic stimulation with nitrous oxide in the dog. Acta Anaesth Scand 1979: 23: 177–181.

Pagel PS, Kampine JP, Schmeling WT, Wartier DC. Comparison of the systemic and coronary hemodynamic actions of desflurane, isoflurane, halothane, and enflurane in the chronically instrumented dog. Anesthesiology 1991: 74: 539–551. .

Pajewski TN, Difazio CA, Mosciki JC, Johns RA. Nitric oxide synthase inhibitor, 7-nitro indazole and nitro-L-arginine methyl ester dose-dependently reduce the threshold for isoflurane anaesthesia. Anesthesiology 1996: 85: 1111–1119.

Pajewski TN, Cechova S, Johns RA. The soluble guanylyl cyclase inhibitor ODQ dose dependently reduces the threshold of isoflurane anaesthesia in rats (Abstract). Anesthesiology 1998: 89: A800.

Park WK, Pancrazio JJ, Suh CK, Lynch III C. Myocardial depressant effects of sevoflurane. Anesthesiology 1996: 84: 1166–1176.

Patel PM, Mutch WAC. The cerebral pressure-flow relationship during 1.0 MAC isoflurane anesthesia in the rabbit: The effect of different vasopressors. Anesthesiology 1990: 72: 118–124.

Patel PM, Drummond JC, Cole DJ, et al. Isoflurane and pentobarbital reduce the frequency of transient ischemic depolarizations during focal ischemia in rats. Anesth Analg 1998: 86: 773–780.

Pelligrino DA, Miletich DJ, Hoffman WE, Albrecht RF. Nitrous oxide markedly increases cerebral cortical metabolic rate and blood flow in the goat. Anesthesiology 1984: 60: 405–412.

Perouansky M, Baranov D, Salman M, Yaari Y. Effect of halothane on glutamate receptor-mediated excitatory postsynapnic currents. Anesthesiology 1995: 83: 109–119.

Petersen KD, Landsfeldt U, Cold GE, et al. ICP during three anaesthetics for elective craniotomy. J Neurosurg Anesthesiol 2000: 12: 167.

Peterson DO, Drummond JC, Todd MM. Effects of halothane and isoflurane on somatosensory evoked potentials in man. Anesthesiology 1984: 61: A344.

Pfeifer G, Oehmen S, Limberg NJ, Schultheiss R. Die Wirkung von Isofluran auf den intrakraniellen Druck. Anästh Intensivther Notfallmed 1987: 22: 214–220.

Plougmann J, Astrup J, Pedersen J. Effect of stable xenon inhalation on intracranial pressure during measurement of cerebral blood flow in head injury. J Neurosurg 1994, 81: 822–828. .

Quinlan JJ, Firestone S, Firestone LL. Isoflurane´s enhancement of chloride flux through rat brain -aminobutyric acid

type A receptors is stereoselective. Anesthesiology 1995: 83: 611–615.
Ramani R, Todd MM, Warner DS. The influence of a cryogenic brain injury on the cerebrovascular response to isoflurane in the rabbit. J Cereb Blood Flow Metab. 1991: 11: 388–397.
Rampil IJ, Laster M, Dwyer RC, et al. No EEG evidence of acute tolerance to desflurane in swine. Anesthesiology 1991a: 74: 889–892.
Rampil IJ, Lockhart SH, Eger II EI, et al. The Electroencephalographic effect of desflurane in humans. Anesthesiology 1991b: 74: 434–439.
Rampil IJ, Kim J-S, Lenhardt R, Negishi C. Bispectral EEG index during nitrous oxide administration. Anesthesiology 1998: 89: 671–677. .
Ratcheson RA, Bilezikjian L, Ferrendelli JA. Effects of nitrous oxide anesthesia upon cerebral energy metabolism. J Neurochem 1977: 28: 223–225.
Ravussin P, de Tribolet N, Wiler-Smith HG. Total intravenous anesthesia is best for neurological surgery. J Neurosurg Anesthesiol 1994: 6: 285–289.
Ray KF, Kohlenberger RW, Shapiro HM. Local cerebral blood flow and metabolism during halothane and enflurane. Anesthesiology 1979: 51: S10.
Reasoner DK, Warner DS, Todd MM, McAllister A. Effects of nitrous oxide on cerebral metabolic rate in rats anaesthetized with isoflurane. Br J Anaesth 1990: 65: 210–215.
Reasoner DK, Todd MM, Scamman FL, Warner DS. The incidence of pneumocephalus after supratentorial craniotomy. Observations of the disappearance of intracranial air. Anesthesiology 1994: 80: 1008–1012.
Rehberg B, Xiao Y-H, Duch DSD. Central nervous system sodium channels are significantly suppressed at clinical concentrations of volatile anesthetics. Anesthesiology 1996: 84: 27A.
Reinhold M, DeRood M, Capon A, et al. The Action of enflurane (Ethrane) on cerebral blood flow. Acta Anaesthesiol Belg 1974: 25: 257–265.
Reinhold H, DeRood M. Cerebral blood flow under enflurane anesthesia. Acta Anaesthesiol Belg 1976: 27 (suppl): 250–258.
Reinstrup P, Uski T, Messeter K. Influence of halothane and isoflurane on the contractile response to potassium and prostaglandin F 2_a in isolated human pial arteries. Br J Anaesth 1994: 72: 581–586.
Reinstrup P, Ryding E, Algotsson L, et al. Effects of nitrous oxide on human regional cerebral blood flow and isolated pial arteries. Anesthesiology 1994: 81: 396–402.
Reinstrup P. The effects of halothane, isoflurane and N_2O on human cerebrovascular contractility and circulation. Modulation by carbon dioxide tension. Thesis, Grahns Boktryckeri, Lund 1994.
Reinstrup P, Ryding E, Algotsson L, et al. Regional cerebral blood flow (SPECT) during anesthesia with isoflurane and nitrous oxide in humans. Br. J Anaesth 1997: 78: 407–411.
Rengasamy A, Pajewski TN, Johns RA. Inhalation anesthetic effects on rat cerebellar nitric oxide and cyclic guanosine monophosphate production. Anesthesiology 1997: 86: 689–698.
Roald OK, Forsman M, Steen PA. Partial reversal of the cerebral effects of isoflurane in the dog by benzodiazepine antagonist flumazenil. Acta Anaesthesiol Scand 1988: 32: 209–212.
Roald OK, Forsman M, Steen PA. The effect of prolonged isoflurane anaesthesia on cerebral blood flow and metabolism in the dog. Acta Anaesthesiol Scand 1989: 33: 210–213.
Roald OK, Forsman M, Heier MS, Steen PA. Cerebral effets of nitrous oxide when added to low and high concentrations of isoflurane in the dog. Anesth Analg 1991: 72: 75–79.
Rolly G, VanAken J. Influence of enflurane on cerebral blood flow in man Acta Anaesthesiol Scand 1979: 71, (Suppl), 59–63.
Ropper AH, Kofke WA, Bromfield EB, Kennedy SK. Comparison of isoflurane, halothane, and nitrous oxide in status epilepticus. Ann Neurology 1986: 19: 98–99.
Roth S, Jones SC, Ebrahim Z, et al. Cerebral blood flow and metabolism during isoflurane-induced hypotension. Anesthesiology 1986: 65: A572.
Saintz JJG, Camiruaga JAE, Cano FF, De la Herran JL. Effects of isoflurane on intravenitricular pressure in neurosurgical patients. Br J Anaesth 1988: 61: 347–349.
Saito R, Graf R, Hübel K, et al. Halothane, but not alphachoralose, blocks potassium-evoked cortical spreading depression in cats. Brain Res 1995: 699: 109–115.
Saito R, Graf R, Hübel K. et al. Reduction of infract volume by halotahne: effect on cerebral blood flow or perifocal spreading depression-like depolarizations. J Cereb Blood Flow Metab 1997: 17: 857–864.
Sakabe T. Effect of enflurane (Ethrane) on canine cerebral metabolism and circulation. Masui 1975: 24: 323.
Sakabe T, Kuramoto T, Inoue S, Takeshita H. Cerebral responses to the addition of nitrous oxide to halothane in man. Br J Anaesth 1976: 48: 957–961.
Sakabe T, Kuvamoto T, Kumagae S, Takeshita H. Cerebral effects of nitrous oxide in the dog. Anesthesiology 1978: 48: 195–200.
Sakabe T, Maekawa T, Fujii S, et al. Cerebral circulation and metabolism during enflurane anesthesia in humans. Anesthesiology 1983: 59: 532–536.
Sakabe T, Tsutsui T, Maekawa T, et al. Local cerebral glucose utilization during nitrous oxide and pentobarbital anesthesia in rats. Anesthesiology 1985: 63: 262–266.
Sano T, Drummond JC, Patel PM, et al. A comparison of the cerebral protective effect of isoflurane and mild hypothermia in a model of incomplete forebrain ischemia in the rat. Anesthesiology 1992: 76: 221–228.
Sakaki T, Abe K, Hoshida T, et al. Isoflurane in the management of status epilepticus after surgery for lesion around the motor area. Acta Neurochir (Wien) 1992: 116: 38–43.
Sarraf-Yazdi S, Sheng H, Miura Y, et al. Relative neuroprotective effects of dizocilpine and isoflurane during focal cerebral ischemia in the rat. Anesth Analg 1998: 87: 72–78.
Sarraf-Yazdi S, Sheng H, Brinkhous AD, Pearlstein RD, Warner DS. J Neurosurg Anesthesiol 1999: 11: 1–36.
Satapathy GC, Dash HH. Tension pneumocephalus after nuerosurgery in the supine position. Br J Anaesth 2000: 84: 115–117.
Sato K, Shirane R, Kato M, Yoshimoto T. Effect of inhalational anesthesia on cerebral circulation in Moyamoya disease. J Neurosurg Anesthesiol 1999: 11: 25–30.
Scheller MS, Todd MM, Drummond JC. The effects of halothane and isoflurane on cerebral blood flow at various levels of $PaCO_2$ in rabbits. Anesthesiology 1984: 61: A528.
Scheller MS, Todd MM, Drummond JC. Isoflurane, halothane, and regional cerebral blood flow at various levels of $PaCO_2$ in rabbits. Anesthesiology 1986: 64: 598–604.

Scheller MS, Todd MM, Drummond JC, Zornow MH. The intracranial pressure effects of isoflurane and halothane administered following cryogenic brain injury in rabbits. Anesthesiology 1987: 67: 507–512.
Scheller MS, Tateichi A, Drummond JC, Zornow MH. The effects of sevoflurane on cerebral blood flow, cerebral metabolic rate for oxygen, intracranial pressure and electroencephalogram are similar to those of isoflurane in the rabbit. Anesthesiology 1988: 68: 548196551.
Scheller MS, Zornow M, Fleischer J, et al. The noncompetitive N-methyl-D-aspartate receptor antagonist MK-801 profoundly reduces volatile anesthetic requirements in rabbits. Neuropharmacology 1989: 28: 677–681.
Scheller MS. Nakakimura K, Fleischer JE, Zornow MH. Cerebral effects of sevoflurane in the dog: Comparison with isoflurane and enflurane. Br J Anaesth 1990: 65: 388–392.
Schettini A, Moreshead G. Effects of halothane and sodium thipentone on surface brain pressure and brain electrical impedance in dogs with normal intracranial tension. Br J Anaesth 1978: 50: 1003–1012.
Schettini A, Furniss WW. Brain water and electrolyte distribution during the inhalation of halothane. Br J Anaesth 1979: 51: 1117–1123.
Schregel W, Geissler C, Schäfermeyer H, Cunitz G. Diameters of large cerebral arteries - relevant for patients with brain disorders? Eur J Anaesth 1991: 8: 321–323.
Schregel W, Schäfermeyer H, Müller C, et al. Einfluss von Halothan, Alfentanil und Propofol auf Flussgeschwindigkeiten, "Gefässquerschnitt" und "Volumenfluss" in der a. cerebri media. Anaesthesist 1992: 41: 21–26.
Schulte am Esch J, Thiemig I, Pfeifer G, Entzian W. Die Wirkung einiger Inhalationsanaesthetika auf den Intrakraniellen Druck unter besonderer Berücksichtigung des Stickoxydul. Anaesthesist 1979: 28: 136–141.
Schwartz AE, Tuttle RH, Poppers PJ. Electroencephalographic burst suppresion in elderly and young patients anesthetized with isoflurane. Anesth Analg 1989: 68: 9–12.
Sebel PS, Ingram DA, Flynn PJ, et al. Evoked potentials during isoflurane anaesthesia. Br J Anaesth 1986: 58: 580–585.
Segal IS, Walton JR, Irwin I, et al. Modulating role of dopamine on anesthetic requirement. Eur J Pharmacol 1990: 186: 9–15.
Seo K, Maekawa T, Takeshita H, Okuda Y. Cerebral energy state and glycolytic metabolism during enflurane anesthesia in the rat. Acta Anaesthesiol Scand 1984: 28: 215–219.
Seyde WC, Longnecker DE. Cerebral oxygen tension in rats during deliberate hypotension with sodium nitroprusside, 2-chloroadenosine or deep isoflurane anesthesia. Anesthesiology 1986: 64: 480–485.
Seyde WC, Ellis JE, Longnecker DE. The addition of nitrous oxide to halothane decreases renal and splanchnic flow and increases cerebral blood flow in rats. Br J Anaesth 1986: 58: 63.
Shah NK, Long CW, Marx W, et al. Cerebrovascular response to CO_2 in edematous brain during either fentanyl or isoflurane anesthesia. Anesthesiology 1988: 69: A620.
Shah NK, Long C, Marx W, et al. Cerebrovascular response to CO_2 in edematous brain during either fentanyl or isoflurane anesthesia. J Neurosurg Anesthesiol 1990: 2: 11–15.
Shapira Y, Paez A, Lam AM, Pavlin EG. Influence of traumatic head injury on halothane MAC in rats. Anesth Analg 1992: 74: S282.
Shapiro HM, Wyte SR, Harris AB, Galindo A. Acute intraoperative intracranial hypertension in neurosurgical patients. Anesthesiology 1972a: 37: 399–405.
Shapiro HM, Greenberg JH, Reivich M, et al. Local cerebral glucose uptake in awake and halothane-anaesthetized primates. Anesthesiology 1978: 48: 97–103.
Sharbrough FW, Messick JM, Sundt TM Jr. Correlation of continuous electroencephalograms with cerebral blood flow measurements during carotid endarterectomy. Stroke 1973: 4: 674–683.
Shimosato S, Carter JG, Kemmotsu O, Takahashi T. Cardio-circulatory effects of prolonged administration of isoflurane in normocarbic human volunteers. Acta Anaesthesiol Scand 1982: 26: 27–30.
Sigmon DH, Florentino-Pineda I, Van Dyke RA, Beierwaltes WH. Halothane impairs the hemondynamic influence of endothelium-derived nitric oxide. Anesthesiology 1995: 82: 135–143. .
Slater SJ, Cox KJA, Lonbardi JV, et al. Inhibition of protein kinase C by alcohols and anesthetics. Nature (Lond) 1993: 364: 82–84.
Smiley RM, Ornstein E, Matteo RS, et al. Desflurane and isoflurane in surgical patients: comparison of emergency time. Anesthesiology 1991: 74: 425–428.
Smith AL, Neigh JL, Hoffman JC, Wollman H. Effects of general anesthesia on autoregulation of cerebral blood flow in man. J Appl Physiol 1970: 29: 665–669.
Smith AL, Wollman H. Cerebral blood flow and metabolism. Effects of anesthetic drugs and techniques. Anesthesiology 1972: 36: 378–400.
Smith AL. The mechanism of cerebral vasodilatation by halothane. Anesthesiology 1973: 39: 581–587.
Smith A, Hoff J, Nielsen S, Larson C. Barbiturate protection in focal cerebral ischemia. Stroke 1974: 5: 1–7.
Smith AL, Marque JJ. Anesthetics and cerebral oedema. Anesthesiology 1976: 45: 64–72.
Smith EH, Rees JMV. The effects of naloxone on the analgesic activities of general anesthetics. Experientia 1981: 37: 289–290.
Soonthon-Brant V, Patel P, Drummond CJ et al. Fentanyl does not increase brain injury after focal cerebral ischemia in rats. Anesth Analg 1999: 88: 49–55.
Stahle L, Collin AK, Ungerstedt U. Effects of halothane anesthesia on extracellular levels of dopamine, dihydroxy phenylacetic acid, homovanillic acid and 5-hydroxylindolacetic acid in rat striatum: A microdialysis study. Arch Pharmacol 1990: 342: 136–140.
Statler KD, Kochanek PM, Dixon CE, et al. Isoflurane improves long-term neurological outcome versus fentanyl after traumatic brain injury in rats. J Neurotrauma 2000: 17: 1179–1189.
Stauton M, Drexler C, Schmid PG, et al. Neuronal nitric oxide synthase mediates halothane-induced cerebral microvascular dilation. Anesthesiology 2000: 92: 125–132.
Steen PA, Michenfelder JD. Barbiturate protection in tolerant and nontolerant hypoxic mice. Anesthesiology 1979: 50: 404–408.
Stevens WC, Cromwell TH, Halsey MJ, et al. The cardiovascular effects of a new inhalation anesthetic, forene , in human volunteers at constant arterial carbon dioxide tension. Anesthesiology: 1971: 35: 8–16.
Stockard JJ, Bickford R. The neurophysiology of anesthesia. In: Gordon E, ed. A basis and practice of neuroanesthesia. Amsterdam:Excerpta Medica 1975: 3–46.

Stone DJ, Johns RA. Endothelium-dependent effects of halothane, enflurane, and isoflurane on isolated rat aortic vascular rings. Anesthesiology 1989: 71: 126–132.
Strebel S, Kaufmann M, Aselmi L, Schaefer HG. Nitrous oxide is a potent cerebrovasodilator in humans when added to isflurane. Acta Anaesthesiol Scand 1995: 39: 653–658.
Study RE. Isoflurane inhibits multiple voltage-gated calcium currents in hippocampal pyramidal neurons. Anesthesiology 1994: 81: 104–116.
Stullken EH, Sokoll MD. Anesthesia and subarachnoid intracranial pressure. Anesth Analg 1975: 54: 494–500.
Stullken EH, Sokoll MD. Intracranial pressure during hypotension and subsequent vasopressor therapy in anesthetized cats. Anesthesiology 1975: 42: 425–431.
Stullken AH, Milde JH, Michenfelder JD, Tinker JH. The nonlinear responses of cerebral metabolism to low concentrations of halothane, enflurane, isoflurane and thiopental. Anesthesiology 1977: 46: 28–34.
Sturaitis MK, Moore LE, Kirsch JR, McPherson RW. A cholinergic agonist induces cerebral hyperemia in isoflurane- byt not pentobarbital-anesthetized dogs. Anesth Analg 1994: 78: 876–883.
Stånge K, Lagerkranser M, Sollevi A. Effect of isoflurane-induced hypotension on cerebral autoregulation in the anesthetized pig. J Neurosurg Anesthesiol 1990: 2: 114–121.
Summors AC, Gupta AK, Matta BF. Dynamic cerebral autoregulation during sevoflruane anesthesia: A comparison with isoflurane. Anesth Analg 1999: 88: 341–345.
S¢ndergård W. Intracranial pressure during general anaesthesia. Dan Med Bull 1961: 8: 18–26.
Takahashi H, Murada K, Ikeda K. Sevoflurane does not increase intracranial pressure in hyperventilated dogs. Br J Anaesth 1993: 71: 551–555.
Takasaki M. The effects of enflurane on canine cerebral oxygen consumption and blood flow. Jap J Anaesthesiol 1974: 23: 806.
Takahashi H, Kirsch JR, Okada T, Traystman RJ. Intensity of halothane- and hypercapnia-induced cerebral hyperemia is strain dependent in rats. Anesth Analg 1996: 83: 359–365.
Talke P, Caldwell J,Dodson B, Richardson CA. Desfluran and isoflurane increase lumbar cerebrospinal fluid pressure in patients undergoing transsphenoidal hypophysectomy. Anesthesiology 1996: 85: 999–1004.
Talke P, Caldwell JE, Richardson CA. Sevoflurane increases lumbar cerebrospinal fluid pressure in normocapnic patients undergoing transsphenoidal hypophysectomy. Anesthesiology 1999: 91: 127–130.
Tambuniello G, Munari C, Gianesi GC. The behaviour of intracranial pressure during anesthesia with enflurane and oxygen alone. Minerva Anesthsiol 1978: 44: 923.
Tao Y-X. Hassan A, Johns RA. Intrathecally administration of cGMP-dependent protein kinase Iα inhibitor significantly reduced the threshold for isoflurane anaesthesia. Anesthesiology 2000: 92: 493–499.
Tempelhoff R. The new inhalational anesthetics desflurane and sevoflurane are valuable additions to the practice of neuroanesthesia: con. J Neurosurg Anesthesiol 1997: 9: 69–71.
Theye RA, Michenfelder JD. The effect of halothane on canine cerebral metabolism. Anesthesiology 1968a: 29: 1113–1118.
Theye RA, Michenfelder JD. The effect of nitrous oxide on canine cerebral metabolism. Anesthesiology 1968b: 29: 1119–1124.
Thornton C, Catley DM, Jordan C, et al. Enflurane anaesthesia causes graded changes in the brainstem and early cortical auditory evoked response in man. Br J Anaesth 1983: 55: 479–485.
Tinker JH, Sharbrough FW, Michenfelder JD. Anterior shift of the dominant EEG rhythm during anesthesia in the Java monkey: Correlation with anesthetic potency. Anesthesiology 1977: 46: 252–259.
Tobin JR, Martin LD, Breslow MJ, Traystman RJ. Selective anesthetic inhibition of brain nitric oxide synthase. Anesthesiology 1994: 81: 1264–1269.
Toda H, Nakamura K, Hatano Y, et al. Halothane and isoflurane inhibit endothelium-dependent relaxation elicited by acetylcholine. Anesth Analg 1992: 75: 198–203.
Todd MM, Drummond JC, Sang UH. The hemodynamic consequences of high-dose methohexital anesthesia in humans. Anesthesiology 1984a: 61: 495–501.
Todd MM, Drummond JC. A comparison of the cerebrovascular and metabolic effects of halothane and isoflurane in the cat. Anesthesiology 1984b: 60: 276–282.
Todd MM. The effects of $PaCO_2$ on the cerebrovascular response to nitrous oxide in the halothane-anaesthetized rabbit. Anest Analg 1987: 66: 1090–1095.
Todd MM, Warner DS. A comfortable hypothesis reevaluated (editorial). Anestheiology 1992: 76: 161–164.
Todd MM, Warner DS, Sokoll MD, et al. A prospective, comparative trial of three anesthetics for elective supratentorial craniotomy. Anesthesiology 1993: 78: 1005–1020.
Todd MM, Wu B, Warner DS, Maktabi M. The dose-related effects of nitric oxide sunthase inhibition on cerebral blood flow during isoflurane and pentobarbital anesthesia. Anesthesiology 1994: 1128–1136.
Todd MM, Weeks J. Comparative effects of propofol, pentobarbital, and isoflruane on cerebral blood flow and blood volume. J Neurosurg Anesthesiol 1996: 8: 296–303.
Toung T, Donham RT, Lehner A, et al. Tension pneumocephalus after posterior fossa craniotomy: report of four additional cases and review of postoperative pneumocephalus. Neurosurgery 1983: 12: 164–168.
Tsai SK, Lee C, Kwan W-F, Chen B-J. Recovery of cognitive functions after anaesthesia with desflurane or isoflurane and nitrous oxide. Br J Anaesth 1992: 69: 255–258.
Tsai Y-C, Lin S-S, Lee K-C, Chang C-L. Cerebral effects of nitrous oxide during isoflurane-induced hypotension in the pig. Br J Anaesth. 1994: 73: 667–672.
Turner CR, Losasso TJ, Muzzi DA, Weglinski MR. Brain relaxation and cerebrospinal fluid pressure during craniotomy for resection of supratentorial mass lesions. J Neurosurg Anesthesiol 1996: 8: 126–132.
Uggeri MJ, Proctor GJ, Johns RA. Halothane, enflurane, and isoflurane attenuate both receptor- and non-receptor-mediated EDRF production in rat thoracic aorta. Anesthesiology 1992: 76: 1012–1017.
Van Aken J, Hautekiet A, Rolly C. Influence of enflurane on cerebral blood flow in man. Acta Anaesthesiol Belg 1977, 28: 133–140.
Van Aken H, Fitch W, Graham DI, et al. Cardiovascular and cerebrovascular effects of isoflurane-induced hypotension in the baboon. Anesth Analg 1986: 65: 565–574.
Verhaegen M, Todd M, Warner D. A comparison of cerebral ischemic flow thresholds during halothane/N20 and isoflurane/N_2O anesthesia in rats. Anesthesiology 1992.

Verhaegen M, Todd MM, Warner DS. Ischemic-depolarization during halothane-nitrous oxide and isoflurane-nitrous oxide anesthesia. Anesthesiology 1994: 81: 965–973.

Virtue RW, Lund LO, Phleps M, et al. Difluoromethyl 1,1,2-trifluoro-2-chloroethyl ether as an anaesthetic agent: results with dogs and a preliminary note on observations in man. Can Anaesth Soc J 1966: 13: 233–241.

Waaben J, Husum B, Hansen AJ, Gjedde A. Hypocapnia prevents the decrease in regional cerebral metabolism during isoflurane-induced hypotension. J Neurosurg Anesthesiol 1989: 1: 29–34.

Wallin RF, Regan BM, Napoli MD, Stern IJ. Sevoflurane: a new inhalation anaesthetic agent. Anesth Analg 1975: 54: 758–766.

Warner DS, Boarini DJ, Kassell NF. Cerebrovascular adaptation to prolonged halothane anesthesia is not related to cerebrospinal fluid pH. Anesthesiology 1985: 63: 243–248.

Warner DS, Deshpanda JK, Wieloch T. The effect of isoflurane on neuronal necrosis follwing near-complete forebrain ischaemia in the rat. Anesthesiology 1986: 64: 19–23.

Warner DS, Zhou J, Ramani R, Todd MM. Reversible focal ischemia in the rat: Effects of halothane, isoflurane, and methohexital anesthesia. J Cereb Blood Flow Metab 1991: 11: 794–802.

Warner DS, Ludvig PS, Pearlstein R, Brinkhous AD. Halothane reduces focal ischemic injury in the rat when brain temperature is controlled. Anesthesiology 1995: 82: 1237–1245.

Warner DS. Isoflurane neuropretection (editorial). Anesthesiology 2000: 92: 1226–1228.

Watanabe K, Arai T, Aoki M, et al. Effects of halothane on the synthesis of neurotransmitter amino acids in mous brain. Acta Anaesthesiol Scand 1993: 37: 706–709.

Watts ADJ, Herrick IA, McLachlan RS, et al. The effect of sevoflruane and isoflurane anesthesia on interictal spile activity among patients with refractory epilepsy. Anesth Analg 1999: 89: 1275–1281.

Weeks J, Todd MM, Warner DS, Katz J. Volatile anesthetics and cerebral blood volume. J Cereb Blood Flow Metab. 1989: 9: suppl 1, S 474.

Wollman H, Alexander SC, Cohen PJ, et al. Cerebral circulation of man during halothane anesthesia. Effects of hypocarbia and of d-tubocurarine. Anesthesiology 1964: 25: 180–184.

Wollman H, Alexander SC, Cohen PJ, et al. Cerebral circulation during general anesthesia and hyperventilation in man. Thiopental induction to nitrous oxide and d-tubocuranine. Anesthesiology 1965: 26: 329–334.

Wollman H, Smith AL, Neigh JL, Hoffman JC. Cerebral blood flow and oxygen consumption in man during electroencephalographic seizure patterns associated with ethrane anesthesia. In: Cerebral blood flow-clinical and experimental results. (eds) Brock M, Fieschi C, Ingvar D, et al. Springer, New York. 1969: 246–248.

Woodcock TE, Murkin JM, Farrar K, et al. Pharmacologic EEG suppression during cardiopulmonary bypass: Cerebral hemodynamic and metabolic effects of thiopental or isoflurane during hypothermia and normothermia. Anesthesiology 1987: 67: 218–224.

Wyrwicz AM, Pszenny MH, Schofield JC, et al. Noninvasive observations of fluorinated anaesthetics in rabbit brain by fluorine-19 nuclear magnetic resonance. Science 1983: 222: 428–430.

Yamamoto M, Hatano Y, Ogawa K, et al. Halothane and isoflurane attenuate the relaxant response to nonadrenergic and noncholinergic nerve stimulation of isolated canine cerebral arteries. Anesth Analg 1998: 86: 552–526.

Yamamura T, Fukuda M, Takeya H, et al. Fast oscillatory EEG activity induced by analgesic concentrations of nitrous oxide in man. Anesth Analg 1981: 60: 283–288.

Yang JC, Clark WC, Ngai SH. Antagonism of nitrous oxide by naloxone in man. Anesthesiology 1980: 52: 414–417.

Yli-Hankala A, Vakkuri A, Särkelä M, et al. Epileptiform electroencephalogram during mask induction of anesthesia with sevoflurane. Anesthesiology 1999: 91: 1596–1603.

Young Kwon J, Bacher A, Deyo DJ, et al. Effects of pentobarbital and isoflurane on conditioned learning after transient global cerebral ischemia in rabbits. Anesthesiology 2000: 92: 171–177.

Young WL, Prohovnik I, Correll JW, et al. A comparison of the cerebral hemodynamic effects of sufentanil and isoflurane in humans undergoing carotid endarterectomy. Anesthesiology 1989a: 71: 863–869.

Young WL, Prohovnik I, Correll JW, et al. Cerebral blood flow and metabolism in patients undergoing anesthesia for carotid endarterectomy. Anesth Analg 1989b: 68: 712–717.

Young WL, Prohovnik I, Correll JW, et al. A comparison of cerebral blood flow reactivity to CO_2 during halothane versus isoflurane anesthesia for carotid endarterectomy. Anesth Analg 1991: 73: 416–421.

Young WL, Barkai AI, Prohovnik I, et al. Effect of $PaCO_2$ on cerebral blood flow distribution during halothane compared with isoflurane anaesthesia in the rat. Br J Anaesth 1991: 67: 440–446.

Zattoni J, Siani C, Rivano C. Effects of ethrane on intracranial pressure. In: Lawin P, Beer R (eds) Ethrane: Proceedings of the first European Symp on modern Anaesthetic Agents. Springer Verlag, Berlin, Heidelberg, New York 1974: 272.

Hypnotic agents

Receptor action

The effects of hypnotic agents are complex. They produce loss of consciousness, loss of memory, changes in spontaneous activity, attenuation of protective reflexes, loss of postural reflexes and unfavourable side effects such as hallucinations, euphoria, and amnesia. Theoretically many of these effects are mediated through changes in the homeostasis of neurotransmitters in the brain, such as dopamine, norepinephrine, acetylcholine, and γ-aminobutyric acid (GABA).

Acetylcholine

Acetylcholine was the first neurotransmitter to be described. Cholinergic neurones are distributed widely through the brain (Lydic et al. 1993, Iversen 1997). Microdialysis studies indicate that several anaesthetic agents affect acetylcholine release in various brain regions (Sato et al. 1996, Kikuchi et al. 1997, Damsma and Fibiger 1991, Taguchi et al. 1993). Cholinergic mechanisms are known to be important in the striatum, where balance between acetylcholine and dopamine release ensures normal motor output. In the hippocampal and frontal cortex acetylcholine plays an important role in the regulation of consciousness, learning and memory (Lydia et al. 1993). In rats propofol has a powerful, and region-selective depressant effect on acetylcholine release from the frontal cortex and hippocampus, but not from the striatum. In human volunteers physiostigmine reverses the propofol-induced unconsciousness and associated depression of the auditory steady state response and bispectral index. These effects were blocked by pretreatment with scopolamine, suggesting that the loss of consciousness produced by propofol is mediated, at least in part, via interruption of central cholinergic muscarinic transmission (Meuret et al. 2000).

GABA (γ-aminobutyric acid)

Electrophysiological and neurochemical studies indicate that most general anaesthetics potentiate inhibitory transmission mediated by GABA, the major inhibitory neurotransmitter in mammals. Clinically relevant concentrations of volatile anaesthetics and propofol potentiate GABA-activated Cl^- currents in the rat hippocampal pyramide neurones (Jones et al. 1992, Hales and Lambert 1991).

Low concentrations of propofol, etomidate, pentobarbital and alphaxalone facilitate GABA release from cortical nerve terminals, suggesting that these drugs may facilitate inhibitory GABA-ergic synaptic transmission by a presynaptic mechanism (Murugaiah and Hemmings 1998)

The inhibitory effects of propofol in the rat hippocampus involve "intra" hippocampal $GABA_A$ receptors while the inhibitory effects in the rat frontal cortex are mediated by $GABA_A$ receptors other than "intra" frontal GABA receptors (Kikuchi et al. 1998).

Potentiation of inhibitory neurotransmission occurs *via* enhancement of $\alpha_1\ \beta_2\ \gamma_{25}GABA_A$-mediated chloride conductance, prolonging and enhancing inhibitory postsynaptic potentials (Franks and Lieb 1994, Jones et al. 1992, Tanelian et al. 1993). Other data indicate that thiopental, propofol and ketamine inhibit K^+-evoked glutamate release from rat cerebrocortical slices. The inhibition produced by thiopental and propofol is mediated by activation of $GABA_A$ receptors, revealing a subtle interplay between GABA-releasing and glutamatergic transmission in anaesthetic action (Buggy et al. 2000).

Excitatory amino acids

Glutamate is a major excitatory neurotransmitter in the central system. The AMPA subtype of glutamate receptor mediates the fast component of excitatory postsynaptic currents. AMPA receptors consist of protein subunits that assemble into pentameric or tetrameric structures that contain an intrinsic channel pore. Based on sequence homology, four subunit genes have been identified and are referred to as *GlutR1* to *GlutR4*. AMPA receptors critically depend on the subunit composition. For example, the presence of the *GlutR2* subunit confers a ninefold to 30-fold decrease in calcium (Ca^{2+}) permeability to AMPA receptors. This reduced calcium permetability is attributed to a positively charged arginine residue in the menbrane reentry pore loop of the *GlutR2* subunit. AMPA receptors that contain the *GlutR2* subunit are further characterized by a reduced sensitivity to endogenous and exogenous polyamines. Recombinant receptors that lack the *GlutR2* subunit demonstrate a fivefold reduced sensitivity to pentobarbital (Taverna et al. 1994), suggesting that neurones deficient of the *glutR2* subunit would be less sensitive to barbiturate inhibition. *GlutR2* null mutant mice, however, are more sensitive to pentobarbital anesthesia despite a reduced sensitivty of *GlutR2*-deficient AMPA receptors to barbiturate blockade (Joo et al. 1999). This finding suggests that the inhibition of AMPA receptors does not correlate with the anaesthetic effects of barbiturates. On the contrary, the result suggests that the increase in sensitivity to anaesthetics results from a global suppression of excitatory neurotransmission in *GlutR2*-deficient mice.

Norepinephrine

Norepinephrine released from noradrenergic nerve terminals stimulates α_1-adrenergic receptors, activates guanine nucleotide binding (G protein), and subsequently enhances phosphatidylinositol turnover. It has been postulated that anaesthetics affect the phsophatidylinositol turnover in the central nervous system. In the rat cerebral cortex norepinephrine-induced inositol monophosphate formation was inhibited by droperidol, fentanyl, diazepam and thiamylal in a dose-dependent manner, suggesting that the effects on phosphatidylinositol turnover in the cortex may be related to these drugs pharmacological action (Makita et al. 1994).

Barbiturate, experimental studies

Effects on systemic blood flow.

In rats doses of barbiturate sufficient to create burst-suppression on EEG are accompanied by a fall in cardiac output and a decrease in flow to muscle and fat. After few minutes cardiac output is normalised. This change coincides with an increase in intestinal flow and a decrease in intestinal resistance (Wada et al. 1996).

Cerebral kinetics

It has been assumed that a high CBF is associated with a more rapid uptake into the brain, and a higher peak concentration after bolus administration (Upton et al. 1996). A diffusion barrier, however, has also been proposed, indicated by a decrease in permeability by barbiturates with a low lipophilicity (Igari et al. 1982). In sheep the cerebral kinetics of thiopental were examined over a range of CBF using chronically instumentation. The cerebral kinetics of thiopental after bolus injection were dependent on CBF, despite partial diffusion limitation. A high CBF produced higher peak cerebral concentrations and shorter time to reach this concentration (Upton et al. 2000).

CBF and $CMRO_2$

In dogs and rats a dose-dependent decrease in CBF and $CMRO_2$, associated with an increase in CVR has been observed after bolus injection of thiopentone (Michenfelder 1974, Carlsson et al. 1975b, Stullken et al. 1977. Björkman et al. 1994), and phenobarbitone (Nilsson and Siesjö 1975). Through the action of barbiturate on CVR and CBV, ICP will decrease. The suppression of $CMRO_2$ by thiopentone injection reaches a plateau of 50% of control, when EEG is isoelectric (Michenfelder 1974, Kassell et al. 1980, Steen et al. 1983). In dogs subjected to thiopentone combined with hypothermia to 30°C, $CMRO_2$ decreases to about 70% of control values (Lafferty et al. 1978). At an even higher degree of hypothermia (14–18°C), EEG becomes isoelectric, and $CMRO_2$ is reduced to 7–14% of control. Under these circumstances $CMRO_2$ is unaffected by barbiturate (Steen et al. 1983). During continuous thiopentone infusion in dogs and goats, loss of consciousness occurs when CBF and $CMRO_2$ are reduced by 23–30%, and emergence from anaesthesia is observed while $CMRO_2$ is still depressed by about 20% (Stullken et al. 1977, Albrecht et al. 1977). In dogs subjected to prolonged deep barbiturate anaesthesia for 90 min until burst suppression on EEG, methohexitone and thiopentone induce the same decrease in CBF and $CMRO_2$; however, when the barbiturate infusion was discontinued, recovery occurred earlier with methohexitone than with thiopentone and $CMRO_2$ and CBF returned more rapidly toward control values (Boardine et al. 1984).

In vitro studies of brain endothelium permeability indicate that thiopental in high doses showed no effects on permeability. Only the passage of α-aminoisobutyric acid was increased (Fischer et al. 1995).

Regional CBF

With the iodoantipyrine technique variation of local CBF in response to pentobarbitone has been studied in the rat. Pentobarbitone more strongly decreased local CBF in the forebrain than in the hindbrain and produced different patterns of changes in local CBF than in local cerebral glucose utilisation, measured with the 2-deoxyglucose technique. The patterns of the CBF variations were columnar in the cerebral cortex and the hippocampus but were patchy in the caudate-putamen, thalamus and inferior colliculus (Otsuka et al.1991). In dogs a shifting of percentage contribution of flow to slow compartment (white matter) was observed after phenobarbitone infusion, suggesting that selective shunting of blood to white matter might explain the fall in ICP and protection of deep white matter observed by many authors (Laurent et al. 1982).

CO_2 reactivity

During high dose thiopentone infusion in dogs until burst suppression level in the EEG, a profound degree of vasoconstriction, equivalent to that produced by hypocapnia at $PaCO_2$ 20 mm Hg occurs. Under these circumstances the CO_2 reactivity is low in the $PaCO_2$ level ranging from 30–40 mm Hg, and absent in the range of 20–30 mm Hg, suggesting that hyperventilation to levels of $PaCO_2$ less that 30 mm Hg does not effectively increase the degree of vasoconstriction (Kassell et al. 1981).

Blood-brain barrier function

In vivo studies have alternately reported decreases and increases of the blood-brain barrier permeability by barbiturates (Saija et al. 1989, Gjedde and Rasmussen 1980, Otsuda et al. 1991, Stewart et al. 1988). *In vitro* studies indicate that barbiturates do not affect brain endothelial permeability (Fischer et al. 1995). However, it has been reported that barbiturates attenuate a hypoxia-induced increase in the permeability of brain-derived microvascular endothelial cells (Fischer et al. 1996). Another study indicates that when the blood-brain barrier is disrupted by hyperosmolar solution, pentobarbitone attenuates the degree of leakage of the blood-brain barrier. Systemic hypotension caused by pentobarbital plays a major role in decreasing the leakage (Chi et al. 1998).

NO

Pretreatment with nitric oxide synthase inhibition reduces CBF during pentobarbital anaesthesia. Nitric oxide under this circumstance seems to influence background vascular tone, and is not the primary mediator of barbiturates effect upon CBF (Todd et al. 1994). Barbiturates inhibit cGMP-mediated endothelium-dependent and independent relaxation of isolated canine mesenteric and rat aorta (Terasako et al. 1994).

Vasodilation

It has been shown that barbiturate in anaesthetically effective doses, exerts a vasodilatory action on vascular smooth muscle cells in systemic vessels and large cerebral arteries (Altura et Altura 1975, Edvinsson and Mc Culloch 1981, Marin et al. 1981). Gross and Abel (1985) in a rabbit basilar artery model found that at a concentration of 3 x 10^{-5} thiopental caused relaxation of norepinephrine-induced contractions. In the monkey Tsuji and Chiba (1986) found that thiopentone showed a biphasic vascular response, with an initial vasoconstriction followed by vasodilation in a dose-dependent manner. In a study by Ogura et al. (1991) it was found that intracerebral venules are relatively less responsive to pentobarbitone than cerebral arterioles and peripheral veins. In the same study it was suggested that barbiturate redistributes blood volume from cerebral veins to more responsive peripheral veins, thereby decreasing intracranial blood volume. It is important to stress that the contractile/dilatatory responses of isolated cerebral arteries might depend on the choice of barbiturate. Thus, it has been found that thiobarbiturates are more potent vasoconstrictors than oxybarbiturates (Hatano et al. 1989). For thiamylal the inhibition of contraction is mediated through the release in intracellular stored Ca^{2+} as well as influx of extracellular Ca^{2+} (Nakamura et al. 1991). The same group found that thiopentone inhibited contractions elicited by Ca^{2+}-influx and Ca^{2+} release to the same extent, whereas pentobarbitone inhibited contractions elicited by Ca^{2+} influx selectively (Yakushiji et al. 1992).

Peripheral circulation

In the peripheral circulation of cat skeletal muscle thiopental in low doses increases the peripheral vascular resistance. The vasoconstriction dominated in large arterioles. In high doses thiopental decreases the peripheral resistance, predominantly owing to dilation of small arterioles (Grände et al. 1990).

Tolerance and age

In dogs, pre-treatment with thiopentone immediately before induction of anaesthesia is associated with acute tolerance of $CMRO_2$ in spite of higher concentrations of thiopentone in CSF and blood (Altenburg et al. 1969). Chronic thiopentone infusion for 24 hours in dogs, is followed by sustained increase in $CMRO_2$ occurring after 3 hours in spite of unchanged blood levels of thiopentone (Gronert et al. 1981). In rats the effects of thiopentone on CBF and $CMRO_2$ are similar in young and elder animals (Baughman et al. 1986).

Energy metabolism

Following a high dose of thiopentone in dogs and rats until isoelectric EEG $CMRO_2$ is reduced by 50%. Under these circumstances the concentrations of ATP, ADP and AMP are unchanged, while the concentrations of glycogen and phosphocreatine are increased, indicating an unchanged or increased energy charge level, and that the cerebral metabolic effect of barbiturate is secondary to functional effects (Michenfelder 1974, Carlsson et al. 1975b). Studies in rats indicate an inhibition of cerebral phosphofructokinase activity by barbiturate. Endogenous substrates are mobilised from existing carbohydrate and amino-acid pools, and thiopentone solubilises bound hexokinase activity, thereby inhibiting energy metabolism (Nilsson and Siesjö 1974, Chapman et al. 1978, Krieglstein et al. 1981).

Glucose metabolism

Studies of regional glucose utilisation in rats indicate that barbiturates induce a universal metabolic depression, partly excluding nucleus interpeduncularis, nucleus habenula and tractus habenulo-interpeduncularis (Herkenhan 1981, Hodes et al. 1983). In comparison with the cerebral cortex, the depression of glucose utilisation in the spinal cord is much less (Crosby et al. 1984). During combined use of nitrous oxide and thiopentone at levels with EEG activity, glucose utilisation is higher in many structures, including the midbrain reticular formation, than that observed with thiopentone alone. These changes were not observed with high thiopentone injection with isoelectric EEG. The findings indicate that nitrous oxide acts as a cerebral metabolic stimulant in the presence of EEG activity during thiopentone anaesthesia (Sakabe et al. 1985).

Local cerebral glucose utilisation in stimulated rats sedated with thiopental is increased in cortical regions responsible for processing of noxious stimuli (Archer et al. 1995).

EEG

Barbiturate initially produces fast EEG activity of 15–30 Hz, with the largest amplitudes frontally. The dominant frequency of these fast waves and the rate at which this dominant frequency is attained, both decrease as the total cumulative dose of barbiturate is augmented. The polymorphic delta waves which initially alternate with the fast activity become more constant as the cumulative dosage rises and become associated with 10–15 Hz spindles. Further increase in total dose causes bursts of activity alternating with runs of suppression and at an even higher dose total electric silence occurs (Stockard and Bickford 1975). It has been demonstrated *in vivo* and *in vitro* that both neocortex and hippocampus exhibit burst suppression and isoelectric activity during thiopental anaesthesia. Thiopental-induced synchronised burst activity, however, was depressed by progressively higher doses of barbiturate (MacIver et al. 1996, Lukatch et al. 1996). Using a computer-controlled infusion pump it is possible to establish a constant serum thiopentone concentration rapidly, and characterise the concentration versus EEG drug effect relationship (Bührer et al. 1992). However the biphasic thiopentone concentration-EEG relationship and the isoelectric EEG at high serum thiopentone concentrations needed to prevent purposeful movement responses, limit the utility of the EEG as a measure of anaesthetic depth when thiopentone is used alone (Hung et al. 1992).

Inverse steal

In baboons subjected to MCAO, the ultra-short acting barbiturate, methohexitone, produce an elevation of CBF in regions of cortical ischaemia. This inverse flow increase most likely results from a reduction in flow in relatively well-perfused cortical regions, as a consequence of a reduction in metabolic rate and vasoconstriction by the barbiturate. Blood flow is therefore diverted into relatively ischaemia regions (Branston et al. 1979). In cats subjected to MCAO, pentobarbitone infusion increases cerebral oxygen availability in poorly perfused cerebral cortex (Feustel et al. 1981).

Hypoxia

During hypoxic studies in mice, barbiturate improves survival and decreases mortality (Arnfred and Secher 1962). During *In vitro* studies of slices from hippocampus tissue exposed to periods of hypoxia the addition of thiopentone to the perfusion medium increases the duration of hypoxia that was survived by CA1 pyramidal cells (Aitken and Schiff 1986). The survival time in hypoxic mice is increased by mild hypothermia and decreased by hyperthermia. When mild hypothermia is combined with pentobarbitone, survival time was generally further increased (Artru and Michenfelder 1981). However, it is important to stress that temperature control was not performed during the early experimental studies of hypoxia. Thus, a fall in cerebral temperature could explain the protective effect of barbiturate (Artru 1988b). Indeed, when temperature is controlled no protective effect of barbiturate was found in the hypoxic mouse model (Milde 1988).

It has been postulated that the protective effect of barbiturate is related to the anaesthetic effect, which is distinct from the anticonvulsant effect (Steen and Michenfelder 1979). As judged by metabolic criteria by measurements of cerebral tissue ATP, phosphocreatine and lactate in rats subjected to unilateral carotid ligation, hypothermia offers better cerebral protection than does phenobarbitone that elicits the same decrease in CBF and CMRO2 (Hägerdal et al. 1978).

ICP hypertension

In cats subjected to ICP hypertension by inflation of an epidural balloon, the increase in ICP during inflation was less in animals pre-treated with barbiturate than untreated animals. In the post- deflation period, the untreated animals developed higher ICP than pre-treated animals, suggesting a protective effect against post compression brain swelling (Bricolo et al. 1981). In a study of dogs subjected to intracranial hypertension by inflation of an epidural balloon there was no benefit from the addition of barbiturate therapy to hyperventilation. Barbiturate under this condition reduced CBF without providing further relief from increased ICP (Louis et al. 1993).

Ischaemia and protection

Several experimental studies of focal cerebral ischaemia in cats, dogs and monkeys have shown that pretreatment with barbiturate offers a brain protective effect by improving survival and diminishing neuropathological changes (Hoff et al. 1973, Smith et al. 1974, Hankinson et al. 1974, Hoff et al. 1975, Corkill et al. 1976, Safar et al. 1976), Michenfelder et al. 1976, Corkill et al. 1978, Bleyart et al. 1978, Todd et al. 1982, Gelb et al. 1986). In rats subjected to asphyxia and arterial hypotension (Nilsson 1971) and dogs subjected to hypoxia (Michenfelder and Theye 1973), barbiturate preserves the cerebral energy charge and the lactate production is decreased. In gerbils subjected to unilateral carotid ligation for one hour, neuropathological examination revealed less extensive neuronal ischaemic cell changes in animals allocated to thiopentone injected one hour after removal of the arterial clamp (Levy and Brierley 1979). In baboons and dogs subjected to temporary MCAO (Selman et al. 1981, Yonas et al. 1981) or extracranial-intracranial by-pass operations (Spetzler et al. 1982), it has been demonstrated that sufficient reperfusion after focal cerebral ischaemia is of utmost importance in the protection against cerebral ischaemic damage.

Studies of intracellular brain pH in monkeys subjected to MCAO in either halothane or thiopentone anaesthesia indicate that the decrease in pH is less pronounced in barbiturate anaesthetized animals. After CBF was restored, brain pH returned towards normal values during thiopentone anaesthesia but continued to deteriorate under halothane anaesthesia (Anderson and Sundt 1983).

Other experimental studies in dogs and monkeys subjected to complete global ischaema have stated that barbiturates do not protect the brain (Steen et al. 1979, Snyder et al. 1979, Gisvold et al. 1984, Koch et al. 1984). Under these circumstances barbiturates if at all (Steen et al. 1978) only induce a very moderate delay in the depletion of cerebral energy reserves (Nordström and Siesjö 1978). Thus, experimental studies do not at present support the use of barbiturate in the treatment of global ischaemia (Shapiro 1985).

It is important to stress that in many studies performed before 1982 brain temperature was not sufficiently monitored. In these studies a brain protective effect can be effected by hypothermia elicited by barbiturate. According to Matsumoto et al. (1997) mild and moderate hypothermia provides better protection than burst-suppression dose of thiopental against ischaemic spinal cord injury in rabbits.

The protective effect upon brain ischaemia by barbiturate and other hypnotics is not caused by an attenuation of the cerebral oxygen consumption. Isoflurane, which possesses a cerebral metabolic depressor effect like thiopental, does not elicit the same cerebral protection against ischaemia. Recently it was found that thiopental attenuates ischaemia-induced $[Ca^{2+}]_I$ increases in the hippocampus and cortex of rats, probably caused by an inhibition of both voltage-gated calcium channels and NMDA receptors. The same study suggested that the regional difference in inhibition by thiopental of NMDA receptors is related to its region-specific action against ischaemia (Zhan et al. 1998).

Free radicals

It has been postulated that free radicals are released in ischaemic cerebral tissue, giving rise to irreversible tissue damage (Michenfelder et al. 1976), and that barbiturate acts as a free radical scavenger. Hypothetically this effect might explain its protective effect (Smith et al. 1974, Flamm et al. 1977). This hypothesis, however, has been rejected (Smith et al. 1980, Siesjö 1984), and it has been accepted that the protective effect of barbiturate, if present at all, is caused by the suppression of cerebral metabolism alone (Astrup 1982, Siesjö 1984). Nevertheless, recent studies of the effect of barbiturates on hydroxyl radicals, lipid peroxidation and hypoxic cell deaths in human neurones indicate that pentobarbital, phenobarbital, methohexital and thiopental dose-dependently inhibited the formation of 2,3, dihydrxybenzoic acid and iron-stimulated lipid peroxidation. However, differences in antioxidant action between the barbiturates were observed. While phenobarbital and pentobarbital increased lactate dehydrogenase release after combined oxygen and glucose deprivation, thiopental and methohexital protected the neurones at all tested concentrations. At high concentration pentobarbital also protected the neurones (Almaas et al. 2000).

Excitatory amino acids

Contrary to what was to be expected, thiopental in burst-suppression doses increases glutamate release during ischaemia. This result indicates that the protective effect of barbiturate does not involve a reduction of excitatory amino acids during ischaemia (Goskowicz et al. 1993). On the other hand, in cortical cell culture barbiturate attenuates excitotoxicity in concentration-dependent fashion (Giffard et al. 1993).

Using postsynaptic-evoked population spike recorded from the CA1 pyramidal cell layer of rat hippocampal slices the following findings were revealed. Thiopental attenuates NMDA- and AMPA-mediated glutamate excitotoxity. Propofol enhanced the NMDA-induced neuronal damage (Zhu et al. 1997).

Serotonin

In rats subjected to cryogenic brain injury, the pentobarbital concentration required to prevent pain stimulus was reduced. The cortical serotonin concentration was increased in injured rats, and inhibition of 5-hydroxytryptamine synthesis abolished the increase in serotonin concentration and normalised the dose of pentobarbitone required to prevent a pain stimulus. This study indicates that serotonergic mechanism influences the pharmacodynamics of pentobarbitone in cryogenic brain injury (Archer et al. 1991).

Barbiturate, human studies

CBF, CVR, $CMRO_2$ and ICP

The experimental data concerning the effect of barbiturates on cerebral circulation and metabolism have been confirmed in clinical studies. Thus, barbiturate induces an associated decrease in CBF and $CMRO_2$ and an increase in CVR (Wechsler et al. 1951, Pierce et al. 1962). These effects are associated with a decrease in ICP (S¢ndergård 1961, Gordon 1970).

EEG

The EEG changes produced by thiopentone injection have been divided into five patterns by Kiersey et al. (1951). The first pattern is characterised by high amplitudes and fast activity of mixed frequencies varying between 10–30 Hz. The second pattern is a complex of many frequencies but with the presence of predominantly slower waves and much variation in voltages. In the third pattern, progressive suppression of cortical activity is separated by bursts of activity. In the fourth pattern the periods with inactivity are further prolonged, ranging between 3 and 10 seconds. During the fifth pattern, the amplitudes fall below 25 microvolt and long periods with isoelectric EEG are recorded.

Clinical studies and craniotomy

Studies of barbiturate treatment in brain ischaemia and high dose barbiturate therapy in neurosurgery and intensive care have been published (Shapiro 1985, Piatt and Schiff 1984). In the following clinical studies of barbiturate in the neuroanaesthetic practice and in the care of neurointensive patients will be referred.

In the neuroanaesthesiological practice, thiopentone has been used during induction of anaesthesia before the use of inhalation agents (Hunter 1972, Astrup et al. 1984, Madsen et al. 1987a) and before neurolept anaesthesia (Arnér and Gordon 1976, Cold et al. 1988). In clinical studies of ICP hypertension, peroperative loads of thiopentone (1.5–3.0 mg/kg) induce a significant decrease in ICP (Shapiro et al. 1973). Although studies of thiopentone supplemented anaesthesia for craniotomy have been promising, the postoperative recovery is prolonged (Hunter 1972). After opening of the dura, thiopentone in a dose of 4–8 mg/kg during maintenance of anaesthesia with nitrous oxide, halothane 0.5% gives rise to a small but significant decrease in $CMRO_2$ by 8%. It has been suggested that although small, this decrease in metabolism may have some protective effect (Astrup et al. 1984).

Aneurysm

In uncontrolled studies, peroperative thiopentone loads have been advocated in surgery for cerebral aneurysm (Hoff et al. 1977, Sokoll et al. 1982, Bendtsen et al. 1984, Belopavlovic et al. 1985). Uncontrolled studies suggest that the frequency of cerebral spasms in patients with cerebral aneurysms might be reduced after deep barbiturate anaesthesia (Belopavlovic et al. 1985). Studies of central haemodynamics during aneurysm surgery with a thiopentone dose of 20–34 mg/kg indicate a reduction of cardiac output and MABP, without generalised evidence of compromised tissue perfusion (Sokoll et al. 1982, Bendtsen et al. 1983, Todd et al. 1985). Similar conclusions were drawn during methohexitone anaesthesia (Todd et al. 1984a) and pentobarbitone anaesthesia (Traeger et al. 1983, Todd et al. 1987).

A–V malformation

Surgery for arterio-venous malformation might be complicated by massive multifocal bleeding and/or oedema. This phenomenon, called normal perfusion pressure breakthrough, has been studied experimentally by Spetzler et al. (1978). Diversion of blood from the arterio-venous malformation into adjacent maximally dilated and non autoregulated small vessels is the pathophysiological reason. The occurrence of this complication might be catastrophic. Preliminary studies, however, indicate that deep thiopentone anaesthesia with loading doses of 10–20 mg/kg can prevent this complication and reduce the formation of oedema (Day et al. 1982, Marshall and Sang U 1983).

Carotid surgery

In patients subjected to carotid end-arterectomy (Moffat et al. 1983, Hicks et al. 1986) and extracranial-intracranial by-pass operations (Lawner and Simeone 1979, Lobe and Brauer 1983), barbiturate anaesthesia has also been advocated, and it has been argued that barbiturate might protect the brain.

Head injury

In patients with severe head injury with persistent ICP hypertension in spite of hyperventilation, thiopentone induces a rapid decrease in ICP accompanied by an increase in CPP. Sustained ICP reduction could be maintained for several days by combining thiopentone therapy and hypothermia to 30° C. (Shapiro et al. 1974). Other clinical studies support these findings (Sidi et al. 1983). Barbiturate sedation together with hyperventilation have been advocated in the control of ICP hypertension, and this regime has been claimed to improve outcome in patients with severe head injury (Saul and Ducker 1982). Uncontrolled (Rockoff et al. 1979), and controlled studies (Eisenberg et al. 1988) seem to support this view Other uncontrolled studies (Yano et al. 1986), and controlled studies (Ward et al. 1985) did not confirm this finding. It has repeatedly been found that cerebral oxygen uptake is reduced in severe head injury (Bruce et al. 1973, Cold et al. 1978) and a fairly good correlation between the level of consciousness and $CMRO_2$ has been demonstrated (Obrist et al. 1979). Barbiturate reactivity, as measured by the fall in $CMRO_2$ after a bolus dose of thiopental 5 mg/kg, is reduced when cerebral oxygen uptake is reduced (Cold 1989). In another study it was found that the barbiturate reactivity is reduced the first four days after severe head injury. However, great inter- and intraindividual differences in barbiturate reactivity may exist (Dahl et al. 1994). It is supposed that poor clinical effect of barbiturate coma treatment to some extent is coupled to the suppression of cerebral metabolism and lost barbiturate reactivity.

By-pass operation

In patients subjected to a cardiopulmonary by-pass operation for open cardiac surgery a preliminary controlled study indicated that thiopentone reduced postoperative neuropsychiatric dysfunction, supposed to be caused by microembolization (Nussmeier et al. 1986). This observation has given rise to optimism. It has been proposed that thiopentone treatment during open heart surgery should not be denied the patients (Michenfelder 1986). However, the issue has been debated (Scheller et al. 1986), and it has been suggested that other factors like hypocapnia might decrease the risks of air embolization, owing to the general reduction in CBF during a by-pass operation (Henriksen 1986). Furthermore, in a later study by Nussmeier and Fish (1987), the changes in neuropsychiatric function after cardiopulmonary by-pass operation were not mitigated by thiopentone or prostaglandin (PGI-2) injection. Only the age of the patients was found to be a predictor of postoperative decrements in performance. In another study thiopentone did not reduce the number of strokes in patients undergoing coronary artery surgery. Thus 1.3% in the placebo against 3.7% of the patients in the thiopentone group experienced stroke (Zaidan et al. 1991). Recently, it was stated that barbiturate offers no proven protective effect (Todd et al. 1991).

Cardiac arrest

In a controlled study of thiopentone treatment after cardiac arrest no improvement of outcome was disclosed (Abramson et al. 1983).

Methohexitone, experimental studies

CBF, $CMRO_2$ and EEG

Methohexitone acts like thiopentone and gives rise to an associated decrease in CBF and $CMRO_2$. In rabbits subjected to global ischaemia, pretreatment with methohexitone at the onset of isoelectric EEG provides protection from ischaemic damage and the animals recovered dramatically (Yatsu et al. 1972). In baboons subjected to MACO, methohexitone induces an inverse steal phenomenon (Branston et al. 1979).

Methohexitone, human studies

CBF

Clinical studies indicate that after intravenous bolus injection of methohexitone the maximal reduction of CBF occurs within 30 sec, and CBF is normalised within 10 min (Herrschaft et al. 1975).Methohexitone gives rise to EEG electroencephalographic activation in patients with psychomotor epilepsy (Musella et al. 1971), and enhances electroencephalographic delineation of epileptogenic foci during surgery for uncontrollable epilepsy (Ford et al. 1982). In a clinical study by Todd et al. (1984a) where continuous infusion of methohexitone was used for patients undergoing operation for arterio-venous malformation, postoperative seizures occurred in 3 out of 11 patients. Although methohexitone is a chemical convulsant (Musella et al. 1971), this finding is suggested to be caused by acute methohexitone withdrawal.

Althesin

This hypnotic agent, consisting of a mixture of alphaxalone and alphadolone acetate dissolved in an emulsifying agent (Cremophor EL), is presently not in use in the Scandinavian countries because of the relative high frequency of anaphylactoid reaction. However, the effects of the drug on cerebral circulation and metabolism have been carefully studied and shall therefore be cited.

Althesin, experimental studies

CBF, $CMRO_2$ and ICP

Animal experiments have shown that a bolus injection of althesin gives rise to an associated decrease in CBF and $CMRO_2$ and a reduction in ICP (Pickerodt et al. 1972, Takahashi et al. 1973, Fitch et al. 1978, Keaney et al. 1978). These changes are followed by suppression of the EEG (Prior et al. 1978). The decrease in CBF, effected by a bolus injection, occurs after 30 seconds and subsides after 10–15 min. (Pickerodt et al. 1972). Other experimental studies in baboons indicate that the decrease in CBF occurred two seconds after slowing of the EEG, while cortical extracellular fluid pH began to increase about 10 sec after the EEG changes, indicating that the change in extracellular pH cannot have initiated the decrease in blood flow which follows the suppression in cerebral metabolism (McDowall et al. 1979). Comparative studies of pentobarbitone and althesin anaesthesia in cats suggest that the two drugs depress neocortical function in a similar manner, but in the hippocampus the EEG spikes were less prominent during pentobarbitone than during althesin anaesthesia (Kayama 1974).

CO_2 reactivity

The CO_2 reactivity is preserved during althesin anaesthesia (Fitch et al. 1978).

Glucose metabolism

In studies of regional cerebral glucose utilisation in rats regional differences have been found. Thus, the glucose utilisation was reduced considerably in the forebrain (cerebral cortex), while the decrease in the hindbrain was much less. These observations suggest that naturally occurring alphaxalone receptors might be present in the brain (Davis et al. 1984).

Althesin, human studies

CBF and $CMRO_2$ and ICP

Human studies have confirmed the experimental findings. Thus, a dose-dependent decrease in CBF and $CMRO_2$ occurs (Renou et al. 1976, Sari et al. 1976, Rasmussen et al. 1978), associated with a decrease in ICP (Turner et al. 1973). Controversy concerning the effect on ICP exists. Thus, Moss (1992) found an increase in ICP accompained by a fall in MABP in five patients with normal pressure hydrocephalus, and Puhringer et al. (1997) found an increase in cerebrospinal fluid pressure in human volunteers.

EEG

Simultaneously with the suppression of cerebral oxygen uptake the EEG is changed. First low frequency activity is obserbed, later on burst suppression activity, and finally isoelectric recording (Prior et al. 1978, Henderson et al. 1982). Accordingly, althesin infusion has been proposed in the treatment of status epilepticus (Munari et al. 1979).

Head injury

In patients with severe head injury an inverse CBF increase has been demonstrated after bolus injection of althesin (Rasmussen et al. 1978). Heavy althesin sedation has been shown to be more effective in controlling ICP hypertension compared with barbiturates, although the clinical outcome is not improved (Bullock et al. 1986). Other studies in severe head injury suggest that althesin bolus injection is especially effective in the treatment of ICP-hypertension (Procaccio et al. 1988).

Craniotomy

During craniotomy for cerebral tumours, althesin induces a dose-dependent decrease in $CMRO_2$ and suppression in EEG. These changes correlated to the concentration of plasma alfaxolone. However, great inter- and intraindividual differences in response were observed making conclusion concerning the level of oxygen uptake from the EEG recordings or plasma alphaxalone impossible (Bendtsen et al. 1985).

Etomidate, experimental studies

CBF and $CMRO_2$

Etomidate, like barbiturate and althesin, decreases CBF and $CMRO_2$ and suppresses the EEG. In dogs the EEG changes elicited by etomidate are similar to barbiturate (Wauquier et al. 1978). During continuous infusion of etomidate in dogs $CMRO_2$ decreases, until there is cessation of neuronal function as reflected by the onset of isoelectric EEG. This occurred when $CMRO_2$ was 48% of control. In the same study CBF initially decreased precipitously and independently of the changes in $CMRO_2$ (Milde et al. 1985). In moderately hypothermic dogs etomidate does not further decrease $CMRO_2$ despite decreasing brain hemisphere electrical activity. In the same study etomidate with or without hypothermia blunts hypotension-induced increase in $AVDO_2$ (Frizzell et al. 1993).

ICP

In anaesthetized dogs thiopentone and etomidate produce comparable decreases in CSF pressure and changes in estimated intracranial compliance and pressure-volume index (Artru 1989).

Glucose metabolism

In rats etomidate has a marked effect on glucose utilisation of the brain. This effect is most pronounced in the forebrain, while the hindbrain is minimally affected, suggesting that the anaesthetic effect of these drugs might be mediated by receptors. Furthermore, the decrease in glucose utilisation was not dose-dependent, thus 1 and 12 mg/kg depressed the glucose utilisation equally (Davis et al. 1986).

Protection

During hypoxia and global ischaemia in mice and dogs, etomidate has a brain protective effect (Wackier et al. 1981, Wackier 1982). Metabolic studies by magnetic resonance spectroscopy in cats during hypoxia indicate that etomidate decreases ICP and reduces glucose-utilisation, CMR(lactate), and the phosphocreatine/Pi ratio (Yoshida et al. 1993). In neurohistological studies in rats subjected to lethal cyanide dosages, and in models of global ischaemia a brain protective effect of etomidate has been documented (Ashton et al. 1981, VanReempts et al. 1982). In rats subjected to forebrain ischaemia reduction in the severity of the ischaemic injury was observed in the CA3 area of the hippocampus and in the ventral portion of the CA1 area (Watson et al. 1992). In dogs subjected to incomplete cerebral ischaemia, the concentrations of ATP and phosphocreatine were maintained at higher levels than in untreated dogs, suggesting that etomidate improves tolerance of the brain to ischaemia (Milde and Milde 1986, Smith et al. 1989). Maintenance of high energy metabolites has also been demonstrated in experiments of severe hypoxia in rats (Keykhah et al. 1986). In a canine model the cerebral oxygen extraction did not change during hypotension with high-dose etomidate, suggesting that etomidate may preserve the cerebral metabolic state under these circumstances (Frizzell et al. 1991). However, in rats subjected to incomplete ischemia, high dose, in contrast to low dose etomidate provokes spiking EEG activity without further depression of $CMRO_2$, and a worsening of outcome following cerebral ischaemia (Baugmann et al. 1989a). The potential neuroprotective effect of etomidate is not mediated through the augmentation of collateral flow during ischaemia (Roberson et al. 1998).

In a recent study of rats the effect of etomidate on *in vivo* ischaemia-induced dopamine release by microdialysis was analysed. Etomidate reduced the magnitude of ischaemia-induced dopamine release, whereas dopamine metabolism was preserved. These findings may be related to etomidates brain protective profile (Koorn et al. 1994).

Etomidate, human studies

CBF, $CMRO_2$, CPP and ICP

Etomidate induces an associated decrease in CBF and $CMRO_2$ (Herrschaft et al. 1975, van Aken and Rolly 1976, Renou et al. 1978), and a decrease in ICP (Cunitz et al. 1973, Schulte an Esch et al. 1978, Moss et al. 1979). When etomidate is administered to early burst suppression pattern on EEG in patients with space-occupying lesions, minimal changes in CPP occur during induction of anaesthesia, and a marked reduction in ICP is maintained following tracheal intubation (Modica and Tempelhoff 1992).

EEG

In spite of involuntary movements during etomidate induction, a dose-dependent suppression of the EEG activity occurs (Ghomein and Yamada 1977, Doenicke et al. 1982). At deep etomidate anaesthesia the EEG is isoelectric. However, seizure activity has been observed during etomidate anaesthesia (Krieger et al. 1985), during prolonged etomidate sedation (Grant and Hutchison 1983) and in patients undergoing craniotomy for surgical removal of their seizure focus (Gancher et al. 1984), indicating a selective activation of the cerebral cortex by etomidate. Consequently, some authors suggest that etomidate should be avoided in patients with epilepsy(Ebrahim et al. 1986).

Craniotomy

During induction of anaesthesia with etomidate in patients with intracranial space-occupying lesions ICP is well controlled (Belopavlovic and Buchthal 1983). Thus, continuous infusion of etomidate has been recommended for neuroanaesthesia (Sear et al. 1984, Batjar et al. 1988). During continuous etomidate infusion, monitoring of EEG indicates an increased sensitivity to etomidate in the elderly patients (Arden et al. 1986). In patients subjected to craniotomy for small supratentorial cerebral tumours, continuous etomidate infusion supplemented with nitrous oxide and fentanyl gives rise to a dose dependent decrease in CBF and $CMRO_2$, and the relative CO_2 reactivity is preserved (Cold et al. 1985). In individual patients a fairly good correlation between the changes in $CMRO_2$, the EEG and the plasma concentration of etomidate was found. However, great inter- and intra-individual differences were observed, making statements concerning the suppression of cerebral oxygen uptake from the EEG recordings impossible (Cold et al. 1986). In comparison with halothane anaesthesia, patients subjected to craniotomy in etomidate supplemented with fentanyl recovered consciousness more rapidly (Cold 1992).

Head injury

In patients with severe head injury, continuous infusion of etomidate in doses of 5–25 g/kg/min. partially seems to control ICP hypertension. Additional doses of 0.2 mg/kg always reduce acutely elevated ICP (Prior et al. 1983). However, the effect on ICP hypertension is only observed in patients with spontaneous EEG activity (Bingham et al. 1985). The attenuating effect upon ICP has also been observed during alphaxalone sedation. In a controlled study, the two drugs appeared equipotent in decreasing ICP and preserving the CPP (Dearden and McDowall 1985).

Adrenocortical function

Early experimental studies showed that etomidate suppresses adrenocortical response to surgical stress in rats (Preziosi and Vacca 1982), and low concentrations of cortisol have been observed in the postoperative period (Finley and McKee 1982). In studies of postoperative ACTH stimulation, the cortisol and aldosterone responses are decreased in patients subjected to etomidate anaesthesia (Klausen et al. 1983, Wagner and White 1984, Fragen et al. 1984). Etomidate inhibits adrenal steroidogenesis by producing a concentration-dependent blockade of the cholesterol side-chain cleavage enzyme and 11-β-hydroxylase (Wagner et al. 1984). In preliminary studies by Ledingham and Watt (1983) the duration of the adrenocortical suppression after a bolus injection of etomidate is about 8–10 h. The suppressive effect of etomidate in patients on treatment with corticosteroids has not been studied.

The above-mentioned effects of etomidate on the adrenocortical axis have raised discussion concerning the use of etomidate in clinical practice. On one hand, the attitude is advanced that there is no strong evidence against the continued availability of etomidate as an induction agent (Owen and Spence 1984). On the other hand, it has been argued that etomidate should be restricted only to those situations where it offers a clinical advantage compared with other available drugs (Wagner and White 1984), or should be omitted totally (Longnecker 1984). In comparison with thiopentone, the use of etomidate has two striking advantages; the stability of the central haemodynamics (Criado et al. 1980) and the minimal histamine release (Doenicke et al. 1973).

Ketamine

Ketamine anaesthesia is accompanied by an increase in blood pressure, heart rate and total oxygen consumption. These effects are not caused by an increase in plasma concentration of epinephrine or norepinephrine. Oxygen consumption is normalised after additional application of pancuronium (Hensel et al. 1972).

Receptor action

Ketamine has been shown to bind to a phencyclidine receptor in animals and man (Weir et al. 1992).

Ketamine can directly dilate cerebral arteries by acting as a calcium channel antagonist. The uptake of calcium is inhibited through both potential-operated (potassium) and receptor-operated (thromboxane A2) channels in cerebrovascular smooth muscle (Wendling et al. 1994). The heterogeneity of oxygen supply in the cerebral microcirculation is not affected by ketamine (Chi et al. 1994). In the pig midazolam antagonises the ketamine-induced increase in $CMRO_2$ (Åkesen et al. 1993).

Ketamine is known as a non-competitive antagonist of NMDA receptors (Thomson et al. 1985). Because ketamine blocks excitation of NMDA receptors, it influences nitric oxide production in the brain. Several reports have demonstrated that ketamine affects the glutamate receptor-nitric-oxide-cGMP pathway *in vitro* (Shimaoka et al. 1996, Li et al. 1997, Galley and Webster 1996). In a study using *in vivo* brain microdialysis coupled with online analysis of total nitric oxide oxidation products (NOx-) it was demonstrated that ketamine produced an increase in NOx- concentrations in the hippocampus and striatum in both anesthetized and non-anesthetized rats. Inhibition of NOS activity by L-NAME, however, attenuated this effect of ketamine without diminishing the anaesthetic effects of ketamine (Wu et al. 2000).

Ketamine, experimental studies

CBF, $CMRO_2$ and cerebral autoregulation

Ketamine is a cerebral vasodilator, which induces an increase in CBF, $CMRO_2$ and ICP. In dogs ketamine increases CBV simultaneous with an increase in CSF pressure (Artru and Katz 1989). In rats Hickey et al. (1989) found that ketamine impaired cerebral autoregulation. However, later studies in rat indicate that autoregulatory cerebrovascular dilation is preserved with low as well as high doses of ketamine, but during low-dose ketamine infusion the autoregulatory curve shifts towards higher MABP values (Engelhard et al. 1997). In rabbits the cerebral vasodilatation is blocked by scopolamine, a cholinergic antagonist. The increase in CBF after ketamine is additive to the cerebral vasodilator actions of CO_2 and of physostigmine, suggesting that ketamine activates a cholinergic cerebral vasodilator system (Reicher et al. 1987).

The metabolic effect of ketamine is influenced by pH in arterial blood. Experiments in rabbits indicate that the increase in $CMRO_2$ is more pronounced in acidotic animals, and the increase in oxygen uptake under this circumstance might enhance the extent of vasodilatation (Oren et al. 1987).

The effect of ketamine on cerebral circulation is influenced by the anaesthetic procedure applied before ketamine injection. Thus, in paralysed N_2O anaesthetized goats CBF and $CMRO_2$ are unchanged (Schwedler et al. 1982), and in barbiturate anaesthetised canines ketamine does not increase CBF (Dawson et al. 1971).

ICP

A significant ICP increase was found in spontaneous breathing piglets subjected to ICP-hypertension by inflation of an epidural balloon, whilst ICP was unchanged in artificially ventilated piglets subjected to the same procedure (Pfenninger et al. 1985). In dogs with normal CSF pressure and no cerebrovascular damage, pre- or posttreatment with diazepam reverse ketamine-induced increase of CBV and CSF pressure (Artru and Katz 1989).

Glucose metabolism

Studies of cerebral glucose utilisation in rats have shown a pronounced increase by 70% in the limbic system, especially in the hippocampus, a less pronounced increase by 20–40% in the extrapyramidal system and a decreased metabolism in the somatosensory and auditory systems, with the greatest reduction in the inferior colliculus (40%) (Nelson et al. 1980, Crosby and al. 1982, Cavazzuti et al. 1987). During withdrawal from a bolus injection a stimulation of the glucose utilisation has been observed throughout the brain with regional differences ranging between 21 and 78% (Davis et al. 1988). Pretreatment with diazepam decreases the glucose uptake by 20% in the hippocampus, an observation which is explained by the epileptogenic character of ketamine (Oguchi et al. 1982). In one study the increase in glucose-utilisation in the limbic system was completely prevented by diazepam (Eintrei et al. 1999).

EEG

In the cat, ketamine induces epileptic EEG of continuous hypersynchronous activity (Kayama and Iwama 1972). In the same animal, painful stimulation during ketamine, unlike barbiturate, is accompanied by increased EEG activity in the reticular formation and the limbic system (Tamasy et al. 1975).

Gene expression

Ketamine-induced c-Fos expression in the rat posterior cingulate and retrosplenial cortices is inhibited by Xenon, whereas nitrous oxide enhanced the c-Fos expression (Nagata et al. 2001).

Protection

In gerbils subjected to ketamine anaesthesia Lightfoote and coworkers (1977) found that cerebral infarction after unilateral carotid ligation exceeded that occurring with barbiturates. Albin et al. (1989) found that the survival time in rats subjected to hypoxia was shortened. Other studies in rats subjected to hypoxia indicate that pre-treatment with ketamine reduces CBF during the period of acute hypoxia. However, eight minutes after hypoxia these animals experienced a period with hyperperfusion, which subsequently decreased to pre-hypoxic levels over the next 30 minutes (Hamilton et al. 1992). Outcome study of rats subjected to ketamine-exposure during the recovery period of spinal cord injury indicates a deterioration (Grissom et al. 1994).

In contrast, studies in rats subjected to near-complete forebrain ischaemia indicate that ketamine administration over several hours provides significant protection in the hippocampal CA1 region. Ketamine acts as an antagonist to N-methyl-D aspartate (NMDA) receptors, the activation of which has been found to be implicated in cerebral ischaemic damage. It is suggested that the brain-protective effect of ketamine under these circumstances is mediated through this effect (Church et al. 1988). Furthermore, S(+) ketamine up-regulates regeneration of proteins following glutamate injury in cultured rat hippocampus neurones (Himmelseher et al. 2000).

In experimental head injury ketamine decreases brain tissue Calcium accumulation and restores Magnium levels to normal levels at 48 hours following injury. These changes are correlated to improvement in neurologic survival and a decrease in infarct volume (Shapira et al. 1992, Shapira et al. 1994).

In experimental studies in rats subjected to controlled haemorrhagic hypotension of 40 mm Hg during 60 minutes, better survival rates were found when the animals were anaesthetised with ketamine as compared with halothane, fluroxene and pentobarbitone (Longnecker and Sturgill 1976).

Ketamine, human studies

CBF, $CMRO_2$ and ICP

Ketamine was initially introduced as an anaesthetic agent for neuroradiological procedures (Corssen et al. 1969b): However, clinical studies showed that ketamine is a cerebral vasodilator. A bolus dose of 263 mg/kg induces an increase in CBF by 50–70% and an increase in $CMRO_2$ by 10–15% (Takeshita et al. 1972, Hougaard et al. 1974), and an increase in ICP has repeatedly been observed (Evans et al. 1971, Gardner et al. 1971, List et al.1972, Gibbs 1972, Shapiro et al. 1972b). The increase in CBF, measured by transcranial Doppler, is not blocked by maintaining arterial blood pressure at baseline values with esmolol. On the other hand, the increase in flow velocity is prevented by prior administration of midazolam (Strebel et al. 1995). It has been argued that in many studies ketamine was administrated to patients on spontaneous respiration where an increase in $PaCO_2$ partly may be responsible for the increase in ICP (Pfenninger and Reith 1990). Studies in artificially ventilation patients with head injury indicate that ketamine can be administered intravenously without any increase in ICP (Hase and Dick 1981). However, in other studies an increase in ICP has been observed in intubated and artificially ventilated patients (Schulte am Esch et al. 1978), and in infants with open fontanelle (Crumrine et al. 1975).

To some extent hyperventilation (Shapiro et al. 1972b) and barbiturates inhibit the increase in ICP (Wyte et al. 1972, Belopavlovic and Buchthal 1982). Furthermore, studies of middle cerebral artery flow velocity and CO_2 reactivity with Doppler technique in patients without neurological disease indicate that flow velocity and CO_2 reactivity are not affected when ketamine is administered during propofol anaesthesia (Sakai et al. 2000).

EEG

Ketamine anaesthesia is followed by increased EEG activity (Corssen et al. 1969a, Thompson 1972, Bennett et al. 1973). In patients with implanted cortical, limbic and thalamic electrodes, ketamine bolus injection provokes seizure activity in the limbic and thalamic areas, but not always from the cortical electrodes(Ferrer-Allado et al. 1973). It has been suggested that ketamine is not a direct cerebral vasodilator, but the increase in CBF is secondary to the increase in neuronal activity and the increase in $CMRO_2$ (Hougaard et al. 1974). This suggestion is in accordance with studies in healthy adults where ketamine causes a dose-dependent transient shift in the EEG with an increase in total power. This change is associated with an increase in mean blood flow velocity suggesting that the before mentioned increase in CBF is correlated to an increase in neuronal activity and not secondary to changes in systemic haemodynamic variables (Kochs et al. 1989).

Evoked potential

Ketamine enhances the cortical component of the somatosensory evoked potential. However, when nitrous oxide is introduced, the ketamine enhanced cortical amplitude is reduced by 50% (Schubert et al. 1990).

Clinical application

As a consequence of the cerebral activation ketamine should be avoided in patients with epilepsy (Winters 1972). The increase in ICP, CBF and $CMRO_2$, indicates that ketamine should be avoided in neuroanaesthetic practice when used alone in patients with decreased intracranial compliance or intracranial hypertension. One exception being the use of ketamine in small doses for induction of anaesthesia in the emergency of haemorrhage shock (Klose et al. 1982). When used in combination with propofol, however, ketamine does not alter middle cerebral artery flow velocity and CO_2 reactivity assessed with transcranial Doppler (Sakai et al. 2000). In patients undergoing craniotomy for tumour or cerebral aneurysm anaesthesia was maintained with isoflurane/nitrous oxide. Ketamine 1 mg/kg did not change MAP, CPP and $AVDO_2$. ICP and flow velocity decreased significantly (Mayberg et al. 1995). The contrasting results found during experimental and clinical studies are summarised by Werner et al. (1997). They argue that the cerebrovascular effects of ketamine are related to the pre-existing cerebrovascular tone induced by the background anaesthesia.

Diazepam, experimental studies

GABA

In pharmacological studies benzodiazepines potentiate the action of gamma-amino butyric acid (GABA), which is an inhibitory neurotransmitter, that exerts its actions at specific bindings sites (Braestrup and Squires 1977, Möhler and Okada 1977). Benzodiazepine receptors appear to interact closely with certain kinds of GABA receptors (Choi et al. 1977). In rats subjected to transient ischaemia an increase in GABA binding receptors in the caudate-putamen has been disclosed (Francis and Pulsinelli 1983). However in gerbils subjected to forebrain ischaemia a marked difference in the distribution between GABA and benzodiazepine binding sites has been found (Onodera et al. 1987).

CBF and $CMRO_2$

In rats subjected to heavy diazepam sedation a 20–30% decrease in CBF has been observed, while

$CMRO_2$ is unchanged. In comparison, supplement of nitrous oxide gives rise to a 50% reduction of both CBF and $CMRO_2$ (Carlsson et al. 1976b). In similar animal experiments the energy charge of the cerebrum and the concentrations of ATP and phosphocreatine were unchanged (Carlsson and Chapman 1981). In dogs subjected to lidocaine induced seizures, diazepam reduces CBF and $CMRO_2$ by 50–60% (Maekawa et al. 1974).

Glucose-utilisation

Diazepam decreases glucose-utilisation in the brain as a whole, and in most areas of the cerebral cortex, thalamus and the limbic system. The dramatic increase in glucose-utilisation in the limbic system observed with ketamine is completely prevented by treatment with diazepam (Eintrei et al. 1999).

In rats subjected to ketamine anaesthesia, pretreatment with diazepam reduces the glucose utilisation in the hippocampus (Oguchi et al. 1982).

ICP

In normal dogs ICP is unchanged after diazepam (Campan and Lazorthes 1976). Other studies in rabbits suggest that specific benzodiazepine binding sites in choroid plexus serve to modulate CSF formation without affecting the levels of cAMP and ATPase (Williams et al. 1990).

Protection

Experiments in rats suggest that diazepam does not protect the brain from hypoxic insults (Berntman et al. 1979).

Diazepam, human studies

CBF and $CMRO_2$

Clinical studies of the effects of diazepam on CBF and metabolism are few. In comatose patients with severe head injury diazepam 15 mg intravenously decreases CBF from 45 to 34 ml/100g/min, and $CMRO_2$ from 1.6 to 1.2 ml O2/100g/min (Cotev and Shalit 1975). In patients without organic brain disease, anaesthesia with fentanyl 10 g/kg, diazepam 10 mg and nitrous oxide 67% decreased CBF and $CMRO_2$ by 35%. Under these circumstances the CO_2 reactivity is preserved (Vernhiet et al. 1978). Similar results have been obtained in patients subjected to a coronary by-pass operation in high-dose fentanyl anaesthesia supplemented with diazepam 0.5 mg/kg (Murkin and Farrar 1989).

Midazolam, experimental studies

Receptor

Midazolam augments both the duration of GABA-mediated synaptic current and the amplitude of GABA-induced current by acting on the $GABA_A$-benzodiazepine receptor in substantia gelatinosa neurons (Kohno et al. 2000).

Structurally distinct benzodiazepines inhibit nucleoside transport to different degrees. Midazolam selectively augments A_2- but not A_1-receptor-mediated effects of adenosine by inhibiting nucleotide transporter (Seubert et al. 2000).

CBF and $CMRO_2$. Effect of Nitrous oxide and age

In rats midazolam produces a 40–45% decrease in CBF and a 55% decrease in $CMRO_2$. When the rats were ventilated with nitrous oxide/oxygen instead of nitrogen oxygen, $CMRO_2$ only decreased by 35%, suggesting that nitrous oxide slightly stimulates cerebral metabolism during midazolam anaesthesia (Hoffman et al. 1986). Using the venous outflow technique, similar results have been obtained in dogs (Fleischer et al. 1988). Compared with young rats the cerebral metabolic depression effected by midazolam is more pronounced in aged rats (Baughman et al. 1987a).

Protection

In the hypoxic mouse model, midazolam provides greater cerebral protection from hypoxia than diazepam but less protection compared with barbiturates (Nugent et al. 1982). In rat hippocampal slices midazolam improves electrophysiologic recovery after anoxia, and reduces the changes in ATP levels and calcium influx during anoxia (Abramowicz et al. 1991). In rats subjected to ischaemia by carotid arterial occlusion and hypotension to 30 mm Hg, the mortality rate and neurologic deficit score were identical in midazolam and methohexitone pretreated animals. In the same study supplements of nitrous oxide increased the mortality rate and neurologic deficit score (Baughman et al. 1987b). In the same model high dose midazolam in contrast to etomidate provides better cerebral protection (Baughman et al. 1989a).

CSF dynamics

In dogs, comparative studies of the rate of CSF formation and resistance to reabsorption of CSF following the administration of thiopentone, midazolam and etomidate were performed. The rate of CSF formation decreased at high doses of all three drugs, however, the resistance to reabsorption was elevated at high doses of midazolam but decreased at high doses of etomidate and thiopentone (Artru 1988a).

Effect of antagonist (flumazenil)

In dogs and goats the benzodiazepine antagonist flumazenil converts the decrease in CBF, $CMRO_2$ and CPP (Fleischer et al. 1988, Kochs et al. 1988). These antagonistic effects are dose-dependant (Artru 1989). In cats investigated with the cranial window technique midazolam alone does not affect the diameter of cerebral arterioles and venules. However, flumazenil results in vasodilation of larger arterioles accompanied by an elevation of MAPB, and an increase in CBF (Kumano et al.1993).

In dogs the rate of CSF formation and the resistance to outflow are unchanged by flumazenil. However, flumazenil given in the presence of midazolam may increase resistance to reabsorption of CSF and thereby increase CSF pressure (Artru 1990). In a later study the responses to flumazenil were not seen in the absence of pre-existing benzodiazepine effect (Artru 1991).

Midazolam, human studies

CBF and $CMRO_2$

Human studies confirm the results of the animal experiments. Thus, a dose-dependent decrease in CBF and $CMRO_2$ has been disclosed (Larsen et al. 1981, Hilfiker and Kettler 1981, Forster et al. 1982). Even during sedation (20 or 40 g/kg midazolam) a decrease in CBF has been found (Cheng et al. 1993). PET studies in sedated volunteers indicate a rCBF decrease in the insula, the cingulate gyrus, multiple areas in the prefrontal cortex, tha thalamus, and parietal and temporal association areas. Relative rCBF was increased in the occipital areas (Veselise et al. 1997).

In studies of continuous midazolam anaesthesia supplemented with fentanyl and nitrous oxide for patients subjected to craniotomy for supratentorial cerebral tumours, CBF and $CMRO_2$ were well sustained during unchanged midazolam infusion. A dose-dependent decrease in CBF and $CMRO_2$ was not found (Knudsen et al. 1990). Studies with Doppler technique in patients without cerebral disease indicate preserved CO_2 reactivity during midazolam anaesthesia (Strebel et al. 1994).

Like diazepam midazolam is an anticonvulsant drug and appears to be effective in terminating status epilepticus, when other drugs including barbiturate, diazepam, lorazepam and phennytoin failed (Kumar and Bleck 1992).

ICP

In patients with severe head injury, midazolam administered as continuous infusion reduces ICP (Cottrell et al. 1982).

Flumazenil

Injection of flumazenil during midazolam anaesthesia gives rise to a CBF increase (Forster et al. 1987), and provokes an increase in ICP (Chiolero et al. 1986a). However, in another study flumazenil did not increase CBF or $CMRO_2$ (Knudsen et al. 1991). Other studies indicate that injection of flumazenil at the end of anaesthesia is associated with a rapid recovery (Chiolero et al. 1986b). Evoked potential amplitude is attenuated by midazolam, but reversed by flumazenil (Kochs and Schulte am Esch 1988).

Flumazenil reverses the memory effects of midazolam. On the other hand, flumazenil by itself has no effect upon memory (Ghoneim et al. 1993).

Propofol, experimental studies

Propofol is used for induction and maintenance of anaesthesia and for sedation. The rapid recovery offers advantages over other hypnotic agents and sedative drugs. For review see Smith et al. 1994, Orser 1994).

GABA

Studies of hippocampal pyramidal neurons from rat brain slice (Hara et al. 1994), and studies with implanted electrodes in the hippocampal dentate gyrus (Albertson et al. 1991) indicate that propofol enhances GABA-mediated inhibition. In a recent study, however, with selectively bred mice no difference in sensitivity of $GABA_A$ receptors in two distinct breeds of mice was found, despite differences in their clinical sensitivity to propofol (Simpson and Blednov 1996).

In a recent study, including a model of aggregating rat brain cell cultures, it was found that propofol given at clinically relevant concentrations might cause irreversible lesions to GABAergic neurones (Honegger and Matthieu 1996). In another study dissociated neonatal cell cultures of newborn rat cortex were investigated. Propofol induced dose-dependent lesions of GABAergic neurones and of glial cells. In contrast, no evidence for neurotoxic effects of propofol was found after long-term treatment of organotypic slice cultures from hippocampus (Spahr-Schopfer et al. 2000).

Excitatory amino acids

Propofol inhibits glutamate-mediated neurotransmission. Using patch clamp technique, propofol selectively inhibits NMDA currents by allosterically modulating the NMDA receptor/channel complex (Bertlik et al. 1994).

Dopaminergic system

Evidence has emerged, suggesting that propofol treatment has potentials in abuse (Zacny et al. 1993). Many drugs of abuse are thought to act preferentially via dopamine within the limbic system (Di-Chiara and Imperato 1986), causing either the release of dopamine or mimicking its action at the receptor level. Propofol has also been reported to bind to dopamine D_2 receptors (Appadu et al. 1994). In a recent study, however, it was demonstrated that propofol inhibited dopamine release in the rat nucleus accumbens in a manner dependent neither on dopamine D_2, $GABA_A$ nor NMDA receptors, suggesting that propofol may be acting not through receptor mechanisms, but by blockade of ion channels (Schulte et al. 2000).

Other channels

In addition to the effects of $GABA_A$ -activated chloride channels, propofol has been shown to have several molecular actions on various receptors including modification of voltage-dependent sodium channels (Frenkel and Urban 1991, Ratnakumari and Hemmings 1997), potassium channels (Baum 1993), and calcium channels (Xuan and Glass 1996). Examination of propofol interactions with sodium channels using ion-flux measurements and toxin binding studies indicates that propofol suppresses glutamate release by blocking sodium currents both in the presence and absence of these activators (Ratnakumari and Hemmings 1997, Ratnakumari and Hemmings 1996). In recent experiments with pharmacologically unaltered sodium channels, propofol inhibition of currents occurred at concentrations achieved clinically in the brain (Rehberg and Duch 1999).

Free radical scavenger function

In a recent study propofol had a direct scavenging activity against HOCl, superoxide-hydrogen peroxide, and hydroxyl radical (Demiryürek et al. 1998).

CBF, $CMRO_2$ and ICP

In experimental studies propofol is known to reduce both CBF and $CMRO_2$ (Vandesteene et al. 1988, Werner et al. 1992). A dose related decrease in CBF and $CMRO_2$ under conditions where blood pressure is maintained has been found (Ramani et al. 1992). However, in the same study a direct drug-related cerebral vasodilation cannot be excluded at excessive propofol concentrations. In dogs low and moderate doses of propofol decrease EEG activity and $CMRO_2$, causing an associated decrease of CBF and CSF pressure (Artru et al. 1992).

In a study of rabbits subjected to ICP-hypertension by an extradural balloon, propofol had a greater effect on ICP-hypertension than hyperventilation, and the two treatments were additive (Watts et al. 1998).

Cerebral kinetics

In sheep the cerebral kinetics of propofol were examined over a range of CBF using chronically instumentation. The cerebral kinetics of propofol after bolus injection were dependent on CBF, despite partial diffusion limitation. A high CBF produced higher peak cerebral concentrations and shorter time to reach this concentration (Upton et al. 2000). The influence of hypovolemia on the pharmacokinetics and the EEG effect of propofol have been studied in the rat. An increased hypnotic effect of propofol was supposed to be attributed to changes in both pharmacokinetics and end organ sensitivity (Paepe et al. 2000).

CO_2 reactivity and cerebral autoregulation

In dogs subjected to low and moderate doses of propofol autoregulation and CO_2 reactivity were preserved. In contrast, high-dose propofol decreases CPP below the lower point of cerebral autoregulation (Artru et al. 1992). In rabbits cerebrovascular reactivity of blood flow and cerebral blood volume are markedly decreased during hypocapnia, but are maintained during hypercapnia (Cenic et al. 2000). In rats propofol reduces CBF in cerebrum and spinal cord (Werner et al. 1990). In the rat and pig autoregulation is present during propofol anaesthesia (Werner et al. 1990, Lagerkranser et al. 1997).

CSF dynamics

In rabbits propofol does not alter the rate of CSF formation or resistance to reabsorption of CSF (Artru 1993).

Glucose metabolism

Studies of glucose utilisation in the rat indicate that forebrain structures showed a greater degree of depression than did the hindbrain regions. The only structures in which the glucose utilisation was spared, were nuclei related to the auditory-vestibular system (Dam et al. 1990). The pattern of metabolic changes produced by propofol thus resembles that observed with barbiturate, althesin and etomidate. In the same animal propofol induction with 8 mg/kg and maintenance with bolus doses of 6 mg/kg induced a depression of glucose utilisation in the sensory-, motor-, the limbic systems, and the spinal cord grey matter. Mean percentage decreases ranged from 40% in the vestibular nucleus to 76% in the cingulate cortex (Cavazzuli et al. 1991).

EEG

The relationship between EEG suppression and $CMRO_2$ is qualitatively similar to that observed with barbiturates (Ramani et al. 1992).

Protection

In mice propofol in low doses afforded a greater degree of protection against pentylenetetrazol-induced seizure than did thiopentone. At greater doses both propofol and thiopental caused marked protection (Lowson et al. 1990). Other experimental studies support these findings (De Riu et al. 1992). In primary cortical cell cultures extracellular acidification rates are attenuated by propofol (Abrahams et al. 1999), and in cultures of rat cerebral astrocytes propofol mitigates the effects of oxidative stress and retention of glutamate (Peters et al. 2001). In the rat propofol improves neurohistopathological outcome following incomplete cerebral ischaemia. This effect is not dependent on plasma glucose, and an improved neurologic outcome is indicated by early postischaemic EEG recovery (Kochs et al. 1992).

In other studies in rats (Redinour et al. 1992) and cats (Weir et al. 1989) the cerebral protective effect of propofol is absent. Thus, in cats subjected to MCAO, neither propofol nor thiopental produced significant reduction in the ischaemic area (Gelb et al. 1993). In contrast to etomidate and barbiturates propofol does not decrease dopamine level in rats subjected to reversible forebrain ischemia (Kahn et al. 1993).

Propofol, human studies

CBF and $CMRO_2$

In human studies propofol given as a bolus injection suppresses CBF, $CMRO_2$ and the cerebral uptake of amino acids. (Stephan et al. 1987, Stephan et al. 1988). Similar changes in CBF and $CMRO_2$ have been observed during continuous infusion with propofol (Vandesteene et al. 1988).

In patients with large malignant brain tumours studies with transcranial Doppler indicate reduced and even paradoxical effects of propofol (Schregel et al. 1993). Studies of transcranial Doppler sonography indicate that propofol does not alter the vessel diameter in the middle cerebral artery (Schregel et al. 1992).

CO_2 reactivity and cerebral autoregulation

After propofol bolus injection the CO_2 reactivity was preserved (Stephan et al. 1987). This finding was also confirmed in studies with Doppler technique (Jansen and Kagenaar 1993, Strebel et al. 1994, Ederberg 1998). In a study including healthy adults the slope of the CBF versus $PaCO_2$ was 1.56 ml/100g/min/ mm Hg $PaCO_2$ (Fox et al. 1992). During continuous propofol infusion in patients without brain disorders the CO_2 reactivity was also found to be intact (Craen et al. 1992, Harrison et al. 1999). Also cerebral autoregulation, evaluated by the transient hyperaemic method, seems to improve (Harrison et al. 1999). In comparison with 1.5 MAC isoflurane and desflurane anaesthesia cerebral autoregulation is preserved with propofol (Strebel et al. 1995). In patients anaesthetised with propofol until EEG silence CO_2 reactivity and autoregulation remain intact (Matta et al. 1995). During propofol/fentanyl anaesthesia nicardipine-, nitroglycerin- and prostaglandin E_1-induced hypotension attenuate the CO_2 reactivity (Endoh et al. 1999).

In healthy subjects the effect of graded hypercapnia upon cerebral autoregulation was tested during sevoflurane and propofol anaesthesia. The threshold of $PaCO_2$ to significantly impair cerebral autoregulation averaged 56 mm Hg during sevoflurane and 61 during propofol anaesthesia (McCulloch et al. 2000).

Microdialysis

During anaesthesia with either propofol or isoflurane for fossa posterior surgery microdialysis catheters were inserted into the frontal cerebral cortex. Baseline values of glucose, lactate, pyruvate, glycerol, glutamate and urea were obtained during awakefulness. Marked increases in the levels of all chemical markers were observed at the beginning and at the end of anaesthesia (Reinstrup et al. 2000).

Craniotomy

In patients subjected to craniotomy for supratentorial lesions and given anaesthesia with continuous propofol infusion supplemented with fentanyl, a dose dependent decrease in $CMRO_2$ was found, while CBF was unchanged (Madsen et al. 1989). In normocapnic patients subjected to craniotomy propofol in doses of 0.35 and 0.8 mg/kg effectively reduces ICP (Zattoni et al. 1986). In patients with space-occupying intracranial lesions, propofol induction (1 mg/kg) did not cause any ICP increase and CPP was unchanged, indicating that propofol can be used safely as an induction agent (Hartung 1987, Ravussin et al. 1988a). In other studies a bolus dose of 2.5 mg/kg produced a significant decrease of CPP, due to a marked decrease in MABP (Hemelrijck et al. 1988). Propofol provides good conditions for intracranial surgery by reducing brain retractor pressure (Moss and Price 1990). In a randomised study including patients with supratentorial cerebral tumours subjected to craniotomy in propofol/fentanyl, isoflurane or nitrous oxide/fentanyl anaesthesia, epidural ICP measured through the first burr hole was compared. No significant differences between the three anaesthetic techniques were disclosed (Todd et al. 1993). In a recent non-randomised study (Bundgaard et al. 1997) ICP during propofol/fentanyl anaesthesia, isoflurane and sevoflurane were compared. ICP was measured with subdural technique described recently just before opening of dura (Cold et al. 1996). ICP during propofol/fentanyl anaesthesia was significantly lower compared with isoflurane and seveflurane. Furthermore, the number of patients with ICP 10 mm Hg, which according to Bundgaard et al. (1997) indicate a high risk of cerebral swelling/herniation after opening of dura was lower in propofol/fentanyl anaesthetised patients. These findings have been confirmed in a recent randomised study, in which ICP during propofol/fentanyl anaesthesia was lower compared with isoflurane- and sevoflurane anaesthesia (Petersen et al. 2000).

Nitrous oxide

In patients subjected to non-neurological surgery the addition of nitrous oxide to continuous propofol infusion does not influence the vasoconstrictor effect nor the CO_2 reactivity (Eng et al. 1992).

Blood pressure

In comparison with thiopentone and etomidate a significant decrease in arterial pressure follows intubation with propofol anaesthesia (Harris et al.1988). In studies of patients subjected to intracranial surgery propofol induction, in comparison with thiopentone-isoflurane induction, was accompanied by less MABP reaction to intubation and application of pin head-holder (Ravussin et al. 1988b).

Total intravenous anaesthesia

Combined with alfentanil, total intravenous anaesthesia with propofol has been investigated in patients with brain tumours. Stable haemodynamics, excellent operating conditions and rapid recovery were documented (Merckx et al. 1988). The same conclusion has been drawn in a clinical study of 30 patients subjected to neurosurgical procedures (van Aken et al. 1990). The recovery is faster with total intravenous propofol anaesthesia compared with midazolam, both supplemented with alfentanil (Vuyk et al. 1990). In another study propofol anaesthesia for craniotomy was supplemented with an infusion of remifentanil, alfentanil or fentanyl. There were no significant differences among groups in the dose required during propofol maintenance, heart rate or mean arterial pressure. However, the time to eye opening was significantly shorter in the remifentanil compared to the alfentanil group but not the fentanyl group (Coles et al. 2000).

Total intravenous anaesthesia with propofol and fentanyl has been used for cerebral aneurysm surgery. Combined with arterial hypertension, in order to prevent cerebral ischaemia, this anaesthetic technique seems to be an alternative to isoflurane-hypertensive anaesthesia (Ravussin and de Trilobite 1993).

The combination of propofol and ketamine has been recommended for total intravenous anaesthesia because the opposing effects of the individual anesthetics result in stable intraoperative haemodynamics (Guit et al. 1991). In patients without neurologic disease ketamine does not influence middle cerebral artery flow velocity or the CO_2 response during propofol administration (Sakai et al. 2000).

EEG

During total intravenous anaesthesia with propofol and fentanyl titration of propofol infusion as assessed by ability to produce a predictable EEG pattern (4 sec interval of burst and suppression) was found to be a useful method for determining maintenance infusion rate (Hemelrijck et al. 1992). The EEG changes are related to the plasma concentration of propofol (Bendriss et al. 1990).

In patients sedated with propofol EEG monitoring may be useful. Memory impairment coincidence with increases in high frequency EEG activity (Veselis et al. 1992).

In children dystonic and choreiform spontaneous movement are elicited by propofol. These movements coincide with the appearance of delta waves on the EEG. The dystonic nature of these movements and the absence of other EEG abnormalities suggest subcortical origin and argue against associated cortical epileptic activity (Borgeat et al. 1991).

Protection

In a recent study of patients undergoing valve-surgery randomisation to either sufentanil or sufentanil plus propofol was performed. Propofol was administered in doses to enectroencephalographic burst suppression. The use of propofol did not reduce the incidence and the severity of neurologic or neuropsychological dysfunction (Roach et al. 1999).

Epilepsy

In patients undergoing cortical resection for intractable epilepsy propofol did not elicit epileptic activity. On the contrary, inter-ictal spikes decreased significantly after propofol 2 mg/kg intravenously (Ebrahim et al. 1994). In another study, including epileptic patients undergoing temporal lobe resection in nitrous oxide isoflurane anesthesia, electrocorticograms were recorded after boluses of thiopental 25 mg or propofol 20 mg iv until burst suppression. Activation occurred more frequently with thiopental than with propofol, but the difference was not significant (Hewitt et al. 1999). In contrast another study indicated that small doses of propofol produced activation of the electrocorticogram in 17 of 20 patients during surgery for intractable epilepsy (Smith et al. 1996). The issue has been debated in an editorial, which summarized that propofol should be avoided in patients with epilepsy who hold a current driving license or have a reasonable prospect of doing so. In other epileptics and in status epilepticus its use can easily be justified (Sneyd 1999).

Head injury

In patients with head injury propofol decreases ICP. MABP and CPP, however, decreases making the use of propofol in patients with head injury controversial (Hartung 1987). In another study it was concluded that propofol 1–2 mg/kg decreased ICP, that the hypotensive effect on blood pressure was mild and that no inadvertent CPP changes were observed (Weinstabl et al. 1990). Other studies in severe head injury indicate a coupled reduction by about 30% in CBF and cerebral metabolism and a significant decrease in CPP by 26% (Pinaud et al. 1988). In head injury propofol infusion rate of about 3 mg/kg/h provides satisfactory sedation, and recovery from propofol sedation was rapid (Farling et al. 1989). Pharmacokinitic studies under these circumstances indicate a long terminal phase with T/2 of 1878 min, a volume of distribution of 1666 l, and a body clearance of 1.57 l/min (Albanese et al. 1990).

Clinical application

From the experimental and clinical studies it is clear that propofol produces a dose related decrease in EEG activity, CBF and $CMRO_2$. Propofol is recommended for induction and maintenance of anaesthesia in neurosurgical patients. Blood pressure should be carefully monitored and CPP maintained (Hoffman and Kochs 1992).

In patients without intracranial disorders the recovery of mental and psychomotor abilities is faster after propofol anaesthesia as compared with midazolam and isoflurane anaesthesia (Motet et al. 1992).

Life-threatening anaphylactoid reactions have been described after the first propofol administration (Laxenaire et al. 1988), and after repeated anaesthetic inductions with propofol (De Leon-Casasola et al. 1992). These reactions occur in patients with a history of drug allergy. It is therefore justified to avoid the use of propofol in those patients in whom other anaphylactoid reactions have occurred (Laxenaire et al. 1992).

Droperidol, experimental studies

CBF and $CMRO_2$

Using the venous outflow technique in dogs, Michenfelder and Theye (1971) found that droperidol in dose of 0.3 mg/kg produced a decrease in CBF by 40%, primarily due to a 30–40% increase in CVR. These effects persisted for the period of observation

(60 min.). No significant change in $CMRO_2$ was found. In the same study droperidol combined with fentanyl (6 g/kg) resulted in a 23% decrease in $CMRO_2$, CBF was decreased by 50% and CVR increased by 85%. During studies in dogs subjected to neurolept anaesthesia a decrease of $CMRO_2$ from 5.2 ml to 3.0 ml O_2/100g/min was observed (Kreuscher 1967). In spontaneously breathing rabbits droperidol combined with fentanyl gives rise to an increase in CBF. However, the change in CBF is correlated to the increase in $PaCO_2$ caused by respiratory depression (deValois and Peperkamp 1971).

In the rat droperidol increases the glucose utilisation, especially in the lateral habenula (Oguchi et al. 1982).

Brain oedema

In dogs subjected to cryogenic lesion, the water content in cerebral tissue close to the lesion is low during neurolept anaesthesia. The same low water content was observed during barbiturate anaesthesia, while the content was considerably higher during halothane, enflurane or isoflurane anaesthesia (Smith and Marque 1976).

Droperidol, human studies

CBF, $CMRO_2$ and ICP

Human studies of thalamonal (droperidol and fentanyl) in sedative doses during normocapnia indicate unchanged CBF and $CMRO_2$ (Barker et al. 1968, Sari et al. 1972). In patients subjected to controlled ventilation, the combination of droperidol and fentanyl gives rise to a small decrease in ICP (Fitch et al.1969) or unchanged ICP (Miller et al. 1975).

Craniotomy

Considering experimental studies and the clinical studies of CBF and ICP, neurolept anaesthesia with barbiturate induction has been advocated in surgery for space-occupying intracranial lesions (Marshall 1973, Arnér and Gordon 1976). In patients subjected to craniotomy for supratentorial tumours during anaesthesia with thiopentone induction, nitrous oxide 67%, fentanyl and droperidol 0.2 mg/kg during moderate hypocapnia, CBF and $CMRO_2$ decreased by 35% in comparison with values obtained in normal awake subjects. The relative CO_2 reactivity was preserved Another finding was a significant negative correlation between plasma droperidol and $CMRO_2$ (Cold et al. 1988). In comparison, during anaesthesia with nitrous oxide, halothane 0.5%, fentanyl, hyperventilated to the same level of $PaCO_2$, the perioperative values of $AVDO_2$ during neurolept anaesthesia were higher, while MABP was at the same level. These findings suggest that halothane anaesthesia in comparison with neurolept anaesthesia gives rise to a relative luxury perfusion state (Engberg et al. 1989).

γ-Hydroxybutyrate (GHB) and γ-Aminobuturate (GABA)

GABA

γ-hydroxybutyrate is an intermediary product in the metabolism of GABA. As such this drug is of interest, since it may act as both a precursor and metabolite of GABA (Vayer et al. 1985). According to Mandel et al. (1987) GABA may act as a neurotransmitter.

CBF and $CMRO_2$

GABA has been used as a hypnotic agent. A decrease in cerebral metabolism has been disclosed in conscious rats (Kuschinsky et al. 1985). However, in anaesthetized cats CBF and $CMRO_2$ are unchanged, whilst glucose utilisation is significantly reduced (Haller et al. 1990). The same investigator found that the sensitivity to pial arteries to H^+ and adenosine is increased by GHB (Haller et al. 1986).

In the hypoxic mouse model GHB increases survival time by 85%. Compared with other studies employing the same hypoxic model, this increase was less than that observed with barbiturate, and equal to that observed with other anaeshtetics. In dogs $CMRO_2$ is depressed by a maximum of 48%. The decrease in CBF, however, exceeds the reduction in $CMRO_2$, and the administration of these high dosages of GHB was accompanied with a reduction in cardiac output. Brain biopsies taken under these circumstances showed a trend towards lower phosphocreatine levels and higher lactate and lactate/pyruvate levels than in untreated dogs (Artru et al. 1980).

In clinical studies flow velocity is unaltered and CO_2 reactivity is maintained by an anaesthetic dose of GHB (Detch et al. 1999). During GHB anaesthesia changes in the EEG resembling a state of non-convulsant epilepsy have been observed (Snead et al. 1976, Depaulis et al. 1988). Consequently, GBH has only attained theoretical interest as hypnotic agent.

Etanolone

CBF and $CMRO_2$

Etanolone, a naturally occurring metabolite of progesterone, has hypnotic properties. In a study of healthy volunteers etanolone reduced CBF and $CMRO_2$ like barbiturate, etomidate and propofol. Coupling was present and a small decrease in MABP was observed (Wolff et al. 1994).

References

Abramowicz AE, Kass IS, Chambers G, Cottrell JE. Midazolam improves electrophysiologic recovery after anoxia and reduces the changes in ATP levels and calcium influx during anoxia in the rat hippocampal slice. Anesthesiology 1991: 74: 1121–1128.

Abrahams M, Eriksson H, Björnström K, Eintrei C. Effects of propofol on extracellular acidification rates in primary cortical cell cultures: application of silicon microphysiometry to anaesthesia. Br J Anaesth 1999: 83: 467–469.

Abramson NS, Safar P, Detre K et al. Results of a randomized clinical trial of brain resuscitation with thiopental. Anesthesiology 1983: 59: A101.

Aitken PG, Schiff SJ. Barbiturate protection against hypoxic neuronal damage in vitro. J Neurosurg 1986: 65: 230–232.

Albanese J, Martin C, Lacarelle B, et al. Pharmacokinitics of long-tern propofol infusion used for sadation in ICU patients. Anesthesiology 1990: 73: 214–217.

Albertsom TE, Tseng C-C, Joy RM. Propofol modification of evoked hippocampal dentate inhibition in urethane.anesthetized rats. Anesthesiology 1991: 75: 82–90.

Albin MS, Bunegin L, Rasch J, et al. Ketamine hydrochloride fails to protect against acute global hypoxia in the rat. Anesth Analg 1989: 68: S8.

Albrecht RF, Miletich DJ, Rosenberg R, Zahed B. Cerebral blood flow and metabolic changes from induction to onset of anesthesia with halothane or pentobarbital. Anesthesiology 1977: 47: 252–256.

Almaas R, Saugstad OD, Pleasure D, Footwelt T. Effect of barbiturates on hydroxyl radicals, lipid peroxidation, and hypoxic cell death in human NT2-N neurons. Anesthesiology 2000: 92: 764–774.

Altenburg BM, Michenfelder JD, Theye RA. Acute tolerance to thiopental in canine cerebral oxygen consumption studies. Anesthesiology 1969: 31: 443–448.

Altura BT, Altura BM. Barbiturates and aortic and venous smooth-muscle function. Anesthesiology 1975: 43: 432–444

Anderson RE, Sundt TM. Brain pH in focal cerebral ischaemia and the protective effects of barbiturate anesthesia. J Cereb Blood Flow Metab 1983: 3: 493–497.

Appadu BL, Strange PG, Lanbert DG. Does propofol interact with D_2 dopamine recectors? Anesth Analg 1994: 79: 1191–1192.

Archer DP, Priddy RE, Tang TKK, et al. The influence of cryogenic brain injury on the pharmacodynaics of pentobarbital. Anesthesiology 1991: 75: 634–639

Archer DP, Froelich J, McHugh M, Pappius HM. Local cerebral glucose utilization in stimulated rats sedated with thiopental. Anesthesiology 1995: 83: 160–168.

Arden JR, Holley FO, Stanski DR. Increased sensitivity to etomidate in the elderly: Initial distribution versus altered brain response. Anesthesiology 1986: 65: 19–27.

Arnér S, Gordon E. The antagonist effect of naloxone hydrochloride after neuroleptanaesthesia during neurosurgery. Acta Anaesth Scand 1976: 20: 201–206.

Arnfred I, Secher O. Anoxia and barbiturates. Arch Int Pharmacodyn Ther 1962: 139: 67–74.

Artru AA, Steen PA, Michenfelder JD. γ-hydroxybuturate: Cerebral metabolic, vascular, and protective effects. J Neurochem 1980: 35: 1114–1119.

Artru AA, Michenfelder JD. Influence of hypothermia or hyperthermia alone or in combination with pentobarbital or phenotoin on survival time in hypoxic mice. Anesth Analg 1981: 60: 867–870.

Artru AA. Dose-related changes in the rate of cerebrospinal fluid formation and resistance to reabsorption of cerebrospinal fluid following administration of thiopental, midazolam, and etomidate in dogs. Anesthesiology 1988a: 69: 541–546.

Artru AA. Survival time during hypoxia: Effects of nitrous oxide, thiopental, and hypothermia. Anesth Analg 1988B: 67: 913–196.

Artru AA, Katz RA. Cerebral blood volume and CSF pressure following administration of ketamine in dogs; modification by pre- or posttreatment with hypocapnia or diazepam. J Neurosurg Anesthesiol 1989: 1: 8–15.

Artru AA. Flumazenil reversal of midazolam in dogs: Dose-related changes in cerebral blood flow, metabolism, EEG, and CSF pressure. J Neurosurg Anesthesiol 1989a: 1: 46–55.

Artru AA. Intracranial volume-pressure relationship following thiopental or etomidate. Anesthesiology 1989b: 71: 763–768.

Artru AA. The rate of CSF formation, resistance to reabsorption of CSF, and aperiodic analysis of the EEG following administration of flumazenil to dogs. Anesthesiology 1990: 72: 111–117.

Artru AA. Intracranial volue-pressure relationship following flumazenil in anesthetized dogs. J Neurosurg Anesthesiol 1991: 3: 107–116.

Artru AA, Shapira Y, Bowdle A. Electroencephalogram, cerebral metabolism, and vascular responses to propofol anesthesia in dogs. J Neurosurg Anesthesiol 1992: 4: 99–109.

Artru AA. Propofol combined with halothane or with fentanyl/halotahne does not alter the rate of CSF formation or resistance to reabsorption of the CSF in rabbits. J Neurosurg Anesthesiology 1993: 5: 250–257.

Ashton D, VanReempts J, Wauquier A. Behavioral, electroencephalographic and histological study of the protective effect of etomidate against histotoxic dysoxia produced by cyanide. Arch Intern Pharmacodynamie Therapie 1981: 254: 196–213.

Astrup J. Energy-requiring cell functions in the ischaemic brain. Their critical supply and possible inhibition in protective therapy. J Neurosurg 1982: 56: 482–497.

Astrup J, Rosen¢rn J, Cold GE, et al. Minimum cerebral blood flow and metabolism during craniotomy. Effect of thipental loading. Acta Anaesthesiol Scand 1984: 28: 478–481.

Barker J, Harper AM, McDowall DG, et al. Cerebral blood flow, cerebrospinal fluid pressure and EEG activity during neuroleptanalgesia induced with dehydrobenzperidol and phenoperidine. Br J Anaesth 1968: 40: 143–144.

Batjar HH, Frankfurt AI, Purdy PD, et al. Use of etomidate, temporary arterial occlusion, and intraoperative angiography in surgical treatment of large and giant cerebral aneurysms. J Neurosurg 1988: 68: 234–240.

Baughman VL, Hoffman WE, Miletich DJ, Albrecht RF. Effects of phenobarbital on cerebral blood flow and metabolism in young and aged rats. Anesthesiology 1986: 65: 500–505.

Baughman VL, Hoffman WE, Albrecht RF, Militich DJ. Cerebral vascular and metabolic effects of fentanyl and midazolam in young and aged rats. Anesthesiology 1987a: 67: 314–319.

Baughman VL, Hoffman WE, Miletich DJ, Albrecht RF. Neurologic outcome following regional cerebral ischemia with methohexital, midazolam, and etomidate. Anesthesiology 1987b: 67: A582.

Baughman VL, Hoffman WE, Miletich DJ, Albrecht RF. Cerebral metabolic depression and brain protection produced by midazolam and etomidate in the rat. J Neurosurg Anesthesiol 1989: 1: 22–28.

Baum VC. Distinctive effects of the three intravenous anaesthetics on the inward rectifier (IKI) and the delayed rectifier (IK) potassium currents in myocardium: implications for the mechanisms of action. Anesth Analg 1993: 76: 18–23.

Belopavlovic M and Buchthal A. Modification of ketamine-induced intracranial hypertension in neurosurgical patients by pretreatment with midazolam. Acta Anaesth scand 1982: 26: 458–462.

Belopavlovic M, Buchthal A. Intracranial pressure changes during the induction of anaesthesia with etomidate in neurosurgical patients. Intracranial Pressure V (eds) Isshii S, Nagai H, Brock M. Springer Verlag, Berlin Heidelberg 1983: 834–837.

Belapavlovic M, Buchthal A, Beks JWF. Barbiturates for cerebral aneurysm surgery. Acta Neurochir 1985: 76: 73–81.

Bedriss P, Stoiber HP, Bendriss-Brusset AC, et al. Propofol effects on EEG and relationship with plasma concentration during neurosurgery. Anesthesiology 1990: 73: A203.

Bendtsen AO, Cold GE, Saaby Lomholt B, et al. Central haemodynamic during thiopental load and sodium nitroprusside induced hypotension. Acta Anaesthesiol Scand 1983, suppl 78: 82: Abstract no 123.

Bendtsen AO, Cold GE, Astrup J, Rosen¢rn J. Thiopental loading during controlled hypotension for intracranial aneurysm surgery Acta Anaesthesiol Scand 1984: 28: 473–477.

Bendtsen A, Kruse A, Madsen JB, et al. Use of a continuous infusion of althesin in neuroanaesthesia. Changes in cerebral blood flow, cerebral metabolism, the EEG and plasma alphaxalone concentration. Br J Anaesth 1985: 57: 369–374.

Bennett DR, Madsen JA, Jordan WS, Wiser WC. Ketamine anaesthesia in brain-damaged epileptics: electroencephalographic and clinical observations Neurology (Minneap.) 1973: 23: 449–460.

Berntman L, Welch FA, Bian Rosa IJ, Harp JR. Diazepam fails to protect brain tissue in hypoxic stress. Anesthesiology 1979: 51: S202.

Bertlik M, Orser BA, Yang L-W, MacDonald JF. Propofol selectively inhibits the NMDA sub-type of glutamate receptor. Can J Anaesth 1994: 41 (suppl, part u): A6

Bingham RM, Procaccio F, Prior PF, Hinds CJ. Cerebral electric activity influences the effects of etomidate on cerebral perfusion pressure in traumatic coma. Br J Anaesth 1985: 57: 843–848.

Björkman S, Nilsson F, Åkeson J, et al. The effect of thiopental on cerebral blood flow, and its relation to plasma conentration, during simulated induction of anaesthesia in a porcine model. Acta Anaesthsiol Scand 1994: 38: 473–478.

Bleyaert AL, Nemoto EM, Safar P, et al. Thiopental amelioration of brain damage after global ischaemia in monkeys. Anesthesiology 1978: 49: 390–398.

Boardini DJ, Kassell NF, Coenter HC. Comparison of sodium thiopental and methohexital for high-dose barbiturate anesthesia. J Neurosurg 1984: 60: 602–608.

Borgeat A, Dessibourg C, Popovic V, et al. Propofol and spontaneous movements: An EEG study. Anesthesiology 1991: 74: 24–27.

Braestrup C, Squires RF. Specific benzodiazepine receptors in rat brain characterized by high affinity (3H)diazepam binding. Proc Natl Acad Sci USA 1977: 74: 3805–3809.

Branston NM, Hope DT, Symon L. Barbiturates in focal ischaemia of primate cortex: effects on blood flow distribution, evoked potential and extracellular potassium. Stroke 1979: 10: 647–653.

Bricolo AP, Glick RP. Barbiturate effects on acute experimental intracranial hypertension. J Neurosurg 1981: 55: 397–406.

Bruce DA, Langfitt TW, Miller JD, et al. Regional cerebral blood flow, intracranial pressure, and brain metabolism in comatose patients. J Neurosurg 1973: 38: 131–145.

Buggy DJ, Nicol B, Rowbotham DJ, Lambert DG. Effects of intravenous anesthetic agents on glutamate release. Anesthesiology 2000: 92: 1067–1073.

Bühler M, Maitre PO, Hung OR, et al. Thiopental pharmacodynamics. I. Defining the pseudo-steady-state serum concentration-EEG effect relationship. Anesthesiology 1992: 77: 226–236.

Bullock R,van Dellen JR, Cambell D, et al. Experience with althesin in the manage ment of persistently raised ICP following severe head injury.J Neurosurg 1986: 64: 414–419.

Bundgaard H, Cold GE. A prospective comparative study of ICP during three anesthetics for elective craniotomy. Acta Anaesthesiol Scand 1997: suppl 110: 166

Bundgaard H, Landsfeldt U, Cold GE. Subdural monitoring of ICP during craniotomy: Thresholds of cerebral swelling/herniation. Acta Neurochir 1998: suppl 71: 276–278.

Campan L, Lazorthes Y. Note sur les effects compares des benzodiazepines et de la chlorpromazine sur la pression intracranienne du chien. Ann Anaesthsiol Fr 1976: 17: 1193–1198.

Carlsson C. Harp JR, Siesjo BK. Metabolic changes in the cerebral cortex of the rat induced by intravenous pentothalsodium. Acta Anaesthesiol Scand 1975b: suppl 57: 7–17.

Carlsson C, Hagerdal M, Kaasik AE, Siesjo BK. The effects of diazepam on cerebral blood flow and oxygen consumption in rats and its synergistic interaction with nitrous oxide. Anesthesiology 1976b: 45: 319–325.

Carlsson C, Chapman AG. The effects of diazepam on the cerebral metabolic state in rats and its interaction with nitrous oxide. Anesthesiology 1981: 54: 488–495.

Cavazzuti M, Porro CA, Biral GP, et al. Ketamine effects on local cerebral blood flow and metabolism in the rat. J Cereb Blood Flow Metab. 1987: 7: 806–811.

Cavazzuti M, Porro CA, Barbieri A, Galetti A. Brain and spinal cord metabolic activity during propofol anaesthesia. Br J Anaesth. 1991: 66: 490–495.

Cenic A, Craen RA, Howard-Lech VL, et al. Cerebral blood volume and blood flow at varying arterial carbon dioxide tension levels in rabbits during propofol anaesthesia. Anesth Analg 2000: 90: 1376–1383.

Chapman AG, Nordstrôm C-H, Siesjö BK. Influence of phenobarbital anesthesia on carbohydrate and amino-acid metabolism in rat brain. Anesthesiology 1978: 48: 175–182.

Cheng MA, Hoffman WE, Baughman VL, Albrecht RF. The effects of midazolam and sufentanil sedation on middle cerebral artery blood flow velocity in awake patients. J Neurosurg Anesthesiol 1993: 5: 232–236.

Chi OZ, Wei HM, Klein SL, Weiss HR. Effect of ketamine on heterogeneity of cerebral microregional venous O_2 saturation in the rat. Anesth Analg 1994: 79: 860–866.

Chi OZ, Chun TW, Liu X, Weiss H. The effects of pentobarbital on blood-brain barrier dusruption caused by intracarotid injection of hyperosmolar mannitol in rats. Anesth Analg 1998: 86: 1230–1235.

Chiolero RL, Ravussin P, Anderes JP, et al. Midazolam reversal with RO-15-1788 in patients with severe head injury. Anesthesiology 1986a: 65: A358.

Chiolero RL, Ravussin P, Chassot PG, et al. RO 15-1788 for rapid recovery after craniotomy. Anesthesiology 1986b: 65: A466.

Choi DW, Farb DH, Fischbach GD. Chlordiazepoxide selectively augments GABA action in spinal cord cultures. Nature 1977: 269: 342–344.

Church J, Zeman S, Lodge D. The neuroprotective action of ketamine and MK-801 after transient cerebral ischaemia in rats. Anesthesiology 1988: 69: 702–709.

Cold GE. Cerebral metabolic rate of oxygen ($CMRO_2$) in the acute phase of head injury. Acta Anaesthesiol Scand 1978: 22: 249–256.

Cold GE, Eskesen V, Eriksen H, et al. CBF and $CMRO_2$ during continuous etomidate infusion supplemented with N_2O and fentanyl in patients with supratentorial cerebral tumours. A dose response study. Acta Anaesthesiol Scand 1985: 29: 490–494.

Cold GE, Eskesen V, Eriksen H, Blatt Lyon B. Changes in $CMRO_2$, EEG and concentration of etomidate in serum and brain tissue during craniotomy with continuous etomidate supplemented with N_2O and fentanyl. Acta Anaesthesiol Scand 1986: 30: 159–163.

Cold GE, Christensen KJS, Nordentoft J, et al. Cerebral blood flow, cerebral metabolic rate of oxygen and relative CO_2 reactivity during neurolept anesthesia in patients subjected to craniotomy for supratentorial cerebral tumours. Acta Anaesthesiol Scand 1988. 32: 310–315.

Cold GE. Measurement of CO_2 reactivity and barbiturate reactivity in patients with severe head injury. Acta Neurochir (Wien) 1989: 98: 153–163.

Cold GE. Etomidate used for brain neurosurgical anaesthesia. The effect upon cerebral circulation and metabolism. Agressologie 1992.

Cold GE, Tange M, Jensen TM, Ottesen S. Subdural pressure measurement during craniotomy. Corrrelation with tactile estimation of dural tension and brain herniation after opening of dura. Br J Neurosurg 1996: 10: 69–75.

Coles JP, Leary TS, Monteiro JN, et al. Propofol anesthesia for craniotomy: A double-blind comparison of remifentanil, alfentanil, and fentanyl. J Neurosurg Anesthesiol 2000: 12: 15–20.

Corkill G, Chikovanni OI, McLeish I, McDonald LW, Youmans JR. Timing of pentobarbital administration for brain protection in experimental stroke. Surg Neurol 1976: 5: 147–149.

Corkill G, Sivalingham S, Reital JA, et al. Dose dependency of the post-insult protective effect of pentobarbital in the canine experimental stroke model. Stroke 1978: 9: 10–12.

Corssen G, Domino EF, Bree RL. Electroencephalographic effects of ketamine anesthesia in children. Anesth Analg 1969a: 48: 141–147.

Corssen G, Groces EH, Gomez S, Allen RJ. Ketamine: its place in anaesthesia for neurosurgical diagnostic procedures. Anesth Analg 1969b: 48: 181–188.

Cotev S, Shalit MN. Effects of diazepam on cerebral blood flow and oxygen uptake after head injury. Anesthesiology 1975: 43: 117–122.

Cottrell JE, Giffin JP, Lim K, et al. Intracranial pressure, mean arterial pressure and heart rate following midazolam or thipental in humans with incracranial masses. Anesthesiology 1982: 57: A323.

Craen RA, Gelb AW, Murkin JM, Chong KY. CO_2 responsiveness of cerebral blood flow is maintained during propofol anaesthesia. Can J Anaesth 1992, A7.

Criado A, Maseda J, Navarro E, et al. Induction of anaesthesia with etomidate: Haemodynamic study of 36 patients. Br J Anaesth 1980: 52: 803–805.

Crosby G, Crane AM, Sokoloff L. Local changes in cerebral glucose utilization during ketamine anaesthesia. Anesthesiology 1982: 56: 437–443.

Crosby G, Crane AM, Sokoloff L. A comparison of local rates of glucose utilization in spinal cord and brain in conscious and nitrous oxide- or pentobarbital-treated rats. Anesthesiology 1984: 61: 434–438.

Cunitz G Danhauser I, Wickbold J. Comparative investigations on the influence of etomidate, thiopentone and methohexitone on the intracranial pressure of the patient. Anaesthesist 1973: 22: 357–366.

Dahl B, Cold GE, Astrup J, Jensen K, Mosdal B, Plougman J. Dynamic changes in barbiturate- and CO2 reactivities in severe head injury. Acta Neurochir (Wien) 1993 (submitted).

Dam M, Pizzolato G, Ricchieri GL, et al. The effects of propofol anaesthesia on local cerebral glucose utilization in the rat. Anesthesiology 1990: 73: 499–505.

Damsma G, Fibiger HC. The effects of anaesthesia and hypothermia in interstitial concentrations of acetylcholine and choline in the striatum. Life Sciences 1991: 48: 2469–2474.

Davis DW, Hawkins RA, Mans AM, et al. Regional cerebral glucose utilization during althesin anesthesia. Anesthesiology 1984: 61: 362–368.

Davis DW, Mans AM, Biebuyck JF, et al. Regional brain glucose utilization in rats during etomidate anaesthesia. Anesthesiology 1986: 64: 751–757.

Davis DW, Mans AM, Biebuyck JF, et al. The influence of ketamine on regional brain glucose use. Anesthesiology 1988: 69: 199–205.

Dawson B, Michenfelder JD, Theye RA. Effect of ketamine on canine cerebral blood flow and metabolism: modification by prior administration of thiopental. Anesth Analg 1971: 5O: 443-447.

Day AL, Friedman WA, Sypert GW, Mickle JP. Successful treatment of the normal perfusion pressure breakthrough syndrome. Neurosurgery 1982: 11: 625–630.
Dearden NM, McDowall DG. Comparison of etomidate and althesin in the reduction of increased intracranial pressure after head injury. Br J Anaesth 1985: 57: 361-368.
DeLeon-Casasola OA, Weiss A, Lema MJ, Anaphylaxis due to propofol. Anesthesiology 1992: 77: 384–386.
Demiryürek AT, Cinel I, Kahraman S, et al. Propofol and intralipid interact with reactive oxygen species: A chemiluminescens study. Br J Anaesth 1998: 80: 649–654.
Depaulis A, Bourguignon J-J, Marescaux C, et al. Effects of gamma-hydroxybuturate and gamma-butyrolactone derivates on spontaneous generalized non-convulsive siezures in the rat. Neuropharmacology 1988: 27: 683–689.
DeRiu PL, Petruzzi V, Testa C, et al. Propofol anticonvulsant activity in experimental epileptoc status. Br J Anaesth 1992: 69: 177–181.
Detsch O, Erkens U, Schneck H, et al. Cerebral blood flow velocity and carbon dioxide vasoreactivity during gamma-hydroxobutyrate/fentanyl anaesthesia in non-neurosurgical patients. Eur J Anaesthesiol 1999: 16: 195–200.
DeValois JC, Peperkamp JPC. The influence of some drugs upon the regulation of cerebral blood flow in the rabbit. In: Ross Russell (ed) Brain and Blood Flow. Pitman Medical and Scientific Publishing Co LTD London 1971: 254–257.
DiChiara G, Imperato A. Preferential stimulation of dopamine release in the nucleus accumbens by opiates, alcohol, and barbiturates: studies with transcerebral dialysis in freely moving rats. Ann NY Acad Sci 1986: 373: 367–381.
Doenicke A, Lorenz W, Beigl R, et al. Histamine release after intravenous application of short-acting hypnotics. A comparison of etomidate, althesin and propanidid. Br J Anaesth 1973: 45: 1097–1104.
Doenicke A, Kugler J, Penzel G et al. Hirnfunktion und Toleranzbreite nach Etomidate, einem neuen, Barbituratfreien i.v. applizierbaren Hypnotikum. Anaesthesist 1973: 22: 357–366.
Doenicke A, Loffler B, Kugler J, et al. Plasma concentration and EEG after various regimens of etomidate. Br J Anaesth 1982: 54: 393–400.
Ebrahim ZY, DeBoer GE, Luders H, et al. Effect of etomidate on the electroencephalogram of patients with epilepsia. Anesth Analg 1986: 65: 1004–1006.
Ebrahim ZY. Schubert A, van Ness P, et al. The effect of propofol on the electroencephalogram of patients with epilepsy. Anesth Analg 1994: 78: 275–279.
Ederberg S, Westerlind A, Houltz E, et al. The effects of propofol on cerebral blood flow velocity and cerebral oxygen extraction during cardiopulmonary bypass. Anest Analg 1998: 86: 1201–1206.
Edvinsson L, Mc Culloch J. Effects of pentobarbital on contractile reponses of feline cerebral arteries. J Cereb Blood Flow Metab 1981: 1: 437–440
Eintrei C, Sokoloff L, Smith CB. Effects of diazepam and ketamine administered individually or in combination on regional rates of glucose utilization in rat brain. Br J Anaesth 1999: 82: 596–602.
Eisenberg HM, Frankowski RF, Contant CF, et al. High-dose barbiturate control of elevated intracranial pressure in patients with severe head injury. J Neurosurg 1988: 69: 15–23.
Endoh H, Honda T, Komura N, et al. Effects of nicardipine-, nitroglycerin- and prostaglandin E1-induced hypotension on human cerebrovascular carbon dioxide reactivity during propofol-fentanyl anesthesia. J Clin Anesth 1999: 11: 545–549.
Eng C, Lam A, Mayberg T. The influence of propofol with and without nitrous oxide on cerebral blood flow velocity and CO_2 reactivity in man. Anesth Analg 1992: 74: S87
Engberg M, Öberg B, Christensen KS, et al. The arterio-venous oxygen content differences ($AVDO_2$) during halothane and neuroleptanaesthesia in patients subjected to craniotomy. Acta Anaesthiol Scand 1989: 33: 642–646.
Engelhard K, Werner C, Lu H, et al. Effect of S-(+)-ketamine on autoregulation of cerebral blood flow. Anasthesiol Intensivmed Notfallmed Schmerzther 1997: 32: 721–725.
Evans J, Rosen M, Weeks RD, Wise C. Ketamine in neurosurgical procedures. Lancet 1971: i: 40–41.
Farling PA, Johnston JR, Coppel DL. Propofol infusion for sedation of patients with head injury in intensive care. Anaesthesia 1989: 44: 222–226.
Ferrer-Allado T, Brechner VL, Dymond A, et al. Ketamine-induced electroconvulsive phenomena in the human limbic and thalamic regions. Anesthesiology 1973: 38: 333–344.
Feustel PJ, Ingvar MC, Severinghaus JW. Cerebral oxyggen availability and blood flow during middle cerebral artery occlusion: Effects of pentobarbital. Stroke 1981: 12: 858–863.
Finlay WEI, McKee JI. Screen cortisol levels in severely stressed patients. Lancet 1982: i: 1414–1415.
Fischer S, Renz D, Schaper W, Karloczek GF. In vitro effects of fentanyl, methoxital, and thiopental on brain edothemial permeability. Anesthesiology 1995: 82: 451–458.
Fischer S. Renz D, Schaper W, Karliczek GF. Effects of barbiturates on hypoxic cultures of brain derived microvascular endothelial cells. Brain Res 1996: 707: 47–53.
Fitch W, McGeorge AP, MacKenzie ET. Anaesthesia for studies of the cerebral circulation: A comparison of phencyclidine and althesin in the baboon. Br J Anaesth 1978: 50: 985–990.
Flamm ES, Demopoulos HB, Seligman ML, Ransohoff J. Possible molecular mechanisms of barbiturate-mediated protection in regional cerebral ischaemia. Acta Neurol Scand 1977 (suppl 64): 150–151.
Fleischer JE, Milde JH, Moyer TP, Michenfelder JD. Cerebral effects of high-dose midazolam and subsequent reversal with Ro 15–1788 in dogs. Anesthesiology 1988: 68: 234–242.
Ford EW, Morrell F, Whisler WW. Methohexital anesthesia in the surgical treatment of uncontrollable epilepsy. Anesth Analg 1982: 61: 997–1001.
Forster A, Juge O, Morel D. Effects of midazolam on cerebral blood flow in human volunteers. Anesthesiology 1982: 56: 453–455.
Forster A, Juge O, Louis M, Nahory A. Effects of a specific benzodiazepine antagonist (RO 15–1788) on cerebral blood flow. Anesth Analg 1987: 66: 309–313.
Fox J, Gelb AW, Enns J, Murkin JM, et al. The responsiveness of cerebral blood flow to changes in arterial carbon dioxide in maintained during propofol-nitrous oxide anesthesia in humans. Anesthesiology 1992: 77: 453–456.
Francis A, Pulsinelli WA. Increased binding of (3H)GABA to striatal membranes following ischemia J Neurochem 1983: 40: 1497–1499.
Franks NP, Lieb WR. Molecular and cellular mechanisms of anaesthetics. Nature 1994: 367: 607–614.
Fragen RJ, Shanks CA, Molteni A, Avram MJ. Effects of etomidate on hormonal responses to surgical stress. Anesthesiology 1984: 61: 652–656.

Frenkel C, Urban BW. Human brain sodium channels as one of the molecular target sites for the new intravenous anaesthetic propofol (2,6-diisopropylphenol) Eur J Pharmacol 1991: 208: 75–79.
Frizzell RT, Meyer YJ, Borchers DJ, et al. The effects of etomidate on cerebral metabolism and blood flow in a canine model for hypoperfusion. J Neurosurg 1991: 74: 263–269.
Frizzell RT, Fichtel FM, Jordan MB, et al. Effects of etomidate and hypothermia on cerebral metabolism and blood flow in a canine model of hypoperfusion. Journal of Neurosurgical Anesthesiology 1993: 5: 104–110.
Galley HF, Webster NR. Brain nitric oxide synthase activity is decreased by intravenous anesthetics. Anesth Analg 1996: 83: 591–594.
Gancher S, Laxer KD, Krieger W. Activation of epileptogenic activity by etomidate. Anesthesiology 1984: 61: 616–618.
Gardner AE, Olson BE, Lichtiger M. Cerebrospinal-fluid pressure during dissociative anaesthesia with ketamine. Anesthesiology 1971: 35: 226–228.
Gelb AW, Floyd P, Lok P, et al. A prophylactic bolus of thiopentone does not protect against prolonged focal ischaemia. Can Anesth Soc J 1986: 33: 173–177.
Gelb AW, Zhang C, Henderson SM. A comparison of the cerebral protective effects of propofol, thiopental, and halothane in temporary feline focal cerebral ischemia. Anesth Analg 1993: 76: S115.
Ghoneim MM, Yamada T. Etomidate: A clinical and electroencephalographic comparison with thiopental. Anesth Analg 1977: 56: 479–485.
Ghoneim MM, Block RI, Ping S, et al. The interactions of midazolam and flumazenil on human memory and cognition. Anesthesiology 1993: 79: 1183–1192.
Gibs JM. The effect of intravenous ketamine on cerebrospinal fluid pressure. Br J Anaesth 1972: 44: 1298–1302.
Giffard RG, Weiss JH, Swanson RA, Choi DW. Secobarbital attenuates excitotoxicity but potentiates oxygen-glucose deprivation neuronal injury in cortical cell culture. J Cereb Blood Flow Metab 1993: 13: 803–810.
Gisvold SE, Safar P, Hendrickx HHL, et al. Thiopental treatment after global ischemia in pigtailed monkeys. Anesthesiology 1984: 60: 88–96.
Gjedde A, Rasmussen M. Pentobarbital anesthesia reduces blood-brain glucose transfer in the rat. J Neurochem 1980: 35: 1382–1387.
Gordon E. The action of drugs on intracranial contents. In: Boulton TB, Bryce-Smith R et al. (eds); Progress in Anaesthesiology, Excerpta Medica, Amsterdam 1970: 60.
Goskowicz R, Patel P, Drummond J, et al. Ischemia induced release of glutamate in the rat brain: The effect of etomidate and thiopental. Anesthesiology 1993: 76: S123.
Grant IS, Hutchison G. Epileptiform seizures during prolonged etomidate sedation. Lancet 1983: ii: 511–512.
Grände P-O, Gustafsson D, Lindberg L. Effects of thiopental on resistance vessels in cat skeletal muscle. Intensive Care Med 1990: 16: 399–404.
Grissom TE, Mitzel HC, Bunegin L, Albin MS. The effect of anesthetics on neurologic outcome during the recovery period of spinal cord injury in rats. Anesth Analg 1994: 79: 66–74.
Gronert GA, Michenfelder JD, Sharbrough FW, Milde JH. Canine cerebral metabolic tolerance during 24 hours deep pentobarbital anesthesia. Anesthesiology 1981: 55: 110–113.
Gross CE, Abel PW. Contraction and relaxation of rabbit basilar artery by thiopental. Neurosurgery 1985: 17: 433–435
Guit JBM, Koning HM, Cosster ML, et al. Ketamine as analgetic for total intravenous anaesthesia with propofol. Anaesthesia 1991: 46: 24–27.
Hagerdal M, Welch FA, Keykhah MM, et al. Protective effects of combinations of hypothermia and barbiturates in cerebral hypoxia in the rat. Anesthesiology 1978: 49: 165–169.
Hales TG, Lambert JJ. The actions of propofol on inhibitory amino acid receptors of bovine adrenomedullary chromaffin cells and rodent central neurons. Br J Pharmacol 1991: 104: 619–628.
Haller C, Kuschinsky W, Reimnitz P. The effect of gamma-hydroxybuturate on the reactivity of pial arteries before and after ischemia. J Cereb Blood Flow Metab 1986: 6: 658–666.
Haller C, Mende M, Schuier F, et al. Effect of γ-hydroxybuturate on local and global glucose metabolism in the anesthetized cat brain. J Cereb Blood Flow Metab 1990: 10: 493–498.
Hamilton K, Bunegin L, Albin MS. The effect of ketamine hydrochloride (KH) on cerebral blood flow (CBF) during acute hypoxia in the rat. Anesth Analg 1992: 74: S128
Hankinson HL, Smith AL, Nielsen SL, Hoff JT. Effect of thiopental on focal cerebral ischaemia in dogs. Surg Forum 1974: 25: 445–447.
Hara M, Kai Y, Ikemoto Y. Enhancement by propofol of the γ-aminobutyric acid response in dissociated hippocampal pryramidal neurons of the rat. Anesthesiology 1994: 81: 988–994.
Harris CE, Murray AM, Anderson JM, et al. Effects of thiopentone, etomidate and propofol on the haemodynamic response to tracheal intubation. Anaesthesia 1988: 43 (suppl): 32–36.
Harrison JM, Girling KJ, Mahajan RP. Effects of target-controlled infusion of propofol on the transient hyperaemic response and carbon dioxide reactivity in the middle cerebral artery. Br J Anaesth 1999: 83: 839–844.
Hartung HJ. Beeinflussung des Intrakraniellen Druckes durch Propofol (disoprivan). Anaesthesist 1987: 36: 66–68.
Hartung HJ. Intrakranielles Druckverhalten bei Patienten mit Schädel Hirn-Trama nach Propofol- bzw Thiopental-Applikation. Anaesthesist 1987: 36: 285–287.
Hase U, Dick W. Zum Verhalten des Intrakraniellen Drucks bei Schädel-Hirn-tramatisierten Patienten nach Ketaminapplikation. In Ketamin (Ketanest) in Notfall- und Katastrophenmedizin. Dick W (ed). Perimed Fachbuch, Erlangen, 1981: 77–81
Hatano Y, Nakamura K, Moriyama S, et al. The contractile responses of isolated dog cerebral and extracerebral arteries to oxybarbiturates and thiobarbiturates. Anesthesiology 1989: 71: 80–86.
Hemelrijck JV, Tempelhoff R, White PF, Jellish WS. EEG-assisted titration of propofol infusion during neuroanesthesia: effect of nitrous oxide. J Neurosurg Anesthesiol 1992: 4: 11–20
Henderson JJ, McGeorg A, Teasdale GM. Pharmacodynamics of althesin infusion: Electroencephalographic studies. Sixth European Congress of Anesthesiology, London, Anaesthesia 1982: 143.
Henriksen L. Brain luxury perfusion during cardiopulmonary bypass in humans. A study of the cerebral blood flow response to changes in CO_2, O_2, and blood pressure. J Cereb Blood Flow Metab 1986: 6: 366–378.

Hensel I, Braum U, Kettler D, et al. Untersuchungen über Kreislauf- und Stoffwechselveränderungen unter Ketamine-Narkose. Anaesthesist: 1972: 21: 44–49.

Herkenham M. Anesthetics and the habenulo-interpeduncular system: selective sparing of metabolic activity. Brain Researce 1981: 210: 461–466.

Herrschaft H, Schmidt H, Gleim F, Albus G. The response of human cerebral blood flow to anesthesia with thiopentone, methohexitone, propanidide, ketamine and etomidate. In: Penzholz H, Brock M, et al. (eds); Advances in Neurosurgery, Springer Verlag, Berlin, Heidelberg, New York, 1975: 120–133.

Hewitt PB, Chu DLK, Polkey E, Binnie CD. Effect of propofol on the electrocorticogram in epileptic patients undergoing cortical resection. Br J Anaesth 1999: 82: 199–202.

Hickey R, Albin MS, Bunegin L. Ketamine abolishes central nervous autoregulation in the rat. Anesth Analg 1989: 68: S120.

Hicks RG, Kerr DR, Horton DA. Thiopentone cerebral protection under EEG control during carotid endarterectomy Anaesth Intens Care 1986: 14: 22–28.

Hilfiker O, Kettler D. Die Wirkung von Midazolam auf die Hirndurchblutung beim Tier und beim Mensch. Arzneim Forsch 1981: 31: 2236–2237.

Himmelseher S, Pfenninger E, Kochs E, Auchter M. S(+) ketamine up-regulates neuronal regeneration associated proteins following glutamate injury in cultured rat hippocampal neurons. J Neurosurg Anesthesiol 2000: 12: 84–94.

Hodes JE, Soncrant TT, Larson DM, et al. Selective changes in local cerebral glucose utilization induced by phenobarbital in the rat. Anesthesiology 1983: 63: 633–639.

Hoff J, Schmith A, Nielsen S, Larson P. Effects of barbiturate and halothane anaesthesia on focal cerebral infarction in the dog. Surg Forum 1973: 24: 449–452.

Hoff JT, Smith AL, Hankinson HL, Nielsen SL, Barbiturate protection from cerebral infarction in primates. Stroke 1975: 6: 28–33.

Hoff JT, Pitts LH, Spetzler R, Wilson CB. Barbiturates for protection from cerebral ischaemia in aneurysm surgery. Acta Neurol Scand 1977: 56: 158–159.

Hoffman WE, Miletich DJ, Albrecht RF. The effects of midazolam on cerebral blood flow and oxygen consumption and its interaction with nitrous oxide. Anesth Analg 1986: 65: 729–733.

Hoffman WE, Kochs E. Propofol: An intravenous anesthetic for neuroanesthetic practice? J Neurosurg Anesthesiol 1992: 4: 75–77.

Honegger P, Matthieu JM. Selective toxicity of the general anesthetic propofol for GABAergic neurons in rat brain cell cultures. J Neurosc Res 1996: 45: 631–636.

Hougaaard K, Hansen A, Brodersen P. The effect of ketamine on regional cerebral blood flow in man. Anesthesiology 1974: 41: 562–567.

Hung OR, Varvel JR, Shafer SL, Stanski DR. Thiopentone pharmacodynamics. II. Quantitation of the clinical and electroencephalographic depth of anesthesia. Anesthesiology 1992: 77: 237–244.

Hunter AR. Thiopentone supplemented anaesthesia for neurosurgery. Br J Anaesth 1972: 44: 506–510.

Iragi Y, Sugiyama Y, Awazu S, Hanano M. Comparative physiologically based pharmacokinetics of hexobarbital, phenobarbital, and thiopental in the rat. J Pharmacokin Biopharm 1982: 10: 53–55.

Iversen SD. Behavioral evaluation of cholinergic drugs. Life Sciences 1997: 60: 1145–1152.

Jansen GFA, Kagenaar D. Effects of propofol in the relation between CO_2 and cerebral blood flow velocity. Anesth Analg 1993: 76: S163.

Jones MV, Brooks PA, Harrison NL. Enhancement of γ aminobutyric acid activated Cl^- currents in cultured rat hippocampal neurones by three volatile anaesthetics. J Physiol 1992: 449: 279–293.

Joo DT, Xiong Z, MacDonald JF. et al. Blockade of glutamate receptors and barbiturate anesthesia. Anesthesiology 1999: 91: 1329–1341.

Kahn R, Martinez-Tica J, Reich DL, et al. The effect of propofol infusion on dopamine release in rat corpus striatum during reversible forebrain ischeia. Anesth Analg 1993: 76: S175.

Kassell NF, Hitchon PW, Gerk MK, et al. Alterations in cerebral blood flow, oxygen metabolism, and electrical activity produced by high dose sodium thiopental. Neurosurgery 1980: 7: 598–603.

Kassell NF, Hitchon PW, Gerk MK, et al. Influence of changes in arterial pCO_2 on cerebral blood flow and metabolism during high-dose barbiturate therapy in dogs. J Neurosurg 1981: 54: 615–619.

Kayama Y, Iwama K. The EEG, evoked potentials, and single-unit activity during ketamine anaesthesia in cats. Anesthesiology 1972: 36: 316–328.

Kayama Y. Comparison of the effects of althesin and barbiturates on the neocortex and hippocampus in cats. Br J Anaesth 1974: 46: 912–917.

Keaney NP, McDowall DG, Pickerodt VWA, et al. Time course of the cerebral circulatory response to metabolic depression. Am J Physiol 1978: 234: H74–H79.

Keykhah MM, Smith DS, O`Neil JJ, et al. The influence of etomidate on brain metabolites during severe hypoxia. Anesthesiology 1986: 65: A251.

Kiersey DK, Bickford RD, Faulconer A. Electroencephalographic patterns produced by thiopental sodium during surgical operations: Description and classification. Br J Anaesth 1951: 23: 141–152.

Kikuchi T, Wang Y, Shinbori H, et al. Effects of ketamine and pentobarbitone on the acetylcholine release from the rat frontal cortex in vivo: Measurement by brain microdialysis. Br J Anaesth 1997: 79: 128–130.

Kikuchi T, Wang Y, Sato K, Okumura F. *In vivo* effects of propofol on acetylcholine release from the frontal cortex, hippocampus and striatum studied by intracerebral microdialysis in freely moving rats. Br J Anaesth 1998: 80: 644–648.

Klausen NO, Moesgaard J, Ferguson AH, et al. Negative synacthen test during etomidate infusion. Lancet 1983: ii: 848.

Klose R, Hartung HJ, Kotsch R, Walz T. Experimentelle Untersuchungen zur Intracraniellen Drucksteigerung durch Ketamine beim Hämorrhagischen Schock. Anaesthesist 1982: 31: 33–38.

Knudsen L, Cold GE, Holdgård HO, et al. The effect of midazolam on cerebral blood flow and oxygen consumption. Interaction with nitrous oxide in patients undergoing craniotomy for supratentorial cerebral tumours. Anaesthesia 1990: 45: 1016–1019.

Knudsen L, Cold GE, Jensen S, et al. Effects of flumazenil on cerebral blood flow and oxygen consumption after midazolam anaesthesia for craniotomy. Br J Anesth 1991: 67: 277–280.

Koch KA, Jackson DL, Schmiedl M, et al. Effect of thiopental therapy on cerebral blood flow after total cerebral ischaemia. Critical Care Med 1984: 12: 90–95.

Kochs E, Roewer N, Peter A, Schulte am Esch J. Wirkungen von Flumazenil auf den Globalen Zerabralen Blutfluss und den Intrakraniellen Druck in der Reperfusionsphase nach Globaler inkompletter Zerebraler Ischämie. Anästh Intensivther Notfallmed 1988: 23: 159-162.

Kochs E, Schulte am Esch J. Antagonism of midazolam sedation by RO 15–1788: Effect on acustical evoked responses. Anesthesiology 1988: 65: A359.

Kochs E, Werner C, Hoffman WE, et al. Concurrent increases in brain electrical activity and intracranial blood flow velocity during low-dose ketaminc anaesthesia. Can J Anaesth 1991: 38: 826–830.

Kochs E, Hoffman WE, Werner C, et al. The effect of propofol on brain electrical activity, neurologic outcome, and neuronal damage following incomplete ischemia in rats. Anesthesiology 1992: 76: 245-252

Kohno T, Kumamoto E, Baba H, et al. Actions of midazolam on GABAergic transmission in substantia gelatinosa neurons of adult rat spinal cord slices. Anesthesiology 2000: 92: 507-515.

Koorn R, Brannan TS, Matinez-Tica J, et al. Effect of etomidate on in vivo ischemia-induced dopamine release in the corpus striatum of the rat: A study using cerebral microdialysis: Anesth Analg 1994: 78: 73–79.

Krieger W, Copperman J, Laxer KD. Seizures with etomidate anesthesia. Anesth Analg 1985: 64: 1226–1227.

Kreuscher H. Die Hirndurchblutung unter Neuroleptanaethesie. Springer Verlag Berlin Heidelberg New York 1967.

Krieglstein J, Sperling G, Twietmeyer G. Effects of thiopental on regulatory mechanisms of brain energy metabolism. Arch Pharmacol 1981: 318: 56–61.

Kumano H, Shimomura T, Furuya H, et al. Effects of flumazenil during administration of midazolam on pial vessel diameter and regional cerebral blood flow in cats. Acta Acaesthesiol Scand 1993: 37: 567–570.

Kumar A, Bleck TP. Intraavenous midazolam for the treatment of refractory status epilepticus. Critical Care Medicine 1992: 20: 483–488.

Kuschinsky W, Suda S, Sokoloff L. Influence of gamma-hydroxybuturate on the relationship between local cerebral glucose utilization and local cerebral blood flow in the rat brain. J Cereb Blood Flow Metab 1985: 5: 58–64.

Lagerkranser M, Stånge K, Sollevi A. Effects of propofol on cerebral blood flow, metabolism, and cerebral autoregulation in the anesthetized pig. J Neurosurg Anesthesiol 1997: 9: 188–193.

Lafferty JJ, Keykhah MM, Shapiro HM, et al. Cerebral hypometabolism obtained with deep pentobarbital anesthesia and hypothermia (30 C). Anesthesiology 1978: 49: 159–164.

Larsen R, Hilfiker O, Radle J Sonntag H. Midazolam: Wirkung auf allgemeine Hämodynamik, Hirndurchblutung und Cerebralen Sauerstoffverbrauch bei Neurochirurgischen Patienten. Anaethesist 1981: 30: 18–21.

Laurent JP, Lawner P, Simeone FA, Fink E. Pentobarbital changes compartmental contribution to cerebral blood flow J Neurosurg 1982: 56: 504–510.

Lawner PM, Simeone FA. Treatment of intraoperative middle cerebral artery occlusion with pentobarbital and extracranial-intracranial bypass. J Neurosurg 1979: 51: 710–712.

Laxenaire M-C, Gueant J-L, Bermejo E, Mouton C. Anaphylactic shock due to propofol. Lancet 1988: 2: 739–740.

Laxenaire M-C, Mata-Bermejo E, Moneret-Vautrin DA, Gueant J-L. Life-threatening anaphylactoid reactions to propofol (Diprivan). Anesthesiology 1992: 77: 275–280.

Ledingham IM, Watt I. Influence of sedation on mortality in critically ill multiple trauma patients. Lancet 1983: i: 1270.

Levy DE, Brierley JB. Delayed pentobarbital administration limits ischemic brain damage in gerbils. Ann Neurol 1979: 5: 59–64.

Li CY, Chou TC, Wong CS, et al. Ketamine inhibits nitric oxide synthase in lipopolysaccharide-treated rat alveolar macrophages. Can J Anaesth 1997: 44: 989–995.

Lightfoote WE, Molinari GF, Chase TN. Modification of cerebral ischemic damage by anaesthetics. Stroke 1977: 8: 627–628.

List WF, Crumrine RS, Cascorbi HF, Weiss F. Increased cerebrospinal fluid pressure after ketamine (Correspondance) Anesthesiology 1972: 36: 98.

Lobe DP, Brauer FS. Barbiturate protection in extracranial-intracranial anastomosis. Anesthesiology 1983: 59: A 331.

Longnecker DE, Sturgill BC. Influence of anesthetic agent on survival following hemorrhage. Anesthesiology 1976: 45: 516–521.

Longnecker DE. Stress free: To be or not to be? (editorial) Anesthesiology 1984: 61: 643–644.

Louis PT, Goddard-Finegold J, Fishman MA, et al. Barbiturates and hyperventilation during intracranial hypertension. Critical Care Medicine 1993: 21: 1200–1206.

Lowson S, Gent JP, Goodchild CS. Anticonvulsant properties of propofol and thiopentone: comparison using two tests in laboratory mice. Br J Anaesth 1990: 64: 59–63.

Ludic R, Keifer JC, Baghdoyan HA, Becker L. Microdialysis on the pontine reticular formation reveals inhibition of acetylcholine release by morphine. Anesthesiology 1993: 79: 1003–1012.

Lukatch HS, MacIver MB. Synaptic mechanisms of thiopental-induced anterations in synchronized cortical activity. Anesthesiology 1996: 84: 1425–1434.

MacIver MB, Mandema JW, Stanski DR, Bland BH. Thiopental uncouples hippocampal and cortical synchronized electroencephalographic activity. Anesthesiology 1996: 84: 1411–1424.

Madsen JB, Cold GE, Hansen ES, Bardrum B.Cerebral blood flow, cerebral metabolic rate of oxygen and relative CO_2 reactivity during craniotomy for supratentorial cerebral tumours in halothane anaesthesia. A dose-response study. Acta Anaesthesiol Scand 1987a: 31: 454–457.

Madsen JB, Guldager H, Jensen FM. CBF and $CMRO_2$ during neuroanaesthesia with continuous infusion of propofol. Acta Anaesthesiol Scand 1989: suppl 91: 33: 143.

Maekawa T, Sakabe T, Takeshita H. Diazepam blocks cerebral metabolic and circulatory responses to local anesthetic-induced seizures. Anesthesiology 1974: 41: 389–391.

Makita T, Shibata O, Tsujita T, et al. Effects of intravenous anesthetics on phosphoidylinositol turnover in rat cerebral cortical prisms. Anesth Analg 1994: 79: 252–256.

Mandel P, Maitre M, Vayer P, Hechler V. Function of gamma-hydroxybuturate: a putative neurotransmitter. Biochem Soc Trans 1987: 15: 215–217.

Marin J, Lobato RD, Rico ML, et al. Effect of pentobarbital on the reactivity of isolated human cerebral arteries. J Neurosurg 1981: 54: 521–524

Marshall LF, SangU H. Treatment of massive intraoperative brain swelling. Neurosurgery 1983: 13: 412–414.
Marchall BM. Neuroleptanesthesia in neurosurgery. In. Oyama T (ed) International Anesthesiology Clinics. Little Brown and Company 1973: 103–125.
Matsumoto M, Iida Y, Sakabe T, et al. Mild and moderate hypothermia provide better protection than a burst-suppression dese of thiopental against ischemic spinal cord injury in rabbits. Anesthesiology 1997: 86: 1120–1127.
Matta BF, Lam AM, Strebel S, Mayberg TS. Cerebral pressure autoregulation and carbon dioxide reactivity during propofol-induced EEG suppression. Br J Anaesth 1995: 74: 159–163,
Mayberg TS, Lam AM, Matta BF, et al. Ketamine does not increase cerebral blood flow velocity or intracranial pressure during isoflurane/nitrous oxide anaesthesia in patients undergoing craniotomy. Anesth Analg 1995: 81: 84–89.
McCulloch TJ, Visco E, Lam AM. Graded hypercapnia and cerebral autoregulation during sevoflurane or porpofol anaesthesia. Anesthesiology 2000: 93: 1205–1209.
McDowall DG, Heuser D, Okuda Y, et al. Relationship between cerebral blood flow changes and cortical extracellular fluid pH during cerebral metabolic depression induced by althesin. Br J Anaesth 1979: 51: 1109–1115.
Merckx L, Van Hemelrijck J, van Aken H, et al. Total intravenous anesthesia using propofol and alfentanil infusion in neurosurgical patients. Anesthesiology 1988: 69: A576.
Meuret P, Backman SB, Bonhomme V, et al. Physiostigmine reverses propofol-induced unconsciousness and attenuation of the auditory steady state response and bispectral index in human volunteers. Anesthesiology 2000: 93: 708–717.
Michenfelder JD, Theye Ra, Effects of fentanyl, droperidol, and innovar on canine cerebral metabolism and blood flow. Br J Anaesth 1971: 43: 630–636.
Michenfelder JD, Theye RA. Cerebral protection by thiopental during hypoxia. Anesthesiology 1973: 39: 510–517.
Michenfelder JD. The interdependency of cerebral functional and metabolic effects following massive doses of thiopental in the dog. Anesthesiology 1974: 41: 231–236.
Michenfelder JD, Milde JH, Sundt JM jr. Cerebral protection by barbiturate anesthesia. Use after middle cerebral artery occlusion in Java monkeys. Arch Neurol 1976: 33: 345–350.
Michenfelder JD. A valid demonstration of barbiturate-induced brain protection in man-At last. Anesthesiology 1986: 64: 140–142.
Milde LN, Milde JH, Michenfelder JD. Cerebral functional, metabolic, and hemodynamic effects of etomidate in dogs. Anesthesiology 1985: 63: 371–377.
Milde LN, Milde JH. Preservation of cerebral metabolites by etomidate during incomplete cerebral ischemia in dogs. Anesthesiology 1986: 65: 272–277.
Milde LN. The hypoxic mouse model for screening cerebral protective agents: a re-examination. Anesth Analg 1988: 67: 917–922.
Miller JD. Barbiturates and raised intracranial pressure. Ann Neurol 1979: 6: 189–193.
Miller R, Tausk HC, Stark DCC. Effect of innovar, fentanyl and droperidol on the cerebrospinal fluid pressure in neurosurgical patients. Can Anaesth Soc J 1975: 22: 502–508.
Modica PA, Tempelhoff R. Intracranial pressure during induction of anaesthesia and tracheal intubation with etomidate-induced EEG burst suppression. Can J Anaesth 1992: 39: 236–241.
Moffat JA, McDougall MJ, Brunet D, et al. Thiopental bolus during carotid endarterectomy-rational drug therapy? Can Anaesth Soc J 1983: 30: 615–622.
Möhler H, Okada T. Benzodiazepines receptor: demonstration in the central nervous system. Science 1977: 198: 849–851.
Moss E, Powell D, Gibson RM, McDowall DG. Effect of etomidate on intracranial pressure and cerebral perfusion pressure. Br J Anaesth 1979: 51: 347–351.
Moss E, Price DJ. Effect of propofol on brain retraction pressure and cerebral perfusion pressure. Br J Anaesth 1990: 65: 823–825.
Moss E. Alfentanil increases intracranial pressure when intracranial compliance is low. Anaesthesia 1992: 47: 134–136.
Motsch J, Brietbarth J, Salzmann R, et al. Kognitive und Psychomotorische Leistungsfähigkeit nach Isofluran-, Midazolam/Alfentanil- und Propofol Anästhesie – Eine vergleichende Untersushung. Anaesthesist 1992: 41: 185–191.
Munari C, Casaroli D, Matteuzzi G, Pacifico L. The use of althesin in drug-resistant status epilepticus. Epilepsia 1979: 20: 475–483.
Murkin JM, Farrar JK. The influence of high dose fentanyl-diazepam anesthesia on cerebral blood flow and cerebral oxygen consumption. Anesth Analg 1989: 68: S205.
Murugaiah KD, Hemmings HC. Effect of intravenous general anesthetics on [^{3}H]GABA release from rat cortical synaptosomes. Anesthesiology 1998: 89: 919–928.
Musella L, Wilder BJ, Schmidt RP. Electroencephalographic activation with intravenous methohexital in psychomotor epilepsia. Neurology 1971: 21: 594–602.
Nagata A, Nakao S, Nishizawa N, et al. Xenon inhibits but N_2O enhances ketamine-induced c-Fos expression in the rat posterior cingulate and retrosplenial cortices. Anesth Analg 2001: 92: 362–368.
Nakamura K, Hatano Y, Nishiwada M, Mori K. The vasodilator effect of thiamylal in dog mesenteric artery. Can J Phar 1991: 69: 1163.
Nelson SR, Howard RB, Cross RS, Samson F. Ketamine-induced changes in regional glucose utilization in the rat brain. Anesthesiology 1980: 52: 330–334.
Nilsson L. The influence of barbiturate anesthesia upon the energy state and upon acid-base parameters of the brain in arterial hypotension and in asphyxia. Acta Neurol Scand 1971: 47: 233–253.
Nilsson L, Siesjö BK. Influence of anesthesia on the balance between production and utilization of energy in the brain. J Neurochem 1974: 23: 29–36.
Nilsson L, Siesjö BK. The effect of phenobarbitone anaesthesia on blood flow and oxygen consumption in the rat brain. Acta Anaesthesiol Scand 1975: suppl 57: 18–24.
Nordström CH. Siesjö BK. Influence of phenobarbital on changes in the metabolites of the energy reserve of the cerebral cortex following complete ischemia. Acta Physiol Scand 1978: 104: 271–280.
Nugent M, Artru AA, Michenfelder JD. Cerebral metabolic, vascular and protective effects of midazolam maleate. Anesthesiology 1982: 56: 172–176.
Nussmeier NA, Arlund C, Slogoff S. Neuropsychiatric complications after cardiopulmonary bypass: Cerebral protection by barbiturate. Anesthesiology 1986: 64: 165–170.
Nussmeier NA, Fish KJ. Neuropsychologic dysfunction after cardiopulmonary bypass: A comparison of two institutions. Anesthesiology 1987: 67: A 14.

Obrist WD, Gennarelli TA, Segawa H, et al. Regulation of cerebral blood flow to neurological status and outcome in head-injured patients. J Neurosurg 1979: 51: 292–300.

Oguchi K, Arakawa K, Nelson SR, Samson F. The influence of droperidol, diazepam and physiostigmine on ketamine-induced behavior and brain regional glucose utilization in rat. Anesthesiology 1982: 57: 353–358.

Ogura K, Takayasu M, Decey RG. Differential effects of pentobarbital on intracerebral arterioles and venules of rats in vitro. Neurosurgery 1991: 28: 537–541.

Ong BY, MacIntyre CJ, Bose D, et al. Phenobarbital prevents loss of cerebral blood flow autoregulation after asphyxia in newborn lambs. Anesth Analg 1986: 65: S115.

Onodera H, Sato G, Kogure K. GABA and benzodiazepine receptors in the gerbil brain after transient ischaemia: Demonstration by quantitative receptor autoradiography. J Cereb Blood Flow Metab 1987: 7: 82–88.

Oren RE, Rasool NA, Rubinstein EH. Effect of ketamine on cerebral cortical blood flow and metabolism in rabbits. Stroke 1987: 18: 441–44.

Orser B. Propofol-induced neuroexcitation and receptor desensitization. Can J Anaesth 1994: 41: 366–371.

Otsuka T, Wei L, Acuff VR, et al. Variation in local cerebral blood flow response to high-dose pentobarbital sodium in the rat. Am J Physiol 1991: 261: H110–H120.

Otsuka T, Wei L, Bereczki D, et al. Pentobarbital produces dissimilar changes in glucose influx and utilization in brain. Am J Physiol 1991: 261: R265–75.

Owen H, Spence AA. Etomidate (editorial). Br J Anaesth 1984: 56: 555–556.

Paepe PD, Belpaire FM, Rosseel MT, et al. Influence of hypovolemia on the pharmacokinetics and the electroencephalographic effect of propofol in the rat. Anesthesiology 2000: 93: 1482–1490.

Peters CE, Korcok J, Gelb AW, Wilson JX. Anesthetic concentrations of propofol protect against oxidative stress in primary astrocyte cultures. Anesthesiology 2001: 94: 313–321.

Petersen KD, Landsfeldt U, Cold GE, Pedersen CB, Mau S, Rasmussen G, Pedersen HS. A prospective, randomized study of ICP during three anesthetics for elevtive craniotomy. A multicenter study. Acta Anaesthesiol Scand 1999: (suppl) 114: 101.

Pfenninger E, Grünert A, Bowdler I, Kilan J. The effect of ketamine on intracranial pressure during haemorrhagic shock under the conditions of both spontaneous breating and controlled ventilation. Acta Neurochir 1985: 78: 113–118.

Pfenninger E, Reith a. Ketamine and intracranial pressure. In Status of Ketamine in Anesthesiology, Domino EF (ed), NPP Books 1990: 109–118.

Piatt JH, Schiff SJ. High dose barbiturate therapy in neurosurgery and intensive care. Neurosurgery 1984: 15: 427–444.

Pickerodt VWA, McDowall DG, Coroneos NJ, Keaney NP. Effect of althesin on cerebral perfusion, cerebral metabolism and intracranial pressure in the anaesthetized baboon. Br J Anaesth 1972: 44: 751–758.

Pierce EC, Lambertsen CJ, Deutsch S, et al. Cerebral cinculation and metabolism during thiopental anesthesia and hyperventilation in man. J Clin Invest 1962: 41: 1664–1671.

Pinaud m, Lelausque JN, Fauchoux N, Chetanneau A. Effects of propofol on cerebral hemodynamics and metabolism in patients with head trauma. Anesthesiology 1988: 69: A569.

Preziosi P, Vacca M. Etomidate and corticothropic axis. Arch Intern Pharmacodyn 1982: 256: 308–310.

Prior PF, Maynard DE, Brierley JB. EEG monitoring for the control of anaesthesia produced by the infusion of althesin in primates. Br J Anaesth 1978: 50: 993–1001.

Prior JGL, Hinds CJ, Williams J, Prior PE. The use of etomidate in the management of severe head injury. Intensive Care Med 1983: 9: 313–320.

Procaccio F, Bingham RM, Hinds CJ, Prior PF,. Continuous EEG and ICP monitoring as a guide to the administration of althesin sedation in severe head injury. Intensive Care Med 1988: 14: 148–155.

Puhringer F, Hormann CH, Langmayr J, et al. The effect of alfentanil on cerebrospinal fluid pressure in human volunteers. Eur J Anaesthesiol 1997: 14: 211–214.

Ramani R, Todd MM, Warner DS. A dose-response study of the influence of propofol on cerebral blood flow, metabolism and the electroencephalogram in the rabbit. J Neurosurg Anesthesiol 1992: 4: 110–119.

Rasmussen NJ, Rosendal T, Overgaard J. Althesin in neurosurgical patients: Effects on cerebral haemodynamics and metabolism. Acta Anaesthesiol Scand 1978: 22: 257–269.

Ratnakumari L, Hemmings HC. Inhibition by propofol of [H]-batrachotoxinin-A 20-(benzoate binding to voltage-dependent sodium channels in the rat cortical synaptosomes. Br J Pharmacol 1996: 119: 1498–1504.

Ratnakumari L, Hemmings HC. Effects of propofol on sodium channel-dependent sodium influx and glutamate release in rat cerebrocortical synaptosomes. Anesthesiology 1997: 86: 428–439.

Ravussin P, Guinard JP, Ralley F, Thorin D. Effect of propofol on cerebrospinal fluid pressure and cerebral perfusion pressure in patients undergoing craniotomy. Anaesthesia 1988a: 43 (suppl): 37–41.

Ravussin P, Berger-Bayer M, Nydegger M, Freeman J. Thiopentone-isoflurane vs propofol in neuroanesthesia for intracranial surgery. Anesthesiology 1988b: 69: A577.

Ravussin P, de Tribolet N. Total intravenous anesthesia with propofol for burst suppression in cerebral aneurysm surgery: Preliminary report of 42 patients. Neurosurgery 1993: 32: 236–240.

Rehberg B, Duch DS. Suppression of central nervous system sodium channels by propofol. Anesthesiology 1999: 91: 512–520.

Reicher D, Bhalla P, Rubinstein EH. Cholinergic cerebral vasodilator effect of ketamine in rabbits. Stroke 1987: 18: 445–449.

Reinstrup P, Ståhl N, Mellergård P, et al. Intracerebral microdialysis in clinical practice: baseline values for chemical markers during wakefulness, anesthesia, and neurosurgery. Neurosurgery 2000: 47: 701–710.

Renou AM, Vernhiet J, Orgogozo JM, Caille JM. Effets de l'alfatesine (CT 1341) sur le debit sanguin et le metabolisme cerebral chez l'homme, modifications globales er regionales. Ann Anesthesiol Fr 1976: 17: 1247–1254.

Renou AM, Vernhiet J, Macrez P et al. Cerebral blood flow and metabolism during etomidate anaesthesia in man. Br J Anaesth 1978: 50: 1047–1051.

Roach GW, Newman MF, Murkin JM, et al. Ineffectiveness of burst suppression therapy in mitigating perioperative cerebrovascular dysfunction. Anesthesiology 1999: 90: 1255–1264.

Robertson SC, Brown III P, Loftus CM. Effects of etomidate administration on cerebral collateral flow. Neurosurgery 1998: 43: 317–324.

Rockoff MA, Marchall LF, Shapiro HM. High-dose barbiturate therapy in humans: A clinical review of 60 patients. Ann Neurol 1979: 6: 194–199.

Sato K, Wu J, Kikuchi T, Wang Y, et al. Differential effects of ketamine and pentobarbitone on acetylcholine release from the rat hippocampus and striatum. Br J Anaesth 1996: 77: 381–384.

Safar P, Stezoski W, Nemoto EM. Amelioration of brain damage after 12 minutes cardiac arrest in dogs. Arch Neurol 1976: 33: 91–95.

Saija A, Princi P, DePasquale R, Costa G. Modifications of the permeability of the blood-brain barrier and local cerebral metabolism in pentobarbital- and ketamine-anaesthetized rats. Neuropharmacology 1989: 28: 997–1002.

Sakabe T, Tsutsui T, Maekawa T, et al. Local cerebral glucose utilization during nitrous oxide and pentobarbital anesthesia in rats. Anesthesiology 1985: 63: 262–266.

Sakai K, Cho S, Fukusaki M, et al. The effects of propofol with and without ketamine on human cerebral blood flow velocity and CO_2 response. Anesth Analg 2000: 90: 377–382.

Sari A, Okuda Y, Takeshita H. The effects of thalamonal on cerebral circulation and oxygen consumption in man. Br J Anaesth 1972: 44: 330–334.

Sari A, Maekawa T, Tohjo M, et al. Effects of althesin on cerebral blood flow and oxygen consumption in man. Br J Anaesth 1976: 48: 545–550.

Saul TG, Ducker TB. Effect of intracranial pressure monitoring and aggressive treatment on mortality in severe head injury. J Neurosurg 1982: 56: 498–503.

Scheller MS, Drummond JC, Todd MM, et al. Are recommendations regarding barbiturate protection during bypass justified? Anesthesiology 1986b: 65: 230–231.

Schregel W, Schäfermayer H, Müller C, et al. Einfluss von Halothan, Alfentanil und Propofol auf Flussgeschwindigkeiten, "Gefässquerschnit" und "Volumenfluss" in der a. Cerebri Media. Anaesthesist 1992: 41: 21–26.

Schregel W, Geisser S, Winkling M, Schaefermayer H, Cunitz G. Transcranial Doppler monitoring during induction of anesthesia: Effects of propofol, thiopental, and hyperventilation in patients with large malignant brain tumors. J Neurosurg Anesthesiol. 1993: 5: 86–93.

Schubert A, Licina MG, Lineberry PJ. The effect of ketamine on human somatosensory evoked potentials and its modification by nitrous oxide. Anesthesiology 1990: 72: 33–39.

Schulte am Esch J, Pfeiffer G, Hiemig I, Entzian W. The influence of intravenous anaesthetic agents on primarily increased intracranial pressure. Acta Neurochir 1978: 45: 15–25.

Schulte D, Callado LF, Davidson C, et al. Propofol decreases stimulated dopamine release in the rat nucleus accumbens by a mechanism indipendent of dopamine D_2 $GABA_A$ and NMDA receptors. Br J Anaesth 2000: 84: 250–253.

Schwedler M, Miletich DJ, Albrecht RF. Cerebral blood flow and metabolism following ketamine administration. Can Anaesth Soc J 1982: 29: 222–226.

Sear JW, Walters FJM, Wilkins DG, Willatts SM. Etomidate by infusion for neuroanaesthesia. Kinetic and dynamic interactions with nitrous oxide. Anaesthesia 1984: 39: 12–18.

Selman RW, Spetzler RF, Roessmann UR, et al. Barbiturate infusion coma therapy for focal cerebral ischaemia. J Neurosurg 1981: 55: 220–226.

Seubert CN, Morey TE, Martynyik AE, et al. Midazolam selectively potentiates the A_{2A}-but not A_1-receptor-mediated effects of adenosine. Anesthesiology 2000: 92: 567–577.

Shapira Y, Artru AA, Lam AM. Ketamine decreases cerebral infarct volume and improves neurological outcome following experimental head injury in rats. J Neurosurg Anesthesiol 1992: 4: 231–240.

Shapira Y, Lam AM, Artru AA, Eng C, Soltow L. Ketamine alters calcium and magnesium in brain tissue following experimental head trauma in rats. J Neurosurg Anesthesiol 1993: 13: 962–968.

Shapiro HM, Wyte SR, Harris AB, Galindo A. Acute intraoperative intracranial hypertension in neurosurgical patients. Anesthesiology 1972a: 37: 399–405.

Shapiro HM, Wyte SR, Harris AB. Ketamine anaesthesia in patients with intracranial pathology. Br J Anaesth 1972b: 44: 1200–1204.

Shapiro HM, Galindo A, Wyte SR, Harris AB. Rapid intraoperative reduction of intracranial pressure with thiopental Br J Anaesth 1973: 45: 1057–1061.

Shapiro HM, Wyte SR, Loeser J. Barbiturate augmented hypothermia for reduction of persistent intracranial hypertension J Neurosurg 1974: 40: 90–100.

Shapiro HM. Barbiturates in brain ischaemia. Br J Anaesth 1985: 57: 82–95.

Shapiro HM. Anaesthesia effects upon cerebral blood flow, cerebral metabolism, electroencephalogram, and evoked potentials. In: Miller DR (ed) Anesthesia, Churchill Livingstone, New York, Edinburgh, London, 1986: 2: 1249–1288.

Shimaoka M, Iida T, Ohara A, et al. Ketamine inhibits nitric oxide production in mouse-activated macrophage-like cells. Br J Anaesth 1996: 77: 238–242.

Sidi A, Cotev S, Hadani M, et al. Long-term barbiturate infusion to reduce intracranial pressure. Critical Care Medicin 1983: 11: 478–481.

Siesjö BK. Cerebral circulation and metabolism. J Neurosurg 1984: 60: 883–908.

Simpson VJ, Blednov Y. Propofol produces differences in behavior but not choride channel function between selected lines of mice. Anesth Analg 1996: 82: 327–331.

Smith AL, Hoff JT, Nielsen SL, Larson CP. Barbiturate protection in acute focal cerebral ischaemia. Stroke 1974: 5: 1–7.

Smith AL, Marque JJ. Anesthetics and cerebral edema. Anesthesiology 1976: 45: 64–72.

Smith DS, Rehncrona S, Siesjö BK. Inhibitory effects of different barbiturates on lipid peroxidation in the brain tissue in vitro: Comparison with the effects of promethazine and chlorpromazine. Anesthesiology 1980: 53: 186–194.

Smith DS, Keykhah MM, O'Neill JJ, Harp JR. The effect of etomidate pretreatment on cerebral high energy metabolites, lactate, and glucose during severe hypoxia in the rat. Anesthesiology 1989: 71: 438–443.

Smith I, White PF, Nathanson M, Gouldson R. Propofol. An update of its clinical use. Anesthesiology 1994: 81: 1005–1043.

Smith M, Sneyd JR, Ross DA, Henry TR. Effects of propofol sedation or seizures and intracranially recorded epileptiform activity in pateints with partial epilepsy. Anesthesiology 1995: 82: 843–851.

Snead OC, Yu RK, Huttenlocher PR. Gammahydroxybuturate: correlation of serum and cerebrospinal fluid levels with electroencephalographic and behavioral effects. Neurology 1976: 26: 51–56.

Sneyd JR. Propofol and epilepsy. Br J Anaesth 1999: 82: 168–169.

Snyder BD, Ramirez-Lassepas M, et al. Failure of thiopental to modify global anoxic injury. Stroke 1979: 10: 135–141.

Sokoll MD, Kassell NF, Davles LR. Large dose thiopental anesthesia for intracranial aneurysm surgery. Neurosurgery 1982: 10: 555-562.

Spahr-Schopfer I, Vutskits L, Toni N, et al. Differential neurotoxic effects of propofol on dissociated cortical cells and organotypic hippocampal cultures. Anesthesiology 2000: 92: 1408-1417.

Spetzler RF, Wilson CB, Weinstein P, et al. Normal perfusion pressure breakthrough theory. In: Clinical Neurosurgery, Williams and Wilkins Company, 1978: 26: 651-672.

Spetzler RF, Selman WR, Roski RA, Bonstelle C. Cerebral revascularization during barbiturate coma in primates and humans. Surg Neurol 1982: 17: 111-115.

Steen PA, Milde JH, Michenfelder JD. Cerebral metabolic and vascular effects of barbiturate therapy following complete global ischaemia. J Neurochem 1978: 31: 1317-1324.

Steen PA, Milde JH, Michenfelder JD. No barbiturate protection in a dog model of complete cerebral ischaemia Ann Neurol 1979: 5: 343-349.

Steen PA, Michenfelder JD. Barbiturate protection in tolerant and nontolerant hypoxic mice. Anesthesiology 1979: 50: 404-408.

Steen PA, Michenfelder JD. Neurotoxicity of Anaesthetics. Anesthesiology 1979: 50: 437-453.

Steen PA, Newberg L, Milde JH, Michenfelder JD. Hypothermia and barbiturates: Individual and combined effects on canine cerebral oxygen consumption. Anesthesiology 1983: 58: 527-532.

Stephan H, Sonntag H, Schenk HD, Kohlhausen S. Einfluss von Disoprivan (Propofol) auf die Durchblutung und Sauerstoffverbrauch des Gehirns and die CO_2 Reaktivität der Hirngefässe beim Menschen. Anaesthetist 1987: 36: 60-65.

Stephan H, Sonntag H, Seyde WC, Henze T, Textor J. Energie- und Aminosäurenstoffwechsel des Menschlichen Gehirns unter Desoprivan und verschiedenen $paCO_2$- Werten. Anaesthesist 1988: 37: 297-304.

Stewart PA, Hayakawa EM, Carlen PL. Ethanol and pentobarbital increase blood-brain barrier permeability to horseradish peroxidase. Brain Res 1988: 443: 12-20.

Stockard JJ, Bickford R. The neurophysiology of anesthesia. In: Gordon E (ed), A Basis and Practice of Neuroanesthesia. Amsterdam:Excerpta Medica 1975: 3-46.

Strebel S, Kaufmann M, Guardiola P-M, Schaefer H-G. Cerebral vasomotor responsiveness to carbon dioxide is preserved during propofol and midazolam anaesthesia in humans. Anaesth Analg 1994: 78: 884-888.

Strebel S, Kaufmann M, Maitre L, Scgaefer HG. Effects of ketamine on cerebral blood flow velocity in humans. Influence of pretreatment with midazolam or esmolol. Anaesthesia 1995: 50: 223-228.

Strebel S, Lam AM, Matta B, et al. Dynamic and static cerebral autoregulation during isoflurane, desflurane, and propofol anesthesia. Anesthesiology 1995: 83: 66-76.

Stullken AH, Milde JH, Michenfelder JD, Tinker JH. The nonlinear responses of cerebral metabolism to low concentrations of halothane, enflurane, isoflurane and thiopental. Anesthesiology 1977: 46: 28-34.

S¢ndergård W. Intracranial pressure during general anaesthesia. Dan Med Bull 1961: 8: 18-26.

Taguchi K, Hagiwara Y, Suzuki Y, Kubo T. Effects of morphine on release of acetylcholine in the rat striatum: An in vivo microdialysis study. Naunyn-Schmiedbergs Archives of Pharmacology 1993: 347: 9-13.

Takeshita H, Okuda Y, Sari A. The effects of ketamine on cerebral circulation and metabolism in man. Anesthesiology 1972: 36: 69-75.

Takahashi T, Takasaki M, Namiki A, Dohi S. Effects of althesin on cerebrospinal fluid pressure. Br J Anaesth 1973: 45: 179-184.

Tamasy V, Koranyi L, Tekeres M. EEG and multiple unit activity during ketamine and barbiturate anaesthesia. Br J Anaesth 1975: 47: 1247-1251.

Tanalian DL, Kosek P, Mody I, MacIver MB. The role of the $GABA_A$ receptor/chloride channel complex in anesthesia. Anesthesiology 1993: 78: 757-776.

Taverna FA, Cameron RB, Hampson DL, et al. Sensitivity of AMPA receptors to pentobarbital. Eur J Pharmacol 1994: 267: R3-5.

Terasako K, Nakamura K, Toda H, et al. Barbiturates inhibit endothelium-dependent and independent relaxations mediated by cyclic GMP. Anesth Analg 1994: 78: 823-830.

Thompson GE. Ketamine-induced convulsions. Anesthesiology 1972: 37: 662-663.

Thomson AM, West DC, Lodge D. An N-methylaspartate receptor-mediated synapse in rat cerebral cortex: a site of action of ketamine? Nature 1985: 313: 479-481.

Todd MM, Chadwick HS, Shapiro HM, et al. The neurologic effects of thiopental therapy following experimental cardiac arrest in cats. Anesthesiology 1982: 57: 76-86.

Todd MM, Drummond JC, SangU H. The hemodynamic consequences of high-dose methohexital anesthesia in humans. Anesthesiology 1984a: 61: 495-501.

Todd MM, Drummond JC. A comparison of the cerebrovascular and metabolic effects of halothane and isoflurane in the cat. Anesthesiology 1984b: 60: 276-282.

Todd MM, Drummond JC, SangU H. The hemodynamic consequences of high-dose thiopental anesthesia. Anesth Analg 1985: 64: 681-687.

Todd MM, Drummond JC, Sang H. Hemodynamic effects of high dose pentobarbital: Studies in elective neurosurgical patients. Neurosurgery 1987: 20: 559-563.

Todd MM, Hindman BJ, Warner DS. Barbiturate protection and cardiac surgery: A different result (editorial). Aneesthesiology 1991: 74: 402-405.

Todd MM, Wu B, Warner DS, Maktabi M. The dose-related effects of nitric oxide synthase inhibition on cerebral blood flow during isoflurane and pentobarbital anesthesia. Anesthesiology 1994: 80: 1128-1136.

Traeger SM, Henning RJ, Doblin W, et al. Hemodynamic effects of pentobarbital therapy for intracranial hypertension. Critical care Medicine 1983: 11: 697-701.

Turner JM, Coroneos NJ, Gibson RM, et al. The effect of althesin on intracranial pressure in man. Br J Anaesth 1973: 45: 168-171.

Tsuji T, Chiba S. Responses of isolated canine and simian basilar arteries to thiopentone by a newly designed pharmacological method for measuring vascular responsiveness. Acta Neurochirurgica 1986: 80: 57-61

Upton RN, Ludbrook GL, Grant C, Gray EC. In *vivo* relationships between the cerebral pharmacokinetics and pharmacodynamics of thiopentone in sheep after short-term administration. J Pharmacokinet Biopharm 1996: 24: 1-18.

Upton RN, Ludbrook GL, Grant C, Doolette DJ. The effect of altered cerebral blood flow on the cerebral kinetics of thiopental and propofol in sheep. Anesthesiology 2000: 93: 1085-1094.

van Aken J, Rolly G. Influence of etomidate, a new short acting anaesthetic agent, on cerebral blood flow in man. Acta Anaesthesiol Belg 1976: suppl 27: 175–180.
van Aken J, Rolly G, Van Weehaeghe X, De Deyne C. Can nitrous oxide be replaced by propofol in neuroanaesthesia? Preliminary results. Eur J Anaesthesiol 1990: 7: 483–491.
Vandesteene A, Trempont V, Engelman E, et al. Effect of propofol on cerebral blood flow and metabolism in man. Anaesthesia 1988: 43 (suppl): 42–43.
van Hemelrijck J, van Aken H, Plets C, Goffin J. The effects of propofol on ICP and cerebral perfusion pressure in patients with brain tumors. Anesthesiology 1988: 69: A570.
van Hemelrijck J, Tempelhoff R, Jellich WS, White PF. Comparison of thiopental isoflurane-N_2O, propofol-N_2O and propofol alone for neuroanesthesia. Anesthesiology 1990a: 73: No3A A167.
van Hemelrijck J, Fitch W, Mattheussen M, et al. Effect of propofol on cerebral circulation and autoregulation in the babbon. Anesth Analg 1990b: 71: 49–54.
van Hemelrijck J, Tempelhoff R, Jellich WS, White PF. Use of EEG for determining propofol requirement during neuroanesthesia. Anesthesiology 1990c: 73: No 3A: A202.
van Hemelrijck J, Fitch W, Mattheussen M, et al. Effect of propofol on cerebral circulation and autoregulation in the baboon. Anesth Analg 1990d: 71: 49–54.
van Reempts J, Borgers M, van Eyndhoven J, Hermans C. Protective effects of etomidate in hypoxic-ischaemic brain damage in the rat. A morphologic assessment. Experimental Neurology 1982: 76: 181–195.
Vayer P, Mandel P, Maitre M. Conversion of gamma-hydorxybutyrate to gamma-aminobutyrate in vitro. J Neurochem 1985: 45: 810–814.
Vernhiet J, Renou AM, Orgogozo JM, et al. Effects of a diazepam-fentanyl mixture on cerebral blood flow and oxygen consumption in man. Br J Anaesth 1978: 5O: 165–169.
Veselis RA, Reinsel RA, Wronski M, et al. EEG and memory effects of low-dose infusions of propofol. Br J Anaesth 1992: 69: 246–254.
Veselis RA, Reinsel RA, Beattie BJ, et al. Midazolam changes cerebral blood flow in discrete brain regions: an $H_2{}^{15}O$ positron emission tomography study. Anesthesiology 1997: 87: 1106–1117.
Vuyk J, Hennis PJ, Burm AGL, et al. Comparison of midazolam and propofol in combination with alfentanil for total intraveneous anesthesia. Anesth Analg 1990: 71: 645–650.
Wada DR, Harashima H, Ebling WF, et al. Effects of thiopental on regional blood flows in the rat. Anesthesiology 1996: 84: 596–604.
Wagner RL, White PF, Kan PB, et al. Inhibition of adrenal steroidogenesis by the anaesthetic etomidate N Engl J Med 1984: 310: 1415–1421.
Wagner RL, White PF. Etomidate inhibits adrenocortical function in surgical patients. Anesthesiology 1984: 61: 647–651.
Ward JD, Becker DP, Miller JD, et al. Failure of prophylactic barbiturate coma in the treatment of severe head injury. J Neurosurg 1985: 62: 383–388.
Watson JC, Drummond JC, Patel PM, Sano T, Akrawi W, Sang U H. An assessment of the cerebral protective effects of etomidate in a model of incomplete forebrain ischemia in the rat. Neurosurgery 1992: 30: 540–544.
Watts ADJ, Eliasziw M, Gelb AW. Propofol and hyperventilation for the treatment of increased intracranial pressure in rabbits. Anesth Analg 1998: 87: 564–568.
Wauquier A, Van den Broeck WAE, Verheyen JL, Janssen PAJ. Electroencephalographic study of the short-acting hypnotics etomidate and methohexital in dogs. Europ J Pharmacol 1978: 47: 367–377.
Wauquier A, Achton D, Clincke G, Niemegers CJE. Anti-hypoxic effects of etomidate, thiopental and methohexital. Arch Int Pharmacodyn Ther 1981: 249: 330–334.
Wauquier A. Brain protective properties of etomidate and flunarizine. J Cereb Blood Flow Metab 1982: 2 (suppl 1) S53–S56.
Wechsler RL, Dripps RD, Kety SS. Blood flow and oxygen consumption of the human brain during anesthesia produced by thiopental. Anesthesiology 1951: 12: 308–313.
Weinstabl C, Mayer N, Hammerle AF, Spiss CK. Effekte von Propofolbolusgaben auf das Intrakranielle Druckverhalten beim Schädel-Hirn-Trauma. Anaesthesist 1990: 39: 521–524.
Weir DL, Goodchild CS, Graham DI. Effects on indices of cerebral ischemia. J Neurosurg Anesthesiol 1989: 1: 284–289
Weir P, Wu J, Tremper K, Buchsbaum M, et al. Ketamine induced changes in cerebral glucose utilization in man as measured by PET scan. Anesth Analg 1992: 74: S344.
Wendling WW, Daniels FB, Chen D, et al. Ketamine directly dilates bovine cerebral arteries by acting as a calcium entry blocker. J Neurosurg Anesthesiol 1994: 6: 186–192.
Werner C, Hoffman WE, Segil LJ, et al. Effects of propofol on cerebral and spinal cord blood flow autoregulation in rats. Anesthesiology 1990: 73: No 3A, A 694.
Werner C, Hoffman WE, Kochs E, et al. The effects of propofol on cerebral blood flow in correlation to cerebral blood flow velocity in dogs. J Neurosurg Anesthesiol 1992: 4: 41–46
Werner C, Reeker W, Engelhard K, et al. Ketamin acemate and S-(+)-ketamine. Cerebrovascular effects and neuroprotection following focal ischemia. Anaesthesist 1997: 46 (suppl 1): S55–60.
Wiklund L. Reversal of sedation and respiratory depression after anaesthesia by the combined use of physiostigmine and nalaxone in neurosurgical patients. Acta Anaesthesiol Scand 1986: 30: 374–378.
Williams GL, Pollay M, Seale T, Hisey B, Roberts RA. Benzodiazepine receptors and cerebrospinal fluid formation. J Neurosurg 1990: 72: 759–762.
Winters WD. Epilepsia or anaesthesia with ketamine. Anesthesiology 1972: 36: 309–312.
Wolff J, Carl P, Hansen PB, H¢gskilde S, et al. Effects of eltanolone on cerebral blood flow and metabolism in healthy volunteers. Anesthesiology 1994: 81: 623–627.
Wolfson LI, Sakurada O. Sokoloff L. Effects of γ-butyrolactone on local cerebral glucose utilization in the rat. J Neurochem 1977: 29: 777–783.
Wu J, Kikuche T, Wang Y, et al. Nox- concetrations in the rat hippocampus and striatum have no direct relationship to anaesthesia induced by ketamine. Br J Anaesth 2000: 84: 183–189.
Wyte SR, Shapiro HM, Turner P, Harris AB. Ketamine-induced intracranial hypertension. Anaesthesiology 1972: 36: 174–176.
Xuan Y-T, Glass PSA. Propofol regulation of calcium entry pathways in cultured A10 and rat aortic smooth muscle cells. Br J Pharmacol 1996: 117: 5–12.
Yakushiji T, Nakamura K, Hatano Y, Mori K. Conparison of the vasodilator effects of thiopentone and pentobarbitone. Can J Anaesth 1992: 39: 604–609.

Yano M, Ikeda Y, Kobayshi S, et al. The outcome with barbiturate therapy in severe head injuries. In: Miller JD, Teasdale GM, Rowan JO, Galvraith SL, Mendelow AD (eds), Intracranial Pressure VI, Springer Verlag, Berlin, Heidelberg 1986: 769–773.

Yatsu FM, Diamond I, Graziano C, Linquist P. Experimental brain ischaemia: Protection from irreversible damage with a rapid-acting barbiturate (methohexital). Stroke 1972: 3: 726–732.

Yonas H, Dujovny M, Nelson D, et al. The controlled delivery of thiopental and delayed cerebral revascularization. Surg Neurol 1981: 15: 27–34.

Yoshida K, Marmarou A, Furuse M. The metabolic protection of hypoxia by etomidate evaluated by magnetic resonance spectroscopy. In: Intracranial Pressure VIII. Avezaat CJJ, van Eijndhoven JHM, Maas AIR, Tans JThJ (eds). Springer Verlag 1993: 273–275.

Zacny JP, Lichtor JL, Thompson W, Apfelbaum JL. Propofol at a subanesthetic dose may have abuse potential i healthy volunteers. Anesth Analg 1993: 77: 544-552.

Zaiden JR, Klochany A, Martin WM, et al. Effect of thiopental on neurologic outcome following coronary artery bypass grafting. Anesthesiology 1991: 74: 406–411.

Zattoni J, Siani C, Balestrero MA et al. Effetto ipotensivo intracranico ed arterioso sistemico di 0.35 e 0.80 mg/kg ev di Diprivan durante neuroanestesia in ventilazione controllata. In: Atti 3rd Riunione Italo-Francece di Neuroanestesia e Rianimazione. Capri, 1986: 54

Zhan RZ, Fujiwara N, Endoh H, et al. Thiopental inhibits increases in $[Ca^{2+}]_I$ induced by membrane depolarization, NMDA receptor activation, and ischemia in rat hippocampal and cortical slices. Anesthesiology 1998: 89: 456–466.

Zhu H, Cottrell JE, Kass IS. The effect of thiopental and propofol on NMDA- and AMPA-mediated glutamate excitotoxicity. Anesthesiology 1997: 87: 944–951

Åkesen J, Björkman S, Messeter K, Rosén I. Low-dose midazolam antagonizes cerebral metabolic stimulation by ketamine in the pig.. Acta Anaesthesiol Scand 1993: 37: 521–531.

Analgesics

Opioids are strong respiratory depressors. As such their place in neuroanaesthesia and neurointensive care should be carefully evaluated. Warnings against opioids in spontaneous breathing patients with cerebral mass expanding lesions are justified. Even 3 mg morphine intravenously can result in hypercapnia that might lead to luxury perfusion and ICP increase (Cold and Felding 1995). Opioids, however, create unparalleled haemodynamic stability and blunt neuroendocrine responses to surgery. Opioid-based induction is complicated by muscular rigidity and difficult ventilation (Hamilton and Cullen 1953, Comstock et al. 1981). The sequelas of difficult ventilation are clinically important and include hypertension, hypoxaemia, pulmonary hypertension, respiratory acidosis and increased ICP (Benthuysen et al. 1986, Benthuysen et al. 1988, Mets and James 1992). The incidence of these complications varies depending on the opioid and dosage used, and the rate at which it is administrated. The incidence of difficult ventilation after a moderate dosage of sufentanil ranges from 84 to 100% (Horrow et al. 1991, Weinger 1993). The common opinion is that difficult ventilation is caused by rigidity of the abdominal or thoracic musculature. Recently, closure of glottis has been proposed to be responsible (Abrams et al. 1996, Bennett et al. 1997).

Action of receptors and transmitters

Morphine and other central analgesics are known to decrease cholinergic neurotransmission in many brain regions. Opioid inhibition of acetylcholine release is relevant to anaesthesia because acetylcholine plays a key role in the central nervous system regulation of arousal, respiratory control, and perception of painful stimuli (Lambert and Appadu 1995, Durieux 1996, Lydic and Baghdoyan 1997).

The median pontine reticular formation is a cholinoceptive region that receives its cholinergic input from more rostral laterodorsal tegmental nuclei and peduncolopontine tegmental nuclei.

Studies in cats indicate that morphine inhibits acetylcholine at the cholinergic cell body region of the laterodorsal tegmental nuclei, and the terminal field in the medial pontine reticular formation. Acetylcholine in the medial pontine reticular formation was not altered by remifentanil, but was significantly decreased by fentanyl (Mortazavi et al. 1999).

It is well known that high concentrations of various opioid agonists and antagonists protect neurones against cerebral ischaemia and neurotoxicity caused by exogenously applied N-methyl-D-aspartate. Electrophysiologic and receptor binding studies indicate that some opioid agonists (meperidine, methadone and ketobemidone) reduce NMDA-induced depolarisation in rat-brain slice preparations and inhibit dizocilpine binding in rat cortical and forebrain membranes. These studies suggest that some opioids have NMDA receptor antagonist properties. Other studies indicate that low-affinity NMDA receptor antagonist activity is a common characteristic of various opioid compounds, and that the inhibition is a result of channel-blockade mechanisms at the site, which partially corresponds with those of Mg^{++} and ketamine (Yamakura et al. 1999).

Morphine, experimental studies

CBF and $CMRO_2$

In dogs subjected to incremental doses of morphine up to 1.2 mg/kg a progressive decrease of $CMRO_2$ and CBF to 85% and 45% of control has been found. A single dose of morphine 2 mg/kg had the same effect. These effects were reversed by pain stimulation (Kuramoto et al. 1979) and nalorphine, which initially produce an overshoot in both CBF and $CMRO_2$ (Takeshita et al. 1972). In the same animal morphine 1 mg/kg intravenously reduces CBF and spinal blood flow to 73% of control. This change is associated with a decrease in $CMRO_2$ (Matsumiya and Dohi 1983). In another study of artificially ventilated cats CBF, oxygen extraction, and consumption were not altered by 1.5 mg/kg morphine (Buchweitz et al. 1984).

Regional CBF

In cats CBF and oxygen extraction in the hypothalamus and thalamic decreased. The study indicates that morphine produces changes in cerebral neuronal and synaptic activity which lowers oxygen consumption in regions rich in opioid receptors, while brain oxygen supply or oxygen consumption were not affected (Buchweitz et al. 1984).

ICP

When morphine is administered to artificially ventilated dogs CSF pressure is unchanged. Under these circumstances nalorphine increases CSF pressure (Weitzner et al. 1963).

Blood-brain barrier

Studies in rats suggest that morphine may be effective in reducing the blood-brain barrier disruption by hyperosmolar mannitol without significant effects on systemic blood pressure (Chi et al. 2000).

Hypocapnia

In dogs hypocapnia decreases plasma clearance and increases brain concentration of morphine (Nishitateno et al. 1979).

Morphine, human studies

ICP, CBF and $CMRO_2$

Studies in healthy volunteers during nitrous oxide and normocapnia indicate that morphine in doses ranging from 1–3 mg/kg, did not change CBF, $CMRO_2$ or CMR-glucose, but decreased MABP and CVR, leaving CBF unchanged (Jobes et al. 1977). During spontaneous respiration morphine, like all central analgesics, induces respiratory depression with hypercapnia, which secondarily decreases CVR and increases CBV, CBF and ICP, leaving $CMRO_2$ unchanged. The respiratory depression after 10 mg morphine is not significantly altered in elderly patients (Daykin et al. 1986). However, in critically ill patients with renal failure morphine clearance is impaired, and a prolonged effect upon ICP might be expected (Bion et al. 1986). Even small doses of morphine provokes increase in $AVDO_2$ in the postoperative period after craniotomy (Cold and Felding 1993).

In patients with severe head injury intravenous morphine (2μg/kg) induced a moderate increase in ICP and decrease in MABP and CPP, without any significant change in $AVDO_2$ and middle cerebral artery flow velocity (de Nadal et al. 2000).

Cerebral autoregulation

The cerebral autoregulation (CA) is not affected by morphine (Jobes et al. 1975).

EEG

Morphine administered for premedication has little effect on the EEG activity. However, in dosages of 1–2 mg/kg, some decrease in frequency occurs, and a more frontal distribution of activity is observed. During nitrous oxide anaesthesia intravenous morphine elicits changes in EEG with desynchronising, an increase in beta activity, and drop out of frontal theta activity (Stockard and Bichford 1975).

Pethidine

CBF and $CMRO_2$

Pethidine gives rise to a small decrease in CBF and $CMRO_2$ (Messick and Theye 1969). Like morphine, pethidine given during nitrous oxide anaesthesia provokes excitatory EEG effects (Pearcy et al. 1957, Stockard et al. 1972).

Shivering

Pethidine is used for postoperative shivering. It effectively reduces the elevated metabolic demand (Macintyre et al. 1987). The anti-shivering property is not fully mediated by m-receptors. Stimulation of k-receptors seems a likely alternative explanation for the anti-shivering action (Kurz et al. 1993).

Phenoperidine

CBF and ICP

Phenoperidine, has been used combined with droperidol for neuroanaesthesia. Given together with droperidol to patients with normal CSF-pathway,

ICP is unchanged (Fitch et al. 1969). In patients with normal arteriography, CBF is unchanged during the combined use of droperidol and phenoperidine (Wilkinson and Brown 1970). However, given alone, to patients with severe head injury and intracranial hypertension, an increase in ICP occurs (Grummitt and Goat 1984). In another study of traumatic coma, phenoperidine did not change ICP, but a significant decrease in MABP and CPP was observed, suggesting that bolus administration of phenoperidine should be avoided in traumatic coma (Bingham and Hinds 1987). Whether autoregulatory mechanisms regulating CVR are responsible for ICP changes have not been investigated.

Fentanyl, experimental studies

CBF and $CMRO_2$

In cats, fentanyl induces an increase in CBF and $CMRO_2$ (Nilsson and Ingvar 1965, Freeman and Ingvar 1967). In comparison, studies of venous outflow in dogs during nitrous oxide, indicate a 18% decrease in $CMRO_2$ and a 47% decrease in CBF after fentanyl in doses of 0.006 mg/kg (Michenfelder and Theye 1971). Milde et al. (1989) studied the effect of fentanyl 50 and 100 mg/kg upon CBF and $CMRO_2$ in dogs, and found that these doses had minimal effect on CBF, oxygen uptake, and the energy state of the brain. In studies of pigs subjected to fentanyl/nitrous oxide and relaxed with pancuronium CBF, $CMRO_2$, CO_2 reactivity and EEG were stable throughout a 100 min period (Åkeson et al. 1993). Thus species, dosage, and rate of administration must play a role.

CO_2 reactivity and cerebral autoregulation (CA)

In dogs, the CO_2 reactivity is unaffected by fentanyl, and the drug does not change cerebral CA (McPherson and Traystman 1984). Neither is the CA affected during fentanyl-nitrous oxide anaesthesia (Hoffman et al. 1992).

In the dog hypocapnia decreases the plasma concentration and increases the brain concentration of fentanyl (Ainslie et al. 1979).

EEG

The discrepancy in CBF response might be explained by the fact that fentanyl in some species induces epileptic EEG changes and metabolic activation (DeCastro et al. 1979, Sebel et al. 1981, Safwat and Daniel 1983, Tommasino et al. 1984, Kofke et al. 1996). In rats fentanyl in small dosages decreases CBF and suppresses the EEG, while higher dosages induce epileptic activity and augment CBF as well as $CMRO_2$ (Safo et al. 1983). During fentanyl-induced epileptic seizure the percentage increase in $CMRO_2$ is higher than that of CBF, suggesting that the increase in flow does not follow the metabolic demand, and thus creates a state of imminent ischaemia (Carlsson et al. 1982).

Limbic system

In rats subjected to fentanyl-induced epileptoid activity a relative hypermetabolism in the limbic system, coupled with a significant reduction of glucose utilisation in the rest of the brain has been observed. These findings suggest a role of the limbic system in the genesis of seizure activity during fentanyl administration (Tommasino et al. 1984).

Energy charge

Although high-dose fentanyl suppresses global $CMRO_2$, studies in rats indicate that fentanyl does not prevent the reduction in high energy phosphate and the accumulation of lactate in brain tissue during hypoxia (Keykhah et al. 1988).

CSF formation

In dogs fentanyl, in comparison with halothane induces a reduction of the resistance against resorption of CSF (Artru 1984d).

Tolerance

In dogs, acute tolerance for the effects of fentanyl-evoked cardiovascular responses occurs within 3 hrs., and rebound withdrawal effects have been observed within 4–5 hrs. (Askitopoulou et al. 1985).

A_2 agonist

A_2 agonists potentiate the analgesic properties of fentanyl. This effect appears to be independent of the routes of administration (Meerts and Kock 1994).

Traumatic brain injury

Fentanyl infusion, in cats subjected to fluid percussion injury, led to a significant decrease in blood pressure when compared with control. Even so, there was no difference in CBF associated with this hypotension, unlike the reduction in CBF observed during haemorrhagic hypotension. The study suggests the possibility of restoration of cerebral autoregulation with infusion of fentanyl (Bedell et al. 1998).

Ischaemia and protection

In many species fentanyl is a pro-convulsant drug. Fentanyl theoretically might provoke adverse effects in the ischaemic brain. However, although fentanyl caused pre-ischaemic evidence of epileptoid activity, it does not adversely affect outcome from forebrain ischaemia (Morimoto et al. 1997), and from focal cerebral ischaemia in the rat (Soonthon-Brant et al. 1999). With the rat hippocampal slice model fentanyl is neither neurotoxic nor protective against anoxic injury to neurones when used in concentrations comparable to those used in clinical practice (Charchaflieh et al. 1998).

In rabbits subjected to focal brain injury, brain tissue PO_2 was better preserved with isoflurane than with fentanyl in areas distant from the lesion. Greater heterogeneity in PO_2 was also observed with fentanyl (Murr et al. 1993).

Fentanyl, human studies

ICP

In patients with space-occupying lesions fentanyl might increase ICP (Miller et al. 1975). In many cases the increase in ICP is secondary to hypercapnia, caused by pulmonary hypoventilation, but an increase in CSF-pressure has also been observed in normocapnic volunteers (Benzer et al. 1992). In contrast, some studies indicate that during induction of anaesthesia with thiopentone, followed by fentanyl and controlled hyperventilation ICP is unchanged (Moss et al. 1978). This finding is in contrast to newer studies in patients with severe head injury, where fentanyl in doses of 2 µg/kg is accompanied by a moderate increase in ICP and a fall in MABP and CPP, but unchanged $AVDO_2$ (de Nadal et al. 1998, de Nadal et al. 2000).

CBF and $CMRO_2$

Studies with Doppler technique indicate that fentanyl during normocapnia increases flow velocity (Trindle et al. 1993). This effect is completely abolished during hypocapnia (Kolbitsch et al. 1997). During induction of anaesthesia with fentanyl 100 µg/kg and diazepam 0.4 mg/kg for cardiac surgery a 25% decrease in CBF was observed, while $CMRO_2$ was unchanged. Under certain circumstances fentanyl administration during controlled ventilation is accompanied by an increase in ICP and a decrease in blood pressure (Knüttgen et al. 1989). This reaction is supposed to be caused by vasodilation secondary to autoregulation challenge. However, histamine-induced vasodilation is also a possible explanation.

Regional CBF.

According to PET studies in humans fentanyl activates regional CBF in cerebral regions associated with pain-related behaviours (cingulus, orbitofrontal, medial prefrontal and caudate nuclei). A decrease in rCBF is noted in both frontal, temporal areas, and the cerebellum (Freestone et al. 1996, Adler et al. (1997)

CO_2 reactivity

In a study including patients with brain tumour rCBF was measured during two levels of $PaCO_2$ using Doppler Laser flowmetry. The probe was placed over cerebral cortex known to be oedematous. The anaesthetic procedures used were isoflurane 0.56% or fentanyl, both maintained with nitrous oxide. During isoflurane anaesthesia there was a wide variety of responses to hypocapnia including patients whose flow indices increased markedly (inverse reaction). The mean flow during fentanyl was lower than it was with isoflurane (Shah et al. 1990).

Hyperventilation decreases the plasma clearance of fentanyl. This effect may give rises to prolonged respiratory depression (Cartwright et al. 1983).

EEG

During high-dose fentanyl anaesthesia (50–70 µg/kg) a massive increase in delta power in the EEG has been observed (Sebel et al. 1981). Increased power in the delta band correlates well with increased dose of fentanyl (Lien et al. 1990).

In accordance with the experimental studies, epileptic seizures have been described after fentanyl injection (Rao et al. 1982, Sebel and Bovill 1983). In patients with complex partial seizure recorded perioperatively for epileptic surgery fentanyl in doses ranging from 18–36 µg/kg administered over 2–7 min was accompanied by seizure activity in the perihippocampal region (Tempelhoff et al. 1992). In another clinical study of patients with temporal lobe epilepsy, both alfentanil and fentanyl induced an increase in spike activity in all patients. Alfentanil (50 µg/kg) was more potent than fentanyl 10 µg/kg. However, alfentanil had a shorter duration of action (Manninen et al. 1999).

Evoked potential

Somato-sensory evoked potentials (EP) remain consistently recordable and interpretable during high dose fentanyl anaesthesia (Schubert et al. 1986).

Clinical application

High dosages fentanyl- and sufentanil anaesthesia have been found to be satisfactory for neurosurgery (Shupak et al. 1983, Shupak et al. 1985). On the other hand, in severe head injury fentanyl as well as sufentanil increase ICP and decrease blood pressure (Sperry et al 1992). When high dosages of these narcotics are used postoperative respiratory treatment or postoperative administration of naloxone might be required. Skilled nursing care must be available for many hours after surgery (Shupak et al. 1985). It is important to stress that during prolonged anaesthesia or sedation with fentanyl the anaesthetic effect might be markedly reduced, suggesting the development of tolerance (Novack et al. 1978, Colpaert et al. 1980, Shafer et al. 1983).

Neurolept anaesthesia

CBF and $CMRO_2$

The combined use of droperidol and fentanyl with nitrous oxide has been advocated for neurosurgical operation. When both drugs are administered a decrease in CBF and $CMRO_2$ are observed in dogs as well as in some human studies (Michenfelder and Theye 1971, Kreuscher 1967). In contrast, other clinical studies have shown that CBF and oxygen uptake are unchanged (Barker et al. 1968, Sari et al. 1972). In a study of patients subjected to craniotomy for cerebral tumours in neurolept anaesthesia supplemented with nitrous oxide during moderate hypocapnia, both CBF and $CMRO_2$ were reduced, 30 ml/100g/min and 2.3 ml O_2 /100g/min respectively. The CO_2 reactivity was preserved (Cold et al. 1988).

ICP

Studies of ICP in patients with space-occupying lesions indicate that ICP is well controlled (Fitch et al. 1969).

EEG

During neurolept anaesthesia slow wave activity of EEG is observed. The prerequisite for this activity seems to be a depression of brain-stem activity. This depression is produced by droperidol (Nilsson and Ingvar 1967). In contrast, in mice the combination of fentanyl and droperidol lowered the threshold for electroshock and pentetrazole-induced convulsions (Hashem and Frey 1988).

Oedema

In experimental studies the total water content close to induced cryogenic injury decreases during neurolept anaesthesia (Smith and Marque 1976).

Naloxone

Studies during recovery after craniotomy suggest that even a small single dose of naloxone (1 μg/kg) effectively antagonises the postoperative respiratory depression without eliminating the immediate postoperative analgesic effect of neurolept anaesthesia (Arnér and Gordon 1976).

Physiostigmin

Wiklund (1986) documented that the combined use of naloxone and physostigmine might reverse sedation and respiratory depression more effectively.

Sufentanil, experimental studies

Pharmacodynamic

In human sufentanil and fentanyl have similar pharmacodynamic profiles. The half-life of brain-barrier equilibrium did not differ (Scott et al. 1991). Intrathecal administration of sufentanil undergoes rapid clearance from CSF and absorption to plasma (Hansdottir et al. 1991).

CBF, $CMRO_2$ and EEG

In rats sufentanil decreases CBF and $CMRO_2$. In studies using the open window technique a bolus injection or continuous infusion of sufentanil decrease pial arteries diameter dose-dependently (Lu et al. 1987). In dogs subjected to isoflurane, nitrous oxide anaesthesia sufentanil decreased CBF and $CMRO_2$ by 35% while ICP was unchanged (Werner et al. 1991). In monkeys a dosage dependent fall in CBF and $CMRO_2$ was observed. In the same study cerebral autoregulation was intact (Bunegin et al. 1990).

Sufentanil produces an EEG pattern of deep anaesthesia, but without burst-suppression periods.

This depression was accompanied by a decrease in $CMRO_2$ below baseline levels (Milde et al. 1990). In rats high doses of sufentanil provoke epileptic seizure activity (Keykhah et al. 1985), and studies of regional glucose utilisation in rats have shown a selective increase in glucose utilisation in subcortical limbic nuclei, particularly the amygdala, suggesting that the EEG pattern of seizure activity might reflect subcortical rather than cortical activation (Young et al. 1984).

ICP

Using the venous outflow technique in the dog sufentanil in doses of 10–200 μg/kg increased CBF that lasted for about 20 min. The CBF then gradually decreased so that it was below baseline levels by the end of a 60 min study period. The transient increase in CBF was accompanied by an equally transient decrease in CVR. ICP did not change (Milde and Milde 1989). In rabbits subjected to acute cryogenic brain injury neither fentanyl nor sufentanil increased CBF or ICP (Sheehan et al. 1992). In dogs subjected to inflation of an epidural balloon, sufentanil produced an increase in CBF and ICP and a fall in ATP and phosphocreatine in the area of the balloon (Milde and Milde 1989).

Sufentanil, human studies

CBF, $CMRO_2$ and CO_2 reactivity

In patients undergoing coronary artery surgery (Murkin et al. 1998) and in a study by Stephan et al. (1991) high dose sufentanil (10 mg/kg) induced a fall in CBF and $CMRO_2$ and an increase in CVR. In healthy volunteers CBF, measured with the Xe^{133} clearance technique, did not change after sufentanil 0.5 mg/kg administered intravenously (Mayer et al. 1990). In elderly patients undergoing carotid endarterectomy in either isoflurane/nitrous oxide or sufentanil/nitrous oxide anaesthesia, both anaesthetic practices had similar effects on CBF, $AVDO_2$, $CMRO_2$ and CO_2 reactivity (Young et al. 1989).

ICP and cerebral autoregulation

In one study of patients with neurosurgical disorders sufentanil did not increase ICP whether baseline ICP was increased or not (Weinstabl et al. 1991). In a study of head injury sufentanil in a dosage of 2 μg/kg decreased ICP and MABP, but did not change CPP (Scholz et al. 1994). In another study of severe head injury a modest dosage of sufentanil increased ICP and decreased blood pressure (Sperry et al 1992). In patients undergoing craniotomy in nitrous oxide, isoflurane anaesthesia a low dosage fentanyl or sufentanil infusion induce significantly better cerebral relaxation than without narcotics (Bristow et al. 1987). In accordance with these observations no difference in brain retractor pressure was found between fentanyl and sufentanil used for analgesia during isoflurane maintenance of aneurysm surgery (Herrick et al. 1990).

In one study sufentanil in a small dosage did not increase ICP. However, in high dosages an increase in ICP was observed (Slee et al. 1990). In another study Werner et al. (1995) investigated patients with severe head injury sedated with midazolam and fentanyl. A bolus of 3 mg/kg sufentanil was injected. In 12 of 30 patients MABP did not decrease after sufentanil, and ICP was unchanged. In 18 patients MABP decreased accompanied by an increase in ICP but with unchanged flow velocity in the middle cerebral artery. The results suggest that the increase in ICP observed with sufentanil might be due to an autoregulatory mechanism. Thus, the decrease in CVR and increase in ICP are secondary to systemic hypotension.

Hypocapnia

It has been demonstrated that hypocapnia prolongs the elimination of sufentanil (Schwartz et al. 1989), and hypocapnia intensifies the EEG response to sufentanil (Matteo et al. 1992).

CPP

No significant difference in CPP was found between alfentanil, sufentanil and fentanyl (Cuillerier et al. 1990).

Adverse effect

Benzel et al. (1990) observed that sufentanil might exacerbate neurological dysfunction. In four patients they found severe deficits after intravenous sufentanil. Naloxone reversed the deficits in three patients.

EEG

Studies of EEG during sufentanil anaesthesia have shown high voltage and slow delta wave activity (Bovill et al. 1982). The intrinsic potency of sufentanil as measured by the serum concentration needed to cause half the maximum EEG slowing, was 12-fold greater than that of fentanyl (Scott et al. 1991).

Alfentanil, experimental studies

CBF, CO_2 reactivity and autoregulation

In dogs alfentanil induces a dose-related decrease in CBF, the CO_2 reactivity is preserved and the upper limit of autoregulation is at a higher pressure (McPherson et al. 1982). In another study of alfentanil anaesthetised rabbits, exposure to 5% CO_2 initially increased CBF to about 160% of baseline, but CBF then decreased to about 130% while $PaCO_2$ was still rising. Under this circumstance it is supposed that mechanisms other than perivascular hydrogen ion concentration mediate the CBF response (Ludbrook et al. 1992).

Rigidity and ICP

In rats subjected to mechanical ventilation, alfentanil increases muscle rigidity, leading to hypercapnia and a significant increase in ICP, which rapidly normalises after non depolarizating relaxants (Benthuysen et al. 1985). Other studies in rats indicate that ICP-hypertension caused by rigidity can be treated effectively with non-depolarizating muscular relaxants and that ICP-hypertension only occurs if rigidity is absent (Benthuysen et al. 1988).

CSF formation

In dogs the formation rate of CSF and resistance to reabsorption of CSF were determined during fentanyl, sufentanil or alfentanil administration. It was concluded that among these narcotics reduction of CSF volume is favoured most by fentanyl, and ease of CSF volume contraction is favoured most by alfentanil (Artru 1991).

Propofol.

In vitro studies of isolated liver microsome obtained form pig and human liver suggest that propofol in clinically relevant concentrations interferes with oxidative metabolic degradation of alfentanil and sufentanil (Janicki et al. 1992).

Alfentanil, human studies

ICP and CPP

In a comparative study in patients with supratentorial tumours fentanyl did not change lumbar CSF pressure, while sufentanil and especially alfentanil injection were followed by an increase in lumbar CSF pressure, and a decrease in MABP and CPP (Marx et al. 1989). In another human study of brain tumour patients CSF-pressure remained unchanged in patients who received nitrous oxide with or without fentanyl for maintenance of anaesthesia. By contrast, in those who received alfentanil, a gradual increase in ICP was found (Jung et al. 1990). This is consistent with the observation by Moss (1992), who found that alfentanil increased ICP in patients with suspected normal pressure hydrocephalus. The increase in ICP occurred immediately after alfentanil administration and was accompanied by a fall in blood pressure. It is supposed that cerebral autoregulatory mechanisms, leading to vasodilation and an increase in ICP, were secondary to the fall in arterial pressure.

In contrast, alfentanil did not change ICP in children undergoing shunt revision (Marcovitz et al. 1990). In another study, where alfentanil was used together with thiopentone for induction of anaesthesia in patients with supratentorial tumours, ICP remained stable without significant difference from pre-anaesthetic levels (Hung et al. 1992). In artificially ventilated patients with closed head injury pre-treatment with alfentanil before suction did not change ICP. In this study a decrease in blood pressure and cerebral perfusion pressure were observed (Hanowell et al. (1993). These findings are also in accordance with studies of transcranial Doppler sonography, indicating that alfentanil did not alter the vessel diameter in the middle cerebral artery (Schregel et al. 1992).

Awake craniotomy

In a report alfentanil was used successfully for awake craniotomy in patients undergoing resection of epileptogenic foci (Welling and Donegan 1989). In another study, however, of awake craniotomy alfentanil or sufentanil did not offer any benefit over fentanyl (Gignac et al. 1993).

Sedation

Continuous intravenous alfentanil sedation has recently been proposed in the intensive care of patients subjected to controlled ventilation (Yate et al. 1984, Cohen and Kelly 1987, Sinclair et al. 1988). However, when administrated together with propofol, the specific activity of each drug (MABP decrease) is potentiated (Gepts et al. 1988).

Remifentanil, experimental studies

CBF

During isoflurane anaesthesia in dogs remifentanil decreased regional CBF in cortex, hippocampus, and the caudate by 50%. In the lower brain regions changes in rCBF were modest or absent (Hoffman et al. 1993).

EEG

The recovery of EEG changes occurs sooner following remifentanil than alfentanil (Hoffman et al. 1993).

CSF formation

Studies of rate of CSF formation and resistance to reabsorption during remifentanil in rabbits indicate that remifentanil does not alter these parameters (Artru and Momota 2000).

Remifentanil, human studies

CBF and CO_2 reactivity

Healthy volunteers were subjected to remifentanil infusion (0,1 μg/kg/min) and subjected to MRI to measure rCBF, rCBV, regional mean transit time, and regional CVR. Rimifentanil increased rCBF and rCBV in white and grey matter (striatal, thalamic, occipital, parietal, frontal) regions with a parallel decrease in transit time in those regions with the exception of occipital grey matter. Regional CVR was decreased in all regions studied. The authors conclude that these findings are consistent with cerebral excitement and/or disinhibition (Lorenz et al. 2000a).

In patients subjected to coronary by-pass graft surgery remifentanil (3 μg/kg/min) reduced flow velocity by 31%. 1μg/kg/min did not change flow velocity (Paris et al. 1998).

In patients undergoing craniotomy in remifentanil, nitrous oxide anaesthesia CBF increased from 21 to 31 ml/100g/min as the $PaCO_2$ increased form 27 to 36 mm Hg. The relative CO_2 reactivity was 3.6%/mm Hg CO_2 (Baker et al. 1997). In patients scheduled for supratentorial tumour surgery remifentanil and fentanyl had similar effects on absolute CBF, and CO_2 reactivity is maintained (Ostapkovich et al. 1998).

ICP and CPP

Awake volunteers were subjected to assessment of cerebral capacity non-invasively by means of phase-contrast magnetic resonance imaging. Measurement of systolic cerebrospinal fluid peak velocity in the aquaduct of Sylvius before and during infusion of remifentanil was performed. Remifentanil did not influence cerebral capacity in these healthy, awake volunteers (Lorenz et al. 2000b).

Four clinical studies of remifentanil for patients undergoing craniotomy for cerebral tumours are available. 1) In a clinical study of patients undergoing supratentorial craniotomy a dosage dependent decrease in CPP was observed. However, ICP did not change, and the effects of remifentanil did not differ from that of equipotent doses of alfentanil (Hindman et al. 1994). 2) In another study of patients subjected to craniotomy for supratentorial tumours the effects of remifentanil 0.5 μg/kg and alfentanil 1.0 μg/kg upon ICP and MABP were compared. Neither opioids caused significant changes in ICP, but both drugs were associated with a dosage-dependent decrease in MABP (Warner et al. 1996). 3) Continuous infusion with remifentanil 0.03μg/kg/min or fentanyl 0.2 μg/kg/min were compared. Anaesthesia included thiopental induction and maintenance with nitrous oxide supplemented with one of the opioids. ICP and CPP were identical in the two groups. MABP was highest in the fentanyl group (Guy et al. 1997). 4) Anaesthesia supplemented with remifentanil (0.2 μg/kg/min), alfentanil 20 μg/kg/h, and fentanyl 2 μg/kg/h) was compared in patients undergoing craniotomy. There were no differences among the groups of heart rate and MABP (Coles et al. 2000).

Dose-response studies

In patients undergoing intracranial surgery under desflurane anaesthesia remifentanil infusions at 0.0625, 0.125 and 0.250 μg/kg/min were compared. The overall quality of the haemodynamic control was superior during infusion of 0.125 μg/kg/min compared with the two other groups (Gesztesi et al. 1999).

EEG

In a study presented by Baker et al. (1997) EEG remained stable with spectral edge frequency of about 25 Hz. The spectral pattern was unchanged during hypocapnia.

Remifentanil and neurosurgical anaesthesia

In a comparative study remifentanil or fentanyl were used as supplement to isoflurane/nitrous oxide in patients undergoing surgery for intracranial mass lesions. The results indicate that remifentanil-based anaesthesia provides stable and similar hemodynamics during the induction, maintenance and emergency phase of anaesthesia when compared with fentanyl-based anaesthesia. The frequencies of adverse event rates for the two opioids were similar. Remifentanil, although not altering the rate of emergency for at least 50% of the patients, did reduce the probability of a slow emergency. Remifentanil decreased the amount of concomitant anaesthesia, and the emergency from anaesthesia was more predictable with remifentanil (Balakrishnan et al. 2000).

The safety profile of remifentanil seems to be similar to that of fentanyl in patients undergoing supratentorial craniotomy. The haemodynamic qualities are identical with fentanyl except during the period between intubation and skin incision, where more remifentanil-anaesthetised patients experience hypotension, and during the early recovery period, where remifentanil-treated patients are more likely to experience hypertension (Warner 1999).

Comparative studies of central analgesics

Recovery

Coles et al. (2000) compared remifentanil, alfentanil and fentanyl as maintenance in patients subjected to craniotomy. Propofol infusion was used in all patients. The time to eye opening was shorter in the remifentanil group compared with the alfentanil, but no difference was observed between the remifentanil and the fentanyl groups.

CBF

In patients scheduled for coronary by pass fentanyl 25 µg/kg, sufentanil 3 µg/kg and sufentanil 6 µg/kg were used for induction of anaesthesia. Flow velocity did not change with fentanyl or low dose of sufentanil. With high dose sufentanil flow velocity decreased by 30%, suggesting that sufentanil decreases blood flow in a dose-related fashion with a threshold effect (Hänel et al. 1997).

ICP

sufentanil in small doses did not increase ICP. However, during high doses an increase in ICP was observed. This reaction appeared to result from indirect vasodilation as part of the autoregulatory response, secondary to systemic hypotension (Slee et al. 1990). This hypothesis was tested by Jamali et al. (1996) who studied CSF-pressure with or without blood pressure stabilisation with phenylephedrine in patients with supratentorial mass lesions. They found that injections of fentanyl or sufentanil, despite producing rapidly corrected decreases in MABP of 18 to 25%, were not associated with any change in CSF-pressure.

MABP

In a randomized study comparisons of alfentanil, fentanyl and sufentanil were performed in patients subjected to craniotomy for supratentorial tumours. In this study alfentanil-treated patients received ephedrine more frequently before intubation. In the recovery period respiratory rate and pH in blood were lowest in sufentanil-treated patients. However, these patients were more alert (From et al. 1990).

In a recent study anaesthesia supplemented with remifentanil (0.2 µg/kg/min), alfentanil (20 µg/kg/h) and fentanyl (2 µg/kg/h) were compared in patients undergoing craniotomy. There were no differences among the groups of heart rate and MABP. However, the time to eye opening was significantly shorter in the remifentanil group compared with the alfentanil group, but not the fentanyl group (Coles et al. 2000).

EEG

Comparative studies of EEG activity during fentanyl, alfentanil, and sufentanil injection, indicate activation of EEG after all three drugs, without any significant difference (Ty Smidt et al. 1986). In another study EEG was analysed. During induction of anaesthesia with fentanyl, sufentanil or alfentanil epileptic EEG activity was never detected, and there was no EEG evidence of a postictal state in any patient. The authors emphasise that rigidity is often explosive in onset and mimics epileptic seizures (Smith et al. 1987).

Naloxone, experimental studies

CBF and $CMRO_2$

This n-allyl derivate of oxymorphine is widely used by anaesthetists to reverse opioid-induced respiratory depression. Given intravenously during halothane anaesthesia in dogs, naloxone does not change CBF or $CMRO_2$ (Artru et al. 1980). However, in rats subjected to nitrous oxide or nitrous oxide supplemented with sufentanil naloxone induces a significant increase in CBF as well as $CMRO_2$ suggesting that these effects are mediated by opioid receptors, and that the depressant effects of N_2O on CBF and metabolism are mediated by opioid receptors as well (Keykhah et al. 1985).

Protection

Experimental studies suggest that naloxone improves neurological outcome after spinal injury (Faden et al. 1981a, Faden et al. 1982a, Flamm et al. 1982). Naloxone improves spinal cord blood flow in the injured region (Faden et al. 1981b, Young et al. 1981). However, no human trials have been performed, and the clinical use in spinal cord injury has not been established.

In gerbils subjected to carotid occlusion, intraperitoneal injection of naloxone reverses the stroke for up to 30 min (Hosobuchi et al. 1982), and in naloxone treated stroked animals, CBF is maintained in all cerebral regions above a critical threshold, and a substantially better cortical somato-sensory-evoked response recovery was observed (Faden et al. 1982). Temperature changes during the experiments might have influenced the results.

Naloxone, human studies

Although naloxone in clinical studies has been reported to completely reverse neurological deficits in patients with cerebral ischaemia (Baskin and Hosobuchi 1981), no controlled studies are yet available. In this context it must be stressed that clinical use of naloxone is not without risk as it can provoke hypertensive reactions (Tanaka 1974, Azar and Turndorf 1979), and even acute pulmonary oedema (Flacke et al. 1977. Concerning the use of naloxone in the postoperative period after craniotomy (see fentanyl).

References

Abrams JT, Horrow JC, Bennett JA, et al. Upper airway closure: a primary source of difficult ventilation with sufentanil induction of anesthesia. Anesth Analg 1996: 83: 629–632.

Adler LJ, Gyulai FE; Diehl DJ,et al. Regional brain activity changes associated with fentanyl analgesia elucidated by positron emission tomography. Anesth Analg 1997: 84: 120–126.

Ainslie SG, Eisele JH, Corkill G. Fentanyl concentrations in brain and serum during respiratory acid-base changes in the dog. Anesthesiology 1979: 51: 293–297.

Arnér S, Gordon E. The antagonist effect of naloxone hydrochloride after neurolept- anaesthesia during neurosurgery. Acta Anaesth Scand 1976: 20: 201–206.

Artru AA, Steen PA, Michenfender JD. Cerebral metabolic effects of nalaxone administered with anaesthetic and subanaesthetic concentrations of halothane in the dog. Anesthesiology 1980: 52: 217–220.

Artru AA. Effects of halothane and fentanyl anesthesia on resistance to reabsorption of CSF. J Neurosurg 1984d: 60: 252–256.

Artru AA. Dose-related changes in the rate of CSF formation and resistance to reabsorption of CSF during administration of fentanyl, sufentanil, or alfentanil in dogs. J Neurosurg Anesthesiol 1991: 3: 283–290.

Artru AA, Momota Y. Rate of CSF formation and resistance to reabsorption of CSF during sevoflurane or remifentanil in rabbits. J Neurosurg Anesthesiol 2000: 12: 37–43.

Askitopoulou H, Whitwam JG, Al-Khudhairi D, et al. Acute tolerance to fentanyl during anaesthesia in dogs. Anesthesiology 1985: 63: 255–261.

Azar I, Turndorf H. Severe hypertension and multiple atrial premature contractions following nalaxone administration. Anesth Analg 1979: 58: 524–525.

Balakrishnan G, Raudzens P, Samra SK, et al. A comparison of remifentanil and fentanyl in patients undergoing surgery for intracranial mass lesions. Anest Analg 2000: 91: 163–169.

Baker KZ, Ostapkovich N, Sisti MB, et al. Intact cerebral blood flow reactivity during remifentanil/nitrous oxide anesthesia. J Neurosurg Anesthesiol 1997: 9: 134–140.

Barker J, Harper AM, McDowall DG, et al. Cerebral blood flow, cerebrospinal fluid pressure and EEG activity during neurolept analgesia induced with dehydrobenzperidol and phenoperidine. Br J Anaesth 1968: 40: 143–144.

Baskin DS, Hosobuchi Y. Nalaxone reversal of ischaemic neurological deficits in man. Lancet 1981: ii: 272–275.

Bedell EA, DeWitt DS, Prough DS. Fentanyl infusion preserves cerebral blood flow during decreased arterial blood pressure after traumatic brain injury in cats. J Neurotrauma 1998: 15: 985–992.

Bennett JA, Abrams JT, van Riper DF, Horrow JC. Difficult or impossible ventilation after sufentanil-induced anesthesia is caused primarily by vocal cord closure. Anesthesiology 1997: 87: 1070–1074.

Benthuysen JL, Kien ND, Quam DD, Martucci RW. The influence of narcotic-induced rigidity on intracranial pressure. Anesthesiology 1985: 63: A393.

Benthuysen J, Smith N, Sanford T, et al. Physiology of alfentanil-induced rigidity. Anesthesiology 1986: 64: 440–446.

Benthuysen J, Kien N, Quam D, Martucci R. Intracranial pressure increases during alfentanil-induced rigidity. Anesthesiology 1988: 68: 438–440.
Benzel EC, Hadden TA, Nossaman, et al. Does sufentanil exacerbate marginal neurological dysfunction? J Neurosurg Anesthesiol 1990: 2: 50–52.
Benzer A, Gottardis M, Russigger L, et al. Fentanyl increases cerebrospinal fluid pressure in normocapnic volunteers. Eur J Anesthesiol 1992: 9: 473–477.
Bingham RM, Hinds CJ. Influence of bolus doses of phenoperidine on intracranial pressure and systemic arterial pressure in traumatic coma. Br J Anaesth 1987: 59: 592–595.
Bion JF, Logan BK, Newman PM, et al. Sedation in intensive care: morphine and renal function. Intensive Care Med 1986: 12: 359–365.
Bovill JG, Sebel PS, Wauquier A, Rog P. Electroencephalographic effects of sufentanil anaesthesia in man. Br J Anaesth 1982: 54: 45–52.
Bristow A, Shalev D, Rice B, et al. Low-dose synthetic narcotic infusions for cerebral relaxation during craniotomies. Anesth Analg 1987: 66: 413–416.
Buchweitz E, Grandison L, Weiss HR. Effect of morphine on regional cerebral oxygen consumption and supply. Brain Reseach 1984: 291: 301–308.
Bunegin L, Albin MS, Ernst PS, Garcia C. Cerebrovascular responses to sufentanil citrate (SC) in primates with and without intracranial hypertension. Anesth Analg 1990): 70: S42.
Carlsson C, Smith DS, Keykhah MM, et al. The effects of high-dose fentanyl on cerebral circulation and metabolism in rats. Anesthesiology 1982: 57: 375–380.
Cartwright P, Prys-Roberts C, Gill K, et al. Ventilatory depression related to plasma fentanyl concentrations during and after anaesthesia in humans. Anesth Analg 1983: 62: 966–974.
Charchaflieh J, Cottrell JE, Kass IS. The effect of fentanyl on electrophysiologic recovery of CA 1 pyramide cells from anoxia in the rat hippocampal slice. Anesth Analg 1998: 87: 68–71.
Chi OZ, Lee DI, Liu X, Weiss HR. The effects of morphine on blood-brain barrier disruption caused by intracarotid injection of hyperosmolar mannitol. Anest Analg 2000: 90: 603–608.
Cohen AT, Kelly DR. Assessment of alfentanil by intravenous infusion as long-term sedation in intensive care. Anaesthesia 1987: 42: 545–548.
Cold GE, Christensen KJS, Nordentoft J, et al. Cerebral blood flow, cerebral metabolic rate of oxygen and relative CO_2 reactivity during neurolept anaesthesia in patients subjected to craniotomy for supratentorial cerebral tumours. Acta Anaesthesiol Scand 1988: 32: 310–315.
Cold GE, Felding M. Even small doses of morphine might provoke "Luxury Perfusion" in the postoperative period after craniotomy. Neurosurgery 1993: 32: 327.
Coles JP, Leary TS, Monteiro JN, et al. Propofol anesthesia for craniotomy: A double-blind comparison of remifentanil, alfentanil, and fentanyl. J Neurosurg Anesthesiol 2000: 12: 15–20.
Colpaert FC, Niemegeers CJE, Janssen PAJ, Maroli AN: The effects of prior fentanyl administration and of pain on fentanyl analgesia. Tolerance to the enhancement of narcotic analgesia. J Pharmacol Exp Ther 1980: 213: 418–424.
Comstock M, Scamman F, Moyers J, Stevens W. Rigidity and hypercarbia associated with high dose fentanyl induction of anesthesia. Anesth Analg 1981: 60: 362–363.
Cuillerier DJ, Manninen PH, Gelb AW. Alfentanil, sufentanil, and fentanyl: effect on cerebral perfusion pressure. Anesth Analg 1990: 70: S75.
Daykin AP, Bowen DJ, Sauders DA, Norman J. Respiratory depression after morphine in the elderly. Anaaesthesia 1986: 41. 910–914.
DeCastro J, VandeWater A, Wouters L, et al. Comparative study of cardiovascular neurological and metabolic side-effects of eight narcotics in dogs. Acta Anaesthesiol Belg 1979: 30: 5–99.
De Nadal M, Austina A, Sahuquillo J. et a. Effects on intracranial pressure of fentanyl in severe head injured patients. Acta Neurochir 1998 (suppl) 71: 10–12.
De Nadal M, Munar F, Poca MA, et al. Cerebral hemodynamic effects of morphine and fentanyl in patients with severe head injury. Anesthesiology 2000: 92: 11–19.
Durieux ME. Muscarinic signaling in the central nervous system: Recent developments an anesthetic implications. Anesthesiology 1996: 84: 173–189.
Faden AI, Jacobs TP, Holaday JW. Opiate antagonist improves neurologic recovery after spinal injury. Science 1981a: 211: 493–494.
Faden AI, Jacobs TP, Mougey E, Holoday JW. Endorphins in experimental spinal injury: Therapeutic effect of nalaxone Ann Neurol 1981b: 10: 326–332.
Faden AI, Jacobs TP, Holady JW. Comparison of early and late nalaxone treatment in experimental spinal injury. Neurology 1982a: 32: 677–681.
Faden AI, Hallenbeck JM, Brown CQ. Treatment of experimental stroke: comparison of nalaxone and thyreotropin releasing hormone. Neurology 1982b: 32: 1083–1087.
Firestone LL, Gyulai F, Mintun M, et al. Human brain activity response to fentanyl imaged by positron emission tomography. Anesth Analg 1996: 82: 1247–1251.
Fitch W, Barker J, Jennett WB, McDowall DG. The influence of neuroleptanalgesic drugs on cerebrospinal fluid pressure. Br J Anaesth 1969: 41: 800–806.
Fitch W, Barker J, Jennett WB, McDowall DG. The influence of neurolept analgesic drugs on cerebrospinal fluid pressure. Br J Anaesth 1969: 41: 800–806.
Flacke JW, Flacke WE, Williams GD. Acute pulmonary edema following nalaxone reversal of high-dose morphine anesthesia. Anesthesiology 1977: 47: 376–378.
Flamm ES, Young W, Demopoulus HB, Decrescito V, Tomasula JJ. Experimental spinal cord injury: treatment with nalaxone. Neurosurgery 1982: 10: 227–231.
Freeman J, Ingvar DH. Effects of fentanyl on cerebral cortical blood flow and EEG in the cat. Acta Anaesth Scand 1967: 11: 381–391.
From RP, Warner DS, Todd MM, Sokoll MD. Anesthesia for craniotomy: A double-blind comparison of alfentanil, fentanyl, and sufentanil. Anesthesiology 1990: 73: 896–904.
Gepts E, Jonckheer K, Maes V, et al. Disposition kinetics of propofol during alfentanil anaesthesia. Anaesthesia 1988: 43 (suppl): 8–13
Gesztesi Z, Mootz BL, White PF. The use of remifentanil infusion for hemodynamic control during intracranial surgery. Anesth Analg 1999: 89: 1282–1287.
Gignac E, Manninen PH, Gelb AW. Comparison of fentanyl, sufentanil and alfentanil during awake craniotomy for epilepsy. Can J Anaesth 1993: 40: 421–424.

Grummitt RM, Goat VA. Intracranial pressure after phenoperidine. Anaesthesia 1984: 39: 565–567.

Guy J, Hindman BJ, Baker KZ, et al. Comparison of remifentanil and fentanyl in patients undergoing craniotomy for supratentiral space-occupying lesions. Anesthesiology 1997: 86: 514–524.

Hamilton W, Cullen S. Effect of levallorphan tartrate upon opoid-induced respiratory depression. Anesthesiology 1953: 14: 550–555.

Hänel F, Werner C, von Knobelsdorff G, et al. The effect of fentanyl and sufentanil on cerebral hemodynamics. J Neurosurg Anesthesiol 1997: 9: 223–227.

Hanowell LH, Thurston JD, Behrman KH, Disbrow EA (1992) Alfentanil administered prior to endotracheal suctioning reduces cerebral perfusion pressure. J Neurosurg Anesthesiol 1993: 5: 31–35.

Hansdottir V, Hedren T, Woestenborghs R, Nordberg G. The CSF and plasma pharmacokinetics of sufentanil after intrathecal administration. Anesthesiology 1991: 74: 264–269.

Hashem A. Frey H-H. Einfluss einiger Neuroleptika und Neuroleptika/Anangetika-Kombinationen auf die Krampfempfindlischkeit bei Mäusen. Anaesthesist 1998: 37: 631–635.

Herrick IA, Gelb AW, Manninen PH, et al. The effect of fentanyl and sufentanil on brain retractor pressure. Anesth Analg 1990: 70: S155.

Hindman B. Warner D, Todd M, et al. ICP and CPP effects of remifentanil and alfentanil. J Neurosurg Ansthesiol 1994: 6: 304.

Hoffman WE, Werner C, Kochs E, et al. Cerebral and spinal cord blood flow in awake and fentanyl-N20 anaesthetized rats: Evidence for preservation of blood flow autoregulation during anesthesia. J Neurosurg Anesthesiol 1992: 4: 31–35.

Horrows JC, Abrams JT, van Riper DF, et al. Ventilatory compliance after three sufentanil-pancuronium induction sequences. Anesthesiology 1991: 75: 969–974.

Hosobuchi Y, Baskin DS, Woo SK. Reversal of neurological deficits by opiate antagonist nalaxone after cerebral ischaemia in animals and humans. J Cereb Blood Flow Metab 1982: suppl 1: 98–100.

Hung OR, Hope CE, Laney G, et al. The effect of alfentanil on intracranial dynamics and hemodynamics in patients with brain tumours undergoing craniotomy. Can J Anesth 1992.A4

Jamali S, Ravussin P, Archer D, et al. The effect of bolus administration of opoids on cerebrospinal fluid pressure in patients with supratentorial lesions. Anesth Analg 1996: 82: 600–606.

Janicki PK, James MFM, Erskine WAR (1992) Propofol inhibits enzymatic degradation of alfentanil and sufentanil by isolated liver microsomes in vitro. Br J Anaesth 68: 311–312

Jobes DR, Kennell E, Bitner R, et al. Effects of morphine-nitrous oxide anesthesia on cerebral autoregulation. Anesthesiology 1975: 42: 30–34.

Jobes DR, Kennell EM, Buch GL, et al. Cerebral blood flow and metabolism during morphine-nitrous oxide anesthesia in man. Anesthesiology 1977: 47: 16–18.

Jung R, Shah N, Reinsel R, et al. Cerebrospinal fluid pressure in patients with brain tumors: Impact of fentanyl versus alfentanil during nitrous oxide-oxygen anesthesia. Anesth Analg 1990: 71: 419–422.

Keykhah MM, Smith DS, Carlsson C, et al. Influence of sufentanil on cerebral metabolism and circulation in the rat. Anesthesiology 1985: 63: 274–277.

Keykhah MM, Smith DS, O'Neil JJ, Harp JR. The influence of fentanyl upon cerebral high-energy metabolites, lactate, and glucose during severe hypoxia in the rat. Anesthesiology 1988: 69: 566–570.

Knüttgen D, Doehn M, Eymer D, Müller M-R. Hirndruckstreigerung nacn fentanyl. Anaesthesist 1989: 38: 73–75.

Kolbitsch C, Hörmann C, Schmidauer C, et al. Hypocapnia reverses the fentanyl-induced increase in cerebral blood flow velocity in awake humans. J Neurosurg Anesthesiol 1997: 9: 313–315.

Kofke W, RH G, Janosky J et al. Opoid neurotoxocity: neuropathologic effects in rats of different fentanyl congeners and the effect of hexamethonium-induced normotension. Anesth Analg 1996: 83: 141–146.

Kreuscher H. Die Hirndurchblutung unter Neuroleptanaestesie. Berlin, Heidelberg, New York, Spriger Verlag, 1967.

Kuramoto T, Oshita S, Takeshita H, Ishikawa T. Modification of the relationship between cerebral netabolism, blood flow, and electroencephalogram by stimulation during anaesthesia in the dog. Anesthesiology 1979: 51: 211–217.

Kurz M, Belani KG, Sessler DI, Kurz A, Larson MD; Schroeder M, Blanchard D. Naloxone, meperidine, and shivering. Anesthesiology 1993: 79: 1193–1201.

Lambert DG, Appadu BL. Muscarinic receptor subtypes: Do they have a place in clinical anaesthesia. Br J Anaesth 1995: 74: 497–499.

Lien C, Matteo RS, Ornstein E, et al. Dose-encephalographic response to fentanyl in man. Anesth Analg 1990: 70: S239.

Lorenz IH, Kolbitsch C, Schocke M, et al. Low-dose remifentanil increases regional cerebral blood flow and regional cerebral blood volume, but decreases regional mean transit time and regional cerebrovascular resistance in volunteers. Br J Anaesth 2000a: 85: 199–204.

Lorenz IH, Kolbitch C, Hörmann C, et al. The effects of remifentanil on cerebral capacity in awake volunteers. Anest Analg 2000b: 90: 609–613.

Lu GP, Prinscott J, Frost EAM, et al. Different response of bolus or continuous infusion of sufentanil on brain microcirculation. Anesthesiology 1987: 67: A 89.

Ludbrook GL, Helps SC, Gorman DF. Cerebral blood flow response to increases in arterial CO_2 tension during alfentanil anesthesia in the rabbit. J Neurosurg Anesthesiol 1992: 12: 529–532.

Lydic R, Baghdoyan HA. Cholinergic contributions to the control of consciousness. Anesthesia: Biologic Foundations: Yaksh TL, et al. (eds) Pliladelphia, Lippencott-Raven Publishers 1997: 433–450.

Macintyre PE, Pavlin EG, Dwersteg JF. Effect of meperidine on oxygen consumption, carbon dioxide production, and respiratory gas exchange in postanaestesia shivering. Anesth Analg 1987: 66: 751–755.

Manninen PH, Burke SJ, Wennberg R, et al. Intraoperative localization of an epileptogenic focus with alfentanil and fentanyl. Anesth Analg 1999: 88: 1101–1106.

Markovitz PB, Cohen DE, Duhaime A, Sutton L. Effects of alfentanil in intracranial pressure in children undergoing ventriculo-periodoneal shunt revision. Anesthesiology 1990: 73: A213.

Marx W, Shah N, Long C, et al. Sufentanil, alfentanil, and fentanyl: Impact on cerebrospinal fluid pressure in patients

with brain tumours. Journal of Neurosurgical Anesthesiology 1989: 1: 3-7.
Matsumiya N, Dohi S. Effects of intravenous or subarachnoid morphine on cerebral and spinal cord hemodynamics and antagonism with naloxone in dogs. Anesthesiology 1983: 59: 175-181.
Matteo RS, Ornstein E, Schwartz AE, et al. Effects of hypocarbia on the pharmacodynamics of sufentanil in humans. Anesth Analg 1992: 75: 186-192.
Mayer N, Weinstabl C, Podreka I, Spiss CK. Sufentanil does not increase cerebral blood flow in healthy human volunteers. Anesthesiology 1990: 73: 240-243.
McPherson RW, Johnson RM, Traystman RJ. The effects of alfentanil on the cerebral vasculature. Anesthesiology 1982: 57: A354.
McPherson RW, Traystman RJ. Fentanyl and cerebral vascular responssitivity in dogs. Anesthesiology 1984: 60: 180-186.
Meert TF, Kock MD. Potentiation of the analgetic properties of fentanyl-like opoids with alpha$_2$-adrenoceptor agonists in rats. Anesthesiology 1994: 81: 677-688.
Messick JM, Theye RA. Effects of pentobarbital and meperidine on canine cerebral and total oxygen consumption rates.Can Anaesth Soc J 1969: 16: 321-330.
Mets B, James MFM. Another complication of opoid-induced chest wall rigidity. S Afr Med J 1992: 81: 385-386.
Michenfelder JD, Theye Ra, Effects of fentanyl, droperidol, and innovar on canine cerebral metabolism and blood flow. Br J Anaesth 1971: 43: 630-636.
Milde LN, Milde JH. Cerebral effects of sufentanil in dogs with reduced intracranial compliance. Anesth Analg 1989: 68: S196.
Milde LN, Milde JH, Gallagher WJ. Cerebral effects of fentanyl in dogs. Br J Anaesth 1989: 63: 710-715.
Milde LN, Milde JH, Gallagher WJ. Effects of sufentanil on cerebral circulation and metabolism in dogs. Anesth Analg 1990: 70: 138-146.
Miller R, Tausk HC, Stark DCC. Effect of innovar, fentanyl and droperidol on the cerebrospinal fluid pressure in neurosurgical patients. Can Anaesth Soc J 1975: 22: 502-508.
Morimoto Y, Morimoto Y, Bart RD, et al. High-dose fentanyl does not adversely affect outcome from forebrain ischemia in the rat. J Neurosurg Anesthesiol 1997: 9: 316-323.
Mortazavi S, Thompson J, Baghdoyan HA, Lydic R. Fentanyl and morphine, but not remifentanil, inhibit acetylcholine release in pontine regions modulating arousal. Anesthesiology 1999: 90: 1070-1077.
Moss E, Powell D, Gibson RM, McDowall DG. Effects of fentanyl on intracranial pressure and cerebral perfusion pressure during hypocapnia. Br J Anaesth 1978: 50: 779-784.
Moss E Alfentanil increases intracranial pressure when intracranial compliance is low. Anesthesia 1992: 47: 134-136
Murkin JM, Farrar JK, Tweed WA, et al. Relationship between cerebral blood flow and 02 consumption during high-dose narcotic anesthesia for cardiac surgery. Anesthesiology 1985: 63: A44.
Murr R, Schürer L, Berger S, et al. Effects of isoflurane, fentanyl, or thiopental anesthesia on regional cerebral blood flow and brain surface PO2 in the presence of a focal lesion in rabbits. Anesth Analg 1993: 77: 898-907.
Nilsson E, Ingvar DH. Cerebral blood flow during neuroleptanalgesia in the cat. Acta Anaesth Scand 1965: 10: 47-54.
Nielsson E, Ingvar DH. EEG findings in neuroleptanalgesia. Acta Anaesth Scandinav 1967: 11: 121-127.
Nishitateno K, Ngai SH, Finch AD, Berkowitz BA. Pharmacokinetics of morphine: concentrations in the serum and brain of the dog during hyperventilation. Anesthesiology 1979: 50: 520-523.
Novack GD, Bullock JL, Eiseli JH. Fentanyl: cumulative effects and development of short-term tolerance. Neuropharmacology 1978: 17: 77-82.
Ostapkovich ND, Baker KZ, Fogarty-Mack P, et al. Cerebral blood flow and CO_2 reactivity is similar during remifentanil/N_2O and fentanyl/N_2O Anesthesia. Anesthesiology 1998: 89: 358-363.
Paris A, Scholz J, von Knobelsdorff G, et al. The effect of remifentanil on cerebral blood flow velocity. Anesth Analg 1998: 87: 569-573.
Pearcy WC, Knott JR, Bjurstrom RO. Studies on nitrous oxide, meperidine and levallorphan with unipolar electroencephalography. Anesthesiology 1957: 18: 310-315.
Rao TLK, Mummaneni N, El-Etr AA. Convulsions: an unusual response to intravenous fentanyl administration. Anesth Analg 1982: 61: 1020-1021.
Safo Y, Greenberg J, Young M, et al. Effects of high dose fentanyl on regional cerebral blood flow. Anesthesiology 1983: 59: A306.
Safwat AM, Daniel D. Grand mal seizures after fentanyl administration. Letter to editor. Anesthesiology 1983: 59: 79.
Sari A, Okuda Y, Takeshita H. The effects of thalamonal on cerebral circulation and oxygen consumption in man. Br J Anaesth 1972: 44: 330-334.
Scholz J, Bause H, Schulz M, et al. Pharmacokinetics and effects on intracranial pressure of sufentanil in head trauma patients. Br J Clin Pharmacol 1994: 38: 369-372.
Schregel W, Schäfermeyer H, Müller C, et al. Einfluss von halothan, alfentanil und propofol auf der flussgeschwindigkeiten, "gefässquerschnitt" und "volumenfluss" in der a. cerebri media. Anaesthesist 1992: 41: 21-26.
Schubert A, Peterson DO, Drummond JC; Saidman LJ. The effect of high-dose fentanyl on human median nerve somatosensory evoked responses. Anesth Analg 1986: 65: S136.
Schwartz AE, Matteo RS, Ornstein E, et al. Pharmacokinitics of sufentanil in neurosurgical patients undergoing hyperventilation. Br J Anaesth 1989: 63: 385-388.
Scott JC, Cooke JE, Stanski DR. Electroencephalographic Quantitation of opoid effect: Comparative pharmacodynamics of fentanyl and sufentanil. Anesthesiology: 1991: 74: 34-42.
Sebel AM, Bovill JG, Fentanyl and convulsions Anesth Analg 1983: 62: 858-859.
Sebel PS, Bovill JG, Wauquier A, Rog P. Effects of high-dose fentanyl anesthesia on the electroencephalogram. Anesthesiology 1981: 55: 203-211.
Shafer A, White PF, Schüttler J, Rosenthal MH. Use of a fentanyl infusion in the intensive care unit: Tolerance to its anesthetic effects. Anesthesiology 1983: 59: 245-248.
Shah NK, Long C, Marx W, et al. Cerebrovascular response to CO2 in edematous brain during either fentanyl or isoflurane anesthesia. J Neurosurg Anesthesiol 1990: 2: 11-15.
Sheehan PB, Zornow MH, Scheller MS, Peterson BM. The effect of fentanyl and sufentanil on intracranial pressure and cerebral blood flow in rabbits with an acute cryogenic brain injury. J Neurosurg Anesthesiol 1992. 4: 261-267.
Shupak RC Harp JR, Stevenson-Smith W. et al. High-dose fentanyl for neuroanesthesia. Anesthesiology 1983: 58: 579-582.

Shupak RC, Harp JR. Comparison between high-dose sufentanil-oxygen and high dose fentanyl-oxygen for neuroanesthesia. Br J Anaesth 1985: 57: 375–381.

Sinclair ME, Sear JW, Summerfield RJ, Fisher A. Alfentanil infusions in the intensive therapy unit. Intensive Care Med 1988: 14: 55–59.

Slee TA, Lam AM, Winn HR. Cerebral blood flow velocity and intracranial pressure response to sufentanil- A dose sponse study. Anesthesiology 1990: 73: No 3A, A 176.

Smith AL, Marque JJ. Anesthetics and cerebral edema. Anesthesiology 1976: 45: 64–72.

Smith NT, Bickford RG, Sanford TJ, Dec-Silver H, Blasco TA. Do seizures occur during clinical induction with opiates? Anesthesiology 1987: 67: A385.

Soonthon-Brant V, Patel PM, Drummond JC, et al. Fentanyl does not increase brain injury after focal cerebral ischaemia in rats. Anesth Analg 1999: 88: 49–55.

Sperry RJ, Bailey PL, Reichman MV, et al. Fentanyl and sufentanil increases intracranial pressure in head trauma patients. Anesthesiology 1992: 77: 416–420.

Stephan H, Gröger P, Weyland A, et al. Effects of high-dose sufentanil-O2 anesthesia on cerebral blood flow, metabolism, and the cerebrovascular response to carbon dioxide in man. Anaesthesist 1991: 40: 153–160.

Stockard JJ, Schauble JF, Bickford RG. On-line computer analyses of the electroencephalogram during anesthesia. In: Scientific abstracts of the 1972 Meeting Am Ass Anaesth 1962: 193–194.

Stockard JJ, Bickford R. The neurophysiology of anesthesia. In: Gordon E, ed. A basis and practice of neuroanesthesia. Amsterdam:Excerpta Medica 1975: 3–46.

Takeshita H, Michenfelder JD, Theye RA. The effects of morphine and N-allylnormorphine on canine cerebral metabolism and circulation. Anesthesiology 1972: 37: 605–612.

Tanaka GY. Hypertensive reaction to nalaxone. JAMA 1974: 228: 25–26.

Tempelhoff R, Modica PA, Bernardo KL, Edwards I. Fentanyl-induced electrocorticographic seizures in patients with complex partial epilepsy. J Neurosurg 1992: 77: 201–208.

Tommasino C, Maekawa T, Shapiro HM. Fentanyl-induced seizures activate subcortical brain metabolism. Anesthesiology 1984: 60: 283–290.

Trindle MR, Dodson BA, Rampil IJ. Effects of fentanyl versus sufentanil in equianesthetic doses on middle cerebral artery blood flow velocity. Anesthesiology 1993: 78: 454–460.

TySmith N, Quinn ML, Westover JC, et al. The EEGs of alfentanil, sufentanil, and fentanyl: A quantitative comparison. Anesth Analg 1986: 65: S145.

Warner DS, Hindman BJ, Todd MM, et al. Intracranial pressure and hemodynamic effects of remifentanil versus alfentanil in patients undergoing supratentorial craniotomy. Anesth Analg 1996: 83: 348–353.

Warner DS. Experience with remifentanil in neurosurgical patients. Anesth Analg 1999: 89: 533–539.

Weinger MB. Opoid induced nuscle rigidity clinical implication and patophysiology. Progress in Anesthesiology. San Antonio Texas, Dannemiller Memorial Education Foundation 1993: 8: pp 198–210.

Weinstabl C, Mayer N, Richling B, et al. Effect of sufentanil on intracranial pressure in neurosurgical patients. Anaesthesia 1991: 46: 837–840.

Weitzner SW, McCay GT, Binder LS. Effects of morphine, levallorphan, and respiratory gases on increased intracranial pressure. Anesthesiology 1963: 24: 291–298.

Welling EC, Donegan J. Neuroleptanalgesia using alfentanil for awake craniotomy. Anesth Analg 1989: 68: 57–69.

Werner C, Hoffman WE, Baughmann VL, et al. Effects of sufentanil on cerebral blood flow, cerebral flow velocity, and metabolism in dogs. Anesth Analg 1991: 72: 177–181.

Werner C, Kochs E, Bause H, et al. Effects of sufentanil on cerebral hemodynamics and intracranial pressure in patients with brain injury. Anesthesiology 1995: 83: 721–726.

Wilkinson IMS, Browne DRG. The influence of anaesthesia and of arterial hypocapnia on regional blood flow in the normal human cerebral hemisphere. Br J Anaesth 1970: 42: 472–482.

Yamakura T, Sakimura K, Shimoji K. Direct inhibition of N-methyl-D-aspartate receptor channel by high concentrations of opioids. Anesthesiology 1999: 91: 1053–1063.

Yate PM, Thomas D, Sebel P. Alfentanil infusion for sedation and analgesia in intensive care. Lancet 1984: ii: 396–397.

Young ML, Smith DS, Greenberg J, et al. Effects of sufentanil on regional cerebral glucose utilization in rats. Anesthesiology 1984: 61: 564–568.

Young W, Flamm ES, Demopoulus HB, et al. Effect of nalaxone on posttraumatic ischaemia in experimental spinal contusion. J Neurosurg 1981: 55: 209–219.

Young WL, Prohovnik I, Correll JW, et al. A comparison of the cerebral hemodynamic effects of sufentanil and isoflurane in humans undergoing carotid endarterectomy. Anesthesiology 1989a: 71: 863–869.

Åkeson J. Messeter K, Rosén I, Björkman S. Cerebral haemodynamic and electrocortical CO_2 reactivity in pigs anaesthetized with fentanyl, nitrous oxide and pancuronium. Acta Anaesthesiol Scand 1993: 37: 85–91.

Neuromuscular blocking agents and local analgesics

Succinylcholine, experimental studies

ICP

In animal experiments succinylcholine increases ICP (Cottrell et al. 1983, Lanier et al. 1986). The increase in ICP is also observed after pre-treatment with thiopentone (Thiagarajah et al. 1988). In dogs subjected to succinylcholine injection, CBF increases within a few CBF minutes, and this hyperperfusion is accompanied by EEG activation (Mori et al. 1973, Lanier et al. 1986), and an increase in $PaCO_2$ (Hagan et al. 1983). Thus, the increase in CBF and ICP might partly be caused by the metabolic activation and partly by the increase in $PaCO_2$. However, the increase in ICP ends when $PaCO_2$ is still increasing, making the $PaCO_2$ increase as the offending challenge unlikely (Artru 1990). Fasciculation in the muscles of the neck, causing stasis in the jugular veins, is also thought to be a factor attributing to the increase in ICP (Cottrell et al. 1983). However, in dogs it was demonstrated that it was not the presence of or absence of fasciculation per se that determined the cerebral response to succinylcholine; instead, it is the effect of succinylcholine on the muscle afferent that correlates with the peak increase in CBF (Lanier et al. 1989). In another study by Artru (1990) it was found that the succinylcholine-induced increase in CSF pressure is without temporal relationship to the increase in $PaCO_2$ or MABP. Consequently, the increase in CSF-pressure cannot be abolished by preventing those changes. Disruption of the blood-brain barrier with mannitol does not enhance the cerebral stimulating effect of succinylcholine (Lanier et al. 1990).

It has been questioned if succinylcholine alone or the preservatives in the solutions had effect on cerebral circulation and metabolism. *In vitro* studies of basilar artery rings from dogs and guinea pigs, however, have shown that paraben, and not succinylcholine is a cerebral vasodilator (Hamilton et al. 1990). On the other hand, Pompy et al. (1991) showed that paraben preservatives do not increase intracranial pressure in cats.

Millis et al (1985) studied ICP in dogs subjected to ICP hypertension. Dogs with decerebrate posturing exhibited larger decreases in arterial oxygen tension. Succinylcholine increased oxygen tension and decreased ICP.

Succinylcholine, human studies

ICP

In human studies without (Halldin and Wåhlin 1959, Marx et al. 1962), and with intracranial space-occupying lesions, an increase in ICP has been observed (March et al. 1980, Minton et al. 1986c). In patients scheduled for craniotomy, induction of anaesthesia with thiopentone pancuronium followed by light enflurane anaesthesia allows successful control of ICP, while the use of succinylcholine for intubation gives rise to an increase in ICP (McLeskey et al. 1974).

During induction of anaesthesia pre-treatment with vecuronium (Minton et al. 1986c), or metocuronium (Stirt et al. 1987) attenuates the increase in ICP. Of some interest is a study by White et al. (1982) indicating that pre-treatment with succinylcholine before suction procedures in severely injured head injury patients, attenuates the ICP increase better than that obtained with thiopentone 3 mg/kg, lidocaine 1.5 mg/kg intravenously or intratracheally and fentanyl 1 g/kg. It must be emphasized that it is impossible to predict in advance which patients will suffer from ICP increase after succinylcholine. Thus, the increase in ICP is not correlated to fasciculation (Minton et al. 1986) or increase in blood pressure. Studies in humans indicate that CBF and flow velocity are unchanged after intravenous administration of the preservatives methylparaben and propylparaben (Gelb et al. 1992).

In patients with severe head injury ICP and CPP are unchanged following succinylcholine administration (Brown et al. 1996). Kovalik et al. (1994) found that susccinylcholine (1 mg/kg) did not alter flow velocity, ICP or CPP in mechanically ventilated patients. In another study pretreatment with a defasciculating dose of metocurine prevented an increase in ICP (Stirt et al. 1987).

In patients with cerebral aneurysm succinylcholine injection provokes hyperkalaemia (Iwatsuki et al. 1980). In patients undergoing early surgery (less than 4 days) following subarachnoid haemorrhage, critical hyperkalaemia after succinylcholine was not observed (Manninen et al. 1989), neither was hyperkalaemia observed in patients with brain tumours (Minton et al. 1986a).

Non depolarising muscular relaxants

Patients with upper motor neurone lesion are relatively resistant to non-depolarising muscular relaxants (Graham 1980, Moorthy and Hilgenberg 1980). In experimental studies immobilisation and disuse atrophy are associated with a decreased sensitivity to these drugs (Gronert 1981, Waud and Waud 1986), and resistance to vecuronium has been observed in patients with cerebral palsy (Moorthy et al. 1991). Furthermore, patients in treatment with carbamazepine (Roth et al. 1988), phenytoin (Ornstein et al. 1987) aminophylline and steroid (Azar et al. 1982) have also decreased sensitivity to non-depolarising muscular relaxants.

D-Tubocuranine, experimental studies

In rats d-tubocuranine induces an increase in CBF, but only when the blood-brain barrier has been opened with urea. The increase in CBF can be antagonised with cimitidine (Vesely et al. 1986). In this context, studies by Gross et al. (1981) indicate that histamine might increase CBF only when the blood-brain-barrier is defect. This observation therefore suggests that the effect of d-tubocuranine on CBF is not caused by a direct effect on cerebral vessels, but is effected by histamine, either through a direct vasodilating effect by histamine (Tindall and Greenfield 1973, Martins et al. 1980), or as a result of histamine-induced increases in $PaCO_2$ (Weiss et al. 1977).

D-tubocuranine, human studies

In patients scheduled for stereotaxic intervention, d-tubocuranine provokes an increase in ICP and a decrease in the average thalamic baseline impedance, suggesting cerebral vasodilatation (Tarkkanen et al. 1974). However, the only human study concerning the effect of d-tubocuranine on CBF indicates unchanged CBF after d-tubocuranine injection (Wollman et al. 1965). In new-born piglets it has been demonstrated that neuromuscular blocking agents with ganglion blocking activity (d-tubocuranine and high dosage pancuronium) as well as the specific ganglion blocker hexamethonium enhance the cerebral autoregulation response. This effect was not observed with vecuronium and low-dosage of pancuronium (Chemtob et al. 1992).

Pancuronium

In dogs pancuronium does not affect ICP, CBF, CMRO2 or EEG (Lanier et al. 1985). In new-born pigs CBF is unchanged after pancuronium, and during bicuculline-induced seizure pancuronium does not attenuate the increase in CBF (Pourcyrous et al. 1992). In neonates with respiratory distress pancuronium attenuates the fluctuations in the CBF velocity pattern (Peabody 1981, Perlman et al.1985). Since fluctuations in CBF are supposed to predispose to intraventricular haemorrhage (Ment et al. 1983), neuromuscular blockers are supposed to prevent the development of neurologic insults.

Atracurium, experimental studies

In cats atracurium does not influence ICP (Giffin et al. 1985). However, in the same animal this drug activates the EEG without changing CBF or $CMRO_2$ (Lanier et al. 1985). Laudanosine, a metabolite of atracurium provokes epileptic seizures (Mercier and Mercier 1955), and an increase in the concentration of laudanosine has been observed after the use of atracurium (Fahey et al. 1984, Boheimen et al. 1984). Atracurium and its metabolite, laudanoside produces two distinct effects upon hippocampal slices. An enhancement of excitatory transmission and neuronal excitability, and blockade of inhibitory GABA-mediated synaptic responses (Chiodini et al. 1998). However, in rabbits subjected to cortical application of the epileptogenic drug cefazoline during craniotomy, no increased incidence of seizure activity could be detected in those animals receiving laudanosine at rates sufficient to produce plasma levels similar to what might be seen following the clinical use of atracurium (Tateishi et al. 1989). Accordingly, it has been argued that the concentrations of laudanosine after neuromuscular blockade with atracurium are incapable of producing neurological or cardiovascular disturbances (Chapple et al. 1987). In studies in mice nitrous oxide antagonises the CNS stimulating action of laudanosine (Arramov and Mori 1990).

Atracurium, human studies

Human studies indicate that atracurium does not influence ICP (Minton et al. 1985, Rosa et al. 1986a, Unni and Young 1986). A maximum dose of atracurium by infusion was accompanied with a laudanosine plasma concentration of 0.34 g/ml. In another study a concentration between 200 and 300 ng/ml at 2 min after atracurium administration for intubation was found (Nigrovic and Fox 1991). It has been proposed that stimulation by laudanosine might accelerate awakening (Beemer et al. 1989).

The incidence of hypotension, cutaneous reaction, and bronchospasm is 3.4, 4.6 and 0.2% respectively after atracurium administration (Beemer et al. 1988).

Cisatracurium

In mechanically ventilated patients with severe head injury cisatracurium does not cause any significant changes in flow velocity, ICP, MABP and CPP (Scramm et al. 1997).

Vecuronium

Like pancuronium, vecuronium does not provoke an increase in ICP in cats (Giffin et al. 1986) or in humans (Minton et al. 1986b, Rosa et al. 1986b).

Pipecuronium

In a randomised study in patients with supratentorial cerebral tumours Shaheen et al. (2000) found that the increase in ICP during intubation was more pronounced after pancuronium compared with pipecuronium. In contrast, Thiel et al. (1996) studied cerebrospinal fluid pressure in neurosurgical patients, and found no significant difference in pressure during intubation between pancuronium and pipecuronium.

Comparative studies

In a primate model of intracranial hypertension, neither atracurium nor succinylcholine elevate ICP when given following a defasciculating dose of succinylcholine (Haigh et al. 1986).

Ducey et al. (1989) compared the effects of succinylcholine, atracurium and vecuronium on intracranial haemodynamics in swine subjected to ICP hypertension by inflation of an epidural balloon. Neither atracurium nor vecuronium changed ICP or CPP. Succinylcholine, however, produced an early decrease in ICP, followed by a rapid increase above preinfusion level.

In neurosurgical patients undergoing mechanical ventilation the effects of rocuronium and vecuronium upon ICP and CPP were compared. No significant difference in ICP and CPP between the two drugs was disclosed (Schramm et al. 1996).

Lidocaine, experimental studies

Receptor actions

Lidocaine, like other local anaesthetics, is a Na^+ channel blocker. Kim-Lee et al. (1994) found that short exposure to hypocalcia in glial cells prompts subsequent, potentially lethal, sodium-dependent calcium entry via the reverse phase of the Na^+/Ca^{2+} exchanger, and that lidocaine is able to block intracellular calcium increases when added at the time of reperfusion.

GABA-induced inhibition of cortical neurones is not affected by lidocaine (Warnick et al. 1971). Competitive NMDA receptor antagonist increases the lidocaine-induced seizure threshold in the rat (McFarlane et al. 1994). Administration of procaine, another Na^+ channel blocker before forebrain ischaemia suppresses ischaemic glutamate release, and reduces neuronal damage in the gerbil hippocampus (Adachi et al. 1999). Like central analgesics, inhalation anaesthetics and hypnotics, lidocaine decreases the utilisation of acetylcholine in the brain (Ngai et al. 1979).

Antiepileptogenic and epileptogenic characters

In monkeys intravenous infusion of lidocaine is associated with diffuse slowing of the EEG activity. Accordingly, lidocaine has anticonvulsive properties in experimental epilepsy. On the other hand, lidocaine might elicit epileptic seizures and an arterial threshold concentration has been defined. Convulsive doses of lidocaine are followed by marked increases in heart rate, mean arterial pressure, pulmonary artery pressure, cardiac output, systemic vascular resistance, left ventricular end diastolic pressure, and myocardial contractility (Rutten et al. 1989). The mechanism of death during toxic intravenous doses of lidocaine is respiratory depression with bradycardia and hypotension without arrhytmias (Nancarrow et al. 1989). It is supposed that seizure activity may result from a selective depression of inhibitory control, normally exerted over excitatory input (DeJong et al. 1969).

It is well known that the acid-base balance affects the threshold of lidocaine toxicity (DeJong et al. 1967, Englesson 1974). Adding vasoconstrictors (epinephrine, norepinephrine) to local anaesthetics may decrease peak plasma concentration of local anaesthetics and increase the duration of the block. Surprisingly, it was found that intravenous injection of lidocaine with epinephrine decreased the convulsing as well as the lethal doses of lidocaine in rats (Yagiela 1985, Torbiner et al. 1989). The greater the concentration of added epinephrine, the lower the cumulative convulsing dosage of lidocaine. And the greater the increase in mean arterial blood pressure the lower the threshold of lidocaine-induced convulsants in rats (Yokoyama et al. 1993). A later study indicates that acute hypertension induced by either epinephrine, norepinephrine or phenylephrine does not influence convulsant thresholds of lidocaine equally. By offsetting the vasoconstricting effect by sodium nitroprusside convulsant threshold was normalised. The authors argue that difference in - and -adrenergic effect might play a role, as might hypertension-induced break down of the blood-brain barrier (Yokoyama et al. 1995).

During lidocaine-induced convulsion *c-Fos* protein was markedly induced in the piriform cortex and amygdala, and slightly induced in the neocortex and thalamus. In contrast, *c-Fos* expression following generalised convulsions induced by non-anaesthetic convulsants was markedly enhanced in the hippocampal region too (Nakao et al. 1994).

CBF and $CMRO_2$

In dogs, lidocaine in a non seizure-producing dosage of 3 mg/kg, reduces $CMRO_2$ by 10% after 2–3 min. $CMRO_2$ is normalised within 5 min. CBF is unchanged. After 15mg/kg $CMRO_2$ is decreased by 27% and CBF is decreased as well. The metabolic depression is of 20 min. duration (Sakabe et al. 1974). In cats lumbar subarachnoid application of local anaesthetics (lidocaine, mepivacaine, or tetracain) does not change CBF or spinal cord blood flow (Porter et al. 1985). In dogs subjected to local application of lidocaine, Dohi et al. (1984) found similar results. When mixtures of phenylephrine and lidocaine were injected, however, spinal blood flow decreased significantly.

During continuous lidocaine infusion until EEG seizures were induced, $CMRO_2$ increased by 12% of control, and CBF increased disproportionally more than the increase in $CMRO_2$. With the determination of seizures $CMRO_2$ returned to control levels within 90 min (Sakabe et al. 1974). In rats neither non-seizure or seizure doses of lidocaine cause any reduction in cerebral energy charge, or other evidence of increased anaerobic metabolism in the cerebral cortex (Maekawa et al. 1981). However, studies using electrodes in the deep cerebral structures (Wagman et al. 1967), and studies of regional glucose utilisation in rats during EEG activation have shown increased glucose utilisation within the limbic system and a simultaneous reduction in glucose utilisation in the rest of the brain (Ingvar and Shapiro 1981). Correlated studies of local CBF and glucose utilisation have shown an uncoupling of local brain metabolism from blood flow during lidocaine-induced subcortical epileptic discharges in areas recognised to be prone to irreversible damage following prolonged seizure activity (Tommasino et al. 1986).

Protection

Lidocaine has been shown to inhibit perturbations of endothelial cell surface membrane. In rabbits lidocaine pre-treatment has a prophylactic effect upon endotoxin-mediated lung injury (Mikawa et al. 1994). In a later study in the same animal, however, it was found that lidocaine did not influence the concentration of activated complement components, cytokines and arachidonic acid metabolites in bronchoalveolar lavage fluid, and the attenuation of endotoxin-induced lung oedema was only slight and likely to be of little clinical significance (Nishina et al. 1995)

In rabbits lidocaine 0.05 mg/kg/min accelerates the time course of EEG recovery after global ischaemia (Sustch and Rubinstein 1991). In dogs lidocaine prolongs the safe duration of circulatory arrest during hypothermia (Zhou et al. 1998). In dogs subjected to deep barbiturate anaesthesia or hypothermia, leading to isoelectric EEG, the addition of lidocaine in a dose of 160 mg/kg caused an additional metabolic inhibition of 15–20%, suggesting that lidocaine under these circumstances might provide some protection of the brain (Astrup et al. 1981b). Lidocaine also caused reduction in the potassium efflux rate of about 50% probably by reducing membrane ion permeability in accordance with its local anaesthetic action (Astrup et al. 1981a). Other studies indicate that lidocaine reduces the increase in extracellular concentration of excitatory amino acids in transient forebrain ischaemia (Fujitani et al. 1994), and influences the action of ryanodine receptors which regulate the efflux of CA^{2+} from the endoplasmic reticulum to the cytosol (Martin et al. 1993). Lidocaine administered 30 min after moderate injury also attenuates the trauma-induced suppression of motor function in the rat (Hamm et al. 1996). These results indicate that lidocaine might have some protective effects against cerebral ischaemia. During forebrain ischaemia in gerbil lidocaine delayed the onset of the ischaemic-induced membrane depolarisation and improved histologic outcome. *In vitro* studies of hippocampal slices indicated that lidocaine inhibited the release of Calcium from intracellular Ca^{2+} stores and inhibited the influx from extracellular space (Liu et al. 1997). In cats subjected to spinal cord injury a certain protective effect has indeed been observed (Kobrine et al. 1984, Chang et al. 1986). In cats subjected to MCAO, a bolus dose of 5 mg/kg followed by continuous infusion, gave better preservation of evoked potentials, smaller infarct size and higher CBF in the peripheral region of the infarct (Shokunbi et al. 1987). A protective effect has not been observed in other studies of cats subjected to spinal injury and monitored with spinal evoked responses (Haghighi et al. 1987), in rats subjected to near complete global ischaemia (Warner et al. 1988), in cats subjected to MCAO (Shokunbi et al. 1986, Gelb et al. 1988), and in rats subjected to radiation-induced brain injury (Oldfield et al. 1990).

From studies in rabbits subjected to reversible ischaemia it has been hypothesised that lidocaine facilitates recovery of EEG and evoked potential only when an ischaemic episode is below a certain combined level of duration and severity (Sustch and Rubinstein 1991).

In studies of asphyxiated pre-term lamb lidocaine led to a significant increase in $PaCO_2$, a decrease in arterial blood-pH, and a decrease in blood flow to the brain. The study suggested that the immature fetus loses its cardiovascular adaptation to asphyxia when exposed to lidocaine obtained from the mother (Morishima et al. 1989). Studies in dogs during isoflurane anaesthesia, where lidocaine in a dose of 15 mg/kg was given, have shown a decrease in the concentration of ATP in cerebral tissue, suggesting a detrimental effect of lidocaine on cerebral metabolism (Milde and Milde 1987). However, low concentration of ATP in cerebral tissue before lidocaine administration makes this conclusion questionable.

Air embolism

In cats subjected to cerebral ischaemia induced by air embolism, lidocaine stabilises blood pressure (Evans et al. 1984), and pre-treatment with lidocaine attenuates the intracranial hypertension caused by the air embolism (Evans et al. 1989), and improves recovery of somatosensory evoked potential (Dutka et al. 1992). Furthermore, lidocaine given after the air embolus is effective in reducing ICP hypertension (Evans and Kobrine 1987).

Lidocaine, human studies

In healthy subjects CBF decreased 12% during lidocaine infusion (5 mg/kg). In contrast, diabetic patients had identical CBF levels before and after lidocaine (Kastrup et al. 1990).

Systematically administered lidocaine, at therapeutic plasma levels, depresses the amplitude and prolongs the latency of somato-sensory evoked potentials (Schubert et al. 1992). Pain of central origin appears to be affected favourably by intravenous lidocaine, whereas pain of peripheral origin is unaffected, except at blood concentrations which approach toxic values (Boas et al. 1982). Lidocaine in clinical doses suppresses the cough reflex (Poulton et al. 1979).

Endotracheal intubation

During endotracheal intubation (Bedford et al. 1980b, Hamill et al. 1981), scalp incision (Bedford et al. 1980a) and suction procedures in neurointensive patients (Donegan et al. 1980, White et al. 1982, Yano et al. 1986), intravenous lidocaine (1.5 mg/kg) inhibits or attenuates the ICP increase. In normal muscle the increase in oxygen consumption obtained by succinylcholine is attenuated by lidocaine (Fukuda et al. 1987). During induction of anaesthesia and intubation, lidocaine (1–2 mg/kg) attenuates the cardiovascular response of hypertension and tachycardia (Abou Medi et al. 1977). In another study lidocaine 1.5 mg/kg was given 1,2,3, and 5 min before intubation. Lidocaine attenuated the increase in heartrate and blood pressure only when given 3 min. before intubation (Tam et al. 1987). In a recent study aerosolised lidocaine, when administered with a semiclosed breathing system in a dose of 0.2 ml/kg of a 5% solution, prevented haemodynamic changes during intubation without signs of lidocaine toxicity (Baronia et al. 1992).

However, other studies indicate that these effects were of minor degree or absent. Thus, lidocaine did not prevent the rate-pressure-product to reach levels which might be dangerous in patients with ischaemic heart disease (Chraemmer-J¢rgensen et al. 1986). In a clinical study by Laurito et al (1987) aerosolised or intravenous lidocaine was not more effective than placebo for the control of haemodynamic response to intubation. Furthermore, in a controlled study of patients with intracranial malformation or brain tumour lidocaine (1.5 mg/kg) administered 2–3 min prior to intubation together with a sleep dose of thiopentone, did not protect against hypertensive pressure peaks in MABP, whereas fentanyl 6 g/kg did so (Bachofen 1988).

Other drugs used for intubation

The effects of other drugs on the pressure response during intubation have been investigated. The -blocking agent labetalol has been studied in a double blind clinical trial. In a dose of 0.25 mg/kg within one minute before intubation, this drug blunts the increase in heart rate and attenuates the increase in blood pressure (Inada et al. 1987, Bernstein et al. 1987). In dosages greater than 0.75 mg/kg it produces a significant reduction of MABP as well (Leslie et al. 1987). Samaha et al. (1996) compared the effects of esmolol (1.5 mg/kg) and lidocaine (1.5 mg/kg) during intubation in neurosurgical patients. Lumbar CSF pressure increased, and CPP decreased in both groups, without any intergroup differences.

Procaine

Procaine has been studied experimentally in the gerbil. During forebrain ischaemia procaine decreases excitatory amino acid release, and improves histological outcome in the hippocampus (Adachi et al. 1999).

During procaine treatment EEG activation in the temporal and occipital lobes correlates with rCBF increase in amygdala (Parkh et al. 1995). In humans procaine yields emotional and psychosensory experiences combined with temporal lobe fast activity. In healthy volunteers studies with PET indicate that procaine increases global CBF, and to a greater extent blood flow in the anterior paralimbic region. Subjects with intense procaine-induced fear, compared with those with euphoria, had greater CBF increase in the anterior amygdala. Procaine-induced visual hallucinations appeared associated with greater global and occipital CBF increases (Ketter et al. 1996). During cardiopulmonary by-pass the cardioplegic procaine-containing solution of Bretschneider resulted in a decrease in CBF (Henriksen et al. 1986).

Tetracaine

In dogs lumbar subarachnoid application of tetracaine does not change CBF or spinal cord blood flow, and the CBF response to hypercapnia is intact (Dohi et al. 1987).

Ropivacaine

Using Laser-Doppler flowmetry ropivacaine decreases spinal blood flow in rats (Kristensen et al. 1996)s and decreases epidural blood flow in humans (Dahl et al. 1990).

Topical application of ropivacaine constricts cerebral pial arteries (Ishiyama et al. 1997). This effect is not inhibited by Yohimbine, a central $_2$-inhibitor (Ishiyama et al. 1997).

References

Abou-Madi MN, Keszler H, Yacoub JM. Cardiovascular reactions to laryngoscopy and tracheal intubation following small and large doses of lidocaine. Canad J Anesth 1977: 24: 12–19.

Adachi N, Chen J, Nakanishi K, Arai T. Pre-ischaemic administration of procaine suppresses ischaemic glutamate release and reduces neuronal damage in the gerbil hippocampus. Br J Anaesth 1999: 83: 472–474.

Artru AA. Succinylcholine-induced increases in CSF pressure are not affected by PaCO2 or mean arterial pressure in dogs. J Neurosurgical Anesthesiology 1990b: 2: 4–10.

Astrup J, Skovsted P, Gjerris F, S¢rensen HR. Increase in extracellular potassium in the brain during circulatory arrest: Effects of hypothermia, lidocaine, and thiopental. Anesthesiology 1981a: 55: 256–262.
Astrup J, M¢ller S¢rensen P, S¢rensen HR, Inhibition of cerebral oxygen and glucose consumption in the dog by hypothermia, pentobarbital, and lidocaine. Anesthesiology 1981b: 55: 263–268.
Avramov MN, Mori K. Nitrous oxide antagonizes CNS stimulation by laudanoside in mice. Br J Anaesth 1990: 65: 704–707.
Azar I, Kumar D, Betcher AM. Resistance to pancuronium in an asthmatic patient treated with amoniphylline and steroids. Can Anaesth Soc J 1982: 29: 280–282
Bachofen M. Dämfung des Blutdruckanstieges bei der Intubation: lidocain oder Fentanyl? Anaesthesist 1988: 37: 156–161.
Baronia AK, Singh PK, Maheshwari A, et al. Inhaled lidocaine for prevention of hemodynamic changes in laryngoscopy and intubation. J Neurosurg Anesthesiol 1992: 4: 154–159.
Bedford RF, Persing JA, Pobereskin L, Butler A. Lidocaine or thiopental for rapid control of intracranial hypertension? Anesth Analg 1980a: 59: 435–437.
Bedford RF, Winn HR, Tyson G, et al. Lidocaine prevents increased ICP after endotracheal intubation. In: Shulman K, Marmarou A, Miller JD, Becker DP, Hochwald GM, Brock M (eds); Intracranial Pressure IV, Springer Verlag, Berlin Heidelberg, New York 1980b: 595–598.
Beemer GH, Dennis WL, Platt PR, et al. Adverse deactions to atracurium and alcuronium. Br J Anaesth 1988: 61: 680–684.
Beemer GH, Bjorksten AR, Dawson PJ, Crankshaw DP. Prduction of laudanosine following infusion of atrachurium in man and its effects on awakening. Br J Anaesth 1989: 63: 76–80.
Bernstein JS, Nelson MA, Ebert TJ, et al. Beat-by-beat cardiovascular responses to rapid sequence induction in humans: Effects of labetamol. Anaesthesiology 1987: 67: A 32.
Boas RA, Covino BG, Shahnarian A. Analgesic responses to i.v. lignocaine. Br J Anaesth 1982: 54: 501–504.
Boheimer N, Ward S, Dopson T, et al. Pharmacokinetics of laudanosine and a quaternary alcohol after an i.v. bolus dose of atracurium in patients with impaired renal function. Br J Anaesth 1984: 57: 345.
Brown MM, Parr MJ, Manara AR. The effect of suxamethonium on intracranial pressure and cerebral perfusion pressure in patients with severe head injuries following blunt trauma. Eur J Anaesthesiol 1996: 13: 474–477.
Chang JL, Chang GL, Nemoto EM, et al. Protective effect of i.v. lidocaine in acute experimental spinal cord injury. Anesthesiology 1986: 65: A319.
Chapple DJ, Miller AA, Ward JB, Wheatley PL. Cardiovascular and neurological effects of laudanosine. Br J Anaesth 1987: 59: 218–225.
Chemtob S, Barna T, Beharry K, et al. Enhanced cerebral blood flow autoregulation in the newborn piglet by d-tubocuranine and pancuronium but not by vecuronium. Anesthesiology 1992: 76: 236–244
Chraemmer-J¢rgensen B, H¢llund-Carlsen PF, Marving J, Christensen V. Lack of effect of intravenous lidocaine on hemodynamic responses to rapid sequence induction of general anesthesia: A double-blind clinical trial. Anesth Analg 1986: 65: 1037–1041.
Cottrell JE, Hartung J, Giffin JP, Shwiry B. Intracranial and hemodynamic changes after succinylcholine administration in cats. Anesth Analg 1983: 62: 1006–1009.
Dahl JB, Simonsen L, Mogensen T, et al. The effect of 0.5% ropivacaine on epidural blood flow. Acta Anaesthesiol Scand 1990: 34: 308–310.
DeJong RH, Robles R, Corbin RW. Central actions of lidocaine-synaptic transmission. Anesthesiology 1969: 30: 19–23.
DeJong RH, Wagman IH, Prince DA. Effect of carbon dioxide on the cortical seizure threshold to lidocaine. Experi Neurol 1967: 17: 221–232.
Dohi S, Matsumiya N, Takeshima R, et al. The effects of subarachnoid lidocaine and phenylephidrine on spinal cord blood flow in dogs. Anesthesiology 1984: 61: 238–244.
Dohi S, Takeshima R, Naito H. Spinal cord blood flow during spinal anesthesia in dogs: the effects of tetracaine, epinephrine, acute blood loss, and hypercapnia. Anesth Analg 1987: 66: 599–606.
Donegan MF, Bedford RF. Intravenously administered lidocaine prevents intracranial hypertension during endotracheal suctioning. Anesthesiology 1980: 52: 516–518.
Ducey JP, Deppe SA, Foley KT. A comparison of the effects of suxamethonium, atracurium and vecuronium on intracranial haemodynamics in swine. Anaesth Intensive Care 1989: 17: 448–455.
Dutka AJ, Mink R, McDemott J, et al. Effect of lidocaine on somatosensory evoked response and cerebral blood flow after canine cerebral air embolism. Stroke 1992: 23: 1515–1521.
Englesson S. The influence of acid-base changes on central nervous system toxicity of local anaesthetic agents. Acta Anaesthesiol Scand 1974: 18: 79–87.
Evans DE, Kobrine AI, Legrys DC, Bradley ME. Protective effect of lidocaine in acute cerebral ischaemia induced by air embolism. J Neurosurg 1984: 60: 257–263.
Evans DE, Kobrine AI. Reduction of experimental intracranial hypertension by lidocaine. Neurosurgery 1987: 20: 542–547.
Evans DE, Catron PW, McDermott JJ, et al. Effect of lidocaine after experimental cerebral ischaemia induced by air embolism. J Neurosurg 1989: 70: 97–102.
Fahey MR, Rupp SM, Fisher DM, et al. The pharmacokinetics and pharmacodynamics of atracurium in patients with and without renal failure. Anesthesiology 1984: 61: 699–714.
Fujitani T, Adachi N, Miyazaki H, et al. Lidocaine protects hippocampal neurons agianst ischemic damage by preventing increase of extracellular excitatory amino acids: a microdialysis study in Mongolian gerbils. Neurosci Lett 1994: 179: 91–94.
Fukuda S, Wakuta K, Ischikawa T, et al. Lidocaine midofies the effect of succicholine on muscle oxygen consumption in dogs. Anesth Analg 1987: 66: 325–328.
Gelb AW, Steinberg GK, Lam AM, et al. The effects of a bolus of lidocaine in focal cerebral ischaemia. Can J Anaesth 1988: 35: 489–493.
Gelb AW, Gignac E, Manninen PH, et al. Methylparaben and propylparaben do not alter cerebral blood flow in humans. Can J Anaesth 1992: 39: 691–694.
Giffin JP, Litwak B, Cottrell JE, et al. Intracranial pressure, mean arterial pressure and heart rate after rapid paralysis with atracurium in cats. Can Anesth Soc J 1985: 32: 618–621.

Giffin JP, Hartung J, Cottrell JE, et al. Effect of vecuronium on intracranial pressure, mean arterial pressure and heart rate in cats. Br J Anaesth 1986: 58: 441–443.
Graham DH. Monitoring neuromuscular block may be unreliable in patients with upper motor neuron lesions. Anesthesiology 1980: 52: 74–75
Gronert GA (1981) Disuse atrophy with resistance to pancuronium. Anesthesiology 55: 567–569
Gross PM, Harper AM, Teasdale GM. Cerebral circulation and histamin: 1. Participation of vascular H1 and H2 receptors in vasodilatatory responses to carotid artery infusion. J Cereb Blood Flow Metab 1981: 1: 97–108.
Haigh JD, Nemoto EM, DeWolf AM, Bleyaert AL. Comparison of the effects of succinylcholine and atracurium on intracranial pressure in monkeys with intracranial hypertension. Can Anaesth Soc J 1986: 33: 421–426.
Halldin M, Wåhlin Å. Effect of succinylcholine on the intraspinal fluid pressure. Acta Anaesth Scand 1959: 3: 155–161.
Hamilton JT, Zhou Y, Gelb AW. Paraben preservatives but not succinylcholine are cerebral vasodilators in vitro. Anesthesiology 1990: 73: 1252–1257.
Hamm RJ, Temple MD, Pike BR, Ellis EF. The effect of postinjury administration of polyethylene glycol-conjugated superoxide dismutase or lidocaine on behavioral function following fluid-percusion brain injury in rats. J Neurotrauma 1996: 13: 325–331.
Hamill JF, Berford RF, Weaver DC, Colohan AR. Lidocaine before endotracheal intubation: Intravenous or laryngotracheal? Anesthesiology 1981: 55: 578–581.
Henriksen L, Barry DI, Rygg IH, Skovsted P. Cerebral blood flow during early cardiopulmonary by-pass in man. Effect of procaine in cardioplegic solutions. Thorac Cardiovasc Surg 1986: 34: 116–123.
Inada E, Cullen DJ, Nemeskal R, Teplick R. Effect of labetalol on the hemodynamic response to intubation: A Controlled radomized double-blind study. Anesthesiology 1987: 67: A 31.
Ingvar M, Shapiro HM. Selective metabolic activation of the hippocampus during lidocaine-induced pre-seizure activity. Anesthesiology 1981: 54: 33–37.
Ishiyama T, Dohi S, Iida H, Watanabe Y. The effect of topical and intravenous ropivacaine on canine pial miccrosirculation. Anesth Analg 1997: 85: 75–81.
Iwatsuki N, Kuroda N, Amaha K, Iwatsuki K. Succinylcholine-induced hyperkalemia in patients with ruptured cerebral aneurysms. Anesthesiology 1980: 53: 64–67.
Kastrup J, Petersen P, Dejgard A. Intravenous lidocaine and cerebral blood flow: impaired microvascular reactivity in diabetic patients. J Clin Pharmacol 1990: 30: 318–323.
Ketter TA, Andreason PJ, Georgs MS, et al. Anterior paralimbic mediation of procaine-induced emotional and psychosensory experiences. Arch Gen Psychiatry 1996: 53: 59–69.
Kim-Lee MH, Stokes BT, McDonold JS. Procaine, lidecaine, and hypothermia inhibits calcium paradox in glial cells. Anesth Analg 1994: 79: 728–733.
Kobrine AI, Evans DE, LeGrys DC, et al. Effects of intravenous lidocaine on experimental spinal cord injury. J Neurosurg 1984: 60: 595–601.
Kovarik WD, Mayberg TS, Lam AM, et al. Succinylcholine does not change intracranial pressure, cerebral blood flow velocity, or the electroencephalogram in patients with neurologic injury. Anesth Analg 1994: 78: 469–473.
Kristensen JD, Karlssten R, Gordh R. Spinal cord blood flow after intrathecal injection of ropivacaine: a screening for neurotoxic effects: Anesth Analg 1996: 82: 636–640.
Lanier WL, Milde JH, Michenfelder JD. The cerebral effects of pancuronium and atracurium in halothane-anesthetized dogs. Anesthesiology 1985: 63: 589–597.
Lanier WL, Milde JH, Michenfelder JD. Cerebral stimulation following succinylcholine in dogs. Anesthesiology 1986: 64: 551–559.
Lanier WL, Iazzo PA, Milde JH. Cerebral function and muscle afferent activities following intravenous succinylcholine in dogs anesthetized with halothane: The effects of pretreatment with a defasciculating dose of pancuronium. Anesthesiology 1989: 71: 87–95.
Lanier WL, Milde JH, Sharbrough FW. Effects of suxamethonium on cerebrum following disruption of the blood-brain barrier in dogs. Br J Anaesth 1990: 65: 708–712.
Laurito CE, Baugman VL, Polek WV, et al. Aerosolized and intravenous lidocaine are no more effective than placebo for the control of hemodynamic response to intubation. Anesthesiology 1987: 67: A 29.
Leslie JB, Kalayjian RW, McLoughlin TM, et al. Ablation of the hemodynamic responses to tracheal intubation with preinduction intravenous labetalol. Anesthesiology 1987: 67: A 30.
Liu K, Adachi N, Yanase H, Kataoka K, Arai T. Lidocaine suppresses the anoxic depolarization and reduces the increase in the intracellular Ca^{2+} concentration in gerbil hippocampal neurons. Anesthesiology 1997: 87: 1470–1478.
Maekawa T, Oshibuchi T, Takeshita H, Imamura A. Cerebral energy state and glycolytic metabolism during lidocaine infusion in the rat. Anesthesiology 1981: 54: 278–283.
Manninen PH, Mahendran B, Gelb AW, Merchant R. The effect of succinylcholine on serum potassium in patients with acutely ruptured cerebral aneurysms. Anesth Analg 1989: 68: S180.
March ML, Dunlop BJ, Shapiro HM, et al. Succinylcholine-intracranial pressure effects in neurosurgical patients. Anesth Analg 1980: 59: 550–551.
Martin C, Ashley R, Shoshan-Barmatz V. The effect of local anesthetics on the ryanodine receptor/Ca^{2+} release channel of brain microsomal memebranes. FEBS Lett 1993: 328: 77–81.
Martins AN, Doyle TF, Wright SJ Jr, Bass BG. Response of cerebral circulation to topical histamine. Stroke 1980: 11: 469–476.
Marx GF, Andrews IC, Orkin LR. Cerebrospinal fluid pressures during halothane anesthesia. Can Anaesth Soc J 1962: 9: 239–245.
McFarlane C, Warner DS, Dexter F, Todd MM. Glutamatergic antagonism: effect on lidocaine-induced seizures in the rat. Anesth Analg 1994: 79: 701–705.
McLeskey CH, Cullen BF, Kennery RD, Galindo A. Control of cerebral perfusion pressure during induction of anesthesia in high-risk neurosurgical patients. Anesth Analg 1974: 53: 985–992.
Ment LR, Stewart WB, Duncan CC, et al. Beagle puppy model of intraventricular hemorrhage: Effect of indomethacin on cerebral blood flow. J Neurosurg 1983: 58: 857–862
Mercier J, Mercier E. Action de quelques alcaloides secondaires de l'opium sur l'electrocorticogramme du chien. C R Soc Biol 1955: 149: 760.

Mikawa K, Maekawa N, Nishina K, et al. Effect of lidocaine pretreatment on endotoxin-induced lung injury in rabbits. Anesthesiology 1994: 81: 689–699.
Milde LN, Milde JH. The detrimental effect of lidocaine on cerebral metabolism measured in dogs anesthetized with isoflurane. Anesthesiology 1987: 67: 180–184.
Millis RM, Wood DH, Trouth CO. Amelioration of hypoxemia by neuromuscular blockade following brain injury. Life Sci 1985: 26: 739–747.
Minton MD, Stirt JA, Bedford RF, Hawworth C. Intracranial pressure after atracurium in neurosurgical patients. Anesth Analg 1985: 64: 1113–1116.
Minton MD, Stirt JA, Bedford RF. Effect of succinylcholine on serum potassium in patients with brain tumors. Anesth Analg 1986a: 65: S100.
Minton MD, Stirt JA, Bedford RF. Vecuronium and intracranial pressure in man. Anesth Analg 1986b: 65: S101.
Minton MD, Grosslight K, Stirt JA, Bedford RF. Increases in intracranial pressure from succinylcholine: Prevention by prior nondepolarizing blockade. Anesthesiology 1986c: 65: 165–169.
Monin P, Hascoet JM, Vert P. Autoregulation of cerebral blood flow. Effect of phenobarbital and pancuronium in the newborn piglet. Dev Pharmacol Ther 1989: 13: 121–128.
Moorthy SS, Hilgenberg JC. Resistance to nondepolarizing muscle relaxants in paretic upper extremities of patients with residual hemiplegia. Anesth Analg 1980: 59: 624–627
Moorthy SS, Krishna G, Dierdorf SF. Resistance to vecuronium in patients with cerebral palsy. Anesth Analg 1991: 73: 275–277
Mori K, Iwabuchi K, Fujito M. The effects of depolarizing muscle relaxants on the electroencephalogram and the circulation during halothane anesthesia in man. Br J Anaesth 1973: 45: 604–610.
Morishima HO, Pedersen H, Santos AC, et al. Adverse effects of maternally administered lidocaine on the asphyxiated preterm fetal lamb. Anesthesiology 1989: 71: 110–115.
Nakao S, Kurata J, Arai T, et al. Lidocaine-induced convulsion does not induced c-fos protein (c-Fos) in rat hippocampus. Acta Anaesthesiol Scand 1994: 38: 845–851.
Nancarrow C, Rutten AJ, Runciman WB, et al. Myocardial and cerebral drug concentrations and the mechanisms of death after fatal intravenous doses of lidocaine, bupivacaine, and ropivacaine in the sheep. Anesth Analg 1989: 69: 276–283.
Nigrovic V, Fox JL. Atracurium decay and the formation of laudanosine in human. Anesthesiology 1991: 74: 446–454.
Ngai SH, Shirasawa R, Cheney DL. Changes in motor activity and acetylcholine turnover induced by lidocaine and cocaine in brain regions of rats. Anesthesiology 1979: 51: 230–234.
Nishina K, Mikawa K, Maekawa N, et al. Does early posttreatment with lidocaine attenuate endotoxin-induced acute lung injury in rabbits. Anesthesiology 1995: 83: 169–177.
Oldfield EH, Friedman R, Kinsella T, et al. Reduction in radiation-induced brain injury by use of pentobarbital or lidocaine protection. J Neurosurg 1990: 72: 737–744.
Ornstein E, Matteo RS, Schwartz AE, et al. The effect of phenytoin on the magnitude and duration of neuromuscluar block following atracurium and vecuronium. Anesthesiology 1987: 67: 191–196
Peabody JL. Mechanical ventilation of the newborn. Good news- bad news. Crit Care Med 1981: 9: 710–713
Parekh PI, Spencer JW, George MS, et al. Procaine-.induced increases in limbic rCBF correlate positively with increases in occipital and temporal EEG fast activity. Brain Topog 1995: 7: 209–216.
Peabody JL. Mechanical ventilation of the newborn. Crit Care Med 1981: 9: 710–713.
Perlman JM, Goodman S, Kreusser KL, Volpe JJ. Reduction in intraventricular hemorrhage by elimination of fluctuating cerebral blood flow velocity in preterm infants with respiratory distress syndrome. N Engl J Med 1985: 312: 1353–1357
Pompy L, Karlin A, Capuano CM, et al. Paraben preservatives do not increase intracranial pressure in cats. Anesthesiology 1991: 75: 669–672.
Porter SS, Albin MS, Watson WA, et al. Spinal and cerebral blood flow responses to subarachnoid injection of local anesthetics with and without epinephrine. Acta Anaesthesiol Scand 1985: 29: 330–338.
Poulton TJ, James FM. Cough suppression by lidocaine. Anesthesiology 1979: 50: 470–472.
Pourcyrous M, Leffler CW, Bada HS, et al. Effects of pancuronium bromide on cerebral blood flow changes during seizures in newborn pigs. Pediatr Res 1992: 31: 636–639.
Rosa G, Orfie P, Sanfilippo M, et al. The effects of atracurium besylate (Tracrium) on intracranial pressure and cerebral perfusion pressure. Anesth Analg 1986a: 65: 381–384.
Rosa G, Sanfilippo M, Vilardi V, et al. Effects of vecuronium bromide on intracranial pressure and cerebral perfusion pressure. Br J Anaesth 1986b: 58: 437–440.
Roth S, Ebrahim Z, Subichin S. Resistance to pancuronium in patients receiving carbamazepine. Anesthesiology 1988: 65: A286
Rutten AJ, Nancarrow C, Mather LE, et al. Hemodynamic and central nervous system effects of intravenous bolus doses of lidocaine, bupivacaine, and ropivacaine in sheep. Anesth Analg 1989: 69: 291–299.
Sakabe T, Maekawa T, Ishikawa T, Takeshita H. The effects of lidocaine on canine cerebral metabolism and circulation related to the electroencephalogram. Anesthesiology 1974: 40: 433–441.
Samaha T, Ravussin P, Claquin C, Ecoffey C. Prevention of increase of blood pressure and intracranial pressure during endotracheal intubation in neurosurgery: esmolol versus lidocaine. Ann Fr Anesth Reanim 1996: 15: 36–40.
Schramm WM, Strasser K, Nartunek A, et al. Effects of rocuronium and vecuronium on intracranial pressure, mean arterial pressure and heart rate in neurosurgical patients. Br J Anaesth 1996: 77: 607–611.
Schramm WM, Jesenko R, Barrunek A, Gilly H. Effects of cisatracurium on cerebral and cardiovascular hemodynamics in patients with severe brain injury. Acta Anaesthesiol Scand 1997: 41: 1319–1322.
Schramm WM, Papousek A, Michalek-Sauberer A, et al. The cerebral and cardiovascular effects of cisatracurium and atracurium in neurosurgical patients. Anesth Analg 1998: 86: 123–127.
Schubert A, Licina MG, Glazo GM, Paranandi L. Systemic lidocaine and human somato-sensory evoked potentials during sufentanil-isoflurane anaesthesia. Can J Anaesth 1992: 39: 569–575.
Shaheen B, Wig J, Grewal S, Tewari MK. Effect of pipecuronium and pancuronium on intracranial pressure and cardiovascular parameters in patients with supratentorial tumours. Neurol India 2000: 48: 37–42.

Shokunbi MT, Gelb AW, Peerless SJ, et al. An evaluation of the effect of lidocaine in experimental focal cerebral ischemia Stroke 1986: 17: 962–966.
Shokunbi MT, Gelb AW, Miller DJ, Wu XM. A continuous infusion of lidocaine protects in temporary focal cerebral ischaemia. Anesthesiology 1987: 67: A580.
Stirt JA, Grosslight KR, Bedford RF, Vollmer D. Pretreatment with a defascilulating dose of metocurine prevents succinylcholine-induced increases in intracranial pressure. Anesthesiology 1986: 65: A302.
Stirt JA, Grosslight KR, Bedford RF, Vollmer D. "Defasciculation" with metocurine prevents succhinylcholine-induced increases in intracranial pressure. Anesthesiology 1987: 67: 50–53.
Stirt JA. Muscle relaxants in neurosurgical anesthesia: What should we do when the pressure's on. J Neurosurgical Anesthesiology 1990: 2: 1–2.
Sustch G, Rubinstein EH. Minor effect of lidocaine on brain electrical recovery after 5 minutes of almost complete cerebral ischemia in the rabbit. J Neurosurg Anesthesiol 1991: 3: 39–46.
Sustch G, Rubinstein EH. Lidocaine accelerates recovery of brain electrical activity after 3 minutes of complete ischaemia in the rabbit. J Neurosurg Anesthesiol 1991: 3: 124–131.
Tam S, Chung F, Campbell M. Intravenous lidocaine: Optimal time of injection before tracheal intubation. Anesth Analg 1987: 66: 1036–1038.
Tarkkanen L, Laitinen L, Johansson G. Effects of d-tubocuranine on intracranial pressure and thalamic electrical impedance. Anesthesiology 1974: 40: 247–251.
Tateichi A, Zornow MH, Scheller MS, Canfell PC. Electroencephalographic effects of laudanosine in an animal model of epilepsy. Br J Anaesth 1989: 62: 548–552.
Thiagarajah S, Sophie S, Azar I, Lear E. Effect of succinylcholine on the ICP of cats with and without thiopentone pretreatment. Br J Anaesth 1988: 60: 157–160.
Thiel A, Wyderka T, Wagner RM, et al. Effects of pipecuronium and pancuronium on cerebrospinal fluid pressure in neurosurgical patients. Acta Anaesthesiol (Belg) 1996: 47: 59–65.
Tindall GT, Greenfield JC Jr. The effects of intra-arterial histamine on blood flow in the internal and external carotid artery in man. Stroke 1973: 4: 46–49.
Tommassino C, Maekawa T, Shapiro HM. Local cerebral blood flow during lidocaine-induced seizures in rats. Anesthesiology 1986: 64: 771–777.
Torbiner ML, Yagiela JA, Mito RS. Effect of midazolam pretreatment on the intravenous toxocity of lidocaine with and without epinephrine in rats. Anesth Analg 1989: 68: 744–749.
Unni VKN, Young HSA. Effects of atracurium on intracranial pressure in man. Anaesthesia 1986: 41: 1047–1049.
Vesely R, Hoffman WE, Gil KSL. Cerebrovascular effects of curare and histamine in the rat. Anesthesiology 1986: 65: A336.
Wagman IH, DeJong RH, Prince DA. Effects of lidocaine on the central nervous system. Anesthesiology 1967: 28: 155–172.
Warner DS, Godersky JC, Smith M-L. Failure of pre-ischaemic lidocaine administration to ameliorate global ischaemic brain damage in the rat. Anesthesiology 1988: 68: 73–78.
Warnick JE, Kee RD, Yim GKW. The effects of lidocaine on inhibition in the cerebral cortex. Anesthesiology 1971: 34: 327–332.
Waud B, Waud DR (1986) Tubocuranine sensitivity of the diaphragm after limp immobilization. Anesth Analg 65: 493–495
Weiss MH, Wertman N, Apuzzo MLJ, et al. The influence of myoneural blockers in intracranial dynamics. Bull Los Angl Neurologic Soc 1977: 42: 1–7.
White PF, Schlobohm RM, Pitts LH, Lindauer JM. A randomized study of drugs for preventing increases in intracranial pressure during endotracheal suctioning. Anesthesiology 1982: 57: 242–244.
Wollman H, Alexander SC, Cohen PJ, et al. Cerebral circulation during general anesthesia and hyperventilation in man. Thiopental induction to nitrous oxide and d-tubocuranine. Anesthesiology 1965: 26: 329–334.
Yagiela JA. Intravascular lidecaine toxocoty: influence of epinephrine and route of administration. Anesthesia Progress 1985: 32: 57–61.
Yano M, Nishiyama H, Yokota H, et al. Effect of lidocaine on ICP response to endotracheal suctioning. Anesthesiology 1986: 64: 651–653.
Yakoyama M, Goto H, Ueda W, et al. Modification of intravenous lidocaine-induced convulsions by epinephrine in rats. Can J Anaesth 1993: 40: 251–256.
Yokayama M, Hirakawa M, Goto H. Effect of vasoconstrictive agents added to lidocaine on intravenous lidocaine-induced convulsions in rat. Anesthesiology 1995: 82: 574–580.
Zhou Y, Wang D, Du M, et al. Lidocaine prolongs the safe duration of circulatory arrest during deep hypothermia in dogs. Can J Anaesth 1998: 45: 692–698.

Drugs used for control of blood pressure

Aim

Controlled hypotension in neurosurgical practice has been used for decades, the aims being 1) to decrease blood loss during surgery, 2) to provide a dry surgical field and 3) to diminish the risk of intraoperative aneurysm rupture. The benefits of controlled hypotension must be discussed in connection with the risks of development of cerebral ischaemia.

Cerebral autoregulation and lower point of cerebral autoregulation

Generally, induced hypotension to MABP levels of 50–60 mm Hg, which traditionally indicate the lower level of cerebral autoregulation in normotensive subjects is advocated (Strandgaard and Paulson 1984). Recently studies in healthy volunteers indicate that the lower point of cerebral autoregulation is higher, about 65–85, median 75 mm Hg (Schmidt et al. 1990, Schmidt et al. 1991). In chronic arterial hypertension in baboons (Strandgaard et al. 1975, Jones et al. 1976) and rats (Barry et al. 1982) the autoregulation curve is shifted to a higher level and similar findings have been observed in man (Strandgaard 1976). Studies in baboons have shown that sympathetic vasoconstriction shifts the lower level of autoregulation towards higher pressures (Fitch et al. 1975). Accordingly, the hypotensive level under these circumstances must be at a higher level.

Cerebral ischaemia and oedema

The lower level of CBF at which cerebral ischaemia threatens is supposed to be about 20 ml/100g/min. Below this level the content of brain water increases. The increase in brain water is supposed to be a result of an increase in osmotic active molecules produced by anaerobic metabolism. It is a cytotoxic oedema and is usually reversible on restoration of MABP (Symon et al. 1979). If the degree of ischaemia is more severe so that CBF decreases to the threshold for failure of cell membrane ion hemostasis at about 10 ml/100g/min, further cytotoxic oedema occurs as a result of sodium passage into the cells. This is a cytotoxic oedema as well and it is reversible unless the cell has been severely damaged (Hossmann 1976, Iannotti and Hoff 1983).

Rebound phenomenon

A point of concern is the period immediately after controlled hypotension. If MABP is allowed to increase rapidly and/or overshoot pre-hypotensive levels resulting in a rebound hypertensive period, plasma proteins and water are forced through the dilated capillary vessels to produce vasogenic oedema and it is suggested that the presence within the circulation of vasodilator agents such as sodium nitroprusside or nitroglycerin might accentuate the vasogenic oedema (Forster et al. 1978).

CBF

Studies by Farrar et al. (1981) indicate that patients without angiographic evidence of cerebral spasms did not have any significant change in CBF during controlled hypotension to MABP 40–50 mm Hg, whilst patients with preoperative angiographic evidence of vasospasm had a significant reduction of CBF. Furthermore, experimental studies during nitroprusside-induced hypotension in animals with MCAO indicate that histopathological damage occurs after 30 min of hypotension (Boisvert et al. 1989), whilst these changes do not occur in normotensive animals subjected to a 2 hour occlusion period (Crowell et al. 1970). This observation has been confirmed in other experimental studies (Cole et al. 1990).

Cerebral spasm

Angiographic evidence of cerebral spasms may be present in 45% of patients within 3 days of subarachnoid haemorrhage (Allcock and Drake 1965). The cerebral autoregulation is generally impaired or abolished in unanaesthetized patients (Heilbrun et al. 1972, Voldby et al. 1985), and the degree of impairment of autoregulation is related to the presence of arterial vasospasms and the severity of the patients clinical condition as evaluated from the Hunt and Hess classification (Voldby et al. 1985).

Brain retractors

The cerebral perfusion pressure during application of brain retractors is reduced during controlled hypotension (Bennett et al. 1977, Albin et al. 1979), and a relationship between low cerebral perfusion pressure and the development of focal infarction as evaluated by CT scanning has been outlined (Rosen¢rn 1989).

Agents

In neuroanaesthesiological practice, a wide range of intravenous agents have been advocated to achieve a state of controlled hypotension. Most popular are drugs with a fast effect on systemic vascular resistance and drugs which are metabolised quickly. Sodium nitroprusside (SNP), nitroglycerin (NG), act as NO donor. Adenosine triphosphate (ATP) and adenosine (A) dilate cerbral arterioles via activation of adenosine A2A and A2B receptors, which agian activate ATP-sensitive K^+ channels. Trimethaphan (TMP), calcium blockers like diltiazem, nifidipine and nicardipine, α and β blockers like propranolol, esmelol, labetalol, urapidil, serotomin blockers like ketanserin, central α_2 blockers like clonidine and dexmedetomidine, angiotensin converting enzyme inhibitors (captopril) and prostaglandins have been investigated experimentally and in clinical studies.

Baroreflex activity and flow distribution

Generally, these drugs exert their effects on preload and afterload. However, baroreflex activity modifies their actions (Chen et al. 1982). Studies in neurally deafferented dogs undertaken with constant cardiac output and constant venous pressure using cardiopulmonary bypass, have shown that SNP- and ATP-induced hypotension caused flow redistribution from splanchnic to extra splanchnic vascular beds, suggesting that redistribution should be taken into consideration in evaluating the haemodynamic changes during induced hypotension (Hoka et al. 1987).

Sodium Nitroprusside (SNP), experimental studies

Action

SNP is a fast acting and potent vasodilator, which predominantly acts on resistance vessels. The vasodilator effect of SNP and related drugs like nitroglycerin are mediated directly through release of NO resulting in activation of guanylate cyclase, and accumulation in intracellular levels of cyclic GMP (Schultz et al. 1977, Katsuki et al. 1977). Amoniphylline potentiates the vasodilatatory effects of SNP (Pearl et al. 1983a)

Toxicity

The toxicity of SNP is based on its metabolic degradation to cyanide. Cyanide is transformed into the relatively nontoxic thiocyanate, mediated by a hepatic and renal enzyme system, rhodanase, a sulfuryl transferase. The rhodanase enzyme system is a mitochondrial enzyme system, localised close to cytochrome oxidase (Schubert and Brill 1968). In dogs subjected to SNP administration, cyanide toxicity occurs at dosages exceeding 1–1.5 mg/kg (Michenfelder 1977). In human initial dosage rates between 0.5–1.5 μ/kg/min are recommended as starting points for very careful titration. Total injected intraoperative dosage should not exceed 3 mg/kg (Tinker and Michenfelder 1976, Vesey et al. 1976, Wildsmith et al. 1979). Acute toxicity leading to death during SNP-induced hypotension has repeatedly been described (Jack 1974, Merrifield and Blundell 1974, Davis et al. 1975). Thiosulfate is effective in dogs and humans in maintaining a safe blood cyanide concentration, when high dosages of SNP are required and without altering the SNP induced haemodynamic effects (Ivankovich et al. 1982, Schulz et al. 1982). In humans hydroxocobalamine has the same effect (Cottrell et al. 1978).

Rebound phenomenon

Discontinuation of SNP infusion is followed by an increase in plasma renin activity, vasopressin and catecholamine (Zubrow et al. 1983). These changes are associated with an overshoot or rebound arterial and pulmonary hypertension. Studies in dogs have shown that the rebound hypertension can be prevented partially or completely by pre-treatment with captopril, an inhibitor of angiotensin converting enzyme (Khambatta et al. 1982). Experiments with saralasin a competitive inhibitor of angiotensin II have given the same result (Delaney and Miller 1980).

Pulmonary shunt fraction

In dogs with artificially induced atelectasis SNP prevents the hypoxic mediated pulmonary vasoconstriction and mediates an increase in Qs/Qt (Colley and Cheney 1977). However, if lung function is normal, experiments in dogs indicate that the shunt fraction is practically unaffected by SNP (Hodges et al. 1977).

CBF and $CMRO_2$

Experiments in rats, cats, dogs and monkeys indicate that the effect of SNP-induced hypotension on CBF differs with species and experimental conditions. Generally, CBF is unchanged, even at very low levels of MABP (Stoyka and Schutz 1975, Grubb and Raichle 1982, de Guerra et al. 1986), or slightly decreased (Carter and Atkinson 1973, Crockard et al. 1976, Ishikawa and McDowall 1980). An increase in CBF has been documented in halothane anaesthetised cats, where SNP was delivered by *in vivo* microdialysis into the cortical tissue (Ohta et al. 1997). In dogs CBF, ICP and $CMRO_2$ were measured, SNP alone dilates cerebral capacitance vessels. On the other hand, SNP in combination with isoflurane also dilates resistance vessels. However the latter effect is not reflected by increased CBF or ICP during hypotension because of isoflurane-induced abolished cerebral autoregulation (Michenfelder and Milde 1988).

Studies by Grubb and Raichle (1982) have shown an increase in cerebral oxygen utilisation in baboons during SNP infusion. This effect is supposed to be a disadvantage but concurrent anaesthesia with halothane or other volatile agents is supposed to block the increase in oxygen requirements.

Cerebral vessels

SNP is a cerebral vasodilator, whether bolus or continuous infusion are used (Ivankovich et al. 1976). Using the open window technique in rats, SNP infusion results in a dosage-related hypotension combined with pial arteriolar dilatation and a prolongation of the cerebral microcirculation transit time without any change in venous diameter (Lu et al. 1982).

CO_2 reactivity

In dogs, the CO_2 reactivity during SNP-induced hypotension is decreased (Gregory et al. 1981) or absent (Artru and Colley 1984). Hypocapnia does not intensify anaerobic metabolism even during MABP of about 40 mm Hg (Artru 1986).

Cerebral autoregulation

The changes in CBF during SNP-infusion are influenced by the capacity of cerebral autoregulation and a left shift of the cerebral autoregulation curve has repeatedly been demonstrated (Stoyka and Schutz 1975, Fitch et al. 1976, Michenfelder and Theye 1977, Maekawa et al. 1979, Crozier et al. 1986). Studies in chronic hypertensive rats have shown that SNP-induced hypotension within the normal range of autoregulation provokes a decrease in both CBF and $CMRO_2$ (Hoffman et al. 1982b).

Blood-brain barrier

The dilatation of cerebral resistance vessels during SNP-induced hypotension is associated with blood-brain barrier dysfunction (Ishikawa et al. 1983). Under the circumstances of dilatation of cerebral vessels vasopressor and especially norepinephrine may increase ICP critically. A gradual return of MABP to baseline values at the end of a period of induced hypotension seems advisable and the prevention of hypertensive episodes immediately after operation desirable (Fitch 1977).

ICP

Experiments in cats (Stullken and Sokoll 1975, March et al. 1979b) and dogs (Todd et al. 1980, Prough et al. 1983a) have shown an increase in ICP associated with SNP-induced hypotension. As regards the ICP increase, studies in cats with ICP hypertension suggest that slow SNP administration should be preferred under conditions of hypocapnia and hyperoxia (March et al. 1979b)

Tissue oxygen tension

Studies in cats of the pattern of the brain-surface oxygen tensions during SNP-induced hypotension did not indicate any shift from control, suggesting well maintained cerebral perfusion (Maekawa et al. 1979).

Sodium Nitroprusside (SNP), human studies

Rebound phenomenon and baroreflex activity

Human studies of SNP-induced hypotension support the experimental findings. SNP infusion is followed by an increase in plasma renin activity, vasopressin (Khambatta et al. 1979) and catecholamine (Fahmy and Gavras 1983, Knight et al. 1983). These changes are associated with rebound arterial and pulmonary hypertension (Shibutani et al. 1983) and resetting of baroreflex sensitivity (Chen et al. 1982). During morphine anaesthesia, the baroreflex sensitivity is greater than during halothane anaesthesia. It is supposed that this difference might explain the difference in dose requirements for SNP in patients anaesthetized with either morphine or halothane (Chen et al. 1982).

Human studies have shown that the rebound hypertension can partially be prevented by pre-treatment with captopril, which simultaneously decreases the dose requirement of SNP (Woodside et al. 1982, Fahmy and Gavras 1983). β-blocking agents have the same effect (Luben and Hempelmann 1982, Khambatta et al. 1984).

Elimination

After SNP-infusion the decay of SNP concentration occurs rapidly. The concentration of SNP is closely correlated to MABP and plasma-HCN (Vesey et al. 1990).

Hypoxia and pulmonary shunt

During SNP-infusion, an increase in Qs/Qt occurs; however, if the lung function is normal, the pulmonary shunt fraction is unaffected (Stone et al. 1976).

CBF and $CMRO_2$

In human studies CBF and $CMRO_2$ are unchanged during SNP-induced hypotension to MABP levels of 50–55 mm Hg, or an average decrease in MABP of 32–42% from baseline level (Griffith et al. 1974, Larsen et al. 1982, Henriksen et al. 1983, Pinaud et al. 1989, Bünemann et al. 1987). Patient with acute stroke were examined with SPECT during SNP administration causing a 10 mm Hg decrease in MABP. RCBF in the penumbral area increased in three og four patients. Besides SNP inhibited expression of platelet aggregation and platelet adhesion molecule (Butterworth et al. 1998).

Rebound CBF changes

In patients subjected to aneurysm surgery during SNP induced hypotension to MABP 40 mm Hg, CBF increased following discontinuation of SNP infusion and the reestablishment of MABP (Henriksen et al. 1983, Pinaud et al. 1989) This observation suggests a redistribution of blood flow to the brain in the presence of impaired cerebral autoregulation or the influence of local brain acidosis (Pinaud et al. 1989).

ICP

In patients subjected to SNP-induced hypotension, an increase in ICP was observed when MABP was decreased to 70% of baseline level. If MABP was decreased further, ICP returned towards baseline values and decreased steadily with further decrease in MABP (Turner et al. 1977). In other studies including patients with hydrocephalus secondary to fossa posterior tumours SNP-induced hypotension resulted in an increase in ICP, associated with a decrease in the level of consciousness and complaint of dizziness and headache (March et al. 1979a).

Nitroglycerin (NG), experimental studies

Action

In dogs NG predominantly exerts its hypotensive effect on capacitance vessels. In comparison with SNP its effect is more inconsistent, the decrease in blood pressure is less rapid, and rebound hypertension is seldom observed.

CBF and $CMRO_2$

In dogs CBF and $CMRO_2$ were unchanged until MABP about 40 mm Hg (Colley and Sivarajan 1984, Artru et al. 1986). However, when ICP was increased artificially, the reduction in CPP was sufficient to lead to a decrease in CBF (Rogers et al. 1979). Hypocapnia during NP-induced hypotension does not give rise to disturbances of cerebral metabolism or EEG alteration (Artru et al. 1986). During NP-induced hypotension spinal CBF did not change (Spargo et al. 1987).

ICP

Like SNP, NP-induced hypotension in cats is associated with an increase in ICP (Rogers et al. 1979b). In dogs, the effect of NP on ICP is dependent on the choice of bolus or continuous infusion. When administered as a continuous infusion the impact on ICP is minimal. In contrast, bolus injection of NG causes a dramatic increase in ICP (Prough et al. 1983b). The same group has compared the effect of SNP and NP in dogs, with or without ICP hypertension by inflation of an epidural balloon and demonstrated that the presence of ICP hypertension diminishes the systemic vasodilating effect of SNP. In contrast, the decrease in MABP and CPP by NG is unaffected by the presence of increased ICP (Prough et al. 1983a).

Pulmonary function

Studies in dogs indicate that NP in comparison with SNP normalizes pulmonary vascular resistance and pulmonary artery pressure in animals with oleic acid pulmonary hypertension. This effect of NP seems to be related to its ability preferentially to dilate the pulmonary vascular bed (Pearl et al. 1983b).

Nitroglycerin, human studies

ICP and CBF

Human studies have shown that NG predominantly acts on capacitance vessels (Gerson et al. 1982).

During fentanyl/midazolam anaesthesia NG induces an increase in CBF averaging 96% during moderate hypocapnia and 69% during hypercapnia (Weyland et al. 1996). During continuous infusion of NG a dosage-related decrease in MABP and an increase in ICP have been observed. Simultaneously, a decrease in intracranial compliance was found (Ghani et al. 1983). NG administered as a bolus injection produces a marked increase in ICP associated with a decrease in MABP. The maximum decrease in MABP occurred 1–2 min following NG, and ICP returned to normal within 2–3 min (Dohl et al. 1981).

In patients subjected to craniotomy, NG-induced hypotension to MABP averaging 69 mm Hg was followed by an increase in ICP from 14 to 31 mm Hg and a decrease in CPP from 90 to 38 mm Hg, suggesting dilatation of capacitance vessels within the relatively non-compliant cranial cavity (Cottrell et al. 1980).

In healthy volunteers sublingual nitroglycerin reduces blood flow velocity without concurrently changing CBF in the perfusion territory of the involved vessels (Dahl et al. 1989).

CO_2 reactivity

In patients without cerebral diseases the CO_2 reactivity was attenauted during NG-induced hypotension to MABP 55 to 60 mm Hg (Endoe et al. 1999). In another study patients were subjected to coronary by-pass operation in midazolam/fentanyl anaesthesia. NG-induced hypotension did not change the CO_2 reactivity (Weyland et al. 1996).

Pulmonary function

In patients with normal lung function, NG like SNP-induced hypotension is associated with an increase in pulmonary artery pressure (Casthely et al. 1982).

Potency

Studies in patients subjected to aneurysm surgery indicate that NG appears to be inferior to SNP for the production of induced hypotension, the reason being a greater decrease in cardiac index and mixed central venous saturation produced by NP (Maktabe et al. 1985).

The introduction of isoflurane for controlled hypotension has to some degree rendered NG superfluous. As stated by Lagerkranser (1992) vasodilators with less effects on ICP, such as isoflurane which also may afford a cerebral protective effect, might be preferable during neuroanesthesia.

Other NO donors

Glycerol trinitrate at clinically relevant doses was studied in healthy volunteers using PET, ultrasonic colour velocity flow imaging, and transcranial Doppler. There was no significant change in either global or regional CBF, and no change in common or internal carotid artery flow velocities (White et al. 2000).

Trimetphaphan (TMP), experimental studies

Action

Trimethaphan (TMP) produces a ganglionic blockade (Nakamura et al. 1980). Recent findings indicate that TMP acts on the motor endplate, but unlike d-tubocurarine TMP does not interact with the recognized site of acetylcholine receptors; the action of TMP appears to be associated with the blockade of end plate ionic channels (Nakamura et al. 1988).

CBF

In comparison with SNP and NG, studies in cats indicate that CBF is significantly lower during TMP-induced hypotension (Ishikawa and McDowall 1980, Gregory et al. 1981) In baboons rendered hypotensive with SNP, TMP or acute hemorrhage with a 50% decrease in MABP, CBF decreased by about 20%. In the same study an increase in cerebral oxygen utilization was observed in animals subjected to SNP or hemorrhage but not during TMT induced hypotension. The authors suggest that the increase in cerebral oxygen uptake observed with SNP and during hemorrhage is due to stimulation of the sympathetic nervous system with release of catecholamine (Grubb and Raichle 1982).

CO_2 reactivity

Studies in cats and dogs have shown that the CO_2 reactivity during TMP-induced hypotension is abolished (Gregory et al. 1981, Artru and Colley 1984). Other studies in dogs have shown that hypocapnia does not intensify the cerebral impact of TMP-induced hypotension on CBF (Artru 1986b).

Cerebral autoregulation

During TMP-induced hypotension in baboons the cerebral autoregulation curve is shifted to the left, and CBF is maintained until MABP 50 mm Hg (Fitch et al. 1976).

ICP

Studies in cats and dogs have demonstrated that TMP, especially rapid induction of hypotension, produces a significant but transient increase in ICP (Stullken and Sokoll 1975, Bunegin et al. 1984, Karlin et al. 1988).

Comparative studies

Several studies concerning the cerebral effects of TMP, SNP and NG indicate that TMP is inferior to SNP and NG. Rats were subjected to induced hypotension by haemorrhage, SNP or TMP. A level of MABP 30 mm Hg for 30 min was achieved. Local CBF was reduced in the neocortex and telencephalon by all three methods, but SNP preserved local CBF significantly better than TMP and haemorrhage (Tsutsui et al. 1995). The pattern of brain surface oxygen tension is moved to lower values during TMT-induced hypotension; an observation not found during SNP-induced hypotension (Maekawa et al. 1979). It has been demonstrated that electrical activity, measured by the cerebral function monitor, is depressed at higher values of MABP during TMP- compared with NP- and SNP-induced hypotension (Ishikawa and McDowall 1980). Furthermore, it has been demonstrated that the MABP threshold for K^+ escape into the extracellular fluid in the central cortex is higher during TMP-induced hypotension than during hypotension induced by NP; and extracellular fluid acidosis is less severe during NP- compared with TMP-induced hypotension (Morris et al. 1983). Other studies in dogs subjected to TMP- or SNP-induced hypotension to 50 mm Hg have shown metabolic alterations by TMP (Michenfelder and Theye 1977).

On the other hand, studies in baboons with intracranial hypertension provoked by inflation of an epidural balloon indicate that moderate hypotension by SNP (20% fall in blood pressure) in comparison with NG and TMP provokes higher ICP levels during inflation and exflation of the balloon and that the CO_2 reactivity is more reduced (Hartmann et al. 1989).

Trimethaphan (TMP), human studies

Catecholamines and renin

Human studies indicate that TMP- in comparison with SNP-induced hypotension results in less increase in circulatory catecholamine, and no activation of plasma-renin (Knight et al. 1983).

ICP

Studies in patients subjected to deliberate hypotension by SNP or TMP indicate that TMP does not usually produce ICP increase, except when intracranial compression is severe (Turner et al. 1977).

SNP plus TMR

The use of SNP 25 mg and TMP 250 mg mixtures for deliberate hypotension has been proposed. In a report, blood cyanide levels were significantly lower with this mixture than with SNP alone (Wildsmith et al. 1983), and studies in humans indicate that the use of this mixture allows for a more rapid decrease of MABP, lower dose requirements for SNP and TMP and diminished or absent sympathetic activation (Fahmy 1985, Fahmy et al. 1986). In studies of mongrel dogs SNP/trimethaphan ratios of 1/2.5 and 1/5 produce induced hypotension with stable reflex sympathetic reflex activity (Nakazawa et al. 1991).

Comparative studies

Kuroda et al. (1997) studied the effect of TMP, NG and diltiazem on CBF in patients with hypertensive intracerebral haemorrhage. A slight decrease in rCBF was found after administration of NG or diltiazem, and a more pronounced decrease during TMP.

Clinical application

The use of TMP has waned recently, partly owing to comparative experimental studies of TMP, SNP and NG, indicating that TMP is inferior to the other drugs and partly owing to clinical studies indicating that other drugs are to be preferred. Thus, it has been demonstrated that the cerebral electrical activity as monitored by cerebral function monitor is depressed at higher values of MABP during TMP compared with SNP-induced hypotension (Thomas et al. 1985).

ATP and adenosine (A), experimenal studies

Action

Changes in rat pial artery diameter were observed directly through a closed cranial window. Adenosin-induced vasodilation of the pial arteries was mediated via activation of adenosine A2A and A2B receptors, but not by the A1 receptor subtype. Activation of the adenosine A2A receptor preferentially contributed to vasodilation via activation of ATP-sensitive K^+ channels, and through the production of nitric oxide (Shin et al. 2000a, Shin et al. 2000b).

Pharmacology

ATP given intravenously in dogs is rapidly degraded to A during transpulmonary passage and the hypotensive effect of ATP is related to the arterial adenosine concentration (Sollevi et al. 1984b). ATP- and A-induced hypotension is characterized by rapid induction (Fukunaga et al. 1982, Lagerkranser et al. 1984, Lagerkranser et al. 1985), and a stable blood pressure level without tachycardia or posthypotensive rebound hypertension (Satinover et al. 1981, Fukunaga et al. 1982, Kassell et al. 1983a, Sollevi et al. 1984b). Accordingly, plasma renin activity is not increased during or following ATP- or A-induced hypotension (Tagawa and Vander 1970, Lagerkranser et al. 1984).

Regulation of CBF

In rats, the concentration of A in the brain increases during hypoxia (Winn et al. 1981), hypotension (Winn et al. 1980b), ischaemia (Berne et al. 1974, Winn et al. 1979), during the recirculation period after transient ischaemia (Du et al. 1989) and during bicuculline-induced seizures (Winn et al. 1980a). Other studies indicate the presence of A receptors (Huang and Drummond 1979) suggesting that A is involved in the maintenance of resting cerebrovascular tone, and that A plays an important role in the regulation of CBF (Berne et al. 1974, Forrester et al. 1979, Winn et al. 1981, Phillis et al. 1987), the regulation of CBF autoregulation under physiological conditions (Morii et al. 1989), and the regulation of CBF during hypoxic hypoxia (Laudignon et al. 1990). This has also been demonstrated during hypotension in newborn piglets (Laudignon et al. 1991).

CBF and $CMRO_2$

In baboons ATP-induced hypotension produces an initial CBF increase followed by a progressive decrease as MABP decreases to 40 mm Hg or 60% of the baseline value (Van Aken et al. 1984a). Studies in rats (Satinover et al. 1981) and dogs (Kassell et al. 1983a, Kien et al. 1987) indicate unaltered CBF unless MABP is markedly decreased. In dogs ATP-induced hypotension to MABP 40 mm Hg induces a CBF decrease by 54–65% and under these circumstances, the cerebral circulation was inadequate to meet unchanged cerebral oxygen demands, resulting in anaerobic metabolism with accumulation of lactate (Newberg et al. 1985).

In dogs subjected to A-induced hypotension (61% decrease in MABP) rCBF was heterogenous, leaving the cerebral cortex and corpus callosum most affected and the brain stem least (Kassell et al. 1983b). In dogs, pigs and monkeys $CMRO_2$ is unchanged during ATP or A-induced hypotension (Kassell et al. 1983b, Van Aken et al. 1984a, Newberg et al. 1985, Stånge et al. 1989). However, in baboons, intracarotid ATP increases $CMRO_2$. This effect was attributed to an elevation of the cellular cyclic AMP level (Forrester et al. 1979).

Rebound phenomenon

Studies in pigs and baboons subjected to A-induced hypotension indicate an increase of CBF in the early post-hypotension period unrelated to rebound hypertension (Van Aken et al. 1984b, Eintrei and Carlsson 1986, Stånge et al. 1989). It is supposed that A may have an effect on the cerebrovascular tone even after termination of its administration, but the mechanism behind this effect is unknown (Stånge et al. 1989).

Glucose utilization

In rats the combination of hypocapnia to $PaCO_2$ 20 mm Hg, and A-induced hypotension to MABP 50 mm Hg leads to a homogenous decline of glucose utilization, the decrease ranging from 20 to 40%. It is supposed that the decrease of glucose utilization may be the result of synaptic inhibition, probably because of impairment of the presynaptic coupling between excitation and transmitter release (Waaben et al. 1989).

Cerebral vessels

In rats, pigs, cats and dogs, adenosine is a potent dilator of cerebral vessels (Berne et al. 1974, Wahl and Kuschinsky 1976, Morii et al. 1986, Stånge et al. 1989). This effect is blocked by theophylline (Wahl and Kuschinsky 1976).

Cerebral autoregulation and CO_2 reactivity

Studies in dogs indicate that the cerebral autoregulation is intact and the CO_2 reactivity is unchanged during adenosine-induced hypotension, as long CPP remains above the lower limit of cerebral autoregulation (Lam and Artru 1992).

Blood-brain barrier

Osmotic disruption of the blood-brain barrier does not affect the vasodilatory effect of ATP (Forrester et al. 1979).

ICP

The effects of adenosine (A) and ATP on ICP have been studied repeatedly. In the study by Thiagarajah et al. (1983), cats were subjected to sodium nitroprusside (SNP) or ATP-induced hypotension to MABP 38% of control. In animals with normal ICP, ATP did not increase ICP, while ICP increased by 86% during SNP. Similar results were obtained in cats with ICP hypertension due to an inflation of an epidural balloon.

In dogs with normal ICP ATP induces an increase in ICP. If ICP, however, is increased by inflation of an epidural balloon prior to ATP administration, the initial ICP increase is followed by a decrease in ICP (Puchstein et al. 1983). Similar results have been obtained in dogs by van Aken et al. (1984b), who also found an ATP-induced decrease in intracranial compliance as evaluated by the volume-pressure curves.

CSF formation and dynamics

In rabbits the rate of formation and resistance to reabsorption of CSF are preserved and unchanged during adenosine-induced hypotension (Shapira et al. 1992).

Protection

Studies in rats subjected to hypoxia have shown that ATP has a protective effect (Kraynack et al. 1981). In dogs topical application of 2-chloroadenosine increases blood flow to outer layers of collateral-dependent brain tissue, and the normal cerebrum (Muhonen et al. 1995).

Comparative studies

In rats, measurements of brain oxygen tensions during SNP, deep isoflurane or 2 chloroadenosine indicated impairment of oxygenation during 2-chloroadenosine induced hypotension, but not during deep isoflurane or SNP-induced hypotension (Longnecker and Seyde 1984). Using the microsphere technique, the same authors have studied rCBF without finding any differences between the three drugs (Monk et al. 1987). If hemorrhage, however, was instituted during the hypotensive period rCBF was best preserved during SNP-hypotension (Sperry et al. 1987). In sheep subjected to A- or SNP-induced hypotension to MABP 30 mm Hg brain surface oxygen tensions were decreased equally (Laycock et al. 1986), and in rabbits subjected to ATP- or SNP-induced hypotension to MABP 50 mm Hg for 3 hours, ATP in comparison with SNP caused minimal metabolic aberration and all animals survived (Chiache et al. 1983).

ATP and adenosine (A), human studies

In human studies ATP- and A-induced hypotension is characterized by rapid induction, stabilized hypotensive level and lack of rebound hypertension (Fukinaga et al. 1983, Lagerkranser et al. 1988). Accordingly, A has recently been introduced as an agent to induce controlled hypotension during aneurysm surgery (Sollevi et al. 1984a, öwall et al. 1984).

Central hemodynamic

Studies of central hemodynamics in patients undergoing cerebral aneurysm surgery or operation for peripheral vascular disease indicate, that A-induced hypotension produces a hyperkinetic circulation in the systemic as well as in the myocardial vascular bed.(Öwall et al. 1988a, Öwall et al. 1988b).

In hypotensive dosages adenosine provokes reversible atrioventricular conduction disturbances (Zäll et al. 1990).

CBF, $CMRO_2$ and cerebral autoregulation

In patients undergoing surgery for cerebral aneurysm in neurolept anaesthesia, and subjected to A-induced hypotension with MABP decrease to 46 mm Hg, systemic vascular resistance was reduced by 61%, but CBF did not change. $AVDO_2$ decreased by 28% and $CMRO_2$ by 17%. In the posthypotensive period MABP was increased by 10% and CBF by 15%. It was concluded that A-induced hypotension at these levels did not unfavorably affect cerebral oxygenation and even might offer a protective effect by reducing oxygen demand. The slight CBF increase in the posthypotensive period was supposed to be secondary to an increase in MABP together with a blunted cerebral autoregulation (Lagerkranser et al. 1989).

From the same group studies by PET in patients with a–v malformation have shown that A produces marked cerebral vasodilation in normocapnic subjects, and that this response can be counteracted by hypocapnia (Sollevi et al. 1987).

Indicator of cerebral ischaemia

In patients undergoing carotid endarterectomy, carotid clamping induced significant increases in jugular venous adenosine, especially in patients with inadequate collateral blood flow. In the same study focal cerebral ischemia was reflected by changes in adenosine concentrations (Weigand et al. 1999).

Theophylline

Four effects on the central nervous system have been demonstrated with theophylline and other methylxanthines. 1) An inhibitor effect upon cAMP- and cGMPdiesterase (Morii et al. 1984). This inhibitory effect is least in the cerebellum (26%) and most markedly in the brain stem (68%) (Uzonov et al. 1975). The inhibitory effect is dependent on dose of theophyllamine. In rats subjected to theophyllamine 10 mg/kg a decrease in cAMP and cGMP were observed. With a dose of 35 mg/kg or higher of theophyllamine an increase in cAMP and cGMP was found (Stefanovich 1979). 2) Release of catecholamines. 3) Calcium mobilization. 4) Blocking of adenosine receptor (P_1 purinoceptor). In contrast to the other effects adenosine receptor blockade occurs at 10^{-4} M or lower. Theophylline has been shown to decrease the effect of electrical stimulation on the increase of cAMP in brain cortex slices (Satin and Rall 1970). In mouse subjected to stab wound injury a sevenfold increase in cAMP was blocked by prior treatment with theophyllamine (Watanaba and Passonneau 1975).

At low concentration of theophyllamine CBF decreases, whereas hyperemia has been observed at high levels (Morii et al. 1987).

Earlier studies with the Kety and Smith method indicated a decrease of CBF after iv. injection (Gottstein 1962). ICP is also reduced (Rich et al. 1953). In human studies Skinhøj and Paulson (1970) found that the decrease in CBF was not elicited by hypocapnia. Intraarterially injected theophyllamine in very small doses is followed by a CBF decrease as well (Gottstein and Paulson 1972). In patients with apoplexy an inverse flow distribution has been found (Skinhøj and Paulson 1970), and clinical improvement has been observed after theophyllamine administration (Olivarius 1961).

Dipyridamole

Dipyridamole pre-treatment decreases dose requirements by its inhibitory effect on A uptake (Kolassa and Pfleger 1975, Wu and Phillips 1982), and is recommended during A-induced hypotension (Sollevi et al. 1984a, Lagerkranser et al. 1988). In piglets subjected to cerebral ischaemia dipyridamole increases extracellular adenosine levels (Park and Gidday 1990).

Isoflurane

CBF and $CMRO_2$

Isoflurane has been used for controlled hypotension in surgery for cerebral aneurysms. During hypotension to MABP levels of 50–60 mm Hg, cardiac output is unchanged (Lam and Gelb 1983), and the pulmonary shunt fraction is unaffected (Nicholas and Lam 1984).Three studies of CBF and $CMRO_2$ during isoflurane-induced controlled hypotension for cerebral aneurysm surgery have been published (Newman et al. 1986, Roth et al. 1986, Madsen et al. 1987).

In all studies CBF was unchanged during the hypotension period, while $CMRO_2$ was reduced by 9–58%. CBF was considerably higher compared with the threshold of cerebral ischemia of 10 ml/100g/min found by Messick et al. (1987) in patients subjected to carotid endarterectomy. Studies of CO_2 reactivity during SNP- and isoflurane-induced hypotension indicate that the CO_2 reactivity was attenuated during isoflurane- as well as during SNP-induced hypotension. This attenuation was most pronounced during SNP-induced hypotension (Matta et al. 1995).

α and β blocking agents

Propranolol

Studies in cats subjected to MCAO suggest a cerebral protective effect of the β-adrenergic receptor blocking agent propranolol (Little et al. 1982, Standefer and Little 1986). Premedication with propranolol attenuates the haemodynamic changes in blood pressure and heart rate during tracheal intubation (Allberry and Drake 1990).

Esmolol

CBF and CPP

Esmolol, an ultra short acting cardioselective β-blocker, has been studied experimentally and clinically. In dogs subjected to esmolol infusion during haemorrhagic hypotension, hypovolaemia and under circumstances of low intracranial compliance, a decrease in CBF is related to a decrease in CPP, suggesting an impairment of cerebral autoregulation (Bunegin et al. 1987).

In patients subjected to surgery for arterio-venous malformation in isoflurane anaesthesia, esmolol in doses of 100–300 mcg/kg/min reduces MABP by 15% from baseline level, without associated reflex tachycardia or rebound hypertension (Ornstein et al. 1986). In patients undergoing craniotomy requiring controlled hypotension, the same group found that the decay in heart rate, blood pressure and plasma-renin activity had different onset time (Ornstein et al. 1995). During SNP-induced hypotension esmolol reduces plasma renin activity dose-dependently and prevents rebound hypertension (Edmondson et al. 1988). In comparison with SNP, other studies indicate that esmolol-induced hypotension is not associated with reflex tachycardia or rebound hypertension (Ornstein et al. 1987). On emergency from generel anesthesia in patients undergoing neurosurgery esmolol was found to be effective in controlling arterial hypertension (Gibson et al. 1988).

Intubation

Esmolol in bolus dosages of 100 mg combined with fentanyl 2–3 μg/kg results in effective control of haemodynamic response to tracheal intubation (Miller et al. 1991). The same effect was obtained with metoprolol (Coleman et al. 1980) and pindolol (Mikawa et al. 1991).

Labetalol

In experimental studies labetalol (a combined α- and β-adrenoceptor blocker) results in a decreased requirement for isoflurane.

CBF and ICP

In the dog with or without intracranial hypertension labetalol did not affect ICP or intracranial compliance (van Aken et al. 1982).

Studies in normotensive subjects indicate that labetalol, given in moderate but clinically relevant doses, does not affect CBF nor CO_2 reactivity (Schroder et al. 1991). PET studies in healthy volunteers confirm these results, indicating that labetalol does not influence global or regional CBF or $CMRO_2$, and cerebral autoregulation is preserved (Olsen et al. 1995). In comparison with deep isoflurane-induced hypotension CBF is unchanged, but a restoration of renal and hepatic blood flow to values observed during normotensive anaesthesia is observed (Durieux et al. 1988). In patients with cerebral disorders subjected to craniotomy with SNP-induced hypotension labetalol permitted withdrawal or reduction of SNP dosage. Labetalol significantly improved CPP and reduced ICP compared with SNP therapy (Orlowski et al. 1988). In the postoperative period after craniotomy labetalol effectively controls arterial hypertension. Simulaneously an increase in cardiac index is found. CBF decreased sligtly from 67 to 57 ml/100g/min (Dubois et al. 1992). In elderly patients both esmolol and labetalol effectively produce reduction of blood pressure. However, esmolol might produce a substantial bradycardia (Singh et al. 1992).

Combined with isoflurane

Intravenous labetalol decreases the induction time of hypotension and the recovery time after anaesthesia, and the concentration of isoflurane needed to maintain hypotension is decreased. Furthermore, the combination of isoflurane and labetalol has a favourable effect on renal function (Toivonen et al. 1992). A significant effect upon postoperative cognitive function, however, has not been detected (Toivonen et al. 1993).

Urapidil

Urapidil is a selective α-adrenoreceptor antagonist which decreases blood pressure by lowering peripheral resistance. Reflex tachycardia does not usually occur, except immediately after bolus injection. Urapidil binds to central serotonin receptors (Kolassa et al. 1989). It is supposed that the sympaphetic counterregulation is suppressed by this effect. Urapidil passes the blood-brain barriere in healthy volunteers (Castor and Schmidt 1994), as well as in patients with compromized blood-brain barrier function, where the drug does not increase ICP (Anger et al. 1988).

Ketanserin

Ketanserin, experimental studies

Ketanserin, an antiserotonergic agent with affinity for both 5-hydroxytryptamine- and α_1-adrenoreceptors, has recently been suggested in the control of perioperative blood pressure control. In humans ketanserin has a terminal half-life of 12 to 25 hours, and is eliminated by the liver.

Serotonin constricts blood flow in collateral vessels, increases collateral resistance in large arteries and collateral vessels, and decreases perfusion pressure (Muhonen et al. 1997). In studies of pial arterioles ketanserin completely blocks the constrictive effect of serotonin. The constrictive effect of aggregated platelet supernatant is blocked by ketanserin (Thompson et al. 1984). In dogs with or without ICP-hypertension ketanserin does not affect ICP (van Aken et al. 1984).

Ketanserin, human studies

In studies of human brain cortex [^{3}H]Ketanserin binds in the nanomolar concentration range both to 5-HT_2 and α_1-adrenergic receptors. Similar results are obtained in rat and pig brain membranes (Hoyer et al. 1987)

Cerebral circulation

In subjects without brain disease autoregulation is not affected by ketanserin (Schmidt et al. 1991). CBF, flow velocity over middle cerebral artery and $CMRO_2$ are unchanged and the CO_2 reactivity and the cerebral autoregulation are preserved (Olsen et al. 1992, Olsen et al. 1993, Weyland et al. 1995). These observations also apply to patients subjected to midazolam-fentanyl or isoflurane anaesthesia (Olsen et al. 1994). In patients with normal-pressure hydrocephalus (Olsen et al. 1996), and head injury (Heytens et al. 1988) ketanserin did not change ICP.

Blood pressure control

Administrated orally to hypertensive patients ketanserin causes a sustained reduction in blood pressure, compared to that obtained with either β-adrenergic blockers or diuretics. Another study indicates a greater efficacy in old than in young patients (Vanhoutte et al. 1988). In patients with essential hypertension ketanserin does not alter creatinin clearence or the plasma level of noradrenalin, renin, and aldesteron (Woittiez et al. 1986).

Postoperative period

In the postoperative period after craniotomy, transitory arterial hypertension often occurs (Engberg et al. 1990, Asmussen et al. 1991). In a clinical study increasing doses of esmolol or labetalol were equally effective in controlling this postanaesthetic hypertension (Muzzi et al. 1990). In another study labetalol appeared safe and effective by providing a long lasting effect with no evidence of rebound hypertension or cardiac dysfunction (Dubois et al. 1992). The hypertensive reaction also can be blocked with intravenous ketanserin (Felding et al. 1995), while metoprolol often is accompanied by bradycardia which compromises its use (Felding et al. 1992). Studies in patients with severe head injury indicate that metoprolol does not affect CBF or cerebral oxygen metabolism (Asgeirsson et al. 1995).

Calcium blockers

Diltiazem

Diltiazem, a calcium blocker possessing vasodilatory properties, has been studied experimentally. In cats with normal ICP and subjected to 30% decrease in MABP, diltiazem did not increase ICP. In animals with artificially raised ICP by inflation of an epidural balloon, diltiazem-induced hypotension was associated with an ICP increase (Thiagarajah et al. 1986). In dogs with or without ICP hypertension by mock CSF infusion, diltiazem-induced hypotension (40% decrease in MABP) increased ICP very little. However, serious cardiac disturbances occurred (Mazzoni et et al. 1985).

Nifedipine

Under certain circumstances the calcium blocking agents nifedipine and nicardipine have cerebral protective effects; consequently both drugs have been proposed for controlled hypotension.

In experimental studies and in human with arterial hypertension nifidipine produces an increase in ICP (Giffin et al. 1983, Tateishi et al. 1988). In patients subjected to maxillofacial surgery with halothane or isoflurane anaesthesia, nifedipine is an effective drug to use for controlled hypotension, provided reflex tachycardia is prevented (Spiss et al. 1985). In dogs the hypotensive action of adenosine remains unimpaired after pretreatment with nifedipine (Rooney et al. 1989).

Nicardipine

In humans without intracranial disorders nicardipine induces a rise in ICP (Nishikawa et al 1986). Experiments in dogs subjected to nicardipine-induced hypotension to MABP 40 mm Hg indicate a significant reduction in rCBF which persists despite return of normal blood pressure (Lam et al. 1988).

During propofol/fentanyl anaesthesia, deliberate hypotension with nicardipine attenuates the CO_2 reactivity (Endoe et al. 1999). In a clinical study of diazepam/fentanyl/nitrous oxide anaesthetised patients nicardipine increased flow velocity, whereas the CO_2 reactivity was preserved and unchanged (Kawaguchi et al. 1991). In another study of patients without cerebral diseases the cerebral autoregulation was tested during propofol/fentanyl anaesthesia. The autoregulation was impaired during nicardipine-induced hypotension to MABP 60–65 mm Hg (Endoe et al. 2000).

During prolonged use nicardipine may result in prolonged periods of hypotension. This effect is unclear and was not caused by an increase in the concentration of nicardipine (Bernard et al. 1992).

Central α_2 agonists

Transmembrane signaling

In neuronal tissue α_2 agonists carry their signal by changes in transmembrane voltage and hence neuronal excitability. For the α_2-adrenergic responses, the transmembrane signaling system involves coupling of three seperate components; a receptor protein, a guanine nucleotide binding protein (G protein), and an effector mechanism.

The α_2-adrenoceptor is a member of the G protein-coupled family. This protein waves forwards and backwards through the membrane, with hydrophobic regions forming alpha helices embeded in the membrane. Negatively charged aspartic acid residues are of crucial importance for agonist binding as they channel the possitively charged ligands into the center of the receptor. More than 10 G proteins are classified, with subunits designated as alpha, beta and gamma. All alpha subunits have a high affinity for guanine nucleotides, and possess an intrinsic GTPase activity, and are substrat for ADP-ribosylation.

The α_2 agonists fall into three main classes: Phenylethylamines (e.g. α-methylnoradrenalin), the imdazolines (e.g. clonidine) and oxalozepines (e.g. azepexole).

α_2 receptors are widespread distributed throughout the central nervous system. α_2 agonists exert many effects including sedation, anxiolysis, antisialagogue effects, analgesia, reduction of anaesthetic requirement during surgery, reduction of intraocular pressure caused by inhibition of ADH release and antagonism of ADH tubular effects. The cardiovascular effects, caused by inhibition of norepinephrine release from prejunctional peripheral nerve endings and centrally elicited effects, include bradycardia and hypotension. The analgetic effect of α_2 agonists is in part caused by spinal release of acetylcholine (Klimscha et al. 1997) and nitric oxide release. α_2 agonist-induced analagesia is enhanced by subarachnoid neostigmine (Bouaziz et al. 1995), but inhibited by blockers of NO synthase. An increased secretion of growth hormone and inhibition of insulin release and platelet aggregation have been demonstrated.

At least five seperate effector mechanisms are directly modulated by activation of α_2 receptors. 1) Inhibition of adenylate cyclase. The resulting decrease in cAMP will attenuate the stimulation of cAMP-dependent protein kinase and hence, phosphorylation of target regulatory proteins. 2) Acceleration of Na^+/H^+ exchange. This reaction may in turn stimulate phospholipase A_2 to initiate the arachidonic pathway, and leads to formation of thromboxane A_2. 3) Activation of K^+ channels. This reaction hyperpolarizes membranes and provides effective means of suppressing neuronal firing. 4) Inhibition of voltage-sensitive Ca^{2+} channels which suppress Ca^{2+} entry into the nerve terminals. The channel is coupled to the α_2 receptor through a G protein. For review (Maze and Tranquilli 1991, Sandler 1996, Eisenach et al. 1996, Dowlatshari and Yaksh 1997).

Clonidine

Action

Clonidine is rapidly absorbed after oral administration, with peak plasma concentrations within 60–90 min. The elimination half-life is between 9 and 12 hours with about 50%, being metabolized in the liver. The rest is excreted unchanged in the kidney.

The site of action of α_2 agonists is supposed to be locus coeruleus, which receives afferents mainly from the nucleus paragigantocellularis, the nucleus prepositus hypoglossi, the hypothalamic and the spinal cord. Efferents from the locus coeruleus project to the reticular formation and several cranial nerve nuclei (Scheinin 1992). Also the dorsal raphe nucleus in the midline of the lower brainstem is influenced by clonidine. Thus, the activity of the dorsal raphe nucleus is enhanced by noradrenaline, and the effect is attenuated by clonidine (Alojado et al. 1994).

The rostral ventrolateral medulla, which controls the tonus of the vascular system comprises adrenergic cardiovascular neurons. Studies in rats treated with clonidine or mivazerol indicate that during emergency from anaesthesia a near total suppression of chatecholamine activation occurs. Pretreatment with idaxolan, an α_2 antagonist blunted this effect (Bruandet e tal. 1998).

Central hemodynamics

Given as premedication clonidine effectively blunts the haemodynamic responses to surgery and hemorrhage. Thus, oral clonidine attenuates the heart rate response to intravenous atropine (Nishikawa and Dohi 1991). In ewes intrathecal clonidine attenuates blood pressure and heart rate adjustments during hemorrhage (Eisenach et al. 1992). In other studies it provokes bradycardia or atrioventricular conduction disturbance (Kibler and Gazes 1977, Abiuso and Abelow 1978, Byrd et al. 1988).

CBF and CO_2 reactivity

In volunteers clonidine (5 µg/kg orally) decreases flow velocity and slightly attenuates the CO_2 reactivity. Clonidine reduces the slope of the $PaCO_2$-CBF response function, but does not affect the cerebral autoregulation (Kanawati et al. 1986).

In patients with severe head injury clonidine decreases blood pressure and CVR without affecting CBF or $CMRO_2$ (Asgeirsson et al. 1995).

Protection

Clonidine improves outcome from incomplete ischaemia in rats (Hoffman et al. 1991).

Anaesthetic requirement

In patients subjected to surgery for cerebral tumour clonidine has a sparing effect upon anaesthetic requirement. In the same study suppression of the central haemodynamics, of adrenal cortical response to surgery, and a lower blood glucose level were found (Gaulmann et al. 1990).

The hypertensive response during laryngoscopy and application of Mayfield clamp were much less in clonidine pretreated patients (Chadha et al. 1992).

Oxygen uptake and CO_2 elimination

During the postoperative period the increase in total body oxygen consumption and CO_2 production were attenuated and a reduction in shivering was observed (Delaunay et al. 1991). Other studies indicate that postoperative pain is ameliorated (Bernard et al. 1991).

Sympathetic outflow

Administered intrathecally or intravenously clonidine has a depressant effect on both the spontaneous sympathetic outflow and the afferent A- and C-fiber-mediated somatosympathetic reflexes (Wang et al. 1994).

Dexmedetomidine, experimental studies

Action

Dexmedetomidine is a superselective α_2-agonist with a α_2 /α_1 binding ratio of 1620/1. Dexmedetomidine reduces the dose requirement of anaesthetics (Peden and Prys-Roberts 1993) and central analgetics (Meert and Kock 1994). Dexmedetomidine injection into the locus ceruleus in rats produces antinociception (Guo et al. 1996). Simultaneously it increases the incidence of intraoperative hypotension and bradycardia (Scheinin et al. 1993).

Alteration of the hypnotic reponse is coupled to inhibition of ion conductance through L and P type calcium channels, and facilitation of conductance through voltage-gated or calcium-activated potassium channels (Nacif-Coelho et al. 1994). Furthermore, activation of K^+ channels, the Na^+/H^+ antiporer, functions associated with depression of neuronal excitability, and the NO-cGMP pathway are involved (Vulliemoz et al. 1996).

In addition to the central inhibitory effect dexmedetomidine has *in vitro* studies indicate a potent inhibitory effect on the peripheral sympathetic nervous system. This effect is reversed by yohimbine, a α_2 antagonist, and was supposed to be modulated by presynaptically calcium-mediated neurotransmitter release (Schedewie et al. 1992). In sheep intrathecal dexmedetomidine decreases blood pressure within one minut. Epidural application has a slower onset of 11 minutes (Eisenach et al. 1994).

CBF, $CMRO_2$ and ICP

In dogs subjected to halothane anaesthesia dexmedetomidine caused reduction in CBF without influencing the metabolic rate of oxygen (Karlsson et al. 1990). Intraventricular dexmedetomidine decreases CBF during normoxia and hypoxia McPherson et al. 1997). In the the dog oral dexmedetomidine also alters the haemodynamic response observed during intravenous ketamin induction (Proctor et al. 1992). α_2 stimulation decreases normocapnic and hypercapnic CBF by a mechanism dependant on anaesthesia, but not related to change in $CMRO_2$. The changes in CBF are completely reversed after administration of the α_2 receptor antagonist, atipamezole (Fale et al. 1994).

In rabbits subjected to ICP-hypertension produced by a cryogenic lesion dexmedetomidine did not change ICP (Zornow et al. 1992).

Big arteries and pial vessels

Stimulation of α_2 adrenoceptors with the agonist UK 14,303 produced dilation in the rat middle cerebral artery. This effect is dependent on intact endothelium, and involve NO pathway (Bryan et al. 1996).

In dogs studies with the cranial window technique indicate that topical application of dexmedetomidine constricts both pial arterial and venous vessels in a concentration dependend manner. The vasoconstictive effect is blunted by yohimbin a α_2 antagonist, and mediated through activation of α_2-adrenoceptors. This action is accompanied by activation ATP sensitive K^+ channels, which excert a counter balancing vasodilatory effect (Ishiyama et al. 1995).

In the same animal dexmedetomidine attenuates the dilation of cerebral vessels induced by isoflurane and sevoflurane in pentobarbital-anesthetized animals (Ohata et al. 1999). The same group has compared spinal and cerebral pial vessels during application of dexmedetomidine and clonidine, and found that both drugs constricted spinal vessels in a concentration-dependent manner (Iida et al. 1999).

Rabbits were prepared for measurement of pial vessel diameters using a closed window preparation. The pial arteriolar dilator response to hypercapnia was significantly attenuated after intrathecal administration of dexmedetomidine. Pretreatment with yohimbine completely blocked the decreased reactivity to hypercapnia. Intrathecal dexmedetomidine did not affect the vasodilation of pial arterioles induced by mild or moderate hypoxia (Takenaka et al. 2000).

EEG

Dexmedetomidine decreases seizure threshold during pentylenetetrazol-induced seizure. This effect is dose-dependent, and is blocked by the selective α_2 antagonist atipamezole (Mirski et al. 1994).

Protection

In the rat dexmedetomidine improves neurological outcome from incomplete cerebral ischaemia (Hoffman et al. 1991, Schultz et al. 1993) and in focal ischaemia (Maier et al. 1993). It is likely that this effect is mediated centrally, possibly by action in the locus ceruleus (Williams et al. 1985, Aghajanian and Wang 1986). Other mechanisms include decreased evoked glutamate release as found in hippocampal rat brain slices during depolarization or hypoxia (Talke and Bickler 1996). This effect, however, was not demonstrated in rabbits after transient global ischaemia (Kim et al. 1996).

Dexmedetomidine, human studies

Chatecholamine release

In volunteers premedication with dexmedetomidine effectively attenuates the cardiostimulatory and postanesthetic delirium effects of ketamine (Levänen et al. 1995).

Dexmedetomidine decreases isoflurane requirement in a dose-dependent manner, and reduces heart rate, systolic and diastolic pressures in healthy volunteers (Khan et al. 1999).

ICP

In patients with normal ICP (patients subjected to transsphenoidal hypophysectomy) spinal CSF pressure is unchanged after dexmedetomidine (Talke et al. 1997)

Cognition

In healthy volunteers sedation and slight impairment of cognitive function persist for several hours after anaesthesia (Khan et al. 1999).

Angiotensin converting enzyme inhibitors

Captopril and Enalaprilat

Captopril and enalaptrilat, both angiotensin converting enzyme inhibitors, give rise to a reset of cerebral autoregulation to lower blood pressure levels in rats (Barry et al. 1984, Jarden et al. 1984) and humans (Waldemar et al. 1989). Cerebral autoregulation is well preserved during captopril treatment of chronic heart failure (Paulson et al. 1986).

In patients subjected to controlled hypotension for non-cerebral reasons, premedication with captopril 1 mg/kg combined with SNP in dosages ranging from 0.16 to 3.23 μg/kg/min reduced MABP to 46 mm Hg without affecting CBF or $CMRO_2$ (Thomsen et al. 1989).

In neurosurgical patients enalaprilat reduces blood pressure within 15 minutes, and the effect lasted for 4 hours. The authors found iv. enalaprilat effective and safe (Tohmo and Karanko 1995).

In rats subjected to incomplete cerebral ischaemia captopril improves neurologic outcome (Werner et al. 1990).

Prostaglandin E_1

Prostaglandin E_1 (PGE_1) has been used clinically for induction of controlled hypotension (Goto et al.1982, Yamamura et al. 1987, Watanabe and Nomiyama 1982).

Olesen et al. (1976) found that intraarterially administered PGE_1 increased CBF in healthy volunteers. Local CBF was unchanged and CO_2 reactivity preserved during Prostaglandin E_1-induced hypotension in patients with subarachnoid hemorrhage (Abe et al. 1992a). In contrast, in patients without cerebral disease and anaesthetised with propofol/fentanyl, the CO_2 reactivity was attenuated during prostaglandin E1-induced hypotension to MABP 55–60 mm Hg (Endoe et al. 1999).

PGE_1 does not change cerebral artery diameter in patients with subarachnoid hemorrhage and cerebral spasms (Steiner et al. 1972).

In patients without cerebral disorders controlled hypotension to 70% of baseline values was induced with PGE_1 or nitroglycerin. Baseline value of jugular oxygen saturation was not affected by either drugs. Both nitroglycerin and PGE_1 increased cerebral oxygen saturation as measured by near infrared spectroscopy. This might be explained by local hyperaemia without mayor alteration in flow/metabolism coupling of the brain. The onset of the changes was slower, and the duration of the effect after discontinuation of the drugs was more prolonged with PGE_1 (Kadoi et al. 1997). In another study including patients undergoing cerebral aneurysm surgery under neurolept anesthesia, local CBF was unchanged during PGE_1 administration, adjusted to maintain MABP at 70 mm Hg. During TMP administration blood pressure decreased to the same level, and a decrease in local CBF was observed. The authors concluded that PGE_1 may be preferable to TMP for hypotensive anaesthesia in patients with cerebral aneurysm, because CBF was maintained (Abe et al. 1991). In other studies by the same group presurgical neurological status and outcome correlated with the CO_2 reactivity and CBF measured during PGE_1-induced aneurysm clipping (Abe et l. 1992b, Abe et al. 1992c).

Clinical application

Although controlled hypotension has been used for aneurysm surgery, controlled outcome studies have never been performed. After the introduction of temporary clipping of the cerebral arteries the use of controlled hypotension has been debated. Clinical data suggest that this technique can be used safely and when applied preclude the use of controlled hypotension (Gianotta et al. 1982, Samson et al. 1994). The major concern during controlled hypotension being development of focal ischaemia.

On the one hand, Lagerkranser (1991) concludes that controlled hypotension should not be used indiscriminately as a routine procedure, but only in carefully selected cases. The physical state of the patient, as judged by the anesthesiologist should be weighed against the need for facilitation of the surgical approach, as judged by the surgeon, and each one must respect the decision reached by the other. The surgeon must not impose his will on the anesthesiologist, and the anesthesiologist should not refuse controlled hypotension for other than medical reasons. In patients without cerebral disorders controlled hypotension is considered safe. MABP should be maintained above 50 mm Hg. The level of $PaCO_2$ is not considered important because the CO_2 reactivity is impaired or lost. The use of direct acting vasodilators such as SNP or isoflurane which shift the cerebral autoregulation to the left are advocated (Moss 1995).

On the other hand, Ruta and Mutch (1991) conclude that controlled hypotension may be potentially hazardeous to the brain and other vital organs. The authors advocate the use of temporary clipping over controlled hypotension during aneurysm surgery. In this context, several clinical studies support the safety of temporary vessel occlusion (Ljunggren et al. 1983, McDermott et al. 1989) which according to Suzuki et al. (1984) can be tolerated in upto 40 min. Other authors stress that myocardial ischemia during controlled hypotension might occur (Kindor and Warner 1991).

As stated by Tietjen et al. (1996) treatment of acute hypertension in patients with threathening or manifest cerebral ischaemia or with space-occupying pathology requires an understanding of the pathophysiology of hypertension and determinants of cerebral perfusion pressure. Individual agents should be selected based on their ability to promtly and reliably decrease blood pressure, while considering effects on CBF and ICP. Comparative studies of central haemodynamic indicate that adenosine is superior to SNP, NG and TMP as it improves cardiac output and preserves CVP. Furthermore, A is a fast acting, non-toxic drug, and tachyphylaxis or rebound hypertension are not observed. However, A like SNP and NG is a cerebral vasodilator and may give rise to ICP hypertension and a dangerous decrease in CPP. A certain degree of brain protection has experimentally been found in A-treated animals, and in clinical studies a small decrease in $CMRO_2$ has been observed. In comparison with isoflurane, A-induced hypotension does not imply any significant advantage. Isoflurane-induced hypotension is associated with a profound suppression of $CMRO_2$ and probably better brain protection and therefore might be considered more safe.

Experimental studies of calcium blocking drugs and combined α- and β-blocking agents are promising, but only few human studies are available, and the effects of these drugs on cerebral circulation and metabolism both experimentally and clinically are rare.

Hypertensive drugs

Hypertensive drugs are used perioperatively to maintain blood pressure. On one hand, hypotensive periods might be prevented in patients with threathening cerebral ischemia. On the other hand hypertensive therapy is used in the treatment of subarchnoid hemorrhage and in patients with severe head injury. Furthermore, septic episodes and hypovolemia are often recorded in neurointensive patients. In both situations hypertensive drugs might stabilize the central haemodynamic.

Adrenoreceptor effect

Both α- and β-adrenoceptors are present in the brain. Sympathomimetic agents contract feline and human pial arteries in a concentration-dependent manner. This action is blocked by α adrenoceptor antagonists. α_1 type adrenoceptors in cerebral vessels are present in man, monkey, sheep, guiney pig and rat. Typical α_1 agonists are phenylephrine and norepinephrine. In feline and dog the α_2 type dominates. Dependency on extracellular Ca^{2+} for contraction of cerebral vessels is a general phenomenon. Thus, the contractile response of the cat middle cerebral artery to potassium, norepinephrine and 5-HT is reduced to 10% in a calcium-free medium.

As both cerebral arteries and veins are sympathetic innervated, sympathetic tone, theoretically might influence capacitance vessels and thus reduce intracranial pressure. Furthermore CSF formation and choroid plexus perfusion are increased after sympathetic denervation.

Normally the effects of circulating catacholamines on CBF and cerebral metabolism are prevented by the intact blood-brain barrier. However, if the barrier is disrupted cateholamines increase CBF and $CMRO_2$ (Clawson et al. 1966).

Epinephrine

Epinephrine has predominantly β_1 agonist effect. In rabbits drugs with β_1 adrenoceptor effect increase CBF and $CMRO_2$. These effects are supposed to be enhanced by increased permeability of the blood-brain barrier. Thus, intracarotid infusion of epinephrine (2–10 µg/min for 4–12 minutes), a dose that caused no increase in MABP, does not change rCBF (Olesen 1972). Similar findings were observed by others (Sensenbach et al. 1953, Greefield and Tindall (1968). However, in another study where epinephrine (37 µg/min) was injected intravenously MABP rose from 91 to 109 mm Hg, and CBF and $CMRO_2$ rose 22% and 24% respectively (King et al. 1951). A similar pattern was found in rats, where epinephrine 2 µg/kg/min had no effect on CBF and cerebral oxygen uptake, while 8 µg/kg/min caused increase in CBF and $CMRO_2$ (Berntman et al. 1978). Blood-brain barrier defect is supposed to enhance the effect of β agonists (MacKenzie et al. 1976, Artru et al. 1981, Abdul-Rahman et al. 1979). Thus, after disruption of BBB by urea increases in CBF and $CMRO_2$ are observed (MacKenzie et al. 1976), and Artru et al. (1981) found that epinephrine only caused $CMRO_2$ increase when BBB permeability to Evan's blue was present.

Norepinephrine

Receptor

Norepinephrine is an endogenous catecholamine with mixed α- and β-agonist properties but with predominantly α_1-adrenergic effects that can produce intense arterial and venous vasoconstriction.

Anatomical studies indicate a high concentration of norepinephrine-containing terminals in the superficial laminae of the spinal cord. They originate in the brain stem, and inhibit the transmission of nociceptive signals. It has been reported that α_2 receptors are concentrated in the substantia gelatinosa. Membrane hyperpolarization of substantia gelatinosa neurons by norepinephrine acting on the α_2-receptors accounts for depression of pain transmission. Experimental studies, however, indicate that norepinephrine also enhances inhibitory synaptic transmission in the substantia gelatinosa through activation of presynaptic α_1 receptors, thus providing a mechanism underlying the clinical use of α_1 agonists with local anesthetics in spinal anaesthesia (Baba et al. 2000a). Other studies suggest that GABA-ergic interneurons possess somatodendrite α_1 receptors, and activation of these receptors excites inhibitory interneurons. This action may comtribute to the analgesic action of norepinephrine (Baba et al. 2000b).

CBF and $CMRO_2$

Pial arterioles and veins display marked vasoconstriction after microapplication of norepinephrine. When blood-brain barrier is intact norepinephrine does not alter CBF or oxygen metabolism. However, if the blood-brain barrier was compromized, an increase in CBF and $CMRO_2$ was found. The norepinephrine-induced increase in CBF can be blocked completely by propranolol.

During intracarotid infusion of norepinephrine (0.25–2 µg/min for 4–12 minutes) rCBF is unchanged (Olesen 1972). Similar findings were obtained by others (Sensenbach et al. 1953, Greenfield and Tindall 1968). An intact blood-brain barrier is prerequisite. If the blood-brain barrier, however, is disrupted, or mean arterial blood pressure is increased above the upper level of cerebral autoregulation, norepinephrine increases CBF and $CMRO_2$ (Clawson et al. 1966, MacKenzie et al. 1976, Strandgaard et al. 1974, Tuor et al. 1986). An increase of norepinephrine after endotoxin is correlated to an increase in $CMRO_2$ (Ekstöm-Jodal et al. 1982). During mild hypothermia supplemented with thiopental-induced isoelectric EEG in rats norepinephrine increased basal $CMRO_2$, suggesting that norepinephrine nullifies the protective effect of hypothermia (Nemoto et al. 1996).

Phenylephrine

Phenylephrine is a selective α_1-adrenergic agonist with essentially no β-adrenergic activity. Phenylephrine does not directly affect intracranial haemodynamics in anaesthetized patients, but might provoke changes in CBF when cerebral autoregulation is impaired (Strebel et al. 1998).

Dopamine (experimental studies)

The brain posesses two dopamine receptors. The dopamine D_1 receptor mediates dilation of cerebral vessels. The dopamine D_2 mediates an increase in glucose utilization (Sharkey and McCulloch 1986). With intact blood brain barrier brain the uptake of dopamine is very low (Oldendorff 1971).

Blood-brain barrier, CBF and $CMRO_2$

In dogs a triphasic effect upon CBF has been disclosed. At low dosage (<2 µg/kg/min), and moderate to high dosages (7–20 28Mmg/kg/min) a CBF reduction has been disclosed. An increase in CBF occurred at intermediate dosages (2–6 μg/kg/min). The CBF reduction was blocked by phentolamine, and was therefore effected by an α-adrenoceptor effect. On the other hand, the CBF increase was blocked by haloperidol and pimazide, both dopamine receptor antagonists. There were no changes in $CMRO_2$ (von Essen 1972, von Essen 1974, von Essen et al. 1980).

In other experimental studies where the blood-brain barrier was disrupted dopamine increases CBF and $CMRO_2$ (Carlsson et al. 1975, Mc Culluch and Harper 1977, Bertman et al.1978, Mc Culloch and Teasdale 1979, von Essen 1974, Sharkey and Mc Culloch 1985). These effects are blocked by dopamine receptor antagonists that alone have very little effect on cerebral oxygen metabolism (Carlsson et al., 1975, Bertman et al. 1978). A close correlation between CBF and $CMR_{glucose}$ was found by Tuor et al. (1986). The regions that display a marked increase in glucose utilization are the caudate nucleus, globus pallidus, subthalamic nucleus, substantia nigra, ventral thalamus, and sensory-motor cortex. Bandres et al. (1992) studied the effect of dopamine on CBF and $CMRO_2$ in unanesthetized monkey. With dosages below the threshold for MABP increase CBF and CMRO2 were unchanged. When MABP increased by 15 to 30 percent CBF and CMRO2 increased 20 and 30% respectively.

In dogs subjected to *E Coli* endotoxin shock dopamine infusion of only 5 μg/kg/min increases CBF and $CMRO_2$ (Ekström-Jodal and Larsson 1982). Also in barbiturate anaesthetized cats an increase in glucose utilization has been demonstrated (Sato et al. 1991).

Direct effect on cerebral vessels

In *in vitro* studies dopamine has contractile effects on major cerebral arteries. This effect exceeds that produced by norepinephrine under the same conditions (Toda 1976, Edvinsson et al. 1978, Hamel et al. 1988). The contractile effect is the result of α-adrenoceptor and of 5-HT receptors, and can be blocked, non-competitively by phentolamine or methysergide (White et al. 1976, Altura et al. 1980, Edvinsson et al. 1985).

Dopamine (human studies)

In humans a dopamine-induced increase in CBF without a change in $CMRO_2$ has been found (Niimi et al. 1982). In other studies dopamine and other dopaminergic acting drugs did not increase $CMRO_2$ (Ehrmantraut et al. 1957, Shenkin 1951, Leenders et al. 1985).

Angiotensin

In has been proposed that angiotensin plays a role in the regulation of the cerebral microcirculation (Paulson et al. 1988, Waldemar and Paulson 1989). Also degradation fragments of angiotensin (angiotensin-(1–7) could be involved in this regulation. Studies of piglet pial arteries suggest that both angiotensin (1–7) and angiotensin II are modest dilators in the cerebral circulation (Meng and Busija 1993).

Olesen (1972) studied the effect of intracarotid angiotensin (0.15–2 μg/min for 4–12 minutes) and found no change in rCBF measured with Xe^{133} technique. This finding was confirmed by Greenfield and Tindall (1968) using electromagnetic flowmetry and implies that angiotensin does not pass the blood-brain barrier.

Ergot alkaloids and dihydroergotamine (DHE)

Olesen and Skinhøj (1972) found that intracarotid injection of hydergine, being composed of three hydrogenated ergot alkaloids i.e. dihydroergocornine, dihydroergocristine and dihydroergocryptine, did not influence rCBF in patients with intact cerebral autoregulation. In contrast, in patients with defect cerebral autoregulation a rCBF increase was disclosed.

Based on studies of peripheral circulation a cerebral venoconstrictive effect of DHE has been proposed (Asgeirsson 1995, Nilsson 1995). Studies in pigs indicate that DHE elicits an increase in MABP, whilst CBF and cerebral oxygen uptake are well maintained (Nielsson et al. 1995).

DHE has been introduced in the treatment of ICP-hypertension in patients with severe head injury (Grände 1989). In patients with intractable ICP-hypertension DHE, together with β blockade and α_2 agonist effectively, reduces ICP, and improves outcome when compared with a historical control (Asgeirsson et al. 1994). On the other hand, DHE does not reduce ICP in patients subjected to craniotomy for cerebral tumours in isoflurane, nitrous oxide anesthesia (Bundgaard et al. 1999). This study indicates that an intact cerebral autoregulation is a prerequisite if an ICP reducing effect is to be expected. On the other hand, when cerebral autoregulation is abolished DHE administration is accompanied by an increase in ICP.

References

Abe K, Demizu A, Kamada K, et al. Local cerebral blood flow with prostaglandin E1 or trimethaphan during cerebral aneurysm clip ligation. Can J Anaesth 1991: 38: 831–836.

Abe K, Demizu A, Yoshiya I. Effect of prostaglandin E1-induced hypotension on carbon dioxide reactivity and local cerebral blood flow after subarachnoid haemorrhage. Br J Anaesth 1992a: 68: 268–271.

Abe K, Demizu A, Mima T, et al. Carbon dioxide reactivity during prostaglandine E1 induced hypotension for cerebral aneurusm surgery. Can J Anaesth 1992b: 39: 253–259.

Abe K, Demizu A, Kamada K, et al. Prostaglandin E1 and carbon dioxide reactivity during cerebral anuerysm surgery. Can J Anaesth 1992c: 39: 247–252.

Abdul-Rahman A, Dahlgren N, Johansson BB, et al. Increase in local cerebral blood flow induced by circulating adrenaline: involvment of blood-brain barrier dysfunction. Acta Physiol Scand 1979: 107: 227.

Abiuso P, Abelow G Atrioventricular dissociation in a patient recieving clonidine. JAMA 1978: 240: 108–109.

Aghajanian GK, Wang YY. Pertussis toxin blocks the outward current evoked by opiate and alpha2-agonist in locus coeruleus neurons. Brain Res 1986: 371: 390–394.

Allberry RAW, Drake HF, Peroperative beta blockade for patients undergoing craniotomy: a comparison between propanolol and atenolol. Can J Anaesth 1990: 37: 448–451.

Allcock JM, Drake CG. Ruptured intracranial aneurysms- the role of arterial spasm. J Neurosurg 1965: 22: 21–29.

Alojado ME, Ohta Y, Kemmotsu O. The effect of clonidine on the activity of neurons in the rat dorsal raphe nucleus in vivo: Anesth Analg 1994: 79: 257–260.

Altura BM, Gebrewold A, Lassoff S. Biphasic responsiveness of rat pial arterioles to dopamine: direct observations on the microcirculation. Br J Pharmacol 1980: 69: 543–544.

Anger C, van Aken H, Feldhaus P, et al. Permeation of the blood-brain barriere by irupadil and its influence on intracranial pressure in man in the presence of compromized intracranial dynamics. J Hypertension 1988: 6: (suppl 2): 63–64.

Artru A, Nugent M, Michenfelder JD. Anaesthetics affect the cerebral metabolis response to circulatory catecholamines. J Neurochem 1981: 36: 1941.

Artru AA, Colley PS. Cerebral blood flow responses to hypocapnia during hypotension. Stroke 1984: 15: 878–883.

Artru AA. Cerebral metabolism and the electroencephalogram during hypocapnia plus hypotension induced by sodium nitroprusside or trimethaphan in dogs. Neurosurgery 1986: 18: 36–44.

Artru AA, Wright K, Colley PS. Cerebral effects of hypocapnia plus nitroglycerin-induced hypotension in dogs. J Neurosurg 1986: 64: 924–931.

Asgeirsson B, Grände PO, Nordström C-H. A new therapy of post-trauma brain edema based on haemodynamic principles for brain volume regulation. Intensive Care Med 1994: 20: 260–267.

Asgeirsson B, Grände PO, Nordström C-H, et al. Effect of hypotensive treatment with α_2-agonist and β_1 -antagonist on cerebral haemodynamics in severely head injured patients. Acta Anaesthesiol Scand 1995: 39: 347–351.

Asgeirsson B. Post-traumatic brain oedema therapy. Grahns Boktryckeri AB, Lund (thesis) 1995.

Asmussen J, Cold GE, Elkjæk S, et al. Changes in $AVDO_2$ in the postoperative period in patients subjected to craniotomy for supratentorial tumors. Acta Neurochir 1989: 101: 9–17.

Baba H, Shimoji K, Yoshimura M. Norepinephrine facilitates inhibitory transmission in substantia gelatinose of adult rat spinal cord (Part 1) Effect on axon terminals of GABAergic and glycinergic neurons. Anesthesiology 2000a: 92: 473–484.

Baba H, Goldstein PA, Okamoto M, et al. Norepinephrine facilitates inhibitory transmission in substantia gelatinose of adult rat spinal cord (Part 2) Effects on somatodendrites sites of GABAergic neurons. Anesthesiology 2000b: 92: 485–492.

Bandres J, Yao L, Nemoto EM, et al. Effects of dobutamine and dopamine on whole brain blood flow and metabolism in unanesthetized monkeys. J Neurosurg Anesthesiol 1992: 4: 250.

Barry DI, Strandgaard S, Graham DI, et al. Cerebral blood flow in rats with renal and spontaneous hypertension: Resetting of the lower limit of autoregulation. J Cereb Blood Flow Metab 1982: 2: 347–353.

Barry DI, Jarden JO, Paulson OB, et al. Cerebrovascular aspects of converting-enzyme inhibition: I. Effects of intravenous captopril in spontaneously hypertensive and normotensive rats. J Hypertens 1984: 2: 589–597.

Bernard J-M, Hommeril J-L, Passuti N, Pinaud M. Postoperative analgesia by intravenous clonidine. Anesthesiology 1991: 75: 577–582.

Bernard J-M, Passuti N, Pinaud M. Long-term hypotensive technique with nicardipine and nitroprusside during isoflurane anesthesia for spinal surgery. Anesth Analg 1992: 75: 179–185.

Berne RM, Rubio R, Curnish RR. Release of adenosine from ischaemic brain. Effect on cerebral vascular resistance and incorporation into cerebral adenine nucleiotides. Circ Res 1974: 35: 262–271.

Berntman L, Carlsson C, Hägerdal M, Siesjö BK. Circulatory and metabolic effects in the brain induced by amphetamine sulphate. Acta Physiol Scand 1978: 102: 310–323.

Berntman L, Dahlgren N, Siesjö BK. Influence of intravenously administered catecholamines on cerebral oxygen consumption and blood flow in the rat. Acta Physiol Scand 1978: 104: 101.

Boisvert DP, Gelb AW, Tang C, et al. Brain tolerance to middle cerebral artery occlusion during hypotension in primates. Surg Neurol 1989: 31: 6–13.

Bouaziz H, Hewitt C, Eisenach JC, Subarachnoid neostigmine potentiation of alpha 2-adrenergic agonist analgesia. Dexmedetomidine versus clonidine. Reg Anesth 1995: 20: 121–127.

Bruandet N, Rentero N, Debeer L, Quintin L. Catecholamine activation in the vasomotor center on emergency from anesthesia: The effect of a α_2 Agonist. Anesth Analg 1998: 86: 240–245.

Bryan RM, Eichler MY, Swafford MWG, et al. Stimulation of α_2 adrenoceptors dilates the rat middle cerebral artery. Anesthesiology 1996: 85: 82–90.

Bundgaard H, von Oettingen G, Jørgensen HA, Cold GE. The effects of dihydroergotamine on ICP, CBF and cerebral metabolism in patients with cerebral tumours. Acta Anaesthesiol Scand (suppl 114) 1999: 98

Bunegin L, Albin MS, Ruiz M. Intracranial pressure responses following rapid induction of hypotension with trimethapan. Anesthesiology 1984: 61: A369.

Bunegin L, Albin MS, Gelineau EF. Effect of esmolol on cerebral blood flow during intracranial hypertension and hemorrhagic hypovolemia. Anesthesiology 1987: 67: A424.
Bünemann L, Jensen K, Thomsen L, Riisager S. Cerebral blood flow and metabolism during controlled hypotension with sodium-nitroprusside and general anaesthesia for total hip replacement a.m. Charnley. Acta Anaesthesiol Scand 1987: 31: 487–490.
Butterworth RJ, Cluckie A, Jackson SH, et al. Pathophysiological assessment of nitric oxide (given as sodium nitroprusside) in acute ischaemic stroke. Cerebrovasc Dis 1998: 8: 158–165.
Byrd BF III, Collins HW, Primm RK. Risk factors for severe bradycardia during oral therapy for hypertension. Arch Intern Med 1988: 148: 729–733.
Carlsson C, Hägerdal M, Siesjö BK. Influence of amphetamine sulphate on cerebral blood flow and metabolism. Acta Physiol Scand 1975: 94: 128–129.
Carter LP, Atkinson JR. Cortical blood flow in controlled hypotension as measured by thermal diffusion. J Neurol Neurosurg Psychiat 1973: 36: 906–913.
Casthely PA, Lear S, Cottrell JE, Lear E. Intrapulmonary shunting during induced hypotension. Anesth Analg 1982: 61: 231–235.
Castor G, Schmidt U. Uradipil permeates the intact blood-brain barrier. Intensive Care Med 1994: 20: 278–281.
Chadha R, Padmanabhan V, Joseph A, Mohanda K. Oral clonidine pretreatment for haemodynamic stability during craniotomy. Anaesth Intens Care 1992: 2: 341–344.
Chen RYZ, Matteo RS, Fan F, et al. Resetting of baroreflex sensitivity after induced hypotension. Anesthesiology 1982: 56: 29–35.
Chiache M, Fukunaga AF, Bloor BC, van Etten A. A comparative study on the sympathetic and the metabolic activities during induced hypotension with adenosine triphosphate and sodium nitroprusside. Anesthesiology 1983: 59: A10.
Clawson CC, Hartmann JF, Vernier RL. Electron microscopy on the effect of gram-negative endotoxin on the blood-brain barrier. J Comp Neurol 1966: 127: 183.
Cole DJ, Drummond JC, Shapiro HM, Zornow MH. Influence of hypotension and hypotensive technique on the area of profound reduction in cerebral blood flow in the rat. Br J Anaesth 1990: 64: 498–502.
Colley PS, Cheney FW. Sodium nitroprusside increases Qs/Qt in dogs with regional atelectasis. Anesthesiology 1977: 47: 338–341.
Colley PS, Sivarajan M. Regional blood flow in dogs during halothane anesthesia and controlled hypotension produced by nitroprusside or nitroglycerin. Anesth Analg 1984: 63: 503–510.
Cottrell JE, Casthely P, Brodie JD, et al. Prevention of nitroprusside-induced cyanide toxicity with hydroxocobalamin. N Engl J Med 1978: 298: 809–811.
Cottrell JE, Gupta B, Rappaport H, et al. Intracranial pressure during nitroglycerin-induced hypotension. J Neurosurg 1980: 53: 309–311.
Crockard HA, Brown FD, Mullan JF. Effect of trimethapan and sodium nitroprusside on cerebral blood flow in rhesus monkeys. Acta Neurochir 1976: 35: 85–89.
Crowell RM, Olsson Y, Klatzo I Ommaya A (1970) Temporary occlusion of the middle cerebral artery in the monkey: clinical and pathological observations. Stroke 1: 439–448.
Crozier WC, Henney JB, Rogers MC, Traystman RJ. Persistence of cerebral blood flow autoregulation during nitroprusside administration. Anesthesiology 1986: 65: A574.
Dahl A, Russell D, Nyberg-Hansen R, Rootwelt K. Effect of nitroglycerin on cerebral circulation measured by transcranial Doppler and SPECT. Stroke 1989: 20: 1733–1736.
Davies DW, Kadar D, Steward DJ, Munro IR. A sudden death associated with the use of sodium nitroprusside for induction of hypotension during anaesthesia. Can Anaesth Soc J 1975: 22: 547–552.
DeGuerra O, Bunegin L, Albin MS. Changes in cerebral blood flow (CBF) following rapid induction of hypotension with sodium nitroprusside. Critical Care Med 1986: 388.
Delaunay L, Bonnet F, Duvaldstin P. Clonidine decreases postoperative oxygen consumption in patients recovering from general anaesthesia. Br. J Anaesth 1991: 67: 397–401.
Dohl S, Matsumoto M, Takahashi T. The effects of nitroglycerin on cerebrospinal fluid pressure in awake and anaesthetized humans. Anesthesiology 1981: 54: 511–514.
Dowlatshahi P Yaksh TL. Differential effects of two intraventricularly in jected alpha-2 agonists, ST-91 and dexmedetomidine, on electroencephalogram, feeding, and electromyogram. Anesth Analg 1997: 84: 133–138.
Dubois M, Caputy A, MacCosbe P, et al. Cerebral blood flow measurements during blood pressure control with labetalol following craniotomy. J Neurosurg Anesthesiol 1992: 4: 176–181.
Durieux ME, Monk CR, Sperry RJ, Matthern GE. Labetalol preserves blood flow to vital organs during deliberate hypotension induced by isoflurane. Anaesthesiology 1988: 69: A899.
Dux E, Fredholm B, Rudolphi K. Adenosine in the ischaemic-induced changes in the gerbil hippocampus. J Cereb Blood Flow Metab 1989: 9: suppl 1: S271.
Edmondson RH, Delvalle OE, Shah N, et al. Esmolol infusion during nitro- prusside- induced hypotension: Impact on the cardiovascular, renin-angiotensin and sympathetic nervous systems. Anesthesiology 1988: 69: A36.
Edvinsson L, Hardebo JE, McCulloch J, Owman CH. Effects of dopaminergic agonists and antagonists on isolated cerebral blood vessels. Acta Physiol Scand 1978: 104: 349–359.
Edvinsson L, McCulloch J, Sharkey J. Vasomotor responses of cerebral arterioles in situ to putative dopamine receptor agonists. Br J Pharmacol 1985: 85: 403–410.
Ehrmantraut WR, Shea JG, Ticktin HE, Fazekas JF. Influence of promazine and methylphenidate on cerebral hemodynamics and metabolism. Arch Int Med 1957: 100: 66–69.
Eintrei C, Carlsson C. Effects of hypotension induced by adenosine on brain surface oxygen pressure and cortical cerebral blood flow in the pig. Acta Physiol Scand 1986: 126: 463–469.
Eisenach JC, Tong C, Limauro D. Intrathecal clonidine and the response to hemorrhage. Anesthesiology 1992: 77: 522–528.
Eisenach JC, Shafer SL, Bucklin BA, et al. Pharmacokinitics and pharmacodynamics of intraspinal dexmedetomidine in sheep. Anesthesiology 1994: 80: 1349–1359.
Eisenach JC, de Kock M, Klinscha W. α_2-adrenergic agonists for regional anesthesia. Anesthesiology 1996: 85: 655–674.
Ekstöm-Jodal B, Häggendal J, Larsson LE, et al. Cerebral hemodynamics, oxygen uptake and cerebral arteriovenous differences of catecholamines following *E Coli* endotoxin in dogs. Acta Anaesthesiol Scand 1982: 26: 446–452.

Ekström-Jodal B, Larsson LE. Effects of dopamine on cerebral circulation and oxygen metabolism in endoxic shock: an experimental study in dogs. Crit Care Med 1982: 10: 375–377.

Endoe H, Honda T, Komura N, et al. Effects of nicardipine-, nitroglycerin-, prostaglandin E1-induced hypotension on human cerebrovascular carbon dioxide reactivity during propofol-fentanyl anaesthesia. J Clin Anesth 1999: 11: 545–549.

Endoe H, Honda T, Komura N, et al. The effects of nicardipine on dynamic cerebral autoregulation in patients anaesthetised with propofol and fentanyl. Anesth Analg 2000: 91: 642–646.

Engberg M, Öberg B, Christensen KS,et al. The arterio-venous oxygen content differences ($AVDO_2$) during halothane and neuroleptanaesthesia in patients subjected to craniotomy. Acta Anaesthiol Scand 1989: 33: 642–646.

Engberg M, Melsen NC, Herlevsen P, et al. Changes of blood pressure and cerebral arterio-venous oxygen content differences ($AVDO_2$) with and without bupivacain scalp infiltration during craniotomy. Acta Anaesthiol Scand 1990: 34: 346–349.

Fahmy NR, Gavras HP. Captopril decreases nitroprusside requirements and prevents rebound hypertension following cessation of nitroprusside infusion in humans. Anesthesiology 1983: 59: A359.

Fahmy NR. Nitroprusside vs. a nitroprusside-trimethaphan mixture for induced hypotension: Haemodynamic effects and cyanide release. Clin Pharmacol Ther 1985: 37: 264–270.

Fahmy NR, Bottros M, Dimedale J, et al. A comparison of the haemodynamic and hormonal effects of a nitroprusside-trimethaphan mixture with nitroprusside or tripethapan alone for induced hypotension. Anesthesiology 1986: 65: A70.

Fale A, Kirsch JR, McPherson RW. Alpha-2-adrenergic agonist effecton normocapnic and hypercapnic cerebral blood flow in the dog are anaesthetic dependent. Anesth Analg 1994: 79: 892–898.

Farrar JK, Gamache FW, Ferguson GG, et al. Effects of profound hypotension on cerebral blood flow during surgery for intracranial aneurysms. J Neurosurg 1981: 55: 857–864.

Felding M, Jacobsen C-J, Cold GE, et al. The effect of metoprolol upon blood pressure, cerebral blood flow, and oxygen consumption in patients usbjected to craniotomy for cerebral tumours. Avta Anaesthesiol Scand 1994: 38: 271–276.

Felding M, Cold GE, Cacopsen C-J, et al. The effects of ketanserin upon cerebral blood flow, and oxygen cpnsumption in patients subjected to craniotomy for cerebral tumours. Acta Anaesthesiol Scand 1995:39: 582–585.

Fitch W, MacKenzie ET, Harper AM. Effects of decreasing arterial blood pressure on cerebral blood flow in the baboon: Influence of sympathetic nervous system. Circ Res 1975: 37: 550–557.

Fitch W, Ferguson GG, Sengupta D, et al. Autoregulation of cerebral blood flow during controlled hypotension in baboons. J Neurol Neurosurg Psychiat 1976: 39: 1014–1022.

Fitch W. Editorial. Sodium nitroprusside and the cerebral circulation. Br J Anaesth 1977: 49: 399–400.

Forrester T, Harper AM, MacKenzie ET, Thomson EM. Effect of adenosine trophosphate and some derivates on cerebral blood flow and metabolism. J Physiol 1979: 296: 343–355.

Forster A, VanHorn K, Marshall LF, Shapiro HM. Anesthetic effects on blood-brain barrier function during acute arterial hypertension. Anesthesiology 1978: 49: 26–30.

Fukunaga AF, Olewine SK, van Etten AP. Haemodynamic effects of ATP and nitroprusside. Anesthesiology 1981: 53: A13.

Fukunaga AF, Flacke WE, Bloor BC. Hypotensive effects of adenosine and adenosine Triphsiophate compared with sodium nitroprusside. Anesth Analg 1982: 61: 273–278.

Fukunaga AF, Sodeyama O, Matsuzaki Y. Haemodynamic and metabolic changes of ATP-induced hypotension during surgery. Anesthesiology 1983: 59: A 12.

Gaumann D, Tassonyi E, Rivest RW, et al. Cardiovascular and endocrine effects of clonidine premedication in neurosurgical patients. Can J Anaesth 1991: 38: 837–843.

Gerson JI, Allen FB, Seltzer JL, et al. Arterial and venous dilation by nitroprusside and nitroglycerin-Is there a difference? Anesth Analg 1982: 61: 256–260.

Gianotta JI, Allen FB, Seltzer JL, et al. Arterial and venous dilation by nitroprusside and nitroglycerin. Is there a difference? Anesth Analg 1982: 61: 256–260.

Gibson BE, Black S, Maass L, Cucchiara RF. Esmolol for the control of hypertension after neurologic surgery. Clin Pharmacol Ther 1988: 44: 650–653.

Giffin JP, Cottrell JE, Hartung J, Shwiry B. Intracranial pressure during nifedipine-induced hypotension. Anesth Analg 1983: 62: 1078–1080.

Goto F, Otani E, Kato S, Fujita T. Prostaglandin E1 as a hypotensive drug during general anaesthesia. Anaesthesia 1982: 37: 530–535.

Gottstein U. Der Hirnkreislauf unter dem Einfluss vasoaktiver Substanzen. Hütlig Verlag, Heidelberg 1962

Gottstein U, Paulson OB. The effect of intracarotid aminophylline infusion on the cerebral circulation. Stroke 1972: 3: 560–565.

Grände PO. The effects of dihydroergotamine in patients with head injury and raised intracranial pressure. Intensive Care Med 1989: 15: 523–527.

Greenfield JC, Tindall GT. Effect of norepinephrine, epinephrine, and angiotensin on blood flow in the internal carotid artery of man. J Clin Invest 1968: 47: 1672–1684.

Gregory P, Ishikawa T, McDowall DG. CO_2 responses of the cerebral circulation during drug-induced hypotension in the cat. J Cereb Blood Flow Metab 1981: 1. 195–201.

Griffith DPG, Cummins BH, Greenbaum R, et al. Cerebral blood flow and metabolism during hypotension induced with sodium nitroprusside. Br J Anaesth 1974: 46: 671–679.

Grubb RL, Raichle ME. Effect of hemorrhagic and pharmacologic hypotension on cerebral oxygen utilization and blood flow. Anesthesiology 1982: 56: 3–8.

Guo T-Z, Jiang J-Y, Buttermann AE, Maze M. Dexmedetomidine injection into the locus ceruleus produces antinociception. Anesthesiology 1996: 84: 873–881.

Hamel E, Edvinsson L, MacKenzie ET. Heterogenous vasomotor responses of anatomically distict feline cerebral arteries. Br J Pharmacol 1988: 94: 423–436.

Hartmann A, Buttinger C, Rommel T, et al. Alteration of intracranial pressure, cerebral blood flow, autoregulation and carbondioxide-reactivity by hypotensive agents in baboons with intracranial hypertension. Neurochirurgica (Stuttg.) 1989: 32: 37–43.

Heilbrun MP, Olesen J, Lassen NA. Regional cerebral blood flow studies in subarachnoid hemorrhage. J Neurosurg 37: 1972: 36–44.

Henriksen L, Thorshauge C, Harmsen A, et al. Controlled hypotension with sodium nitroprusside: Effects on cerebral blood flow and cerebral venous blood gases in patients operated for cerebral aneurysms. Acta Anaesthesiol Scand 1983: 27: 62–67.

Heytens L, Verlooy J, Van Vyve M, et al. Influence of ketanserin on intracranial pressure. In Janssen J (ed) Prospects and Strategies in Cardiovascular Research. Assen/Maastricht: Van Gorcum, 1988; 41.

Hodges MR, Stanley TH, Johansen RK. Pulmonary shunt and cardiovascular responses to CPAP during nitroprusside-induced hypotension. Anesthesiology 1977: 46: 339–341.

Hoffman WE, Albrecht RF, Militich DJ. Cerebrovascular and metabolic effects of SNP-induced hypotension in young and aged hypertensive rats. Anesthesiology 1982b: 56: 427–430.

Hoffman WE, Cheng MA, Thomas C, et al. Clonidine decreases plasma catecholamines and improves outcome from incomplete ischemia in the rat. Anesth Analg 1991a: 73: 460–464.

Hoffman WE, Kochs E, Werner C, et al. Dexmedetomidine improves neurologic outcome from incomplete ischemia in the rat. Anesthesiology 1991b: 75: 328–332

Hoka S, Siker D, Bosnjak ZJ, Kampine JP. Alteration of blood distribution and vascular capacitance during induced hypotension in deafferented dogs. Anesthesiology 1987: 66: 647–652.

Hossmann KA. Development and resolution of ischaemic brain swelling. In Pappius HM, Feindal W (eds); Dynamics of brain edema. Springer Verlag, Berlin, Heidelberg, New York 1976: 219–228.

Hoyer D, Vos P, Closse A, et al. [^{3}H] Ketanserin labels serotonin 5-HT_2 and α_1-adrenergic receptors in human brain cortex. J Cardiovasc Pharmacol 1987: 10 (suppl 3): S48–S50.

Huang M, Drummond GI. Adenylate cylase in cerebral microvessels: Action of guanine nucleotides, adenosine and other agonists. Mol Pharmacol 1979: 16: 462–472.

Iannotti F, Hoff J. Ischemic brain edema with and without reperfusion: An experimental study in gerbils. Stroke 1983: 14: 562–567.

Iida H, Ohata H, Iida M, et al. Direct effects of α_1 and α_2-adrenergic agonists on spinal and cerebral pial vessels in dogs. Anesthesiology 1999: 91: 479–485.

Ishikawa T, McDowall DG. Electrical activity of the cerebral cortex during induced hypotension with sodium nitroprusside and trimethaphan in the cat. Br J Anaesth 1980: 53: 605–611.

Ishikawa T, Funatsu N, Okamoto K, et al. Blood-brain barrier function following drug-induced hypotension in the dog. Anesthesiology 1983: 59: 526–531.

Ishiyama T, Dohi S, Iida H, et al. Mechanisms of dexmedetomidine-induced cerebrovascular effects in canine *In vivo* Experiments. Anesth Analg 1995: 81: 1208–1215.

Ivankovich AD, Miletich DJ, Albrecht RF, Zahed B. Sodium nitroprusside and cerebral blood flow in anesthetized and unanesthetized goat. Anesthesiology 1976: 44: 21–26.

Ivankovich AD, Braverman B, Shulman M, Klowden AJ. Prevention of nitroprusside toxicity with thiosulfate in dogs. Anesth Analg 1982: 61: 120–126.

Jack RD. Toxicity of sodium nitroprusside. Br J Anaesth 1974: 46: 952.

Jarden JO, Barry DI, Juhler M, et al. Cerebrovascular aspects of converting-enzyme inhibition: II. Blood-brain varrier permeability and effect of intracerebroventricular administration of captopril. J Hypert 1984: 2: 599–604.

Jones JV, Fitch W, MacKenzie ET, et al. Lower limit of cerebral blood flow autoregulation in the baboon. Circ Res 1976: 39: 555–557.

Kadoi Y, Saito S, Morita T, et al. The differential effects of prostaglandin nitroglycerin on regional cerebral oxygenation in anesthetized patients. Anesth Analg 1997: 85: 1054–1059.

Kanawati IS, Yakch TL, Anderson RE, March RW. Effects of clonidine on cerebral blood flow and the response to arterial CO_2. J Cereb Blood Flow Metab 6: 1986: 358–365

Karlin A, Hartung J, Cottrell JE. Rate of induction of hypotension with trimethaphan modifies the intracranial pressure response in cats. Br J Anaesth 1988: 60: 161–166.

Karlsson BR, Forsman M, Roald OK, et al. Effect of Dexedeetomidine, a selective and potent α_2-agonist, on cerebral blood flow and oxygen consumption during halothane anesthesia in dogs. Anesth Analg 1990: 71: 125–129.

Kassell NF, Boarini DJ, Olin JJ, Sprowell JA. Cerebral and systemic circulatory effects of arterial hypotension induced by adenosine. J Neurosurg 1983a: 58: 69–76.

Kassell NF, Boarini DJ, Sprowell JA, Olin JJ. Pharmacologically induced profound arterial hypotension in the anaesthetized dog. J Neurosurg 1983b: 58: 77–83.

Katsuki S, Arnold W, Murad F. Effects of sodium nitroprusside, nitroglycerin, and sodium azide on levels of cyclic nucleotides and mechanical activity of various tissues. J Cyclic Nucleotides Res 1977: 3: 239–246.

Kawaguchi M, Furuya H, Kurehara K, Yamada M. Effect of nicardipine on cerebral vascular responses to hypocapnia and blood blow velocity in the middle cerebral artery. Stroke 1991: 22: 1170–1172.

Khambatta HJ, Stone JG, Khan E. Hypertension during anaesthesia on discontinuation of sodium nitroprusside-induced hypotension. Anesthesiology 1979: 51: 127–130.

Khambatta HJ, Stone JG, Khan E. Captopril attenuates vasoactive hormonal release during nitroprusside-induced hypotension. Anesthesiology 1982: 57: A62.

Khambatta HJ, Stone JG, Matteo RS, Khan E. Propranolol premedication blunts stress response to nitroprussde hypotension. Anesth Analg 1984: 63: 125–128.

Khan ZP, Munday IT, Jones RM, et al. Effects of dexmedetomidine on isoflurane requirements in healthy volunteers. 1: Pharmacodynamic and pharmacokinetic interactions. Br J Anaesth 1999: 83: 372–380.

Kibler LE, Gazes PC (1977) Effect of clonidine on atrioventricular conduction. JAMA 238: 1930–1932.

Kien ND, White DA, Reitan JA. Eisele JH. Cardiovascular function during controlled hypotension induced by adenosine triphosphate or sodium nitroprusside in the anesthetized dog. Anesth Analg 1987: 66: 103–110.

Kim HK, Zornow MH, Strnat MAP, Maze M. Dexmedetomidine does not attenuate increases in excitatory amino acids after transient global ischemia in the rabbit. J Neurosurg Anesthesiology 1996: 8: 230–235.

King BD, Sokoloff L, Wechsler RL. The effects of l-epinephrine and l-norepinephrine upon cerebral circulation and metabolism in man. J Clin Invest 1951: 31: 273.

Kinkor RD, Warner DS. Unexpected myocardial complications after controlled hypotension. J Neurosurg Anesthesiology 1991: 2: 136–141.

Klimscha W, Tong C, Eisenach JC. Intrathecal alpha 2-adrenergic agonists stimulate acetylcholine and norepinephrine

release from sipnal cord dorsal horn in sheep. An in vivo micrdialysis study. Anesthesiology 1997: 110-116.
Knight PR, Lane GA, Hensinger RN, et al. Catecholanmine and renin-angiotensin response during hypotensive anesthesia induced by sodium nitroprusside or trimethaphan camsylate. Anesthesiology 1983: 59: 248-253.
Kolassa N, Pfleger K. Adenosine uptake by eruthrocytes of man, rat, and guinea-pig and its inhibition by hexobendine and dipyridamole. Biochem Pharmacol 1975: 24: 154-156.
Kolassa N, Beller KD, Sanders KH. Evidence for the interaction of urapidil with (5-HT 1A)-receptors in the brain leading to a decrease in blood pressure. Am J Cardiol 1989: 63: 36C-39C.
Kraynack BJ, Gintautas J, Hinshaw J. Adenosine triphsophate increases survival time during hyoxia. Neuropharm 1981: 20: 887-890.
Kuroda K, Kuwata N, Sato N, et al. Changes in cerebral blood flow accompanied with reduction of blood pressure treatment in patients with hypertensive intracerebral hemorrhage. Neurol Res 1997: 19: 169-173.
Lagerkranser M, Irestedt L, Sollevi A, Andreen M. Central and splanchnic hemodynamics in the dog during controlled hypotension with adenosine. Anesthesiology 1984: 60: 547-552.
Lagerkranser M, Sollevi A, Irestedt L, et al. Renin release during controlled hypotension with sodium nitroprusside, nitrogycerin and adenosine: A comparative study in the dog. Acta Anaesthesiol Scand 1985: 29: 45-49.
Lagerkranser M, Bergstrand G, Gordon E, et al. Cerebral blood flow and metabolism during adenosine-induced hypotension in patients undergoing cerebral aneurysm surgery. Acta Anaestheiol Scand 1989: 33: 15-20.
Lagerkranser M. Controlled hypotension in neurosurgery: Pro. J Neurosurg Anesthesiol 1991: 3: 150-152
Lagerkranser M. Effects of nitroglycerin on intracranial pressure and cerebral blood flow. Acta Anaesthesiol Scand 1992: 36 [suppl 97]: 34-36
Lam AM, Gelb AW. Cardiovascular effects of isoflurane-induced hypotension for cerebral aneurysm surgery. Anesth Analg 1983: 62: 742-748
Lam AM, Wu X, Gelb AW. Regional cerebral blood flow during nicardipine and nitroprusside induced hypotension. Anesth Analg 1988: 67: S 125.
Lam A, Artru AA. Autoregulation of cerebral blood flow in response to adenosine-induced hypotension in dogs. J Neurosurg Anesthesiol 1992: 4: 120-127.
Larsen R, Teichmann J, Hilfiker O, et al. Nitroprusside-hypotension: Cerebral blood flow and cerebral oxygen consumption in neurosurgical patients. Acta Anaesth Scand 1982: 26: 327-330.
Laudignon N, Farri E, Beharry K, Rex J, Aranda JV. Influence of adenosine on cerebral blood flow during hypoxic hypoxia in the newborn piglet. J Appl Physiol 1990: 68: 1534-1541.
Laudignon N, Beharry K, Farri E, Aranda JV. The role of adenosine in the vascular adaptation of neonatal cerebral blood flow during hypotension. J Cereb Blood Flow Metab 1991: 11: 424-431
Laycock JRD, Coakham HB, Silver IA, Walters FJM. Changes in brain surface oxygen tension during profound hypotension induced with sodium nitroprusside or adenosine in the sheep. Br J Anaesth 1986: 58: 1422-1426.
Lee H-W, Caldwell JE, Dodson B, Talke P. The effect of clonidine on cerebral blood flow velocity, carbon dioxide cerebral vasoreactivity, and response to increased arterial pressure in human volunteers. Anesthesiology 1997: 87: 553-558.
Leenders KL, Wolfson L, Gibbs JM, et al. The effect of L-DOPA on regional cerebral blood flow and oxygen metabolism in patients with Parkinson´s disease. Brain 1985: 108: 171-191.
Levänen J, Mäkelä M-J, Scheinin H. Dexmedetomidine premedication attenuates ketamine-induced cardiostimulatory effects and postanesthetic delirium. Anesthesiology 1995: 82: 117-1125.
Ljunggren B, Säveland H, Brandt L, et al. Temporary clipping during early operation of ruptured aneurysm: preliminary report. Neurosurgery 1983: 12: 525-530
Longnecker DE, Seyde WC. Cerebral oxygen tension during deliberate hypotension with sodium nitroprusside, 2-C1-adenosine, or deep isoflurane anesthesia in rats. Anesthesiology 1984: 61: A366.
Lu GP, Chi OZ, Kaul DK, et al. Effects of nitroprusside on cerebral microcirculation. Anesthesiology 1982: 57: A49.
Lüben V, Hempelmann G. Improved deep controlled hypotension in aneurysmal surgery. Acta Neurochir 1982: 60: 201-214.
MacKenzie ET, MCCulloch J, O'Keane M, et al. Cerebral circulation and norepinephrine: relevance of the blood brain barrier. Am J Physiol 1976: 231: 483.
Madsen JB, Cold GE, Hansen ES, et al. Cerebral blood flow and metabolism during isoflurane-induced hypotension in patients subjected to surgery for cerebral aneurysms. Br J Anaesth 1987: 59: 1204-1207
Maekawa T, McDowall DG, Okuda Y. Brain surface oxygen tension and cerebral cortical blood flow during hemorrhagic and drug-induced hypotension in the cat. Anesthesiology 1979: 51: 313-320.
Maier C, Steinberg GK, Sun GH, et al. Neuroprotection by the alpha-2-adrenoceptor agonist dexmedetomidine in a focal model of cerebral ischemia. Anesthesiology 1993: 79: 306-312.
Maktabi M, Warner D, Boarini D, et al. A comparison of nitroprusside, nitroglycerin and deep isofluran anesthesia for induced hypotension. Anesthesiology 1985: 63: A403.
Maktabi M, Warner DS, Sokoll MD. The effects of hypotension induced by sodium nitroprusside and isoflurane on serum catecholamines and plasma renin activity. Anesthesiology 1986: 65: A578.
March ML, Shapiro HM, Smith RW, Marshall LF. Changes in neurologic status and intracranial pressure associated with sodium nitroprusside administration. Anesthesiology 1979a: 51: 336-338.
March ML, Aidinis SJ, Naughton KVH, et al. The technique of nitroprusside administration modifies the intracranial pressure response. Anesthesiology 1979b: 51: 538-541.
Matta BF, Lam AM, Mayberg TS, et al. Cerebrovascular response to carbon dioxide during sodium nitroprusside- and isoflurane-induced hypotension. Br J Anesth 1995: 74: 296-300.
Maze M, Tranquilli W. Alpha-2 adrenoceptor agonists: defining the role in clinical anesthesia. Anesthesiology 1991: 74: 581-605.
Mazzoni P, Giffin JP, Cottrell JE, et al. Intracranial pressure during diltiazem-induced hypotension in anesthetized dogs. Anesth Analg 1985: 64: 1001-1004.
Mc Culloch J, Harper AM. Cerebral circulation: effect of stimulation and blockade of dopamine receptors. Am J Physiol 1977: 233: H222-H227.

Mc Culloch J, Teasdale G. Effects of apomorphine upon local cerebral blood flow. Eur J Pharmacol 1979: 55: 99–102.

McDowall GD. Induced hypotension and brain ischaemia. Br J Anaesth 1985: 57: 110–119.

McDermott MW, Durity FA, Borozny M, Mountain MA. Temporary vessel occlusion and barbiturate protection in cerebral aneurysm surgery. Neurosurgery 1989: 25: 54–62

McPherson RW, Koehler RC, Kirsch JR. Intraventricular dexmedetomidine decreases cerebral blood flow during normoxia and hypoxia in dogs. Anesth Analg 1997: 84: 139–147.

Meert TF, Kock MD. Potentiation of the analgetic properties of fentanyl-like opioids with alpha-2-adrenoceptor agonists in rat. Anesthesiology 1994: 81: 677–688.

Meng W, Busija DW. Comparative effects of angiotensin-(1–7) and angiotensin II on piglet pial arterioles. Stroke 1993: 24: 2041–2045.

Merrifield AJ, Blundell MD. Toxicity of sodium nitroprusside. Br J Anaesth 1974: 46: 324.

Messick JM, Casement B, Sharbrough FW, et al. Correlation of regional cerebral blood flow (rCBF) with EEG changes during isoflurane anesthesia for carotid endarterectomy: Critical rCBF. Anesthesiology 1987: 66: 344–349

Michenfelder JD, Theye RA. Canine systemic and cerebral effects of hypotension induced by hemorrhage, trimethaphan, halothane or nitroprusside. Anesthesiology 1977: 46: 188–195.

Michenfelder JD. Cyanide release from sodium nitroprusside in the dog. Anesthesiology 1977: 46: 196–201.

Michenfelder JD, Milde JH. The interaction of sodium nitroprusside, hypotension, and isoflurane in determining cerebral vasculature effects. Anesthesiology 1988: 69: 870–875.

Mikawa K, Maekawa N, Goto R, et al. Effects of pindolol on the cardiovascular response to tracheal intubation. British Journal Anaesthesia 1991: 67: 416–420.

Miller DR, Martineua J, Wynands JE, Hill J. Bolus administration of esmolol for controlling the haemodynamic response to tracheal intubation: The Canadian multicentre trial. Can J Anaesth 1991: 38: 849–858.

Mirski MAZ, Rossell LA, McPhersom RW, Traystman RJ. Dexmedetomidine decreases seizure threshold in a rat model of experimental generalized epilepsy. Anesthesiology 1994: 81: 1422–1428.

Monk CR, Sperry RJ, Durieux ME, et al. The regional haemodynamic effects of induced hypotension with isoflurane, sodium nitroprusside or 2-chloroadenosine. Anesthesiology 1987: 67: A34.

Morii S, Nagai AC, Berne RM, Winn HR. Attenuation of hypoxic hyperemia by theophylline: the role of adenosine in cerebral blood flow regulation. Surg Forum 1984: 35: 504–507.

Morii S, Ngai AC, Winn HR. Reactivity of rat pial arterioles and venules to adenosine and carbon dioxide: With detailed description of the closed cranial window technique in rats. J Cereb Blood Flow Metab 1986: 6: 34–41.

Morii S, Nagai AC, Ko KR, Winn HR. Role of adenosine in regulation of cerebral blood flow: effects of theophylline during normoxia and hypoxia. Am J Physiol 1987: 253: H165–175.

Morii S, Wang R, Ohtaka H, et al. Possible involvment of adenosine in vasodilatory reponse of the rat pial arterioles to hypotension. J Cereb Blood Flow Metab 1989: 9: suppl 1, S487.

Morris PJ, Heuser D, McDowall DG, Hashiba M, Myers D. Cerebral cortical extracellular fluid H^+ and K^+ activities during hypotension in cats. Anesthesiology 1983: 59: 10–18.

Moss E. Cerebral blood flow during induced hypotension (editorial) Br J Anaesth 1995: 74: 635–637.

Muhonen MG, Loftus CM, Heistad DD. Effect of adenosine and 2-chloroadenosine on cerebral collateral vessels. J Cereb Blood Flow Metab 1995: 15: 1075–1081.

Muhonen MG, Robertson C, Gerdes JS, Loftus CM. Effects of serotonin on cerebral circulation after middle cerebral artery occlusion. J Neurosurg 1997: 87: 301–306.

Muzzi DA, Black S, Lasasso J, Cucchiara RF. Labetalol and esmolol in the control of hypertension after intracranial surgery. Anest Analg 1990: 70: 68–71.

Nacif-Coelho C, Correa-Sales C, Chang LL, Maze M. Perturbation of ion channel conductance alters the hypnotic response to the alpha-2-adrenergic agonist dexmedetomidine in the locus coereleus of the rat. Anesthesiology 1994: 81: 1527–1534.

Nakamura K, Koide M, Imanaga T, et al. Prolonged neuromuscluar blockade following trimethaphan infusion: A case report and in vitro study of cholinesterase inhibition. Anaesthesia 1980: 35: 1202–1207.

Nakamura K, Hatano Y, Mori K. The site of action of trimethaphan-induced neuromuscular blockade in isolated rat and frog muscle. Acta Anaesthesiol Scand 1988: 32: 125–130.

Nakazawa K, Hatano Y, Mori K. The site of action of trimethaphan-induced neuromuscular blockade in isolated rat and frog muscle. Acta Anaesthesiol Scand 1991: 73: 59–63.

Nemoto EM, Klementavicius R, Melick JA. Norepinephrine activation of basal cerebral metabolic rate for oxygen ($CMRO_2$) during hypothermia in rats. Anesth Analg 1996: 83: 1262–1267.

Newberg LA, Milde JH, Michenfelder JD. Cerebral and systemic effects of hypotension induced by adenosine or ATP in dogs. Anesthesiology 1985: 62: 429–436.

Newman B, Gelb AW, Lam AM. The effect of isoflurane-induced hypotension on cerebral blood flow and cerebral metabolic rate for oxygen in humans. Anesthesiology 1986: 64: 307–310

Nicholas JF, Lam AM. Isoflurane-induced hypotension does not cause impairment in pulmonary gas exchange. Can Anaesth Soc J 1984: 31: 352–358

Niimi T, Sawada T, Kuriyama Y, et al. The effect of dopamine on cerebral circulation and metabolism in man. Jpn J Stroke 1981: 3: 318–325.

Nilsson F. Cerebral vasoconstriction as treatment of intracranial hypertension. Aspects based on experimental investigations (thesis), ESSatryck, Malmö 1995.

Nishikawa T, Omote K, Namiki A, Takahashi T. The effect of nicardipine on cerebrospinal fluid pressure in humans. Anesth Analg 1986: 65: 507–510.

Nishikawa T, Dohi S. Oral clonidine blunts the heart rate response to intravenous atropine in humans. Anesthesiology 1991: 75: 217–222

Ohata H, Iida H, Dohi S, Watanabe Y. Intravenous dexmedetomidine inhibits cerebrovascular dilation induced by isoflurane and sevoflurane in dogs. Anesth Analg 1999: 89: 370–377.

Ohta K, Rosner G, Graf R. Nitric oxide generation from sodium nitroprusside and hydroxylamine in brain. Neuroreport 1997: 8: 2229–2235.

Oldendorff WH. Brain uptake of radiolabeled amino acids, amines, and hexoses after arterial injection. Am J Physol 1971: 221: 1229–1639.

Olesen J. The effect of intracarotid epinephrine, norepinephrine, and angiotensin on regional cerebral blood flow in man. Neurology 1972: 22: 978–987.

Olesen J, Skinhøj E. Effects of ergot alkaloids (hydergine) on cerebral haemodynamic in man. Acta Pharmacol Toxicol 1972: 31: 75–85.

Olesen J. Effect of intracarotid prostaglandin E1 on regional cerebral blood flow in man. Stroke 1976: 7: 566–569.

Olivarius B. Behandling af friske cerebrale infarter med theophyllamin. UfL 1961: 123: 376–382.

Olsen KS, Henriksen L, Dige-Petersen H, et al. Effect of ketanserin on global cerebral blod flow and cerebral oxygen metabolism during midazolam-fentanyl or isoflurane anaesthesia. Br J Anaesth 1992: 69: 263–268.

Olsen KS, Videbaeck C, Schmidt JF, Paulson OB. The effect of ketanserin on cerebral blood flow and cerebrovascular CO_2 reactivity in healthy volunteers. Acta Neurochir 1992: 119: 7–11.

Olsen KS, Madsen PL, Børme T, Schmidt JF. The effect of ketanserin on cerebral blood flow and oxygen metabolism in healthy volunteers. Acta Neurochir 1993: 125: 83–85.

Olsen KS, Henriksen L, Owen-Falkenberg A, et al. Effect of 1 and 2 MAC isoflurane with or without ketanserin on cerebral blood flow autoregulation in man. Br J Anaesth 1994: 72: 66–71.

Olsen KS, Svendsen LB, Larsen FS, Paulson OB. Effect of labetalol on cerebral blood flow, oxygen metabolism and autoregulation in healthy humans. Br J Anaesth 1995: 75: 51–54.

Olsen KS, Albeck M, Agerlin N, Schmidt JF. The effect of ketanserin in ICP and CBF in patients with normal-pressure hydrocephalus. J Neurosurg Anesthesiol 1996: 8: 216–219.

Orlowski JP, Shiesley D, Vidt DG, Barnett GH, Little JR. Labetalol to control blood pressure after cerebrovascular surgery. Crit Care Med 1988: 16: 765–768.

Ornstein E, Matteo RS, Schwartz AE. The use of esmolol for deliberate hypotension. Anesthesiology 1986: 65: A575.

Ornstein E, Matteo RS, Winstein JA, Schwartz AE. A randomised controlled trial of esmolol for deliberate hypotension. Anesthesiology 1987: 67: A423.

Ornstein E, Young WL, Ostapkovich N, et al. Are all effects of esmolol equally rapid in onset? Anesth Analg 1995: 81: 297–300.

Öwall A, Gordon E, Lagerkranser M, et al. Clinical experience with adenosine for controlled hypotension during cerebral aneurysm surgery. Anesth Analg 1984: 66: 229–234.

Öwall A, Järnberg P, Brodin L, Sollevi A. Effects of adenosine-induced hypotension on myocardial hemodynamics and metabolism in fentanyl anesthetized patients with peripheral vascular disease. Anesthesiology 1988a: 68: 416–421.

Öwall A, Lagerkranser M, Sollevi A. Effects of adenosine-induced hypotension on myocardial hemodynamics and metabolism during cerebral aneurysm surgery. Anesth Analg 1988b: 67: 228–232.

Park TS, Didday JM, Effect of dipyridamole on cerebral extracellular adenosine levels in vivo. J Cereb Blood Flow Metab 1990: 10: 424–427.

Paulson OB, Jarden JO, Vorstrup S, et al. Effect of captopril on the cerebral circulation in chronic heart failure. Eup J Clin Invest 1986: 16: 124–132.

Paulson OB, Waldemar G, Andersen AR, et al. Role of angiotensin in regulation of cerebral blood flow. Circulation 1988: 77 (suppl 1): I55–I58.

Pearl RG, Rosenthal MH, Ashton JPA, Murad F. Aminophylline potentiates sodium nitroprusside-induced hypotension. Anesthesiology 1983a: 59: A126.

Pearl RG, Rosenthal MH, Achton JPA. Pulmonary vasodilator effects of nitroglycerin and sodium nitroprusside in canine oleic acid-induced pulmonary hypertension. Anesthesiology 1983b: 58: 514–518.

Peden CJ, Prys-Roberts C. The role of alpha-1 agonist in generel anesthesia. Curr Opinion Anesthesiology 1993: 6: 653–658.

Phillis JW, Walter GA, O'Regan MH, Stair RE. Increases in cerebral cortical perfusate adenosine and inosine concentrations during hypoxia and ischaemia. J Cereb Blood Flow Metab. 1987: 7: 679–686.

Pinaud M, Souron R, Lelausque J, et al. Cerebral blood flow and cerebral oxygen consumption during nitroprusside-induced hypotension to less than 50 mm Hg. Anesthesiology 1989: 70: 255–260.

Proctor LT, Schmeling WT, Warltier DC. Premedication with oral dexmedetomidine alters hemodynamic actions of intravenous anesthetic agents in chronically instrumented dogs. Anesthesiology 1992: 77: 554–562.

Prough DS, Stullken EH, Scuderi PE, Johnson JC. Intracranial hypertension limits the systemic hypotensive effect of nitroprusside, but not nitroglycerin. Anesthesiology 1983a: 59: A354.

Prough DS, Stullken EH, Scuderi PE. Technique of administration alters increases in intracranial hypertension produced by nitroglycerin but not by nitroprusside. Anesthesiology 1983b: 59: A353.

Puchstein C, van Aken H, Anger C, et al. Influence of ATP-induced hypotension on intracranial pressure and intracranial compliance. Anesthesiology 1983: 59: A356.

Rich M, Scheinberg P, Belle MS. Relationship between cerebrospinal fluid pressure changes and cerebral blood flow. Circ Res. 1953: 21: 517–525.

Rogers MC, Traystman RJ. Nitroglycerin and nitroprusside induced changes in cerebral hemodynamics Anesthesiology 1979a: 51: S199.

Rogers MC, Hamburger C, Owen K, Epstein MH. Intracranial pressure in the cat during nitroglycerin-induced hypotension. Anesthesiology 1979b 51: 227–229.

Rooney MW, Crystal GJ, Salem R. Influence of nifedipine on systemic and regional hemodynamics during adenosine-induced hypotension in dogs. Anest Analg 1989: 68: 261–269.

Rosen¢rn J (1989) The risk of ischaemic brain damage during the use of self-retaining brain retractors. Acta Neurol Scand [suppl 120] vol 79

Roth S, Jones SC, Ebrahim Z, et al. Cerebral blood flow and metabolism during isoflurane-induced hypotension. Anesthesiology 1986: 65: A572

Ruta TS, Mutch WAC. Controlled hypotension for cerebral aneurysm surgery: Are the risks woth the benefits?. J Neurosurg Anesthesiol 1991: 2: 153–156

Samson D, Batjar HH, Bowman G. A clinical study of the parameters and effects of temporary arterial occlusion in the management of intracranial aneurysms. Neurosurgery 1994: 34: 22–29.

Sandler AN. The role of clonidine and alpha-2-agonists for postoperative analgesia (editorial). Can J Anaesth 1996: 43: 1191–1194.
Satin A, Rall TW. The effect of adenosine and adenine nucleotides on the cyclic adenosine 3',5'-phosphate content of guinea pig cerebral cortex slices. Mol Pharmacol 1970: 6: 13–23.
Satinover I, Hoffman WE, Albrecht RF, et al. Controlled hypotension with ATP and sodium nitroprusside. Anesthesiology 1981: 55: A10.
Sato M, Niiyama K, Kurado R, Oiku M. Influence of dopamine on cerebral blood flow and metabolism for oxygen and glucose under barbiturate administration in cats. Acta Neurochir 1991: 110: 174–180.
Scheinin M. The locus coeruleus (editorial). Anesthesiology 1992: 76: 873–875.
Scheinin M, Jaakola M-J, Sjövall S, et al. Intramuscular dexmedetomidine as premedication for generel anesthesia. Anesthesiology 1993: 78: 1065–1075.
Schedewie H, Boban N, Schmeling WT, Bosnjak ZJ. Dexmedetomidine inhibits synaptic transmission in the canine stellate ganglion. Anesth Analg 1992: 74: S261.
Schmidt JF, Waldemar G, Vorstrup S, et al. Computerized analysis of cerebral blood flow autoregulation in humans: Validation of a method for pharmacological studies. J Cardiovasc Pharmacol 1990: 15: 983–988.
Schmidt JF, Olsen KS, Waldemar G, et al. The effect of ketanserin on the autoregulation of cerebral blood flow in healthy volunteers. Acta Neurochirurgica 1991: 111: 138–142.
Schroeder T, Schiebeck J, Howardy P, et al. Effect of labetalol on cerebral blood flow and middle cerebral arterial flow velocity in healthy volunteers. Neurol Res 1991: 13: 10–13.
Schubert J, Brill WA. Antagonism of experimental cyanide toxicity in relation to the in vivo activity of cytochrome oxidase. J Pharmacol Exp Ther 1968: 162: 352–359.
Schultz KD, Schultz K, Schultz G. Sodium nitroprusside and other smooth muscle relaxants increase cyclic GMP levels in art ductus deferens. Nature 1977: 256: 750–751.
Schutz JA, Hoffman WE, Albrecht RF. Sympathetic stimulation with physiolostigmine worsens outcome from incomplete brain ischemia in rats. Anesthesiology 1993: 79: 114–121.
Schulz V, Gross R, Pasch T, et al. Cyanide toxicity of sodium nitroprusside in therapeutic use with and without sodium thiosulphate. Klin Wochenschr 1982: 60: 1393–1400.
Sensenbach W, Madison L, Ochs L. A comparison of the effect of l-norepinephrine, synthetic l-epinephrine, and USP epinephrine upon cerebral blood flow and metabolism in man. J Clin Invest 1953: 32: 226–232.
Shapira Y, Artru AA, Lam AM. Changes in the rate of formation and resistance to reabsorption of cerebrospinal fluid duirng deliberate hypotension induced with adenosine or hemorrhage. Anesthesiology 1992: 76: 432–439.
Sharkey J, Mc Culloch L. Relationship between local cerebral blood flow and glucose utilization with selective dopamine receptor agonists. J Cereb Blood Flow Metab 1985: 5: (suppl): 537–538.
Sharkey J, Mc Culloch J. Dopaminergic mechanism in the regulation of cerebral blood flow and metabolism: role of different receptor subtypes. In Owaman C, Hardebo JE (eds) Neural regulation of brain circulation, Elsevier. Science 1986: 111-127.
Shenkin HA. Effects of various drugs upon cerebral circulation and metabolism in man. J Appl Phsiol 1951: 3: 465–471.
Shibutani K, Komatsu T, Bhalodia R, et al. Rebound hemodynamic responses after the withdrawal of nitroprusside in anesthetized patients. Anesthesiology 1983: 59: A16.
Shin HK, Park SN, Hong KW. Implication of adenosine A2A receptors in hypotension-induced vasodilation and cerebral blood flow antoregulation in rat pial arteries. Life Sci 2000a: 67: 1435–1445.
Shin HK, Shin YW, Hong KW. Role of adenosine A(2B) receptors in vasodilation of rat pial artery and cerebral blood flow autoregulation. Am J Physiol: 2000: 278: H339–344.
Singh PP, Dimich I, Sampson I, Sonnenklar N. A comparison of esmelol and labetalol for the treatment of perioperative hypertension in geriatric ambulatory surgical patients. Can J Anaesth 1992: 39: 559–562.
Skinhøj E, Paulson OB. The mechanism of action of aminophylline upon cerebral vascular disorders. Acta Neurol Scand 1970: 46: 129–140.
Sollevi A, Lagerkranser M, Irestedt L, et al. Controlled hypotension with adenosine in cerebral aneurysm surgery. Anesthesiology 1984a: 61: 400–405.
Sollevi A, Lagerkranser M, Andreen M, Irestedt L. Relationshhip between arterial and venous adenosine levels and vasodilatation during ATP- and adenosine-infusion in dogs. Acta Physiol Scand 1984b: 120: 171–176.
Sollevi A, Ericson K, Eriksson L, et al. Effect of adenosine on human cerebral blood flow as determined by positron emission tomography. J Cereb Blood Flow Metab 1987: 7: 673–678.
Spargo PM, Tait AR, Knight PR, Kling TF. Effect of nitroglycerin-induced hypotension on canine spinal cord blood flow. Br J Anaesth 1987: 59: 640–647.
Sperry RJ, Monk CR, Durieux ME, et al. Regional cerebral blood flow during deliberate hypotension complicated by hemorrhage. Anesthesiology 1987: 67: A575.
Spiss CK, Zadrobilek E, Weindlmayr-Goettel M, et al. Nifedipine induced hypotension in man: hemodynamic response during isoflurane and halothane anesthesia. Anesthesiology: 1985: 63: A 93.
Standefer M, Little JR. Improved neurological outcome in experimental focal cerebral ischemia treated with propranolol. Neurosurgery 1986: 18: 136–140.
Stefanovich V. Influence of theophylline on concentration of cyclic 3'.5'-adenosine monophosphate and cyclic 3',5'-guanosine monophosphate of rat brain. Neurochem Res 1979: 4: 587–594.
Steiner L, Forster DMC, Bergvall U. Effect of prostaglandin E1 on cerebral circulatory disturbances following subarachnoid hemorrhage in man. Neuroradiol 1972: 4: 20–24.
Stone JG, Khambatta HJ, Matteo RS. Pulmonary shunting during anesthesia with deliberate hypotension. Anesthesiology 1976: 45: 508–515.
Stoyka WW, Schutz H. The cerebral response to sodium nitroprusside and trimethaphan controlled hypotension. Can Anaesth Soc J 1975: 22: 275–283.
Strandgaard S, Jones JV, MacKenzie ET, Harper AM. Upper-limit of cerebral blood flow autoregulation in experimental renovascular hypertension in the baboon. Circ Res 1975: 37: 164–167.
Strandgaard S. Autoregulation of cerebral blood flow in hypertensive patients. The modifying influence of profound an-

tihypertensive treatment on the tolerance to acute, drug-induced hypotension. Circulation 1976: 53: 720–727.
Strandgaard S, Paulson OB. Cerebral autoregulation. Stroke 1984: 15: 413–416.
Strandgaard S, MacKenzie ET, Sengupta D. et al. Upper limit of autoregulation of cerebral blood flow in the baboon. Circ Res 1974: 34: 435–440.
Stullken EH, Sokoll MD. Intracranial pressure during hypotension and subsequent vasopressor therapy in anesthetized cats. Anesthesiology 1975: 42: 425–431.
Stånge K, Lagerkranser M, Rudehill A, Sollevi A. Effect of adenosine-induced hypotension on cerebral blood flow and metabolism in the pig. Acta Anaesthesiol Scand 1989: 33: 199–203.
Stånge K, Lagerkranser M, Sollevi A. Effect of isoflurane-induced hypotension on cerebral autoregulation in the anesthetized pig. J Neurosurg Anesthesiol 1990: 2: 114–121.
Suzuki J, Yoshimoto T, Kayama T (1984) Surgical treatment of middle cerebral artery aneurysms. J Neurosurg 61: 17–23
Symon L, Branston NM, Chikovani O. Ischemic brain edema following middle cerebral artery occlusion in baboons: Relationship between regional cerebral water content and blood flow at 1 and 2 hours. Stroke 1979: 10: 184–191.
Tagawa H, Vander AJ. Effects of adenosine compounds on renal function and renin secretion in dogs. Circ Res 1970: 26: 327–338.
Takenaka M, Iida H, Iida M, Dohi S. Intrathecal dexmedetomidine attenuates hypercapnic but not hypoxic cerebral vasodilation in anesthetized rabbits. Anesthesiology 2000: 92: 1376–1384.
Talke P, Bickler PE. Effects of dexmedetomidine on hypoxia-evoked glutamate release and glutamate receptor activity in hippocampal slices. Anesthesiology 1996: 85: 551–557.
Talke P, Tong C, Lee H-W, et al. Effect of dexmedetomidine on lumbar cerebrospinal fluid pressure in humans. Anesth Analg 1997: 85: 358–364.
Tateishi A, Sano T, Takeshita H, et al. Effects of nifedipine on intracranial pressure in neurosurgical patients with arterial hypertension. J Neurosurg 1988: 69: 213–215.
Thiagarajah S, Azar I, Lear E, Suazo J. Comparative evaluation of intracranial pressure changes in cats during adenosine triphosphate and nitroprusside induced hypotension. Anesthesiology 1983: 59: A352.
Thiagarajah S, Azar I, Lear E, Rudolf D. Effect of diltiazem-induced hypotension on normal and increased intracranial pressure of cats. Can Anaesth Soc J 1986: 33: 578–582.
Thomas WA, Cole PV, Etherington NJ, et al. Electrical activity of the cerebral cortex during induced hypotension in man. Br J Anaesth 1985: 57: 134–141.
Thompson JA, Wei EP, Kontos HA. Inhibition by ketanserin of serotonin induced cerebral arteriolar constriction. Stroke 1984: 15: 1021–1024.
Thomsen LJ, Riisager S, Jensen KA, Bünemann L. Cerebral blood flow and metabolism during hypotension induced with sodium nitroprusside and captopril. Can J Anaesth 1989: 36: 392–396.
Tietjen CS, Hurn PD, Ulatowski JA, Kirsch JR. Treatment modalities for hypertensive patients with intracranial pathology: options and risks. Crit Care Med 1996: 24: 311–322.
Tinker JH, Michenfelder JD. Sodium nitroprusside: Pharmacology, toxicology and therapeutics. Anesthesiology 1976: 45: 340–353.
Toda N. Influence of dopamine and noradrenaline on isolated cerebral arteries of the dog. Br J Pharmacol 1976: 58: 121–126.
Todd MM, Morris PJ, Philbin DM. Acute neurologic changes caused by nitroprusside-induced intracranial hypertension. Anesth Analg 1980: 59: 561–562.
Tohmo H, Karanko M. Enalaprilat controls postoperative hypertension while maintaining cardiac function and systemic oxygenation after neurosurgery. Int Care Med 1995: 21: 651–656.
Toivonen J, Virtanen H, Kaukinen S. Labetalol attenuates the negative effects of deliberate hypotension induced by isoflurane. Acta Anaesthesiol Scand 1992: 36: 84–87.
Toivonen J, Kuikka P, Kaukinen S. Effect of deliberate hypotension induced by labetalol with isoflurane on neuropsychological function. Acta Anaesthesiol Scand 1993: 37: 7–11.
Tsutsue T, Maekawa T, Goodchild C, Jones JG. Cerebral blood flow distribution during induced hypotension with haemorrhage, trimetaphan or nitroprusside in rats. Br J Anaesth 1995: 74: 686–690.
Tuor UI, Edvinsson L, Mc Culloch J. Catecholamines and the relationship between cerebral blood flow and glucose use. Am J Physiol 1986: 251. H824–833.
Turner JM, Powell D, Gibson RM, McDowall DG. Intracranial pressure changes in neurosurgical patients during hypotension induced with sodium nitroprusside or trimethaphan. Br J Anaesth 1977: 49: 419–425.
Uzunov P, Petkov V, Stancheva S. Differential inhibition of phosphodiesterase according to the organ origin of the enzyme. Acta Neurobiol Exp (Warzawa) 1975: 35: 159–164.
Van Aken H, Puchstein C, Schweppe M-L, Heinecke A. Effect of labetalol on intracranial pressure in dogs with and without intracranial hypertension. Acta Anaesthesiol Scand 1982: 26: 615–619.
Van Aken H, Puchstein C, Fitch W, Graham DI. Haemodynamic and cerebral effects of ATP-induced hypotension. Br J Anaesth 1984a: 56: 1409–1415.
Van Aken H, Puchstein C, Anger C, et al. Changes in intracranial pressure and compliance during adenosine triphosphate-induced hypotension in dogs. Anesth Analg 1984b: 63: 381–385.
Van Aken H, Anger C, Puchstein C, Thijs J, Lawin P. Influence of ketanserin, an antihypertensive agent with specific 5-HT_2-receptor blocking activity, on intracranial pressure. Crit Care Med 1984c: 12: 4–7.
Vanhoutte P, Amery A, Birkenhäger W, et al. Serotoninergic mechanisms in hypertension. Focus on the effect of ketanserin. Hypertension 1988: 11: 111–133.
Vesey CJ, Cole PV, Simpson PJ. Cyanide and thiocyanate concentrations following sodium nitroprusside infusion in man. Br J Anaesth 1976: 48: 651–660.
Vesey CJ, Sweeney B, Cole PV. Decay of nitroprusside. II: In vivo. Br J Anaesth 1990: 64: 704–709.
Voldby B, Enevoldsen EM, Jensen FT. Cerebrovascular reactivity in patients with ruptured intracranial aneurysms. J Neurosurg 1985: 62: 59–67
Von Essen C. Effects of dopamine on cerebral blood flow in the dog. Acta Neurol Scand 1974: 50: 39–52.
Von Essen C. Effects of dopamine, noradrenaline and 5-hydroxytryptamine on the cerebral blood flow in the dog. J Pharm Phramacol 1972: 24: G68.

Von Essen C, Zervas NT, Brown DR, et al. Local cerebral blood flow in the dog during intravenous infusion of dopamine. Surg Neurol 1980: 13: 181.

Vulliemoz Y, Shen H, Virag L. Alpha-2 adrenoceptor agonists decrease cyclic guanosine 3',5'-monophosphate in the mouse brain. Anesthesiology 1996: 85: 544–550.

Waaben J, Husum B, Hansen AJ, Gjedde A. Hypocapnia prevents the decrease in regional cerebral metabolism during isoflurane-induced hypotension. J Neurosurg Anesthesiol 1989: 1: 29–34.

Waaben J, Husum B, Hansen AJ, Gjedde A. Regional cerebral blood flow and glucose utilization during hypocapnia and adenosine-induced hypotension in the rat. Anesthesiology 1989: 70: 299–304.

Wahl M, Kuschinsky W. The dilatory action of adenosine on pial arteries of cats and its inhibition by theophylline. Pflûgers Arch 1976: 362: 55–59.

Waldemar G, Paulson OB. Angiotensin converting enzyme inhibition. A review. Br J Clin Pharmacol 1989: 28: 177S–182S.

Waldemar G, Schmidt JF, Andersen AR, et al. Angiotensin converting enzyme inhibition and cerebral flow autoregulation in normotensive and hypertensive man. J Hypertens 1989: 7: 229–235.

Wang C, Knowles MG, Chakrabarti MK, Whitman JG. Clonidine has comparable effects of spontaneuous sympathetic activity and afferent A- and C-fiber-mediated somatosympathetic reflexes in dogs. Anesthesiology 1994: 81: 710–717.

Watanabe H, Passoneau J. Cyclic adenosine monophosphate in cerebral cortex: alteration following trauma. Arch Neurol 1975: 32: 181–184.

Watanabe H, Nomiyama S. Study of hypotension anaesthesia with Prostaglandin E1. Japanese J of Anesthesiology 1982: 31: 820–824.

Weigand MA, Michel A, Eckstein HH, et al. Adenosine. A sensitive indicator of cerebral ischemia during carotid endarterectomy. Anesthesiology 1999: 91: 414–421.

Werner C, Hoffman WE, Kochs E, et al. The angiotensin converting enzyme inhibitor captopril improves neurologic outcome from incomplete ischemia in rats. Anesthesiology 1990: 73: A695.

Weyland A, Stephan H, Grüne F, et al. Effect of ketanserin on global cerebral blood flow and middle cerebral artery velocity. Anesth Analg 1995: 80: 64–70.

Weyland A, Grune F, Buhre W, et al. The effect of nitroglycerin on cerebrovascular circulation, cerebrovascular CO_2 reactivity and blood flow rate in basal cerebral arteries. Anaesthesist 1996: 45: 1037–1044.

White RP, Hagen A, Robertson JT. Experimental evaluation of the spasmogenicity of dopamine on the basilar artery. J Neurosurg 1976: 44: 45–49.

White RP, Deans C, Hindley C, et al. the effect of nitric oxide donor glycerol trinitrate on global and regional cerebral blood flow in man. J Neurol Sci 2000: 178: 23–28.

Wildsmith JAW, Drummond GB, MacRae WR. Metabolic effects of induced hypotension with trimethaphan and sodium nitroprusside. Br J Anaesth 1979: 51: 875–879.

Williams JT, Henderson G, North RA. Characterization of $alpha_2$-adrenoreceptors which increased potassium conductance in rats locus coeruleus neurones. Neuroscience 1985: 14: 95–102

Winn HR, Rubio R, Berne RM. Brain adenosine production in the rat during 60 seconds of ischemia. Circ Res 1979: 45: 486–492.

Winn HR, Welsh JE, Rubio R, Berne RM. Changes in brain adenosine during bicuculline-induced seizures in rats. Circ Res 1980a: 47: 568–577.

Winn HR, Welsh JE, Rubio R, Berne RM. Brain adenosine production in the rat during sustained alteration in systemic blood pressure. Am J Physiol 1980b: 239: H 636–641.

Winn HR, Rubio R, Berne RM. The role of adenosine in the regulation of cerebral blood flow. J Cereb Blood Flow Metab 1981: 1: 239–244.

Woittiez AJJ, Wenting GJ, van den Meiracker AH, et al. Chronic effect of ketanserin in mild to moderate essential hypertension. Hypertension 1986: 8: 167–173.

Woodside JR, Garner L, Bedford RF, et al. Captopril reduces the dose requirement for SNP-induced hypotension. Anesthesiology 1982: 57: A61.

Wu PH, Phillis JW. Uptake of adenosine by isolated rat brain capillaries. J Neurochem 1982: 38: 687–690.

Yamamura H, Inada Y, Fujita T, et al. The safety of Prostaglandin E1 (G511) in induced hypotension during surgery in patients complicated with ischemia heart disease. Japanese J of Anesthesiology 1987: 36: 537–541.

Zäll S, Edén E, Winsö I, et al. Controlled hypotension with adenosine or sodium nitroprusside during cerebral aneurysm surgery: Effect on renal hemodynamics, excretory function, and renin release. Anesth Analg 1990: 71: 631–636.

Zornow MH, Scheller MS, Sheehan PB, et al. Intracranial pressure effects of dexmedetomidine in rabbits. Anesth Analg 1992: 75: 232–237.

Zubrow AB, Daniel SS, Stark RI, et al. Plasma renin, catecholamine, and vasopressin during nitroprusside-induced hypotension in ewes. Anesthesiology 1983: 58: 245–249.

CHAPTER 9

The sitting position

From a surgical aspect, the sitting position improves access to infratentorial structures, reduces blood loss, and improves venous drainage. On the other hand, the hydrostatic difference between cerebral veins and the right atrium augments the risk of air embolism. Furthermore, the change in position might provoke postural hypotension.

The potential for serious complications after venous air embolism and successful malpractice liability claims are the principle reasons for the dramatic decline in the use of the sitting position in neurosurgical practice. Although there have been several studies substantiating the relative safety compared with the prone or park bench positions, its use will continue to decline as neurosurgeons abandon its application and trainees in neurosurgery are not exposed to its relative merits (Porter et al. 1999).

In this review, two aspects of the sitting position are discussed: The influence of the sitting position upon systemic blood pressure and consequently cerebral perfusion pressure (CPP). In this respect hypotension might provoke a dangerous decrease in CPP and jeopardise cerebral oxygenation. The other issue is the occurrence of air embolism with special reference to its prevention, diagnosis, and treatment.

Cardiovascular effects

The effects of change in position from supine to the sitting position on the cardiovascular performance have been studied repeatedly (Ward et al. 1966, Albin et al. 1974, Dalrymple et al. 1979). In healthy conscious volunteers, the stroke volume and cardiac output might decrease, and the heart rate and systemic vascular resistance will increase, leaving MABP unchanged or increased.

Anaesthesia

Marshall et al. (1983) compared the cardiovascular effects of four different anaesthetic techniques and found that morphine/nitrous oxide anaesthesia compared with enflurane, halothane, and neurolept anaesthesia resulted in the least impairment when positioning was changed from supine to the sitting position. During anaesthesia the decrease in MABP is not always apparent (Tausk and Miller 1983). In a study by Albin et al. (1976) 32% of the patients had a 10–20% drop in blood pressure in reaching the sitting position, while 11% became temporarily hypertensive. In other studies, the incidence of hypotension is between 5 and 10% (Millar 1972, Young et al. 1986).

In anaesthetised patients the change from supine to sitting position is accompanied by a 14% decrease in intrathoracic blood volume, whereas total circulating blood volume remained constant. Concomitant changes in arterial pressure and stroke volume index are thus caused primarily by a reduction in cardiac preload (Buhre et al. 2000).

ECG

Electrocardiographic monitoring has been recommended especially in hypertensive patients where myocardial ischaemia may occur. However, myocardial ischaemic complication also has been observed after controlled hypotension in apparently healthy patients (Kinkor and Warner 1991).

Treatment

Intravenous infusion of crystalloid before change in position from supine to the sitting position has been recommended. Matjasko et al. (1985) recommended doses between 7–14 ml/kg. Nevertheless, vasopressors are often necessary to prevent or treat postural hypotension (Millar 1972, Tinker and Vandam 1972). The use of bandages on the legs to promote venous return might to some degree prevent hypotension (Tinker and Vandam 1972, Dalrymple et al. 1979). Geevarghese (1977) observed that this precaution not always prevented postural hypotension. Other studies indicate the importance of abdominal compression to protect against gravitational acceleration (Wood and Lambert 1952, Burton and Krutz 1975). Thus, the antigravity suit has been recommended by several authors (Burton and Krutz 1975, Geevarghese 1977). With an inflation pressure of 25 mm Hg in the antigravity suit, the necessary volume of intravenous fluid and the use of vasopressors were less in patients supplied with an antigravity suit, compared with patients only supplied with elastic leg bandages (Freuchen 1959). In a recent study of the antigravity suit (G suit, aviation type) inflation of the suit to 3.3 kPa (25 mm Hg) in the sitting position was followed by a significant increase in systolic blood pressure and CVP. The addition of 5 mm Hg PEEP during suit inflation was accompanied by a further increase in CVP (Brodrick and Ingram 1988).

Pneumocephalus

Intracranial air entrance might occur as a consequence of the sitting position. Postoperative neurological deterioration is an early sign, and intracranial air by CT scan is diagnostic (Suri et al. 2000).

Sitting position and seizures

In an analysis of 511 patients undergoing fossa posterior surgery it was found that postoperative seizures occurred more often in patients operated in the sitting position, especially when associated with venous air embolism or pneumocephalus (Suri et al. 1998).

Cerebrovascular and spinal cord dynamics

CBF

In dogs subjected to intracranial hypertension by inflation of an epidural balloon a decrease in cerebral and spinal CBF occurred in the sitting position, while $CMRO_2$ remained fairly constant (Ernst et al. 1988).

In a study Jensen et al. (1989) with the intravenous Xe^{133} technique did not find any decrease in CBF after change to the sitting position. In another study changes in transcranial Doppler blood velocity indicated a relative change in CBF in the area supplied by the middle cerebral artery. This result suggests a dose-dependent decrease in CBF for at least 2 min presumably due to anaesthetic-induced impairment of cerebral compensatory mechanisms (Werner et al. 1990). Tindall et al. (1967) found that hypocapnia in the sitting position decreased carotid artery flow by 48% and increased CVR.

Air embolism and CBF

In rabbits air injected intraarterially caused arteriolar dilation and reduced CBF. These effects were independent of dosage, whereas the detrimental effect of air embolism on brain function was dosage dependent (Helps et al. 1990).

Brain oxygenation

In a recent study brain oxygenation was studied with near-infrared spectroscopy. In awake volunteers no changes in brain oxygenation during change from the supine to the sitting position were observed. In sevoflurane/nitrous oxide anaesthetised patients, however, brain oxygenation decreased significantly (Fuchs et al. 2000).

Air embolism

Venous pressure

A pressure gradient of 5 cm between the upper pole of a wound and the right atrium is sufficient to allow air to pass into the venous system (Albin et al. 1983). Patients in the sitting position, where a gradient of 30 cm is usual, are therefore especially vulnerable to air embolism. The clinical effects of air embolism are determined by several factors. Butler and Hills (1979) stated that a large volume of air must exceed the lungs capacity to dissipate the air. Experimental studies indicate that the rate of air entry is related to the morbidity (Wollfe and Robertson 1935, Richardson et al. 1937).

Studies in dogs subjected to continuous air infusion indicate a progressive increase in central venous pressure (CVP), an abrupt increase in pulmonary arterial pressure, a progressive decrease in peripheral resistance and a compensatory increase in cardiac output. Blood pressure decreased moderately until compensation was exceeded, at which point blood pressure decreased sharply. The electrocardiographic changes involve peaking of the p waves and later on depression of the ST segment. Changes in heart sounds occur when significant cardiovascular decompensation has already occurred (Adornato et al. 1978). The same authors studied the effects of a bolus injection of air and found an increase in CVP but a decrease in pulmonary arterial pressure, ST depression on ECG, and shock.

The increase in pulmonary vascular resistance during a pulmonary embolism is caused by pulmonary arterial obstruction to blood flow and by the release of vasoactive substances. $Endothelin_1$ is involved in the humorally mediated component of vasoconstriction and cardiodepression during pulmonary air embolism (Dschietzig et al. 1998). Abnormalities in endothelin$_1$ metabolism ensue (Sofia et al. 1997). The resulting higher circulating levels of endothelin reflect the pulmonary endothelial cell dysfunction which occurs in acute pulmonary embolism (Stewart et al. 1991) In an experimental study in dogs the haemodynamic effects of an endothelin receptor antagonist were studied during venous air embolism. An attenuation of pulmonary perfusion pressure and the pulmonary vascular resistance were found. The same study indicated a lower serum level of thromboxane A_2 in antagonist treated animals (Tanus-Santos et al. 2000).

Threshold

The threshold for the lung to filter air is 0.30 ml/kg/min (Butler and Hills 1979, Butler and Hills 1985).This threshold is reduced during halothane and isoflurane anaesthesia (Katz et al. 1985) but increased during nitrous oxide anaesthesia and PEEP (Butler et al. 1985, Butler et al. 1986). In dogs subjected to halothane anaesthesia, the threshold of transpulmonary passage of venous air was 0,04 ml/kg/5 sec, but about 1 ml/kg/5 sec during pentobarbitone anaesthesia with or without halothane (Yahagi and Furuya 1987).

Fate

The fate of air emboli in the pulmonary circulation has been studied in dogs with a thoracic window. The findings indicate that venous air emboli are eliminated primarily in the pulmonary arterioles, as a result of molecular diffusion of gas across the arteriolar wall into alveolar spaces (Presson et al. 1989).

Surgical procedure

Episodes of air embolism occur predominantly early during the operative procedure (Albin et al. 1976, Standefer et al. 1984), especially during stripping of muscles and fascia (Leivers et al. 1971), drilling of the skull (Ericsson 1964), and during fascial layer closure (O'Higgins 1970). Tension pneumocephalus occurring very often after craniotomy (Reasoner et al. 1994), also can be a source of venous air embolism (Olympio and Bell 1994).

Venous air embolism as a cause of haemodynamic instability has been reported during craniectomy for craniosynostosis repair (Cuchiara 1982, Harris et al. 1986, Harris et al. 1987, Joseph et al. 1985). In a prospective study of 23 children undergoing surgery 83% of the patients demonstrated 64 episodes of venous air embolism, and six patients had hypotension associated with venous air embolism (Faberowski et al. 2000).

Air embolism very often is detected in patients breathing spontaneously. However, controlled ventilation is presently used during surgery in the sitting position. With this technique the incidence of air embolism theoretically should be smaller. The introduction of stereotaxic surgery in awake or sedated patients breathing spontaneously increases the risk of air embolism. Recently air embolism was detected in two patients undergoing elective pallidotomy while lightly sedated and breathing spontaneously. No haemodynamic changes were detected. Both patients developed coughing and became tachypneic (Suarez et al. 1999).

Nitrous oxide

The difference in blood-gas solubility between nitrous oxide and nitrogen results in enlargement of intravascular air bubbles when nitrous oxide is applied. The lethal volume of intravenously administered air is significantly less in animals receiving nitrous oxide compared to oxygen/air mixtures (Munson and Merrick 1966). From the same group it has been suggested that nitrous oxide is best avoided (Munson et al. 1975). Losasso et al. (1992), however, studied the incidence of air embolism in 300 neurosurgical patients operated in the sitting position, and found that 50% nitrous oxide had no measurable effect on the incidence or severity of venous air embolism if its administration was discontinued immediately upon Doppler detection of air embolism.

Foramen ovale and systemic air embolism

The occurrence of air embolism in the sitting position might be fatal, partly because the air obstructs venous return to the heart and consequently reduces blood pressure and provokes hypoxia, and partly because the embolus passes into the general circulation, either through the lungs (Singbartl et al. 1990) or through a patent foramen ovale.

At postmortem examination a patent foramen ovale is present in about 20% of the population (Edwards 1968). Preoperative contrast-enhanced echocardiography provides a safe method of detection of right-to-left shunts (Higgins et al. 1984). With this method Guggiare et al. (1985) found an incidence of 13% of right-to-left shunts and it has been argued that if a right-to-left shunt is detected, surgery in the sitting position should be avoided (Brodrick 1987). In another study 23% of patients subjected to fossa posterior surgery, and 10% of patients subjected to cervical surgery had patent foramen ovale (Papadopoulos et al. 1994). In a recent study transcranial Doppler sonography was compared with contrast-enhanced transesophageal echocardiography. It was concluded that transcranial Doppler sonography was a highly sensitive and highly specific method for detecting a patent foramen ovale (Stendel et al. 2000). Other studies with contrast-enhanced transcranial Doppler indicate that it is necessary to standardise the procedure to permit comparable quantitative assessment of the shunt volume during the Valsalva manoeuvre. Thus, 10 ml of contrast medium should be injected with the patient in the supine position, and the Valsalva manoeuvre is to be performed 5 seconds after the start of the injection (Schwarze et al. 1999).

The occurrence of right-to-left embolization of air is dependent on a right-to-left pressure gradient over the heart. Studies in dogs have shown that venous air embolism causes an increase in pulmonary pressure and CVP and an increase in the right-to-left pressure gradient (Adornato et al. 1978, Perkins-Pearson et al. 1982).

Systemic air embolism occurred in about 2% of all patients having venous air embolism, and in 0.5% of all patients subjected to the sitting position (Matjasko et al. 1985). Coronary air embolism might present itself with ST elevation or depression or widening of the ORS complex, and after cerebral artery air embolism epileptogenic activity has been observed (Clayton et al. 1985). Postoperatively, cerebral deterioration as a result of cerebral ischaemia might occur (Gronert et al. 1979).

PEEP

Although PEEP has been used clinically in the prevention of air embolism (Voorhies et al. 1983), the effect of PEEP on the right-to-left pressure gradient is still debated. Studies in sheeps and dogs (Metha and Sokoll 1981, Pfitzer and McLean 1987), and humans (Perkin and Bedford 1984) indicate an increase in the pressure gradient, when PEEP or active lung inflation for 10 sec. are applied, while other studies indicate an unchanged pressure gradient, in the presence of PEEP (Pearl and Lawson 1986, Zasslow et al. 1986). In one study of patients undergoing neurosurgery of the posterior fossa, the right-to-left pressure gradients were calculated during application of PEEP and compared with the pressures obtained with pneumatic anti shock garments. It was found that both procedures increased right atrial pressure without any difference in the right-to left pressure gradient (Tassani et al. 1992). Furthermore, PEEP raises the threshold of the lung for the filtration of air, and it is consequently unlikely that PEEP will increase the incidence of paradoxical air embolism (Butler et al. 1986). In another study in dogs PEEP at 15 cm H_2O was compared with neck compression at 40 mm Hg. Neither manoeuvre affected CBF measured by microsphere technique or $CMRO_2$. In canine, neck vein compression elevates sagital sinus pressure above atmospheric pressure, but PEEP does not, suggesting that neck compression used as a prophylactic measure is superior to PEEP (Toung et al. 1988). Another experimental study of sagital sinus pressure in piglets confirms that PEEP does not increase sinus pressure, whereas volume load increases this pressure, although not enough to compensate for the effects of the upright position (Gaida et al. 1992). In pigs the effects of intravascular volume expansion and of three patterns of ventilation were studied (intermittent positive pressure ventilation with zero end-expiratory pressure, intermittent positive pressure ventilation with 10 cm water PEEP, and spontaneous ventilation). The incidence of paradoxical air embolism was not different in any of the three situations (Black et al. 1989).

Venous pressure

Studies of jugular venous bulb pressure in patients subjected to neck compression and/or PEEP in the sitting position show that neck compression elevates jugular bulb venous pressure to positive values, an effect not observed with PEEP up to 20 cm H20 (Sinding et al. 1991). Studies of transverse sinus pressure during fossa posterior surgery in the sitting position support that PEEP does not increase sinus pressure. It was shown that hyperventilation might be dangerous in the sitting position as sinus pressure is reduced. On the other hand, hypercapnic ventilation increased sinus pressure and mean arterial blood pressure (Zentner et al.1991).

Diagnosis

The incidence of air embolism in the sitting position depends on the methods used to detect embolization and the type of operation, suboccipital craniectomies being particularly susceptible (Matjasko et al. 1985, Standefer et al. 1984). Precordial Doppler devices introduced by Michenfelder et al. (1972) are sensitive to the quantity of air in the range of 0.12–0.24 ml/kg (English et al. 1978, Glenski et al. 1986). Real-time wavelet analysis of the precordial Doppler ultrasound has been used experimentally. With this technique it was possible to correlate the volume of the air embolism with the cumulative embolic power of the embolic heart sounds (Lui et al. 1998).

Even more sensitive is transoesophageal Doppler with a sensitivity of 0.05–0.2 ml/kg (Martin and Colley 1983), transoesophageal echocardiography with a sensitivity of 0.05–0.19 ml/kg (Glenski et al. 1986, Couture et al. 1994) and catheter tip Doppler transducer mounted on a flexible indwelling central venous catheter with a sensitivity of 0.05–0.06 ml/kg (Solanki et al. 1990). End-tidal CO_2 analysis detects air embolisms of 0.18–0.63 ml/kg (Edmonds-Seal et al. 1971, Glenski et al. 1986), while changes in CVP, ECG, MABP and oxygen tension are detected at even greater air embolisms (English et al. 1978, Glenski et al. 1986). In a recent study of 21 patients operated in the sitting position venous air embolism was monitored by cardiac two-dimensional 4-chamber view using transoesophageal echocardiography. Micro bubbles in the right atrium were detected in all patients. Paradoxical air embolism occurred in three patients (Mammoto et al. 1998).

Studies in the upright sheep of venous pressure in the jugular bulb suggest that an increase in pressure provides an earlier and more reliable warning than did a Doppler probe (Pfitzner et al. 1987). In another study in dogs end-tidal nitrogen and pulmonary arterial pressure increased earlier than did the change in end-tidal CO_2. The changes, however, were simultaneously recorded after large infusion dosages (Matjasko et al. 1987). Monitoring of mixed venous saturation does not offer advantageous as compared with end-tidal CO2 (Russell and Graybeal 1992).

Morbidity

As stated by Standefer et al. (1984) and Matjasko et al. (1985) the sitting position is safe indicated by low morbidity and mortality. In a retrospective study of 579 patients undergoing the sitting or prone position for fossa posterior surgery venous air embolism occurred more often in the sitting position (45% versus 12%). However, no morbidity or mortality were attributed to venous air embolism and the incidence of hypotension or perioperative cardiopulmonary complications were not increased in the sitting position suggesting that selection of a head-down surgical position solely to decrease perioperative complications is not justified (Black et al. 1988). The same conclusion was drawn in a study of 432 consecutive operations for vestibular Schwannoma in either sitting or prone position (Duke et al. 1998). In another study the incidence of air embolism in the sitting position was 28% measured with Doppler. (Sørensen et al. 1990). Nevertheless, the number of neurosurgical centres using the sitting position routinely has decreased considerably (Elton and Howell 1994).

Prone position

There are only few reports of fatality owing to air embolism in the prone position. One patient was subjected to fossa posterior surgery for a large arterio-venous malformation (Shenkin and Goldfedder 1969). Fatal complication has also been described in two patients subjected to the prone position for lumbar laminectomy (Albin et al. 1991). Placement of Doppler probe on the anterior part of chest can lead to displacement or pressure sores. However, in children < 10 kilograms the Doppler probe can be placed between the right scapula and spine (Soriano et al. 1994).

Other positions

The lateral sitting position is superior as compared with the conventional sitting position, because it is possible to change to the lateral supine position without disturbing the surgical procedure (Garcia-Bengochea et al. 1976). In a clinical study the lateral sitting position with 45 degree elevation of the head and thorax was investigated. CPP and ICP were more stable compared to the upright sitting position and the lateral position with 20 degree elevation of the head and thorax (Calliauw et al. 1987).

Treatment of air embolism

Mandatory to a successful resuscitation of patients with air embolism is the speed of diagnosis and treatment (Ericsson et al. 1964). To assess the point of entry of air and start treatment immediate alertness and communication between the neurosurgeon and the anaesthesiologist are important, as soon as air embolization is diagnosed (Michenfelder et al. 1969). Bimanual neck compression by hand has been recommended (Michenfelder et al. 1969, Tausk and Miller 1983), or inflation of an inflatable neck tourniquet or neck tie (Hewer and Logue 1962, Buckland and Manners 1976, Sale 1984). Manual positive pressure ventilation with a long inspiratory hold has been recommended. This manoeuvre should prevent further air aspiration and assist in the early localization of the air entrapment site (Sharma and Tripathi 1994). However, brief periods of this procedure decrease CBF, and therefore should be used cautiously (Wending et al. 1994).

Although the use of nitrous oxide does not influence the incidence of air embolism in some studies (Knüttgen et al. 1989), immediate withdrawal of nitrous oxide and the administration of pure oxygen will control and reduce the expansion of air bubbles in the blood (Nunn 1959, Munson 1971). Aspiration through a central caval catheter or a Swan Ganz catheter may remove some of the air (Bedford et al. 1981), but this attempt is often disappointing because it is difficult to secure the ideal position of the catheter (Sink et al. 1976). A special pulmonary artery catheter has been studied experimentally. Air aspiration through this catheter is more effective compared with pulmonary catheters, and improves survival (Bowdle and Artru 1988). Other catheter prototypes (Arrow, Bunegin-Albin) have been introduced (Colley and Artru 1987, Noel 1989). One catheter 70 cm in lenght, with a balloon tip, end hole, and eight side holes has been used successfully in a case of air embolism with retrieval of 35 ml of air (Noel 1989). Experimental studies with the same catheter indicate that the catheter is effective for aspiration of venous air in the seated position, and success rate of resuscitation was significantly increased (Artru 1992). However, with air entrance through the femoral vein neither position of a multiorified catheter in the superior nor inferior portion of the atrium are effective for retrieval of venous air embolism (Artru 1992, Artru 1994).

Durant

Left lateral position, either horizontal or head down has been recommended in the treatment of air embolism. The effect of this change in position, known as "Durant's manoeuvre", is based on animal studies showing this position to be superior to other body positions as regards outcome after air embolism (Durant et al. 1947). Repositioning in the left lateral position might improve circulation by its gravity effect on the position of the air embolism in the heart (Hamby and Terry 1952, Marshall 1965, Alvaran et al. 1978). However, studies in the dogs indicate that this change in body position does not affect the haemodynamic response to venous embolism (Mehlhorn et al. 1994).

Hypotension

Hypotension should be treated with a rapid infusion of crystalloid and colloid (Matjasko et al. 1985). During persistence of hypotension vasopressors such as ephedrine or dopamine might be necessary.

Lidocaine and perfluorocarbon

Experiments with cats have demonstrated that pretreatment with intravenous lidocaine increases the recovery of neural function after acute cerebral ischaemia induced by air embolism (Evans et al. 1984, Dutka et al. 1992). Other experimental studies have shown that pre-treatment with perfluorocarbon, which increases solubilities of oxygen, nitrogen and carbon dioxide, may potentially protect against the effects of air embolism (Spiess et al. 1986), and attenuate some of the detrimental cardiovascular effects of the air embolism (Tuman et al. 1986).

Deoxycycline

Deoxycycline, a member of the tetracycline family of antibiotics, inhibits leukocyte activities including chemotaxis, adhesion, degranulation, superoxide generation, and metalloproteinase activity. *In vitro* studies in rabbits suggest that pre-treatment with deoxycycline reduced leukocyte adherence and increased tolerance to temporary spinal cord ischaemia (Clark et al. 1994). *In vivo* studies in rabbits indicate that deoxycycline improves somatosensory potentials after cerebral air embolism. This effect is observed 1 hour after air embolism. The results of somatosensory potentials correlate with neurologic impairment, suggesting that deoxycycline inhibits a key process in the pathophysiology of cerebral air embolism (Reasoner et al. 1997).

Clinical application

In the hands of a skilled neurosurgeon and anaesthesiologist overall mortality and morbidity are comparable in the prone and the sitting position. Patients with ischaemic heart disease, severe hypertension and known right-to-left shunts should not be placed in the sitting position.

The presence of a patent foramen ovale is an absolute contraindication. Preoperative contrast echocardiography should be used as a screening technique to detect the population at risk of paradoxical air embolism caused by the presence of a patent foramen ovale (Porter et al. 1999).

A prophylactic regime including anti-G suit, intravenous crystalloid combined with reasonable monitoring for detection of venous air embolism should be available for securing a safe procedure. Intravenous as well as inhalation anaesthetics can be used. Nitrous oxide 50% can be used safely, but avoidance of nitrous oxide has also been recommended. However, if air embolism occurs, nitrous oxide, when used, should immediately be discontinued.

The sitting position should remain in the neurosurgeons armamentarium. However, several caveats must be emphasised. Assessment of the relative risk-benefit, based on the individual patients physical status and surgical implications for the particular intracranial pathology, is of paramount importance. The patients should be informed of the specific risks of venous air embolism, quadriparesis and peripheral nerve palsies. Appropriate charting of patient information, provided and special consent issues are essential (Porter et al. 1999).

References

Adornato DC, Gildenberg MD, Ferrario CM, et al. Pathophysiology of intravenous air embolism in dogs. Anesthesiology 1978: 49: 120–127.

Albin MS, Jannetta PJ, Maroon JC, et al. Anaesthesia in the sitting position. IV, Europ Congress Anaesth. Madrid: Excerpta Medica, Amsterdam 1974, pp 775–778.

Albin MS, Babinski MF, Maroon JC, Jannetta PJ. Anaesthetic management of posterior fossa surgery in the sitting position. Acta Anaesth Scand 1976: 20: 117–128.

Albin MS, Babinski M, Gilbert J, Smith SL. Venous air embolism is not restricted to neurosurgery. Anesthesiology 1983: 59: 151.

Albin MS, The paradox of paradoxic air embolism-PEEP, Valsalva and patent foramen ovale. Should the sitting position be abandoned. Anesthesiology 1984: 61: 222–223.

Albin MS, Ritter RR, Pruett CE, Kalff K. Venous air embolism during lumbar laminectomy in the phrone position: report of three cases. Anesth Analg 1991: 73: 346–349

Alvaran SB, Toung JK, Graff TE, Benson DW. Venous air embolism: Comparative merits of external cardiac massage, intracardiac aspiration, and left lateral decubitus position. Anesth Analg 1978: 57: 166–170.

Artru AA. Modification of a new catheter for air retrieval and resuscitation from lethal venous air embolism: Effect of nitrous oxide on air retrieval. Anesth Analg 1992: 75: 226–231.

Artru AA. Venous air embolism in prone dogs positioned with the abdomen hanging freely: percentage of gas retrieval and success rate of resuscitation. Anesth Analg 1992: 75: 715–719.

Artru AA. Placement of a multiorified catheter in the inferior portion of the right atrium; percentage of gas retrieval and success rate of resuscitation after venous air embolism in prone dogs positioned with the abdomen hanging freely. Anesth Analg 1994: 79: 740–744.

Bedford RF, Marshall WK, Butler A, Welsh JE. Cardiac catheters for diagnosis and treatment of venous air embolism. J Neurosurg 1981: 55: 610–614.

Black S, Ockert DB, Oliver WC, Cucchiara RF. Outcome following posterior fossa craniotomy in patients in the sitting or horizontal positions. Anesthesiology 1988: 69: 49–56.

Black S, Cucchiara RF, Nishimura RA, Michenfelder JD. Parameters affecting occurrence of paradoxical air embolism. Anesthesiology 1989: 71: 235–241.

Bowdle TA, Artru AA. Treatment of air embolism with a special pulmonary artery catheter introducer sheath in sitting dogs. Anesthesiology 1988: 68: 107–110.

Brodrick PM. The sitting position; monitoring, diagnosis and treatment of air embolism. In Jewkes DA (ed.) Bailliere's Clinical Anesthesiology. Anaesthesia for Neurosurgery. WB Saunders 1987, pp 419–440.

Brodrick PM, Ingram GS. The antigravity suit in neurosurgery. Anaesthesia 1988: 43: 762–765.

Buckland RW, Manners JM. Venous air embolism during neurosurgery. Anaesthesia 1976: 31: 633–643.

Buhre W, Weyland A, Buhre K, et al. Effects of the sitting position on the distribution of blood volume in patients undergoing neurosurgical procedures. Br J Anaesth 2000: 84: 354–357.

Burton RR, Krutz RW. G tolerance and protection with anti-G suit concepts. Aviation Space Environm Med 1975: 46: 119–124.

Butler BD, Hills BA. The lung as a filter for microbubbles. J Appl Physiol 1979: 47: 537–543.

Butler BD, Hills BA. Transpulmonary passage of venous air emboli. J Appl Physiol 1985: 59: 543–547.

Butler BD, Luehr S, Hills B, Katz J. Nitrous oxide anaesthesia and pulmonary air embolism. Anesthesiology 1985: 63: A422.

Butler BD, Leiman BC, Luehr S, Katz J. Effects of PEEP on the incidence of paradoxical air embolism in the absence of ASD in dogs. Anesthesiology 1986: 65: A81.

Calliauw L, VanAken J, Rolly G, Verbeke L. The position of the patient during neurosurgical precedures on the posterior fossa. Acta Neurochir (Wien) 1987: 85: 154–158.

Clark WM, Calcagno FA, Gabler WL, et al. Reduction of central nervous system reperfusion injury in rabbits using deoxycycline treatment. Stroke 1994: 25: 1411–1416.

Clayton DG, Evans P, Williams C, Thurlow AC. Paradoxical air embolism during neurosurgery. Anaesthesia 1985: 40: 981–989.

Colley PS, Artru AA. Bunegin-Albin catheter improves air retrieval and resuscitation from lethal venous air embolism in dogs. Anesth Analg 1987: 66: 991–994.

Couture P, Boudreault D, Derouin M, et al. Venous carbon dioxide embolism in pigs: An evaluation of end-tidal carbon dioxide, transesophageal echocardiography, pulmonary artery pressure, and precordial auscultation as monitoring modalities. Anesth Analg 1994: 79: 867–873.

Cuchiara RF. Air embolism in children undergoing suboccipital craniotomy. Anesth Analg 1982: 57: 338–339.

Dalrymple DG, MacGowan SW, MacLeod GF. Cardiorespiratory effects of the sitting position in neurosurgery. Br J Anaesth 1979: 51: 1079–1082.

Dschietzig T, Laule M, Alexiou K, et al. Coronary constriction and consequent cardiodepression in pulmonary embolism are medaited by pulmonary big endothelin and enhanced in early endothelial dysfunction. Crit Care Med 1998: 26: 510–517.

Duke DA, Lynch JJ, Harner SG, et al. Venous air embolism in sitting and supine patients undergoing vestibular Schwannoma resection. Neurosurgery 1998: 42: 1282–1287.

Dutka AJ, Mink R, McDermott J, Clark JB, Hallenbeck JM. Effect of lidocaine on somatosensory evoked response and cerebral blood flow after canine cerebral air embolism. Stroke 1992: 23: 1515–1521

Edmonds-Seal J, Prys-Roberts C, Adams AP. Air embolism, a comparison of various methods of detection. Anaesthesia 1971: 26: 202–208.

Edwards JE. Interatrial communication. In Gould SE (ed.) Pathology of the heart. Illinois: Charles C Thomas 1968, pp 260–261.
Elton RJ, Howell RSC. The sitting position in neurosurgical anaesthesia: a survey of British practice in 1991. Br J Anaesth. 1994: 73: 247–248.
English JB, Westenskow D, Hodges MR, Stanley TH. Comparison of venous air embolism monitoring methods in supine dogs. Anaesthesiology 1978: 48: 425–429.
Ericsson JA, Gottlieb JD, Sweet RB. Closed chest massage in the treatment of venous air embolism. New Eng. J Med 1964: 270: 1353–1354.
Ernst PS, Albin MS, Bunegin L, et al. Cerebrovascular and spinal cord dynamics of the sitting position. Anesthesiology 1988: 69: A554.
Evans DE, Kobrine AI, Legrys DC, Bradley ME. Protective effect of lidocaine in acute cerebral ischaemia induced by air embolism. J Neurosurg 1984: 60: 257–263.
Faberowski LW, Black S, Mickle JP. Incidence of venous air embolism during craniectomy for craniosynostosis repair Anesthesiology 2000: 92: 20–23.
Freuchen IP. The use of an anti gravity suit in neurosurgery. Acta Anaesth Scand 1959: 3: 17–23.
Fuchs G, Schwartz G, Kulier A, Litscher G. The influence of positioning in spectroscopic measurements of brain oxygenation. J Neurosurg Anesthesiol 2000: 12: 75–80.
Gaida B-J, Eberle B, Otto S, et al. Superior sagital sinus pressure in "upright" pigs. Effect of volume load and airway pressure. Anesth Analg 1992: 74: S104
Garcia-Bengochea F, Munson ES, Freeman JV. The lateral sitting position for neurosurgery. Anesth Analg 1976: 55: 326–330.
Geevarghese KP. Anesthetic management of patients undergoing surgery for posterior fossa lesions. Intern Anesth Clin 1977: 15: 165–194.
Glenski JA., Cucchiara RF, Michenfelder JD. Transesophageal echocardiography and transcutaneous O2 and CO2 monitoring for detection of venous air embolism. Anesthesiology 1986: 64: 541–545.
Gronert GA, Messick JM, Cucchiara RF, Michenfelder JD. Paradoxical air embolism from a patent foramen ovale. Anesthesiology 1979: 50: 548–549.
Guggiara M, Lechat PH, Garen C, et al. Prevention of paradoxical air embolism by 2-D contrast echocardiography in neurosurgical patients. Anesthesiology 1985: 63: A425.
Hamby WB, Terry RN. Air embolism in operations done in the sitting position. A report of five fatal cases and one of rescue by a simple maneuver. Surgery 1952: 31: 212–215.
Harris MM, Strafford MA, Rowe RW, et al. Venous air embolism and cardiac arrest during craniectomy in the supine infant. Anesthesiology 1986: 65: 547–550.
Harris MM, Yemen TA, Davidson A, et al. Venous embolism during craniectomy in supine infants. Anesthesiology 1987: 67: 816–819.
Helps SC, Meyer-Witting M, Reilly PL, Gorman DF. Increasing doses of intracarotid air and cerebral blood flow in rabbits. Stroke 1990: 21: 1340–1345.
Hewer AJH, Logue V. Methods of increasing the safety of neuroanaesthesia in the sitting position. Anaesthesia 1962: 17: 476–482.
Higgins JR, Strunk BL, Schiller NB. Diagnosis of paradoxical embolism with contrast echocardiography. Am Heart J 1984: 107: 375–377.
Jensen KA, Bünemann L, Ohrstrom J, et al. CBF in the sitting versus the supine position. J Cereb Blood Flow Metab 1989: suppl 1: S613.
Joseph MM, Leopold GA, Carillo JF. Venous air embolism during repair of craniosynostosis in the lateral position. Anesthesiol Rev 1985: 12: 46–48.
Katz J, Luehr S, Hills BA, Butler BD. Halothane decreases pulmonary filtration of venous air emboli. Anesthesiology 1985: 63: A523.
Kindor RD, Warner DS. Unexpected myocardial complications after controlled hypotension. J Neurosurg Anesthesiol 1991: 3: 136–141.
Knüttgen D, Stölzle U, Köning W, et al. Zur Problematik der Luftembolie bei sitzender Position. Anaesthesist 1989: 38: 490–497.
Leivers D, Spilsbury RA, Young JVI. Air embolism during neurosurgery in the sitting position. Br J Anaesth 1971: 43: 84–90.
Losasso T, Muzzi DA, Dietz NM, Cucchiari RF. Fifty percent nitrous oxide does not increase the risk of venous air embolism in neurosurgical patients operated upon in the sitting position. Anesthesiology 1992: 77: 21–30.
Lui P-W, Chan BCB, Chan FHY, et al. Wavelet analysis of embolic heart sound detected by precordial Doppler ultrasound during continuous venous air embolism in dogs. Anesth Analg 1998: 86: 325–331.
Mammoto T, Hayashi Y, Ohnishi Y, Kuro M. Incidence of venous and paradoxical air embolism in neurosurgical patients in the sitting position: detection by transesophageal echocardiography. Acta Anaesthesiol Scand 1998: 42: 643–647.
Marshall BM. Air embolism in neurosurgical anesthesia, its diagnosis and treatment. Can Anaesth Soc J 1965: 12: 255–261.
Marshall WK, Bedford RF, Miller ED. Cardiovascular responses in the seated position-Impact of four anesthetic techniques. Anesth Analg 1983: 62: 648–653.
Martin JT. Positioning in anesthesia and surgery. Saunders Company 1978, pp 44–79.
Martin RW, Colley PS. Evaluation of transesophageal doppler detection of air embolism in dogs. Anesthesiology 1983: 58: 117–123.
Matjasko J, Petrozza P, Cohen M, Steinberg P. Anesthesia and surgery in the seated position: Analysis of 554 cases. Neurosurgery 1985: 17: 695–702.
Matjasko MJ, Hellman J, MacKenzie CF. Venous air embolism, hypotension, and end-tidal nitrogen. Neurosurgery 1987: 21: 378–382.
Mehta M, Sokoll MD. Relation of right and left atrial pressure during venous air embolism. Anesthesiology 1981: 55: A238.
Mehlhorn U, Burke EJ, Butler BD, et al.. Lit position does not affect the hemodynamic response to venous air embolism in dogs. Anesth Analg 1994: 79: 734–739.
Michenfelder JD, Martins JT, Altenburg BM, Rehder K. Air embolism during neurosurgery: an evaluation of right-atrial catheters for diagnosis and treatment. J Am Med Ass 1969: 298: 1353–1358.
Michenfelder JD, Miller RH, Gronert GA. Evaluation of an ultrasonic device (Doppler) for the diagnosis of venous air embolism. Anesthesiology 1972: 36: 164–167.
Millar RA. Neurosurgical anaesthesia in the sitting position. A report of experience with 110 patients using controlled or spontaneous ventilation. Br J Anaesth 1972: 44: 495–505.

Munson ES. Effect of nitrous oxide on the pulmonary circulation during venous air embolism. Anesth Analg 1971: 50: 785–792.

Munson ES, Merrick HC. Effect of nitrous oxide on venous air embolism. Anesthesiology 1966: 27: 783–787.

Munson ES, Paul WL, Perry JC, et al. Early detection of venous air embolism using Swan-Ganz catheter. Anesthesiology. 1975: 42: 223–226.

Noel TA II. Air embolism removal from both pulmonary artery and right atrium during sitting craniotomy using a new catheter: report of a case. Anesthesiology 1989: 70: 709–710.

Nunn JF. Controlled respiration in neurosurgical anaesthesia. Anaesthesia 1959: 14: 413–414.

O'Higgins JW. Air embolism during neurosurgery. Br J Anaesth 1970: 42: 459–462.

Olympio MA, Bell WO. Venous air embolism after craniotomy closure: Tension pneumocephalus implicated. J Neurosurgical Anesthesiology. 1994: 6: 35–39.

Papadopoulos G, Kuhly P, Brock M, et al.Venous and paradoical air embolism in the sitting position. A prospective study with transoesophageal echocardiography. Acta Neurochir (Wien) 1994: 126: 140–143.

Pearl RG, Lawson CP. Hemodynamic effects of PEEP during continuous venous air embolism in the dog. Anesthesiology 1986: 64: 724–729.

Perkins NAK, Bedford RF. Hemodynamic consequences of PEEP in seated neurological patients implications for paradoxical air embolism. Anesth Analg 1984: 63: 429–432.

Perkins-Pearson NAK, Marshall WK, Bedford RF. Atrial pressures in the seated position. Implication for paradoxical air embolism. Anesthesiology 1982: 57: 493–497.

Pfitzner J, McLean AG. Venous air embolism and active lung inflation at high and low CVP: A study in "Upright" anesthetized sheep. Anesth Analg 1987: 66: 1127–1134.

Pfitzner J, McLean AG, Crawshaw KM. Embolized air collection in the superior vena cava of "upright" sheep. Anesth Analg 1987: 66: 1135–1140.

Porter JM, Pidgeon C, Cunningham AJ. The sitting position in neurosurgery: A critical appraisal. Br J Anaesth 1999: 82: 117–128.

Presson RG, Kirk KR, Haselby KA, Wagner WW. The fate of air emboli in the pulmonary circulation of the dog. Anesth Analg 1989: 68: S227.

Reasoner DK, Todd MM, Scammer FL, Warner DS. The incidence of pneumocephalus after supratentorial craniotomy. Anesthesiology 1994: 80: 1008–1012.

Reasonor DK, Hindman BJ, Dexter F, et al. Deoxycycline reduces early neurologic impairment after cerebral arterial air embolism in the rabbit. Anesthesiology 1997: 87: 569–576.

Richardson HF, Coles BC, Hall GE. Experimental gas embolism: I. Intravenous air embolism. Can Med Ass J 1937: 36: 584–588.

Russell GB, Graybeal JM. Detection of venous air embolism: comparison of oxygenation and ventilation monitoring methods in dogs. J Neurosurg Anesthesiol 1992: 4: 36–40

Sale JP. Prevention of air embolism during sitting neurosurgery. The use of inflatable venous neck tourniquet. Anaesthesia 1984: 39: 795–799.

Schwarze JJ Sander D, Kukla C, et al. Methodological parameters influence the detection of right-to-left shunts by contrast transcranial Doppler ultrasonography. Stroke 1999: 30: 1234–1239.

Sharma K, Tripathi M. Detection of site of air entry in venous air embolism: Role of valsalva maneuver. J Neurosurgical Anesthesiology. 1994: 6: 209–211.

Shenkin HN, Goldfedder P. Air embolism from exposure of posterior cranial fossa in phrone position. J Am Med Ass 1969: 210: 726

Sinding H, Noreng M, Cold GE. Studies of jugular venous bulb pressure (JVB) in the sitting position. Acta Anaesthesiol Scand 1991 (suppl 96), vol 35: 64, p 192.

Singbartl G, Metzger G, Stögbauer R, Haarmann W. Paradoxe Luftembolie bei geschlossenem Foramen ovale. Anaesthesist 1990: 39: 44–49.

Sink JD, Comer BP, James PM, Loveland SR. Evaluation of catheter placement in the treatment of venous air embolism. Ann Surg 1976: 183: 58–61.

Solanki DR, Yearwood TL, Martin RW. Detection of venous air embolism in dogs with a central venous Doppler tipped catheter. Anesth Analg 1990: 70: S381.

Sofia M, Faraone S, Alifano M, et al. Endothelin abnormalities in patients with pulmonary embolism. Chest 1997: 111: 544–549.

Soriano SG, McManus ML, Sullivan LJ, et al. Doppler sensor placement during neurosurgical procedures for children in the phrone position. J Neurosurg Anesthesiol 1994: 6: 153–155.

Spiess BD, Braverman B, Woronowicz A, Ivankovich AD. Protection from cerebral air emboli with perfluorocarbons in rabbits. Anesthesiology 1986: 65: A361.

Standefer M, Bay JW, Trusso R. The sitting position in neurosurgery: A retrospective analysis of 488 cases. Neurosurgery 1984: 14: 649–658.

Stendel R, Gramm HJ, Schröder K, et al. Transcranial doppler ultrasonography as a screening technique for detection of a patent foramen ovale before surgery in the sitting position. Anesthesiology 2000: 93: 971–975.

Stewart DJ, Levy RD, Cernacek P, Langleben D. Increased plasma endothelin-1 in pulmonary hypertension: marker or mediator of disease? Ann Intern Med 1991: 114 464–469.

Suarez S, Ornaque I, Fabregas N, et al. Venous air embolism during Parkinson surgery in patients with spontaneous ventilation. Anesth Analg 1999: 88: 793–794.

Suri A, Mahapatra AK, Bithal P. Seizures following posterior fossa surgery. Br J Neurosurg 1998: 12: 41–44.

Suri A, Mahapatra AK, Singh VP. Posterior fossa tension pneumocephalus. Childs Nerv Syst 2000: 16: 196–199.

Sørensen J, Troelsen S, Kaalund J. Changes in blood gases during venous air embolism. Europ J Anaesthesiology 1990: 7: 467–471.

Tanus-Santos JE, Gordo WM, Udelsmann A, Junior HM. The hemodynamic effects of endothelin receptor antagonism during a venous air infusion in dogs. Anesth Analg 2000: 90: 102–106.

Tassani P, Eberl-Lehmann P, Enzenbach R. Interartrial pressure difference during inflation of pneumatic antishock garments and positive end-expiratory pressure ventilation. J Neurosurg Anesthesiol 1992: 4: 160–166.

Tausk HC, Miller R. Anesthesia for posterior fossa surgery in the sitting position. Bull New York Academy Med 1983: 59: 771–783.

Tindall GT, Craddock A, Greenfield JC. Effects of the sitting position on blood flow in the internal carotid artery of man during general anaesthesia. J Neurosurg 1967: 26: 383–389.

Tinker JH, Vandam LD. How effective is the G Suit in neurosurgical operations? Anesthesiology 1972: 36: 609–611.

Toung TJK, Miyabe M, McShane AJ, et al. Effect of PEEP and jugular venous compression on canine cerebral blood flow and oxygen consumption in the head elevated position. Anesthesiology 1988: 68: 53–58.

Tuman KJ, Spiess BD, McCarthy RJ, Ivankovich AD. Cardiorespiratory effects of venous air embolism in dogs receiving a perfluorocarbon emulsion. J Neurosurg 1986: 65: 238–244.

Voorhies RM, Fraser RAR, Poznak AV. Prevention of air embolism with positive end expiratory pressure. Neurosurgery 1983: 12: 503–506.

Ward RJ, Danziger F, Bonica JJ, et al. Cardiovascular effects of change in posture. Aerospace Medicine 1966: 37: 257–259.

Wending W, Sadel S, Jimenez D, et al. Cardiovascular and cerebrovascular effects of the applied valsalva manoeuvre in anaesthetized neurosurgical patients. Europ J Anaesthesiol 1994: 11: 81–87.

Werner C, Kochs E, Reimer R, et al. Einfluss von Lagerungsvänderungen auf die Zerebrale Hämodynamik unter Allgemeinanaesthesie. Anaesthesist 1990: 39: 429–433.

Wolffe JB, Robertson HF. Experimental air embolism. Ann Int Med 1935: 9: 162–165.

Wood EH, Lambert EH. Some factors which influence protection afforded by pneumatic anti-Gravity suits. J Aviation Med 1952: 23: 218.

Yahagi N, Furuya H. The effects of halothane and pentobarbital on the threshold of transpulmonary passage of venous air emboli in dogs. Anesthesiology 1987: 67: 905–909.

Young ML, Smith DS, Murtagh F, et al. Comparison of surgical and anesthetic complications in neurosurgical patients experiencing venous air embolism in the sitting position. Neurosurgery 1986: 18: 157–161.

Zasslow MA, Pearl RG, Larson CP, Silverberg G. PEEP does not affect left atrial-right atrial pressure gradient in neurosurgical patients. Anesthesiology 1986: 65: A 304.

Zentner J Albrecht T, Hassler W. Prevention of an air embolism by moderate hypoventilation during surgery in the sitting position. Neurosurgery 1991 28: 705–708.

CHAPTER 10

Acute head injury

Severe head injuries place a tremendous burden upon the society, partly because of the high mortality and morbidity, and partly because the economical resources used during the acute phase in the neurosurgical intensive care unit and during rehabilitation are very high. Even with the best results moderate and severe disability may be expected in 20–30% of the patients.

In this survey emphasize is focused on experimental head injury and development of cerebral oedema. On this basis clinical studies of cerebral circulation and metabolism in human head injury and principles of treatment are reviewed.

The dynamic pathophysiological changes which follow head injury are caused by successive events. First, the trauma directly influences the cerebral circulation and metabolism. Later on, the occurrence of intracranial haematoma, brain ischaemia, brain oedema, intracranial hypertension, systemic hypotension and systemic hypertension influences ICP, CBF and $CMRO_2$. Accordingly, studies in experimental models including one or more of these pathogenic factors, are important in the understanding of the dynamic changes following head injury.

Experimental studies

Models of acute head injury have gained considerable interest. These models include the non-impact acceleration device model of Gennarelli (1983), the fluid percussion model in cats (Sullivan et al. 1976), the impact acceleration model in rats (Nilsson et al 1977a), the Remington stunner model in cats (Tornheim et al. 1981), and the Piston-induced cortical contusion model (Madsen and Reske Nielsen 1987). In a model of diffuse brain injury the trauma was based on a weight-dropping device (Marmarou et al. 1994).

Recently the experimental animal models of traumatic brain injury have been described and evaluated (Park et al. 1999).

Correlation

In these models good correlations between trauma intensity and the pathophysiological and biochemical changes in the cerebral tissue have been found (Nilsson et al 1977, Tornheim et al. 1983, Wagner et al. 1985, Gennarelli et al. 1986). The depletion of ATP and phosphocreatine and the increase in lactate are related to the intensity of the trauma. In some experiments the increase in lactate caused by the trauma is unevenly distributed within the brain, the hippocampus being the most vulnerable part of the brain (Young et al. 1985).

Acidosis

The increase in cerebral lactate concentration is of interest, because brain tissue lactic-acidosis is an important factor in the development of cell damage (Siesjö and Wieloch 1985). Furthermore, prevention of the spread of local lactic-acidosis to adjacent normal tissue has a beneficial effect on recovery of brain tissue (Marshall et al. 1975, Becker et al. 1979). Accordingly, experimental studies have shown that treatment of brain acidosis with the weak base tromethapine reduces the incidence of intracranial hypertension and decreases the mortality in cats subjected to controlled ventilation over a 3 days period following fluid percussion injury (Rosner and Becker 1984).

Non-impact acceleration models

Direction of acceleration

Gennarelli (1983) used a single non-impact controlled acceleration device which delivered movement of the head in a single plane. In experimental studies in monkeys the direction of the acceleration was found to be of importance, The sagittal motions produced greater ICP elevations than did coronal plane motions (Gennarelli et al. 1983).

In a later study from the same group demonstrated that for an equal degree of acceleration coronal plane motion produced less ICP change than did sagittal motion, interspersed with horizontal motion in between and that ICP hypertension developed with increasing severity of the injury from concussion to diffuse axonal injury (Gennarelli et al. 1986).

Impact models

Brain energy

An impact acceleration trauma of 7–9 m/sec in rats was followed by an increased metabolic rate and increased neuronal activity (Nilsson and Nordström 1977a, Nilsson et al. 1977). The depletion in brain energy metabolism occurred at 1 min and was most pronounced at 4 min. Restitution was found after 15 min. At acceleration trauma of 9 m/sec the metabolic changes were most pronounced in the brain-stem (Nilsson and Pontén 1977).

CBF and $CMRO_2$

Immediately after the trauma CBF was increased. However, within few minutes a 30–40% decrease was observed and normalisation of CBF occurred over 20–30 min. $CMRO_2$ increased during the first minute. Later on, a decrease in $CMRO_2$ was observed. This decrease correlated with the intensity of the trauma (Nilsson and Nordström 1977a).

In a closed head injury model in rats severe arterial hypertension did not occur following the insult, and blood-brain barrier (BBB) disruption did not occur immediately after the trauma. At 30 seconds after injury, a significant and heterogeneous increase in rCBF was observed, and rCBV increased significantly in several regions. It was suggested that vascular responses in the period immediately after the trauma might result from derangement of cerebral autoregulation (Nawashiro et al. 1994).

In a study in rats the animals were subjected to cortical contusion induced with a pneumonic impactor, and dropping of a brass cylinder. The contusion produced hyperglycosis and ischaemia in the impacted cortical tissue and underlying hippocampus immediately and through a 30 minutes post-injury. CBF and glucose utilisation was depressed throughout the contused cortex, and in the ipselateral subcortical regions, (Sutton et al. 1994). In another study a moderate injury resulted in mean CBF increases of 44% in substantia nigra, and 10% increase in hypothalamus, septal nucleus and pontine grey, while there were a decrease of local CBF in many other regions. A tendency for rCBF to return to control values by 4 hours after the injury was observed. In severe injury local CBF was markedly decreased throughout widespread areas, and none of the areas showed any increase in CBF with time. Glucose metabolism decreased in all structures and the percentage changes from control was more than those of CBF. At 4 hours there was a significant recovery of 5–35% in glucose metabolism in most areas (Shima et al. 1993). Bryan et al. (1995) studied rCBF after controlled cortical impact injury in the rat. In the region of cortical impact they found cortical ischaemia (rCBF < 20 ml/100g/min). In the ipsilateral hemisphere ischaemic flow values were also demonstrated. At 30 minutes the ischaemic zone showed very sharp boundaries with cortical areas of hyperperfusion surrounding the ischaemic zone. After 4 hr the ischaemic boundaries were not as sharp and the hyperperfusion areas were not present. In other regions including the caudate-putamen, hippocampus, and thalamus reductions in rCBF ranging from 50 to 30% of control were demonstrated.

CO_2 reactivity

In rats indicate that within the region of cortical contusion both CBF and the CO_2 reactivity are reduced (Forbes et al. 1997). In other experimental studies, mild traumatic brain injury impairs and severe injury abolishes the CO_2 reactivity in the acute stages after injury (Saunders et al. 1979, Golding et al. 1999). Restoration of CO_2 reactivity during hypocapnia has been documented by the oxygen radical scavenger N-acetylcysteine (Ellis et al. 1991) and by L-Arginine (Golding et al. 2000).

Blood-brain barrier (BBB)

With an impact acceleration trauma disruption of the blood-brain barrier has been found. Unlike percussion trauma where the dura is exposed, BBB disruption occurred in the absence of a dramatic arterial pressure surge. Despite the sealing of the BBB within 4 hours after the trauma, oedema formation continued (van den Brink et al. 1993). Acute inflammation, indicated by E-selectin upregulation and neutrophil accumulation, does not play a role in the BBB disruption (Whalen et al. 1998). In another study immature rats were subjected to impact injury. BBB permeability was observed at 1 h and was largely resolved after 24 h (Adelson et al. 1998).

In a MR imaging study of an impact-acceleration model in rats it was found that injury was associated with a rapid and transient blood-brain barrier opening that begins at the time of the trauma and last no more than 30 minutes. Furthermore, it was documented that hypoxia and hypotension prolongs the time of blood-brain barrier breakdown (Barzó et al. 1996).

Autoregulation

In rats cerebral autoregulation is impaired 24 h after traumatic brain injury (Engelborghs et al. 2000).

Oedema

In an impact acceleration model of rats diffusion-weighted MR imaging was used to detect the type of oedema that develops after traumatic brain injury. It was found that the rise in ICP following trauma coupled with secondary insults of hypoxia and hypotension is predominantly caused by cytotoxic oedema, and that ischaemia plays a major role in the development of brain oedema in this experimental model (Ito et al. 1996).

Uncontrolled haemorrhage and blood pressure

Haemorrhagic hypotension aggrevates the detrimental effects of head trauma on neurologic outcome. In a rat model Talmor et al. (1999) examined whether phenylephrine or normal saline to increase mean arterial blood pressure to 70, 80 and 90 mm Hg during combination of a blunt impact injury and uncontrolled haemorrhage would improve neurologic outcome. The results indicated that that maintaining MABP at these levels with either methods worsened the neurodeficit score and/or survival and did not affect cerebral oedema formation.

Hypoxia

Mild and moderate hypoxia after traumatic impact injury has been studied by Clark et al. (1997). Animals with additional hypoxaemia that were killed 7 days after the trauma had increased motor function deficits together with a greater loss of CA3-neurons.

Brain temperature

Traumatic brain injury causes an immediate reduction in brain temperature, followed by hyperthermia. The rate at which brain temperature returns to normal is negatively correlated with behavioural and anatomical outcome (Weisend and Feeney 1994)

Fluid Percussion, Piston and Weight drop Models

CBV, CBF, and glucose utilisation

In cats subjected to fluid percussion, and studied by cranial window technique, CBV was increased after the blow (Duckrow et al. 1981). In the same model CBF was relatively resistant to the blow (DeWitt et al. 1981, Lewelt et al. 1982). Using microsphere technique DeWitt et al. (1986) observed that within one min of injury an increase in CPP, dilatation of the arterioles, and an increase in CBF occurred. In the same study no evidence of reduced CBF was found in any region studied. These changes returned to pre-injury levels by 30 min. In contrast, studies with laser-Doppler flowmetry in rats indicate that at 5 min post-injury, laser flow decreases bilaterally by 20–30% in the hippocampus and striatum, and remains significantly reduced during a 60 min period. The magnitude of the blood flow changes and the severity of the ensuing neurological impairment were correlated (Long et al. 1996). Studies of fluid percussion in piglets indicated a decrease in CBF and CPP and an increase in ICP within 5 min after the trauma (Pfenninger et al. 1986, Shibita et al. 1993). Studies with microsphere technique have demonstrated that CBF in all regions is reduced in a period of 1 h after fluid percussion (Yamakanii et al. 1989). Qian et al. (1996) used laser Doppler flowmetry in a rat model of percussion injury. They found four patterns of cerebral circulation responses. Little response occurred after percussion pulses of less than 1.33 atm. In animals subjected to pulses greater than 4.3 atm local CBF increased synchronously with blood pressure, and then both parameters decreased continuously, until death. In animals, subjected to pulses of 1.5 to 2.3 atm, a transient increase in rCBF with no synchronous rise in blood pressure was disclosed. In animals, subjected to pulses of 2.7–3.9 atm, rCBF increased with blood pressure immediately following the injury, but rCBF decreased markedly by 60 seconds and remained below the pre-injury baseline

With a rat weight-dropping-model of cortical contusion laser Doppler flow decreased to 60% within 2 min on the ipsilateral side of the trauma. On the contralateral side there was an initial flow increase to 172% at 4 min. This hyperperfusion phase was followed by a mild hypoperfusion phase with a flow of 78% of baseline, lasting approximately 60 min (Nilsson et al. 1996).

In rats glucose uptake is reduced at the centre of the contusion. However, increased glucose utilisation has repeatedly been demonstrated. The increased glucose utilization is supposed to be caused by reestablishment of ionic hemeostasis (Yoshino et al. 1991, Hovda et al. 1992, Kawamata et al. 1992), resulting in an increase in extracellular lactate (Yang et al. 1985, Iano et al. 1988, Dhillon et al. 1999, Prasad et al. 1994, Kawamata et al. 1995). This increase in glycolysis is followed by a period of decreased cerebral metabolism, which is associated with neurological and cognitive deficits resolving spontaneously over the course of weeks depending on the severity of the insult (Yoshino et al. 1991, Hovda et al. 1996, Prins and Hovda 1998). In pup rats fluid percussion injury produces an initial increase in glucose utilisation followed by a shorter period of metabolic depression than seen in adult rats (Thomas et al. 2000). Increased glucose utilisation coincides with patterns of negative shift of DC potentials, suggesting that the increased glucose uptake is due to spreading depression (Sunami et al. 1989). Increased glucose utilisation was especially observed in the ipsilateral hemisphere with 40% increase in the cerebral cortex and 90% increase in the hippocampus. The hypermetabolic state followed immediately after the injury, and was still documented 30 min after. At 6 h after the injury many regions within the ipsilateral hemisphere went into a state of suppressed glucose utilisation which lasted for as long as 5 days (Yoshino et al. 1991).

CO_2

When cerebral percussion trauma was combined with hypoventilation in order to mimic true cerebral contusion, a marked alteration in CBF, CMR-glucose, PCr/P ratio and tissue pH were observed indicating cerebral ischaemia (Andersen et al. 1988). Posttraumatic hypoventilation further augments neuronal damage and produces more extensive brain oedema (Shima and Marmarou 1993). In cats subjected to fluid percussion the CO_2 reactivity is inversely related to the severity of the trauma (Saunders et al. 1979).

Cerebral autoregulation (CA)

The CA is easily abolished by fluid percussion trauma and the degree of impairment is correlated to the intensity of the trauma (Lewelt et al. 1980, Seelig et al. 1983).

Spasm of cerebral arteries

Bukovski et al. (1997) have analysed the contractility of the posterior and middle cerebral arteries *ex vivo* after fluid-percussion trauma. The traumatic insult did not affect the serotonin- and potassium-induced contractility of the blood vessels, and did not impair their sensitivity to serotonin suggesting that traumatic impact in itself did not contribute to the development of spasms. Even disruption of the vascular endothelium did not change contractility of the vessels.

Hypoxemia and hypotension

In rats subjected to impact of 4.9 atmospheres plus hypoxemia to PaO_2 40 mm Hg for 30 min, an increase in morbidity was associated with more widespread and severe cerebral oedema and a decrease in CBF in the ipsilateral hemisphere (Ishige et al. 1987).

Other studies in rats indicate that the brain is extremely vulnerable to hypovolemic hypotension as reflected by the loss of high-energy phosphates in the brain (Ishige et al. 1988). In experiments in cats the trauma was found to attenuate the capacity of CBF to increase during hypoxaemia (Lewelt et al. 1982).

Blood-brain barrier (BBB)

With the fluid percussion model disruption of BBB is observed. Two factors contribute to this disruption. The mechanical deformation of tissue and cerebral vessels upon impact and the hypertensive surge that accompanies the injury. Using radioactive tracer technique the BBB is temporarily damaged due to trauma, but subsequent arterial pressure surge deteriorates the dysfunction of the BBB further (van den Brink et al. 1994).

With the same model, an early and pronounced expression of heat shock protein at the impact site, and a more delayed and less prominent expression in other regions of the brain were found. These findings parallel the temporal and regional pattern of breakdown of the BBB after a similar head injury (Tanno et al. 1993).

Phosphocreatine and ATP

MR spectroscopy has been used in the study of rats subjected to fluid percussion trauma of 1.5–2.5 atmospheres. Following the injury the ratio of phosphocreatine to inorganic phosphate (PCr/P) showed a biphasic decline. The first decline reached nadir at 40 min with recovery at 100 min. At two hours this event was followed by a second decline that persisted for the remaining six hours. The first but not the second decrease in PCr/P ratio was associated with tissue acidosis. These changes suggest an altered mitochondrial energy production and is not caused by CBF reduction (Vink et al. 1987).

Studies by Hashimoto et al. (1986) have shown that a change in phosphorus metabolism occurs over a period of time (15–20 min). In the same study it was demonstrated that ATP peaks were preserved until phosphocreatine was almost entirely depleted.

Lactate and mitochodrial function

In studies of fluid percussion trauma Vink et al. (1997) found, that hypoglycaemia or hyperglycaemia did not change brain tissue pH during a period of 4 h after trauma. Neither did cytosolic phosphorylation nor neurological outcome change. In contrast, studies in cats subjected to fluid percussion trauma indicated that an excess of lactate and a decrease in tissue pH occur. These changes are not accompanied by depletion of ATP or phosphocreatine, and the level of CBF, $CMRO_2$ and CMR-glucose are relatively unchanged. Under these circumstances the authors concluded that the increased lactate was not a function of cerebral ischaemia caused by flow deprivation. Theoretically, these changes might indicate a mild derangement of the brain energy metabolism reflecting altered mitochondrial function (Young et al. 1985, Andersen et al. 1998, Unterberg et al. 1988). Studies with electron microscopy in rats subjected to brain concussion, resulting in unconsciousness for 3–10 min, have shown swelling of the mitochondria. The swelling arises after 30 min, with maximum after one hour, and disappearance after 24 hours (Bakay et al. 1977). In common with these findings other authors suggested that mitochodrial function is depressed after traumatic brain injury, and that anaerobic glycolysis is facilitated (Andersen and Marmarou 1992a, Andersen and Marmarou 1992b, Pellerin and Magistretti 1994). This increased glycolysis might support restoration of ionic homeostasis, and generates extracellular fluid lactate. Schurr et al. (1997), in studies of hippocampal slices, found that lactate, not glucose fuels the recovery of synaptic function from hypoxia upon reoxygenation. Moreover, Chen et al. (2000), in a microdialysis study of rats subjected to fluid percusion brain injury, demonstrated that an increase in plasma-lactate resulted in a more rapid recovery of dialysate glucose, indicating a beneficial role for lactate.

Excitatory amino acids

In rats subjected to fluid percussion injury a marked elevation in extracellular glutamate and aspartate have been documented adjacent to the trauma site. The increase in excitatory amino acids was related to the severety of the injury, and was associated with a reduction in cellular bioenergetic state. Treatment with dextrophane, an NMDA antagonist, limited the neurological dysfunction, and improved the bioenergetic state after trauma (Faden et al. 1989). *In Vitro* studies indicate that increased extracellular fluid glutamate caused lactate production into the extracellular fluid space, by astrocytes (Pellerin and Maggistretti 1994).

Rats subjected to mild closed head injury by dropping a brass weight were subjected to hypoxia. Hypoxia prolonged the glutamate release, which was attenuated by pre-treatment with a NMDA antagonist (Katoh et al. 1998).

Nociceptin orphanin FQ (NOC/oFQ)

NMDA- and glutamate-induced pial artery dilation is reversed to vasoconstriction after fluid percussion injury. This impairment of NMDA-induced pial artery dilation is more pronounced in newborn vs. juvenile pigs. Nociceptin orphanin (NOC/oFQ) is released in CSF after fluid percussion injury. Endothelin-1, in concentrations present in CSF following fluid percussion injury, contributes to the release of CSF NOC/oFQ. This release is greater in newborn vs. juvenile pigs (Armstead 2001). NOC/oFQ released by fluid percussion injury also contributes to impaired dilation to other opioids including methionin enkephalin (Armstead 2000). NOC/oFQ increases O_2^- production in a cyclooxygenase-dependent manner, suggesting that cyclooxygenase-dependent O_2^- generation links NOC/oFQ release to impaired NMDA-induced vasodilation after brain injury (Kulkarni and Armstead 2000).

Nitric oxide (NO) and acetylcholine

An impairment of NO-mediated relaxation after fluid-percussion brain injury has been demonstrated in the cat.

Acetylcholine-induced cerebral vasodilation observed with the open cranial window technique was converted to vasoconstriction (Wei et al. 1980, Dewitt et al. 1986). This impairment is not irreversible but exhibits recovery within 4 h after injury (Ellison et al. 1989).

Adrenoceptor antagonist

In newborn piglets with traumatic brain injury treatment with adrenoreceptor antagonist normalises pial arteriolar diameter, otherwise contracted as a result of brain injury. Adrenergic blockade also normalises CBF (Shibata et al. 1993).

Ethanol intoxication

Rats subjected to ethanol intoxication showed an increased mortality and markedly worsened neurologic deficits at 24 h postinjury. Following injury, free magnium and cytosolic phosphorylation declined, and brain intracellular pH was consistently higher (Yomakami et al. 1995). Studies in immature pigs indicated that in ethanol pretreated animals pulmonary ventilation and the hypercapnic ventilatory response were decreased, and $PaCO_2$ increased (Zink et al. 1995).

In contrast, other studies have demonstrated a beneficial effect of ethanol in experimental traumatic brain injury. Thus, ethanol 3g/kg, reduced lesion volume by 50% (Kelly et al. 1997). A reduction in cognitive impairment has been observed (Janis et al. 1998), and Folkerts et al. (1998) showed a partial neuroprotective effect for motor and cognitive function in rats. In a recent study, Kelly et al. (2000) found that the reduction in CBF typically seen within the contusion core and penumbra is less severe in ethanol treated animals. Furthermore, they found that low-dose ethanol is associated with a marked attenuation of immediate postinjury hyperglycosis and with normalisation of glucose utilisation in the injury penumbra.

The influence of temperature

Rats subjected to delayed brain hyperthermia (39°C) after brain injury showed a significant increased mortality, and increased contusion volume compared with normothermic animals. At 15 minutes after the 3-hour hyperthermic period, the area of haemorrhage and horseradish peroxidase extravasation was increased, and a higher frequency of abnormally swollen myelinated axons was demonstrated in the somatosensory cortex, corpus callosum and internal capsula (Dietrich et al. 1996).

Heat shock protein (hsp) and c-fos

In a model of midline fluid percussive injury, *Fos* protein was found to be increased in the CA1 neurons of the hippocampus as early as 15 min following injury (Phillips and Belardo 1993). Using lateral fluid-percussion brain injury in the rat an increase in the expression of 72-kDA heat shock protein (HSP 72) and mRNA was found (Lowenstein et al. 1994, Tanno et al. 1993, McIntosh et al. 1989).

Raghupathi et al. (1995) demonstrated that lateral fluid-percussion triggers regionally and temporally specific expression of *c-fos* and hsp 72 mRNA. These results may be suggestive of differential neurochemical alterations in neurons and glia following experimental injury.

Fibroblast growth factor

In rats subjected to fluid percussion damage treatment with basic fibroblast growth factor was associated with a significant reduced number of damaged cortical neurones and a reduced contusion volume (Dietrich et al. 1996).

Microglia and Purkinje cells

Experimental studies indicate that even mild traumatic brain injury is followed by cerebellar activation of microglia in the vermis within a few days after forebrain injury. In coronal sections the processes of activated microglia were oriented in stripes perpendicular to the cortical surface. A significant loss of Purkinje cells 7 days postinjury was observed (Fukuda et al. 1996).

The brain stem

Studies of fluid percussion injury in the cat indicate that changes in pressure-volume index (PVI), far-field brain-stem auditory evoked responses (BAER) and CBF correlate well with the degree of brain-stem injury following severe head injury. Thus high-level fluid-percussion injury is predominantly a model of brain-stem injury (Shima and Marmarou 1991).

Transneuronal degeneration and cerebral atrophy

Using a fluid-percussion model in the rat deficits in cognition and neurologic motor function persisting for at least 1 year has been observed. Histopathological examination of rats at various time points up to 1 year following injury has revealed a substantial and progressive brain atrophy, most notable in the cortex ipsilateral to injury (Bramlett et al. 1997). Another study indicated substantial and progressive tissue loss with concomitant ventriculomegaly in the ipsilateral hemisphere. The regions with the most notable atrophy included the cortex, hippocampus, thalamus, and septum (Smith et al. 1997).

Platelet function

Focal platelet accumulation was studied with ^{111}Indium-tropolone-labeled platelets. In autoradiographic images, focal sites of platelet accumulation within the traumatised hemisphere were restricted to the pial surface, the external capsule, and within the CSF compartments. The accumulation of platelets was not correlated to regions with flow deprivation. (Dietrich et al. 1996).

Activation of leukocytes

Isaksson et al. (1997) studied activation of leukocyte-endothelium interaction, with up regulation of intercellular adhesion molecules in a cerebral contusion model. They observed a marked increase in intracellular adhesion molecules expression in cerebral capillaries 6–24 h after trauma. This up regulation was also found in the contralateral hemisphere.

Age

In rats subjected to fluid percussion trauma an age-related increase in mortality rate and greater acute neurological deficits was found (Hamm et al. 1991).

Genetic aspects

After traumatic lesion genetic aspects seems to influence the control of activation of microglia and astrocytes in the central nervous system. Steward and Trimmer (1997) compared mice mutants with a genetically determined delay of Wallerian degeneration with normal wildtype animals. Focal lesion in the wild type animals caused an up regulation of messenger RNA synthesis for glial fibrillary acidic protein (a marker of astrocyte activation) after a characteristic time pattern, whereas the mutants had an attenuated and delayed microglial and astrocyte activation (Schauwecker and Steward 1997).

Piston-induced Cerebral Contusion

This model has been described by Madsen and Reske Nielsen 1987). During CBF measurement by microsphere technique Madsen et al. (1990) in piglets found flow values ranging from 25–33 ml in white matter and hippocampus, intermediate flow values ranging from 40–50 ml in cortical grey and thalamus and high flow values in nucleus caudatus lentiformis and vermis. In the same mode (Madsen and Reske-Nielsen 1987), focal CBF was reduced and the CO_2 reactivity was absent (Madsen 1990a, Madsen 1990c). After pretreatment with barbiturate CBF was reduced as well, and the accumulated change in CBF was most pronounced in the damaged zone. In regions with hyperaemia, in contrast, only small accumulated effects were observed. No inverse flow reactions were found (Madsen 1991b).

In studies with ion-selective microelectrodes in rats contusion produced a transient membrane depolarisation associated with a pronounced cellular release of K^+ and massive Ca^{2+} entry into the intracellular compartment (Nilsson et al. 1993).

Traumatic subarachnoid haemorrhage

CBF

Subarachnoid haemorrhage is a common finding in acute head injury, and experimental studies of blood flow is therefore of interest. Rats were subjected to intercisternal injection of autologous blood. ICP increases to about 50 mm Hg accompanied by a decrease in global CBF of 50%. This flow reduction persisted for several hours and at 24 h, flows were still reduced at 85% of control values (Jackowski et al. 1990).

Acute Subdural Haematoma

Ischaemia

Acute subdural haematoma has been studied in a rat model, where autologous venous blood was injected into the subdural space. Three hours later the subdural haematoma was removed using saline irrigation. In this model the major cause of cerebral swelling observed after removal of the haematoma was enlargement of the zone of focal tissue ischaemia under the haematoma. On the other hand, hyperaemia was only patchy and only found infrequently. Thus, brain swelling after haematoma is more likely to be due to progressive ischaemic oedema than hyperaemia (Kuruda and Bullock 1992).

In the same model rCBF and glucose metabolism were measured autoradiographically. In the core of the infarct below the subdural haematoma rCBF and glucose metabolism were less than 15% of control values. This core was surrounded by a brim in which glucose metabolism was increased by 60%, and rCBF was reduced by the same amount. In the hippocampus a massive increase in metabolism was accompanied by a paradoxical decrease in rCBF. This discrepancy indicates loss of flow/metabolism coupling (Kuroda and Bullock 1992).

The progression of the zone of ischaemia seen in this model is consistent with studies indicating an excitatory process in the peri-ischaemic zone characterised by glutamate release and transient glucose hypermetabolism (Bullock et al. 1994).

Model of Diffuse Brain Injury

Rodents subjected to a weight-drop device on the intact skull develop neuropathological changes resembling diffuse axonal brain injury (Marmarou et al. 1994). The pathological changes involved the corpus callusum, internal capsule, optic tract, cerebral and cerebellar peduncles, and the long tracts in the brain stem (Montasser et al. 1994).

In the immature rats a model of diffuse traumatic brain injury has been investigated (Adelson et al. 1996). Diffuse brain-blood barrier dysfunction has been ducumented with this model, in which acute inflammation, as evidenced by the presence of neurotrophil accumulation nor E-selectin expression, did not occur (Adelson et al. 1998).

Mass Expanding Lesions

CBF, $CMRO_2$ and CPP

The effect of a mass-expanding lesion on CBF has been studied experimentally with subdural or epidural balloons (Johnston et al. 1973, Goodman and Becker 1973, Sullivan et al. 1977). In these models the microscopic and macroscopic changes are related to the expansion of the mass lesion (Goodman and Becker 1973). CBF is well maintained as long as CPP is preserved above the lower level of CA (Johnston et al. 1973).

In studies of acute experimental brain compression and decompression a transient hyperaemia was found after deflation of an epidural balloon. CBF and $CMRO_2$ decreased markedly with low $AVDO_2$ and flat EEG in animals with long inflation period of the balloon. In animals with short inflation a gradual recovery of CBF and $CMRO_2$ with high $AVDO_2$, and reappearance of EEG was found (Xu et al. 1993).

Pressure gradients and PVI

No pressure gradients were present between supratentorial compartments, but pressure differences occurred between infratentorial and supratentorial regions (Johnstone and Rowan 1974b). With an increase in mass effect a progressive increase in pressure-volume index was observed, indicating compromised cerebral compliance (Sullivan et al. 1977).

Mock-CSF infusion Studies

ICP and CBF

The influence of increased ICP on CBF has been studied in a mock-CSF infusion model. In dogs a decrease in CBF was observed when CPP falls below 60 mm Hg, and a further decrease in flow and $CMRO_2$ occurred at CPP values of 40 mm Hg. The changes in CBF follow the principles of regulation of CA (Hamar et al. 1973). In baboons subjected to mock-CSF induced ICP-hypertension CBF remained constant until ICP levels of 50 mm Hg; in the interval of ICP 50–100 mm Hg a marked increase in CBF was associated with systemic hypertension. A further increase in ICP resulted in a progressive decrease in CBF. Prior section of the spinal cord prevented the increase in CBF and the systemic hypertension (Johnston et al. 1972). At CPP levels below the lower range of CA the CBF and CBV dropped sharply, and the CVR gradually increased (Barzó et al. 1991).

ATP, phosphocreatine and lactate

In dogs subjected to CPP reduction to 30–35 mm Hg by mock CSF infusion depletion of ATP and phosphocreatine and an increase in cerebral lactate were observed. Resting energy states were not approached until 30–90 min after restitution of normal CPP. In the same study CSF pressure release was followed by hyperaemia of approximately the same duration (Zwetnow 1970).

MR studies

In cats magnetic resonance spectroscopy has been used during gradually raised ICP by mock CSF. Lactate rose at CPP below 49 mm Hg. The increase in lactate preceeded a threshold decrease in phosphocreatinine, which was observed at an average CPP of 29 mm Hg (Sutton et al. 1987).

$AVDO_2$

Cats were subjected to ICP-hypertension by mock-CSF, and $AVDO_2$ was measured repeatedly. It was found that at an average $AVDO_2$ of 8.4 vol% energy failure occurred. On this point the venous oxygen content averaged 1.45 vol%. When ICP was raised to the threshold of metabolic failure and hyperventilation was instituted ($PaCO_2$ level 10–18 mm Hg), metabolic failure as evidenced by a fall in phosphocreatine was observed (Sutton et al. 1990). These studies are supplemented by Bissonnette et al. (1991) who assessed intracellular oxygen concentration in rabbits. When ICP, during gradual increases in ICP, exceeded 18 cm H_2O intracellular mitochondrial O_2 decreased, but the decline in intracellular oxygenation with elevated ICP was inversely related to FiO_2.

Ischaemia

Incomplete and complete

Cerebral ischaemia is a frequent finding in patients dying after head injury. In rats subjected to cerebral ischaemia even mild concussion potentiates selective ischaemic hippocampal neuronal damage, and mild concussion decreases the threshold for post-ischaemic neuronal excitation (Jenkins et al. 1989). In rabbits Marshall et al. (1975b) induced incomplete (CPP 20 mm Hg), and complete ischaemia of 15 min duration. They found normal brain morphology in oligaemic animals but ischaemic damages in the striatum and hippocampus in complete ischaemia.

In this model high energy metabolism were exhausted within 5 min of the insult. Recovery of ATP and phosphocreatine occurred within 15 min and before EEG activity was observed. Severe lactic acidosis persisted for at least 15 min after the insult (Marshall et al. 1975c). During the oligaemic period CBF was about 20% of control values, but hyperaemia was seen from 1 to 5 min after reestablishment of cerebral circulation. Oligaemic animals had better outcome, and hypocapnia improved neurological outcome (Marshall et al. 1975a).

The changes in cerebral circulation and metabolism during and after incomplete and complete ischaemia have been reviewed (Siesjö 1992a, 1992b). The same author suggests that elective neuronal vulnerability observed after brief periods of ischaemia is elicited by postsynaptic damage to neurons innervated by excitatory amino acids (aspartate and glutamate) which give rise to enhanced calcium influx and osmolytic damage.

CBF and $CMRO_2$

In the immediate postischaemic period $CMRO_2$ is reduced (Snyder et al. 1975, Hossmann et al. 1976, Nordström and Rehncrona 1977). Later, $CMRO_2$ increases towards control values and under certain circumstances $CMRO_2$ might overshoot the control value (Hossmann et al. 1976, Kofke et al. 1979, Levy and Duffy 1977).

pH and oedema

Studies in cats with MR spectroscopy during and after a period of hypoxia or ischaemia indicate that an increase in lactate is accompanied by a decrease in intracellular pH. Furthermore, a delayed recovery of phosphocreatine has been found to be due to metabolic acidosis and not to delayed recovery of ATP and ADP (Gyulai et al. 1987).

In experiments of repeated ischaemic insults in gerbils, a pronounced cumulative effect on the development of cerebral oedema was observed (Tomida et al. 1987). Rats subjected to closed head injury combined with hypoxia and hypotension showed a markedly increase in brain swelling compared with animals subjected only to closed head injury or closed head injury combined with hypotension. The main component of brain swelling was brain water (Kita and Marmarou 1994).

Cerebral oedema

Cerebral oedema is a frequent finding in experimental as well as human head trauma. The development of oedema has been studied experimentally after cold injury lesion and after traumatic brain injury. It has been discussed whether, traumatic oedema was of vasogen or ischaemic, cytotoxic origin. Barzo et al. (1997) studied the development of traumatic oedema in rats subjected to impact-acceleration injury with diffuse weighted MR imaging. They found that posttraumatic oedema is associated with a biphasic pathophysiological response. First, there is a brief period of increased water diffusion distance signifying a predominantly vasogenic oedema formation that occurs immediately after injury. Second, at approximately 45 minutes postinjury, water diffusion distance bigins to decrease because of the formation of a slower and more widespread cellular oedema that becomes dominant and is sustained 1 or 2 weeks postinjury.

Cryogenic lesions

The development of brain swelling and changes in water content has been described in the rat. The devolopment of oedema is caused by breakdown of the blood-brain barrier (Schneider et al. 1994). Development of cryogenic brain swelling and oedema is markedly enhanced in old versus young animals (Unterberg et al. 1994).

CBF

In cats cryogenic lesion elicited a focal CBF decrease, and rCBF was found to be inversely proportional to the water content in the brain tissue (Frei et al. 1973). The decrease in rCBF is attenuated by hyperbaric oxygen (Miller et al. 1970). In monkeys a cryogenic injury resulted in an immediate zone of no/low flow, that progressed in size over time in concert with an expanding zone of oedema. Changes in local CBF in regions remote from the injury were phasic and asynchronous with progressive rises in ICP (Darby et al. 1993).

Glucose utilisation

Generally, local glucose utilisation is decreased in thermally traumatised rat brains (Pappius 1981). However, in the cat model of vasogenic oedema it was found that the increased tissue water level did not alter local CBF, but induced an increase in local glucose uptake, suggesting an increase in anaerobic metabolism (Sutton et al. 1989). Other studies suggest that pentobarbitone reduces local glucose utilisation proportionally to the control values obtained before pentobarbitone administration (Elphinstone et al. 1987).

ICP gradients and mean arterial blood pressure (MABP)

Tissue pressure differences of 13 mm Hg between oedematous and normal brain tissue have been observed (Reulen and Kreysch 1973). In cats subjected to hemispheric cryogenic injury, inter-hemispheric pressure gradients reached about 4 mm Hg within one hour. The transtentorial pressure gradient remained above 10 mm Hg for several hours (Furuse et al. 1981). These differences in pressure promote bulk flow and spread of oedema (Reulen et al. 1977). Cerebral oedema is enhanced by a sudden increase in MABP which also provoke an increase in ICP (Schutta et al. 1968).

Bradykinin

The kallikrein-kinin system eliciting bradykinin also plays a role as mediator of vasogenic oedema (Unterberg and Baethmann 1984, Maier-Hauff et al. 1984). Bradykinin provokes massive vasodilatation of cerebral vessels and opening of the BBB (Wahl et al. 1983, Unterberg et al. 1984). These effects are prevented by aprotinine, a trypsin inhibitor (Unterberg et al. 1986).

Bradykinin B_2 receptors are located on the luminal and abluminal membranes of endothelial cells, om smooth-muscle cells of the cerebral arterioles and on astrocytes and neurones. B_2 antagonists attenuate brain-blood barrier damage and reduce cerebral vasogenic oedema formation following global and focal cerebral ischemia (Kamiya et al. 1993, Raidoo et al. 1996), and reduction in brain swelling by B_2 receptor antagonist after cortical impact injury was observed in the rat (Stover et al. 2000).

Vasopressin

It has been demonstrated that in the cold-injured brain, stimulation of the medullary reticular formation results in an increase in brain water content (Nagao et al. 1989). Other data shows that stimulation of the reticular formation results in an increase in CSF-vasopressin in both normal and cold-injured brains (Kuniyoshi et al. 1993) and that intraventricular vasopressin administration results in an increase in brain water permeability (Raichle and Grupp 1978).

Arginine-vasopressin receptor antagonist suppresses the formation of vasogenic brain oedema after cryogenic injury (Nagao et al. 1994, Bemana et al. 1997). OPC-21268, a non-peptide arginine vasopressin VI receptor antagonist, reduces brain water content, brain swelling and blood-brain barrier permeability in rats subjected to cryogenic injury (Bemana and Nagao 1999). In another study in rats subjected to cryogenic injury it was found that the inhibition of the arginine vasopressin with RU51599, a selective kappa opioid agonist which acts as arginine vasopressin release inhibitor, has a protective effect on cryogenic-induced brain oedema (Ikeda et al. 1997).

Leucotriens

Leucotrienes which are known to increase the permeability of blood vessels do not open blood-brain barrier nor do they induce brain oedema (Unterberg et al. 1991).

Diuretics

Torasemide, a lipophilic diuretic compound which interacts with the $Na^{+}2Cl^{-}K^{+}$ carrier and with chloride channels, reduces ICP in cryogenic oedema of nephrectomized rats (Plangger 1994). In cryogenic brain oedema torasemide attenuates brain swelling (Bewrger et al. 1994).

Mannitol

In studies of cryogenic brain injury multiple doses of mannitol reduces traumatic brain swelling, thus favouring repeated mannitol administration even when the BBB is defective (von Berenberg et al. 1994).

Traumatic brain lesion

CBV

Based on recent studies (Marmarou et al. 1991, Schroeder et al. 1993) it was concluded that blood volume is reduced in areas of ischaemia following traumatic brain oedema, and oedema volume is increased. Thus, oedema is a major contributor to the swelling process in diffuse traumatic injury. As clinical MR studies have not revealed BBB compromise in the presence of swelling, it is considered that other forms of oedema, primarily ischaemic and neurotoxic, make a substantial contribution.

Capillary pressure

In a study of compression-induced ICP-hypertension it was found that ICP needs to increase to a level higher than the cerebral capillary pressure for the progression of localised vasogenic oedema (Hayashi et al. 1993).

Cyclooxygenase-2 induction

Cyclooxygenase-2 (COX2) is an inflammatory mediator that converts arachidonic acid from damage membranes into vasoactive postaglandins and produces reactive oxygen species in the process (Kontos et al. 1980, Ellis et al. 1989). COX2 probably plays a role in secondary responses that may result in increased ICP, vasospasm and cerebral ischaemia, resulting in worsening outcomes. Basal COX2 is regulated by normal glutamatergic synaptic activity in the brain. Neuronal induction of COX2 occurs after traumatic brain injury (Strauss et al. 1997, Strauss et al. 1998). The acute and chronic increase in brain COX2 that follows moderate traumatic brain injury are maximal in areas known to be associated with cognitive deficits (Strauss et al. 2000).

Prostaglandin

In experimental studies of brain trauma evidence has emerged, that release of prostaglandins plays a part in the generation of cerebral oedema (Shohami et al. 1987). In cats subjected to fluid percussion trauma, phospholipase C, a precursor enzyme, responsible for the generation of diacyl to prostaglandins, is elevated (Ellis et al. 1981, Wei et al. 1982).

After blunt head injury in the rat increased rates of prostaglandin and thromboxane synthesis were demonstrated as early as 15 min after injury. The concentrations were maximal at 1–24 h, and gradually resolved by 10 days after injury (Shohami et al. 1987). These events coincided with brain oedema formation and resolution (Shapira et al. 1988). In a study from the same group methylprednisolone did not alter brain tissue levels of eucosanoids or oedema formation (Shapira et al. 1992).

Free radical

Superoxide (Kontos and Wei 1986) and vasopressin (Reeder et al. 1986) may also be responsible for the formation of cerebral oedema after head injury. In a compression-induced ICP-hypertension model superoxide free radical increased immediately in the compressed brain tissue suggesting that free radicals directly cause secondary tissue damage. As sources of these radicals, arachidonic acid release and interventions by intravascular generating factors such as activation of neutrophils are suggested (Hayashi et al. 1993).

Lazaroid and 1,2-bis (nicotinamido)-propane (AVS), both free radical scavengers reduce oedema formation and spreading from cryogenic lesion (Arbit et al. 1993, Kamada et al. 1994), Schneider et al. 1994) Yet, lazaroid did not change the intracranial pressure-volume relationship (Arbit et al. 1993).

In the rat subjected to fluid percussion injury the new inhibitor of lipid peroxidation (LY341122) led to a reduction in overall contusion volume and reduced the frequency of damaged neurons (Wada et al. 1999).

Excitatory amino acid (EAA)

In experimental subdural haematoma in rats EAA antagonist (kynuremic acid) attenuates the increase in brain water (Kinoshita et al. 1994).

Heat shock protein

Long term exposure to heat reduces oedema formation and protects BBB after closed head injury in the rat (Shohami et al. 1994). Generation of heat shock protein is suggested to attenuate oedema formation.

Platelet activating factor (PAF)

There is evidence that PAF is involved in the pathophysiology of brain oedema (Braquet et al. 1987, Kochanek et al. 1988). PAF antagonists have been reported to reduce brain oedema and ischaemic damage (Kochaneh 1987, Panetta 1987, Spinnewyn et al. 1987). In another study of cryogenic oedema in rat pre-treatment with PAF-antagonist (TCV-309) reduced water content and volume of ischaemia (Tokutomi et al. 1994).

Cellular integrity and biochemical disorders

Calcium Homeostasis and Channel Blockers

Recent studies have focused on the pathological significance of calcium accumulation in the central nervous system following traumatic brain injury. Disturbances in neuronal homeostasis may result in the activation of calcium-sensitive enzymes, including kinasis, lipasis, phosphatases and proteases. Activation of calpains, calcium-activated intracellular proteases, may play a major role in the neuro degenerative changes following HI. This is supported by studies of calpain inhibitors, which are able to attenuate neuronal damage, even when administrated in the posttraumatic period (Kampfl et al. 1997).

Brain oedema

Calcium channel blockers exerts a protective effect following cerebral ischaemia and subarachnoid haemorrhage. In the rat subjected to fluid-percussion brain injury the calcium channel blocker (S)-emopamil reduces brain oedema, attenuates memory dysfunction and attenuates deficits in motor function (Okiyama et al. 1992). Another experimental study indicated that combined treatment with nicardipine, phenobarbital and methylprednisolone ameliorates vasogenic brain oedema after cryogenic lesion (Lin et al. 1994).

Glutamate and excitatory amino acid (EAA) antagonists

Glutamate and aspartate

In rats subjected to subdural haematoma, the concentration of EAA increases in the ischaemic cortex underlying the haematoma. In this region CBF averaged 25 ml/100g/min. Hippocampal glutamate levels rose as well, yet CBF was preserved in this region. The study suggests focal hypermetabolism by "excitotoxic processes" after subdural haematoma (Bullock et al. 1991). In the same animal Palmer et al. (1993) used a controlled cortical impact model, and found that the maximal increase in EAA was proportional to the severity of the injury. After moderate injury the EAA concentration was normalised after 20–30 min, and normalisation was disclosed after 60 min.

In rats the release of EAA from contused tissue and non-contused tissue surrounding the lesion was studied. The increase in EAA was attenuated by antagonist through microdialysis, suggesting that release of EAA from the surrounding brain areas appears to be a consequence that is secondary to the release of EAA from the contused brain tissue (Tanaka et al. 1994).

Immediately after concussion glucose utilisation increases, and it is proposed that the induced hypermetabolism reflects the effort of brain cells to restore normal ionic balance disrupted by massive ionic fluxes through transmitter gated ion channels (Kawamata et al. 1992).

Antagonist

In a rodent model pre-treatment with NMDA antagonist reduced the volume of ischaemic brain damage (Chen et al. 1991). In the rat subjected to focal ischaemia similar results have been found with a non-competitive NMDA antagonist, when given 15 minutes after a controlled cortical impact injury in the rat (Kroppenstedt et al. 1998). Concussive brain injury in rats causes a massive increase in extracellular K^+ which occur concomitantly with an increase flux of glutamate. Kynurenic acid, an excitatory amino acid antagonist, effectively attenuated the increase in K^+ flux (Katayama et al. 1990). In experimental subdural haematoma the noncompetitive NMDA blocker dextromethorphan reduces infarction lesion below the haematoma (Duhaime et al. 1996). In rats, subjected to a cortical impact injury, ifenprodil, a polyamine-site NMDA receptor antagonist, inproved blood-brain barrier function, reduced cerebral oedema formation and reduced injury volume (Dempsey et al. 2000). Other studies indicate that NMDA antagonists attenuate spatial memory impairments after fluid-percussion injury in rats (Okiyama et al. 1997).

Ketamine

Ketamine, another NMDA antagonist, decreases cerebral infarct volume and improves neurological outcome following experimental head trauma in rats (Shapira et al. 1992).

Clinical studies

The concentration of EAA in CSF following traumatic brain injury is increased. The high levels of glutamate, combined with the frame over which it was observed suggest that intervention with antagonist is a possibility (Baker et al. 1993).

Critique concerning the role of EAA

Several studies indicate that after moderate brain injury the initial increase in extracellular glutamate is cleared within 5 min (Obrenovitch et al. 1993). The same author found that very high concentrations of exogenous glutamate must be applied extracellularly to induce depolarisation, far in excess of those measured early after traumatic brain injury (Obrenovitch et al. 1997b). Local inhibition of glutamate uptake with L-*trans*-pyrrolidine-2,3,-dicarboxylate increased the extracellular concentration of glutamate 25-fold, but this only produced minor local depolarisations that were not mediated by ionotropic glutamate receptors (Obrenovitch et al. 1997a). Spreading depression requires functional NMDA-operated channels, but high extracellular glutamate does not potentiat its elicitation nor its propagation (Obrenovitch et al. 1996b, Obrenovitch and Zilkha 1995). Intracellular application of L-*trans*-pyrrolidine-2,4,-dicarboxylate increases markedly extracellular glutamate in the hippocampus, striatium, and cortex of rats, but it significantly reduced the latency for anoxic depolarization only in the cerebral cortex (Obrenovitch et al. 1997b).

To explain the beneficial actions of glutamate antagonists in experimental brain injury (Obrenovitch and Urenjak (1997) proposed abnormalities of glutamatergic neurotransmission such as deficient Mg^{2+} blockade of NMDA-receptor ionophore complexes, and phenomenon such as spreading depression, which requires activation of glutamate receptors and is detrimental to neurones in damaged/vulnerable brain regions. Finally, they stress that beneficial effects of glutamate receptor antagonists in experimental models do not necessarily imply the occurrence of excitatoxic processes. Thus, glutamate-receptor antagonist may be protective by reducing the energy demand required to counterbalance Na^+ influx associated with glutamatergic synaptic transmission. In a subdural haematoma model Tsuchida et al. (1996) found that sodium channel blocker is highly neuroprotective, and that this effect, partly, is mediated by the inhibition of glutamate release form ischaemic cortex underneath the haematoma.

Free radical scavenger

Polyethylene glycol (PEG) conjugated superoxide dismutase (SOD) has been shown to be beneficial in several types of experimental ischaemic and traumatic injury when used before fluid percussion lesion (Muir et al. 1995) and after the lesion (Hamm et al. 1996). In traumatic brain injury in the rat exogenous licithinized SOD reduced brain oedema in the periphery of the lesion 6 hrs. after the trauma, confirming the important role of O_2^- in the development of brain oedema (Yunoki et al. 1997). In another study rats were subjected to cortical contusion followed and treatment with the superoxide radical scavenger OPC-14177. The histopathological necrosis and the formation of oedema were attenuated by OPC-14177 (Mori et al. 1998).

Inflammatory response

Experimental studies have shown that reactive microglia and infiltrating monocytes release neurotoxic substances following brain trauma (Giulian et al. 1993). It is supposed that release of cytokines by inflammatory reactions plays an important role by causing blood-brain barrier dysfunction and oedema (Gordon et al. 1990).

The intercellular adhesion molecule-1 (ICAM-1) is expressed by endothelial cells. This molecule is essential for promoting adhesion and transmigration of circulating leukocytes across the blood-brain barrier. In a clinical study the concentration of soluble ventricular fluid ICAM-1 correlates with the extent of cerebral damage and blood-brain barrier damage (Pleines et al. 1998). In experimental studies a maximal inflammatory response at 4–6 days after the trauma is observed (Holmin et al. 1995). After brain contusion in the rat no expression was seen during the first 2 days after the trauma. On day 4–6, however, strong interleukin-1β, and interleukin -6mRNA expression was detected in mononuclear cells surrounding the contusion. Immuno-histochemical double labeling confirmed that mononuclear phagocytes and astrocytes produced interleukin-lβ, and that astrocytes produced tumour necrosis factor (Holmin et al. 1997).

Development of oedema coincides with the maximum inflammatory response (Holmin et al. 1995) suggesting that anti-inflammatory treatment could prevent oedema, and thus secondary neuronal injury. Holmin and Mathiesen (1996) found that colchicine and dexamethasone administered after cerebral trauma in rats reduced inflammation and oedema.

Inflammatory reactions such as leukocytosis with a white blood cell count exceeding 20 10^6/l is associated with a poor clinical grade on admission and with a high mortality (Keskil et al. 1994

Cholinergic receptors

Cholinergic neurones within the ventrobasal forebrain are essential for memory and cognitive function, and central noradrenergic and dopaminergic systems participate in selective attention and motivation. In rats subjected to fluid-percussion injury a selective loss of ventrobasal forebrain cholinergic neurons has been demonstrated (Schmidt and Grady 1995). Studies in the same animal subjected to weight drop contusion indicate that the cholineesterase inhibitor, scopolamine, reversed the decline in CBF of the cerebral cortex (Scremin and Jenden 1997). However, tetrahydroaminoacridine, another cholinesterase inhibitor, does not improve cognitive performance following experimental brain injury (Pike et al. 1997). Activation of pontine cholinergic sites seems to be implicated in unconsciousness following cerebral contusion in the cat (Hayes et al. 1984).

Cytidine-5-diphosphate (CDP)-choline

Administration of CDP-choline has been used extensively as a brain activating factor in different neurodegenerative disorders, such as Alzheimer's decease, memory defects, chronic vascular diseases and after postconcussional trauma (Levin 1991). For review (Dixon et al. 1997). Although de precise mechanism of action of CDP-choline is unknown, two primary rationales have been proposed for the therapeutic use of CDP-choline. The first is that CDP-choline attenuates lipid membrane damage by enhancing brain phospholipid metabolism. The second is that CDP-choline stimulates biosynthesis of acetylcholine by providing additional choline, the rate-limiting factor of acetylcholine synthesis.

Several lines of evidence indicate that rats subjected to traumatic HI produces disturbances in spatial memory function that may be related to a decreased capacity of cholinergic neurones to release acetylcholine. Microdialysis studies 2 weeks following traumatic HI have demonstrated reduced release of acetylcholine evoked by the muscarinic autoreceptor antagonist, scopolamine (Dixon et al. 1996). In another study CDP-choline reduced posttraumatic cerebral oedema and improved blood-brain barrier function in rats (Baskaya et al. 2000). Traumatic HI produces increased sensitivity to disruption of spatial memory function by scopolamine that occurs concurrently with a reduction in scopolamine-evoked acetylcholine release. Traumatic HI produces a time-dependent loss of choline transferase activity. Accordingly, it is possible that reduced acetylcholine neurotransmission is attributable to altered acetylcholine synthesis. In studies of rats subjected to cortical impact injury administration of CDP-choline attenuated posttraumatic motor- and spatial memory performance deficits, and microdialysis studies demonstrated that CDP-choline increased acetylcholine levels in dorsal hippocampus and the neocortex in normal, awake rats (Dixon et al. 1997). In human post-mortem brain from patients who died following head injury, choline acetyltransferase activity was consistently reduced. The presence of subdural haematoma and a prolonged survival period after head injury tended to be associated with lower choline acetyltransferase activity (Murdoch et al. 1998).

γ-aminobutyric acid (GABA)

γ-aminobutyric acid (GABA), the major inhibitory neurotransmitter in the brain, has inhibitory effects on cholinergic neurotransmission. Applied GABA inhibits central acetylcholine release (Bianchi et al. 1982, Stoof et al. 1979). Agonists that facilitate the activity of the $GABA_A$-receptor complex, such as muscimol, have potent cholinergic-inhibiting properties, and impair memory function in animals (Brioni et al. 1990, Miller and Richter 1986, Wood et al. 1979). Therefore, diminishing this inhibitory control over cholinergic activity, or disinhibition, may facilitate cholinergic neurotransmission and in turn enhance cognition (Sater et al. 1988). In a study of chronic post-injury administration of suritozole, a negative modulator at the $GABA_A$ receptor, promoted cognitive recovery (O'Dell and Hamm 1995).

Magnesium

Magnesium is recognised for its importance in a vast variety of critical cellular processes including glycolysis, oxidative phosphorylation, cellular respiration, protein synthesis and ATP-ase function. Magnesium salts have a protective effect after experimental brain trauma (Vink et al. 1988, McIntosh et al. 1989, Smith et al. 1983, Bara et al. 1994). In the rat both $MgSO_4$ and $MgCl_2$ given as a bolus at 30 min after severe closed head injury significantly improved brain intracellular free magnesium concentration and neurological outcome (Heath and Vink 1998). In another study fibroblast growth factor and Mg^{2+} were evaluated separately and in combination to assess their potential additive effects on posttraumatic neurological recovery in rats subjected to fluid precussion injury. No effect of any drug treatment or combination was observed on the extent of the postinjury lesion volume in the injured cortex (Guluma et al. 1999).

Heat shock protein

Heat shock proteins (hsp) are expressed as part of the stress response in cells exposed to a variety of pathologic stimuli. Induction of heat shock proteins protects cells from subsequent lethal stimuli. Hsp72 is generated by traumatic brain injury (Tanno et al. 1993, Lowenstein et al. 1994, Raghupathi et al. 1995). HSP protects cultured neurones from glutamate neurotoxicity (Lowenstein et al. 1991, Rordorf et al. 1991) and stimuli that induces apoptotic cell death (Mailhos et al. 1993). In rats subjected to controlled cortical impact injury it was found that hsp72 was expressed in the ipselateral cortex and hippocampus after cortical impact (Chen et al. 1998).

Primary damage in human head injury

Cerebral contusion and dilaceration

Pressure waves

Impacts associated with human head injury have a translational and rotational component. Passing through the cerebral tissue the pressure wave disrupts axons, gives rise to a diffuse brain lesion, and causes cerebral contusion immediately below the impact and at the contralateral side of the trauma (contracoup).

Contusion of cerebral tissue is localised on the crests of gyri, and may extend into white matter. Contusion is localised below fractures and below the site of impact. Contre coup lesions are localized on the contralateral hemisphere, declive parts of the frontal and temporal lobes, in the cortex above and below the Sylvian fissures, the lateral surface of the temporal lobe and the basal cerebellar hemispheres.

Degree of damage

In accordance with experimental studies by Ommaya and Gennerelli (1974) acceleration trauma with rotational component produces centripetal progression, which is always maximal in the peripheral region. Compared with subcortical regions the cerebral damage therefore is more severe in the cerebral cortex than in subcortical regions. The authors argue that primary brain-stem lesion does not exist. Neuropathological studies in humans support this view (Mitchell and Adams 1973).

Consistent with the centripetal model of progressive brain injury Levin et al. (1988) found that the depth of the brain lesion, evaluated by MR imaging, was positively related to the degree and the duration of impaired consciousness.

Oedema formation

Studies in rats indicate that the osmolality of contused brain tissue increases rapidly. The increase in osmolality is not caused by changes in inorganic ion contents, suggesting a metabolic production of osmoles or release of ideogenic osmoles. Furthermore, the contused brain tissue strongly attracks water, provided that blood supply is maintained (Katayama et al. 1998).

Subdural haematoma

Subdural haematoma is caused by rupture of small veins bridging the subdural space. The incidence varies between 20 and 63%. The initial damage is severe, and the clinical picture is that of an unconscious patient becoming more deeply unconscious. Unilateral brain swelling is often found in patients with subdural haematoma. After evacuation of the haematoma the brain expands to occupy the available intracranial space. However, hypoxic and ischaemic damage is often observed in the involved cerebral cortex.

Late diagnose contributes to a high mortality. Evacuation of haematoma within 4 hours improves prognosis.

Extradural haematoma

The incidence is 5–15%. About 85% have fracture of the skull. The haemorrhage most often results from laceration of the middle meningeal artery. After a lucid interval the patients often deteriorate. The duration of the lucid interval depends on the rapidity by which the haematoma develops.

Most extradural haematomas are localised in the temporal region, but localisation in the frontal, parietal and in the posterior fossa is also seen. The clinical picture is related to increased ICP, tentorial herniation and compression of the brain stem.

Intracerebral haematoma

Is present in 15–22% of the patients. Intracerebral haematoma is localised in the subfrontal and temporal regions, and less frequently in the cerebellum. Often the development is delayed for several days.

Diffuse axonal injury (DAI)

DAI has been described radiologically as changes secondary to shearing injury of the cerebral white matter. These lesions consist of eccentric haemorrhage in the corpus callosum, diffuse cerebral swelling, subarachnoid haemorrhage and haemorrhage around the third ventricular region and in the white matter (Zimmerman et al. 1978).

In a study by Adams et al. (1982) a low incidence of lucid interval, cerebral contusion, intracranial haematoma, and evidence of a high ICP was found. In another study of 414 patients with acute head injury 14 patients were classified as DAI. Parenchymal haemorrhagic lesions were seen in the basal ganglia (50%), midbrain (33%) and corpus callosum (16%). Initially the ICP was below 20 mm Hg in most patients. However, ICP- hypertension developed in 60% of the patients. Mortality was 33% and no patients had a good recovery (Kobayashi et al. 1989). If diffuse brain swelling and associated intracranial mass lesions other than deep white matter haemorrhage are excluded, ICP hypertension is rarely observed and mortality rates of 12% has been found (Sganzerla et al. 1993).

The features of DAI in humans are comparable with DAI produced in primates subjected to angular acceleration trauma of the head.

Traumatic subarachnoid haemorrhage (tSAH)

A grading scale based on CT scanning findings has been proposed. Grade 1 indicate thin tSAH (< 5 mm). Grade 2, thick tSAH (> 5 mm). Grade 3, thin tSAH with mass lesion, and grade 4, thick tSAH with mass lesion. A significant correlation between this grading system and admission GCS and discharged GOS was found (Green et al. 1995). Grading system from tSAH has been proposed by Green et al. (1995) and Marshall et al. (1997).

The presence of tSAH on CT scanning has been shown to confer a worse prognosis than the injury alone (Green et al. 1996, Kakarieka et al. 1995). TSAH patients undergo more chest procedures and their incidence of hypoxia and hypotension is greater. They spent more days in intensive care unit, more total days hospitalised, and had worse GOS at discharge than patients without tSAH (Green et al. 1996). The mechanism by which tSAH results in worse outcomes is unclear. It has been postulated that vasospasm in the presence of tSAH produces ischaemia in this group of patients. On the other hand, studies with Xe-CT scan og rCBF and rCBV indicate that in regions with cerebral ischaemia compromise of the microvasculature is the cause of early ischaemia after severe head trauma, rather than vasospasm of the larger cunductance vessels (Schröder et al. 1998).

Neurogenic pulmonary oedema

The pathogenesis of neurogenic pulmonary oedema is not well understood. Specific destructive lesions in the CNS have been observed to cause pulmonary oedema including the destruction of the medullary solitary tracts, and hypothalamic lesions.

Acute lung injury

In a study from the Coma Data Bank acute lung injury, defined as a ratio of partial pressure of PaO_2 to fractional expired oxygen of 300 mm Hg or less, was analysed. 20% of comatose patients developed acute lung injury, and they were three times more likely to die or survive in a vegetative state. Specific anatomic brain lesions were not associated with acute lung injury. However, patients with more severe lesions (large non-evacuated mass lesions, and those with midline shift) demonstrated a 10-, and 5 -fold increased risk of acute lung injury (Bratton and Davis 1997).

Secondary Damage in Human Head Injury

Jeffreys and Jones (1981) called attention to avoidable factors which contribute to deterioration of HI patients. Avoidable factors contributing to death were identified in 30%, and those possibly contributing to death were identified in 24%. Of the avoidable factors 38% occurred in patients who "talked and died", and 77% in patients with intracranial haematoma. The most common avoidable factors were failure to recognise the development of a haematoma, respiratory difficulties leading to hypoxia/hypercapnia, hypotension, and convulsions. All of these factors might in it self or in combination lead to ICP-hypertension, reduced CPP, progression of cerebral oedema and cerebral ischaemia. It is of vital importance to avoid hypotension and hypoxia (Chesnut et al. 1993, Marmarou et al. 1991) Neuroradiological examination (CT- and MR scans) are the most important tool to diagnose pathological mass ocupying structures. Repeated CT scans combined with miticulous monitoring of cerebral haemodynamic and intracranial pressure are the most important steps in diagnosis and prevention of secondary cerebral damage.

CT and MR-scanning

Haematoma and oedema

CT- and MR scans are the most valuable tools in detection localisation, size and expansion of of intracranial space occupying mass, whether caused by haemorrhage or oedema. Repeated CT scanning with intervals of days is performed as soon as neurological deterioration occurs, or when monitoring of ICP indicate a progressive increase.

Ischaemia and hyperaemia

In a study of dynamic CT performed in 42 patients a hyperaemic state was found in non-fatal injured patients. On the other hand in 17 of 25 fatally injured patients, dynamic CT scans revealed a severely ischaemic state (Yoshino et al. 1985). By measuring Hounsfield units in patients with head injury it has been found that diffuse brain swelling was caused by cerebrovascular congestion in 53% of the patients. Immediate brain swelling without proceeding hyperaemic phase occurred less frequently (32%) (Rózsa et al. 1989).

Mendelow et al. (1983) calculated CBV by CT scanning taken before and after intravenous injection of iodine contrast. They found CBV ranging from 2–8%. An association between high CBV and elevated ICP was not found. Muizelaar et al. (1991) have studied changes in CBF and CBV in patients with cerebral ischaemia. They found that CBV was reduced in patients with ischaemia. By MR studies brain water in these patients was measured, and found to be increased (Marmarou et al. 1994).

Diffuse swelling

The question if diffuse brain swelling after head injury is more malignant in adults than children was investigated by Lang et al. (1994). By CT scan they found that swelling was more common in adults than in children. Features that were associated with deterioration were the presence of prolonged coma after injury, diffuse axonal injury, subarachnoid haemorrhage and episodes of hypotension. In children suffering from severe brain trauma, studies with MR scanning indicate that the depth of brain lesion is directly related to severity of acute impairment of consciousness and inversely related to outcome. This study support the Ommaya-Gennarelli model to paediatric closed HI (Levin et al. 1997).

Ventricular volume

In patients with HI, ventricular volume was measured by CT scanning before and after evacuation of an intracranial haematoma. A correlation between a decrease in ventricles volume and an increase in ICP was observed (Murphy et al. 1983). Other studies including preoperative volumetric analysis of the ventricles in patients with extradural haematoma have shown that an increase in the total volume of the ventricles above normal, a midline shift exceeding 10 mm and obliteration of the third ventricle, and basal cisterns, might contribute to the increase in ICP (Findley et al. 1983). In patients with diffuse injury no relationship between the size of the ventricles and ICP was observed. On the other hand, an association between obliteration of the third ventricle and the basal cisterns and an increase in ICP was observed (Teasdale et al. 1984).

ICP-hypertension (IH) and ICP-monitoring

Several investigations of ICP in patients suffering from severe head injury indicate that intracranial hypertension (IH) often occurs. In a study of 160 patients with severe head injury Miller et al. (1977) found IH (ICP > 10 mm Hg) in 82% of the patients and in 97% of the patients with a mass lesion. Although ICP > 40 mm Hg was only observed in 10% of the patients, IH was found to be the primary reason for death in 50% of the patients. In a later study these findings were confirmed by the same investigators (Miller et al. 1981).

Long term course of ICP monitoring indicate that a subgroup of patients (31%) develops a secondary rise in ICP. This rise develops 3 to 10 days after the trauma. The outcome of patients with a secondary rise was worse when compared with patients without this complication. Delayed intracerebral haemorrhage, traumatic vasospasm, hyponatremia and leukocytosis were diagnosed in some cases, but in many patients the reason for IH could not be identified (Unterberg et al. 1993).

Critical levels

Incarceration is accompanied by a characteristic pattern of sudden ICP rise (Troupp and Vapalahti 1971) and a decrease in CPP to very low levels (Balslev-J¢rgensen et al. 1972).

Pressure levels above 30–40 mm Hg for several hours is associated with a poor outcome (Troupp 1967, Vapalahti et al. 1969, Cold et al. 1975, Changaris et al. 1987). In a study of severe head injury where carotid blood flow was determined by electromagnetic flowmetry. CBF was found to change passively with changes in blood pressure indicating total loss of CA. In the same study ICP levels above 40 mm Hg were associated with flow deprivation (Gobiet et al. 1975).

The level at which ICP indicates anti-hypertensive therapy is debated. ICP of about 20-25 mm Hg is tolerated for short periods of 5–10 min. At pressures above this level for longer periods (20–30 min) re-evaluation as regard respiration, circulation, degree and choice of sedation, and neurological evaluation with special reference to the occurrence of an expanding lesion is mandatory.

If IH persists, and operative intervention is not indicated, the available therapeutic measures include controlled hyperventilation, sedation with barbiturates or other hypnotic agents, the use of analgesics (provided the ventilation is controlled), and osmotic therapy. Moreover, ventricular drainage in selective cases is effective in controlling IH (Johnston et al. 1970); however, continuous drainage for longer periods might increase the compression of the cerebral ventricles and thus negate the effect of drainage.

Indication of ICP monitoring

Based on clinical studies several investigators have argued that ICP should be recorded as it provides a guide to therapy (Johnston et al. 1970, Becker et al. 1977, Papo 1977, Marshall et al. 1979a, Marshall et al. 1979b, Kobayashi et al. 1983, Moss et al. 1983). Moreover, a high level of ICP is correlated to a poor outcome (Kobayashi et al. 1983, Klauber et al. 1984). It has been demonstrated that ICP monitoring might be a guide to aggressive therapy including prolonged hyperventilation, osmotic therapy and barbiturate coma treatment (Becker et al. 1977, Marshall et al. 1979b, Saul and Ducker 1982).

ICP recording is found to be indispensable in patients with abnormal CT scan (mass lesion), patients with posturing, patients over 40 years of age, and patients with a period of arterial hypotension (Narayan et al. 1982, Becker et al. 1983, Teasdale et al. 1986). On the other hand, ICP hypertension might occur in patients without signs of intracranial hypertension on the initial CT-scan (O'Sullival et al. 1994).

Intraventricular pressure recording, besides being a very precise method of ICP recording, also gives the opportunity to perform drainage and withdrawal of ventricular fluid for biochemical studies (lactate etc). However, this technique has been practically abandoned because of the risk of infection which range from 4.7 to 10.3% (Clark et al. 1989). It has been replaced by subarachnoid screw and epidural transducer. Other methods are reviewed in chapter 3.

CSF formation

In a study by Marmarou et al. (1987) it was found that CSF absorption parameters (CSF-formation and outflow resistance) accounted for approximately one-third of the ICP rise after severe HI. The authors suggested that other mechanisms presumably vascular in origin might be a predominant factor in elevation of ICP.

Pressure volume index (PVI)

The pressure volume idenx is defined as the volume necessary to raise the ICP by a factor of 10 mm Hg. The clinical significance of intracranial pressure-volume index (PVI) has been evaluated by Tans and Poortvliet (1983). They concluded that a PVI index < 10 ml (normal value 25 ml) indicates antihypertensive treatment. Maset et al. (1987) found a clear relationship between low PVI values measured soon after the injury and subsequent development of ICP-hypertension. However, in other studies PVI varied independently of the clinical course, outcome and ICP, making any decisions regarding therapeutic interventions difficult (Kosteljanetz 1986, Marmarou et al. 1986). As stated by Gray and Rosner (1987), in experimental studies the PVI is a complex function of CPP varying directly with CPP within the autoregulatory range and indirectly with CPP below the autoregulatory range.

Oedema

The significance of cerebral oedema in IH has been evaluated by Galbraith et al. (1984). They found a striking correlation between high water content in white matter around an intracranial haematoma (determined by gravimetric technique in biopsies taken during operation) and the level of ICP. In patients with diffuse cerebral lesions this correlation was not observed.

Ischaemia

Neuropathological studies of brains from consecutive patients dying as a result of blunt head injury have shown obvious signs of ischaemic damage in 91%. These changes are found in the cerebral cortex in 46%, hippocampus 81%, cerebellum 36% and the basal ganglia in 79% (Graham et al. 1978). Neuropathological findings of brain herniation suggest well-defined ischaemic lesions of parahippocampal and cingulate gyri and infarction in the medial occipital cortex (Adams and Graham 1976). The ischaemic brain damage is probably due to intracranial hypertension caused by mass lesions and brain swelling (Langfitt and Gennarelli 1982).

Water shed areas

Direct impact caused by blunt lesions and secondary events like hypotension might result in localised necrosis at boundary zones between the major cerebral arteries (water shed lesions) (Adams et al. 1966, Adams et al. 1976).

Transneuronal degeneration and cerebral atrophy

Atrophy of the brain has been documented following traumatic brain injury (Teasdale and Hadley 1990, Levin et al. 1981, Timming et al. 1982, Grosswasser-Reider et al. 1993, Gale et al. 1995, Anderson and Bigler 1994). Studies linking traumatic brain injury in humans with the development of Alzheimer's disease demonstrate the potential of brain trauma to initiate or facilitate active neurodegenerative cascades (Tokuda et al. 1991, Roberts et al. 1990, Mortimer et al. 1991, Graham et al. 1995). Other studies indicate that brain trauma exacerbates the decline of cognitive function during the ageing process, even when the trauma occurred many years ago (Stuss et al. 1989, Corkin et al. 1989). MR studies indicate that nonthalamic traumatic lesions result in smaller thalamic volume, suggesting that subcortical brain structures may be susceptible to trans-neuronal degeneration following cortical lesions (Anderson et al. 1996).

In a recent study speciments of brain tissue were excised during emergency craniotomy for evacuation of cerebral contusions. The speciments were analysed for apoptosis-related genes p53, bcl-2 and bax. Bax expression was detected in all patients, whereas bcl-2 expression was noted in six of 31 patients. The study indicate that apoptosis does occur in patients after traumatic brain injury, and it is suggested that apoptotic processes may contribute to secondary injury processes (Ng et al. 2000).

Thalamic lesion

The GABAergic neurones of the thalamus reticular nucleus, have been implicated as important components in attentional processing systems. Neurons in the thalamic reticular nucleus are exquisitely sensitive to degeneration following experimental global ischaemia and closed head injury in primates. In a human study of brains from non-survivors after HI a high incidence of thalamic reticular lesions was found in all age groups. The lesions were characterised by loss of one fourth to three fourths of the neurones from the region of the nucleus associated with the frontal cortex and thalamic medio-dorsal and ventrolateral nuclei. Sparing of the thalamic reticular neurones correlated highly with the presence of extensive frontal cortical lesions, suggesting that an intact corticothalamic projection was necessary for degeneration of the thalamic reticular nucleus (Ross et al. 1993)

Posttraumatic seizure

Clinically evident seizure activity occurs after brain injury. Clinical series report an incidence of 4 to 10%. The peak incidence of early posttraumatic clinically observed seizure activity is during the initial 48 hours, with the high-risk period continuing up to 1 week post-injury. In early studies focal as well as generalised recognised seizures occur with greater frequency (8–10%) in more severely injured patients (Annegers et a. 1980). In a recent study seizure activity, as monitored by continuous EEG, occurred in 20% during the first week after traumatic brain injury in 94 patients with only six patients displaying status epilepticus (Vespa et al. 1999). In a double-blind placebo-controlled trial of 404 patients the incidence of early posttraumatic seizures was effectively reduced by prophyllactic administration of phenytoin for 1 or 2 weeks without drug-related side effects (Haltiner et al. 1999). In another randomized study valproat therapy indicates no benefit over short-term phenytoin therapy for prevention of early seizures (Temkin et al. 1999).

Prognostic indicators

Outcome assessment

Glasgow outcome scale

Since Jennett and Bond (1975) described the Glasgow outcome scale (GOS) it has been used in most clinical outcome trials. This scale is based on the overall social capability of the patient, and takes account of the combined effect of specific mental and neurological deficits. Besides death, four categories of survival are recognised: Vegatative state, severe disability, moderate disability, and good recovery.

In patients who are in a vegetative state at discharge a striking improvement over time has been disclosed. thus, decisions regarding withdrawal of supportive care should be postponed until at least 6 months after injury (Choi et al. 1994). For review (Braakman 1992).

Influenced by the fact that the result of most clinical outcome trials have been negative, the use of the Glasgow outcome scale in clinical trials has been discussed. Maas et al. (1999) call attention to the dichotomized nature of the GOS, and the U-shaped distribution in most outcome studies.

Perhaps there is time for more sensitive psychological tests when different strategies for cerebral protection are investigated (Cottrell 2000).

Factors influencing outcome

The following factors are of prognostic significance: Age of the patients (Overgaard et al. 1973, Jennett 1978, Braakman et al. 1988, Choi et al. 1988), posttraumatic hypertension (Overgaard et al. 1973), low cerebral perfusion pressure (Mendelow et al. 1993), hypotension (Jones et al. 1994, Pigula et al. 1993, Chesnut et al. 1993, Fearnside 1993), periods of hypotension occurring during resuscitation and transport, but also in the intensive care unit (Chesnut et al. 1993), intraoperative hypotension (Pietropaoli et al. 1992), hypoxaemia (Gentleman 1992, Pigula et al. 1993, Chesnut et al. 1993, Jones et al. 1994), abnormal motor activity (Overgaard et al. 1973, Jennett 1978, Choi et al. 1988), Glasgow coma scale (Jennett 1978, Siegel et al. 1991), Glasgow-Liege scale (Born et al. 1985, Born 1988, Choi et al. 1988), intraventricular haemorrhage (Leroux et al. 1992), pupillary response (Jennett 1978, Choi et al. 1988), oculocephalic reflexes (Jennett 1978, Choi et al. 1988), leukocytosis (Keskil et al, 1994), EEG (Rae-Grant et al. 1996) and evoked potential (Lindsay et al. 1981, Sleigh et al. 1999).

In fact a single episode of systolic blood pressure below 90 mm Hg will double mortality (Chesnut et al. 1993).

Gender

Studies of outcome after severe HI indicate that a higher mortalilty in woman as compared with men (Klauber et al. 1981, Kraus et al. 2000). In a metaanalysis, including eight studies, it was found that outcome after traumatic HI was worse in woman than in men (Farace and Alves 2000). The authors suggest that a prospective study of sex differences in traumatic HI outcome is needed.

Outcome in children

Several studies indicate that the outcome in paediatric patients is better than adults (Bruce et al. 1978). However, no difference in outcome in paediatric and adult patients was found in patients with a mass lesion and patients with increased ICP, regardless of whether the ICP was reducible (Alberico et al. 1987). In another study of the traumatic coma data bank it was found that children 0–4 years-old had an increased mortality (Levin et al. 1992). In children intracranial hypertension is especially found in patients with Glasgow coma score < 5. It is concluded that aggressive therapy with ICP monitoring in order to keep ICP < 20 mm Hg seems justified (Bruce et al. 1978). In paediatric head injury controlled lumbar subarachnoid drainage is a useful treatment when aggressive therapy and ventricular CSF-fluid evacuation have failed to control a high ICP (Levy et al. 1995).

Hyperglycaemia

Hyperglycaemia seems to indicate a poor outcome. In one study persistent non-ketotic hyperglycaemia was a grave prognostic sign in head-injured patients (Merguerian et al. 1981). In another study patients who subsequently remained in a vegetative state or died had a higher glucose level both on admission and later on than patients who had a good outcome (Lam et al. 1991). Head injury patients fed on carbohydrate-free diet had lower blood glucose and lactate and higher ketone body concentrations. However, these changes did not influence CSF lactate and cerebral lactate production (Ritter et al. 1996).

Alcohol

Alcohol abusers have a higher incidence of acute subdural haematoma and show increased postoperative morbidity and mortality (Sonne and T¢nnesen 1992).

Chest injury

A high mortality (80%) has been observed in patients with combined cerebral injury and chest trauma. Outcome worsens with the severity of the pulmonary injury and is especially bad in cases with a need of ventilatory support (Kotwica and Brzezinski 1990).

Other factors

In a study of 734 patients form the traumatic coma data bank pulmonary infection, shock, coagulopathy and septicaemia were significant, independent predictors of an unfavourable outcome (Piek et al. 1992).

During intra-hospital transport a significant correlation between increased frequency of insults post-transfer, compared with the pre-transfer situation, and a high injury severity score was observed (Andrews et al. 1990).

Plasma myeloperoxidase is increased and vitamin E levels decreased (Hans et al. 1992). Impairment of helper T-cell function has also been observed (Quattrocchi et al. 1991). Whether these findings are of prognostic significance is unsolved.

CT scanning

Among findings at CT scanning, midline shift out of proportion to the extent of the intracranial haemorrhage is a useful predictor of poor outcome (Quattrocchi et al. 1991).

Delayed or progressive brain injury defined as CT scans which has been classified as worse, because of a new lesion, or an increase in lesions present at the time of admission has been studied in consecutive patients. Delayed injury was found in 44%, and 51% of the patients developed significant CT changes occurring either spontaneously or following surgery. Final outcome is better predicted by using the control CT scans than using initial CT scans. Delayed injury was associated with the presence of coagulopathy, subdural haematoma on the initial CT scan, higher mortality, slower recovery and poorer outcome at 6 months (Stein et al. 1993, Lobato et al. 1997). In a similar study by Servadei et al. (1995) it was found that a significant proportion of post-traumatic patients, particularly those who are unconscious, harbour early evolving intracranial lesions, especially intracerebral and extracerebral haematomas. They concluded that when CT scan is performed within 3 hours after injury, a CT scan should be repeated within 12 hours.

Prediction based on multifactorial premises

Predictive factors for non-recovery of consciousness for at least 1 month include fever of central origin, diffuse body sweating, disturbances in antidiuretic hormone, abnormal motor reactivity and respiratory disturbances (Sazbon and Grosswasser 1990).

In a British study including 315 patients with GCS of 8 or less the presence of cerebral oedema, intraventricular blood, and the degree of midline shift predicted a high mortality. With age of the patients, abnormal motor responses and the CT scanning data an accuracy of 84% was obtained (Fearnside et al. 1993).

By including age, pupillary reaction, ICP, hypotensive periods, GCS, extracranial injuries and CT scan a new prognostic scale has been found to be accurate with no falsely pessimistic predictions (Gibson and Stephenson 1989). Within the population of very severely injured patients (GCS 3–5), the simple combination of age and admission GCS appears to predict accurately non-functional outcome Quigley et al. 1997).

In another study it was not possible to predict or distinguish, with a fair degree of probability, between patients who will remain in a vegetative state from those who will die (Brackman et al. 1988).

Regulation of cerebral circulation and metabolism

During the last decades the dynamic changes in CBF and metabolism have been reviewed repeatedly (Enevoldsen 1980, Jennett and Teasdale 1981, Enevoldsen 1986, Sundbärg 1988, Cold 1990).The implications for therapy, including controlled prolonged hyperventilation, barbiturate coma treatment etc., however, have only sparsely been commented upon and will be discussed in the section therapy in acute head injury.

Cerebral blood volume (CBV)

In a study of 37 head-injured patients (GCS $\leq$ 8) regional CBF and CBV was measured. CBV values ranged from 2.0 to 10.1 ml/100g. There was no relationship with time after injury at which the measurements were performed. CBF did not correlation with CBF in the early posttraumatic period. Patients with raised ICP (> 20 mm Hg) had significantly higher CBV than patients with normal ICP. Yet the presence of signs of brain swelling on CT had no relation to the level of CBV (Bouma et al. 1998).

Hyperaemia

Children

Global hyperaemia is often observed in children and young victims (Kasoff et al. 1972, Muizelaar et al. 1989a) indicating a hyperaemic or hyperperfusion syndrome (Langfitt et al. 1977, Obrist et al. 1979, Cold and Jensen 1980, Obrist et al. 1984). Furthermore, hyperaemia has been observed after hypotensive periods of shock and after evacuation of haematoma (decompression) (Obrist et al. 1984). That development of posttraumatic hyperaemia is age dependent has been documented autoradiographycally in immature, mature, and aged rats (Biagas et al. 1996).

Perifocal hyperaemia

Studies of local CBV by SPECT indicate an increase in local CBF in the medial margin of subdural haematoma (Kuhl et al. 1980), and patchy in the pericontusional region (Bergholt et al. 1996).

Hyperaemia and cognitive function

Neuropsychological studies of outcome within the first year after HI revealed greater impairment of overall intellectual and memory functions in patients with hyperaemia in the acute phase after injury than in patients with reduced flow. In the same study patients with ICP hypertension showed greater memory deficits than did those without ICP elevations (Uzzell et al. 1986). These observations are in contrast to studies performed by Sakas et al. (1995). They followed 53 patients within 3 weeks of brain injury with SPECT, and correlated focal hyperaemic zones with CT and MR scanning studies at 3 months. Hyperaemia was found in structurally normal brain tissue, it persisted for about 10 days, but was never observer within oedematous pericontusional zones. The mortality rate of patients with focal hyperaemia was lower than that of individuals without.

Biochemical mechanisms

Until recently it was believed that reactive hyperaemia was caused primarily by the generation of vasoactive metabolites (lactate, adenosine) which induced vasodilatation through relaxation of vascular smooth muscle. However, it has been established that the release of vasoactive neuropeptides from perivascular sensory nerves, via axon reflex-like mechanisms also has a significant impact upon the hyperperfusion syndrome. Among neuropeptides it is supposed that calcitonin gene-related peptide (CGRP), more than other neuropeptides (substance P, neurokinin) is likely to be the most important mediator of the neurogenic component of cortical hyperaemia (For review: MacFarlane et al. 1991).

Transcranial Doppler

With transcranial Doppler differences in hyperaemic and non-hyperaemic patients after severe head injury has been observed. The transcranial Doppler waveform of non-hyperaemic patients had a diastolic notch, which was absent in hyperaemic patients (Chan et al. 1992).

Reduced CBF

Reduced CBF has been found in elderly patients (Obrist et al. 1979, Cold and Jensen 1980, Obrist et al. 1984), and extremely low CBF values indicate impending brain death (Balslev-J¢rgensen et al. 1972, Overgaard and Tweed 1975, Overgaard et al. 1981, Overgaard et al. 1983), and a poor prognosis (Langfitt et al. 1977, Overgaard and Tweed 1983, Cold 1989a).

Level of consciousness

In deeply comatose patients, recovery of consciousness is followed by an increase or normalisation of CBF (Langfitt et al. 1977, Obrist et al. 1984).

Cerebral contusion

With externally placed detectors hyperaemia is especially observed in regions with cortical contusion. The clearance curves from these regions are characterised by an initial fast component referred to as a tissue peak. Correspondingly, early appearance of veins on arteriographic examination was found (Enevoldsen et al. 1976). Re-perfusion hyperaemia and/or hyperaemia in the pericontusional tissue can explain these findings. In contrast, Alexander et al. (1994) found low CBF in patients with cerebral contusion. Indeed, contused tissue is devitalised with CBF values far below ischaemic threshold and consequently tissue necrosis inevitably supervenes (Schröder et al. 1995, Astrup et al. 1995). Also in pericontusional tissue is flow deprived, oedematous, and with low cerebral blood volume (Stirred et al. 1995).

Subdural haemorrhage

In patients with subdural haematoma CBF was reduced, paralleling a reduction in $CMRO_2$ during the first 48 h after trauma. These changes were not associated with increased $AVDO_2$, suggesting that the reduction in CBF is related to diminished energy requirement or diminished ability for normal oxidative metabolism (Salvant and Muizelaar 1993).

Traumatic subarachnoid haematoma

In traumatic subarachnoid haemorrhage associated with vasospasm a correlation between reduced CBF and high flow velocity has been found (Martin et al. 1992).

Diffuse swelling and mass-lesion

In another study, including 35 comatose patients, CBF was measured within few hours after the injury with the stable xenon-enhanced CT method. In seven patients with diffuse swelling CBF was lower in all brain regions as compared with CBF in patients without diffuse swelling or with focal contusions. In four of the seven patients with diffuse swelling CBF < 18 ml/100g/min was found. Overall, global or regional ischaemia was found in 11 of the 35 patients (Bouma et al. 1992).

Reduced CBF has also been observed in regions adjacent to mass lesions (Bruce et al. 1973)

The acute phase

In a study including 186 patients CBF was measured with the 133-Xe technique. During the first 6 hours after the injury, CBF was low and $AVDO_2$ high. However, CBF increased when measured within 24 hours. CBF below the threshold of infarction (CBF < 18 ml/100g/min) was found in 33% of the studies obtained within 6 hours The incidence rapidly decreased thereafter (Bouma et al. 1991). Low CBF during the initial 48 h after traumatic HI has also been documented by continuous thermal diffusion flowmetry (Sioutos et al. 1995).

Oedema, water shed regions

Reduced CBF seems to indicate brain swelling caused by oedema (Overgaard and Tweed 1976, Bruce et al. 1973, Schröder et al. 1995). In addition severe oligaemia has been observed in the boundary zones between the cerebral arteries, and flow deprivation in these regions is related to a poor outcome (Overgaard and Tweed 1983).

Brain stem lesion

Experimental studies of mesencephalic reticular formation lesions in rats where a marked reduction of rCBF and glucose utilisation was observed (Hawkins et al. 1979).

Other studies in rats with reticular formation lesions indicate, that the reduction in CBF and metabolism persists throughout the four day observation period (Hass et al. 1976).

In patients with impairment of the brain-stem reflexes but without evidence of cortical lesions judged by arteriography and explorative operation CBF might be homogeneously low without indicating a poor prognosis (Cold and Jensen 1980). That CBF might be very low in patients with impaired or abolished brain-stem reflexes suggests that brain-stem lesions per se profoundly reduce cortical CBF and metabolism. This view is supported by reports of very low CBF and $CMRO_2$ in apallic patients and in patients with midbrain infarction (Ingvar and Sourander 1970).

Pupillary dilatation in patients with severe head injury has been associated with decreased brain stem blood flow, suggesting that brain stem ischaemia rather than mechanical compression of the IIIrd cranial nerve, is an important causal factor. Thus, pupil dilation may be an indicator of ischaemia of the brain stem. If cerebral blood flow and CPP can be rapidly restored in patients with severe head injury who has dilated pupils, the prognosis may be good (Ritter et al. 1999).

Mechanisms

Valuable studies on mechanisms underlying the post-traumatic flow decrease were provided by Anthes et al. (1996). They measured cross-sectional areas of arterioles in the spinal cord parenchyma of rats subjected to cord compression injury. Microcirculatory vasospasm and a significant constriction of the arteriolar lumen, that was attributable to an increased width of the smooth muscle layer of media, together with shortening of the smooth muscle cells were found. In view of the paucity of evidence of vasospasm of perenchymal versus extraparenchymal blood vessels, these observation are pertinent.

A concurrent acidosis may support the flow deprivation from trauma. Kempski et al. (1997) have reported that acidosis induces endothelial swelling, and swelling of the glial cells, which may contribute to the failure of the cerebral microcirculation.

Ischaemia

In patients with severe head injury neuropathological studies indicate that ischaemic damage of the brain structures is a fairly common finding (Graham and Adams 1971, Graham et al. 1978). The ischaemic damages might be secondary to hypotensive periods (Adams et al. 1966, Adams and Graham 1976), and the changes may be caused by intracranial hypertension (Langfitt and Gennarelli 1982).

Biochemical studies

The occurrence of cerebral ischaemia is supported by experimental studies indicating a correlation between the severity of the trauma on one hand, and on the other hand, the neuropathological changes, biochemical changes in cerebral tissue and ventricular fluid, with depletion of phosphocreatine and ATP, and increase in lactate (Nilsson et al. 1977, Tornheim et al. 1983, Wagner et al. 1985, Gennarelli et al. 1986, Vink et al. 1987). Accordingly, clinical studies in the acute phase of HI indicate an increase in ventricular fluid lactate. Other studies have shown a persistently high lactate level in the ventricular fluid and these studies suggest a poor outcome (Fieschi et al. 1974, Overgaard and Tweed 1974, Cold et al. 1975b, Enevoldsen et al. 1976, Enevoldsen and Jensen 1978, Cold 1981, DeSalles et al. 1986). An increase in lactate concentration is associated with a decrease in extracellular pH (deSalles et al. 1987b).

ICP level

ICP hypertension is a fairly common finding in the acute phase of HI (Miller et al. 1977). A pressure exceeding 40 mm Hg for hours is therefore associated with a poor outcome (Troupp 1967, Vapalahti et al. 1969, Cold et al. 1975a, Miller et al. 1977, Miller et al. 1981, Changaris et al. 1987). These findings suggest that ICP hypertension might be a factor of importance in the development of cerebral ischaemia. According to guidelines for the management of severe traumatic brain injury, intracranial pressure treatment should be initiated at an upper threshold of 20–25 mm Hg, but in the same guidelines it is stressed that patients can herniate at ICP less than these values. Furthermore, pupillary abnomalities might occur with ICP values as low as 18 mm Hg (Marshall et al. 1983).

CPP

A low CPP (CPP <60 mm Hg) for several hours has been correlated with subsequent a poor outcome This observation suggests that ischaemic damages owing either to ICP-hypertension or to a decrease in CPP are of major importance.

CBF patterns

^{133}Xe studies

The early studies of CBF in HI unveiled an inhomogeneous pattern. During the first days after the trauma CBF differed considerably. High and low CBF values were found, unrelated to the level of $PaCO_2$ and MABP (Fieschi et al. 1974, Overgaard and Tweed 1974, Enevoldsen et al. 1976).

In 21 comatose patients repeated CBF showed some characteristic patterns. In relatively young patients subjected to decompression after cerebral contusion, with or without abnormal brain-stem reflexes, a hyperperfusion phase occurring within 24 hours after the trauma was observed. The duration of this phase differed considerably. In patients with impairment of the brain-stem reflexes this hyperdynamic phase was followed by a period with low CBF. Another pattern with increasing CBF during the first week after the trauma was also observed. In patients with a poor outcome and abnormal brain-stem reflexes, the hyperaemic phase was followed by a period with reduced CBF. In elderly patients with hemispheric cortical lesions and in patients with abnormal brain-stem reflexes but without severe lesions of the cerebral hemispheres, classified as diffuse injury, a low perfusion phase was identified. The duration of the low flow phases might be several weeks (Cold and Jensen 1980).

In a study including 76 patients with HI by Overgaard (1975). The authors found hemispheric ischaemia with CBF < 20 ml in 7 patients, all of whom died or remained apallic. In all patients the brain-stem reflexes were absent or impaired. In 20 patients an initial hemispheric hyperaemia was seen with CBF > 65 ml (initial slope). Other studies indicate that if hyperaemia is present a tendency to normalisation with time occurs (Overgaard and Tweed 1974, Langfitt et al. 1977), whereas persistence of hyperaemia indicates a poor outcome (Fieschi et al. 1974).

In a prospective study of CBF (measured by the ^{133}Xe clearance), $AVDO_2$ and transcranial Doppler in 125 patients with severe HI three distinct haemodynamic phases during the first 2 weeks after injury were documented. Phase 1 (hypoperfusion phase) occurs on the day of injury, and is defined by low CBF, normal flow velocities, normal hemispheric index (ratio between flow velocity in middle cerebral artery and extracranial carotid artery) and normal $AVDO_2$. $CMRO_2$ is approximately 50% of normal during this phase and remains depressed during the second and third phases. In phase 2 (hyperaemic phase, day 1–3), CBF increases, $AVDO_2$ falls, flow velocity rises and the hemispheric index remains low. In Phase 3 (vasospasm phase, Days 4–15), there is a fall in CBF, a further increase in flow velocity, and a pronounced rise in hemispheric index (Martin et al. 1997).

In another study ^{133}Xe flow was performed repeatedly. The lowest flow was observed on the day of injury, and the highest were documented on postinjury days 1 to 5. Patients were divided into three groups based on CBF values obtained during the period of maximum flow. Group 1 had CBF less than 33 ml on all determinations. Group 2 had CBF both less than and greater than or equal to 33 ml. Group 3 and CBF greater than or equal to 33 ml on all measurements. Significant differences across group 1 to 3 regarding mean age, incidence of patients requiring evacuation of intradural haematomas and incidence of abnormal pupils. Favourable neurological outcome at 6 months in group 1 to 3 was 0%, 46% and 59% respectively (Kelly et al. 1997).

Stable Xenon-CT studies

Because methodological errors, especially the "look through" phenomenon may influence the ^{133}Xe measurements, other techniques for CBF measurement in the acute phase of head injury are of interest. CBF has been measured with stable Xenon-computer-tomography within 7 days after the injury. During the first day, patients with an initial GCS score of 3 or 4 and no surgical mass had lower flow than did those with a higher GCS score or mass lesions. In the first 4 hours, those without surgical mass lesions had a mean CBF of 27 ml/100g/min, which rose to 44 ml/100g/min by 24 hours. Patients without surgical mass lesions who died tended to have a lower global CBF than did those with better outcome. Mass lesions were associated with a high global CBF and bi-hemispheric contusions with the lowest flows. By 24 hours after injury global CBF increased in groups that originally had low flows and decreased in those with very high initial flows. By 36–48 hours, most patients had CBF values between 32 and 55 ml/100g/min. Cortical, basal ganglion, and brain-stem blood flow values frequently differed by 25% or more from global averages. Brain-stem CBF varied significantly, but did not correlated with clinical signs of brain-stem dysfunction. Abnormal CO_2 reactivity was found with acute subdural haematoma and diffuse swelling but not with isolated epidural haematoma (Marion et al. 1991).

In a stable Xe-CT study CBF and CBV by mean transit time were measured simultaneously. CBV did not differ from normal values. Generally no correlation between CBF and CBF was found. However, an inverse relationship between CBF and CBV was found. This finding appeared to be consistent with autoregulatory mechanism (Bouma et al. 1993).

Spasms of cerebral vessels

Cerebral spasm

With Doppler technique it has been demonstrated that traumatic subarachnoid haemorrhage is associated with cerebral vasospasm. Thus, middle cerebral artery velocities exceeding 120 cm/sec were observed in 27% of thirty patients (Martin et al. 1992).

High flow velocity is correlated to high CBF, but also to cerebral vasospasm. The ratio between the velocities of blood flow in the middle cerebral artery (V_{MCA}) to the velocity in the internal carotid artery (V_{ICA}) is used as an spasm index. After traumatic brain injury high spasm indices were found in 40% of 35 patients with HI. The increase began as early as 48 h after injury, reached a maximum between days 5 and 7, and lasted until 2 weeks after injury. A significant correlation was found between the occurrence of spasm and the quantity of cisternal or intracerebral blood seen on CT scan (Weber et al. 1990).

In a clinical study of 350 patients with moderate to severe head injury spasms of the intracranial arteries were found in 19%. Narrowing of the internal carotid artery was observed in 18 patients and narrowing of the cerebral arteries at the site of the cerebral contusion was seen in 33 patients (Suwanwela and Suwanwela 1972).

In a series of 96 patients who died after acute head injury there was a relationship between spasm at angiography, the presence of intracranial haematoma, and the ischaemic damage in the ipselateral cortex (MacPherson and Graham 1978). These observation supplement a study by Taneda et al. (1996) who found a close correlation between the main site of the subarachnoid blood and the location of severe vasospasm. Furthermore, development of focal ischaemia in the cerebral territories corresponding to the vasospastic arteries was disclosed. Stepwise logistic regression analysis confirmed that haemodynamically significant vasospasms are a significant predictor of poor outcome, independent of the admission-GCS and age. By combining flow velocity and ^{133}Xe-CBF data the same authors strongly suggest that the important factor influencing outcome is not vasospasm per se, but vasospasm combined with low CBF (Lee et al. 1997).

Cerebral metabolic rate of oxygen ($CMRO_2$)

Level of consciousness

In the acute phase after head injury $CMRO_2$ is low (Bruce et al. 1973, Cold 1978, Obrist et al. 1979, Obrist et al. 1984). A correlation between state of consciousness and $CMRO_2$ has been observed (Langfitt et al. 1979, Muizelaar et al. 1989a). Corte et al. (1997) studied 23 patients with severe HI during the first 48 hours after trauma. CBF varied from 18 to 60 ml/100g/min. $CMRO_2$ was depressed in relation to the severity of injury, ranging from a mean of 0.9 ml/100g/min for GCS 3 to 1.7 ml/100g/min for patients with GCS 6–7.

Outcome

Over a large range on consciousness levels a high $CMRO_2$ indicates a good outcome (Tabaddor et al. 1972, Hass 1976, Jaggi et al. 1990). In a study of 96 patients with severe HI the probability of recovery was correctly predicted in 82% of the patients when age, initial GCS, and occurrence of ICP-hypertension were combined with evaluation of $CMRO_2$ (Jaggi et al. 1990). In deeply comatose patients the correlation between $CMRO_2$ and outcome is poor (Bruce and Langfitt 1976, Cold 1978, Obrist et al. 1984). Thus, values as low as 0.4 ml O_2/100g/min have been found in patients who regained consciousness and recovered (Cold 1978). In one study it was found that patients with the lowest admission GCS and the lowest $CMRO_2$ values, had the poorest 6-months outcome (Corte et al. 1997).

Infarction

In a clinical study $CMRO_2$ and $CMR_{lactate}$ were measured and correlated to CT scanning. It was found that patients showing cerebral infarction at CT scanning exhibited a characteristic cerebral metabolic pattern. A $CMRO_2$ of less that 0.6 γmol O_2/100g/min in one or more studies and a markedly elevated lactate production were observed in these patients (Robertson et al. 1987).

Coupling between CBF and $CMRO_2$

The correlation between $CMRO_2$ and CBF is generally absent (Bruce et al. 1973, Muizelaar et al. 1989a). However, Obrist et al. (1984) found a positive correlation in patients with reduced CBF (below 30 ml). In another study this finding was not documented. Repeated studies at interval of days demonstrated a positive correlation between $CMRO_2$ and CBF in about 50% of the patients. This correlation was found to exist independently of the presence or absence of hyperaemia defined as CBF > 30 ml (Cold 1986).

Estimate of cerebral metabolic rate

Jaggi et al. (1995) used the product of $PaCO_2$ and $AVDO_2$ as an estimate of $CMRO_2$. The estimated $CMRO_2$ was defined as $eCMRO_2 = AVDO_2 \cdot PaCO_2 \cdot CBF/PaCO_2/100$. They argued that the last component equals 100, leaving $eCMRO_2 = AVDO_2 \cdot PaCO_2/100$. In their studies of global $CMRO_2$ and CBF in traumatic brain injury, they found a pretty good correlation between real and estimated $CMRO_2$.

Glucose utilisation

With PET it has been demonstrated that disturbances of glucose metabolism extends beyond the structural abnormalities demonstrated with MR and CT scanning. In a study of three patients anterior temporal dysfunction with decreased glucose metabolism was observed (Langfitt et al. 1986).

Increased CBF relative to $CMRO_2$ could be indicative of increased glycolysis, because normally CBF is coupled functionally to both the cerebral metabolic rate of oxygen and glucose. Using [^{18}F]fluorodeoxyglucose PET technique, hyperglycolysis was found both regionally and globally and was documented in 56% of patients studied within 8 days of injury (Bergsneider et al. 1997). Increased glucose utilisation is considered as a compensatory metabolic response that adjusts an acute energy demand more promptly than oxidative metabolism (Bergsneider et al. 1997). Increased glucose utilisation most likely causes tissue acidosis if oxygen utilisation is inhibited. The severity of these changes depends on the actual blood glucose level, as demonstrated in experimental cerebral ischaemia.

Bergsneider et al. (2000) studied the correlation between $CMR_{glucose}$ and the level of consciousness within the first month following traumatic brain injury in 42 patients. Reduction of glucose utilisation was found in 88% of the studies. The level of consciousness did not correlate with global $CMR_{glucose}$ or severity of the head injury, and intraparenchymal haemorrhagic lesions were associated with either focal $CMR_{gluocse}$ reduction or elevation.

Cerebral autoregulation (CA)

The CA has been found to be impaired in patients with severe HI (Fieschi et al. 1974, Enevoldsen et al. 1976, Cold and Jensen 1978, Enevoldsen and Jensen 1978, Muizelaar et al. 1989b). With a 16 channel cerebrograph placed over the most severely injured hemisphere, regional loss of CA was observed in 83% of the comatose patients. In patients recovering from HI an improvement of CA has generally been observed (Cold and Jensen 1978). Even in patients with mild HI (GCS 13–15) impaired CA is found in 28% (Jürgen et al. 1997). In 31 patients with diffuse brain injury type III global autoregulation was preserved in 32% and abolished in 68% of the patients (Sahuquillo et al. 1998). With laser Doppler flowmetry the relationship between flow velocity and CPP was studied.Changes in this relationship with time was found, indicating improvement or deterioration in autoregulation. Three patterns were identified. 1) intact CA. 2) transient loss; and 3) persistent loss of CA. Patients with intact CA favoured a good outcome, while patients with persistence of impairment had a poor outcome (Lam et al. 1997).

Pressure- and volume controlled studies of CA

In haemorrhagic shock models pressure controlled haemorrhage has been widely used. However, pressure controlled models have been criticised because it is necessary to re-infuse blood in order to keep the pressure constant, and this procedure influences the animals natural homeostatic responses to haemorrhage. In contrast volume-controlled haemorrhagic shock models are more suited to replicate important aspects of the clinical situation of haemorrhagic shock, since the physiological homeostatic responses can take place. In conscious rats subjected to volume-controlled haemorrhage the following results were found. During less severe haemorrhage CBF was significantly higher than in the control group. During severe haemorrhage CBF remained unchanged, although significant increases in rCBF could be detected in many brain structures. The mean coefficient of variation of CBF increased, indicating a larger heterogeneity of CBF (Waschke et al. 1996).

Relationship between CBF and cardiac output

In a series of severely head-injured patients cardiac output and CBF were measured simultaneously. Blood pressure was manipulated with phenylephrine or trimethaphane and blood viscosity by mannitol infusion. No correlation existed between the changes in cardiac output and the changes in CBF, regardless of the status of blood pressure autoregulation. A significant increase in CBF was found after administration of mannitol when autoregulation was defective. The data support the hypothesis that, within broad limits, CBF is not related to cardiac output, even when autoregulation is impaired (Bouma and Muizelaar 1990).

Hypocapnia and cerebral autoregulation

Hypocapnia improves cerebral autoregulation in the acute phase of brain injury. Another study indicate that regions with false" autoregulation is changed to regions with impaired autoregulation (Cold et al. 1981). With transcranial Doppler technique Newell et al. (1996) found that autoregulation improved during hyperventilation, and the degree of improvement of CA was correlated with the CO_2 reactivity.

Tissue peaks

Regions close to cerebral contusion are especially exposed to CBF increase when CPP is augmented. Tissue peaks are provoked in these regions (Enevoldsen et al. 1976, Cold and Jensen 1978, Enevoldsen and Jensen 1978). Later studies with Xe-CT scanning and SPECT indicated that regions with cerebral contusion were more or less ischaemic. So tissue peak indicate hyperaemia in the surrounding tissue.

Lactate and false CA

A biphasic correlation between ventricular fluid lactate and the slope of the CBF/CPP relationship was found in early studies. This finding suggests that hemispheric CA is preserved at low levels of lactate, impaired at levels ranging from 3–5 mmol/l, and preserved at levels above 5 mmol/l (Cold and Jensen 1978). In another study a dissociation between CA and CO_2 reactivity was found. Thus, the CO_2 reactivity was impaired in patients with apparently intact CA, while the CO_2 reactivity was normal in patients with impaired CA (Enevoldsen and Jensen 1978). These observation suggest the occurrence of "false" CA as well. These observations together with findings indicating intact CA during the first days after the trauma have raised the question whether intact CA is a false phenomenon (Fischi et al. 1974).

The mechanism of false CA is explained by an increase in tissue pressure owing to leakage of the blood-brain barrier during angiotensin infusion. In this way an increase in MABP provokes an increase in tissue pressure. The result is an unchanged or even reduced CPP. Clinical studies of CA in patients with severe HI rarely support this view, because the false reaction is not associated allways with an increase in ICP (Fieschi et al. 1974, Cold and Jensen 1978, Enevoldsen and Jensen 1978). That false CA is a fairly common phenomenon is supported by studies of CA during moderate and pronounced hypocapnia. In contradiction to clinical studies of CA in cerebral tumours and apoplexy (Paulson et al. 1972), a decrease in $PaCO_2$ does not improve CA in patients with HI. On the contrary, hypocapnia changes regions with intact ("false") CA to regions with impaired CA, suggesting an improvement from a state of "false" CA to impaired CA (Cold et al. 1981).

Whatever the reason for "false" CA, mechanisms other than an increase in ICP measured as intraventricular pressure might be responsible. It has been proposed that intraventricular pressure rarely outlines brain tissue pressure, and tissue gradients might exist within the brain.

ICP gradients have been documented experimentally (Kuchiwaka et al. 1992, Wolfla et al. 1996) and in clinical studies (Sahuquillo et al. 1999, Bundgaard and Cold 2000). However, bifrontal studies of subarachnoid pressure in severe HI indicate that pressure gradients seldom exists (Yano et al. 1987).

Transient hyperaemic response

Transcranial flow velocity during carotid compression has been used in the evaluation of cerebral autoregulation. In practice two 5-second carotid compressions with an interval of 60 seconds are used. In healthy volunteers sufficient time for the cerebrovascular system to recover from the previous compression occurs (Smielewski et al. 1996). The transient hyperaemic response ratio (THRR: the ratio of the hyperaemic flow velocity recorded after carotid release, and the pre-compression baseline velocity) is used as index. With this technique 47 patients with HI was studied. The hyperaemic response proved to be lower in patients who exhibited a poor clinical grade at admission (GSC < 6), and it was lower in patients achieving a poor outcome. Loss of post-compression hyperaemia occurred when CPP fell below 50 mm Hg (Smielewski et al. 1997).

Pressure-reactivity index

Czosnyka et al. (1998) developed a method based upon slow waves in blood pressure and ICP. A pressure-reactivity index (PRx) was calculated as a moving correlation coefficient between 40 consecutive samples of values for ICP and arterial blood pressure averaged over 5 seconds.A positive PRx correlated with high ICP, low admission GCS and poor outcome at 6 months after injury. During the first two days following injury, PRx was positive in patients with unfavourable outcome.

Level of CPP, vasoreactive cascade

Clinically, it has often been observed that an increase in MABP is followed by a decrease in ICP, the net result being an increased CPP. Rosner (1987) studied this relationship systematically, and defined the vasoreactive cascade where a decrease in MABP elicits a decrease in cerebral vascular resistance given rise to an increase in CBV and ICP, and thus a potential fall in CPP. This cascade only exists when CA is intact. Another study indicates that lowering MABP in patients with intact CA causes a steep increase in ICP, while rising blood pressure did not change the ICP. When CA was impaired, ICP varied directly with blood pressure (Bouma et al. 1992).

CO_2 reactivity

Relation to outcome

CO_2 reactivity is impaired or abolished in the acute phase of HI (Fieschi et al. 1974, Cold et al. 1977a). In a recent study by Sahuquillo et al. (1998) global CO_2 reactivity, measured by the change in $AVDO_2$, was only normal in 2 of 31 patients with diffuse brain swelling. A low CO_2 reactivity indicate a poor outcome (Overgaard and Tweed 1974, Cold et al. 1977a, Messeter et al. 1986, Tenjin et al. 1990). In a study by Shalén and co-workers (1991), three of 16 patients with intact CO_2 reactivity died (19%) and 12 of 16 patients (75%) reached good recovery/moderate disability. In the group of patients with impaired CO_2 reactivity (Δ CBF/$\Delta PaCO_2$ mm Hg < 1.0) 11 of 22 patients (50%) died, and only 3 patients (14%) reached good recovery or moderate disability. An improvement of CO_2 reactivity has been observed in patients who recover the acute phase (Cold et al. 1977a).

Tissue peak

In patients subjected to intraarterially Xe^{133} studies tissue peaks are often localised to regions with cerebral contusion. Hypocapnia abolished these fast compartments (Enevoldsen et al. 1976, Cold et al. 1977b). In these tissue peak regions the CO_2 reactivity is fairly high (Cold et al. 1977b).Tissue peak hyperaemia is not localised to the ischaemic region with contusion, but is supposed to be localised to the surrounding tissue. In other studies high hemispheric or global CBF is associated with a high CO_2 reactivity (Obrist et al. 1984, Cold 1986, Cold 1989b).
Low CBF
In regions with very low hemispheric CBF hypocapnia decreases CBF even further. Clinical studies suggest that hyperventilation even in regions with moderate or severe oligaemia might reduce CBF (Cold 1989a)

Regional differences

In a recent study by Marion and Bouma (1991) Xe-CT scanning was used. They found that hemispheric CO_2 reactivity ranged from 1.3 to 8.5%/mm Hg $PaCO_2$. Lobar, cerebellar, basal ganglia, and brainstem CO_2 reactivities frequently varied from the mean global value by more than 25%. The greatest variability occurred in patients with acute subdural haematoma, and patients with diffuse injuries.

Inverse steal

In hemispheric studies with the intraarterially Xe^{133} method inverse steal reactions was observed in 11% of all regions in the acute phase (Cold et al. 1977b).

Lactate

In patients with cortical contusion a correlation between ventricular fluid lactate and the CO_2 reactivity has been observed. This finding suggest that the increase in lactate, probably caused by ischaemia in the contused region, provokes dilatation of cerebral vessels and hyperaemia in surrounding areas (Cold et al. 1977a).

Relation to "false" CA

Studies of CA and CO_2 reactivity indicate that "false" or inverse reactions to angiotensin-induced MABP increase are found in regions with low or abolished CO_2 reactivity (Enevoldsen and Jensen 1978, Cold et al. 1981).

$CMRO_2$

A negative correlation between $CMRO_2$ and $PaCO_2$ was observed by Gordon and Bergvall (1977). During hypocapnia an increase in $CMRO_2$ despite a decrease in CBF has been observed (Gennarelli et al. 1979). $AVDO_2$ predominantly represents extraction of global oxygen, whereas mean CBF in these studies represents cortical flow in one hemisphere. Thus, CBF in the contralateral hemisphere, and in the deep structures of the brain are not involved. Under these circumstance the accuracy of the measurement is critical. In a study where the calculation of CBF was based on 32 detectors (16 placed over each hemisphere), hypocapnia did not change $CMRO_2$ (Cold 1989b). Generally it is believed that $CMRO_2$ is unchanged during hypocapnia.

Free radical formation

In experimental studies it has been shown that absence of CO_2 reactivity are induced by posttraumatic initiation of arachidonic acid metabolism by cyclooxygenase with formation of oxygen radicals. Treatment with cyclooxygenase inhibitor, indomethacin, and treatment with superoxide dismutase and catalase normalises CO_2 reactivity (Wei et al. 1981, Kontos et al. 1981). N-acetylcystein, another oxygen free radical scavenger has the same effect (Ellis et al. 1991).

Barbiturate reactivity

The effect of barbiturate upon CBF and $CMRO_2$ is reduced in the acute phase of HI. In clinical studies abolished or decreased CO_2- and barbiturate reactivities indicate a poor prognosis. In contrast, preserved CO_2 reactivity is associated with an intact effect of barbiturate on CBF and $CMRO_2$, and indicate a good recovery (Messeter et al. 1986, Nordström et al. 1988).

In another study the barbiturate reactivity, as indicated by the change in $CMRO_2$ or regionally as the change in rCBF after a bolus doses of thiopentone 5 mg/kg was found to depend on the $CMRO_2$ level before barbiturate injection. Levels of $CMRO_2$ ranging from 1.0 and 1.1 ml O_2/100g/min was associated with abolished barbiturate reactivity. However, great inter- and intraindividual differences in barbiturate reactivities were found, prohibiting a general statement. The relationship between CO_2 reactivity and barbiturate reactivity was found to be poor, although highly significant correlations could be found in some patients suffering from severe HI (Cold 1989b). In another study from the same group $CMRO_2$ values and barbiturate reactivity were studied with intervals of 24 hours during the first 4 days after the acute trauma. The $CMRO_2$ values as well as the barbiturate reactivities were depressed in these deeply unconscious patients. Only in a subgroup of patients with relatively high $CMRO_2$ a metabolic suppression by barbiturate was found (**Dahl et al. 1991**).

Neurological assessment and monitoring

Glasgow coma scale (GCS) assessment

GCS was introduced by Teasdale and Jennett (1974). It has now been used for almost three decades as a convenient numerical characterisation of the severity of head injury that can be obtained reliably by physicians, nurses, and other medical personnel (Fielding and Rowley 1990, Braakman et al. 1977). GCS is a powerful independent predictor of outcome (Marshall et al. 1983, Jennett et al. 1977, Marshall et al. 1991).

Prehospital care often involves muscular relaxation, sedation, and intubation. Under these circumstances GCS assessment is difficult. A pseudoscore of 1 for the verbal (eye opening component) portion of the GCS has been proposed. Other have suggested a different scoring system that take into account untestable areas, but still enables the quantification of brain injury severity. In Sweden the reaction level scale (RLS) has been used since 1984. This system allows the assessment of all patients with a head injury, including those who are intubated or have severe periorbital swelling (Stålhammar and Starmark 1986). A 100-point scoring system including information about respiration, blood pressure pulse, temperature, and pupil size and reactivity as well as the variables of the GCS was introduced by Bouzart and Lindemuth (1978). Another screening system is the Maryland Coma Score, in which the result is a fraction calculated by dividing the patients GCS sum score by the total possible points from which that patients could be tested (Salcman et al. 1981).

To overcome the recognized problem in applying the GCS to infants other pediatric coma scales have been described. Many of these scales incorporate motor and verbal responses not appropiate for children less than two years of age or require knowledge of complex brain stem/or ocular responses which are not practical for use. Recently, a new scale (Infant Face Scale") was introduced for children less than 2 years of age. This scale demonstrates improved interrater reliability in comparison to the GCS (Durham et al. 2000).

In a recent survey Marion and Carlier (1994) revealed important inter-centre and intra-centre differences of opinion regarding how the initial GCS scores are obtained. Such differences make it difficult to interpret the results of head injury studies that use the initial GCS scores to describe injury severity. A GCS of 13 to 15 is one of the primary criteria in the classification of mild injury.

In a study of 3370 patients, consecutively admitted to trauma centre with non-missile HI, positive loss of consciousness, and admission GCS of 13 to 15 outcome were analysed. A significant difference between the frequency of positive CT scans and the need for neurosurgical interventions in patients with GCS of 13 versus 14, and 14 versus 15 were found (Culotta et al. 1996).

Assessment according to CT scanning

Marshall et al. (1991) proposed a new classification according to CT findings: According to this classification the following groups are identified. Duffuse injury I: No visible intracranial pathology seen on CT scan; Diffuse injury II: Cisterns are present with midline shift 0–5 mm, and/or high or mixed-density lesions ≤ 25 cc; Diffuse injury III: Cisterns compressed or absent with midline shift 0–5 mm and/or high or mixed density lesions ≤ 25 cc; Diffuse injury IV: Midline shift > 5 mm without high or mixed-density lesions > 25 cc; Evacuated mass lesion: Any lesion surgically evacuated; Nonevacuated mass lesion: High or mixed-density lesion > 25 cc not surgical evacuated.

In a recent study, including 94 patients, none patients in diffuse injury I presented intracranial hypertension. In diffuse group III with bilateral brain swelling had a 62% risk of developing increased ICP. All patients in diffuse injury IV had refractory ICP-hypertension. In the catagory of evacuated mass lesion two thirds of the patients presented an ICP-hypertension. 85% of patients with a non-evacuated mass lesion showed an increased ICP (Poca et al. 1998).

Neuroworsening

Neuroworsening is defined as by the occurrence of one or more of the following objective criteria: A spontaneous decrease in Glasgow Coma Scale motor score of ≥ 2 points, compared with the previous examination, a new loss of pupillary reactivity, interval development of pupillary asymmetry of ≥ 2 mm, or deterioration in neurological status sufficient to warrent immediate medical or surgical intervention (Morris et al. 1998). Juul et al. (2000) recently analysed 427 patients randomized to a selfotel outcome study. They defined neurological deterioration or "neuro worsening" as episodes of one or more of the following: A spontaneous decrease in GCS motor scores of 2 points or more from the previous examination; a further loss of pupillary reactivity; development of pupillary asymmetry greater than 1 mm; deterioration in the neurological status sufficient to warrant immediate medical or surgical intervention. Using these principles they found that treatment protocols for the management of HI should emphasize the immediate reduction of raised ICP to less than 20 mm Hg if possible, and a CPP greater than 60 mm Hg appears to have little influence on the outcome of the patients.

Doppler flow velocity

Flow velocity measurement has gained increasing interest during the acute phase of HI. In one study all patients with infarction had unilateral elevation of mean blood velocity in the territory of the relevant cerebral vessel. On the other hand, infarction never developed in any patients with increased mean blood velocity that was associated with global hyperaemia as evaluated by $AVDO_2$ (Chan et al. 1992). On the other hand, it has been demonstrated that traumatic SAH is associated with cerebral vasospasm. Thus, middle cerebral artery velocity exceeding 120 cm/sec was observed in 27% of thirty patients (Martin et al. 1992).

In a study including 96 patients both internal carotid artery and middle cerebral artery velocities were depressed during the first 3 days after the trauma, and then increased to maximum between day 5 and 7 (Steiger et al. 1994). In patients with severe HI the ratio between velocity in middle cerebral artery (MCA) and the internal carotid artery seems to correlate well with the distribution of CBF studied with SPECT (Romner et al. 1996).

Newell et al. (1997) evaluated haemodynamic responses with transcranial Doppler in 22 HI patients. They found a decrease in flow velocity during A and B waves. Dynamic cerebral autoregulation, and CO_2 reactivity were reduced within 48 h of admission. Mannitol caused an increase in MCA velocity, and changes in flow velocity during barbiturate treatment was correlated to ICP response as well as to the CO_2 reactivity.

Biochemical Studies

Lactate in CSF

Experimental studies

In cats subjected to fluid-percussion trauma the concentration of lactate in brain tissue, CSF, and blood increased in proportion to the severely of the injury. The initial elevation of CSF lactate may reflect the systemic response to trauma; the secondary rise of CSF lactate levels may be due to slow seepage of lactate produced by brain tissue into the CSF space (Iano et al. 1988).

Human studies

In clinical studies of acute HI a high concentration of lumbar CSF lactate (Kurze et al. 1966, Zupping 1970, Crockard and Taylor 1972, King et al. 1974, Sood et al. 1980), suboccipital CSF lactate (Metzel and Zimmermann 1971, Seitz and Ocker 1977) and ventricular fluid lactate (Fieschi et al. 1974, Overgaard and Tweed 1974, Cold et al. 1975, Enevoldsen et al. 1976, Enevoldsen and Jensen 1978a) have been observed during the first days after trauma.

Generally, an initially or persistently high lactate level indicates a poor outcome. In patients with severe head injury, however, the interpretation of increased CSF lactate is difficult owing to contamination by blood (Granholm 1969), hypocapnia (Granholm and Siesjö 1969), Cold et al. 1975), and CNS infection, all of which will increase CSF lactate. In patients with severe HI, subjected to controlled ventilation with $PaCO_2$ ranging from 34–40 mm Hg a high concentration of lactate in ventricular fluid seems of prognostic value (Cold et al. 1975b. Cold 1981). In another study of patients with head injury subjected to moderate hypocapnia, the level of ventricular fluid lactate during the first four posttraumatic days was significantly and persistently higher in patients with a poor outcome. In contrast, the concentration in patients with a good outcome declined rapidly within 48 hours. In the same study lactic-acidosis was found to be associated with a high ICP level (DeSalles et al. 1986). In another study the increase in ventricular fluid lactate correlated to a decrease in extracellular pH (DeSalles et al. 1987b).

Creatine kinase in CSF

Creatine-kinase-BB isoenzyme activity has been shown to rise very rapidly in CSF after parenchymal brain damage (Maas 1977, Rabow and Hedman 1979, Bakay and Ward 1983). An increase in serum creatine kinase-BB and neuron specific enolase have also been demonstrated (Skogseid et al. 1992). The increase in CSF may be due to destruction of cell membranes with release of the enzyme into the extracellular space and seepage into the CSF.

Clinical studies have shown that creatine kinase isoenzyme activity in CSF is of prognostic significance (Kaste et al. 1981, Nordby and Urdal 1982, Rabow and Hedman 1985). Studies by Rabow et al. (1986), however, indicate that no significant correlation between the activity of the enzyme and outcome among surviving patients could be obtained. The same investigators found that the creatine kinase activity reached nadir a few hours after the trauma and the activity of creatine kinase had a monoexponential drop with a half-time of approximately 10 hours. In a later study the relation between contusion volume, as estimated by CT scan and CSF-creatine-kinase-BB was insignificant (Rabow et al. 1989). Other clinical studies show a negative correlation between the activity of cyclic AMP and the coma grade following HI (Fleicher et al. 1977).

Nitric oxide in CSF

Under pathological conditions NO plays a deleterious role, potentially leading to disturbances in cerebral blood flow autoregulation (Faraci and Brian 1994), and direct neurotoxicity and cellular injury (Chao et al. 1992, Merrill et al. 1993, Albina et al. 1993). Nitrite and nitrate concentrations are increased in CSF in patients with meningitis, and reduced in patients with neurodegenerative disorders. Thus, nitric oxide production in the CNS appears to be increased as part of an inflammatory response. In experimental brain trauma local inflammatory responses have been demonstrated, and an increase in CSF nitrite and nitrate concentrations peaking at 30 to 42 h after trauma has been demonstrated in human head injury (Clark et al. 1996).

Hyperglycaemia

Experimental studies

Hyperglycaemia in rats causes secondary ischaemia after cortical impact injury. Thus, the contusion volume increases significantly, and the density of normal appearing neurones in the CA1 area of the hippocampus is reduced (Cherian et al. 1997). Another experimental study indicate that posttraumatic glucose infusion significantly increases the damage caused by controlled cortical impact injury. The adverse effect on neurological outcome could partly, but not completely, be explained by the temperature effects of glucose infusion, which increases brain temperature (Cherian et al. 1998).

Human studies

Short term hyperglycaemia related to stress after the injury coupled with an impaired cerebral oxidative metabolism is supposed to be the reason for the initially high lactate level (Clifton et al. 1981, Clifton et al. 1983). However, the increase in ventricular fluid lactate outlasts the acute response to injury, and the increase in lactate concentration may reflect a dysfunction in cerebral cellular metabolism caused by the injury itself and aggravated by secondary insults (DeSalles et al. 1987a).

S-100B

S-100B, a small demeric cytosolic protein exists in various forms, depending on its and β chain structure. The β-form, which is called S-100B, is found in astroglia and Schwann cells. The protein is highly specific for tissue of the nervous system, as well as for malignant melanom cells. Elevated levels of serum S-100B have been reported in patients after minor head injury (Ingebrigtsen and Romner 1996, Ingebrigtsen et al. 1999). Logistic analysis revealed S-100B as an independent predictor of outcome, and persistent elevation of S-100B levels for 2 to 6 days, even in patients with favourable outcome, may reflect ongoing secondary damage after severe head injury (Raabe et al. 1999). In another study of patients with severe head injury high serum concentrations of neuron specific enolase and S-100 were significantly correlated to poor neurological outcome (KcKeating et al. 1998).

Microdialysis

A new aspect of chemical monitoring of neurosurgical intensive care patients is intracerebral microdialysis. With this technique the concentrations of energy-related metabolites including lactate, pyruvate, hypoxanthine, glutamate, aspartate, taurine and glycine in the extracellular fluid ca be monitored continuously (Persson and Hillered 1992, Landolt et al. 1994). Microdialysis was used in a recent study of HI. Elevated extracellular lactate, reduced glucose and an elevated lactate/glucose ratio were observed with cerebral hypoxia and ischaemia, and elevated lactate and an increased lactate/glucose ratio correlation with death (Goodman et al. 1999). Seizure activity is accompanied by a 90% increase in lactate, lasting 60–90 minutes (During et al. 1994).

During high ICP of low CPP, microdialysis helps in determining how serious it affects brain tissue and the necessity to intervene pharmacologically and/or surgically. After interventions, microdialysis shows the resulting effects on brain chemistry.

Microdialysis studies of patients with severe head injury have demonstrated relative increases in extracellular K^+ and glutamate in the acute phase. Activation of excitoxicity or efflux of potassium ions into the extracellular space leading to spreading depression were considered underlying mechanisms. A strong relationship exists between elevated levels of excitatory amino acids and high ICP after traumatic brain injury (Bullock et al. 1994). In another study, including 83 consecutive severe HI patients it was found that the magnitude of glutamate correlatied with 6-months outcome and with high ICP (Koura et al. 1998).

Multiparametric monitoring

The main monitoring approach currently used in severe head injury is measurement of ICP and MABP combined with intermittent estimate of $PaCO_2$ and PaO_2. New brain function multiprobe systems have been developed combining these classical parameters with tissue oxygen tension, local CBF, brain temperature, microdialysis etc. Mayevsky et al. (1998) described a system, which enabled monitoring of the following parameters continuously in real time from the surface of the cortex: ICP, tissue blood flow and volume, intramitochondrial NADH redox state, direct current steady potential, electrocorticography and tissue temperature. Clear correlations were recorded between haemodynamic, metabolic, ionic and electrical activities under various treatments administered to patients with severe head injury.

In another study combined ICP, CPP, laser Doppler flowmetry was performed. Over the entire interval of continuous monitoring for all patients, 97% of local CBF data was at ischaemic levels below a CPP of 70 mm Hg. For CPP above 70 mm Hg, local CBF data had considerable dispersion, ranging from ischaemia (71%), to normal (19%), and hyperaemic (10%) levels. Autoregulation was found to be impaired or absent in all monitored patients (Miller et al. 1998).

Czosnyka et al. (1996) reviewed the principles of multimodal monitoring and assessment of cerebral haemodynamic reserve after severe head injury. Their experiences are based on measurement of ICP, CPP, flow velocity, jugular bulb saturation, brain tissue oxygenation and microdialysis.

Using a multiparametric monitoring system Mayecsky et al. (1996), in studies of patients with severe HI, found evidence for the occurrence of direct current potential shifts, consistent with spreading depression.

$AVDO_2$ and lactate/oxygen index (LOI)

Correlation between CBF and $AVDO_2$ is generally is poor. However, in a study by Robertson et al. (1989) $AVDO_2$ and $AVD_{lactate}$ were studied together with global CBF, and the lactate-oxygen index ($-AVD_{lactate}/AVDO_2$). When data from all patients were analysed, including those with cerebral ischaemia and those without, $AVDO_2$ had only a modest correlation with CBF. When patients with ischaemia, indicated by an increased $CMR_{lactate}$, were excluded from the analysis, CBF and $AVDO_2$ had a much improved correlation. Most patients with a very low CBF would have been misclassified as having a normal or increased CBF based on the $AVDO_2$ alone. However, when measurements of $AVDO_2$ were supplemented with $AVD_{lactate}$, four distinct CBF patterns could be distinguished. Patients with an ischaemia/infarction pattern typically had LOI of 0.08 or greater and a variable $AVDO_2$. The three non-ischaemic CBF patterns had a LOI of less than 0,08, and could be classified according to the $AVDO_2$: Patients with normal CBF (mean 42 ml/100g/min) had an $AVDO_2$ between 1.3 and 3 γmol/ml. A CBF pattern of hyperaemia (mean CBF 53 ml/100g/min was caracterised by an $AVDO_2$ of less than 1.3 γmol/ml. A compensated hypoperfusion CBF pattern (mean CBF 23 ml/100g/min) was identified by an $AVDO_2$ of more than 3 γmol/min. The study suggests that reliable estimates of CBF may be made from $AVDO_2$ and $AVD_{lactate}$ measurements.

In another study $AVDO_2$ was followed repeatedly in traumatic head injury before and after mannitol treatment and before and after craniotomy for mass expanding hematoma. The results indicate that limited improvement in an elevated $AVDO_2$ after treatment consisting of either craniotomy or mannitol administration for ICP-hypertension was associated with delayed cerebral infarction and poor outcome. By contrast, large improvements in $AVDO_2$ was associated with favourable outcome and no evidence of delayed cerebral ischaemia (leRoux et al. 1997).

The interpretation of AVDO2, however, must be taken with reservation, because in acute anaemia a decreased $AVDO_2$ yields false ischaemic values of LOI, when net global cerebral oxygenation and lactate production are normal (Cruz et al. 1994).

Although it has been argued that a widened $AVDO_2$ combined with a low CBF almost always have been associated with a poor neurological outcome, other investigators do not agree. In a prospective, intervention study including 205 adults with acute, essentially isolated brain trauma initially increased AVDO2 appears to indicate global cerebral viability rather than cerebral ischaemia (Cruz 1996).

CO_2 reactivity and autoregulation determined by $AVDO_2$

When $CMRO_2$ is considered constant, changes in $AVDO_2$ reflects changes in CBF. Under these circumstance relative changes in $AVDO_2$ can be viewed as inverse changes in CBF, and used for evaluation of CO_2 reactivity and cerebral autoregulation. With this technique Sahuquillo et al. (1996) found that of 39 patients with severe head injury 20% were classified as having impaired autoregulation and 18% impaired CO_2 reactivity. All patients with impaired CO_2 reactivity also had impaired autoregulation.

Jugular oxygen saturation

Continuous monitoring of jugular oxygen saturation with fiberoptic oxygen catheters has been practiced for some years. A low jugular oxygen saturation indicate cerebral oligaemia caused by hypocapnia, fall in arterial oxygen content and decrease in CPP. Continuous monitoring of jugular saturation results in rapid detection of these events with the possibility to normalise cerebral circulation (Cruz 1988). Desaturation periods was found very frequently within the first 48 h after trauma. Hypocapnia was associated with 45% of the episodes, hypoperfusion 22% and raised ICP was found in 9% (Lewis et al. 1995).

The use of jugular bulb catheters has been debated. It has been stressed that intraoperative monitoring of venous oxygen saturation is of value for detecting and treating cerebral venous desaturation (Matta et al. 1994). Monitoring of bulb saturation with optimizing cerebral extraction of oxygen, and the level of CPP has been claimed to result in better outcome than when CPP is managed alone (Cruz 1998).

Accuracy of unilateral measurements have been discussed. Thus Metz et al. (1998) found that mean and maximum bilateral venous saturation difference varied between 1,4% to 21% and 8.1% to 44.3% respectively, suggesting that the reliability of unilateral venous bulb saturation is questionable (Metz et al. 1998).

Ischaemic threshold of venous saturation

In experimental studies of non-traumatized cats thresholds for brain energy failure were reported as being associated with cerebral venous oxygen content levels of 2 vol% corresponding to a venous saturation about 30 (Sutton et al. 1990). In a study presented by Cruz (1993) neurological deterioration in patients with severe head injury might occur at jugular venousoxygen content ranging from 3.5 to 4,5 vol% dependent upon the total haemoglobin content.

A clear and definite threshold of jugular desaturation as sign of global cerebral ischaemia has, however, not been defined. Threshold of 55% has been proposed, suggesting that below this level cerebral oxygenation is critical (Dearden 1991). Whether this threshold is of clinical importance were studied recently. In a retrospective study jugular venous saturation was classified as high at ≥ 75% and low at 55% or less. A high venous saturation occurred in 19% of patients. There was no consistent relationship between venous saturation and CBF or CPP. High venous saturation was associated with a higher mortality and a poorer neurological outcome, and it was concluded that high venous saturation is a heterogeneous condition, more than a global phenomenon (Cormio et al. 1999).

Bilateral studies of venous oxygen saturation suggest that the reliability of a single estimation is questionable, and it is not possible to identify the most appropriate side for monitoring (Stocchetti et al. 1994). Moreover, Latronico et al. (2000) evaluated whether bilateral monitoring of saturation, in addition to standard monitoring, results in modification of the management of severe head trauma. They found that discrepancies in simultaneous bilateral samples were substantial and gave rise to relevant interpretation problems, and that imtermittent saturation monitoring did not substantially influence the management of the patients.

Cerebral haemodynamic reserve

Cruz et al. (1991) introduced a new index, the cerebral haemodynamic reserve (CHR). CHR was assessed as the ratio of changes in global cerebral oxygen extraction to changes in CPP as a result of spontaneous increases in ICP. During the course of hyperventilation ($PaCO_2$ in the range of 20 mm Hg) for ICP control below 20 mm Hg observations were made over the initial 48 hours postinjury. Despite normal CPP ICP elevations to 20 mm Hg were associated with compromised CHR, as evidenced by decreases in jugular oxygenation directly attributed to the ICP increases. In 27% of the observations CHR was preserved as evidenced by no changes or increases in jugular oxygenation when ICP increased. The CHR improved on the second day, suggesting an improved tolerance of the cerebral hemodynamics to ICP increases. The authors concluded that under circumstances of profound hyperventilation, ICP elevations within the normal CPP range may result in decreased cerebral oxygenation.

Near-infrared spectroscopy (NIRS)

NIRS is a continuous direct, noninvasive monitoring device of cerebral oxygenation and cerebral blood volume. Near-infrared spectroscopy performed in the emergency room reliably identified the presence of a traumatic intracranial haematoma in each of 40 patients in whom a CT scan also revealed the presence of a haematoma (Gopinath et al. 1993). Based on the difference in absorbency of light at 760 nM between the two hemispheres Gopinath et al. (1995) found that an increase in this difference occurred prior to an increase in ICP in 24 of 27 patients with delayed haematoma. In children NIRS reliable detects changes in cerebral haemodynamics. With this monitoring system earlier detection of the effects of intervention for cerebral oxygen desaturation and/or changes in CBV is possible (Adelson et al. 1998).

Correlation between jugular bulbus oximetry and near-infrared spectroscopy

Tissue oxygen saturation determined by near-infrared spectroscopy does not reflect changes in cerebral oxygenation detected by the jugular bulb oximetry. The discrepancy may be explained by inadequate in the algorithm used to filter out extracranial components (Lewis et al. 1996). In a study of 31 patients with head injury or subarachnoid hemorrage NIRS were compared to ICP and regional brain tissue pO2. Limited correlations and low sensitivity were found (Buchner et al. 2000) In another comparative study of severe closed head injury it was concluded that cerebral oxygen saturation assessed by near-infrared spectroscopy does not adequately reflect changes in jugular venous oxygen saturation. Changes in arterio-venous partitioning, infrared-spectroscopy contamination by extracranial signal, algorithm errors, and dissimilar tissue sampling may explain this discrepancy (Ter Minassian et al. 1999).

Brain tissue oxygen tension

In order to avoid secondary cerebral ischaemia caused by hypotension, hypocapnia and low CPP, brain tissue oxygen tension monitoring is a logical step. Brain tissue oxygen tension reflects the balance between the oxygen offered by the cerebral blood flow and the oxygen consumption by the brain tissue. Using a Clark-type microelectrode placed via a transcranial bolt into the cerebral white matter it is possible to monitor brain tissue PO_2. Dinjs et al. (1997) reported acceptable stability and complication rates for the Clark-type microelectrode used in 70 patients for 1–6 days. Monitoring brain tissue PO_2 with fiberoptic sensor technology also appears feasible (McKinley et al. 1996, Mc Kinley et al. 1997).

In 17 patients with severe head injury brain tissue oxygen tension after initially low values at day zero after the trauma, increased together with an increase in flow velocity. This relative hyperaemic phase on days 3 and 4 was followed by a decrease in oxygen tension the following days. During the first 3 days after the trauma a paradoxical increase in brain tissue oxygen tension was found in some patients subjected to hypocapnia. Thereafter a fall in oxygen tension was observed, indicating an increased risk of ischaemia by hypocapnia (Dinjs et al. 1996).

In another study brain tissue PO_2 measurement with Licox and Paratrend probes were compared. There were no significant difference in brain tissou oxygen tension with the two probes. In pericontusional tissue brain tissue PO_2 is decreased compared to normal. In contusional brain tissue PO_2 was always below the hypoxic threshold (10 mm Hg), and when inspired oxygen fraction was increased to 100%, no change in brain tissue oxygen tension was observed (Sarrafzadeh et al. 1998).

Outcome

Ischaemic periods, defined as brain tissue PO_2 below 10 mm Hg for longer than 15 min, are associated with unfavourable outcome (Kiening et al. 1996, van den Brink et al. 1998). In another study, including 35 patients with GCS $\leq$ 8 56% of the patients with more than 300 min of brain tissue $O_2 < 10$ mm Hg died, 22% had an unfavourable outcome and 22% an favourable outcome (Bardt et al 1998).

CPP

Kiening et al. (1996) studied brain tissue PO_2 during changes of CPP. If CPP dropped to below 40 mm Hg, and was pharmacologically increased to 60 mm Hg, or more, brain tissue PO_2 increased from 13 to 19 mm Hg. If, however, initial CPP was above 60 mm Hg further increase in CPP to above 80 mm Hg had no significant effect on brain tissue oxygen tension. Decompression craniotomy was performed on one patients for persistent ICP-hypertension, and CPP as low as 30 mm Hg. Postsurgical ICP and CPP were 15 and 78 mm Hg respectively, and brain tissue PO_2 increased from the 8–12 mm Hg to 23 mm Hg. In another study a high CPP improved low values of brain tissue PO_2 in focal lesions (Stocchetti et al. 1998).

Head position

Lowering head position from 30° to flat position had no effect on CPP or brain tissue oxygen tension. Meixenberger et al. (1997) reported a similar finding of brain tissue PO_2 with head position.

Hyperventilation

Hyperventilation from a $PaCO_2$ of 29 to 21 mm Hg was associated with a ICP reduction from 34 to 16 mm Hg, and increase in CPP from 62 to 81 mm Hg. Brain tissue PO_2, however, decreased from 31 to 14 mm Hg (Kiening et al. 1997, Unterberg et al. 1997). Suazo et al. (2000) studied 90 patients with severe HI and GSC $\leq$ 8. Hyperventilation was applied, and brain tissue PO_2 monitored. CO_2 reactivity was calcualted as Δ brain tissue $PO_2/\Delta PaCO_2$. The CO_2 reactivity was low on day 1, increasing on subsequent days. Reactivity on days 1 and 2 was not related to outcome. The results indicated that increased hyperventilation causes a reduction in brain tissue PO_2, providing further evidense for possible increased risk of secondary ischaemic damage during hyperventilation.

Increased oxygen fraction

Increased oxygen fraction to higher levels appears to improve the oxygen supply in brain tissue. During the early phase after head injury high oxygen fractions, reduced lactate levels in brain tissue, and increased tissue oxygen tension (Menzel et al. 1999).

Mannitol

Administration of mannitol was not associated with increases in brain tissue PO_2. This was true whether mannitol was given during normal or an elevated ICP. In all situations, however, CPP was above 60 mm Hg before mannitol infusion (Kiening et al, 1997, Unterberg et al. 1997).

Comparison of brain tissue oxygen tension and jugular venous saturation

In a porcine model brain tissue PO_2 was more responsive to physiological variations, and the absolute values were more sensitive than oxygen measurement in the sagital sinus (Menzel et al. 1998). Gopinath et al. (1999) compared the characteristics of jugular venous oxygen saturation and brain tissue oxygen tension as monitors for cerebral ischaemia in 58 patients with severe head injury. The two monitors provided complimentary information, and neither monitor alone identified all episodes of ischaemia. The best strategy for using these monitors was to take advantage of the unique features of each monitor. Jugular venous saturation should be used as a monitor of global oxygenation. Brain tissue oxygen tension should be used as a monitor of local oxygenation, ideally with the catheter placed in an area of the brain that is vulnerable to ischaemia but that may be salvageable with appropriate treatment.

Therapy in acute head injury

The management of severe head injury is based on the concept of preventing, limiting, and treating processes leading to secondary damage. Monitoring and observation of patients with head injury consequently focus on prevention and detection of these insults.

Secondary damage might be of extra- as well as intracerebral origin. Extracerebral reasons include arterial hypotension, hypoxaemia, hyperthermia and infection, all of which might precipitate cerebral ishaemia. Damage of intracerebral origin includes secondary development of intracranial haematoma and ICP-hypertension caused by haematoma, contusion and oedema. As a consequence therapy in the acute phase of head trauma has focused on early detection of intracranial mass expanding lesions by CT/MR scanning and surgery.

Treatment of ICP-hypertension has through many years been a cornerstone in the management of these patients. Besides based on processes occurring at the biochemical level causing cell membrane dysfunction, disturbances of the microvascular circulation other treatment modalities have been investigated.

Unfortunately the results of clinical controlled studies investigating non-surgical treatment have been disappointing. Maas et al. (1999) summarized the results of recent trials of neuroprotective agents in head injury. None of the trials showed efficiency in the general population of patients with severe head injury. A critical analysis of the possible reasons for treatment failure suggests that special attention should be focused on the heterogeneity of the patient population, the importance of baseline prognostic indicators, and the problems caused by the distribution of outcome and the dichotomization of these outcomes in the Glasgow Outcome Scale.

Decompressive craniectomy

Bifrontal decompressive craniectomy for management of posttraumatic cerebral oedema was described by Venes and Collins (1975). In a retrospective study including 28 patients decomprssive craniectomy was performed an average of 68 hours after trauma. ICP decreased below 25 mm Hg in all patients, CPP improved and CBF and microcirculation normalised. The mortality rate was 11% (Kunze et al. 1998).

Ventricular and spinal drainage

Ventricular drainage has been used in several studies for control of ICP hypertension. Ventricular drainage can be effected continuously or intermittently. Combined drainage and ICP recording through the same catheter is often practised. Collapse of the ventricular system and blocking of the catheter by tissue fragments and/or coagulated blood to some degree prevent or restrict its use.

External lumbar drainage in uncontrollable intracranial hypertnesion has been advocated in adults with severe head injury (Willemse and Egeler-Peerdeman 1998).

Controlled hyperventilation

In the acute phase of HI there is no doubt that intubation and controlled ventilation may prevent hypoxia and hypercapnia. Mechanical ventilation may be life-saving if a mass expanding lesion is present.

As regard hypercapnia several studies indicate that the degree of the initial hypoxia or hypercapnia determines, to a large extent, the early mortality (MacIver et al. 1958, Frost et al. 1979, Kohi et al. 1984). The degree of hypoxia and hypercapnia shortly after a neurotrauma correlates fairly well with the degree of unconsciousness as assessed with the Glasgow Coma Scale (Pfenninger and Lindner 1991).

The effect of hyperventilation upon ICP depends on several factors. Thus, prolonged controlled hyperventilation enhances control of ICP-hypertension in stages with a high CBF, and transient moderate hyperventilation temporarily improves the cerebral autoregulation (Cold et al. 1981, Newell et al. 1996). On the other hand, the ICP-reducing effect during phases with reduced CBF (early phase of severe HI, old victims), although present, may be of limited therapeutic value. Owing to a decrease in MABP and CPP controlled hyperventilation may be dangerous, the reason being a decrease in cardiac output effected by positive pressure ventilation. Moreover, hyperventilation may provoke regional decreases in CBF close to or below threshold of ischaemia and synaptic function (Cold 1990), and forced hyperventilation to an end-tidal $PaCO_2$ of 21 mm Hg increases the risk of inducing brain ischaemia (Unterberg et al. 1997). In a prospective study of 33 patients with severe head injury studies of $AVDO_2$ and $AVD_{lactate}$ were performed. According to basal $AVDO_2$ 76% of the patients were considered as hyperaemic and 24% as not hyperaemic. According to $AVDO_2$ and $AVD_{lactate}$, no advserse effects were found during four hours of hyperventilation in hyperaemic patients. Only in one non-hyperaemic patient hyperventilation provoked increased anaerobic cerebral metabolism (Ausina et al. 1998). In another study light hyperventilation provoked marked decrease in brain tissue PO_2, suggesting increased risk of secondary ischaemic damage during hyperventilation (Suazo et al. 2000).

In children controlled hyperventilation has been advocated by Bruce et al. (1978). In a Xe-CT study by Skippen et al. (1997) it was found that hyperventilation reduced CBF to 50 ml (normal value 65 ml/100g/min), $CMRO_2$ was 1.0 ml O2/100g/min and $AVDO_2$ 2.3 vol%. In spite of their relatively high mean CBF, regionally very low CBF was found in many patients, and hypocapnia provoked even lower values.

Manual ventilation with bag is not an adequate treatment of ICP-hypertension. Bagging may cause cerebral oligaemic and frequently precipitates a cerebral hypoperfusion with imminent cerebral ischaemia (Procaccio et al. 1993).

During the last decade the use of hypocapnia in acute HI has been discussed (Cold 1990, Jacobsen and Isaacs 1993, Patel 1993). Miller et al. (1992) have summarised their approach to the management of ICP-hypertension after HI. In patients with cerebral hyperaemia and elevated ICP, CA is lost, $AVDO_2$ is low, and the CO_2 reactivity is preserved. Hyperventilation to a $PaCO_2$ level about 20–25 mm Hg is expected to produce a beneficial effect. On the other hand, in patients with preserved CA and compromised CPP, secondary vasodilation may result in increasing ICP. In these patients hypocapnia increases $AVDO_2$ and decreases cerebral venous saturation. The object has also been discussed by Chesnut (1997), who pointed out that the definition of hyperaemia as CBF that outstrips $CMRO_2$ may be wrong when it is not based on regional studies. The therapeutic goal is a reduction of cerebral blood volume. Cerebral blood volume, however, exists as multiple, interdependent compartments, including such compartments as resistance vessels, the post-parenchymal venous system and a large pial venous system. Each of these compartments may react independently.

In the American and European guidelines for therapy controlled prophylactic hyperventilation is not advocated. This attitude are based on risk of cerebral ischaemia elicited by hypocapnia, and supported by controlled outcome studies of prophylactic hyperventilation indicating that outcome at least is not improved (Muizelaar et al. 1991). In their study they allocated a group of severe HI to moderate hypocapnia ($PaCO_2$ level 32 mm Hg) and hyperventilation ($PaCO_2$ level 25 mm Hg), and a third group with hyperventilation to the same level in addition to treatment with the buffer tromethamine (THAM). At 3 and 6 months after the injury the number of patients with a favourable outcome was lower in the hyperventilated group than in the control- and the THAM groups. However, this occurred exclusively in patients with an initial motor score of 4–5. At 12 months after the trauma this difference was not found.

Adaptation to prolonged hypocapnia

Experimental studies

During prolonged controlled hyperventilation adaptation of CSF-pH and CBF occur (Raichle et al. 1970,

Hansen et al. 1986, Albrecht et al. 1997, Muizelaar et al. 1988). In dogs prolonged hypocapnia does not alter the rate of CSF formation (Artru and Hornhein 1987)

Clinical studies

In apoplexy and other cerebral diseases adaptation of CBF, CSF-pH and CSF-bicarbonate has been observed (Christensen et al. 1974, Ellingsen et al. 1987. In an uncontrolled study patients with severe HI were subjected to controlled hyperventilation for 24 hours in the subacute phase (day 4–6 after the trauma). ICP was well controlled, and ventricular fluid lactate stabilised within 24 hours prior to application of hyperventilation No signs of CSF-pH adaptation was found during the next 6 to 24 hours. This finding suggests that the normal mechanism of CSF-pH adaptation is delayed or abolished in severe HI (Cold et al. 1977a). When hyperventilation is used in the treatment of brain swelling in HI patients, it is not uncommon that unacceptable rises in ICP occur during withdrawal of hyperventilation (Havell 1984).

CPP targeted therapy of ICP-hypertension

Clinical studies by Rosner and Coley (1986) indicate that a low CPP might precipitate ICP-hypertension. Rosner argues that a low CPP is capable of stimulating cerebral vasodilatation and increase CBV and ICP (vasodilatory cascade). According to Rosner and Becker (1984) plateau waves are a result of this cascade. The same author has demonstrated that a MABP decrement often precedes ICP pressure waves. These findings suggest that CA is present even in the acute phase of HI, and the author argues that the optimal CPP is close to 85–90 mm Hg in normotensive patients, at which level the lowest level of ICP is observed (Rosner 1987).

In a later study 34 patients with GCS < 7 were treated following these principles. Overall mortality was 21%, and uncontrollable ICP 8% (Rosner and Daugton 1990). In another study a fall in CPP below 70 mm Hg was associated with a progressive change in transcranial Doppler flow, and a fall in jugular venous oxygen saturation (Chan et al. 1992). Studies with multimodal monitoring including tissue oxygen pressure, jugular venous saturation, MABP, ICP and CPP indirectly support the findings by Rosner. At least a CPP > 60 mm Hg emerges as a crucial factor guarantering sufficient brain oxygenation. Any intervention used to further elevate CPP, however, does not improve cerebral oxygenation. The concept of CPP as a guide to therapy has been supplemented by experimental studies in cats subjected to a controlled cortical impact injury. Under these experimental conditions, CPP should be kept at levels ranging from 70 to 105 mm Hg in order to prevent an increase in traumatic contusion volume. A CPP of 60 mm Hg and lower as well as a CPP of 120 mm Hg and higher was detrimental (Kroppenstedt et al. 1999).

Rosners concept has been criticised. Experimental studies in the cat of traumatic brain swelling indicate that cerebral swelling is provoked by arterial hypertension, and is accompanied by a marked elevation of the sagital sinus pressure, and a fall in $AVDO_2$ (Marshall et al. 1969).

In patients with severe head injury venous saturation rises with increasing perfusion pressure during and after endotracheal suctioning, suggesting impairment or absent of autoregulatory response (Fortune et al. 1994). Simard and Bellafleure (1989) in a review point out, that the occurrence of a hyperadrenergic state, and elevation of blood pressure may damage the blood-brain barrier and promote brain swelling and formation of oedema. Juul et al. (2000) in their analyses of 427 patients chalenged the CPP concept, and document that treatment protocols for the management of HI should emphasize immediate reduction of raised ICP to less than 20 mm Hg. Furthermore, they argue that a greater CPP than 60 mm Hg appears to have little influence on the outcome of the patients. Cruz et al. (1995) studied severe acute head injury with multivariate neurophysiological monitoring including CBF, $CMRO_2$, $AVDO_2$ and CVR. They found that in severe head injury cerebral haemodynamic and oxygen metabolic variables are not necessary correlated with CPP. Moreover, they found that CVR and not CPP was more closely related with different patterns of CBF and metabolism. In a reply Hallifax (1996) and Rosner (1996) stated that in the material of Cruz et al. cerebral autoregulation was preserved, and consequently a poor correlation was found between CPP and CBF. Furthermore it was stressed to be fallacious to make any conclusions based on group data of single patient measurements.

Based on studies of CA, Bouma et al. (1993) summarised as follows: A fall in blood pressure is always detrimental. With impaired CA it may invoke a risk of cerebral ischaemia, while with intact CA it may lead to a dangerous increase in ICP and brain stiffness, due to compensatory vasodilation. Artificially raised blood pressure, if necessary to maintain blood pressure, is only prudent when CA is known to be intact. In these cases induced hypertension has little effect upon ICP and PVI, and may thus be regarded safe. With defective CA, however, this manoeuvre causes a deterioration of the biomechanical status of the brain.

In a recent review Previgliano et al. (1997) summarize the following conclusions. 1) low CPP is harmful for HI patients, no matter what the type of injury or the autoregulatory status, and must be avoided. 2) A CPP of 70–80 mm Hg has been proven to be safe and useful. Rosner´s data are so impressive that a controlled trial between traumatic coma bank data and CPP management should be carried out. 3) jugular venous oxygen saturation and transcranial Doppler are good tools by which to assess the optimal CPP for each patient. Both allow identification of different types of patients with different therapeutic approaches. First there is the nonhyperaemic patient, who usually have low venous saturation, low flow velocity, and a high pulsatility index (PI). In this group osmotic therapy and a CPP around 70–80 mm Hg should be the treatment of choice. Next come the patient with high venous saturation, a constant PI, and a low flow velocity. Hyperventilation can be used, mainly due to its effect on ICP and venous saturation, which enhances CPP. Third comes the patient with high venous saturation, low flow velocity and high PI. In this patient the risk of non-contusion-related infarction is high, so CPP should be elevated. The last group are patients with high venous saturation, high flow velocity, and a constant or high PI. In this group barbiturates and strict CPP control by means of MABP control should be used.

Vasopressor therapy (dopamine, norepinephrine)

In the brain dopamine is acting via Dopamine D_1 receptors, which mediates dilation of cerebral vessels, and D_2 mediating an increase in glucose utilisation (Edvinsson et al. 1978, Kebabian and Calne 1979, von Essen et al. 1990, Sharkey and McCulloch 1986). Normally dopamine does not cross the blood-brain barrier, but if the BBB is defect an increase in CBF, glucose utilisation and oxygen consumption are observed (McCulloch and Harper 1977, Sharkey and McCulloch 1985).

In cats dopamine administrated for blood pressure control together with thiamylal induced anaerobic cerebral glycolysis in spite of maintained CBF and $CMRO_2$ (Sato et al. 1991). In a recent study in unanesthetized monkeys CBF and $CMRO_2$ were unaffected by dobutamine at doses unto 100 γg/kg/min. In the same study dopamine at doses unto 15 γg/kg/min did not affect CBF or $CMRO_2$, but at doses of 50 γg/kg/min CBF and $CMRO_2$ increased (Badres et al. 1992). In an intact cerebral autoregulation model of sheep the effects of norepinephrine, epinephrine and dopamine upon ICP, CBF, $AVDO_2$ and oxygen utilisation were compared. All three drugs increased MABP in a dose-dependent manner. Norepinephrine and epinephrine had no effects upon ICP, CBF, $AVDO_2$ and oxygen utilisation. Infusion of dopamine, upto 60 ug/min resulted in an increase in ICP and CBF, reduction in $AVDO_2$ and i biphasic response in oxygen utilisation (Myburgh et al. 1998).

In 16 patients with severe head injury the adrenergic vasopressors dopmaine, noradrenaline and methoxamine were used to increase MABP. The results indicated that the increase in MABP effectively increased CPP, but without changes in ICP. Compared with dopamine in doses of 10 to 52 γg/kg/min noradrenaline at a dose of 0.5 mg to 5 mg/h was effective and safe and was considered to drug of choice (Biestro et al. 1998).

In patients with preserved cerebral autoregulation CBF is unchanged after norepinephrine-induced MABP increase. In patients with impaired cerebral autoregulation an increase in MABP was found. These findings suggest that CPP management with norepinephrine can be used to increase MABP without potentiating hyperaemia if pressure autoregulation is preserved (Mascia et al. 2000).

CPP-targeted or ICP targeted management

Robertson et al. (1999) studied 189 patients assigned to either CBF-targeted or ICP-targeted management during randomly assigned time blocks. In the CBF targeted protocol, CPP was kept > 70 mm Hg and $PaCO_2$ was kept at approximately 35 mm Hg. In the ICP-targeted grup, CPP was kept at > 50 mm Hg and hyperventilation of 25–30 mm Hg was used to treat intracranial hypertension. The CBF-targeted protocol reduced the frequency of jugular desaturation from 50,6 to 30%. The risk of cerebral ischaemia was 2,4-fold greater with the ICP-targeted protocol. Despite the reduction in secondary ischaemic insults there was no difference in neurologic outcome (Robertson et al. 1999).

Treatment of acidosis with THAM

Experimental studies

Experimental studies in cats indicate that THAM (trishydroxy-methylaminomethan) decreases the production of brain lactate and brain oedema and promotes the recovery of cerebral energy dysfunction. THAM ameliorates the deleterious effects of hyperventilation by minimising energy disturbances, and that it also decreases the formation of brain oedema (Yoshida and Marmarou 1991).

Clinical studies

In a preliminary study Seitz and Ocker (1977) demonstrated that treatment of CSF acidosis by intrathecal injection of bicarbonate improved CBF as well as brain metabolism in patients with severe HI. Intrathecal administration of THAM in patients with severe cerebral acidosis causes an alkaline shift of CSF pH, and secondary efflux of lactate, resulting in a decrease of CSF elastance and a reduction of the risk of ICP elevation (Kuklane et al. 1993). Another study in patients with severe HI indicate that intravenous treatment with THAM effectively controls ICP-hypertension (Pfenninger et al. 1989a), also when compared with mannitol 20% and sorbitol 40% (Gaab et al. 1990). When used prophylactically, a preliminary controlled study revealed lower levels of CSF-lactate and probably improved recovery (Rosner et al. 1989). In another randomized prospective clinical study treatment with THAM versus conventional treatment was compared. The THAM group had fewer episodes of ICP elevation than those in the control group, and the rate of patients needing hyperventilation for control of ICP was higher in the control group (Wolf et al. 1993).

Hypothermia

Treatment with hypothermia is based upon protection against thermo-pooling, non-release of glutamate, lack of synaptic excitation, a low metabolic demand, stabilisation of the vital signs, and a low systemic energy transport into the brain (Hayashi et al. 1994).

Experimental studies

In several models of traumatic brain injury hypothermia has been shown to improve histopathologic and behavioral outcome (Jiang et al. 1991, Clifton et al. 1993, Lyeth et al. 1993, Palmer et al. 1993, Dietrich et al. 1994a, Dietrich et al. 1994b, Bramlett et al. 1995, Globus et al. 1995, Clark et al. 1996). In the cat studies with microdialysis during inflation of an epidural baloon indicate that the increase in extracellular glutamate is attenuated (Mori et al. 1998). Posttraumatic hypothermia has been reported to ameliorate the integrity of the blood-brain barrier (Jaing et al. 1992) and reduce neuronal injury and decrease contusion volume (Dietrich et al. 1990, Palmer et al. 1993). Microtubulo-associated protein has been reported to be protected from traumatic brain injury by hypothermia (Taft et al. 1993). Inflammatory response to injury involving the infiltration and accumulation of polymorphonuclear leukocytes is reduced by hypothermia (Whalen et al. 1977a, Whalen et al. 1997b), and posttraumatic hypothermia reduces myeloperoxidase activity, which has been reported to be a reliable marker of polymorphonuclear leukocyte activity (Chatzipanteli et al. 2000).

In a rat acute subdural model, moderate hypothermia (32 and 34°C) did not affect the ICP or cerebral perfusion pressure, but was associated with a significant lower cortical brain oedema formation beneath the haematoma (Kawai et al. 2000).

In a canine model of epidural brain compression immediate post-insult hypothermia (31°C) for 5 hours prevented the rise in ICP, and decreased cerebral tissue damage. However, hypothermia did not prevent brain herniation during rewarming (Pomeranz et al. 1993). Prolongation of hypothermia to 48 hours maintained a low intracranial pressure during hypothermia, but did not prevent lethal brain swelling and herniation after rewarming (Ebmeyer et al. 1998). Nevertheless, a protective effect of moderate hypothermia on behavioural deficits has been found following cortical impact injury in the rat. This finding was, however, not correlated to a decrease in focal cortical necrosis (Dixon et al. 1998).

In a rodent model of cerebral contusion treatment with moderate hypothermia (32°C for 4 hr), a 21-aminosteroid iv, repeatedly, or both were studied. Axonal injury was equally demonstrated in all groups indicating that combination therapy was no more efficacious than either therapy alone (Marion and White 1996).

Rats subjected to fluid percussion were studied within the 1st hour of injury. Evidence of marked region-specific uncoupling of local glucose metabolism and CBF was found. The finding was characterised by up to 2.5-fold elevations in the local metabolic rate of glucose ($LCMR_{glucose}$)/local CBF ratio in zones known to be pathologically traumatized (Sao et al. 1993, Sao et al. 1995). In the same model it was found that posttraumatic hypothermia (30° C for 3 hours) did not improve cerebral glucose utilisation (Sao et al. 1999).

Clinical studies

It is important to realize that brain temperature and core temperatur are not identical. In a recent study of traumatic brain injury Rumania et al. (1998) reported an average brain temperature that was 1.1° C higher than core (rectal) temperature. In an editorial Dewitt and Plough (1998) concluded that in febrile patients after traumatic brain injury, measurement of core temperature may underestimate brain temperature.

In uncontrolled ICP-hypertension mild hypothermia reduces ICP and increases CPP. Mild hypothermia decreases CBF, $AVDO_2$ and $CMRO_2$ (Shiozaki et al. 1993), and $CMR_{lactate}$ (Metz et al. 1996). In one study patients were subjected to mild hypothermia to 32–33°C within a meantime of 10 hours after injury, and maintained at that temperature for 24 hours. Hypothermia reduced ICP and CBF without rebound increase during rewarming (Marion et al. 1993). In another study of 16 consecutive patients mild hypothermia (34°) did not decrease the CSF concentration of excitatory amino acids and cytokines compared with a normothermic group of patients (Shiozaki et al. 1999).

During moderate hypothermia cardiac index decreases by 18%, but recovered at 24 h of hypothermia, and surpassed baseline values after rewarming. Platelet counts dropped continuously up to 24 h after rewarming. Creatine clearance decreased during cooling, and recovered by 24 h after rewarming. An increased incidence of elevated serum lipase activity with signs of pancreatitis was found. Rewarming normalised the pancreatic alterations (Metz et al. 1996).

Side effects of hypothermia include reduced enzyme activity, altered pharmacokinetics and pharmacodynamics, altered neuromuscular response, change in neuronal electrical activity and evoked response (Sessler 1997). Other complications are impaired resistance to infections (Kurz et al. 1996) and coagulopathy (Resnick et al. 1994). Compensating for these complications might change the outcome of large-scale investigations in a positive way.

Outcome studies have been published. In a phase II study by Clifton et al. (1993) 46 patients with severe HI were studied in a randomized study to either standard management at 37°C or hypothermia to 32–33°C. Cooling began within 6 hours of injury. Rewarming was at a rate of 1°C per 4 h beginning 48 h after the hypothermic level was reached. GOS scores at 3 months after injury showed an absolute increase of 16% (i.e. 36.4–52.2%) in the number of patients in good recovery/moderate disability as compared with severe disability/vegetative survivals/death. Seizure incidence was lower in the hypothermic group. On the other hand, sepsis was observed more commonly in the hypothermic group.

Marion et al. (1997), in a randomized controlled study compared the effect of moderate hypothermia and normothermia in 82 patients. The patients assigned to hypothermia were cooled to 33°C during a mean of 10 hours after injury, and kept at this temperature for 24 hours, and then rewarmed. At 12 months 62% of the patients in the hypothermic group and 38% of those in the normothermic group had good outcomes (moderate, mild or no disabilities. Hypothermia did not improve the outcomes in the patients with a coma score of 3 or 4 on admission. Among the patients with scores of 5 to 7, hypothermia was associated with significant improved outcomes at 3 and 6 months, although not at 12 months.

Jiang et al. (2000) published a study, including 87 patients with GCS $\leq$ 8, where randomisation to 33–35°C or normothermia were applied. One year mortality and favourable outcome (good recovery and moderate disability) in the hypothermic group were 25.6% and 46.1%. respectively. In the normothermic group the mortality rate was 45,6 and favurable outcome was 27,3%.

In a multicentre study of 392 patients with closed head injury the patients were randomised to either normothermia or hypothermia to 33 degrees Celsius initiated within 6 hours and maintained for 48 hours. The hypothermic patients had more hospital days with complications than the normothermic patients. Mortality was 28% in the hypothermic group and 27% in the normothermic group. In conclusion hypothermia did not improve outcome (Clifton 2001). It therefore seems premature to recommend hypothermia for general use.

Barbiturate

Experimental studies

The effect of hypocapnia and barbiturate upon ICP was studied in dogs subjected to ICP-hypertension. It was demonstrated that barbiturate was not more effective in reducing ICP than hyperventilation alone (Louis et al. 1993).

Clinical studies

When barbiturate is administered, continuous EEG monitoring is a better modality than serum or CSF concentration by showing the therapeutic goal of burst-suppression activity. Thus, the minimum necessary dose can be titrated (Winer et al. 1991).

Barbiturate has been used extensively in the control of ICP-hypertension. When ICP-hypertension is present injection of barbiturate often elicits an immediate decrease in ICP (Shaper et al. 1974, Eisenberg et al. 1988). Several studies suggest that barbiturate coma treatment can be used advantageously in comatose patients with HI (Marshall et al. 1979, Saul and Ducker 1982, Hoppe et al. 1981). Studies in children indicate, that even when CPP is reduced, barbiturate administration can be effective in the treatment of resistant ICP-hypertension (Pittman et al. 1989). In a recent microdialysis study of patients with severe ICP-hypertension it was found that thiopental coma was associated with a reduction of lactate, glutamate and aspartate in the extracellular space (Goodman et al. 1996).

Owing to a negative inotropic effect of barbiturate a fall in MABP often occurs. As a consequence CPP remains unchanged or is reduced, even when ICP decreases. In one study arterial hypotension was found in 58% of patients (Schalén et al. 1992). In both uncontrolled (Yano et al. 1986), and controlled studies, barbiturate coma treatment does not improve recovery (Ward et al. 1985). In another study of patients with ICP-hypertension mannitol treatment was compared with that of barbiturate. It was found that barbiturate was less effective than mannitol for control of ICP-hypertension, and that the mortality rate in barbiturate treated patents was higher (Schwartz et al. 1984). As stated by Sawada et al. (1982), tolerance to barbiturate occurs within days of therapy. Accordingly, during chronic barbiturate therapy the metabolic effect of barbiturate on cerebral metabolism is probably also diminished. Barbiturate therapy is not advocated by the American and European guidelines.

It cannot, however, be excluded that in subgroup of patients with intact reactivities for CO_2- and barbiturate, and only a moderate suppression of $CMRO_2$, barbiturate might be effective and perhaps improve outcome (Cold 1990, Moskopp et al. 1991).

Propofol

In a clinical study of sedation for acute HI patients, continuous infusion with propofol was compared with midazolam/morphine sedation. Propofol led to a fall in $AVDO_2$. However, there were no differences in the level of MABP, ICP or CPP, and the outcomes were similar in the two groups (Stewart et al. 1994).

Morphine and fentanyl

In a recent study patients with severe head injury were subjected to morphine (0.2 mg/kg) or fentanyl (2γg/kg). Before the study CO_2 reactivity and cerebral autoregulation were assessed. Both morphine and fentanyl caused an increase in ICP and decrease in MABP and CPP, but estimated $AVDO_2$ and flow velocity remained unchanged. In patients with preserved cerebral autoregulation the opioid-induced ICP increases were not different than in those with impaired autoregulation (deNadal et al. 2000).

Calcium blockers

The effect of nimodipine on outcome has been studied in HI. The study demonstrate that it is unlikely that nimodipine has any effect on outcome. However, in subgroup of patients a modest improvement could not be excluded (Bailey et al. 1991).

Other studies of treatment of cerebral vasospasms in patients with severe head injury with nicardipine (Compton et al. 1990) and nimodipine (Koston et al. 1985) were inconclusive.

A multicenter trial of the efficacy of nimodipine on outcome after severe head injury was published by an European study group (1994). The main hypothesis, that nimodipine would increase the percentage of patients with a favourable outcome from 50 to 60%, was rejected. A trend toward favourable outcome, however, was seen in patients who exhibited traumatic subarachnoid haemorrhage. In a recent controlled study, however, patients treated with nimodipine for traumatic subarachnoid haemorrhage had a significantly less unfavourable outcome at 6 months than placebo-treated patients (Harders et al. 1996).

N-Methyl-D-Aspartate antagonist

In a recent study including 693 patients with severe head injury selfotel, a competitive N-methyl-D-aspartate antagonist, was enrolled in a double-blind trial. Data analysis revealed no statistical significant difference in mortality rate (Morris et al. 1999).

Bradykinin B_2 receptor antagonist

Narotam et al. (1998), in a randomised placebo-controlled, single blind trial involving 20 highly selected patients, found treatment with the B_2 antagonist, CP-0127, prevented pathological rise in ICP and subsequent neurological deterioration, thereby reducing the therapy intensity level. Mamarou et al. (1999) studied Bradycor, another B_2 antagonist, in a phase II, randomised, double blind trial. Although positive trends were observed for both ICP and therapy intensity level, these differences were not significant.

Hyperbar oxygen therapy

Hyperbar oxygen therapy has been studied. In a clinical survey this treatment did not increase the number of patients with a favourable outcome (Rockswold et al. 1992).

Free radical scavenger

Experimental studies

In microdialysis experiments of acute subdural haematoma in rats it was found that free radicals in the brain underlying the acute haematoma was increased. However, prolonged increase in FiO_2 does not lead to further increase in free radical production in the injured brain (Doppenberg et al. 1998).

Rats were subjected to fluid-percussion injury. Superoxide dismutase administrated 15 min after trauma prevented the decrease in CBF otherwise found. This effect is facilitated by L-arginine (DeWitt et al. 1997).

Clinical studies

In a controlled study PEG-SOD was administrated to severely HI patients with GCS < 9. At three months after injury 20% of the patients receiving 10000 U/kg of PEG-SOD were vegetative or had died. In the control group 40% were vegetative or had died (Muizelaar et al. 1993).

Mannitol

Pharmacokinetic

A strong positive correlation between mannitol concentration and serum osmolality has been found. The integrated values of mannitol concentration difference between the cerebral and the peripheral compartment correlates with the decrease in ICP (Kobayashi et al. 1994).

Cerebral circulation

Mannitol gives rise to an increase in CBF and $CMRO_2$ (Bruce et al. 1973, Mendelow et al. 1985, Jafar et al. 1986). Mannitol rapidly counteracts cerebral oligaemia effected by hypocapnia (Cruz et al. 1990). Clinical studies suggest that the increase in CBF is due to a reduction in blood viscosity (Burke et al. 1981, Muizelaar et al. 1983). Other studies suggest that the decrease in ICP is only observed in patients with intact cerebral autoregulation (Muizelaar et al. 1984).

Outcome

In one study mannitol treatment for ICP-hypertension was compared with that of barbiturate. It was found that barbiturate was less effective than mannitol for control of ICP-hypertension, and the mortality rate in barbiturate treated patients was higher (Schwartz et al. 1984).

In another trial 80 patients with GCS of 8 or less were randomized to mannitol treatment for ICP elevations > 25 mm Hg, while another group received mannitol treatment irrespective of ICP readings. No differences in mortality rate or neurological outcome were demonstrated between the two groups (Smith et al. 1986).

Hypertonic saline

Experimental studies

7.2% hypertonic saline/10% dextran versus 20% mannitol for treatment of ICP-hypertension was compared. Both solutions decreased ICP. Hypertonic saline afforded a higher CPP than mannitol. The water content in the traumatised hemisphere, however, was increased, while the contralateral hemisphere was dehydrated. With mannitol no differences in water content were disclosed between the injured and non-injured regions (Berger et al. 1994). Another study support these findings (Freshman et al. 1993).

Pigs were subjected to cryogenic lesion and haemorrhagic hypotension. Small-volume resuscitation with hypertonic saline and dextran and dispirin cross-linked haemoglobin significantly improved MABP and CPP compared with Ringer´s lactate (Shackford 1997). In a microcirculatory study of rabbits equipped with a cranial window, hypertonic saline combined with dextran completely prevented the increase in arteriolar diameter, and prevented the activation of white blood cell without affecting the increased posttraumatic ICP (Härtl et al. 1997).

Clinical studies

In patients with resistant ICP-hypertension hypertonic saline effectively reduces ICP (Worthley et al. 1988), and it lowers raised ICP in children with severe HI (Fisher et al. 1992).

In a cohort analysis of data from previous prospective randomized studies treatment with hypertonic saline resulted in a survival until discharge of 38% compared with 27% with standard care (Wade et al. 1997). In another study, including 27 patients with cerebral oedema of different aetiology (8 patients with head injury), 3% hypertonic saline was used. In head injury patients a reduction in mean ICP within the first 12 hrs correlated with an increase in serum Na^+ (r^2 =.91), and severity of postoperative oedema (r^2 =.82). In patients with head injury the beneficial effect, however, was short-lasting.

After 72 hrs of infusion four of eight patients required intravenous pentobarbital due to poor ICP control (Qureshi et al. 1998).

Nevertheless, in a multicenter study the efficacy of 250 ml 7.5% NaCl solution versus isotonic saline in influencing systemic resuscitation and outcome in patients with multiple injuries was compared. Although hypertonic saline significantly improved blood pressure resuscitation, there were no differences in survival between the groups (Vassar et al. 1993).

On the basis of experimental and clinical studies Chesnut (1997) summarises: Based on the hypertonic salines efficacy and its apparently strongly positive risk/benefit ratio, it is unclear why the administration of hypertonic saline has not become the standard of practice in resuscitation of severe brain trauma. Prough and Zornow (1998) in another editorial argue that rebound ICP-hypertension might occur with hypertonic saline, and suggest controlled, blinded outcome trials. These points of view are supported by a retrospective (Petersen et al. 2000) and a prospective study (Khanna et al. 2000) using 3% hypertonic saline in pediatric patients.

Dihydroergotamine (DHE)

Experimental studies

DHE increases peripheral vascular resistance, mainly by increasing resistance in the venous capacitance vessels.

Clinical studies

In normal adults DHE does not influence CBF (Andersen et al. 1987). In severe head injury DHE decreases ICP and increases CPP, while CBF and CVR are unchanged (Grände 1989, Ryding et al. 1990, Gopinath et al. 1984). In patients subjected to craniotomy for cerebral tumours DHE administration, however, resulted in an increase in MABP, CPP and ICP. The authors argue that abolished cerebral autoregulation might explain why DHE under these circumstances increased ICP (Bundgaard et al. 2000).

The Lund model

A new therapy has been proposed from the group in Lund. The main concept is that opening of the blood-brain barrier upsets the normal brain volume regulation, including oedema formation. Under this circumstance transcapillary fluid fluxes will be controlled by hydrostatic pressure and colloid osmotic pressure, rather than by crystalloid osmotic pressure. To reduce capillary pressure hydrostatic pressure therapy with metoprolol and the $_2$-agonist clonidine is combined with procapillary vasoconstiction with DHE. Although clinical controlled outcome studies have not been performed, preliminary result with this regime seems promising (Asgeirsson et al. 1994, Grände et al. 1997, Naredi et al. 2001).

α_2 agonists (clonidine)

In a clinical study the effect of a 10 minutes clonidine infusion of 25 γg/kg upon $AVDO_2$ and flow velocity was studied. ICP, $PaCO_2$, $AVDO_2$ and flow velocity did not change after clonidine administration. In contrast MABP and CPP decreased, and a transient increase in ICP was found in some patients, suggesting cerebral autoregulatory vasodilation (Minassian et al. 1997). In other clinical studies smaller doses of 1 γg/kg and 2.5 γg/kg had no effect on ICP, CBF or $CMRO_2$ (Asgeirsson et al. 1995, Payen et al. 1990).

Cyclooxygenase inhibitors (indomethacin)

Experimental studies

Indomethacin blocks cyclooxygenase. It acts as an arteriolar vasoconstrictor and increases CVR, decreases CBF, while $CMRO_2$ remains unchanged (Pickard and MacKenzie 1973, Dahlgren et al. 1981). In cats and rats indomethacin reduces cerebral oedema (Dempsey et al. 1985, Yen and Lee 1987). In some animals indomethacin provides cerebral protection against ischaemia (Sasaki et al. 1988, Shigeno et al. 1985, Hallenbeck and Furlow 1979). However, cerebral protection has not been documented in other studies of focal ischaemia (Harris et al. 1982, Awad et al. 1983, Sutherland et al. 1988, Suzuka et al. 1989), and in traumatic HI (Shapira et al. 1988).

The permeability of monolayers of rat cerebral endothelial cells were investigated to assess potential changes in the integrity of the blood-brain barrier. Exposure of the endothelial vells to tumour necrosis factor- and interleukin-1β and interleukin-6 induced a deline in the trans endothelial electrical resistance, which was completely restored by indomethacin (de Vries et al. 1996).

Clinical studies

The vasoconstrictive effect of indomethacin has been used in the treatment of ICP-hypertension in acute HI. A bolus doses of 30 mg indomethacin is followed by an immediately decrease in ICP, accompanied by a decrease in CBF, and an increase in $AVDO_2$, whilst $CMRO_2$ was unchanged (Jensen et al. 1991). In another study, the effect of indomethacin upon ICP and CBF was compared with that of hypocapnia. It was found that indomethacin 30 mg elicited an ICP decrease comparable with a fall in $PaCO_2$ of 1 kPa (Dahl et al. 1996). Indomethacin also effectively decreases ICP during craniotomy (Bundgaard et al. 1996).

Guidelines for intensive care unit management

Recently two guidelines concerning the management of severe head injury in adults have been published. From the European brain injury consortium (EBIC) the need for international collaboration in the conduct of research in the clinical management of head injury has been stressed. Thus, the EBIC has been formed to promote international, multicentre, interdisciplinary research aimed at improving the outcome of patients with severe HI or other kinds of acute brain damage (Teasdale et al. 1997)

Ghajar et al. (1995) published a study of current practice in the monitoring and treatment of patients with severe HI. The survey indicated there was a considerable variation in the management of patients in the United States. Corticosteroids were still used in 64% of trauma centres, and 29% of the centres reported aiming for $PaCO_2$ values of < 25 mm Hg. The establishment of guidelines for the management of severe head injury for the management of head injury was warranted. As a consequence The American guidelines for the management of severe head injury was elaborated and published in 1996, revised in 1998 and published in J of Neurotrauma in 2000.

EBIC-guidelines for intensive care unit management

This guideline has been presented by the EBIC consortium (Maas et al. 1997).

Monitoring and general care

Minimal monitoring requirements include ECG, SaO_2, invasive arterial blood pressure, temperature and end-tidal CO_2, if ventilated. Maintain SaO_2 > 95%, MABP > 90 mm Hg.Give iv. fluids to maintain normovolaemia and normal blood chemistry; There is no indication for fluid restriction, as treatment of cerebral oedema. In selected cases with severe concomitant pulmonary injury/oedema some fluid restriction may be appropriate. CVP monitoring is recommended to ensure normovolaemia. If ICP is monitored then there should also be continuously monitoring of MABP and calculation of CPP. Ventilator parameters: While on intermittent positive pressure ventilation (IPPV), adjust ventilation to maintain: PaO_2> 13 kPa, and $PaCO_2$ 4.0–4.5 kPa. Early institution of nutrition by enteral feeding. General care is aimed at maintaining normal "milieu interne" avoiding hyperthermia, hyperglycaemia, preventing and promptly treating secondary complications. Consider follow-up CT next day or earlier if clinically indicated. A single early initial CT often does not disclose the full extent of intracranial injuries.

Extracranial surgery

There is no general consensus on the time of more elective orthopaedic or craniofacial surgery in the absence of a life threatening disorder. Some clinicians advocate early internal fixation of limb fractures of faciomaxillary deformities; others advocate delayed surgery. If early surgical repair is chosen there should be full cardiovascular monitoring, and preferably also ICP monitoring: procedures should be carried out in accordance with neuroanaesthesia principles, e.g., cerebral vasodilation and episodes of hypotension must be avoided. Preoperative evaluation of the coagulation system is recommended. During surgery monitoring of the neurological condition (pupils) and preferably also ICP and/or neurophysiological monitoring is advocated. However, such monitoring procedures may fail to identify the development of focal mass lesions, with midline shift and for this reason early prolonged extracranial surgery for non life threathening injuries should be avoided.

Management of CPP and ICP

ICP therapy is only definitely indicated if raised ICP has been demonstrated by monitoring, or if there is CT evidence of increased ICP (e.g., absent/compressed basal cisterns) or clinical signs of developing intracranial herniation. Treatment should not only be aimed at reducing ICP, but especially at restoring CPP to appropriate levels (60–70 mm Hg). The precise level of ICP above which treatment should be instituted has not been established, but generally ICP elevations above 20–25 mm Hg should be treated unless other clear local policies have been identified. In the first few days after trauma more active treatment is indicated than in the later posttraumatic phase. There is no consensus whether patients should be nursed flat or with the head up to a maximum of 30° elevation.

Before initiating treatment directed at ICP, check for monitor malfunction, remediable extracranial disorders ($PaCO_2$, blood pressure etc).

Accepted methods of management of ICP and CPP are. Sedation, analgesia and mild to moderate hyperventilation ($PaCO_2$ 4.0–4.5 kPa).

Volume expansion and inotropics or vasopressors when arterial blood pressure is insufficient to maintain CPP in a normavolaemic patient.

Osmotic therapy. Preferably mannitol given repeatedly in bolus infusions or as indicated by monitoring. Serum osmolality should be maintained < 315. Other agents, such as glycerol of Sorbitol are not advocated. If osmotherapy has insufficient effect, furosemide can be given additionally.

If these methods fail more intensive hyperventilation ($PaCO_2$ < 30 mm Hg), preferably with monitoring of cerebral oxygenation to detect cerebral ischaemia, for instance by jugular oxymetry. Alternatively the use of barbiturates, including increased sedation may be considered.

Other ICP-directed therapies are considered to be experimental and should not be instituted in patients enrolled into studies of other forms of treatment. There is no established indication for steroids in the management of acute head injury.

Operative treatment

A surgically significant epidural haematoma, or acute subdural haematoma should be evacuated immediately upon detection. For small haemorrhagic contusions or other small intracerebral lesion: a conservative approach is generally adopted; but operation should be considered urgent for large intracerebral lesions with high or mixed density on CT scan.

Specific indication for operation include.
- Clinical deterioration
- Size: > 1 cm thick extracerebral clot,
- > 25–30 ml intracerebral haematoma
- Midline shift > 5 mm
- Enlargement of contralateral ventricle (temporal horn)
- Obliteration of basal cisterns/third ventricle
- Raised or increasing ICP

Depressed skull fracture. Operation is definitely indicated only if it is a compound (open) fracture (not over sagital sinus) or if the fracture is so extensive that it causes mass effect.

Closed depressed skull fractures are usually treated conservatively, but operation may be appropriate in selected cases to reduce mass effect or correct defigurement.

Decompressive craniotomy: may be considered in exceptional situations.

The American: Guidelines for the management of severe traumativ brain injury.

A joint venture of The Brain Trauma Foundation, The American Association of Neurological Surgeons, The joint Section on Neurotrauma and Critical Care.

Terminology used in the American Guidelines

In assessing the degree of certainty associated with a particular recommendation, the following terminology is the most widely accepted and is used in the document,

Standards. Represent accepted principles of patients management that reflect a high degree of clinical certainty.

Guidelines. Represents a particular strategy or range of management strategies that reflect a moderate clinical certainty.

Options. Are the remaining strategies for patients management for which there is unclear clinical certainty.

When assessing the value of therapies or interventions, the available data are classified into one of three categories according to the following criteria.

Class I evidence. Prospective randomized controlled trials. The gold standard of clinical trials. However, some may be poorly designed, lack sufficient patients number, or suffer from other methodological inadequacies.

Class II evidence. Clinical studies in which the data are collected prospectively, retrospective analysed, and that the data were based on clearly reliable data. Types of studies so classified include observational studies, cohort studies, prevalence studies, and case-control studies.

Class III evidence. Most studies based on retrospectivel collected data. Evidence used in this class indicates clinical series databases or registries, case reviews, case reports, and expert opinion with some support from animal studies.

Standards are generally based on Class I evidence. However, strong Class II evidence may from the basis for a standard, especially if the issue does not lend itself to testing in a randomized format. Conversely, weak or contradictory Class I evidence may not be able to support a standard. Guidelines are usually based on Class II evidence or a preponderance of Class II evidence. Options are usually based on Class III evidence and are clearly much less useful except for educational purposes and in guiding future studies.

Integration of brain-specific treatment into the initial resuscitation of severe HI patients

Standards. There are insufficient data to support standard for this topic.

Guidelines. There are insufficient data to support guidelines.

Options. The first priority for the HI patients is complete and rapid physiologic resuscitation. No specific treatment should be directed at ICP-hypertension in the absence of signs of transtentorial herniation or progressive neurologic deterioration not attributable to extracranial explanations. When either signs of transtentorial herniation or progressive neurologic deterioration not attributable to extracranial explanations are present, however, the physician should assume that ICP-hypertension is present and treat it aggressively. Hyperventilation should be rapidly established. The administration of mannitol is desirable, but only under conditions of adequate volume resuscitation.

Sedation and neuromuscular blockade can be useful in optimising transport of the HI patient. However, both treatments interfere with the neurologic examination. In the absence of outcome-based studies, the choice of sedation is left to the physician. Neuromuscular blockage should be employed when sedation alone proves inadequate, and short-acting agents should be used when possible.

Resuscitation of blood pressure and oxygenation

Standards. There are insufficient data to support a treatment standard for this topic.

Guidelines. Hypotension (systolic blood pressure < 90 mm Hg) or hypoxia (apnoea, or cyanosis or an O_2 saturation < 90% in the field or a pO_2 < 60 mm Hg) must be monitored and scrupulously avoided, if possible, or corrected immediately in severe TBI patients.

Options. The MABP should be maintained above 90 mm Hg through the infusion of fluids throughout the patients course to attempt to maintain perfusion pressure (CPP) > 70 mm Hg. Patients with a GCS<9, who are unable to maintain their airway or who remain hypoxemic in spite of supplemental O_2 require that their airway be secured preferably by endotracheal intubation.

Indications for ICP monitoring

Standards. There are insufficient data to support a treatment standard for this topic.

Guidelines. ICP monitoring is appropriate in patients with severe head injury with an abnormal admission CT scan. Severe HI is defined as a GCS of 3–8 after cardiopulmonary resuscitation. An abnormal CT scan of the head is one that reveals haematoma, contusions, oedema or compressed basal cisterns. ICP monitoring is appropriate in patients with severe HI with a normal CT scan if two or more of the following features are noted at admission: age over 40 years, unilateral or bilateral motor posturing, systolic blood pressure < 90 mm Hg. ICP monitoring is not routinely indicated in patients with mild or moderate HI. However, a physician may chose to monitor ICP in certain conscious patients with traumatic mass lesions.

ICP treatment threshold

Standards. There are insufficient data to support a treatment standard. *Guidelines*: ICP treatment should be initiated at an upper threshold of 20–25 mm Hg.

Options. Interpretation and treatment of ICP based on any threshold should be corroborated by frequent clinical examination and CPP data.

Guidelines for CPP

Standards. There are insufficient data to support treatment standards.

Guidelines. There are insufficient data to support treatment guidelines. Options: CPP should be maintained at a minimum of 70 mm Hg

Guidelines for use of hyperventilation

Standards. In the absence of increased ICP, chronic prolonged hyperventilation therapy ($PaCO_2$ of 25 mm Hg or less) should be avoided after severe traumatic brain injury (TBI).

Guidelines. The use of prophylactic hyperventilation ($PaCO_2$< 35 mm Hg) therapy during the first 24 h after severe HI should be avoided because it can compromise cerebral perfusion during a time when CBF is reduced.

Options. Hyperventilation therapy may be necessary for brief periods when there is acute neurologic deterioration or for longer periods if there is ICP-hypertension refractory to sedation, paralysis, CSF-drainage, and osmotic diuretics. Jugular venous oxygen saturation, $AVDO_2$, brain tissue oxygen monitoring and CBF monitoring may be help to identify cerebral ischaemia if hyperventilation resulting in PaCO2 values less than 30 mmHg, is necessary.

Guidelines for use of mannitol

Standards. There are insufficient data to support treatment standards.

Guidelines. Mannitol is effective for control of raised ICP after severe HI. Effective doses range form 0.25 to 1g/kg body weight.

Options. The indications for use of mannitol prior to ICP monitoring are signs of transtentorial herniation or progressive neurologic deterioration not attributable to extracranial explanations. However, hypovolaemia should be avoided by fluid replacement. Serum osmolality should be kept below 320 mOsm because concern for renal failure. Euvolaemia should be maintained by adequate fluid replacement. A Foley catheter is essential in these patients. Intermittent boluses may be more effective than continuous infusion

Use of barbiturates in the control of ICP-hypertension

Standards. There are insufficient data to support a treatment standard.

Guidelines. High-dose barbiturate therapy may be considered in haemodynamically stable salvageable severe HI patients with ICP-hypertension refractory to maximal medical and surgical ICP-lowering therapy.

Nutritional support of the brain-injured patient

Standards. There are insufficient data to support standards.

Guidelines. Replace 140% of resting metabolism expenditure in non-paralysed patients and 100% of resting metabolism expenditure in paralysed patients using enteral or parenteral formulae containing at least 15% of calories as protein by the seventh day after injury.

Options. The preferable option is the use of jejunal feeding by gastrojejunostomy because of ease and avoidance of gastric intolerance.

As a supplement Taylor et al. (1999) in a prospective randomized study of 82 patients found that enhanced enteral nutrition accelerates neurologic recovery and reduces both incidence of major complications and postinjury inflammatory responses. Skal dette ikke flyttes væk fra guidelines

The role of antiseizure prophylactic therapy

Standards. Prophylactic use of phenytoin, carbamazepine, phenobarbital or valproate is not recommended for preventing late post-traumatic seizures (PTS).

Guidelines. There are no guidelines available.

Options. It is recommended as a treatment option that anticonvulsant may be used to prevent PTS in patients at high risk for seizures following HI. Phenytoin and carbamazepine have been demonstrated to be effective in preventing PTS. However, the available evidence does not indicate that prevention of early PTS improves outcome following HI.

The future

Advances in critical care, neuroradiological imaging and the reorganisation of trauma systems have led to a pronounced reduction in death and disability resulting from traumatic brain injury. Guidelines are made and should be implemented in prehospital and hospital care. Prospective randomised trials should be made to strengthen the recommendations and to close the loop from clinical research to bedside practice (Ghajar 2000).

The main purpose of the treatment of patients with head injury is the functional result after hospital care. It is of utmost importance to see the traumasystem as a continuum reaching from prophylactics to prehospital, intensive care and rehabilitation in order to bring the patient back to as normal a life as possible.

References

Adams JH, Brierley JB, Conner RCR, Treip CS. The effects of systemic hypotension upon the human brain. Clinical and neuropathological observations in 11 cases. Brain1966:89:235–236

Adams JH, Graham DI, The relationship between ventricular fluid pressure and the neuropathology of raised intracranial pressure. Neuropath Appl Neurobiol 1976: 2: 323–332.

Adams JH, Graham DI, Murray LS, Scott G. Diffuse axonal injury due to non-missile head injury in humans. A analysis of 45 cases. Ann Neurol 1982: 12: 557–563.

Adelson PD, Robichaud RJ, Hamilton RL, Kockanek PM. A model of diffuse traumatic brain injury in the immature rat. J Neurosurg 1996: 85: 134–141.

Adelson PD, Nemoto E, Colak A, Painter M. The use of near infrared spectroscopy (NIRS) in children after traumatic brain injury: A preliminary report. Acta Neurochir 1998 (suppl) 71: 250–254.

Adelson PD, Whalen MJ, Kochanek PM, et al. Blood-brain barrer permeability and acute inflammation in two dels of traumatic brain injury in the immature rat: a preliminary report. Acta Neurchir 1998 (suppl) 71: 104–106.

Alberico AM, Ward JD, Choi SC, Marmarou A, Young HF. Outcome after severe head injury. Relationship to mass lesions, diffuse injury, and ICP course in pediatric and adult patients. J Neurosurg 1987: 67: 648–656.

Albina JE, Cui S, Mateo RB, et al. Nitric oxide-mediated apoptosis in murine peritoneal macrophages. J Immunol 1993: 150: 5080–5085.

Albrecht RF, Miletich DJ, Ruttle M. Cerebral effects of extended hyperventilation in unanesthehetized goats. Stroke 1987: 18: 649–655.

Aldrich EF, Eisenberg HM, Saydjari C, Luerssen TG, Foulkes MA, Jane JA, Marshall LF, Marmerou A, Young HF. Diffuse brain swelling in severely head-injured children – A report from til NIH traumatic coma banK. J Neurosurg 1992: 76: 450–454.

Alexander MJ, Martin NA, Khanna R, Caron M, Becker DP. Regional cerebral blood flow trends in head injured patients with focal contusions and cerebral edema. Acta Neurochir [suppl] **Årstal** 60: 479–481.

Andersen AR, Tfeft-Hansen P, lassen NA. The effect of ergotamine and dihydroergotamine on cerebral blood flow in man. Stroke 1987: 18: 120–123.

Andersen BJ, Unterberg AW, Clarke GD, Maramrou A. Effect of posttraumatic hypoventilation on cerebral energy metabolism. J Neurosurg 1988: 68: 601–607.

Andersen BJ, Marmarou A.Functional compartmentalization of energy production in neural tissue. Brain Res. 1992a: 585: 190–195.

Andersen BJ, Marmarou A. Post-traumatic selective stimulation of glycolysis. Brain Res. 1992b: 585: 184–189.

Anderson CV, Bigler ED. The role of caudate nucleus and corpus callosum atrophy in trauma-induced anterior horn dilation. Brain Inj 1994: 8: 565–569.

Anderson CV, Wood D-MG, Bigler ED, Blatter DD. Lesion volume, injury severity, and thalamic integrity following head injury. J Neurotrauma 1996: 13: 59–65.

Andrews PJD, Piper IR, Dearden NM, Miller JD. Secondary insults during intrahospital transport of head-injured patients. Lancet 1990: 335: 327–330.

Annegers JF, Grabow JD, Groover RV, et al. Seizures after head trauma; a population study. Neurology 1980: 30: 683–689.

Anthes DL, Theriault E, Tator CH. Ultrastructural evidence for arteriolar vasospasm after spinal cord trauma. J Neurosurg 1996: 39: 804–814.

Arbit E, DiResta GR, Wronski M, Lee J, Galicich JH. The effect of lazaroid on cerebral elastance and edema in a cryogenic injury model. In Intracranial Pressure VIII. Avezaat CJJ et al. (eds). Springer Verlag 1993: 108–111.

Armstead WM. Role of NOC/oFQ in impaired opioid-induced pial artery dilation following injury. Brain Res 2000: 869: 231–235.

Armstead WM. Age dependent endothelin contributes to NOC(oFQ induced impairment og NMDA cerebrovasodilation after brain injury. Peptides 2001: 22: 39–46.

Artru AA, Hornbein TF. Prolonged hypocapnia does not alter the rate of CSF profuction in dogs during halothane anesthesia or sedation with nitrous oxide. Anesthesiology 1987: 67: 66–71.

Asgeirsson B, Grände PO, Nordström C-H. A new therapy of posttrauma brain edema based on haemodynamic principles for brain volume regulation. Int Care Med 1994: 20: 260–267.

Asgeirsson B, Grände PO, Nordström C-H, et al. Effects of hypotensive treatment with $_2$ -agonist and $\beta_1$antagonist on cerebral haemodynamics in severily head-injured patients. Acta Anesthesiol Scand 1995: 39: 347–351.

Astrup J, Bergholt B, Gyldersted C. Blood flow in cerebral contusions. J Neurotrauma (abstract) 1995: 12: 377.

Ausina A, Baguena M, Nadal M. et al. Cerebral hemodynamic changes during sustained hypocapnia in severe head injurY: can hyperventilation cause cerebral ischemia? Acta Neurochir 1998 (suppl) 71: 1–4.

Awad I, Little JR, Lucas F, et al. Modification of focal cerebral ischemia by prostacyclin and indomethacin. J Neurosurg 1983: 58: 715–719

Bailey I Bell A, Gray J et al. A trial of the effect of nimodipine on outcome after head injury. Acta Neurochir 1991: 110: 97–105.

Bakay L, Lee JC, Lee GC, Peng J. Experimental cerebral contusion. Part I: An electron microscopic study. J Neurosurg 1977: 47: 525–531.

Bakay RAE, Ward AA Jr. Enzymatic changes in serum and cerebrospinal fluid in neurological injury. J Neurosurg 1983: 58: 27–37.

Baker AJ, Moulton RJ, MacMillan V, Shedden PM. Excitatory aminoacids in cerebrospinal fluid following traumatic brain injury in humans. J Neurosurg 1993: 79: 369–372.

Balslev-Jørgensen P, Heilbrun NP, Boysen G, et al. Cerebral perfusion pressure correlated with regional cerebral blood flow, EEG, and aortacervical arteriography in patients with severe brain disorders progressing to brain death. Europ Neurol 1972: 8: 207–212.

Bandres J, Yao L, Nemoto EM, et al. Effects of dobutamine and dopamine on whole brain blood flow and metabolism in unanesthethetized monkeys. J Neurosurg Anesthesiol 1992: 4: 250–256.

Bara M, Guiet-Bara A, Durlach J. Comparative effects of MgCl and $MgSO_4$ on the ionic transfer components through the isolated human amniotoc membrane. Magnes Res 1994: 7: 11–16.

Bardt TF, Unterberg AW, Härtl R. et al. Monitoring of brain PO_2 in traumatic brain injury: Effect of cerebral hypoxia on outcome. Acta Neurochir 1998 (suppl) 71: 153–156.

Baro P, Dóczi T, Csete K, et al. Measurement of regional cerebral blood flow and blood flow velocity in experimental intracranial hypertension: Infusion via the cisterna magna in rabbits. Neurosurgery 1991: 28: 821–825.

Barzó P, Marmarou A, Fatouros P, et al. Magnetic resonance imaging-monitored acute blood-brain barrier changes in experimental traumatic brain injury. J Neurosurg 1996: 85: 1113–1121.

Barzo P, Marmarou AA, Fatouros P et al. Contribution of vasogenic and cellular edema to traumatic brain swelling measured by diffusion-weigthed imaging. J Neurosurg 1997: 87: 900–907.

Baskaya MK, Docal A, Rao AM, Dempsey RJ. Neuroprotective effects of citicoline on brain edema and blood-brain barrier breakdown after traumatic brain injury. J Neurosurg 2000: 92: 448–452.

Becker DP, Miller JD, Ward JD, et al. The outcome from severe head injury with early diagnosis and intensive management. J Neurosurg 1977: 47: 491–502.

Becker DP, Miller JD, Sweet RC, et al. Head injury management. In Neural trauma (ed) Popp AJ, New York, Raven Press 1979: 313–328.

Becker DB. Selecting patients for intracranial pressure monitoring in severe head injury. In Intracranial Pressure V. Ishii S et al. (eds). Springer Verlag, Berlin, Heirdelberg, New York 1983: 512–516.

Bemana I, Takahashi E, Nakamura T. et al. OPC-21268, an orally effective, nonpeptide arginine vasopressin VI receptor antagonist reduces vasogenic brain edema. Acta Neurochir 1997 (suppl): 70: 194–197.

Bemana I, Nagao S. Treatment of brain edema with a nonpeptide arginine vasopressin VI receptor antagonist OPC-21268. Neurosurgery 1999: 44: 148–154.

Berger S, Staub F, Stoffel M, et al. Therapeutical effecacy of a novel chloridew transport blocker and an IP3-analoque in vasogenic brain edema. Acta Neurochir 1994 [suppl] 60: 534–537.

Berger S, Schürer L, Härtl R, et al. 7.2% NaCl/dextran 60 versus 20% mannitol for treatment of intracranial hypertension. Acta Neurochir 1994 [suppl] 60: 494–498.

Bergsneider M, Hovda DA, Shalmon E. et al. Cerebral hyperglycolysis following severe traumatic brain injury in humans: a positron emission tomography study. J Neurosurg 1997: 86: 241–251.

Bergsneider M, Hovda DA, Lee SM, et al. Dissociation of cerebral glucose metabolism and level of consciousness during the period of metabolic depression following human traumatic brain injury. J Neurotraum 2000: 17: 389–401.

Biagas KV, Grundl PD, Kochanek PM, et al. Posttraumatic hyperemia in immature, mature, and aged rats: Auradiographic determination of cerebral blood flow. J Neurotrauma 1996: 13: 189–200.

Bianchi C, Tanganelli S, Marzola G, et al. GABA induced changes in acetylcholine release from slices of guinea-pig brain. Naunyn Schmiedebergs Arch Pharmacol 1982: 318: 253–258.

Biestro A, Barrios E, Baraibar J, et al. Use of vasopressors to raise cerebral perfusion pressure in head injured patients. Acta Neurochir 1998 (suppl) 71: 5–9.

Bissonnette B, Bickler PE, Gregory GA, Severinghaus JW. Intracranial pressure and brain redox balance in rabbits. Can J Anaesth 1991: 38: 654–659.

Born JD. The Galsgow-Liége Scale. Acta Neurochir 1988: 91: 1–11.

Bouma GJ, Muizelaar JP. Relationship between cardiac output and cerebral blood flow in patients with intact and with impaired autoregulation. J Neurosurg 1990: 73: 368–374.

Bouma GJ, Muizallar P, Choi SC, et al. Cerebral circulation and metabolism after severe traumatic brain injury. The elusive role of ischemia. J Neurosurg 1991: 75: 685–693.

Bouma GJ, Muizelaar P, Stringer WA, et al. Ultra-early evaluation of regional cerebral blood flow in severely head-injured pateints using Xenon-enhanced computerized tomography. J Neurosurg 1992: 77: 360–368.

Bouma GJ, Muizelaar JP, Bandoh K, Marmarou A. Blood pressure and ICP dynamics in severe head injury: Relation with CBF autoregulation. In Intracranial Pressure VIII (eds) Avzaat CJJ et al. Springer Verlag 1993: 296–299.

Bouma GJ, Muizelaar JP Schurman R, et al. Cerebral blood volume in acute head injury: Relationship to CBF and ICP. In Intracranial Pressure VIII (eds) Avezaat CJJ et al. Springer Verlag 1993: 429–534.

Bouma GJ, Muizelaar JP, Fatouros P. Pathogenesis of traumatic brain swelling: Role of cerebral blood volume. Acta Neurochir 1998 (suppl) 71: 272–275.

Bouzarth WF, Lindermuth JR. Head injury watch sheet modified for a digital scale. J Trauma 1978: 18: 571.

Braakman R, Avezaat CJ, Maas AI, et al. Interobserver agreement in the assessment of the motor response of the Glasgow coma scale. Clin Neurol Neurosurg 1977: 80: 100.

Braakman R, Jennett WB, Minderhoud JM, Prognosis of posttraumatic vegetative state. Acta Neurochir 1988: 95: 49–52.

Braakman R. Early prediction of outcome in severe head injury. Acta Neurochir 1992: 116: 161–163.

Bramlett HM, Dietrich WD, Green EJ, Busto R. Chronic histopathological consequence of fluid-percussion brain injury in rats: Effects of post-traumatic hypothermia. Acta Neuropathol 1997: 93: 190–199.

Braquet P, Touqui L, Shen TY, Vargaftic BB. Perspectives in platelet-activating factor release. Pharmacol Rev 1987: 39: 9–145.

Bratton SL, Davis RL. Acute lung injury in isolated traumatic brain injury. Neurosurgery 1997: 40: 702–712.

Brioni JD, Decker MW, Gamboa LP, et al. Muscimol injections in the medial septum impair statial learning. Brain Res. 1990: 522: 227–234.

Bryan RM, Cherian L, Robertson C. Regional cerebral blood flow after controlled cortical impact injury in rats. Anesth Analg 1995: 80: 687–695.

Bruce DA, Langfitt TW, Miller JD, et al. Regional cerebral blood flow, intracranial pressure, and brain metabolism in comatose patients. J Neurosurg 1973: 38: 131–145.

Bruce DA, Langfitt TW, The pronostic value of ICP, CPP, CBF, and $CMRO_2$ in head injury. In McLaurin RL (ed) Head Injuries, Grune and Stratton, New York, 1976: 23–25.

Bruce DA, Schut L, Bruno LA, et al. Outcome following severe head injuries in children. J Neurosurg 1978: 48: 679–688.

Buchner K, Meixensberger J, Dings J, Roosen K. Bear-infrared spectroscopy not useful to monitor cerebral oxygenation after severe brain injury. Zentralbl Neurochir 2000:61(2):69–73

Bukoski RD, Wang SH, Bian K, DeWitt DS. Traumatic brain injury does not alter cerebral artery contractility. Am J Physiol 1997: 272: H1406–H1411.

Bullock R, Butcher SP, Chen M-H, et al. Correlation of the extracellular glutamate concentration with extent of blood flow reduction after subdural hematoma in the rat. J Neurosurg 1991: 74: 794–802.

Bullock R, Zauner A; Tsuji O, et al. Excitatory amino acid release after severe human head trauma: eeffect of intracranial pressure and cerebral perfusion pressure changes. In: Nagal H, et al. (eds). Intracranial Pressure IX. Springer Verlag, Berlin Heidelberg New York Tokyo 1994: 264–267.

Bundgaard H, Jensen K, Cold GE, Bergholt B, Frederiksen R, Pless S. Effects of indomethacin on intracranial pressure, cerebral blood flow, and cerebral metabolism in patients subjected to craniotomy for cerebral tumors. J Neurosurg Anesthesiol 1996: 8: 273–279.

Bundgaard H, Cold GE. Studies of regional subdural pressure gradients during craniotomy. Br J Neurosurgery 2000: 14: 229-234.

Bundgaard H, von Oetingen G, Jørgensen HA, Cold GE. The effects of dihydroergotamine on intracranial pressure, cerebral blood flow and cerebral metabolism in patients subjected to craniotomy for brain tumors. J Neurosurg Anesthesiol 2000 (in press).

Burke AM, Greenberg JH, Sladky J, Reivich M. Regional variation in cerebral perfusion during acute hypertension. Neurology 1987: 37: 94-99.

Chan k-H, Dearden NM, Miller JD. The significance of posttraumatic increase in cerebral blood flow velocity. A transcranial Doppler ultrasound study. Neurosrugery 1992: 30: 697-700.

Chan K-H, Miller JD, Dearden NM, et al. The effect of changes in cerebral perfusion pressure upon middle cerebral artery blood flow velocity and jugular bulb venous oxygen saturation after severe brain injury. J Neurosurg 1992: 77: 55-61.

Chan K-H, Dearden NM, Miller JD, et al. Transcranial Doppler waveform differences in hyperaemic and non-hyperaemic patients after severe head injury. Surg Neurol 1992: 38: 433-436.

Changaris DG, McGraw CP, Richardson JD, et al. Correlation of cerebral perfusion pressure and Glasgow Coma Scale to outcome. J Trauma 1987: 27: 1007-1012.

Chao CC, Hu S, Molitor TW, et al. Activated microglia mediate neuronal cell injury via a nitric oxide mechanism. J Immunol 1992: 149: 2736-2741.

Chatzipanteli K, Alonso OF, Kraydieh S, Dietrich D. Importance of posttraumatic hypothermia and hyperthermia on the inflammatory response after fluid percussion brain injury: biochemical and immunocytochemical studies. J Cereb Blood Flow Metab 2000: 20: 531-542.

Chen M, Clark RSB, Kochanek PM, Chen J, Schiding JK, Stetler RA, Simon RP, Graham SH. 72-kDa heat shock protein and mRNA expression after controlled cortical impact injury with hypoxemia in rats. J Neurotrauma 1998: 15: 171-181.

Chen M-H, Bullock R, Graham DI, et al. Ischemic neuronal damage after acute subdural hematoma in the rat: Effects of pretreatment with glutamate antagonist. J Neurosurg 1991: 74: 944-950.

Chen T, Qian Y-Z, Di X, et al. Lactate/glucose dynamics after rat fluid percussion brain injury. J Neurotrauma 2000: 17: 135-142.

Cherian L, Goodman JC, Robertson CS. Hyperglycemia increases brain injury caused by secondary ischemia after cortical impact injury in rats. Crit Care Med 1997: 25: 1378-1383.

Cherian L, Hannay HJ, Vagner G, Goodman JC, Contant CF, Robertson CS. Hyperglycemia increases neurological damage and behavioral deficits from post-traumatic secondary ischemic insults. J Neurotrauma 1998: 15: 307-321.

Chesnut RM, Marshall SB, Piek J, et al. Early and late systemic hypotension as a frequent and fundamental source of cerebral ischemia following severe brain injury in the traumatic coma data bank. Acta Neurochir 1993) (suppl) 59: 121-125.

Chesnut RM, Marshall LF, Klauber MR, et al. The role of secondary brain injury in determining outcome from severe head injury. J Trauma 1993: 34: 216-222.

Chesnut RM. Avoidance of hypotension: Conditio sine qua non of successful severe head-injury management. J Trauma 1997: 42: S4-S9.

Chesnut RM, Hyperventilation in traumatic brain injury: Friend or foe. Crit Care Med 1997: 25: 1275-1278.

Choi SC, Narayan RK, Anderson RL, Ward JD. Enhanced specificity of prognosis in severe head injury. J Neurosurg 1988: 69: 381-385.

Choi SC, Barnes TY, Bullock R, et al. Temporal profile of outcomes in severe head injury. J Neurosurg 1994: 81: 169-173.

Christensen MS. Acidbase changes in cerebrospinal fluid and blood, and blood voluem changes following prologed hyperventilation in man. Br J Anaesth 1974: 46: 348-357.

Christensen MS. Prolonged artificial hyperventialtion in cerebral apoplexy. Acta Anaesthesiol Scand 1976: [suppl]62: 1-24.

Clark RS, Kochanek PM, Marion DW, et al. Mild posttraumatic hypothermia reduces mortality after severe controlled cortical impact in rats. J Cereb Blood Flow Metab 1996: 16: 253-261.

Clark RSB, Kochanek PM, Obrist WD. Et al. Cerebrospinal fluid and plasma nitrite and nitrate concentrations after head injury in humans. Crit Care Med 1996: 24: 1243-1251.

Clark RSB, Kochanek PM, Dixon CE, et al. Early neuropathologic effects of mild or moderate hypoxemia after controlled cortical impact injury in rats. J Neurotrauma 1997: 4: 179-189.

Clark WC, Muhlbauer MS, Lowrey R, et al. Complications of intracranial pressure monitoring in trauma patients. Neurosurgery 1989: 25: 20-24.

Clifton GL, Ziegler MG, Grossman RG. Circulation catecholamines and sympathetic activity after head injury. Neursurgery 1981: 8: 10-14.

Clifton GL, Robertson CS, Kyper K, et al. Cardiovascular responses to severe head injury. J Neurosurg 1983: 59: 447-454.

Clifton GL, Allen S, Barrodale P. et al. A Phase II study of moderate hypothermia in severe brain injury. J Neurotrauma 1993: 10: 263-271.

Clifton GL, Jiang JY, Lyeth BG, et al. Marked protection by moderate hypothermia after experimental traumatic brain injury. J Cereb Blood Flow Metab 1993: 11: 114-121.

Clifton GL, Miller ER, Choi SC et al. Lack of effect of induction of hypothermia after acute brain injury. NEJM 2001:344:556-563.

Cold GE, Enevoldsen E, Malmros R. The prognostic value of continuous intraventricular pressure recording in unconscious brain-injured apteints under controlled ventilation. In Intracranial Pressure II (eds) Lundberg N et al. Springer Verlag, Berlin, Heidelberg, Neyw York, 1975a: 517-521.

Cold GE, Enevoldsen EM, Malmros R. Ventricular fluid lactate, pyruvate, bicarbonate and pH in unconscious patients subjected to controlled hyperventilation. Acta Neurol Scand 1975b: 52: 187-195.

Cold GE, Jensen FT, Malmros R. The cerebrovascular CO_2 reactivity during the acute phase of brain injury. Acta Anaesthesiol Scand 1977a 21: 222-231.

Cold GE, Jensen FT, Malmros R. The effects of $PaCO_2$ reduction on regional cerebral blood flow in the acute phase of brain injury. Acta Anaesthesiol Scand 1977b: 21: 359-367.

Cold GE. Cerebral metabolic rate of oxygen ($CMRO_2$) in the acute phase of brain injury. Acta Anaesthesiol Scand 1978: 22: 249-256.

Cold GE, Jensen FT. Cerebral autoregulation in unconscious patients with brain injury. Acta Anaesthesiol Scand 1978: 22: 270–280.
Cold GE, Jensen FT, Cerebral blood flow in the acute phase after head injury. Part I: Correlation to age of the patients, clinical outcome and localization of the injured region. Acta Anaesthesiol Scand 1980: 24: 245–251.
Cold GE. Cerebral blood flow in the acute phaser after head injury. Part II: Correlation to intraventricular pressure (IVP), cerebral perfusion pressure (CPP), $PaCO_2$, ventricular fluid lactate, lactate/pyruvate ratio and pH. Acta Anaesthesiol Scand 1981: 25: 332–335.
Cold GE, Christensen MS, Schmidt K. Effect of two levels of induced hypocapnia on cerebral autoregulation in the acute phase of head injury coma. Acta Anaesthesiol Scand 1981: 25: 397–401.
Cold GE. The relationship between cerebral metabolic rate of oxygen and cerebral blood flow in the acute phase of head injury. Acta Anaesthesiol Scand 1986: 30: 453–457.
Cold GE. Does acute hyperventilation provoke cerebral oligemia in comatose patients after acute head injury? Acta Neurochir 1989: 96: 100–106.
Cold GE. Measurements of CO_2 reactivity and barbiturate reactivity in patients with severe head injury. Acta Neurochir 1989: 98: 153–163.
Cold GE. Cerebral blood flow in acute head injury. Acta Neurochir 1990 [suppl] 49: 1–66.
Compton JS, Lee T, Jones NR, et al. A double blind placebo controlled trial in the calcium entry blocking drug, nicardipine, in the treatment of vasospasm follwoing severe head injury. Br J Neurosurg 1990: 4: 8–15.
Corkin S, Rosen JT, Sullivan EV, Clegg RA. Penetrating head injury in young adulthood exacerbates cognitive decline in later years. J Neurosci 1989: 9: 3876–3883.
Cormio M, Valadka AB, Robertson CS. Elevated jugular venous oxygen saturation after severe head injury. J Neurosurg 1999: 90: 9–15.
Corte FD, Giordano A, Pennisi MA, et al. Quantitative cerebral blood flow and metabolism determination in the first 48 hours after severe head injury with a new dynamic SPECT devise. Acta Neurochir 1997: 139: 636–642.
Cottrell JE. Brain care in the new millennium. Will anything change. Europ J Anaesthesiol 2000:17 (suppl 118) 1–5
Crockard HA, Taylor AR. Serial CsF lactate/pyruvate values as a guide to prognosis in head injury coma. Europ Neurol 1972: 8: 151–157.
Cruz J. Continuous versus serial global cerebral hemometabolic monitoring: Apllications in acute brain trauma. Acta Neurochir 1988 [suppl 42], 35–39.
Cruz J, Miner ME, Allen SJ, et al. Continuous monitoring of cerebral oxygenation in acute brain injury: Injection of mannitol during hyperventilation. J Neurosurg 73: 725–730.
Cruz J, Miner ME, Allen SJ, Alves WM, Gennarelli TA. Continuous monitoring cerebral oxygenation in acute brain injury: Assessment of cerebral hemodynamic reserve. Neurosurgery 1991: 29: 743–749.
Cruz J. On-line monitoring of global cebral hypoxia in acute brain injury. Relationship to intracranial hypertension. J Neurosurg 1993: 79: 228–233.
Cruz J, Hoffstad OJ, Jaggi JL. False cerebral ischemia in acute brain injury with acute anemia. Crit Care Med 1994: (abstract) A58.
Cruz J, Jaggi JL, Hoffstad OJ. Cerebral blood flow, vascular resistance, and oxygen metabolism in acute brain trauma: Redefining the role of cerebral perfusion pressure? Crit Care Med 1995: 23: 1412–1417.
Cruz J. Relationship between early patterns of cerebral extraction of oxygen and outcome from severe acute traumatic brain swelling: Cerebral ischemia or cerebral viability? Crit Care Med 1996: 24: 953–956.
Cruz J. The first decade of continuous monitoring of jugular bulb oxyhemoglobine saturation: Management strategies and clinical outcome. Crit Care Med 1998: 26: 344–351.
Culotta VP, Sementilli ME, Gerold K, Watts CC. Clinicopathological heterogeneity in the classification of mild head injury. Neurosurgery 1996: 38: 245–250.
Czosnyka M, Kirkpatrick PJ, Pickard JD. Multimodal monitoring and assessment of cerebral haemodynamic reserve after severe head injury. Cerebrovasc Brain Metab Rev 1996: 8: 273–295.
Czosnyka M, Smielewski P, Kirkpatrick P et al. Continuous monitoring of cerebrovascular pressure-reactivity in head injury. Acta Neurochir 1998 (suppl) 71: 74–77.
Dahl B, Jensen K, Cold GE, Astrup J. Studies of barbiturate reactivity in patients with severe head injury. Acta Anaesthesiol Scand (suppl 96) 1991 (abstract) p201.
Dahl B, Bergholt B, Cold GE, Astrup J, Mosdal B, Jensen K. Kjærsgaard JO. CO_2- and indomethacin vasoreactivity in patients with head injury. Acta Neurochir 1996: 138: 265–273.
Dahlgren N, Nilsson B, Sakabe T, Siesjö BK. The effect of indomethacin on cerebral blood flow and oxygen consumption in the rat at normal and increased carbon dioxide tensions. Acta Physiol Scand 1981: 111: 475–485.
Darby JM, Nemoto EM, Yonas H, et al. Local cerebral blood flow measured by Xenon-enhanced CT during cryogenic brain edema and intracranial hypertension in monkeys. J Cereb Blood Flow Metab 1993: 13: 763–772.
Dempsey RJ, Roy MW, Meyer KL, Donaldson DL. Indomethacin-mediated improvement following middle cerebral artery occlusion in cats. Effects of anesthesia. J Neurosurg 1985: 62: 874–881.
Dempsey RJ, Baskaya MK, Dogan A. Attenuation of brain edema, blood-brain barrier breakdown, and injury volume by ifenprodil, a polyamine.site N-Methyl-D-Aspartate receptor antagonist, after experimental traumatic brain injury in rats. Neurosurgery 2000: 47: 399–406.
DeNadal M, Munar F, Poca MA, et al. Cerebral hemodynamic effects of morphine and fentanyl in patients with severe head injury: absence of correlation to cerebral autoregulation. Anesthesiology 2000: 92: 11–19.
DeSalles AAF, Kontos HA, Becker DP et al. Prognostic significance of ventricular fluid CSF lactic acidosis in severe head injury. J Neurosurg 1986: 65: 615–624.
DeSalles AAF, Muizellar P, Young HF. Hyperglycemia, cerebrospinal fluid lactic acidoses, and cerebral blood flow in severely head-injured patients. Neurosurgery 1987: 21: 45–50.
DeSalles AAF, Kontos HA, Ward JD, et al. Brain tissue pH in severely head-injured patients: A report of three cases. Neurosurgery 1987: 20: 297–301.
DeVries HE, Blom-Roosemalen MCM, van Oosten M, de Boer AG, van Berkel TCJ, Breimer DD, Kuiper J. The influence of cytokines on the integrity of the blood-brain barrier in vitro. J Neuroimmunology 1996: 64: 37–43.

DeWitt DS, Jenkins LW, Lutz H, et al. Regional cerebral blood flow following fluid percussion injury. J Cereb Blood Flow Metab 1981: (suppl 1): 579–580.
DeWitt DS, Jenkins LW, Wei EP, et al. Effects of fluid percussion brain injuryon regional cerebral blood flow and pial artriolar diameter. J Neurosurg 1986: 64: 787–794.
DeWitt DS, Smith TG, Deyo DJ, et al. L-arginine and superoxide dismutase prevents or reverse cerebral hypoperfusion after fluid-percussion traumatic brain injury. J Neurotrauma 1997: 14: 223–233.
DeWitt DS, Prough DS. Accurate measurement of brain temperature. Crit Care Med 1998: 26: 431–432.
Dhillon HS, Carman HM, Zhang D, et al. Severity of experimental brain injury on lactate and free fatty acid accumulation and Evans blue extravasation in the rat cortex and hippocampus. J Neurotrauma 1999: 16: 455–469.
Dietrich WD, Busto R, Valdes I Halley M. The importance of brain temperature in alterations of the blood-brain barrier during brain ischemia J Neuropathol Exp Neurol 1990: 49: 486–497.
Dietrich WD, Alonso O, Halley M. Early microvascular and neuronal consequences of traumatic brain injury: a light and electron microscopic study in rat. J Neurotrauma 1994a : 11: 289- 301.
Dietrich WD. Alonso O, Busto R. et al. Posttraumatic brain hypothermia reduces histopathological damage following concussive brain injury in the rat. Acta Neuropath 1994b: 87: 250–258.
Dietrich WD, Alonso O, Busto R, Finklestein SP. Posttreatment with intravenous basic fibroblast growth factor reduces histopathological damage following fluid-percussion brain injury in rats. J Neurotrauma 1996: 13: 1996.
Dietrich WD, Alonso O, Busto R, et al. Widespread hemodynamic depresssion and focal platelet accumulation after fluid percussion brain injury: A double-label autoradiographic study in rats. J Cereb Blood Flow Metab 1996: 16: 481–489.
Dietrich WD, Alonso O, Halley M, Busto R. Delayed posttraumatic brain hyperthermia worsens outcome after fluid percussion brain injury: a light and electron microscopic study in rats. Neurosurgery 1996: 38: 533–541.
Dinjs J, Meixensberger J, Amschler J, et al. Brain tissue pO_2 in relation to cerebral perfusion pressure, TCD findings and TCD-CO_2-reactivity after severe head injury. Acta Neurochir 1996: 138: 425–434.
Dinjs J, Meixensberger J, Roosen K. Brain tissue PO_2-monitoring catheter stability and complications. Neurol Res 1997: 19: 241–245.
Dixon CE, Bao J, Long DA, Hayes RL. Reduced evoked release of acetylcholine in the rodent hippocampus following traumatic brain injury. Pharm Biochem and Behav 1996: 53: 679–686.
Dixon CE, Ma X, Marion DW. Effects of CDP-choline treatment on neurobehavioral deficits after TBI and on hippocampal and neocortical acetylcholine release. J Neurotrauma 1997: 14: 161–168.
Dixon E, Markgraf CG, Angileri F, Pike BR, Wolfson B, Newcomb JK, Bismar MM, Blanco AJ, Clifton GL, Hayes RL. Protective effects of moderate hypothermia on behavioral deficits but not necrotic cavitation following cortical impact injury in the rat. J Neurotrauma 1998: 15: 95–103.
Doppenberg EMR, Rice MR, Di X, Young HF, Woodward JJ, Bullock R. Increased free radical production due to subdural hematoma in the rat: Effect of increased inspired oxygen fraction. J Neurotrauma 1998: 15: 337–347.
Duckrow RB, LaManna JC, Rosenthal M, Levasseur JE. Oxydative metabolic activity of the cerebral cortex after fluid percussion injury in the cat. J Neurosurg 1981: 54: 607–614.
Duhaime A-C, Gennarelli LM, Boradman C. Neuroprotection by dextromethorphan in acute experimental subdural hematoma in the rat. J Neurotrauma 1996: 13: 79–85.
Durham SR, Clancy RR, Leuthardt E. et al. CHOP infant coma scale ("infant face scale"): A novel coma scale for children less than two years of age. J Neurotrauma 2000: 17: 730–737.
During MJ, Fried I, Leone P, et al. Direct measurement of extracellular lactate in the human hippocampus during spontaneous seizures. J Neurochem 1994: 62: 2356–2361.
Ebmeyer U, Safar P, Radovsky A, Obrist W, Alexander H, Pomeranz S. Moderate hypothermia for 48 hours after temporary epidural brain compression injury in a canine outcome model. J Neurotrauma 1998: 15: 323–336.
Edvinsson L, Hardebo JE, McCulloch J, Owman CH. Action of dopamine agonists on brain vessels *in vitro* and after *in vivo* microapplication. Acta Physiol Scand 1978: 104: 349–359.
Eisenberg HM, Frankowski RF, Contant CF, et al. High-dose barbiturate control of elevated intracranial pressure in patients with severe head injury. J Neurosurg 1988: 69: 15–23.
Ellingsen I, Hauge A, Nicolaysen G, et al. Changes in human cerebral blood flow due to step changes in PaO_2 and $PaCO_2$. Acta Physiol Scnad 1987: 129: 157–163.
Ellis EF, Weight KF, Wei EP, et al. Cyclooxygenase products of arachidonic acid metabolism in cat cerebral cortex after experimental concussive brain injury. J Neurchem 1981: 37: 892–896.
Ellis EF, Police RJ, Rice LY, et al. Increased plasma PGE2, 6-keto-PGF1 alpha, and 12-Hete levels following experimental concussive brain injury. J Neurotrauma 1989: 6: 31–37.
Ellis EF, Dodson LY, Police RJ. Restoration of cerebrovascular responsiveness to hyperventilation by the oxygen radical scavenger N-Acetylcysteine following experimental traumatic brain injury. J Neurosurg 1991: 75: 774–779.
Ellison MD, Erb DE, Kontos HA., Povloshock JT. Recovery of impaired endothelium-dependent relaxation after fluid-percussion brain injury in cats. Stroke 1989: 20: 911–917.
Elphinstone MG, Archer DP, Pappius HM. The effect of pentobarbitone anesthesia on glucose metabolism in traumatized rat brain. Can J Anaesth 1987: S102–203.
Enevoldsen EN, Cold GE, Jensen FT, Malmros R. Dynamic changes in regional CBF, intraventricular pressure, CSF-pH and lactate levels during the acute phase of head injury. J Neurosurg 1976: 44: 191–214.
Enevoldsen EM, Jensen FT. Cerebrospinal fluid lactate and pH in patients with severe head injury. Clin Neurol Neurosurg 1978: 80: 213–225.
Enevoldsen EM, Jensen FT. Autoregulation of CO_2 responses of cerebral blood flow in patients with severe head injury. J Neurosurg 1978: 48: 689–703.
Enevoldsen Em. Dynamic changes in regional cerebral blood flow, cerebral ventricular pressure, cerebrospinal pH and lactate during the acute phase of severe head injury. 1981. FADL´s forlag, København, Århus,
Enevoldsen EM, CBF in head injury. Acta Neurochir 1986 (suppl 36): 133–136.
Engelborghs K, Haseldonckx M, Reempts van J, et al. Impaired autoregulation of cerebral blood flow in an experimental

model of traumatic brain injury. J Neurotrauma 2000: 17: 667–677.

European Study Group on Nimodipine in Severe Head Injury. A multicenter trial of the efficacy of nimodipine on outcome after severe head injury. J Neurosurg 1994: 80: 797–804.

Faden AI, Demediuk P, Panter SS, Vink R. The role of exci tory amino acids and NMDA receptors in traumatic injury. Science 1989: 244: 798–800.

Faraci E, Alves WM. Do woman fare worse: A metaanalysis gender differences in traumatic brain injury outcome. J Neurosurg 2000: 93: 539–545.

Fearnside MR, Cook RJ, McDowall P, McNeil RJ. The Westmead head injury project outcome in severe head injury. A comparative analysis of pre-hospital, clinical and CT variables. Br J Neurosurg 1993: 7: 267–279.

Feraci FM, Brian Je Jr. Nitric oxide and the cerebral circulation. Stroke 1994: 25: 692–703.

Fielding K, Rowley G. Reliability of assessment by skilled observers using Glasgow coma scale. Aust J Adv Nurs 1990: 7: 13.

Fieschi C, Battistini N, Beduschi A, et al. Regional cerebral blood flow and intraventricular pressure in acute head injuries. J Neurol Neurosurg Psychiat 1974: 37: 1378–1388.

Findley G, Kohi Y, Matheson M, et al. Volumetric analysis of the contralateral dilated ventricle. J Neuro Neurosurg Psychiat 1983: 46: 368–372.

Fineman L, Hovda DA, Smith M, et al. Concussive brain injury is associated with a prolonged accumulation of calcium: A 45-calcium autoradiographic study. Brain Rec 1993

Fleischer AS, Rudman DR, Fresh CB, Tindall GT. Concentration of 3`5`cyclic adenosine monophosphate in ventricular CSF of patients following severe head trauma. J Neurosurg 1977: 47: 517–524.

Folkerts MM, Berman RF, Muizelaar JP. Moderate acute ethanol intoxication provides partial neuroprotection in a rat model of diffuse brain injury. J Neurotrauma (abstract) 1998: 15: 870.

Fortune JB, Feustel PJ, Weigle CG, Popp AJ. Continuous measurement of jugular venous oxygen saturation in response to transient elevations of blood pressure in head-injured patients. J Neurosurg 1994: 80: 461–468.

Frei HJ, Wallenfang T, Poll W, et al. Regional cerebral blood flow and regional metabolism in cold induced edema. Acta Neurochir 1973: 29: 15–28.

Freshman SP, Battistella FD, Matteucci M, Wisner DH. Hypertonic saline (7.5%) versus mannitol: A comparison for treatment of acute head injuries. J Trauma 1993: 35: 344–348.

Forbes ML, Hendrich KS, Kochanek PM, et al. Assessment of cerebral blood flow and CO_2 reactivity after controlled cortical impact by perfusion magnetic resonance imaging using **serial** spin-labeling in rats. J Cereb Blood Flow Metab 1997: 17: 865–874.

Frost EAM, Aranciba CU, Shulman K. Pulmonary shunt as a prognostic indication in head injury. J Neurosurg 1979: 50: 768–772.

Fukuda K, Aihara N, Sagar SM; et al. Purkinje cell vulnerability to mild traumatic brain injury. J Neurotrauma 1996: 13: 255

Furuse M, Brick M, Hasuo M, Dietz H. Relationship between brain tissue pressure gradients and cerebral blood flow distribution studied in circumscribed vasogenic cerebral oedema. Neurochirurgica 1981: 24: 10–14.

Gaab MR, Seegers K, Smedema RJ, et al. A compartive analysis of THAM (tris-buffer) in traumatic brain oedema. Acta Neurochir 1990 (suppl 51): 320–323.

Galbraith S, Cardoso E, Patterson J, Marmarou A. The water content of white matter after head injury in man. In Recent progress in the study and therapy of brain oedema. (eds) Go KG, Baethmann AF. Plenum Publishing Corporation. 1984: 323–330.

Gale SD, Johnson SC, Bigler ED, Blatter DD. Trauma-induced degenerative changes in brain injury: A morphometric analysis of three patients with preinjury and postinjury MR scans. J Neurotrauma 1995: 12: 151–158.

Gennarelli TA, Obrist WD, Langfitt TW, et al. Vascular and metabolic reactivity to changes in $paCO_2$ in head injured patients. In Popp AJ, Bourke RS, Nelson LR, Kimelberg HK (eds) Neural trauma, Raven Press, New York 1979; 1–8.

Gennarelli TA. Head injury in man and experimental animals. Clinical aspects. Acta Neurochir (suppl) 1983: 1–13.

Gennarelli TA, Marcincin RP, Thibault LE, Thompson CJ. Effect of direction of head movement on ICP in experimental head injury. In: Intracranial Pressure V (eds) Ishii S, Nagai H, Brock M. Springer Verlag, Berlin 1983: 483–486.

Gennarelli TA, Pastusko M, Sakamoto T. et al. ICP after experimental diffuse head injuries. In: Intracranial Pressure VI (eds) miller JD, Teasdale GM, Rowan JO, Galbraith SL, Mendelow AD. Springer Verlag, Berlin 1986: 15–19.

Gentleman D. Causes and effects of systemic complications among severely head injured patients transferred to a neurosurgical unit. Int Surg 1992: 77: 297–302.

Ghajar J, Hariri RJ, Narayan RK, et al. Survey of critical care management of comatose head-injured patients in the United States. Crit Care Med 1995: 23: 560–567.

Ghajar J. Traumatic brain injury. Lancet 2000:365:923–929

Gibson RM, Stephenson GC. Aggressive management of severe closed head trauma: Time for reappraisal. Lancet ii 1989: 369–370.

Globus MY, Alonso O, Dietrich WD et al. Glutamate release and free radical production following brain injury: effects of posttraumatic hypothermia. J Neurochem 1995: 65: 1704–1711.

Giulian D, Corpus M, Chapman S, et al. Reactive mononuclear phagocytes release neurotoxins after ischemic and traumatic injury to the central nervous system. J Neurosci Res 1993: 36: 681–693.

Gobiet W, Grote W, Bock WJ. The realtion between intracranial pressure, mean arterial pressure, and cerebral blood flow in patients with severe head injury. Acta Neurochir 1975: 32: 13–24.

Golding EM, Steenberg ML, Contant CF Jr et al. Cerebrovascular reactivity to CO_2 and hypotension after mild cortical impact injury. Am J Physiol 1999: 277: H1457–H1466.

Golding EM, Robertson CS, Bryan RM. L-Arginine partially restores the diminished CO_2 reactivity after mild controlled cortical impact injury in theadult rat. J Cereb Blood Flow Metab 2000: 20: 820–828.

Goodman JC, Valadka AB, Gopinath SP, Cormio M, Robertson CS. Lactate and excitatory amino acids measured by microdialysis are decreased by pentobarbital coma in head-injured patients. J Neurotrauma 1996: 13: 549–556.

Goodman JC, Valadka AB, Gopinath SP, Uzura M, Robertson CS. Extracellular lactate and glucose alterations in the brain after head injury measured by microdialysis. Crit Care Med 1999: 27: 1965–1973.

Goodman SJ, Becker DP. Vascular pathology of the brain stem due to experimentally increased intracranial pressure: Changes noted in the micro- and macrocirculation. J Neurosurg 1973: 39: 601–609.

Gopinath SP, Robertson CS, Grossman RG, et al. Near-infrared spectroscopy localization of intracranial hematomas. J Neurosurg 1993: 79: 43–47.

Gopinath SP, Robertson CS, Narayan RK. Cerebrovascular effects of dihydroergotamine in head injury. Crit Care Med 1994 (abstract) A 204.

Gopinath SP, Robertson CS, Contant CF, et al. Early detection of delayed traumatic intracranial hematoma using near-infrared spectroscopy. J Neurosurg 1995: 83: 438–444.

Gopinath SP, Valadka AB, Uzura M, Robertson CS. Comparison of jugular venous oxygen saturation and brain tissue PO_2 as monitors of cerebral ischemia after head injury. Crit Care Med 1999: 27: 2337–2345.

Gordon CR, Merchant RS, Marmarou A, et al. Effect of murine recombinant interleukin-1 on brain edema in the rat. Acta Neurochir 1990 (suppl) 51: 268–270.

Gordon E. Bergvall U. The effect of controlled hyperventilation on cerebral blood flow and oxygen uptake in patients with brain lesions. Acta Anaestheiol Scand 1977: 17: 63–70.

Graham DI, Adams JH. Ischemic brain damage in fatal head injuries. Lancet 1971: i: 265–266.

Graham DI, Adams JH, Doyle D. Ischemic brain damage in fatal non-missile head injury. J Neurol Sci 1978: 39: 213–234.

Graham DI, Gentleman SM, Lynch A, Roberts GW. Distribution of β-amyloid protein in the brain following severe head injury. Neuropath Appl Neurobiol 1995: 21: 27–34.

Grände PO. The effect of dihydroergotamine in patients with head injury and raised intracranial pressure. Int Care Med 1989: 15: 523–527.

Grände PO, Asgeirsson B, Nordström CH. Physiologic principles for volume regulation of a tissue enclosed in a rigid shell with application to the injured brain. J Trauma 1997: 42: S23–S31.

Granholm L, Siesjö BK. The effect of hypercapnia and hypocapnia upon the cerebrospinal fluid lactate and pyruvate concentrations and upon the lactate, pyruvate, ATP, ADP, phsophocreatine and creatine concentrations of the cat brain. Acta Phyiol Scand 1969: 75: 257–266.

Granholm L. The effect of blood in the CSF on the CSF lactate, pyruvate and bicarbonate concentrations. Scand J Clin Lab Invest 1969: 23: 361–366.

Gray WJ, Rosner MJ. Pressure-volume index as a function of cerebral perfusion pressure. Part 2: The effects of low cerebral perfusion pressure and autoregulation. J Neurosurg 1987: 67: 377–380.

Greene KA, Marciano FF, Johnson BA, et al. Impact of traumatic subarachnoid hemorrhage on outcome in nonpenetrating head injury. J Neurosrug 1995: 83: 445–452.

Green KA, Marciano FF, Johnson BA, et al. Impact of traumatic subarachnoid hemorrhage on outcome in nonpenetrating head injury. Part 1: A proposed computerized tomography grading scale. J Neurosurg 1995: 83: 445–452.

Green KA, Jacobowitz R, Marciano FF, et al. Impact of traumatic subarachnoid hemorrhage on outcome in nonpenetrating head injury. Part II: relationship to clinical course and outcome variables during acute hospitalization. J Trauma 1996: 41: 964–971.

Grosswasser-Reider I, Cohen M, Costeff H, Groswasser Z. Late CT findings in brain trauma. Relationship to cognitive and behavioral sequelae and to vocational outcome. AJR 1993: 160: 147–152.

Guidelines for the management of severe head injury (eds) Bullock R, Chesnut RM, Clifton G, Ghajar J, Marion DW, Narayan RK, Newell DW, Pitts LH, Rosner MJ, Wilberger JE. J Neurotrauma 1996: 13: 639–734.

Guluma KZ, Saatman KE, Brown A, Raghupathi R, McIntosh TK. Sequential pharmacotheray with magnesium chloride and basic fibroblast growth factor after fluid percussion brain injury results in less neuromotor efficacy than achieved with magnesium alone. J Neurotrauma 1999: 16: 311–321.

Gyulai L, Schnall M, McLaughlin AC, et al. Simultaneous 31P- and 1H-nuclear magnetic resonance studies of hypoxia and ischemia in the cat brain. J Cereb Blood Flow Metab 1987: 7: 543–551.

Halifax A. Role of cerebral perfusion pressure in acute brain trauma. Crit Care Med 1996: 24: 1273–1274.

Hallenbeck JM, Furlow TW. Prostaglandin I2 and indomethacin prevent impairment of post-ischemic brain reperfusion in the dog. Stroke 1979: 10: 629–637.

Haltiner AM, Newell DW, Temkin NR, Dikmen SS, Winn HR. Side effects and mortality associated with use of phenytoin for early posttraumatic seizure prophylaxis. J Neurosurg 1999: 91: 588–592.

Hamer J, Høyer S, Stoeckel H, et al. Cerebral blood flow and cerebral metabolism in acute increase in intracranial pressure. Acta Neurchir 1973: 28: 95–110.

Hamm RJ, Jenkins LW, Lyeth BG, et al. The effect of age on outcome following traumatic brain injury in rats. J Neurosurg 1991: 75: 916–921.

Hamm RJ, Temple MD, Pike BR, Ellis EF. The effect of postinjury administration of polyethylene glycol-conjugated superoxide (pegorgotein, dismutase) or lidocaine on behavioral function following fluid-percussion brain injury in rats. J Neurotrauma 1996: 13: 325–332.

Hans P, Franssen C, Pincemail J, et al. Plasma myeloperoxidase and vitamine E levels in head injury: Preliminary results related to outcome. J Neurosurg Anesthesiol 1992: 4: 26–30.

Hansen NB, Nowicki PT, Miller RR, et al. Alterations in cerebral blood flow and oxygen consumption during prolonged hypocapnia. Pediatr Res 1986: 20: 147–150.

Harders A, Kakarieka A, Braakman R, et al. Traumatic subarachoid hemorrhage and its treatment with nimodipine. J Neurosurg 1996: 85: 82–89.

Harris RJ, Bayhan M, Branston NM, et al. Modulation of the pathophysiology of primate focal cerebral ischemia by indomethacin. 1982: 13: 17–24.

Härtl R, Medary MB, Ruge M, et al. Hypertonic/hyperoncotic saline attenuates microcirculatory disturbances after traumatic brain injury. J Trauma 1997: 42: S41–S47.

Hashimoto T, Pitts LH, Pogliani L, et al. Changes in brain phosphorus metabolism in rats following fluid percussion injury. In: Intracranial Pressure VI. (eds) Miller JD, et al., Springer Verlag, Berlin, Heidelberg. 1986: 30–34.

Hass WK. Prognostic value of cerebral oxidative metabolism in head trauma. In: McLaurin RL (ed) Head Injuries, Springer Verlag, Grune and Stratton, New York, 1976: 35–37.

Hass WK, Rapaport ZH, Kobayashi M, et al. Temporal effect of reticular formation lesions on rat regional cerebral blood flow (abstract). Stroke 1976: 7: 7.

Havill JH. Prolonged hyperventilation and intracranial pressure. Crit Care Med 1984: 12: 72–74.

Hawkins RA, Hass WK, Ransohoff J. Cerebral blood flow, glucose utilization, oxydative metabolism, and plasticity after mesencephalic reticular formation lesions. In: Popp AJ, et al. (eds) Neural Trauma, Raven Press, New York, 1979: 9–18.
Hayashi N, Hirayama T, Udagawa A, et al. Systemic management of cerebral edema based on a new concept in severe head injury patients. Acta Neurochir 1994 (suppl) 60: 541–543.
Hayes RL, Pechura CM, Katayama Y, et al. Activation of pontine cholinergic sites implicated in unconsciousness following cerebral concussion in the cat. Science 1984: 223: 301–303.
Heath DL, Vink R. Neuroprotective effects of $MgSO_4$ and $MgCl_2$ in closed head injury: a comparative phosphorus NMR study. J Neurotrauma 1998: 15: 183–189.
Holmin S, Mathiesen T. Biphasic edema development after experimental brain contusion in rat. Neurosci Lett 1995: 194: 97–100.
Holmin S, Mathiesen T, Shetye J, Biberfeld P. Intracerebral inflammatory response to experimental brain contusion. Acta Neurochir 1995: 132: 110–119
Holmin S, Mathiesen T, Dexamethasone and colchicine reduce inflammatory and delayed edema following experimental brain contusion. Acta Nerochir 1996: 138: 418–424.
Holmin S, Schalling M, Höjeberg B, et al. Delayed cytokine expression in rat brain following experimental contusion. J Neurosurg 1997: 86: 493–504.
Hoppe E, Christensen L, Christensen KN. The clinical outcome of patients with severe head injuries, treated with high-dose dexamethasone, hyperventilation and barbiturates. Neurochirurgica 1981: 24: 17–20.
Hossmann KA, Sakaki S, Kimoto K. Cerebral uptake of glucose and oxygen in the cat brain after prolonged ischemia. Stroke 1976: 7: 301–305.
Hovda DA, Katayama Y, Yoshida A, et al. Pre- or postsynaptic blocking of glutamatergic functioning prevents the increase in glucose utilization following concussive brain injury. In: The Role of Neurotransmitters in Brain Injury, Globus M, et al. (eds)Plenum Press, New York 1992: 327–332.
Hovda DA, Badie KFH, Samli A, Becker DP. Administration of an omega-comopeptide one hour following traumatic brain injury reduces 45-calcium accumilation. Acta Neurochir 1994: (suppl) 60: 521–523.
Hovda DA. Metabolic dysfunction. In: Neurotrauma. Narayan RK et al. (eds). McGraw-Hill, New York 1996: 1459–1478.
Ikeda Y, Teramoto A, Nakagawa Y, et al. Attenuation of cryogenic induced brain oedema by arginine vasopressin release inhibitor RU51599. Acta Neurochir 1997: 139: 12: 1173–1179.
Inao S, Marmarou A, Clarke GD, et al. Production and clearance of lactate from brain tissue, cerebrospinal fluid, and serum following experimental brain injury. J Neurosurg 1988: 69: 736–744.
Ingebrigtsen T, Romner B, Kongstad P, Langbakk B. Increased serum concentrations of protein S-100 after minor head injury. A biochemical serum marker with prognostic value?. J Neurol Neurosurg Psychiat 1995: 59: 103–104.
Ingebrigtsen T, Romner B. Serial S-100 protein serum measurements related to early magnetic resonance imaging after minor head injury: Case report. J Neurosurg 1996: 85: 945–948.
Ingebrigtsen T, Waterloo K, Jacobsen EA, Langbakk B, Romner B. Traumatic brain damage in minor head injury: Relation of serum S-100 protein measurements to magnetic resonance imaging and neurobehavioral outcome. Neurosurgery 1999: 45: 468–476.
Ingvar DH, Haggendal E, Nilsson E, et al. Cerebral circulation and metabolism in a comatose patients. Arch Neurol 1964: 11: 13–19.
Ingvar DH, Sourander P. Destruction of the reticular core of the brain stem. Arch Neurol 1970: 23: 1–8.
Isaksson J, Lewén A, Hillered L, Olsson Y. Up-regulation of intracellular adhesion molecule 1 in cerebral microvessels after cortical contusion trauma in a rat model. Acta Neuropathol 1997: 94: 16–20.
Ishige N, Pitts LH, Berry I, et al. The effect of hypoxia on traumatic head injury in rats: Alterations in neurologic function, brain edema, and cerebral blood flow. J Cereb Blood Flow Metab 1987: 7: 759–767.
Ishige N, Pitts LH, Berry I, et al. The effects of hypovolemic hypotension in high-energy phsophate metabolism of traumatized brain in rats. J Neurosurg 1988: 68: 129–136.
Ito J, Marmarou A, Barzó P, et al. Characterization of edema by diffusion-weighted imaging in experimental traumatic brain injury. J Neurosurg 1996: 84: 97–103.
Jackowski A, Crockard A, Burnstock G, et al. Time course of intracranial pathophysiological changes following experimetnal subarachnoid haemorrhage in the rat. J Cereb Blood Flow Metab 1990: 10: 835–849.
Jacobsen WK, Isaacs WB. Cerebral injury: Are manipulations of carbon dioxide beneficial? J Neurosurg Anesthesiol 1993: 5: 59–61.
Jaggi JL, Cruz J, Gennarelli TA. Estimated cerebral metabolic rate of oxygen in severely brain-injured patients. A valuable tool for clinical monitoring. Crit Care Med 1995: 23: 66–70.
Jafar JJ, Johs LM, Mullian SF. The effect of mannitol on cerebral blood flow. J Neurosurg 1986: 64: 754–759.
Jaggi JL, Obrist WD, Gennarelli TA, Langfitt TW. Relationship of early cerebral blood flow and metabolism to outcome in acute head injury. J Neurosurg 1990: 72: 176–182.
James HE, Bruce DA, Welch F. Cytotoxic edema produced by 6-Aminonicotinamide and its response to therapy. Neurosurgery 1978: 3: 196–200.
Janis LS, Hoane MR, Conde D, et al. Acute ethanol administration reduces the cognitive deficits assiciated with traumatic brain injury in rats. J Neurotrauma 1998: 15: 105–115.
Jeffreys RV, Jones JJ. Avoidable factors contributing to the death of head injury patients in general hospitals in Mersye region. Lancet 1981, ii, 459–461.
Jenkins LW, Moszynski K, Lyeth BG, et al. Increased vulnerability of the mildly traumatized rat brain to cerebral ischemia. Brain Res 1989: 477: 211–224.
Jennett B, Bond M. Assessment of outcome after severe brain damage. A practical scale. Lancet i: 1975: 480–484.
Jennett B, Teasdale G, Galbraith S. et al. Severe head injuries in three countries. J Neurol Neurosurg Psychiat 1977: 40: 291.
Jennett B. Severe head injury. Prediction of outcome as a basis for management decisions. Int Anesthesiol Clin 1979: 17: 133–152.
Jennett B, Teasdale C. Dynamic pathology. In: Management of head injury (eds) Jennett B, Teasdale C. Davis Company, Philadephia, 1981: 45–75.
Jennett B, Teasdale C. Management of head injuries in the acute state. Philadelphia FA Davis Company 1981: 240–241.

Jensen K, Ohrström J, Cold GE, Astrup J, The effect of indomethacin on intracranial pressure, cerebral blood flow, and cerebral metabolism in patients with severe head injury and intracranial hypertension. Acta Neurochir 1991: 108: 116–121.

Jiang JY, Lyeth BG, Clifton GL, et al. Relationship between body and brain temperature in traumatically brain-injured rodents. J Neurosurg 1991: 74: 492–496.

Jiang JY, Lyeth BG, Kapasi MZ, et al. Moderate hypotehrmia reduces blood-brain barrier disruption following traumatic brain injury in the rat. Acta Neuropathol (Berl) 1992: 84: 495–500.

Jiang JY, Ming-kun Y, Zhu C. Effect of long-term mild hypothermia therapy in patients with severe traumatic brain injury: 1-year follow-up review of 87 cases. J Neurosurg 2000: 93: 546–549.

Johnston IH, Johnston JA Jennett B. Intracranial pressure changes following head injury. Lancet 1970: ii: 433–436.

Johnston IH, Rowan JO, Harper AM, Jennett WB. Raised intracranial pressure and cerebral blood flow. 1: Cisterna magna infusion in primates. J Neurol Neurosurg Psychiat 1972: 35: 285–296.

Johnston IH, Rowan JO, Harper AM, Jennett WB. Raised intracrnial pressure and cerebral blood flow. 2: supratentorial and infratentorial mass lesions in primates. J Neuro Neurosurg Psychiat 1973: 36: 161–170.

Johnston IH, Harper AM. The efffect of mannitol on cerebral blood flow. An experimental study. J Neurosurg 1973: 38: 461–471.

Johnston IH, Rowan JO. Raised intracranial pressure and cerebral blood flow 4: Intracranial pressure gradients and regional cerebral blood flow. J Neurol Neurosurg Psychiat 1974: 37: 585–592.

Jones PA, Andrews PJD, Midfley S. et al. Measuring the burden of secondary insults in head-injured patients during intensive care. J Neurosurg Anesthesiol 1994: 6: 4–14.

Jünger EC, Newell DW, Grant GA, et al. Cerebral autoregulation following minor head injury. J Neurosurg 1997: 86: 425–432.

Juul N, Morris GF, Marshall SB, The executive commitee of the international selfotel trial, Marshall LF. Intracranial hypertension and cerebral perfusion pressure: influence on neurological deterioration and outcome in severe head injury. J Neurosurg 2000: 92: 1–6.

Kakarieka A, Braakman R, Schakel EH. Subarachnoid hemorrhage after head injury. Cerebrovasc Dis 1995: 5: 403–406.

Kamada K, Houkin K, Iwasaki Y, Abe H. A high-field magnetic resonance imaging study of experimental vasogenic brain edema and its response to AVS: 1.2-bis (nicotinamido)-propane. Acta Neurochir 1994 (suppl) 60: 463–470.

Kamiya T, Katayama Y, Kashiwagi F, et al. The role of bradykinin in mediating ischemic brain edema in rats. Stroke 1993: 24: 571–575.

Kampfl A, Posmantur RM, Zhao X, Schmutzhard E, Clifton GL, Hayes RL. Mechanisms of calpain proteolysis following traumatic brain injury: Implications for pathology and therapy: A review and update. J Neurotrauma 1997: 14: 121–134.

Kasoff SS, Zingesser LH, Shulman K. Compartmental abnormalities of regional cerebral blood flow in children with head trauma. J Neurosurg 1972: 36: 463–470.

Kaste M, Hernesniemi J, Somer H, et al. Creatinekinase isoenzymes in acute brain injury. J Neurosurg 1981: 55: 511–515.

Katayama Y, Becker DP, Tamura T, Hovda DA. Massive increases in extracellular potassium and the indiscrimate release of glutamate following concussive brain injury. J Neurosurg 1990: 73: 889–900.

Katayama Y, Mori T, Maeda T, Kawamata T. Pathogenesis of the mass effect of cerebral contusions: Rapid increase in osmolality within the contusion necrosis. Acta Neurochir 1998 (suppl) 71: 289–292.

Kawamata T, Katayama Y, Hovda DA, et al. Administration of excitatory amino acid antagonists via microdialysis attenuates the increase in glucose utilization seen following concussive brain injury. J Cereb Blood Flow Metab 1992: 12: 12–24.

Kawamata T, Katayama Y, Hocda DA, et al. Lactate accumulation following concussive brain injury: The role of ionic fluxes induced by excitatory amino acids. Brain Res 1995: 674: 196–204.

Katoh H, Shima K, Nawashiro H, et al. Selective hippocampal damage to hypoxia after mild closed head injury in the rat. Acta Neurochir 1998 (suppl) 71: 247–249.

Kawai N, Nakamura T, Okauchi M, Nagao S. Effects of hypothermia on intracranial pressure and brain edema formation: studies in a rat acute subdural hematoma model. J Neurotrauma 2000: 17: 193–202.

Kebatian JW, Calne DB, Multiple receptors for dopamine. Nature 1979: 277: 93–96.

Kelly DF, Martin NA, Kordestani R, et al. Cerebral blood flow as a predictor of outcome following traumatic brain injury. J Neurosurg 1997: 86: 633–641.

Kelly DF, Lee SM, Pinanong PA, Hovda DA. Paradoxical effects of acute ethanolism in experimental brain injury. J Neurosurg 1997: 86: 876–882.

Kelly DF, Kozlowski DA, Haddad E. et al. Ethanol reduces metabolic uncoupling following experimental head injury. J Neurotrama 2000: 17: 261–272.

Kempski O, Behmanesh S. Endothelial cell swelling and brain perfusion. J Trauma Injury Infect Crit Care 1997: 42: S38–S40.

Keskil S, Baykaner MK, Ceviker N, Aykol S. Head trauma and leucocytosis. Acta Neurochir 1994: 131: 211–214.

Khanna S, Davis D, Petersen B et al. Use of hypertonic saline in the treatment of severe refractory posttraumatic intracranial hypertension in pediatric traumatic brain injury. Crit Care Med 2000:28:4:1144–1151

Kiening KL, Unterberg AW, Bardt TF, et al. Monitoring of cerebral oxygenation in patients with severe head injuries: brain tissue PO_2 versus jugular vein oxygen saturation. J Neurosurg 1996: 85: 751–757.

Kiening KL, Härtl R, Unterberg AW, et al. Brain tissue PO_2 monitoring in comatose patients: implication for therapy. Neurol Res 1997: 17: 233–240.

King LR, McLaurin RL, Knowles HC. Acid-base balance and arterial and CSF lactate levels following human head injury. J Neurosurg 1974: 40: 617–625.

Kinoshita K, Katayama Y, Hirayama T, Tsubokawa T. Attenuation of hemispheric swelling associated with acute subdural hematomas by excitatory amino acid antagonist in rats. Acta Neurochir 1994: (suppl) 60: 505–507.

Kita H, Marmarou A. The cause of acute brain swelling after the close head injury in rats. Acta Neurchir 1994 (suppl) 60: 452–455.

Klauber MR, Marshall LF, Barrett-Connor E, et al. Prospective study of patients hospitalized with head injury in San Diego County, 1978. Neurosurgery 1981: 9: 236–241.

Klauber MR, Toutant SM, Marshall LF. A model for predicting delayed intracranial hypertension following head injury. J Neurosurg1984: 61: 695–699.

Kobayashi S, Nakazawa S, Yano M, et al. The value of intracranial pressure (ICP) measurement in acute head injury showing diffuse cerebral swelling. In Intracranial Presssure V. (eds) Ishii S, Nagai H, Brock M. Springer Verlag, Berlin, Heidelberg, 1983: 527–531.

Kobayashi S, Yokota H, Yajima K, et al. Diffuse axonal injury in severe head trauma. Neurosurg Rev 1989: 12 (suppl): 451–457.

Kochaneh PM, Dutka AJ, Kumaroo KK, Hallenbeck JM. Platelet activating factor receptor blockade enhances recovery after multifocal brain ischemia. Life Sci 1987: 41: 2639–2644.

Kochaneh PM, Nemoto EM, Melich JA, et al. Cerebrovascular and cerebrometabolic effects of intracarotid infused platelet-activating factor in rats. J Cereb Blood Flow Metab 1988: 8: 546–551.

Kofke WA, Nemoto EM, Hjossman KA, et al. Brain blood flow and metabolism after global ischemia and postinsult thiopental therapy in monkeys. Stroke 1979: 10: 544–560.

Kohi YM, Mendelow AD, Teasdale GM, Allardice GM. Extracranial insults and outcome on patients with acute head injury - relationship to Glasgow Coma Scale. Injury 1984: 16: 25–29.

Kontos HA, Wei EP, Povlishock JT, et al. Cerebral arteriolar damage by arachidonic acid and prostaglandin G2. Science 1980: 209: 1242–1245.

Kontos HA, Wei EP. Superoxide production in experimental brain injury. J Neurosurg 1986: 64: 803–807.

Kuruda Y, Bullock R. Failure of cerebral blood flow-metabolism coupling after acute subdural hematoma in the rat. Neurosurgery 1992: 31: 1062–1071.

Kosteljanetz M. Acute head injury: Pressure-volume relations and cerebrospinal fluid dynamics. Neurosurgery 1986: 18: 17–24.

Koston H, Rumpf E, Stampfl G, et al. Treatment of cerebral vasospasm following severe head injury with the calcium influx blocker nimodipine. Neurchirugica 1985: 28: 103–109.

Kotwica Z, Brzezinski J. Head injuries complicated by chest trauma. A review of 50 consecutive patients. Acta Nerochir 1990: 103: 109–111.

Koura SS, Doppenberg EMR, Marmarou A, et al. Relationship between excitatory amino acid release and outcome after severe head injury. Acta Neurochir 1998 (suppl) 71: 244–246.

Kraus JF, Peek-Asa C, McArthur D. The independent effect of gender on outcomes following traumatic brain injury: A preliminary investigation. Neurosurg Focus (1): Article 5, 2000

Kroppenstedt S-N, Schneider G-H, Thomale U-W, Unterberg AW. Protective effects of aptoganel HCl (Cerestat) following controlled cortical impact injury in the rat. J Neurotrauma 1998: 15. 191–197.

Kroppenstedt S-N, Kern M, Thomale U-W, Schneider G-H, Lanksh WR, Unterberg AW. Effect of cerebral perfusion pressure on contusion volume following impact injury. J Neurosurg 1999: 90: 520–526.

Kuhl DE, Alavi A, Hoffman EJ, et al. Cerebral blood volume in head-injured patients. J Neurosurg 1980: 52: 309–320.

Kuklane M, Eelmäe J, Roose M, Kaasik AE. Correction of CSF acidosis and craniospinal system viscoelastic parameters with intrathecal THAM. In Intracranial Pressure VIII. (eds) Avezaat CJJ et al. Springer Verlag 1993: 620–622.

Kulkarni M, Armstead WM. Superoxide generation links nociceptin/orphanin FQ (NOC/oFQ) release to impaired N-methyl-D-aspartate cerebrovasodilation after brain injury. Stroke 2000: 31: 1990–1996.

Kuniyosho T, Nagao S, Kagawa M, et al. Role of stimulation of medullary reticular formation on centrally released arginine, vasopressine in cold induced edema. In: Intracranial Pressure VIII (eds) Avezaat CJJ et al. Spriger Verlag 1993: 120–123.

Kunze E, Meixenberger J, Janka M, et al. Decompressive craniectomy in patients with uncontrolled intracranial hypertension. Acta Neurochir 1998 (suppl) 71: 16–18.

Kuroda Y, Bullock R. Local cerebral blood flow mapping before and after removal of acute subdural hematoma in the rat. Neurosurgery 1992: 30: 687–691.

Kurz A, Sessler DI, Lenhardt R. Perioperative normothermia to reduce the incidence of surgical wound infection and shorten hospitalization. N Engl J Med 1996:334:1205–1209

Kurze T, Tranquada RE, Benedict K. Spinal fluid lactic acid levels in acute cerebral injury. In: Head Injury, Caveness WF, Walker AE (eds), Philadelphia, Lippencott, 1966: 254–259.

Lam AM, Winn HR, Cullen BF, Sundling N. Hyperglycemia and neurological outcome in patients with head injury. J Neurosurg 1991: 75: 545–551.

Lam JMK, Hsiang JNK, Poon WS. Monitoring of autoregulation using Doppler flowmetry in patients with head injury. J Neurosurg 1997: 86: 438–445.

Landolt H, Langemann H, Mendelowitsch A, Grgatzl O. Neurochemical monitoring and on-line pH measurements using brain microdialysis in patients in intensive care. Acta Neurochir 1994 (suppl) 60: 475–478.

Lang DA, Teasdale GM, Macpherson P, Lawrence A. Diffuse brain swelling after head injury: More often malignant in adults than children. J Neurosurg 1994: 80: 675–680.

Langfitt TW, Obrist WD, Gennarelli TA, et al. Correlation of cerebral blood flow with outcome in head injured patients. Ann Surg 1977: 186: 411–414.

Langfitt TW, Gennarelli TA. Can the outcome from head injury be improved? J Neurosurg 1982: 56: 19–25.

Langfitt TW, Obrist WD, Alavi A. et al. Computerized tomography, magnetic resonance imaging and positron emission tomography in the study of brain trauma. J Neurosurg 1986: 64: 760–767.

Latronico N, Beindorf AE, Rasulo FA, et al. Limits of intermittent jugular bulb oxygen saturation monitoring in the management of severe head trauma patients. Neurosurgery 2000: 46: 1131–1139.

Lee JH, Martin NA, Alsina G. et al. Hemodynamically significant cerebral vasospasm and outcome after head injury: a prospective study. J Neurosurg 1997: 87: 221–233.

LeRoux P, Haglund MM, Newell DW, et al. Intraventricular hemorrhage in blunt head trauma: An analysis of 43 cases. Neurosurgery 1992: 31: 678–685.

LeRoux PD, Newell DW, Lam AM, et al. Cerebral arteriovenous oxygen difference: a predictor of cerebral infarction and outcome in patients with severe head injury. J Neurosurg 1997: 87: 1–8.

Levin HS, Meyers CA, Grossman RG, Sarwar M. Ventricular enlargement after closed head injury. Arch Neurol 1981: 38: 623–629.

Levin HS, Williams D, Crofford MJ, et al. Relationship of depth of brain lesions to consciousness and outcome after closed head injury. J Neurosurg 1988: 69: 861–866.
Levin HS. Treatment of postconcussional symptoms with CDP-choline. J Neurol Sci 1991: 103: S39–S42.
Levin HS, Aldrich EF, Saydjari C, et al. Severe head injury in children. Experience of the tramatic coma data bank. Neurosurgery 1992: 31: 435--444.
Levin HS, Mendelsohn D, Lilly MA, et al. Magnetic resonance imaging in relation to functional outcome of pediatric closed head injury: A test of the Ommaya-Gennarelli model. Neurosurgery 1997: 40: 432-441.
Levy DE, Duffy TE. Cerebral energy metabolism during transient ischemia and recovery in the gerbil. J Neurochem 1977: 28: 63–70.
Levy DI, Rekate HL, Cherny WB. Et al. Controlled lumbar drainage in pediatric head injury. J Neurosurg 1995: 83: 453-460.
Lewelt W, Jenkins LW, Miller JD. Autoregulation of cerebral blood flow after experimental fluid perfusion injury of the brain. J Neurosurg 1980: 53: 500–511.
Lewelt W, Jenkins LW, Miller JD. Effect of experimental fluid-percusion injury of the brain on cerebrovascular reactivity to hypoxia and to hypercapnia. J Neurosurg 1982: 56: 332–338.
Lewis SB, Myburgh JA, Reilly PL. Detection of central venous desaturation by continuous jugular bulb oximetry following acute neurotrauma. Anesth Intens Care 1995: 23: 307–314.
Lewis SB, Myburgh JA, Thornton EL, Reilly PL. Cerebral oxygenation monitoring by near-infrared spectroscopy is not clinically usefull in patients with severe closed-head injury: A comparison with jugular venous bulb oximetry. Crit Care Med 1966: 24: 1334–1338.
Lin SZ, Chiou TL, Chiang YT, Song WS. Combined treatment with nicardipine, phenobarbital and methylprednisolone ameliorates vasogenic brain edema. Acta Nerochir 1994 (suppl) 60: 528–530.
Lindsay KW, Carlin J, Kennedy I, et al. Evoked potentials in severe head-injury- Analysis and relation to outcome. J Neurol Neurosurg Psychiat 1981: 44: 796–802.
Lobato RD, Gomez PA, Alday R, et al. Sequential computerized tomography changes and related final outcome in severe head injury patients. Acta Neurochir 1997: 139: 385–391.
Long JB, Gordon J, Bettencourt JA, Bolt SL. Laser-Doppler flowmetry measurements of subcortical blood flow changes after fluid percussion brain injury in rats. J Neurotrauma 1996: 13: 149–162.
Louis PT, Goddard-Finegold J, Fishman MA, et al. Barbiturates and hyperventilation during intracranial hypertension. Crit Care Med 1993: 21: 1200–1206.
Lowenstein DH, Chan PH, Miles MF. The stress protein response in cultured neurons: characterization and evidence for a protective role in excitatotoxicity. Neuron 1991: 7: 1053–1060.
Lowenstein DH, Gwinn RP, Serens MS, et al. Increased expression of mRNA encoding calcindin-D28K, the glucose-regulated proteins, or the 72 kDA heat shock protein in three models of acute CNS injury. Mol Brain Res 1994: 22: 299–308.
Lyeth BG, Jiang JY, Robinson SE et al. Behavioral protection by moderate hypothermia initiated after experimental traumatic brain injury. J Neurotrauma 1993: 10: 57–64.
Maas AIR. Cerebrospinal fluid enzymes in acute brain injury. Dynamics of changes on CSF enzymes activity after experimental brain injury. J Neurol Neurosurg pschiat 1977: 40: 655–665.
Maas AIR, Dearden M, Teasdale GM, et al. EBIC-guidelines for management of severe head injury in adults. Acta Neurochir 1997: 139: 286–294.
Maas AIR, Steyerberg EW, Murray GD, Bullock R, Baethmann A, Marshall LF, Teasdale GM. Why have recent trials of neuroprotective agents in head injury failed to show convincing efficacy? A pragmatic analysis and theoretical considerations. Neurosurgery 1999: 44: 1286–1298.
MacFarlane R, Moskowitz MA, Sakas DE, et al. The rose of neuroeffector mechanisms in cerebral hyperperfusion syndromes. J Neurosurg 1991: 75: 845–855.
MacIver IN, Frey JCS, Matheson JG, The role of respiratory insufficiency in the mortality of severe head injury. Lancet i 1958: 390–393.
MacPherson P, Graham DI. Correlation between angiographic findings and the ischemia of head injury. J Neurol Neurosurg Psychiat 1978: 41: 122–127.
Madsen FF, Reske-Nielsen E, A simple mechanical method using a piston to produce localized cerebral contusions in pigs. Acta Neurochir 1987: 88: 65–72.
Madsen FF. Regional cerebral blood flow after a localized cerebral contusion in pigs. Acta Neurchir 1990a 105: 150–157.
Madsen FF, Jensen FT, Væth M, Djurhus JC. Regional cerebral blood flow in pigs estimated by microspheres. Acta Neurochir 1990: 103: 139–147.
Madsen FF. Regional cerebral blood flow in the pig after a localized cerebral contusion treated with barbiturates. Acta Neurochir 1990b: 106: 24–31.
Madsen FF, Changes in regional cerebral blood flow after hyperventilation in the pig with an induced focal cerebral contusion. Acta neurochir 1990c: 106: 164–169.
Maier-Hauff K, Baethmann AJ, Lange M, et al. The kallikrein-kinin system as mediator in vasogenic brain edema. J Neurosurg 1984: 61: 97–106.
Mailhos C, Hovard MK, Latchman DS. Heat shock protein neuronal cells form programmed cell death by apoptosis. Neuroscience 1993: 55: 621–627.
Marion DW, Darby J, Yonas H. Acute regional cerebral blood flow changes caused by severe head injuries. J Neurosurg 1991: 74: 407–414.
Marion DW, Bouma GJ, The use of stable xenon-enhanced computed tomography studies of cerebral blood flow to define changes in cerebral carbon dioxide vasoresponsitivity caused by a severe head injury. Neurosurgery 1991: 29: 869–873.
Marion DW, Obrist WD, Carlien PM, et al. The use of moderate therapeutic hypothermia for patients with severe head injuries. A preliminary report. J Neurosurg 1993: 79: 354–362.
Marion DW, Carlier PM. Problems with initial Glasgow coma scale assessment caused by prehospital treatment of patients with head injuries: Results of a national survey. J Trauma 1994: 36: 89–95.
Marion DW, White MJ. Treatment of experimental brain injury with moderate hypothermia and 21-aminosteroids. J Neurotrauma 1996: 13: 139–145.
Marion DW, Penrod LE, Kelsey SF et al. Treatment of traumatic brain injury with moderate hypothermia. New Engl J Med 1997: 336: 540–545.

Marmarou A, Mset AL, Ward JD, et al. Contribution of CSF and vascular factors to elevation of ICP in severely head-injured patients. J Neurosurg 1987: 66: 883–890.

Marmarou A. Traumatic brain edema: An overview. Acta Neurochir 1994 (suppl) 60: 421–424.

Marmarou A, Anderson BL, Ward JD et al. Impact of ICP instability and hypotension on outcome in patients with severe head injury. J Neurosurg 1991: 75: s159–s166.

Marmarou A, Montasser A, Foda AE, et al. New model of diffuse brain injury in rats. Part I: Pathophysiology and biomechanics. J Neurosurg 1994: 80: 291–300.

Marmarou A, Nichols J, Burgess J, et al. Effect of the bradykinin antagonist Bradycor (Deltibant CP-1027) in severe traumatic brain injury: Results of a multi-center, randomized, palcebo-controlled trial. J Neurotraum 1999: 16: 431–444.

Marshall LF, Durity F, Lounsbury R, et al. Experimental cerebral oligemia and ischemia produced by intracranial hypertension. Part I: Pathophysiology, electroencephalography, cerebral blood flow, blood-brain barrier and neurological function. J Neurosurg 1975a 43: 308–317.

Marshall LF, Graham DI, et al. Experimental cerebral oligemia and ischemia produced by intracranial hypertension. Part 2: Brain morphology. J Neurosurg 1975b: 43: 318–322.

Marshall LF, Welch F, Diruty F, et al. Experimental cerebral oligemia and ischemia by intracranial hypertension. Part 3: Brain energy metabolism. J Neurosurg 1975c: 43: 323–328.

Marshall LF, Smith RW, Rauscher LA, Shapiro HM. Mannitol dose requirement in brain-injured patients. J Neurosurg 1978: 48: 169–172.

Marshall LF, Smith RW, Shapiro HM. The outcome with aggressive treatment in severe head injuries. Part I: The significance fo intracranial pressure monitoring. J Neurosurg 1979a: 50: 20–25.

Marshall LF, Smith RW, Shapiro HM. The outcome with aggressive treatment in severe head injuries. Part II: Acute and chronic barbiturate administration in the management of head injury. J Neurosurg 1979b: 50: 26–30.

Marshall LF, Becker DP, Bowers SA, et al. The national traumatic coma data bank.Part 1. Design, purpose, goals. and results. J Neurosurg 1983: 59: 276.

Marshall LF, Barba D, Toole BM, et al. The oval pupil: clinical significance and relationship to intracranial hypertension. J Neurosurg 1983: 58: 566–568.

Marshall LF, Gautille T, Klauber MR, et al. The outcome of severe closed head injury. J Neurosurg 1991: 75: 328.

Marshall LF, Marshall SB, Klauber MR, et al. A new classification of head injury based on computerized tomography J Neurosurg 1991: 75: S14–S20.

Marshall WJS, Jackson JLF, Langfitt TW. Brain swelling caused by trauma and arterial hypertension. Arch Neurol 1969: 21: 545–553.

Martin NA, Doberstein C, Zane C, et al. Posttraumatic cerebral arterial spasm: Transcranial Doppler untrasound, cerebral blood flow, and angiographic findings. J Neurosurg 1992: 77: 575–583.

Martin NA, Patwardhan RV, Alexander MJ, et al. Characterization of cerebral hemodynamic phases following severe head trauma: hypoperfusion, hyperemia, and vasospasm. J Neurosurg 1997: 87: 9–19.

Mascia L, Andrews PJ, McKeating EG, et al. Cerebral blood flow and metabolism in severe brain injury: the role of pressure autoregulation during cerebral perfusion management. Intensive Care med 2000: 26: 202–205.

Maset AL, Marmarou AM, Ward JD, et al. Pressure-volume index in head injury. J Neurosurg 1987: 67: 832–840.

Matta DF, Lam AM, Mayberg TS. A critique of the intraoperative use of jugular venous bulb catheters during neurosurgical procedures. Anesth Analg 1994: 79: 745–750.

Mayevsky A, Doron A, Manor T, et al. Cortical spreading depression recorded from the human brain using a multiparametric monitoring system. Brain Res 1996: 740: 268–274.

Mayevsky A, Manor T, Meilin S, et al. Real-time multiparametric monitoring of the injured human cerebral cortex-a new approach. Acta Neurochir 1998 (suppl) 71: 78–81.

McCulloch J, Harper AM. Cerebral circulation: Effect of stimulation and blockade of dopamine receptors. Am J Physiol 233: H222–H227.

McIntosh TK, Faden AI, Yamakami I, Vink R. Magnesium deficiency exacerbates and pretreatment improves outcome following traumatic brain injury in rats. J Neurotrauma 1988: 5: 17–31.

McIntosh TK, Vink R, Noble L, et al. Traumatic brain injury in the rat. Characterization of a lateral fluid-percussion model. Neurosci 1989: 28: 233–244.

McKeating EG, Andrews PJD, Mascia L. Relationship of neuron specific enolase and protein S-100 concentrations in systemic and jugular venous serum to injury severity and outcome after traumatic brain injury. Acta Neurochir 1998 (suppl) 71: 117–119.

McKinley BA, Morris WP, Parmley CL, Butler BD. Brain parenchyma PO_2, PCO_2, and pH during and after hypoxic, ischemic brain insult in dogs. Crit Care Med 1996: 24: 1858–1868.

McKinley BA, Parmley CL. Brain parenchyma PO_2, PCO_2, and pH following severe closed head injury: Emerging patterns. Acta Neurochir 1998, in press.

Mendelow AD, Teasdale G, Teasdale E, et al. Cerebral blood volume and intracranial pressure in head injured patients. In: Intracranial pressure V. Ishii S, et al. (eds), Springer Verlag, Berlin 1983: 495–500.

Mendelow AD, Teasdale G, Russell T, et al. Effect of mannitol on cerebral blood flow and cerebral perfusion pressure in human head injury. J Neurosurg 1985: 63: 43–48.

Mendelow AD, Allcutt DA, Chanbers IR, et al. Intracranial and cerebral perfusion pressure monitoring in the head injured patients. Which Index?. In: Intracranial Pressure VIII. Avezaat CJJ et al. (eds). Springer Verlag 1993: 544–548.

Menzel M, Rieger A, Roth S. et al. Simultaneous continuous measurement of pO_2, pCO_2, pH and temperature in brain tissue and sagittal sinus in a porcine model. Acta Neurochir 1998 (suppl) 71: 183–185.

Menzel M, Doppenberg EMR, Zauner A, Soukup J, Feinert M, Bullock R. Increased inspired oxygen concentration as a factor in improved tissue oxygenation and tissue lactate levels after severe human head injury. J Neurosurg 1999: 91: 1–10.

Merguerian PA, Perel A, Wald U, et al. Persistent non-ketotic hyperglycemia as a grave prognostic sign in head-injured patients. Crit Care Med 1981: 9: 838–840.

Merrill JE, Ignarro LJ, Sherman MP, et al. Microglial cell cytotoxicity of oligodendrocytes is mediated through nitric oxide. J Immunol 1992: 151: 2132–2141.

Messeter K, Ponten U, Siesjö BK. The influence of deep barbiturate anesthesia upon the regulation of extra- and intracellular pH in the rat brain during hypercapnia. Acta Physiol Scand 1972: 85: 174–182.

Messeter K, Nordstöm C-H, Sundberg G, et al. Cerebral hemodynamics in patients with severe head trauma. J Neurosurg 1986: 64: 231–237.

Metz C, Holzschuh M, Bein T. et al. Moderate hypothermia in patients with severe head injury: Cerebral and extracerebral effects. J Neurosurg 1996: 85: 533–541.

Metz C, Holzschuh M, Bein T, et al. Jugular bulb monitoring of cerebral metabolism in severe head injury: Accuracy of unilateral measurements. Acta Neurochir 1998 (suppl) 71: 324–327.

Metzel E, Zimmermann WE. Changes of oxygen pressure, acitd-base balance, metabolites and electrolytes in cerebrospinal fluid and blood after cerebral injury. Acta Neurochir 1971: 25: 177–188.

Meixensberger J, Baunach S, Amschler J, et al. Influence of body position on tissue PO_2, cerebral perfusion pressure and intracranial pressure in patients with acute brain injury. Neurol Res 1997: 19: 249–253.

Miller JA, Richter JA. Effects of GABAergic drugs *in vivo* on high-affinity choline uptake *in vitro* in mouse hippocampal synaptosomes. J Neurochem 1986: 47: 1916–1918.

Miller JD, Ledingsham IM, Jennett WB. Effects of hyperbaric oxygen on intracranial pressure and cerebral blood flow in experimental cerebral oedema. J Neurol Neurosurg Psychiat 1970: 33: 745–755.

Miller JD, Becker DP, Ward JD. Et al. Significance of intracranial hypertension in severe head injury. J Neurosurg 1977: 47: 503–516.

Miller JD, Butterworth JF, Gudeman SK, et al. Further experience in the management of severe head injury. J Neurosurg 1981: 54: 289–299.

Miller JD, Dearden NM, Piper IR, Chan KH. Control of intracranial pressure in patients with severe head injury. J Neurotrauma 1992 (suppl 1)): S317–326.

Miller JI, Chou MW, Capocelli A, et al. Continuous intracranial multimodality monitoring comparing local cerebral blood flow, cerebral perfusion pressure, and microvascular resistance. Acta Neurochir 1998 (suppl) 71: 82–84.

Minassian AT, Beydon L, Decq P, Bonnet F. Changes in cerebral hemodynamics after a single dose of clonidine in severily head-injured patients. Anesth Analg 1997: 84: 127–132.

Minassian AT, Poirier N, Pierrot M, Menei P, Granry JC, Ursino M, Beydon L. Correlation between cerebral oxygen saturation measured by near-infrared spectroscopy and jugular oxygen saturation in patients with severe closed head injury. Anesthesiology 1999: 91: 985–990.

Mitchell DS, Adams JH. Primary focal impact damage to the brainstem in blunt head injuries. Does it excist? Lancet ii 1973: 215–218.

Montasser A, Foda A-E, Marmarou A. A new model of diffuse brain injury in rats. Part II morphological characterization : J Neurosurg 1994: 80: 301–313.

Mori K, Maeda M, Miyazaki M, Iwase H. Effects of mild and moderate hypothermia on cerebral metabolism and glutamate in an experimental head injury. Acta Neurochir 1998 (suppl) 71: 222–224.

Mori T, Kawamata T, Katayama Y, et al. Antioxidant, OPC-14117, attenuates edema formation, and subsequent tissue damage following cortical contusion in rats. Acta Neurochir 1998 (suppl) 71: 120–122.

Morris GF, Juul N, Marshall SB, et al. Neurological deterioration as a potential alternative endpoint in human clinical trials of experimental pharmacological agents for treatment of severe traumatic brain injuries. Neurosurgery 1998: 43: 1369–1374.

Morris GF, Bullock R, Marshall SB, Marmarou A, Maas A, the selfolol investigators, Marshall LF. Failure of the competitive N-methyl-D-aspartate antagonist selfotel (CGS 19755) in the treatment of severe head injury: Results of a phase III clinical trials. J Neurosurg 1999: 91: 737–743.

Mortimer JA, Van Duijn CM, Chandra L, et al. Head trauma as a risk factor for Alzheimer's disease: A collaborative reanalysis of case-control studies. Int J Epidemiol 1991: 20: S28–S35.

Moskopp D, Rise F, Wassmann H, Nadstawek J. Barbiturates in severe head injuries. Neurosurg Rev 1991: 14: 195–202.

Moss E, Gibson SJ, McDowall DG, Gibson RM. Intensive management of severe head injuries. Anaesthesia 1983: 38: 214–225.

Muir JK, Tynan M, Cadwell R, Ellis EF. Superoxide dismutase improves post-traumatic cortical blood flow in rats. J Neurotrauma 1995: 12: 179–188.

Muizelaar JP, Wei EP, Kontos HA, Becker DP. Mannitol causes compensatory cerebral vasconstriction and vasodilatation in response to blood viscosity changes. J Neurosurg 1983: 59: 822–828.

Muizelaar JP, Lutz HA, Becker DP. Effect of mannitol on ICP and CBF, and correlation with pressure autoregulation in severely head-injured patients. J Neurosurg 1984: 61: 700–706.

Muizelaar JP, Van der Poel HG, Li Z, et al. Pial arteriolar vessel diameter and CO_2 reactivity during prolonged hyperventilation in the rabbit. J Neurosurg 1988: 69: 923–927.

Muizelaar JP, Marmarou A, DeSalles AAF, et al. Cerebral blood flow and metabolism in severely head-injured children. Part 1: Relationship with GCS score, outcome, ICP, and PVI. J Neurosurg 1989a: 71: 63–71.

Muizelaar JP, Ward JD, Marmarou A, Cerebral blood flow and metabolism in severely head-injured children. Part 2: Autoregulation. J Neurosurg 1989b: 71: 72–76.

Muizelaar JP, Marmarou A, Ward JD, et al. Adverse effects of prolonged hyperventilation in patients with severe head injury: A randomized clinical trial. J Neurosurg 1991: 75: 731–739.

Muizelaar JP, Marmarou A, Young HF, et al. Improving the outcome of severe head injury with the oxygen radical scavenger polyethylene glycol-conjugated superoxide dismutase. A phase II trial. J Neurosurg 1993: 78: 375–382.

Murdoch I, Perry EK, Court JA, Graham DI, Dewar D. Cortical cholinergic dysfunction after human head injury. J Neurotrauma 1998: 15: 295–305.

Murphy A, Teasdale G, Matheson M, et al. Relationship between CT indicis of brain swelling and intracranial pressure after head injury. In: Intracranial Pressure V. (eds) Isshi S, et al. Springer Verlag, Berlin, 1983: 562–566.

Myburgh JA, Upton RN, Grant C, Martinez A. A comparison of the effects of norepinephrine, epinephrine, and dopamine on cerebral blood flow and oxygen utilisation. Acta Neurochir 1998 (suppl) 71: 19–21.

Nagao S, Ogawa T, Kuniyoshi T, Ohmoto T. Effect of stimulation of the medullary reticular formation on vasogenic brain edema. Adv Experimental Neurotrauma Res 1989: 1 : 35–40.

Nagao S, Kagawa M, Bemana I, et al. Treatment of vasogenic brain edema with arginine vasopressin receptor antagonist - An experimental study. Acta Neurochir (suppl) 60: 502–504.

Narayan RK, Kishore PRS, Becker DP, et al. Intracranial pressure: To monitor or not to monitor? A review of our experience with severe head trauma. J Neurosurg 1982: 56: 650–659.

Naredi S, Olivecrona M, Lindgren C, et al. An outcome study of severe traumatic head injury using the "Lund therapy" with low-dose prostacyclin. Acta Anaesthesiol Scand 2001: 45: 402–407.

Narotam PK, Rodell TC, Nadvi SS, et al. Traumatic brain contusions: A clinical role for the kinin antagonist CP-0127. Acta Neurochir 1998: 140: 793–803.

Nawashiro H, Shima K, Chigasaki H. Blood-brain barrier, cerebral blood flow, and cerebral plasma volume immediately after head injury in the rat. Acta Neurchir 1994 (suppl) 60: 440–442.

Nelson LR, Auen EL, Bourke RS, et al. A comparison of animal head injury models developed for treatment modalities evaluation. In (eds) Grossman RG et al. Seminars in Neurological Surgery, Head injury: Basic and Clinical Aspects. New York, Raven Press 1982: 117–127.'

Newell DW, Weber JP, Watson R, et al. Effect of transient moderate hyperventilation on dynamic cerebral autoregulation after severe head injury. Neurosurgery 1996: 39: 35–44.

Newell DW, Aaslid R, Stooss R, et al. Evaluation of hemodynamic responses in head injury patients with transcranial Doppler monitoring. Acta Neurochir 1997: 139: 804–817.

Ng I, Yeo T-T, Tang W-Y, et al. Apoptosis occurs after cerebral contusions in humans. Neurosurgery 2000: 46: 949–956.

Nilsson B, Nordström C-H, Experimental head injury in the rat. Rat 3: Cerebral blood flow and oxygen consumption after concussive impact acceleration. J Neurosurg 1977a: 47: 262–273.

Nilsson B, Nordström C-H. Rate of cerebral energy consumption in concussive head injury in the rat. J Neurosurg 1977b: 47: 274–281.

Nilsson B, Ponten U, Voigt G. Experimental head injury in the rat. Part 1: Mechanics, pathophysiology and morphology in an impact acceleration trauma model. J Neurosrug 1977: 47: 241–251.

Nilsson P, Hillered L, Olsson Y, et al. Regional changes in interstitial K^+ and Ca^{2+} levels following cortical compression contusion trauma in rats. J Cereb Blood Flow Metab 1993: 13: 183–192.

Nilsson P, Gazelius B, Carlson H, Hillered L. Continuous measurement of changes in regional cerebral blood flow following cortical compression contusion trauma in the rat. J Neurotrauma 1996: 13: 201–209.

Nordby HK, Urdal P. The diagnostic value of measuring creatine kinase BB activity in cerebrospinal fluid following acute head injury. Acta Neurochir 1982: 65: 93–101.

Nordström C-H, Rehncrona S, Postischemic cerebral blood flow and oxygen utilization rate in rats anesthetized with nitrous oxide or phenobarbital. Acta Phsiol Scand 1077: 101: 230–240.

Nordström C-H, Messeter K, Sundberg G, et al. Cerebral blood flow, vasoreactivity, and oxygen consumption during barbiturate therapy in severe traumatic brain lesions. J Neurosurg 1988: 68: 424–431.

Obrenovitch TP, Zilkha E. High extracellular potassium, and not extracellular glutamate, is required for the propagation of spreading depression. J Neurophysiol 1995: 73: 2107–2114.

Obrenovitch TP, Zilkha E, Urenjak J. Evidence against high extracellular glutamate promoting the elicitation of spreading depression by potassium. J Cereb Blood Flow Metab 1996: 16: 923–931.

Obrenovitch TP, Urenjak J, Zilkha E. Effects of increased extracellular glutamate levels on the local field potential in the brain of anaesthetized rats. Br J Pharmacol 1997a: 121: 372–378.

Obrenovitch TP, Urenjak J. Is high extracellular glutamate the key to excitatoxicity in traumatic brain injury? J Neurotrauma 1997: 14: 677–698

Obrist WD, Gennarelli TA, Segewa H, et al. Relation of cerebral blood flow to neurological status and outcome in head-injured patients. J Neurosurg 1979: 51: 292–300.

Obrist WD, Langfitt TW, Jaggi JL, et al. Cerebral blood flow and metabolism in comatose patients with acute head injury. Relationship to intracranial hypertension. J Neurosurg 1984: 61: 241–253.

O'Dell DM, Hamm RJ. Chronic postinjury administration of MDL 26479 (suritozole), a negative modulator at the $GABA_A$ receptor, and cognitive impairment in rats following traumatic brain injury. J Neurosurg 1995: 83: 878–883.

Okiyama K, Smith DH, White WF, et al. Effects of the novel NMDA antagonists CP-98,113, CP-101,581 and CP-101.606 on cognitive function and regional cerebral edema following experimental brain injury in the rat. J Neurotrauma 1997: 14: 211–218.

Okoyama K, Smith DH, Thomas MJ, McIntosh TK. Evaluation of a novel calcium channel blocker, (s)-emopamil, on regional cerebral edema and neurobehavioral function after experimental brain injury. J Neurosurg 1992: 77: 607–615,

Ommaya AK, Gennarelli TA. Cerebral concussion and traumatic unconsciousness. Correlation of experimental and clinical observations on blunt head injuries. Brain 1974: 97: 633–654.

O`Sullival MG, Statham PF, Jones PA, et al Role of intracranial pressure monitoring in severely head-injured patients without signs of intracranial hypertension on initial computerized tomography. J Neurosurg 1994: 80: 46–50.

Overgaard J, Hvid-hansen O, Land A-M, Pedersen KK, Christensen S. Haase J, Hein O, Tweed WA. Prognosis after head injury based on early clinical examination. Lancet ii, 1973: 631–635.

Overgaard J, Tweed WA. Cerebral circulation after head injury. Part 1: cerebral blood flow and its regulation after closed head injury with emphasis on clinical correlations. J Neurosurg 1974: 41: 531–541.

Overgaard J. Reflections on prognostic determinants in acute head injury. In: McLaurin (ed). Head injuries, Grune and Stratton, New York 1975: 11–23.

Overgaard J, Tweed WA. RCBF in impeding brain death. Acta Neurochir 1975: 31: 167–175.

Overgaard J, Mosdal C, Tweed WA. Cerebral circulation after head injury. Part 3: Does reduced regional cerebral blood flow determine recovery of brain fuction after blunt head injury. J Neurosurg 1981: 55: 63–74.

Overgaard J, Tweed WA. Cerebral circulation after head injury. Part 4: Functional anatomy and boundery-zone flow deprivation in the first week of traumatic coma. J Neurosurg 1983: 59: 439–446.

Palmer AM, Marion DW, Botscheller ML, et al. Traumatic brain injury-induced excitotoxicity assessed in a controlled cortical impact model. J Neurochem 1993: 61: 2015–2024.

Palmer AM, Marion DW, Botscheller ML, Redd EE. Therapeutic hypothermia is cytoprotective without attenuating the traumatic brain injury-induced elevations in interstitiel

concentrations of aspartate and glutamate. J Neurotrauma 1993: 10: 363–372.
Panetta T, Marcheselli VL, Braquet P, et al. Effects of platelet activating factor antagonist (BN-52021) on free fatty acids, diacylglycerols, polyphosphateinositides and blood flow in the gerbil brain: Inhibition of ischemic-reperfusion induced cerebral injury. Biochem Biophys Rec Commun 1987: 149: 580196587.
Papo I, Caruselli G. Long-term intracranial pressure monitoring in comatose patients suffering from head injuries. A critical survey. Acta Neurochir 1977: 39: 187–200.
Pappius HM, Local cerebral glucose utilization in thermally traumatized rat brain. Ann Neurol 1981: 9: 484–491.
Park HK, Fernandez I, Dujovny M, Diaz FG. Experimental animal models of traumatic brain injury: Medical and biomechanical mechanism. Crit Rev Neurosrug 1999: 9: 44–52.
Patel PM, Hyperventilation as a therapeutic intervention: Do the potential benefits outweight the known risks. J Neurosurg Anesthesiol 1993: 5: 62–65.
Paulson OB, Olesen J, Christensen MS,. Restoration of autoregulation of cerebral blood flow by hypocapnia. Neurology 1972: 22: 286–293.
Payen D, Quintin L, Plaisance P, et al. Head injury: clonidine decreases plasma catecholamines. Crit Care Med 1990: 18: 392–395.
Pellerin L, Magistretti PJ. Glutamate uptake into astrocytes stimulates aerobic glycolysis: a mechanism coupling neuronal activity to glucose utilization. Proc Natl Acad Sci USA 1994: 91: 10625–10629.
Petersen B, Khenna S, Fischer B, Marshall L: Prolonged hypothermia controls elevated intracranial pressure in head injured pediatric patients. Crit Care Med 2000:28:4:1136–1143
Pfenninger E,Lindner KH, Ahnefeld FW. Die Infusion con THAM (trishydroxymethyl-aminomethan) als Therapie zur Senkung des erhöhten intrakranielle Druckes beim akuten Schädel-Hirn-Trauma. Anaesthesist 1989a: 38: 189–192.
Pfenninger E, Reith A, Breitig D, et al. Early changes of intracranial pressure, perfusion pressure, and blood flow after acute head injury. J Neurosurg 1989b: 70: 774–779.
Pfenninger E, Lindler K-H. Arterial blood gases in patients with acute head injury at the accident site and upon hospital adminssion. Acta Anaesthesiol Scand 1991: 35: 148–152.
Phillips LL, Belardo ET. Expression of *c-fos* in the hippocampus following mild and moderate fluid percussion brain injury. J Neurotrauma 1993: 9: 323–333.
Pichard JD, MacKenzie ET. Inhibition of prostaglandin synthesis and the response of baboon cerebral circulation to carbon dioxide. Nature 1973: 245: 187–188.
Piek J, Chesnut RM, Marshall LF, et al. Extracranial complications of severe head injury. J Neurosurg 1992: 77: 901–907.
Pietropaoli JA, Rogers FB, Shackford SR. Et al. The deleterious effects of intraoperative hypotension on outcome in patients with severe head injuries. J Trauma 1992: 33: 403–407.
Pigula FA, Wald SL, Shackford SB, Vane DW. The effect of hypotension and hypoxia on children with severe head injuries. J Pediatr Surg 1993: 28: 310–316.
Pike BR, Hamm RJ, Temple MD, Buck DL, Lyeth BG. Effect of tetrahydroaminoacridine, a cholinesterase inhibitor, on cognitive performance following experimental brain injury. J Neurotrauma 1997: 14: 897–905.
Pittman T, Bucholz R, Williams D. Efficacy of barbiturates in the treatment of resistant intracranial hypertension in severely head-injured children. Pediatr Neurosci 1989: 15: 13–17.
Plangger CA. Effects of torasemide on intracranial pressure, mean systemic arterial pressure, and cerebral perfusion pressure in experimental brain edema of the rat. Acta Neurochir 1994 (suppl) 60: 519–520.
Pleines UE, Stover JF, Kossmann T, Trentz O, Morganti-Kossmann MC. Soluble ICAM-1 in CSF coincides with the extent of cerebral damage in patients with severe traumatic brain injury. J Neurotrauma 1998: 15: 399–409.
Poca MA, Sahuquillo J, Baguena M, et al. Incidence of intracranial hypertension after severe head injury. A prospective study using the traumatic coma data bank classification. Acta Neurochir 1998 (suppl) 71: 27–30.
Pomoranz S, Safar P, Radocsky A, et al. The effect of resuscitative moderate hypothermia following epidural compression on cerebral damage in a canine outcome model. J Neurosurg 1993: 79: 241–251.
Prasad MR, Ramaiah C, McIntosh TK, et al. Regional levels of lactate and norepinephrine after experimental brain injury. J Neurochem 1994: 63: 1086–1094.
Previgliano I, Ceraso D, Rozas MC, et al. Cerebral perfusion pressure management in head injury. Crit Rev Neurosurg 1997: 7: 36–44.
Prins ML, Hovda DA. Traumatic brain injury in the developing rat: Effects of maturation on Morris water maze acquisition. J Neurotrauma 1998: 15: 799–811.
Procaccio F, Menasce G, Sacchi L, et al. Ischemic insult due to mannual hypervenitlation in head injured patients with intracranial hypertension. In Intracranial Pressure VIII (eds) Avezaat CJJ, et al. Springer Verlag 1993: 583–588.
Prough DS, Zornow MH. Hypertonic maintenance fluids for patients with cerebral edema: Does the evidence support a "phase II" trial? Crit Care Med 1998: 26: 421–422.
Qian L, Ohno K, Maehara T, et al. Changes in lCBF, morphology and related parameters by fluid percussion injury. Acta Neurochir 1996: 138: 90–98.
Quattrocchi KB, Frank EH, Miller CH, et al. Impairment of helper T-cell function and lymphokine-activated killer cytotoxicity following severe head injury. J Neurosurg 1991: 75: 766–773.
Quattrocchi KB, Prasad P, Willits NH, Wagner FC. Quantification of midline chift as a predictor of poor outcome following head injury. Surg Neurol 1991: 35: 183–188.
Quigley MR, Vidovich D, Cantella D. et al. Defining the limits of survivorship after very severe head injury. J Trauma 1997: 42: 7–10.
Qureshi AI, Suarez JI, Bhardwaj A, et al. Use of hypertonic (3%) saline-**acetate** infusion in the treatment of cerebral edema: Effect on intracranial pressure and lateral displacement of the brain. Crit Care Med 1998: 26: 440–446.
Raabe A, Grolms C, Sorge O, Zimmermann M, Seifert V. Serum S-100B protein in severe head injury. Neurosurgery 1999: 45: 477–483.
Rabow L, Hedman G. CKBB-isoenzymes as a sign of cerebral injury. Acta Neurochir (suppl) 1979: 28: 108–112.
Rabow L, Hedman G. Creatine-kinase BB activity after head trauma related to outcome. Acta Neurochir 1985: 76: 137–139.
Rabow L, DeSalles AAF, Becker DP, et al. CSF brain creatine kinase levels and lactic acidosis in severe head injury. J Neurosurg 1986: 65: 625–629.

Rabow L. Cook D. Lipper et al. Relationship between CT attenuation changes and post-traumatic CSF-CK-BB-activity after severe head injury in man. Acta Neurochir 1989: 100: 155–157.

Rae-Grant AD, Exkert N, Barbour PJ, et al. Outcome of severe brain injury: A multimodality neurophysiologic study. J Trauma 1996: 40: 401–407.

Raghupathi R, Welch FA, Lowenstein DH, et al. Regional induction of *c-fos* and heat shock protein-72 mRNA, following fluid-percussion brain injury in the rat. J Cereb Blood Flow Metab 1995: 15: 467–473.

Raichle ME, Posner JB, Plum F. Cerebral blood flow during and after hyperventilation. Arch Neurol 1970: 23: 294–403.

Raichle ME, Grupp RL, Regulation of brain water permeability by centrally-released vasopressin. Brain Res 1978: 143: 191–194.

Raidoo DM, Ramchurren N, Naidoo Y et al. Visualisation of bradykinin B_2 receptors on human brain neurons. Immunopharmacology 1996: 33: 104–107.

Reeder RF, Nattie EE, North WG. Effect of vasopressin on cold-induced brain edema in cats. J Neurosurg 1986: 64: 941–950.

Resnick DK, Marion DW, Darby JM. The effect of hypothermia on the incidence of delayed traumatic intracerebral hemorrhage. Neurosurgery 1994:34:252–255

Reulen HJ, Kreysch HG, Measurement of brain tissue pressure in cold induced cerebral oedema. Acta Neurchir 1973: 29: 29–40.

Reulen HJ, Graham R, Spatz M, Klatzo I. Role of pressure gradients and bulk flow in dynamics of vasogenic edema. J Neurosurg 1977: 46: 24–35.

Ritter AM, Robertson CS, Goodman JC, et al. Evaluation of a carbohydrate-free diet for paitents with severe head injury. J Neurotrauma 1996: 13: 473

Ritter AM, Muizelaar JP, Barnes T, Choi S, Fatouros P, Ward J, Bullock MR. Brain stem blood flow, pupillary response, and outcome in patients with severe head injuries. Neurosurgery 1999: 44: 941–948.

Roberts GW, Allsop D, Bruton C. The occult aftermath of boxing. J Neurol Neurosurg Psychiat 1990: 53: 373–389.

Robertson CS, Grossman RG, Goodman JC, Narayan RK, The predictive value of cerebral anaerobic metabolism with cerebral infarction after head injury. J Neurosurg 1987: 67: 361–368.

Robertson CS, Narayan RK, Gokaslan ZL, et al. Cerebral arteriovenous oxygen difference as an estimate of cerebral blood flow in comatose patients. J Neurosurg 1989: 70: 222–230.

Robertson CS, Contant CF, Narayan RK, Grossman RG. Cerebral blood flow, $AVDO_2$, and neurologic outcome in head-injured patients. J Neurotrauma 1992a (suppl 1): 9: S349–S358.

Robertson CS, Contant CF, Gokaslan ZL, Narayan RK, Grossman RG. Cerebral blood flow, arteriovenous oxygen difference, and outcome in head injured patients. J Neurol Neurosurg Psychiat 1992b: 55: 594–603.

Robertson CS, Valadka AB, Hannay J, Contant CF, Gopinath SP, Cormio M, Uzura M, Grossman RG. Prevention of secondary ischemic insult after head injury. Crit Care Med 1999: 27: 2086–2095.

Rockoff MA, Marshall LF, Shapiro HM. High-dose barbiturate therapy in humans. A clinical review of 60 patients. Ann Neurol 1979: 6: 194–199.

Rockswold GL, Ford SE, Anderson DC, et al. Results of a prospective randomized trial for treatment of severely brain-injured patients with hyperbaric oxygen. J Neurosurg 1992: 76: 929–934.

Romner B, Bellner J, Kongstad P. Sjöholm H. Elevated transcranial Doppler flow velocities after severe head injury: Cerebral vasospasm or hyperemia? J Neurosurg 1996: 85: 90–97.

Rordorf G, Koroshetz WJ, Bonventre JV. Heat shock protects cultured neurons from glutamate toxicity. Neuron 1991: 7: 1043–1051.

Rosner MJ, Becker DP. Experimental brain injury: Successful therapy with a weak base, tromethamine. With an overview of CNS acidoses. J Neurosurg 1984: 60: 961–971.

Rosner MJ, Becker DP. Origin and evolution of plateau waves. J Neurosurg 1984: 60: 312–324.

Rosner MJ, Coley I. Cerebral perfusion pressure, the ICP and head elevation. J Neurosurg 1986: 65: 636–641.

Rosner MJ, Coley I. Cerebral perfusion pressure: A hemodynamic mechanism of mannitol and postmannitol hemogram. Neurosurgery 1987: 21: 147–156.

Rosner MJ. Cerebral perfusion pressure: Link between intracranial pressure and systemic circulation. In: Wood JH (ed). Cerebral Blood Flow. Physiological and Clinical Aspects 1987: 425–448.

Rosner MJ, Elias KG, Coley I. Prospective randomized trial of THAM therapy in severe brain injury: Preliminary results. In Hoff JT, Betz AL (eds) Intracranial Pressure VII. Springer Verlag, Berlin, Heidelberg, New York, 1989: 611–615.

Rosner MJ, Daughton S. Cerebral perfusion pressure management in head injury. J Trauma 1990: 30: 933–941.

Rosner MJ. Role of cerebral perfusion pressure in acute brain trauma. Crit Care Med 1996: 24: 1274.

Ross DT, Graham DI, Adams JH. Selective loss of neurons from the thalamic reticular nucleus following severe human head injury. J Neurotrauma 1993: 10: 151–165.

Rozsa L, Grote EH, Egan P. Traumatic brain swelling studied by computerized tomography and densitometry. Neurosurg Rev 1989: 12: 133–140.

Rumana CS, Gopinath SP, Uzara M, et al. Brain temperature exceeds systemic temperature in head injured patients. Crit Care Med 1998: 26: 562–567.

Ryding E. Asgeirsson B, Berntman L, Grände PO, Messter K, Nordström C-H, Sjöholm H. Dihydroergotamine treatment of increased ICP following severe head injury. Nordic CBF symposium, Lund 1990, Abstract

Sahuquillo J, Poca MA, Ausina A, et al. Arterio-jugular differences of oxygen (AVDO2) for bedside assessment of CO_2-reactivity and autoregulation in hte acute phase of severe head injury. Acta Neurochir 1996: 138: 435–444.

Sahuquillo J, Munar F, Baguena M, et al. Evaluation of the cerebrovascular CO_2-reactivity and autoregulation in patients with posttraumatic diffuse brain swelling (diffuse injury III). Acta Neurochir 1998 (suppl) 71: 233–236.

Sahuquillo J, Poca M-A, Arribas M, Garnacho A, Rubio E. Interhemispheric supratentorial pressure gradients in head-injured patients. Are they clinically important. J Neurosurg 1999: 90: 16–26.

Sakabe T, Siesjö BK. The effect of indomethacin on blood flow-metabolism couple in the brain under normal, hypercapnic and hypoxic conditions. Acta Physiol Scand 1979: 107: 283–284.

Sakas DE, Bullock MR, Patterson J, et al. Focal cerebral hyperemia after focal head injury in humans: A benign phenomenon? J Neurosurg 1995: 83: 277–284.
Salcman M, Schepp RS. Ducker TB. Calculated recovery rates in severe head trauma. Neurosurgery 1981: 8: 301
Salvant JB, Muizelaar JP. Changes in cerebral blood flow and metabolism related to presence of subdural hematoma. Neurosurgery 1993: 33: 387–393.
Sarrafzadeh AS, Kiening KL, Bardt TF, et al. Cerebral oxygenation in contusioned vs. Nonlesioned brain tissue: Monitoring of $PtiO_2$ with Licox and Paraternd. Acta Neurochir 1998 (suppl) 71: 186–189.
Sarter M, Stephens DN. β-carbolines as tools in memory research: Animal data and speculations, In: Hindmarch I, Ott H (eds) Benzodiazepine receptor ligands, memory and information processing. Springer Verlag 1988: 230–245.
Sato M, Niiyama K, Kuroda R, Ioku M. Influence of dopamine on cerebral blood flow, and metabolism for oxygen and glucose under barbiturate administration in cats. Acta Neurochir 1991: 110: 174–180.
Saul TG, Ducker TB. Effect of intracranial pressure monitoring and aggressive treatment on mortality in severe head injury. J Neurosurg 1982: 56: 498–503.
Saunders ML, Miller DJ, Stablein D, Allen G. The effects of graded experimental trauma on cerebral blood flow and responsiveness to CO_2. J Neurosurg 1979: 51: 18–26.
Sawada Y, Sugimoto H, Kabayashi H, et al. Acute tolerance to high-dose barbiturate in patients with severe head injuries. Anesthesiology 1982: 56: 53–54.
Sazbon L, Groswasser Z, Outcome in 134 patients with prolonged posttraumatic unawareness. J Neurosurg 1990: 72: 75–80.
Schalén W, Messeter K, Nordström C-H. Cerebral vasoreactivity and the prediction of outcome in severe traumatic brain lesions. Acta Anaesthesiol Scand 1991: 35: 113–122.
Schalén W, Messeter K, Nordstöm C-H. Complications and side effects during thiopentone therapy in patients with severe head injuries. Acta Anaeshtesiol Scand 1992: 36: 369–377.
Schauwecker PE, Steward O. Genetic influence on cellular reactions to brain injury: Activation of microgli in the denervated neuropil in mice carrying a mutation (Wld^S) that causes delayed Wallerian degeneration. J Compart Neurol 1997: 380: 82–94.
Schmidt RH, Grady S. Loss of forebrain cholinergic neurons following fluid-percussion injury: Implications for cognitive impairment in closed head injury: J Neurosrug 1995: 83: 496–502.
Scremin OU, Li MG, Jenden DJ. Cholinergic modulation of cerebral cortical blood flow changes induced by trauma. J Neurotrauma 1997: 14: 573–586.
Schneider GH, Underberg A, Lanksch WR, Unterberg A. Dynamics of posttraumatic brain swelling following a cryogenic injury in rats. Acta Neurochir 1994 (suppl) 60: 437–439.
Schröder ML, Muizelaar JP, Bullock MR. Et al. Focal ischemia due to traumatic contusions documented by stable xenon-CT and ultrastructural studies. J Neurosurg 1995: 82: 966–971.
Schröder ML, Muizelaar JP, Fatouros P. et al. Early cerebral blood volume after severe traumatic brain injury in patients with early cerebral ischaemia. Acta Neurochir 1998 (suppl) 71: 127–130.
Schurr A, payne RS, Miller JJ, Rigor BM. Brain lactate, not glucose, fuels the recovery of synaptic function from hypoxia upon reoxygenation: an *in vitro* study. Brain Res. 1997: 744: 105–111.
Schutta HS, Kassell NF, Langfitt TW. Brain swelling produced by injury and aggravated by arterial hypertension. A light and electronic microscopic study. Brain 1968: 91: 281–292.
Schwartz ML, Tator CH, Rowed DW, et al. The University of Toronto head injury treatment study: A prospective randomized comparison of pentobarbital and mannitol. Can J Neurol Sci 1984: 11: 434–440.
Seelig JM, Lewelt W, Jenkins JD, et al. Autoregulation of CBF in response to changes in arterial and intracranial pressure after experimental head injury. In: Intracranial Pressure V. (eds) Ishii S. et al. Springer Verlag, Berlin 1983: 487–489.
Seitz HD, Ockar K. The prognostic and therapeutic importance of cahnges in CSF during the acute stage of brain injury. Acta Neurochir 1977: 38: 211–231.
Servadei F, Nanni A, Nasi MT, et al. Evolving brain lesions in the first 12 hours after head injury: Analysis of 37 comatose patients. Neurosurg 1995: 37: 899–907.
Sesaki T, Nakagomi T, Kirino T, et al. Indomethacin ameliorates ischemic neuronal damage in the gerbil hippocampal CA1 sector. Stroke 1988: 19: 1399–1403.
Sessler DI. Mild perioperative hypothermia. N Engl J Med 1997:336:1730–1737.
Sganzerla EP, Tomei G, Servadei F, et al. Diffuse traumatic axonal injury: A longitudinal study. In: Intracranial Pressure VIII (eds) Avezaat CJJ et al. Springer Verlag 1993: 568–572.
Shackford SR. Effect of small-volume resuscitation on intracranial pressure and related cerebral variables. J Trauma 1997: 42: S48–S53.
Shapira Y, Shohami E, Sidi A. et al. Experimental closed head injury in rats: Mechanical, patophysiological, and neurological properties. Crit Care Med 1988: 16: 258–265.
Shapira Y. Davidson E, Weidenfeld Y, et al. Dexamethasone and indomethacin do not affect brain edema following head injury in rats. J Cereb Blood Flow Metab 1988: 8: 395–402.
Shapira Y, Artru AA, Yadid G, Shohami E. Methylprednisolone does not decrease eicosanoid concentrations or edema in brain tissue or improve neurologic outcome after head trauma in rats. Anesth Analg 1992: 75: 238–244.
Shapira Y, Artru AA, Lam AM. Ketamine decreases cerebral infarct volume and improves neurological outcome following experimental head trauma in rats. J Neurosurg Anesthesiol 1992: 4: 231–240.
Shapiro HH, Wyte SR, Loeser J. Barbiturate augmented hypothermia for reduction of persistent intracranial hypertension. J Neurosurg 1974: 40: 90–100.
Sharkey J, McCulloch J. Dopaminergic mechanism in the regulation of cerebral blood flow and metabolism: Role of different receptor subtypes. In Owman C, hardebo JE (eds). Neural Regulation of Brain Circulation. Elsevier Science Publishers 1985: 111–127.
Sheinberg M, Kanter MJ, Robertson CS, et al. Continuous monitoring of jugular venous oxygen saturation in head-injured patients. J Neurosurg 1992: 76: 212–217.
Shabata M, Einhaus S, Schweitzer JB, et al. Cerebral blood flow decreases by adrenergic stimulation of cerebral vessels in anaesthetized newborn pigs with traumatic brain injury. J Neurosurg 1993: 79: 696–704.
Shigeno S, Fritschka E, Shigeno T, Brock M. Effects of indomethacin on rCBF during and after focal cerebral ischemia in the rat. Stroke 1985: 16: 235–240.

Shima K, Marmarou A. Evaluation of brain-stem dysfunction following severe fluid-perfusion head injury to the cat. J Neurosurg 1991: 74: 270–277.
Shima K, Marmarou A. Effect of posttraumatic hypoventilation. In: Intracranial Pressure VIII. (eds) Avezaat CJJ, et al. Springer Verlag 1993: 476–478.
Shima K, Marmarou A, Roshimae N, et al. Cerebral blood flow and glucose metabolism following experimental head injury. In Intracranial Pressure VIII (eds) Avezaat CJJ, et al. Springer Verlag 1993: 473–475.
Shiozaki T, Sugimoto H, Teneda M, et al. Effect of mild hypothermia in uncontrollable intracranial hypertension after severe head injury. J Neurosurg 1993: 79: 363–368.
Shizaki T, Kato A, Taneda M, Hayakata T, Hashiguchi N, Tanaka H, Shimazu T, Sugimoto H. Little benefit from mild hypothermia therapy for severely head injured patients with low intracranial pressure. J Neurosurg 1999: 91: 185–191.
Shohami E, Sidi A, Cotev S. Head injury induces increased prostaglandin synthesis in rat brain. J Cereb Blood Flow Metab 1987: 7: 58–63.
Shohami E, Novokov M, Horowitz M. Long term exposure to heat reduces edema formation after closed head injury in the rat. Acta Neurochir 1994 (suppl) 60: 443–445.
Siegel JH, Gens DR, Mamantov T, et al. Effect of associated injuries and blood volume replacement on death, rehabilitation needs, and disability in blunt traumatic brain injury. Crit Care Med 1991: 19: 1252–1265.
Siesjö BK, Wieloch T, Brain injury: Neurochemical aspects. In Becker DP, Poloshock JT (eds) Cerebral Nervous System Trauma Report. Williams Byrd Press 1985: 513–532.
Siesjö BK. Pathophysiology and treatment of focal cerebral ischemia. Part !: Pathophysiology. J Neurosurg 1992: 77: 169–184.
Siesjö BK. Pathophysiology and treatment of focal cerebral ischemia. Part II: Mechanisms of damage and treatment. J Neurosurg 1992: 77: 337–354.
Simard JM, Bellefleur M. Systemic arterial hypertension in head trauma. Am J Cardiol 1989: 63: 32C–35C.
Sioutos PJ, Orozco JA, Carter LP. Et al. Continuous regional cerberal blood flow monitoring in head-injured patients. Neurosurgery 1995: 36: 943–950.
Skippen P, Seear M, Poskitt et al. Effect of hyperventilation on regional cerebral blood flow in head-injured children. Crit Care Med 1997: 25: 1402–1409.
Skogseid IM, Nordby HK, Urdal P, et al. Increased serum creatine kinase BB and neuron specific enolase following head injury indicates brain damage. Acta Neurochir 1992: 115-106–111.
Sleigh JW, Havill JH, Frith R, Kersel D, Marsh N, Ulyatt D. Somatosensory evoked potentials in severe traumatic brain injury: A blinded study. J Neurosurg 1999: 91: 577–580.
Smielewski P, Czosnyka M, Kirkpatrick P, et al. Assessment of cerebral autoregulation using carotid artery compression. Stroke 1996: 27: 2197–2203.
Smielewski P, Czosnyka M, Kirkpatrick P, Pickard JD. Evaluation of the transient hyperemic response test in head-injured patients. J Neurosurg 1997: 86: 773–778.
Smith HP, Kelly DL, McWhorter JM, et al. Comparison of mannitol regimens in patients with severe head injury undergoing intracranial monitoring. J Neurosurg 1986: 65: 820–824.
Smith DH, Okiyama K, Gennarelli TA, McIntosh TK. Magnesium and ketamine attenuate cognitive dysfunction following experimental brain injury. Neurosci Lett 1993: 157: 211–214.
Smith DH, Chen X-H, Pierce JES, et al. Progressive atrophy and neuron death for one year following brain trauma in the rat. J Neurotrauma 1997: 14: 715–727.
Snyder JV, Nemoto EM, Carroll RG, Safar P. Global ischemia in dogs. Intracranial pressure, brain blood flow and metabolism. Stroke 1975: 6: 21–27.
Sonne N, Tønnesen H. The influence of alcoholism on outcome after evacuation of subdural hematoma. Br J Neurosurg 1992: 6: 125–130.
Sood SC, Gulati SC, Kumar M, Kak VK. Cerebral metabolism following brain injury II. Lactic acid changes. Acta Neurochir 1980: 53: 47–51.
Spinnewyn B, Blavet N, Clostre F, et al. Involvment of platelet-activating factor (PAF) in cerebral post-ischemic phase in mongolian gerbils. Prostaglandins 1987: 34: 337–349.
Stalhammar D, Starmark JE. Assessment of responsiveness in head injury patients: The Glasgow coma scale and some comments on alternative methods. Acta Neurochir 1986 (suppl) 36: 91.
Steiger H-J, Aaslid R, Stooss R. Seiler RW. Transcranial Doppler monitoring in head injury: Relation between type of injury, flow velocities, vasoreactivity, and outcome. Neurosurgery 1994: 34: 79–86.
Stein SC, Spettell C, Young G, Ross SE. Delayed and progressive brain injury in closed-head trauma. Radiological demonstration. Neurosurgery 1993: 32: 25–31.
Steward O, Trimmer PA. Genetic influences on cellular reactions ot CNS injury: The reactive response of astrocytes in denervated neuropil regions in mice carrying a mutation (Wld^S) that causes delayed Wallerian degeneration. J Comparat Neurol 1997: 380: 70–81.
Stocchetti N, Paparella A, Bridelli F, et al. Cerebral venous oxygen saturation studied with bilateral samples in the internal jugular veins. Neurosurgery 1994: 34: 38–444.
Stocchetti N, Chieregato A, De Marchi M. et al. High cerebral perfusion pressure improves low values of local brain tissue O_2 tension ($PtiO_2$) in focal lesions. Acta Neurochir 1998 (suppl) 71: 162–165.
Stoof JC, Den Breejen EJS, Mulder AH, et al. GABA modulates the release of dopamine and acetylcholine from rat caudate nucleus slices. Eur J Pharmacol 1979: 57: 35–42.
Stover JF, Dohse N-K, Unterberg AW. Significant reduction in brain swelling by administration of nonpeptide kinin B_2 receptor antagonist LF 16-0687Ms after controlled cortical impact injury in rats. J Neurosurg 2000: 92: 853–859.
Strauss K. Raghupathi R, McIntosh TK, Narayan RK. Eicosanoid-related genes are modulated in a rat model of traumatic brain injury. J Neurotrauma 1997: 14: A794.
Strauss K, Cole RW, Metha S, Narayan RK. A dehydroepiandrosterone analog improves behavioral outcome and alters cyclooxygenase-2 gene expression after traumatic brain injury in the rat. J Neurotrauma 1998: 15: A898
Strauss K, Barbe MF, Marshamm RM, et al. Prolonged cyclooxygenase-2 induction in neurons and glia following traumatic brain injury in the rat. J Neurotrauma 2000: 17: 695–711.
Stuss DT, Stethem LL, Picton TW, et al. Traumatic brain injury, aging and reaction time. Canadian J Neurol Sci 1989: 16: 161–167.
Suazo JAC, Maas AIR, Brink van den WA, et al. CO_2 reactivity and brain oxygen pressure monitoring in severe head injury. Crit Care Med 2000: 28: 3268–3274.

Sullivan HG, Martinez J, Becker DP, et al. Fluid percussion model of mechanical brain injury in the cat. J Neurosurg 1976: 45: 520–534.

Sullivan HG, Miller DJ, Becker DP, et al. The physiological basis of intracranial pressure change with progressive epidural brain compression. J Neurosurg 1977: 47: 532–550.

Sunani K, Nakamura T, Ozawa Y. et al. Hypermetabolic state following experimental head injury. Neurosurgical Review 1989: 12: 400–411.

Sundbärg G. Neurosurgical intensive care and the treatment of severe head injuries. Lund, Studentlitteratur (Thesis) 1988.

Sutherland G, Lesiuk H, Bose R, Sima A. Effect of mannitol, nimodipine, and indomethacin singly or in combination on cerebral ischemia. Stroke 1988: 19: 571–578.

Sutton LN, McLaughin AC, Kemp W, et al. Effects of increased ICP on brain phosphocreatine and lactate determined by simultaneous IH and 31P NMR spectroscopy. J Neurosurg 1987: 67: 381–386.

Sutton LN, Baranco D, Greeberg J, et al. Cerebral blood flow and glucose metabolism in experimental brain edema. J Neurosurg 1989: 71: 868–874.

Sutton LN, McLaughin AC, Dante S. et al. Cerebral venous oxygen content as a measure of brain energy metabolism with increased intracranial pressure and hyperventilation. J Neurosurg 1990: 73: 927–932.

Sutton RL, Hovda DA, Adelson PD, et al. Metabolic changes following cortical contusion: Relationship to edema and morphological changes. Acta Neurochir 1994 (suppl) 60: 446–448.

Suwanwela C, Suwanwela N. Intracranial arterial norrowing and spasm in acute head injury. J Neurosurg 1972: 36: 314–323.

Suzuka T, Mabe H, Nagai H. Role of arachidonic acid metabolites on development of ischemia cerebral edema in rat middle cerebral artery occlusion. J Cereb Blood Flow Metab 1989 (Suppl 1): S89.

Tabaddor K, Bhushan C, Pevsner PH, Walker AE. Prognostic value of cerebral blood flow (CBF) and cerebral metabolic rate of oxygen ($CMRO_2$) in acute head trauma. J Trauma 1972: 12: 1053–1055.

Talmor D, Merkind V, Artru AA, Shapiro O, Geva D, Roytblat L, Shapira Y. Treatment to support blood pressure increases bleeding and/or decreases survival in a rat model of closed head trauma combined with uncontrolled hemorrhage. Anesth Analg 1999: 89: 950–956.

Tanaka H, Katayama Y, Kawamata T, Tcubokawa T. Excitatory amino acid release from contused brain tissue into surrounding brain areas. Acta Neurochir 1994 (suppl) 60: 524–527.

Taneda M, Kataoka K, Akai F, et al. Traumatic subarachnoid hemorrhage as a predictable indicator of delayed ischemic symptoms. J Neurosurg 1996: 84: 762–768.

Tanno H, Nockels RP, Pitts LH, Noble LJ. Breakdown of the blood-brain barrier after fluid percussive brain injury in the rat. Part 1. Distribution and time course of protein extravasation. J Neurotrauma 1992: 9: 21–32.

Tanno H, Nockels RP, Pitts LH, Noble LJ. Immunolocalization of heat shock protein after fluid percussion brain injury and relationship to breakdown of the blood-brain barrier. J Cereb Blood Flow Metab 1993: 13: 116–124.

Tans JTJ, Poortcliet DCJ. Intracranial volume-pressure relationship in man. Part 2: Clinical significance of the pressure volume index. J Neurosurg 1983: 59: 810–816.

Taylor SJ, Fettes SB, Jewkes C, Nelson RJ. Prospective, randomized, controlled trial to determine the effect of early enhanced enteral nutrition on clinical outcome in mechanically ventilated patients suffering form head injury. Crit Care Med 1999: 27: 2525–2531.

Teasdale E, Jennett B. Assessment and prognosis of coma after head injury. Acta Neurochir 1976: 34: 45–55.

Teasdale E, Cardoso E, Galbraith E, Teasdale G. CT scan in severe diffuse head injury: Phsiological and clinical correlations. J Neurol Neurosurg Psychiat 1984: 47: 600–603.

Teasdale GM, Mendelow AD, Galbraith S. Causes and consequences of raised intracrnial pressure in head injuries. In: Intracranial Pressure VI (eds) miller JD, et al. Springer Verlag 1986: 3–8.

Teasdale E, Hadley DM. Radiodiagnosis in head injury, In: Handbook of Clinical Neurology (eds) Vinken PJ, et al. Elsevier Science Publisher, Amsterdam 1990: 143–179.

Teasdale GM, Braakman R, Cohadon F, et al. The European brain injury consortium. Acta Neurochir 1997: 139: 797–803.

Temkin NR, Dikmen SS, Anderson GD, et al. Valproat therapy for prevention of posttraumatic seizures: a randomized trial. J Neurosurg 1999: 91: 593–600.

Tenjin H, Yamaki T, Nakagawa Y, et al. Impairment of CO_2 reactivity in severe head injury patients: An investigation using thermal diffusion method. Acta Neurochir 1990: 104: 121–125.

Thomas S, Prins ML, Samil M, Hovda DA. Cerebral metabolic response to traumatic brain injury sustained early in development: A 2-deoxy-D-glucose autoradiographic study. J Neurotrauma 2000: 17: 650–665.

Timming R, Orrison W, Mikula JA. Computerized tomography and rehabilitation outcome after severe head trauma. Arch Phys Med Rehabil 1982: 63: 154–159.

Tokuda T, Ikeda S, Yanagisawa N, et al. Re-examination og exboxers's brains using immunohistochemistry with antibodies to amyloid b-protein and tau protein. Acta Neuropathol 1991: 82: 281–285.

Tokutomi T, Segemori M, Kikuchi T. Hiroshata M. Effect of platelet-activating factor antagonist on brain injury in rats. Acta Neurochir 1994 (suppl) 60: 508–510.

Tomida S, Nowak TS, Vass K, et al. Experimental model for repetitive ischemia attacks in the gerbil: The cumulative effect of repeated ischemic insults. J Cereb Blood Flow Metab 1987: 7: 773–782.

Tomita H, Ito U, Tone H, et al. High colloid oncotic therapy for continuous brain edema. Acta Neurochir 1994 (suppl) 60: 547–549.

Tornheim PA, McLaurin RL. Acute changes in regional brain water content following experimental closed head injury. J Neurosurg 1981: 55: 407–413.

Tornheim PA, Liwnicz BH, Hirsch CS, et al. Acute responses to experimental model and gross pathology. J Neurosurg 1983: 59: 431–438.

Troupp H. Intraventricular pressure in patients with severe brain injuries. J Trauma 1967: 7: 875–883.

Troupp H, Vapalahti M. Intraventricular pressure in the final stages of severe brain injury. Acta Neurochir 1971: 25: 189–195.

Tsuchida E, Harms JF, Woodward JJ, Bullock R. A use-dependent sodium channel antagonist, 619C89, in reduction of ischemic brain damage and glutamate release after acute subdural hematoma in the rat. J Neurosurg 1996: 85: 104–111.

Unterberg A, Baethmann AJ. The kallikrein-kinin system as mediator in vasogenic brain edema. Part 1: Cerebral exposure to bradykinin and plasma. J Neurosurg 1984: 61: 87–96.

Unterberg A, Dautermann C, Baethmann AJ. Et al. The kallikrein-kinin system as mediator in vasogenic brain edema. J Neurosurg 1986: 64: 269–276.

Unterberg A, Andersen BJ, Clarke GD, Marmarou A. Cerebral energy metabolism following fluid percussion brain injury in cats. J Neurosurg 1988: 68: 594–600.

Unterberg A, Schmidt W, Wahl M, et al. Evidence against leukotriens as mediators of brain edema. J Neurosurg 1991: 74: 773–780.

Unterberg A, Kiening K, Schmiedek P, Lanksch W. Long-term observations of intracranial pressure after severe head injury. The phenomenon of secondary rise of intracranial pressure. Neurosurgery 1993: 32: 17–24.

Unterberg A, Schneider GH, Gottschalk J, Lanksch WR. Development of traumatic brain edema in old versus young rats. Acta Neurochir 1994 (suppl) 60: 431–433.

Unterberg AW, Kiening KL, Härtl R, et al. Multimodal monitoring in patients with head injury: Evaluation of the effects of treatment on cerebral oxygenation. J Trauma 1997: 42. S32–S37.

Uzzell BP, Obrist WD, Dolinskas CA, Langfitt TW. Relationship of acute CBF and ICP findings to neurophychological outcome in severe head injury. J Neurosurg 1986: 65: 630–635.

Van den Brink WA, Samtos BO, Marmarou A, Avezaat CJJ. Temporal blood brain barrier damage and continued edema formation in experimental closed head injury in the rat. In: Intracranial Pressure CIII (eds) Avezaat CJJ et al. Springer Verlag 1993: 144–147.

Van den Brink WA, Santos BO, Marmorou A, Avezaat CJJ. Quntitative analysis of blood-brain barrier damage in two models of experimental head injury in the rat. Acta Neurochir 1994 (suppl) 60: 456–458.

Van den Brink WA, van Santbrink H, Avezaat CJJ, et al. Monitoring brain tissue oxygen tension in severe head injury. The Rotterdam Experience. Acta Neurochir 1998 (suppl) 71: 190–194.

Vapalahti M, Troup H, Heiskanen O. Extremely severe brain injuries treated with hyperventilation and ventricular drainage. In: Cerebral Blood Flow. (eds) Brock et al. Springer Verlag 1969: 266–267.

Vassar MJ, Perry CA, Holcroft JW. Prehospital resuscitation of hypotensive trauma patients with 7.5% NaCl versus 7.5% NaCl with added dextran: A controlled trial. J Trauma 1993: 34: 622.

Venes JL, Collins WF. Bifrontal decompressive craniectomy in the management of head trauma. J Neurosurg 1975: 42: 429–433.

Vespa PM, Nuwer MR, Nenov V, et al. Increased incidence and impact of nonconvulsive and convulsive seizures after traumatic brain injury as detected by continuous electroencephalographic monitoring. J Neurosurg 1999: 91: 750–760.

Vink R, McIntosh TK, Weiner MW, faden AI. Effects of traumatic brain injury on cerebral high-energy phosphates and pH: A 31P magnetic resonance spectroscopy study. J Cereb Blood Flow Metab 1987: 7: 563–571.

Vink R, McIntosh TK, Demediuk P, Weiner MW, Faden AI. Decline in intracellular free magnesium concetration is associated with irreversible tissue injury following brain trauma. J Biol Chem 1988: 263: 757–761.

Vink R, Golding EM, Williams JP, McIntosh TK. Blood glucose concentration does not affect outcome in brain trauma: A ^{31}P MRS study. J Cereb Blood Flow Metab 1997: 17: 50–53.

Von Berenberg P, Unterberg A, Schneider GH, Lanksch WR. Treatment of traumatic brain edema by multiple doses of mannitol. Acta Neurochir (suppl) 60: 532–533.

Von Essen C, Zervas NT, Brown DR, et al. Local cerebral blood flow in the dog during intravenous infusion of dopamine. Srug Neurol 1980: 13: 181–188.

Wada K, Alonso OF, Busto R, Panetta J, Clemens JA, Ginsberg MD, Dietrich WD. Early treatment with a novel inhibitor of lipid peroxidation (LY341122) improves histopathological outcome after moderate fluid percussion brain injury in rats. Neurosurgery 1999: 45: 601–608.

Wade CE, Grady JJ, Kramer GC, et al. Individual patient cohort analysis of the efficacy of hypertonic saline/dextran in patients with traumatic brain injury and hypotension. J Trauma 1997: 42: S61–S65.

Wagner KR, Tronheim PA, Eichhold HK. Acute changes in regional cerebral metabolite values following experimental blunt head injury. J Neurosurg 1985: 63: 88–96.

Wahl M, Young AR, Edvinsson L, Wagner F. Effects of bradykinin on pial arteries and arterioles *in vitro* and *in situ*. J Cereb Blood Flow Metab 1983: 3: 231–237.

Ward JD, Becker DP, Miller CD, et al. Failure of prophyllactic barbiturate coma in the treatment of severe head injury. J Neurosurg 1985: 62: 383–388.

Waschke KF, Riedel M, Albrecht DM, et al. Regional heterogeneity of cerebral blood flow response to graded volume-controlled hemorrhage. Intensive Care Med 1996:22:1026–1233.

Weber M, Grolimund P, Seiler RW. Evaluation of posttraumatic cerebral blood flow velocities by transcranial Doppler ultrasongraphy. Neurosurgery 1990: 27: 106–112.

Wei EP, Dietrich WD, Povlishock JT, et al. Functional, morphological, and metabolic abnormalities of the cerebral microcirculation after concussive brain injury in cats. Circ Res 1980: 46: 37–47.

Wei EP, Kontos HA, Dietrich WD, et al. Inhibition by free radical scavengers and by cyclooxygenase inhibitors of pial arteriolar abnomalities from concussive brain injury in cats. Circ Res 1981: 48: 95–103.

Wei EP, Lamp RG, Kontos HA. Increased phospholipase C activity after experimental brain injury. J Neurosurg 1982: 56: 695–698.

Weisend M, Feeney DM. The relationship between traumatic brain injury-induced changes in brain temperature and behavioral and anatomical outcome. J Neurosurg 1994: 80: 120–132.

Whalen MJ, Carlos TM, Clark RS, et al. The relationship between brain temperature and neutrophil accumulation after traumatic brain injury in rats. Acta Neurochir 1997b: 70: 260–261.

Whalen MJ, Carlos TM, Clark RS, et al. The effect of brain temperature on acute inflammation after traumatic brain injury in rats. J Neurochem 1997a: 14: 561–572.

Whalen MJ, Carlos TM, Kochanek PM, Heineman S. Blood-brain barrier permeability, neutrophil accumulation and vascular adhesion molecule expression after controlled cortical impact in rats. A preliminary study. J Neurochir 1998 (suppl) 71: 212–214.

Willemse RB, Egeler-Peerdeman SM. External lumbar drainage in uncontrollable intracranial pressure in adults with severe head injury: a report of 7 cases. Acta Neurochir 1998 (suppl) 71: 37-39.

Winer JW, Rosenwasser RH, Jimenez F. Electroencephalographic activity and serum and cerebrospinal fluid pentobarbitale levels in determining the therapeutic end point during barbiturate coma. Neurosurgery 1991: 29: 739-742.

Wolf AL, Levi L. Marmarou A, et al. Effect of THAM upon outcome in severe head injury: A randomized prospective clinical trial. J Neurosurg 1993: 78: 54-59.

Wolfla C, Luerssen TG, Bowman RM, Putty TK. Brain tissue pressure gradients created by expanding frontal epidural mass lesion. J Neurosurg 1996: 84: 642-647.

Wood PL, Cheney DL, Costa E, et al. An investigation of whether septal gamma-aminobutyric-containing interneurons are involved in the reduction in the turnover rate of acetylcholine elicited by substance P and β-endorphin in the hippocampus. Neurosci 1979: 4: 1479-1484.

Xiong Y, Peterson PL, Muizelaar JP, Lee CP. Amelioration of mitochondrial function by a novel antioxidant U-101033E following traumatic brain injury in rats. J Neurotrauma 1997: 14: 907-917.

Xu BN, Yabuki A, Mishina H, et al. Pathophysiology of brain swelling after experimental brain compression and decompression. Neurosurgery 1993: 32: 289-296.

Yamakami I, McIntosh TK. Effects of traumatic brain injury on regional cerebral blood flow in rats as measured with radiolabeled microspheres. J Cereb Blood Flow Metab 1989: 9: 117-124.

Yamakami I, Vink R, Faden AI, et al. Effect of ethanol intoxication on experimental brain injury in the rat: Neurobihavioral and phosphorus-31 nuclear magnetic resosnance spectroscopy studies. J Neurosurg 1995: 82: 813-821.

Yang MS, Dewitt DS, Becker DP, Hayes RL. Regional brain metabolite levels following mild experimental head injury in the cat. J Neurosurg 1985: 63: 617-621.

Yano M, Ikeda Y, Kobaychi S, Yamamoto Y, Otsuka T. The outcome with barbiturate therapy in severe head injuries. In: Intracranial pressure VI (eds) Miller JD, et al. Springer Verlag, 1986: 769-773.

Yen MH, Lee SH. Effects of cycolooxygenase and lipooxygenase inhibitors on cerebral edema induced by freezing lesions in rats. Europ J Pharmacol 1987: 144: 369-373.

Yoshida K, Marmarou A. Effects of tromethamine and hyperventilation on brain injury in the cat. J Neurosurg 1991: 74: 87-96

Yoshini E, Yamaki T, Higushi T, et al. Acute brain edema in fatal head injury: Analysis by dynamic CT scanning. J Neurosurg 1985: 63: 830-839.

Yoshino A, Hovda DA, Kawamata T, et al. Dynamic changes in local cerebral glucose utilization following cerebral concussion in rats: evidence of a hyper- and subsequent hypometabolic state. Brain Research 1991: 561: 106-119.

Yoshino A, Hovda DA, Katayama Y, et al. Hippocampal CA3 lesion prevents post-concussive metabolic dysfunction in CA1. J Cerebr Blood Flow Metab 1992: 12: 996-1006.

Young M, Rewitts DS, Becker DP, Hayes RL. Regional brain metabolite levels following mild experimental head injury in the cat. J Neurosurg 1985: 63: 617-621.

Yunoki M, Kawauchu M, Ukita N, et al. Effect of lecithinized superoxide dismutase on traumatic brain injury in rats. J Neurotrauma 1997: 14: 739-746.

Zimmerman RA, Bilaniuk LF, Gennarelli T. Computed tomography of shearing injuries of the cortical white matter. Radiology 1978: 127: 393-396.

Zhao W, Young TY, Ginsberg MD. Registration and three-dimentional reconstruction of autoradiographic images by the disparity analysis method. IEEE Trans Med Imag 1993: 12: 782-791.

Zhao W, Ginsberg MD, Smith DW. Three-dimentional quantitative autoradiography by disparity analysis: theory and application to image averaging of local cerebral glucose utilization. J Cereb Blood Flow Metab 1995: 15: 552-565.

Zhao W, Alonso OF, Loor JY, Busto R, Ginsberg MD. Influence of early posttraumatic hypothermia therapy on local cerebral blood flow and glucose metabolisme after fluid percussion brain injury. J Neurosurg 1999: 90: 510-519.

Zink BJ, Feustel PJ. Effects of ethanol on respiratory function in traumatic brain injury. J Neurosurg 1995: 82: 822-828.

Zupping R. Cerebral acid-base and gas metabolism in brain injury. J Neurosurg 1970: 33: 498-505.

Zwetnow NN. The influence of an increased intracranial pressure on the lactate, pyruvate, bicarbonate, phosphocreatine, ATP, ADP and AMP concentrations of the cerebral cortex of dogs. Acta Physiol Scand 1970 (suppl) 339: 1-31.

CHAPTER 11

Aneurysmal subarachnoid haemorrhage

Epidemiology

Prevalence and incidence

The prevalence of saccular cerebral aneurysm at autopsy has been found to range between 0.2 and 9.6%. According to Kassell and Torner (1982) the prevalence is 2.5%, but Sekhar and Heros (1981) found a prevalence of 5%.

The incidence of ruptured cerebral aneurysms in patients admitted to hospital is 5–15 per 100000 per year (Pakarinen 1967, Wiebers et al. 1981, Kassell and Torner 1982). In one study patients with unruptured intracranial aneurysm were followed for several years. Saccular aneurysm less than 10 mm i diameter had a very low probability of subsequent rupture. Among patients with aneurysm 10 mm or larger in diameter a rupture rate of 24% at 7 years after the diagnosis was found for patients younger than 59 years, and a rupture rate of 48% was found for patients of age older than 59 years (Wiebers et al. 1987).

Genetics

Between 5 and 10% of patients with ruptured aneurysm will have one or more first order relatives who had a ruptured aneurysm

Associated disease

In series of cerebral aneurysm about 5% has suffered from polycystic kidney disease. About 1% of patients with aneurysm also have coarctation of the aorta, and 5 % of paitents with coarctation will develope an aneurysm. It has been suggested that patients with arterial hypertension more likely develop multiple aneurysm. In about 30–40% of ruptured aneurysm the patients have preexisting arterial hypertension.

In cocain abusers ruptur of aneurysm seems to happen at an earlier age than would otherwise be expected, and the mortality is higher.

Outcome Studies

Mortality

In series of SAH patients subjected to operation, the mortality rate ranges between 20 and 28% (Fortuny and Prieto-Valiente 1981, Kassell et al. 1990a), with an overall mortality of 46–50%, and a good recovery in about 25–28% (Hijdra et al. 1987b, Rosenørn et al. 1987). In super selective groups of good-grade patients (Hunt and Hess I and II) a surgical favourable result was observed in 87% at six months follow-up (Edner et al. 1992). In patients with unruptured intracranial saccular aneurysm the total operative morbidity and mortality were 15 and 4% respectively (Eskesen et al. 1987). In patients with SAH of unknown aetiology a 55% mortality rate and a 7% risk of rebleeding were found over a 5-year period (Eskesen et al. 1984).

In patients older than 70 years six-month outcomes for unruptured aneurysms were: Excellent, 70%; good, 15%; fair, 5%; poor, 7.5%; and death, 2.5%. In the same study outcomes for ruptured aneurysms were: Excellent 34%; good, 9%; fair 5,6%; poor, 3,4% and death 45% (Chung et al. 2000).

Prognostic indices

A number of factors have been reported to influence the operative results, including sex (McKissock et al. 1962, McKissock et al. 1965), age (O`Laoire 1978, Kassell et al. 1990a), systemic hypertension (Stornelli and French 1964, Krayenbühl et al. 1972, Hollin and Decker 1977, Kassell et al. 1990a), preoperative condition (Drake 1971, Krayenbühl et al. 1972), recurrent haemorrhage (Hijdra et al. 1987), thickness of the subarachnoid clot (Kassell et al. 1990a), Ultra-early evidence of vasospasm at admission (Qureshi et al. 1999), delayed cerebral ischaemia or vasospasm (Stornelli and French 1964, Hijdra et al. 1987), site of the aneurysm (McKissock et al. 1965, Rosenørn et al. 1987, Kassell et al. 1990a), number of aneurysms (Andrews and Spiegel 1979) operative method (Dutton 1969, Rosenørn et al. 1987), and hyperthermia (Weir et al. 1989). The incidence of hydrocephalus and vasospasm and their ultimate effect upon outcome have also been considered (Dutton 1969, Drake 1971, Millikan 1975, Saito et al. 1977).

Poor neuropsychological outcome is associated with the age of the patients, and anterior communicating artery aneurysm (Bornstein et al. 1987). Trapping of the anterior communicating aneurysm, which disrupts blood supply to the dorsal perforating branches from the anterior communicating artery, results in amnestic syndrome in many patients (Gade 1982).

In a recent study, timing of grading was found to be an important factor in outcome prediction. Thus, the patients worst clinical grade is most predictive of outcome, especially when the patients were assessed using the World Federation of Neurological Surgeons Scale or Glasgow Coma Scale (Chiang et al. 2000).

It must be stressed, however, that even in patients of Hunt and Hess grade IV and V aggressive treatment should not be denied. In a retrospective study of 159 patients favourable outcome occurred in 54% of H&H grade IV and 24% of grade V (LeRoux et al. 1996).

Glucose

Elevated glucose levels during the first week after SAH predict a poor outcome. Although experimental data suggest a deleterious effect of hyperglycaemia, a causal link between hyperglycaemia and outcome after delayed cerebral ischaemia has not been established (Lanzino et al. 1993).

Experimental models

Models of pressure thresholds

In a model of aneurysms, constructed by elastic tissue and collagen, an incremental increase in systolic pressure produced a non-linear N-shaped pressure-volume curve with an initial linear enlargement in volume with increased pressure until a pressure threshold was reached. At this pressure there was an abrupt increase in volume to a new stable equilibrium volume, where a further increase in pressure would cause a rupture of the aneurysm. This always occurred in the thinner more compliant part of the wall (Austin et al. 1989).

Models of subarachnoid haemorrhage (SAH)

Models of experimental SAH include cisterna magna injection of autologous blood. In this model CBF is reduced acutely. This model, however does not resemble clinical SAH with respect to leakage of blood from the diseased vessel. A model that provides a better resemblance with clinical SAH is injection of autologous blood into the subarachnoid space at arterial pressure. This model, on the other hand requires craniotomy followed by dural and arachnoid dissection, and often the use of larger animals are required. In certain animal models, a second injection of blood is required to produce more reliable results, especially when investigating delayed vasospasm. To produce histopathological evident cell injury, following cisterna magna injection of autologous blood, the erythrocytes must be "lysed" to release more potent spasmogenic activity. For review (Matz et al. 1996). A model of SAH in rats that does not require craniotomy has been developed. The method is based upon endovascular arterial rupture near the bifurcation of the anterior cerebral artery, and the middle cerebral artery. Endovascular rupture is achieved by advancing a nylon suture through the ipselateral internal carotid artery after introduction through the external carotid artery. This model more closely resembles aneurysmal rupture, and does not require craniotomy. Furthermore, it produces acute cerebral ischaemia following SAH (Veelken et al. 1995, Zea Longa et al. 1989).

Femoral artery model of vasospasm

Okada et al. (1990) found that the response of cerebral arteries to a variety of injuries including subarachnoid haemorhage is analogous to that of systemic arteries. Thus, chronic narrowing of the femoral artery was found to be analogous in terms of degree, specifity, temporal course and histopathological appearance to that observed in cerebral arteries after SAH.

Infusion models

In a recent study a cranial window was implated in rats. Artificial CSF, containing the hemolysis products K^+ and haemoglobin, was superfused topically over the brain. Superfusion with CSF containing haemoglobin combined with either a high concentration of K^+ (35 mmol/L) or a low concentration of glucose reduced CBF gradually. Spreading ischaemia in the cortex appeared when CBF reached 40 to 70% compared with baseline (Dreier et al. 2000).

Intracranial pressure

Peak pressure

During recurring SAH an extreme increase in ICP, developing within one minute and declining over several minutes, has been observed. The peak ICP during this episode is in the range of MABP, and the event is accompanied by Cushing response and eventually cerebral circulatory arrest (Grote and Hassler 1988). In experimental SAH in cats the Cushing response does not improve the cerebral circulation. On the contrary, it resulted in a further increase in ICP (Brinker et al. 1992).

Warning episodes

Before the catastrophic changes of manifest subarachnoid haemorrhage, smaller ICP increases without severe deterioration have been observed. According to Nornes and Magnæs (1972) these "warning episodes" were never seen after the aneurysm was clipped, and the episodes are regarded as forerunners of a life-threatening haemorrhage.

In a consecutive series of 422 patients with SAH 20% had episodes suggesting "warning leak". The proportion of patients with a good neurological condition (Hunt and Hess grades 1 and 2) who had good outcome was 88% in the group with no warning episodes, versus 54% in the group where the SAH was preceded by a warning leak episode (Jakobsson et al. 1996).

Vasoparalysis

It has been proposed that the acute rise in ICP after SAH is caused by a reflex-mediated vasoparalysis, triggered by hypothalamus and the vasomotor centre. The suspected reflex mechanism may be life saving, because the high ICP compresses the ruptured dome of the aneurysm. On the other hand, depending upon its duration, it may cause ischaemic, damage or death (Krasznai and Grote 1994).

ICP level

A close correlation between the height of the ICP level and the level of consciousness or clinical grading according to Hunt and Hess has been demonstrated (Hayashi et al. 1976, Hase et al. 1978, Voldby and Enevoldsen 1982a, Hartmann 1980). ICP greater than 50 mm Hg has uniformly been associated with a poor outcome (Kassell et al. 1976). In another study a mean ICP level exceeding 25 mm Hg for several days was associated with a poor outcome, and in the same study the correlation between ICP level and outcome was poor when severe vasospasm or rebleeding occurred (Voldby and Enevoldsen 1982a).

Pressure waves

In the acute phase ICP tracings in patients with communicating hydrocephalus indicate continuing plateau waves in conjunction with B-waves (Hayashi et al. 1984). In the postoperative period baseline ICP is lower in patients whose outcome was good, and the height of plateau waves and B-waves was less (Kaye and Brownbill 1981).

Drainage

In unconscious patients reduction of ICP by ventricular drainage is accompanied by an increase in CBF to levels of relative hyperaemia (Jakobsen et al. 1990b). Lowering ICP by drainage does not appear to increase the risk of rebleeding (Voldby and Enevoldsen 1982a). However, the same authors suggested that drainage of CSF should be avoided during recurrent haemorrhage, and should not be resumed until a steady-state ICP level was achieved (Voldby and Enevoldsen 1982c).

Vasospasm

During the initial stages of cerebral vasospasm a decrease in ICP has found (Kaye and Brownhill 1981). A secondary increase in ICP thereafter follows due to ischaemic brain swelling or infarction (Hayashi et al.1978).

Hydrocephalus

In 897 patients with SAH 25.9% developed hydrocephalus. Significant associations among the following factors and hydrocephalus were observed: Severity of 3-month post-SAH Glasgow Coma Scale; increased ventricular size at admission; neurological grade severity at admission; pre-existing hypertension; alcoholism; female sex; increased aneurysm size; pneumonia; meningitis; and inraventricular haemorrhage at admission (Sheehan et al. 1999).

In chronic communicating hydrocephalus following SAH fibrosis of the arachnoid villi has been suggested as the cause for obstruction of CSF-flow. Studies at autopsy of arachnoid villi from patients with SAH suggest that proliferation of arachnoidal cells, triggered by inflammatory reaction or blood clotting products results in obstruction of CSF-flow through arachnoid villi into the venous sinuses (Massicotte and Bigio 1999).

Dynamic of CSF

Outflow resistance

After experimental SAH in the cat ICP is slightly elevated, and a decrease in the buffering capacity of the intracranial space and a sharp rise in outflow resistance were found. During constant infusion of blood into the cisterna magna, an extensive and constant increase in ICP was observed (Brinker et al. 1990).

In patients with SAH resistance to outflow of CSF is increased, and a linear correlation between ICP level and outflow resistance has been found (Kosteljanetz 1984). In a recent study resistance to outflow reached its maximum at 4–7 days after SAH and then showed a tendency to decrease. A second peak of increased outflow resistance appeared in the days 12–20 after SAH in Hunt and Hess group IV and V. In the same study a worsening in intracranial compliance at the first week after ictus was observed in Hunt and Hess grade IV and V (Heinsoo et al. 1998). Increased ICP due to a block in the CSF resorption pathways is found in most patients with acute SAH and impairment of consciousness. Usually the CSF pathways clear spontaneously in about 2 weeks, but if CSF resorption is still impaired after 4 weeks a permanent shunt is needed (Sundberg and Pontén 1976).

Fibrinolysis

The effect of intrathecal fibrinolysis on CSF absorption has been investigated in experimental subarachnoid haemorrhage in cats. Intrathecal application of recombinant tissue plasminogen activator resulted in an almost total restoration of CSF outflow resistance (Brinker et al. 1991).

Central and cerebral haemodynamics

Intravascular Blood Volume

Experimental studies

In rhesus monkey subjected to SAH an increase in intravascular blood volume correlates with an increase in CBF (McGillicuddy et al. 1979).

Clinical studies

This is in accordance with clinical data indicating that many patients subjected to aneurysm surgery are in a stage of hypovolaemia (Maroon and Nelson 1979), and other studies indicating that volume expansion can reverse the neurological deficits associated with vasospasm (Pritz et al. 1978). Other clinical studies have demonstrated that an increase in systemic arterial pressure and in intravascular volume can reverse neurological deficits (Kosnik and Hunt 1976, Gianotti et al. 1978).

CBF and $CMRO_2$, experimental studies

In experimental SAH in baboons CBF and $CMRO_2$ increased immediately after SAH in spite of a decrease in CPP, and the occurrence of vasospasm in the larger cerebral arteries as demonstrated angiographically. Two days after SAH, CBF and $CMRO_2$ decreased , and CVR increased. The EEG activity became slow and arterial spasm was still present (Hashi et al. 1972). In contrast to this study an immediate increase in CBF and $CMRO_2$ was not observed. In the Rhesus monkey intracranial hypertension secondary to experimental cisternal SAH is associated with an immediate occurrence of cerebral ischaemia. Under this condition a decrease in $CMRO_2$ and CBF is accompanied by a decrease in cerebral glucose consumption. Regional studies indicate a primary depression of oxidative metabolism unrelated to ischaemia where glucose supply is adequate (Fein 1975). In similar models in cats and rabbits CBF decreased markedly within 5 minutes of SAH, falling by 30–40% of the basal level (Umansky et al. 1983, Diringer et al. 1994). The steep initial decline in CBF was followed by a second phase in which CBF continued to decrease, but at a more moderate rate. From 60 to 90 minutes after SAH, the CBF tended to stabilise at a level below basal values (Umansky et al. 1983). In a recent study the endovascular puncture model was used to create SAH in rats. A fall in the concentration of moving blood cells and a rise in flow velocity implied that acute microcirculatory vasoconstriction was the cause of an immediate decrease in CBF. Interstitiel tissue oxygenation decreased as well, indicating that a change in oxygen delivery rather than in oxygen utilization occurred at the cellular level (Critchley and Bell 2000).

It has been discussed if the acute decrease in CBF after SAH is caused by changes in ICP and CPP. In studies in rats the acute decrease in CBF occurs independently of changes in ICP and CPP. The same study demonstrated that the decrease in CBF is associated with larger haemorrhage size, persistent elevation of extracellular glutamate, and poor outcome. A CBF reduction to less than 40% of baseline for 60 minutes after SAH predicted 24-hour mortality with 100% accuracy (Bederson et al. 1998).

Angiotensin IV and nitric oxide

Angiotensin IV, a natural degradation product of angiotensin II, induces an endothelium dependent dilation of pial arterioles (Haberl et al. 1991). Angiotensin IV reverses the acute CBF reduction after experimental SAH in the rat. This effect is not antagonised by specific angiotensin II antagonists, and studies of nitric synthase activity did not support a role for NO in the action of angiotensin IV (Näveri et al. 1994).

$AVDO_2$

In dogs the decrease in $CMRO_2$ and CBF is accompanied by an initial increase in $AVDO_2$. After the bleeding, however, the $AVDO_2$ became markedly reduced (Steiner et al. 1978).

Glucose utilisation

In a rat-model of SAH the glucose utilisation was diffusely decreased with the largest percentage reduction in regions displaying the highest basal metabolic rate. The decrease of CMR-glucose was related to the presence of blood in the subarachnoid space and to ICP-hypertension (Solomon et al. 1987).

Neurological deficits

A correlation between the severity of neurological deficits and the degree of impaired CBF has been demonstrated in experimental SAH in the monkey (Petruk et al. 1972).

CPP

The importance of reduced CPP has been studied in experimental SAH in the canine. MABP was reduced gradually with trimethaphane to 40 mm Hg in the presence of well documented vasospasm. This procedure, however, did not cause evoked potential change, focal neurological deficits or pathological evidence of cerebral infarction (Kaplan et al. 1986).

CBF and $CMRO_2$, clinical studies

Low CBF

In patients with major neurological deficits, impairment of the consciousness and progressive enlargement in ventricular size a reduction of CBF has been observed (James 1968, Ferguson et al. 1972, Weir et al. 1978, Gelmers et al. 1979, Merory et al. 1980).With intravenous or inhalation technique CBF is higher in patients having a favourable outcome (Géraud et al. 1984), and in conscious patients (Mountz et al. 1991). Old patients seem especially at risk of developing low CBF after SAH (Meyer et al. 1982, Meyer et al. 1983). In a study of 116 patients with SAH CBF was studied with the ^{133}Xe inhalation technique. CBF fell progressively during the first 2 weeks after SAH, and was abnormally low throughout the 3 weeks of investigation after haemorrhage. For unilateral localised aneurysm the changes in CBF also affected the other hemisphere (Meyer et al. 1983).

Comparison of central conduction time or transit time with that of CBF indicate a poor correlation (Zingesser et al. 1968). However, in another investigation CBF studies were superior, because conduction time only tended to increase in grade IV patients (Rosenstein et al. 1985).

Hyperaemia

In other studies of conscious patients with SAH relative hyperaemia with CBF 50 ml/100g/min and reduced $CMRO_2$ at 2.2 ml O_2/100g/min were observed. During the following week CBF decreased to 41 ml, and $CMRO_2$ remained reduced and constant. In unconscious patients $CMRO_2$ was initially 1.3 ml O_2/100g/min, followed by a gradual increase to 1.7 ml after 4–5 days. Simultaneously, CBF increased from 18 ml to 30 ml/100g/min (Jakobsen et al.1990).

During regional CBF studies hyperaemic areas, focal vasoparalysis and global impairment of autoregulation have been observed (Heilbrun et al. 1972, Voldby et al. 1985b). Hyperaemic regions are supposed to be regarded as a reaction to initial ischaemia (Gelmers et al. 1979). In these regions the degree of flow abnormalities correlates fairly well with the clinical grading and the neurological deficits (Heilbrum et al. 1972, Ishii 1979).

Haematoma and hydrocephalus

A marked reduction of CBF has been found in patients with intracerebral haematoma and in patients with ventricular dilation (Ishii 1979, Menon et al. 1981). Communicating hydrocephalus produced a significant decrease in CBF (Hayashi et al. 1984).

SPECT

In patients with anterior communicating artery aneurysm rCBF measured with SPECT dropped in frontal areas, where MR studies indicated cerebral lesion, predominantly in the anterior prefrontal lobe, on the side of the surgical flap. Most of these prefrontal lesions were likely to be due to surgical procedure and not to vasospasm. In the same study rCBF was elevated in the posterior cortical areas and cerebellum. This hyperaemia is supposed to be due to release of a physiological inhibition exerted by the prefrontal cortex (Rouesseaux et al. 1994).

PET

With the PET method, employing radioactive ^{15}O, a decrease in CBF and $CMRO_2$ was observed. Patients with more severe neurological deficits, and patients with a more severe degree of vasospasm had a marked depression of CBF and $CMRO_2$. These changes were accompanied by an increase in CBV. The results suggest that vasospasm is caused by constriction of the large radiographically visible extraparenchymal vessels, accompanied by a massive dilation of intraparenchymal vessels (Grubb et al. 1977). In another PET study patients studied in the pre-spasm stage (2–4 days after SAH) showed CBF averaging 45 ml/100g/min, $CMRO_2$ of 2.7 ml O_2/100ml/min and CBV of 5.5 ml/100ml. During the spasm stage (6–15 days after SAH) CBF was 39 ml/100ml/min, $CMRO_2$ 2.4 ml 0_2/100ml/min and CBV 5.4 ml/100ml. Thus, CBV was considerably elevated, CBF decreased and $CMRO_2$ also tended to decrease, suggesting an effect of vasospasm (Kuwamura et al. 1992).

Clot formation

A significant negative correlation has been found between $CMRO_2$ and the amount of subarachnoid blood, with additional reduction of $CMRO_2$ in case of ventricular bleeding (Jacobsen et al. 1991).

Blood-brain barrier (BBB) dysfunction

Experimental studies

The capillary system during the acute phase of SAH has been studied experimentally. In a rat model BBB changes were assessed by quantitative alpha-aminoisobutyric acid technique. In experimental SAH the BBB damage increased in cerebral cortices and cerebellar grey matter, averaging 1.3 and 1.5 times control values (Germanó et al. 1992). In cats suffering from SAH an early and marked increase in capillary permeability was found. This leakage was correlated to a high blood pressure (Trojanowski 1982). Evans blue extravasation in experimental SAH is correlated to the degree of arterial hypertension (Shigeno et al. 1982). These findings are in concert with studies in rats indicating that brain oedema in the acute phase should be classified as vasogenic oedema (Doczi et al. 1986). In rats subjected to SAH blood-brain barrier permeability dysfunction was detected 36 hours after SAH, peaking at 48 hours, and normalising on day 3 (Germano et al. 2000).

On the other hand, Peterson and Cardoso (1983) in cats subjected to SAH found that vasospasm to some degree prevented extravasation of Evans Blue during hypertension.

Clinical studies

A significant increase in the permeability of the BBB after SAH has been described in clinical studies (Doczi 1985). He found that patients with abnormal enhancement by CT scan are likely to be in less favourable clinical grades, have a high incidence of marked or diffuse spasm, have a poorer outcome independent of surgical or conservative treatment, and develope cerebral infarction more frequently. Furthermore, systemic arterial hypertension was associated with an increased incidence of abnormal enhancement.

Cerebral autoregulation (CA) experimental studies

Changes related to time after SAH

In a dog SAH-model a decreased autoregulatory capacity has been demonstrated (Steiner et al. 1978). Studies of the time course of the impairment of cerebral autoregulation during chronic cerebral vasospasm in primates indicate total loss of autoregulation until 2 weeks after SAH, at which time partial normalisation of CA occurred. However, CA was only found at a very narrow blood pressure range.

(Handa et al.1992). Studies, including MR spectroscopy and rCBF, in primates indicate, that when CA is abolished during chronic vasospasm, changes in cerebral energy metabolism are coupled with changes in CBF. Under these conditions there exists a critical level for ischaemia, below which high-energy phosphorus metabolites become markedly depleted. These changes occurred at MABP less than 60 mm Hg (Handa et al. 1993).

Hyperventilation

In the rat subjected to subarachnoid haemorrhage hyperventilation to $PaCO_2$ levels of about 2,9 to 4.1 kPa restores cerebral autoregulation (Hauerberg et al. 1993). Even hyperventilation to $PaCO_2$ levels ranging from 4.0 to 4.67 kPa restores cerebral autoregulation (Ma et al. 2000).

Cerebral autoregulation (CA), clinical studies

Hunt and Hess

In one study CA was especially disturbed in good grade patients subjected to early operation (Dernbach et al. 1988). In another study CA was intact in patients in good clinical condition, but was impaired in patients in poor clinical condition. In the same study a close correlation between the degree of vasospasm and the degree of CA impairment was found, and ICP-hypertension and CSF-lactic acidosis were commonly found in association with vasoparalysis (Voldby et al. 1985a).

After induced arterial hypotension intact cerebral autoregulation was found before as well as after treatment with nimodipine (Rasmussen et al. 1999).

Transcranial Doppler

In a preliminary study Giller (1990), with a mathematical analysis, has studied the correlation between blood velocity and blood pressure. With this technique autoregulation was found to be impaired in SAH patients. The temporal nature of autoregulation was found to correlate fairly good with the changes in neurological status.

CO_2 reactivity

Experimental studies

In baboons SAH is accompanied by a decrease in CBF and $CMRO_2$, and the CO_2 reactivity is attenuated (Mendelow et al. 1981). In cats subjected to SAH CBF remained within normal range, but CO_2 reactivity to hypercapnia was blunted (Diringer et al. 1993). However, in a recent study of SAH in rabbits with verified basilar artery vasospasm the reactivities to hypercapnia and hypoxia were intact (Diringer et al. 1994).

Clinical studies

CO_2 reactivity is disturbed in good grade patients after early operation (Dernbach et al. 1988). Impaired CO_2 response has been demonstrated in patients with severe neurological deficits, severe degree of vasospasm, CSF-lactic acidosis and patients with marked depression of mean CBF (Ishii 1979, Voldby et al. 1985a). After nimodipine treatment an increase in CO_2 reactivity was observed (Rasmussen et al. 1999).

Vasospasm

The appearance of arterial narrowing on the angiogram after aneurysmal haemorrhage is indicative of radiographic vasospasm. If clinical symptoms and signs of cerebral ischaemia or infarction develop, delayed cerebral ischaemia or delayed ischaemic neurological deficits are diagnosed. This development is secondary to clinical or symptomatic cerebral vasospasm (For review MacDonald 1995)

Experimental studies

Phases

In experimental studies, cerebral vasospasm is a biphasic phenomenon. The acute phase occurs within minutes of the rupture, and lasts less than 10 minutes. The chronic phase occurs 3 to 24 hours after the haemorrhage and lasts for days (Brawley et al. 1968). Thus, *in vitro* studies in a "two haemorrhage" canine model arterial segments excised from the basilar artery revealed a progressive increase in arterial stiffness from day 2 to 7 (Matsui et al. 1994).

Stimulation

Mechanical stimulation and blood in the periarterial region are potential causes of spasm. The mechanical stimulation, in comparison with that induced by blood, only gives rise to spasm of short duration (Kapp et al. 1968a). Another study by the same group demonstrated that prolonged exposure to air and exposure to hypotonic solutions increased cerebral vasospasm (Kapp et al. 1968b).

Ca^{2+}

Delayed cerebral vasospasm is due to a sustained tonic smooth-muscle contraction. This contraction is mediated by a rise in intracellular calcium, and results in a calmodulin-dependent activation of myosin light chain kinase, leading to interaction between actin and phosphorylated light chains of myosin (Marston 1982). It is supposed that vasodilation elicited by calcitonin-gene-related peptide (CGRP) is mediated by cAMP and/or cGMP. However, in long-lasting tonic contraction, phosphorylation of myosin light chains induced by the calmodulin system is temporarily observed only in the initial phase of the contraction, and does not continue.

The initial phase of contraction is followed by a sustained tonic phase, which has not been clearly identified. It could be due to a myosin phosphorylation mechanism (Dillon et al. 1981) or the protein kinase C system (Nishizawa et al. 1992). Recently *in vitro* studies of basilar artery ring strips were performed in a rabbit model of SAH. CGRP-induced vasodilation was attenuated during vasospasm and the vasodilatory response mediated by cAMP and cGMP was intact, although the levels of cGMP in SAH vessels were reduced. Together these observations suggest, that attenuation in the capacity of vessels to dilate in response to CGRP occurs during vasospasm, and the change in CGRP vasoreactivity is a result of modifications prior to, or independent of the elevation of cyclic nuchleotide second messengers (Sutter et al. 1995). In studies of isolated rings of primate cerebral arteries oxyhemoglobin, but not methemoglobin, produced a transient increase in the intracellular levels inositol triphosphate (ITP), which triggers the release of Ca^{2+} from intracellular stores.

The increase in intracellular Ca^{2+} is prevented by neomycin, a phospholipase C inhibitor (Vollrath et al. 1994).

The Ca^{2+}-ATPase, which consumes energy to export intracellular Ca^{2+} to extracellular space is involved in the regulation of Ca^{2+} homeostasis. In the dog two-haemorrhage model, the activity of this enzyme decreases 24 hours after experimental SAH, inversely with basilar artery contraction, suggesting a persistent disturbance of Ca^{2+} homeostasis, and indicating that damage to the plasma membrane in the cerebral arterial smooth-muscle cells proceeds to myonecrosis after SAH (Wang et al.1994).

Energy metabolism

Using high-performance liquid chromatography in studies of canine cerebral arteries subjected to chronic SAH, it was found that the levels of ATP, guanosine triphosphate (GTP), and creatine phosphate were decreased, suggesting serious disturbances in the energy metabolism (Kim et al. 1992).

Free radicals

Other mechanisms involve the formation of free radicals. Because of deficient scavenging mechanisms in the CSF, these free radicals cause lipid peroxidation. Products of lipid peroxidation affect the cerebral arterial wall from the very early stage, probably infiltrating the wall through channels of the wall opening to the CSF space to exhibit inflammatory changes such as subintimal cell proliferation and myonecrosis. Lipid peroxidation also leads to degeneration of membrane phospholipids, such as phosphatidylcholine and phosphatidylethanolamine and to rise in the intracellular level of diacylglycerol, an intrinsic protein kinase C activator. Subsequent release of arachidonic acid stimulates the arachidonic cascade which generates various eicosanoids and free radicals contributing to inflammatory changes in the arterial wall (Sano 1994).

Protein kinase C (PKC)

Calcium mediated stimulation of protein kinase C resulting in a different chain phosphorylation has also been proposed (Park and Rasmussen 1986, Rasmussen et al. 1990). In dogs subjected to SAH protein kinase C activity is remarkably altered (Takuwa et al. 1993). It is suggested that protein kinase C in the vascular smooth muscle is translocated to the membrane from the cytosol, and that this process is activated by SAH (Nishizawa et al. 1992). In studies of canine basilar arteries it was found that tonic contraction of the vessel was dependent on the PKC system. The initiation of the contraction by the calmodulin system was necessary for the subsequent PKC-dependent tonic contraction. Specific calmodulin antagonists like chlorpromazine partially inhibited the tonic contraction associated with PKC activation. Another calmodulin antagonist, trifluoperazine, inhibited the PKC system as well (Nishizawa et al. 1992). Both tonic and spastic contractions of basilar artery of the dog are effectively dilated by inhibition of protein kinase C (Minami et al. 1992). In comparison with nicardipine and papaverine the dilatory effect of protein kinase C inhibitor in a canine "two haemorrhage model" is sustained for a longer period (Matsui et al. 1994). Other experimental studies of two-hemorrhagic models, however, indicate a discrepancy between membrane-bound PKC activity in the basilar artery and angiographic contraction, suggesting that vasospasm after SAH cannot be explained solely on the basis of activation of the PKC pathway (Sako et al. 1993).

Complement system

Most important, blocking of complement activation by the protease inhibitor (FUT-175) has been shown to ameliorate vasospasm both in a rabbit model and in humans in a therapeutic trial. Recently it was shown that specific depletion of complement by systemic administration of cobra venum abrogated the development of experimental vasospasm in rabbits. In another study it was demonstrated that complement activation by aged erythrocytes can result in membrane attack complexes insertion into innocent bystander smooth-muscle cell membranes, and that this mechanism may contribute to development of vasospasm after SAH (Park et al. 1997).

Clinical studies

In clinical studies arterial spasm is the main cause of postoperative morbidity and mortality in patients with SAH (Allcock and Drake 1965). Neither angiographic vasospasm grades nor the incidence of symptomatic vasospasm are influenced by age of the patients (Inagawa 1992).

Complement system

A number of findings indicate that complement system is essential to the development of vasospasm. Activated components of complement have been found in plasma and CSF of patients with SAH whose course is complicated by ischaemia-induced neurological deficits. Complement deposits have been identified in the walls of vasospastic vessels in patients as well as in experimental animals.

Coagulation

Measurement of coagulation factors, hemorrheological variables and cardiolipin immunoreactivity does not predict delayed ischaemic deficit in clinical studies (Ameriso et al. 1992).

Histopathological Changes in Vasospasm

Experimental studies

Histopathological changes in cerebral spastic arteries have been described. In experimental studies media necrosis, subendothelial polymorph infiltration of the arteries and subsequent intimal thickening have been observed (Fein et al. 1974, Alksne et al. 1974, Tanabe et al. 1978), and in arteries from patients with SAH (Crompton 1964, Conway and McDonald 1972, Hughes and Scianchi 1978, Sakai et al. 1979). However, these findings have not been observed in other studies of repeated SAH in dogs and in post-mortem examination of brain vessels from patients with SAH and arterial spasm (Elderik et al. 1981), and studies in monkeys indicate that cerebral vasospasm after SAH was not associated with proliferation of cells in the vessel wall. Nor was the intensity of the limited proliferation changes responsible for narrowing of the vessel diameter(Pluta et al. 1992). *In vitro* studies of arteries from experimental SAH in monkeys indicate large spontaneous irregularities in tone and decreased dispensability. In addition they exhibited large, prolonged spontaneous increases in muscle tone. These changes were supposed to be caused by an inflammatory response (Bevan et al. 1987).

Clinical studies

Histopathological changes in cerebral spastic arteries have also been described in arteries from patients with SAH (Crompton 1964, Conway and McDonald 1972, Hughes and Scianchi 1978, Sakai et al. 1979).

Immunoreactivity

Circulating immunocomplexes and complement activation are elevated in patients with vasospasm (Pellettieri et al. 1981), Østergaard et al. 1987). A high immunocomplex content proceeds the onset of vasospasm, and a low content proceeds clinical improvement (Pellettieri et al. 1986).

CBF and $CRMO_2$ during vasospasm

Experimental studies

In experimental studies vasospasm of the cerebral arteries is accompanied by a reduction in CBF (James 1968, Jakubowski et al. 1976), and an increase in transit time (Kak and Taylor 1967). After SAH combined with mechanical trauma of the arteries, the decrease in CBF after SAH follows a biphasic pattern. Angiographic constriction of the large arteries is not necessarily associated with a decrease in CBF until the vessels constrict to 50% or less of the control calibre (Simeone et al. 1972).

Human studies

In patients with SAH and vasospasm the CBF reduction is correlated to major neurological dysfunction (Ferguson et al. 1972, Yamamoto et al. 1979). A positive correlation between rCBF and the diameter of the major supplying vessels has been observed. In a study of intra-arterially infused ^{133}Xe, angiographic vasospasm was accompanied by global and focal reduction in CBF, but hyperaemic regions with tissue peaks were also observed. CBF in patients with severe diffuse vasospasm averaged 21 ml/100g/min. Many of these patients developed infarction (Voldby et al. 1985b).

In the same study $CMRO_2$ decreased synchronously with the decrease in arterial calibre, and the $CMRO_2$ was more reduced than CBF, indicating an uncoupling between flow and metabolism (Voldby et al. 1985b). This relative luxury perfusion was associated with CSF lactic acidosis and ICP-hypertension. In another study vasospasm of severe degree was accompanied by focal areas of depressed flow below 30 ml/100g/min (Ishii 1979). Studies in patients with focal vasospasm indicate that the reduction of CBF is global and not restricted to the area of the spastic vessels (Jacobsen et al. 1990a). Other studies confirm this observation, and in one study an estimate of CBF seems to be of little use in the prognostic evaluation of patients with SAH (Bergvall et al. 1973). Pickard et al.(1980) found that patients with impaired autoregulatory capacity after SAH ran a much grater risk of developing late ischaemic deterioration, and Mickey et al. (1984) using SPECT demonstrated that delayed neurological deficits were accompanied by large areas of well defined regional flow decrease in the vascular territories of the middle cerebral artery. Concurrent with these studies Davis et al. (1990) found that SPECT facilitates early diagnosis of cerebral tissue hypoperfusion due to vasospasm.

SPECT and PET studies

Studies with SPECT indicate that it is an acceptable technique, that can demonstrate varying degrees of regional hypoperfusion in patients with symptomatic vasospasm (Naderi et al. 1994).

With PET regional reductions in blood flow associated with increase in CBV were observed in the cortical territory corresponding to cerebral vasospasm. A reduction in $CMRO_2$ even in apparently normal cortex despite normal CBF was also found (Hino et al. 1989).

Xe-CT

The Xenon-enhanced method appears very sensitive to the early detection of vasospasm. In a series of 51 patients infarction was not found if CBF remained above 18 ml/100g/min (Yonas et al. 1989).

CO_2 reactivity and cerebral autoregulation

During delayed cerebral ischaemia secondary to vasospasm impaired CO_2 reactivity was observed (Yamamoto et al. 1979). Studies using transcranial Doppler and the transient hyperaemic response test indicate that when the effects of primarily impaired autoregulation are magnified by vasospasm, the risk of delayed ischaemic deficits seems to be very high (Lam et al. 2000). In another clinical study cerebral autoregulation was tested by continuous recording of flow velocity and blood pressure. It was found that cerebral autoregulation impairment preceded vasospasm, and that ongoing vasospasm worsens cerebral autoregulation. Furthermore, it was demonstrated that cerebral autoregulation assessment early after subarachnoid haemorrhage (1–6 days) is predictive of outcome (Lang et al. 2001).

During nimodipine treatment the CO_2 reactivity is impaired (Messeter et al. 1987).

Diamox

In a study of reactivity to acetazolamide (Diamox) it was observed that diamox initially provoked steal phenomenon in the arterial territory of the vasospasm. Later on, the reactivity to diamox changed to subnormal and at last normal reactivity, suggesting that serial CBF measurements plus diamox are useful to determine the most appropriate time for aneurysm surgery (Dinh et al. 1993).

Experimental studies of vasospasm and the adrenogenic system

Nuclei A_1 and A_2

By producing a selective chemical lesion in adult rats prior to experimental SAH, it was demonstrated that the catecholamine nuclei A_1 and A_1 in the mesencephalon, via projections to hypothalamus, including the median eminence are involved in the development of spasm (Dahlström and Fuxe 1964, Svendgaard et al. 1985). These findings suggest that blood in the subarachnoid space does not produce vasospasm via a direct vascular mechanism, but also via a neural or neurochemical pathway.

Treatment with systemic 6-hydroxydopamine (6-OHDA),which causes a depletion of noradrenaline from central sympathetic nerves, prevents the development of delayed spasm, while acute spasm can be prevented by lesions in the mesencephalus of the ascending catecholamine fibers originating in the lower brain stem and projecting to hypothalamus (Delgado et al. 1987). It is suggested that 6-OHDA treatment results in an altered spasm pattern via its effect on catecholamine fibres projecting between the medullary A1 and A2 nuclei and the hypothalamus.

CBF

Lesioning in the medulla oblongata of the ascending fibres from A_1 and A_2 also prevented the development of the global decrease in CBF, together with an increase in glucose utilisation seen in normal animals with SAH, and the focal low-flow areas with markedly elevated glucose utilisation, which develops in normal rats 2 days after SAH disappeared as well (Delgado et al. 1986, Delgado et al. 1986b).

Median eminence

Lesion of the median eminence, but not hypophysectomy, prevents the development of vasospasm. It is suggested that projection from the nucleus A_1 and A_2 to the median eminence is interrupted, and thus the development of vasospasm (Svendgaard et al. 1986, Svendgaard et al. 1987).

Substance P

In a rat model of SAH it has been shown, that depletion of substance P-containing sensory nerves to the cerebral arteries with capsaicin prior to SAH prevents the development of both acute and late spasm. Intrathecal injection of substance P antagonist, spantide, also prevents late vasospasm (Delgado-Zygmunt et al. 1990). The authors suggest that in this model substance P-containing nerve fibres localised on the cerebral arteries could constitute the sensory link in a reflex arc system involved in the development of spasm. In this arc the presence of a clot in the subarachnoid space stimulates substance P-containing nerve fibres on the cerebral arteries including a centripetal impulse to the A_2 nucleus, and secondary the development of vasospasm.

Chatecholamine

Norepinephrine produces cerebral vasoconstriction in normal animals (Frazer et al. 1970, Lobato et al. 1980). In the rat brain norepinephrine is elevated in the cerebral hemisphere, especially in neurones that originate in the locus coeruleus (Solomon et al. 1986). The authors suggest that activation of the nucleus coeruleus during experimental SAH leads to decreased CBF and metabolism.

Denervation

Adrenergic denervation hypersensibility has been proposed to play a role in the development of cerebral vasospasm after SAH (Syon 1971). This theory was supported by studies indicating that catecholamine histofluorescens was diminished in cerebral arteries after experimental SAH (Peerless and Yasargil 1971, Rosenblum and Guiloanti 1973). However, adrenergic denervation of cat basilar arteries by injection of 6-hydroxydopamine into the cisterna magna indicate that denervation is not the cause of cerebral vasospasm (Duff et al. 1987).

Blockade

Parenteral phenoxybenzamine, in experimental SAH in cats, is effective in preventing spasm, but not when provoked by mechanical stimulation (Flamm et al. 1972a). Phentolamine, when topically applicated, also alleviates spasm induced by mechanical manipulation, but only for 15 minutes (Flamm et al. 1972b). These drugs, however, when injected intracisternally, have side effects. Thus, larger doses of phenoxybenzamine cause chemical basilar meningitis and phentolamine causes arterial hypotension (Martins and Wiley 1973). In another study in dogs intrathecally injected phenoxybenzamine was not superior to saline (White et al. 1979), and in cats the effectiveness of isoproterenol, phentolamine and phenoxybenzamine in modifying basilar arterial spasm was studied. None of these agents were effective in inhibiting the initial peak constriction of the arteries (Smigiel and Sundt 1974).

Clinical studies of vasospasm and the adrenogenic system

CSF

The concentration of norepinephrine in CSF of patients with SAH is elevated (Cummins and Lothian 1973, Shigeno et al. 1982). In one study the concentrations of noradrenaline and adrenaline in CSF were increased in patients with delayed focal cerebral ischaemia. Higher catecholamine levels in CSF were found in blood vessels supplying the hypothalamus, and the highest concentrations were found in patients with a poor outcome (Dilraj et al. 1992).

It has been demonstrated that the concentration of norepinephrine in CSF is too low to account for prolonged vasospasm (Shigeno et al. 1982). In another clinical study it was found that the primary vasoconstrictive activity of CSF from patients with SAH is not norepinephrine (Boullin et al. 1981).

Blockade

Intra-carotid injection of phenoxybenzamine has been accompanied by rapid improvement in patients with pronounced neurological disability owing to vasospasm (Cummins and Griffith 1971).

Trigeminal system and vasospasm

Also the trigeminal system seems to be involved in cerebral vasospasm. In monkeys a unilateral postganglionic lesion causes constriction of the cerebral arteries which is sustained after SAH (Shiokawa et al. 1992).

Dopamine and Vasospasm

Wurtman and Zervas (1974) suggested that monoamines, like dopamine, might be released from damaged neurones during the acute phase of SAH. Such loss could be associated with an abnormal amount in the CSF, which in turn might provoke vasospasm. In dogs dopamine given intracisternally generates vasospasm of the basilar artery. However, compared with prostaglandin E_2 and blood, the spasm induced by dopamine was delayed in onset, less in incidence, and usually less intense (White et al. 1976).

CSF Biochemistry

Experimental studies

Neuropeptides

In experimental ischaemia, the proinflammatory cytokine interleukin-1 mediates cellular damage. In addition an interleukin-1 antagonist reduces brain damage after episodes of temporary ischaemia.

Clinical studies

Lactate and pH

In the presence of SAH the CSF is acidotic and lactate concentration is increased. The lactate is derived from glycolysis by the enzyme systems of the shed blood cells (Fromann and Smith 1967). CSF-lactic acidosis is especially observed in patients with impaired consciousness, focal neurological deficits, vasospasm, poor prognosis and in patients with ICP-hypertension (Fujishima et al. 1975, Voldby and Enevoldsen 1982b). In one study a CSF lactate value above 3.5 mmol/l was associated with a poor outcome (Voldby and Enevoldsen 1982b).

Creatine kinase

A biochemical marker of brain cell damage, the BB-isoenzyme of creatine kinase, has been used to evaluate any possible brain injury caused by SAH. It was found that operation caused brain cell damage, even in the absence of any clinical signs of deterioration. The increase in BB-isoenzyme is more pronounced with early compared with late operation (Rabow et al. 1995).

CSF creatine phosphokinase (CP) is increased in SAH. However, the actual value of CP has no diagnostic specificity, although tissue-destructive processes like infarction engenders abnormally high levels (Greenblatt 1976).

Neuropeptides and cytokines

Neuropeptide Y is a well-known cerebral vasoconstrictor (Edvinsson et al. 1984, Allen et al. 1984). Consecutive determinations of this neuropeptide in the ventricular fluid of SAH patients indicate an increase 6–11 days after the onset of SAH, suggesting that neuropeptides may play a role in the pathogenesis of vasospasm (Suzuki et al. 1989).

In a recent study of SAH the level of calcitonin-gene-related peptide (CFRP), substance P, and vasoactive peptide (VIP) were measured in the external jugular vein and in the CSF. The highest CGRP levels were found in patients with the highest velocity index values (Juul et al. 1995).

SAH is accompanied by an increased leukocyte count in blood and low grade fever, indicating a systemic inflammatory process. Interleukin-6, an inflammatory marker, is found to be dramatically elevated in patients with SAH. The highest level is found at day 6 after SAH (Mathiesen et al. 1993). The role of pro-inflammatory and anti-inflammatory cytokines in the development of vasospasm after SAH was recently studied in 15 patients. During development of clinical vasospasm an increase in pro-inflammatory cytokine (IL-6) in the CSF was found. In patients with angiographic vasospasm an increased expression in anito-inflammatory cytokines (IL-10) was present immediately after SAH. In patients without vasospasm the balance between pro- and anti-inflammatory cascade remained stable over time (Mascia et al. 2000).

Tumour necrosis factor- synthesis occurs under circumstances that are similar to interleukin-1 and interleukin-6 syntheses. CSF-Interleukin-1 receptor antagonist (IL-RA) and CSF-tumour necrosis factor- increase after SAH and high cytokine levels correlate with brain damage, suggesting that fever, leukocytosis, and nitric oxide synthesis are mediated by these cytokines (Mathiesen et al. 1997).

Phospholipase and eicosanoids

Phospholipase C is released in CSF from patients with SAH. The activity reflects the extend of brain damage (Nakashima et al. 1993).

The CSF eicosanoids level is raised following SAH but not sufficiently to be vasoactive per se within the cerebral circulation. However, in patients with rebleeding and intraventricular haemorrhage the CSF levels of eicosanoids were raised 250-fold over the normal range. These concentrations are found to be sufficient to have cerebrovascular effects (Pickard et al. 1994).

Cardiac Arrhythmias

Clinical studies

Myocardial lesion

In autopsy study of patients dying from SAH myocardial lesions are frequently found. It is suggested that these subendothelial damages are caused by hypothalamic stimulation leading to an acute increase in tone of the autonomic sympathetic nervous system (Doshi and Neil-Dwyer 1980, Marion et al. 1986). Elevation of catecholamine in plasma in the acute phase of SAH, as demonstrated in several studies, also may play a role (Cruickshank et al. 1974, Loach and Benedict 1980).

ECG

Electrocardiographic changes simulating myocardial ischaemia or infarction have been described in patients with SAH (Cropp and Manning 1960). The frequency of cardiac arrhythmia in patients with SAH has been detected in 91% of patients. In the same study the frequency of serious arrhythmias (torsade de pointe, ventricular flutter or fibrillation) was 41% (Andreoli et al. 1987).These arrhythmias responded to sympathetic blocking agents, which also may have a protective effect on subendothelial ischaemia, but there is no evidence that prophylactic administration of beta-blocking agents alters the outcome in SAH (Neil-Dwyer et al. 1978). Electrocardiographic changes occur more frequently in association with deteriorating levels of consciousness, pyrexia, and diastolic hypertension (Galloon et al. 1972). In a series of 57 patients with SAH echocardiographic signs of ventricular wall motion abnormalities were identified in 8%. Four patients experienced hypotension and three pulmonary oedema. Patients with wall motion abnormalities were more likely to have T wave inversion and severe qTc segment prolongation besides borderline creatine kinase MB elevation (Mayer et al. 1995). In another study of patients with giant aneurysm without SAH abnormal ECG, mostly ST or T wave changes were observed (Manninen et al. 19??).

Nimodipine treatment does not reduce the frequency or type of abnormal ECG tracings (Mee et al. 1988).

Treatment

Haemodilution

Experimental studies

Haemodilution with diaspirin-crosslinked-haemoglobin ameliorates occlusive cerebral ischaemia. In rats subjected to SAH, and treated with diaspirin-crosslinked-haemoglobin, an increase in CBF was demonstrated, and the number of death neurones was less compared with the control group (Cole et al. 1997).

Clinical studies

In some studies early surgery and aggressive management of vasospasms with hypervolemic hemodilution therapy have been recommended (Muizelaar and Becker 1986, Awad et al. 1987). A decrease in blood viscosity seems to promote cerebral circulation, and an inverse correlation has been demonstrated between blood viscosity and level of consciousness in patients with SAH (Schievink et al. 1987). Even liberal fluid intake, at least three litre per day seems to decrease mortality and the incidence of delayed cerebral ischaemia (Hasan et al. 1989). In one study the incidence of preoperative vasospasms was 20% against 60% in the control group, and in the treated group 87% survived to operation, against 53% in the control group (Rosenwasser et al. 1983). This therapy has to be guided by monitoring of central hemodynamics (CH), especially pulmonary wedge pressure (PWP). Thus, neurological deficits can be reversed by increasing PWP, and in individual patients an optimal PWP can be defined, below which neurological deficits reappear. The optimum PWP ranged from 14 to 16 mm Hg (Finn et al. 1986). In other studies a depletion of blood cell volume, more than lowering of the plasma volume, was supposed to be responsible for neurological deterioration. Consequently, repeated monitoring of cerebral blood volume has been recommended (Kodo et al. 1981).

In patients refractory to conventional hypervolemic agent, hyperdynamic therapy with dobutamine in the presence of volume loading resulted in a 52% increase in cardiac index, and a decrease in total peripheral resistance. During this therapy reversal of ischaemic symptoms due to SAH was evident in 78% of patients (Levy et al. 1993).

Blood pressure control and hypervolaemia

Clinical studies

The main aim in the treatment of symptomatic vasospasm is to keep the CPP > 70 mm Hg. To achieve this goal induced hypertension can be necessary. Dopamine 10–20 g/kg/min, dobutamine 2–10 g/kg/min, and phenylephrine 0.5–1g/kg/min are among the vasoactive agents commonly used. These principles of treatment are supplemented with volume expansion, usually crystalloids and 5% albumin, hemodilution, hematocrit of 30–33%, and improved rheology by mannitol infusion (Levy 1990).

In another study intravascular volume expansion with 500 ml 5% albumin did not increase CBF or reverse symptomatic vasospasm (Yamakami et al. 1987).

Pulmonary oedema

In a series of 47 patients early aneurysm surgery was performed during prophylactic hypervolemia. Aggressive volume therapy to the point of cardiovascular collapse, as evidenced by a high rate of pulmonary oedema was applied. The authors concluded that no appreciable decrease in neurological morbidity and mortality was found (Medlock et al. 1982).

Swan-Ganz monitoring

In many centres invasive haemodynamic monitoring with Swan-Ganz technique has become standard in the management of SAH. In a retrospective analysis of 630 Swan-Ganz catheters placed in 184 patients with SAH a 13% incidence of catheter-related sepsis, a 2% incidence of congestive failure, a 1.3% incidence of subclavian vein thrombosis, and a 1% incidence of pneumothorax were found. Pulmonary artery rupture was not observed (Rosenwasser et al. 1995).

Haemorrhagic infarct and hypertensive encephalopathy

Several studies warn against the danger of haemorrhagic infarction that may result from continuing induced hypertension after a delayed ischaemia has resolved (Ohta et al. 1982, Terada et al. 1987). In a study it was concluded that hypervolaemic therapy is contraindicated in a patient with massive abnormality on CT scanning at the time when a delayed ischaemic deficit is manifested, especially when it occurs within 6 days after the SAH. To avoid haemorrhagic infarction, it is also important to discontinue hypervolemic therapy as soon as the delayed ischaemic deficit has resolved (Shimoda et al. 1993).

Two cases of hypertensive encephalopathy have been described following hyperdynamic therapy for cerebral vasospasm (Amin-Hanjani et al. 1999).

Free radical scavengers, experimental studies

When oxyhemoglobin is converted to methemoglobin, superoxide anions are released. Superoxides initiate free radical reactions including peroxidation of polyunsaturated fatty acids in the cell membrane. Hematin, another degradation product of oxyhemoglobin also catalyzes the conversion of polyunsaturated fatty acids to their peroxidized forms. At last leukocytes in the subarachnoid clot produce free radical species. *In vitro* and *in vivo* studies indicate that free radical reactions initiated by clot lysis play an important role in the genesis of chronic vasospasm in SAH (Sano et al. 1980). On the other hand, in monkeys intrathecal superoxide dismutase and catalase do not protect against oxyhemoglobin-induced vasospasms, suggesting that mechanisms mediated by free radicals may not be an important factor in the genesis of vasospasms (Loch Macdonald et al. 1992).

Zanthine oxidase

In the dog the role of Xanthine oxidase (XO) in the liberation of oxygen free radicals have been studied as a cause of tissue damage, secondary to chronic vasospasm. In experimental vasospasm this enzyme is activated. However, treatment with allopurinol, a specific blocker of XO, did not change the morphological changes of the vessels, nor the prostaglandin levels (Kim et al. 1987).

AVS (N,N-propylenedinicotinamide)

AVS is a water-soluble compound which scavenges hydroxyl radicals in aqueous environment at neutral pH. AVS ameliorates vasospasm (Asano et al. 1984), as well as ischaemic damage (Asano et al. 1989) in relevant experimental models. Prophylactic adminsitration of AVS improves CBF and glucose utilisation in the rat brain subjected to SAH (Yamamoto et al. 2000).

Clinical studies of AVS

In a placebo-controlled double-blind trial of 162 patients with SAH, and with GCS between 7 and 15 on admission, AVS-treated patients had significantly less delayed ischaemic neurological deficits due to vasospasms (placebo 54% versus AVS-treated 36%). At one month the GOS was significant improved in treated patients (Asano et al. 1996).

Lazaroids

Experimental studies

In experimental studies the 21-aminosteroid U-74006F has been reported to attenuate chronic vasospasm (Steinke et al. 1989, Vollmer et al. 1989, Zuccarello et al. 1989). In a primate model dosages of 0.3–1.0 mg/kg attenuate vasospasm 7 days after induction of SAH (Kanamura et al. 1990). The same results were found in a two-haemorrhage model of beagle dogs (Matsui and Asano 1994). In another study the peroxidation was studied in subarachnoid haemorrhagic clots, and it was suggested that the salutary effect of U-74006F in vasospasm is mediated by a reduction of lipid peroxidation (Kanamaru et al. 1991).

In rats subjected to SAH both tiralazad and one of the metabolites (U-89678) reduced the blood-brain barrier dysfunction, and both compounds enhanced neuronal survival in a concentration-dependent fashion (Smith et al. 1996).

Clinical studies

In a randomised, double-blind, vehicle-controlled trial of SAH including 1023 patients tiralazad in doses of 0.6. 2 and 6 mg/kg were compared with placebo. All patients were in treatment with nimodipine. Patients receiving 6 mg/kg/day of tiralazad had reduced mortality (P = 0.01) compared with patients treated with placebo. There was non-significant reduction in symptomatic vasospasm in the same group (P = 0.048). The benefits of treatment with tiralazad were primarily shown in men rather than women, and no difference between outcome in the groups treated with 0.6 and 2 mg/kg/day and the group treated with placebo was disclosed (Kassell et al. 1996). In another clinical trial including 245 patients the results suggested that tiralazad 2 mg/kg/day improved 3-month outcome (Haley et al. 1995). Haley et al. (1997), however, performed a second randomised study including 897 patients. The patients were allocated to three groups: placebo, 2 mg/kg/day, and 6 mg/kg/day tirilazad within 48 hrs. of the SAH and continuing through 10 days. At three months post-SAH, there were no significant differences among the groups with regard to mortality rate, favourable outcome, or employment status. When the data were stratified according to gender and neurological status on admission, men with grade IV an V in the 6 mg/kg/day group had a mortality of 5% compared with 33% in the control group. Recently Lazino et al.(1999) and Lanzino and Kassell (1999) performed two parallel randomised studies of high-dose (15 mg/kg/day) tirilazad in women. A significant reduction in the incidence of symptomatic vasospasm was observed in the treatment group, but mortality rate at 3 months was not affected by tirilazad. Sequential analysis, however, revealed a reduction in mortality rates among patients with neurological grades IV and V, favouring the tirilazad group.

Calcium Antagonists

Experimental studies (nimodipine)

In a randomised placebo-controlled study of SAH in monkeys, nimodipine 1 mg/kg every 8 hours reduced vasospasm slightly (Espinosa et al. 1984). In a canine model Zabranski et al. (1986) and Glioia et al. (1985) found a beneficial effect of intrathecal nimodipine as compared with systemic administration in reversing angiographic vasospasm. However, in a primate model of chronic cerebral vasospasm intrathecally applied nimodipine was not effective in prevention of angiographic vasospasm (Lewis et al. 1988). When vasoconstriction is induced by K^+ or serotonin, studies of isolated rabbit basilar artery indicate that the vasodilatory effect of nimodipine is decreased in the presence of haemoglobin (Toshima et al. 1992).

Clinical studies (nimodipine)

Allen et al. (1983), in a double-blind, randomised placebo controlled trial, demonstrated that neurological deficits from vasospasm by the end of 21 days treatment with nimodipine caused death in 8 of 60 patients given placebo, against 1 of 56 patients given nimodipine. This result has also been found in poor-grade aneurysm patients (Petruk et al. 1988). In other studies nimodipine treatment was associated with a significant reduction of cerebral infarcts visualised by CT scans in patients who received intermediate or late surgery (Öhman et al. 1991a); a low incidence of delayed neurological dysfunction (Gilsbach et al. 1990),; and a low incidence of death caused by delayed cerebral ischaemia (Öhman and Heiskanen 1988, Öhman et al. 1991b).

In the British Aneurysm Nimodipine Trial 554 patients were studied in a blind, placebo controlled, randomised trial. The findings indicate that nimodipine treatment was associated with a 34% reduction in the incidence of infarction, and a 40% decrease in the incidence of poor outcome (Pickard et al. 1989). Furthermore, analysis of the amount of basal SAH on CT scans in patients with deficits from spasm showed that an increase in subarachnoid blood was not associated with worsening of neurological outcome among patients in treatment with nimodipine. Other controlled studies confirm these findings (Mee et al. 1988). In a metaanalysis including seven trials, and a total of 1202 patients nimodipine improved outcome. The odds of good, and good plus fair outcomes were improved by ratios of 1.86:1 and 1.67:1 respectively for nimodipine versus control, and the odds for deficits and/or mortality attributed to vasospasms and CT-assessed infarction rate were reduced by ratios of 0.46:1 to 0.58:1 in the nimodipine group (Barker and Ogilvy 1996).

In a retrospective study, however, it has been questioned if calcium antagonists really are useful, whether nimodipine or nicardipine were used (Mercier et al. 1994).

Intrathecal administration

In patients with SAH, intrathecal administration of nimodipine (0.2 mg in 1 ml) via a cisternal catheter caused angiographic vasodilation in 9 of 12 patients (Auer 1985). On the other hand, intra-carotid nimodipine administration did not change cerebral vessel calibre as evaluated angiographically (Grotenhuis et al. 1984).

Oxygen tension

During nimodipine treatment PaO_2 decreases and pulmonary shunt fraction increases. These changes are supposed to be caused by a disproportional decrease in vascular resistance in hypoventilated regions of the lung, and is reversed by increased PEEP (Germann et al. 1987).

Nicardipine

Experimental studies

Nicardipine has been studied experimentally. In rabbits subjected to SAH, basilar artery constricted by serotonin is not relaxed by nicardipine; however, nicardipine does enhance the vasodilatory response to acetylcholine and ATP (Pasqualin et al. 1992).

Clinical studies

In a clinical dose-dependent study a dose of 10 mg/h was used. Symptomatic vasospasm was diagnosed in only 6%, and no death due to vasospasm occurred (Flamm et al. 1988). In another randomised trial the results of high-dose and low-dose nicardipine treatment was virtually equivalent, but administration of low-dose nicardipine was attended by fewer side effects (Haley et al. 1994). The same authors found that high-dose nicardipine was associated with a reduced incidence of symptomatic vasospasm in patients with recent SAH, but not with an improvement in overall outcome at 3 months when compared with standard management (Haley et al. 1993a). High-dose intravenous nicardipine, on the other hand, reduced the incidence and severity of delayed arterial narrowing (Haley et al. 1993b).

Other Ca^{2+} antagonists

Mexiletine is a sodium channel blocker, which also activates ATP-sensitive K^+ channels, and blocks Ca^{2+} channels. Caner et al. (2000) investigated the effects of mexiletine in rabbits and found, that mexiletine induces potent relaxation in cerebral arteries contracted with various agents, and that it prevents and partially reverses SAH-induced vasoconstriction.

In a co-operative Japanese study another calcium antagonist AT877 reduced angiographically demonstrated vasospasm by 38%, and reduced the number of patients with poor outcome associated with vasospasm (Shibuya et al. 1992).

Eicosanoids, experimental studies

Although both prostaglandin E_2 and F_2 contract isolated cerebral arteries, and reduce CBF in the baboon when given by intra-carotid infusion (Pickard et al. 1977), other studies indicate that PGE_1 (Pelofsky et al. 1972) and PGE_2 (Boullin et al. 1979, Chapleau and White 1979, Jarman et al. 1979, Paul et al. 1982, Quintana et al. 1982, von Holst et al. 1982) may function as a cerebral vasodilator, and might be of use in the prevention of cerebral vasospasm.

In delayed cerebral vasospasm the formation of prostacyclin in the canine cerebral arteries was reduced (Maeda et al. 1981, Sasaki et al. 1981, Walker et al. 1983). An imbalance in the formation of constrictor and dilator eicosanoids has been observed in a primate model of vasospasm. This is more likely to arise from a relative lack of the vasodilator component prostacyclin, than from a surplus of the constrictor component thromboxane. In the same study prevention of angiographic vasospasm by early clot removal is associated with an enhanced synthesis of prostacyclin by non-spastic vessels (Nosko et al. 1988).

Eicosanoids, clinical studies

Human pial arteries contracted by PGF_2 , noradrenaline of 5-hydroxytryptamine consistently relax in response to prostacyclin. Prostacyclin, however, is less potent on human pial vessels (Uski et al. 1983). Prostaglandin E_1 has been used for controlled hypotension in aneurysm surgery. rCBF did not change during prostaglandin E1-induced hypotension (Abe et al. 1991).

In patients with SAH the levels of prostaglandin E_2, thromboxane B, and 6-oxy-2-prostaglandin F_1 in CSF were increased. The concentration of these Eucosanoids, however, did not correlate to the amount of subarachnoid clot seen at CT scanning, the presence of vasospasm on angiography nor the clinical outcome (O'Neill et al. 1992).

Aspirin and platelet function

In animal experiments aspirin has been shown to be effective in the secondary prevention of cerebrovascular ischaemic events. Administration of aspirin inhibits experimental vasospasm induced by oxyhaemoglobin when the aspirin infusion is started 1 hour before the intracisternal injection of oxyhaemoglobin.

Some prospective aspirin trials have not been able to confirm whether aspirin increases the risk of vasospasm or reduces the risk of delayed ischaemia after SAH (Antiplatelet trial 1994). In one retrospective study of 291 patients a reduced risk of ischaemic complications with aspirin treatment was found (Juvela 1995).

Leukotrienes

Experimental studies

Cerebral arteries have been shown to produce leukotrienes (Moskowitz et al. 1984). Leukotrien LTD_4 constricts cerebral arteries *in vivo* and *in vitro* (Tagari et al. 1983, Rosenblum 1985). Leukotrienes are produced by leukocytes, mast cells and macrophages, which infiltrate the wall of cerebral vessels after SAH (Hughes and Shiahchi 1978, Faleiro et al. 1981, Liszczak et al. 1983). Leukotrienes also are involved in the generation of cerebral vasospasm. Leukotrien C_4 and D_4 constrict pial arterioles after local application (Mayhan et al. 1986, Rosenblum 1985). In mongrel dogs subjected to "two haemorrhage" ONO-1078, a potent leukotriene antagonist, decreases CSF levels of leukotriene C4 and prevents angiographic vasospasm (Kobayashi et al. 1992).

Clinical studies

Clinical studies indicate that the level of immunoreactive cysteinyl-leukotrienens in CSF after SAH correlates with blood flow velocity (Winkling et al. 1997).

Lipooxygenase

Experimental studies

Blockade of the lipooxygenase products of arachidonic acid has been studied in experimental delayed vasospasm in the canine. With intravenous administration of the selective inhibitor of 5-lipoxygenase, angiographic evidence of vasospasm was not reversed, and CBF was not increased. However, with oral administration vasospasm was reduced, and the contractile property of excised basilar arteries, in response to vasoconstrictor agents was inhibited (Yokota et al. 1987).

Indomethacin, a cyclooxygenase inhibitor, fails to reverse angiographic delayed vasospasm in a canine model (Fukumori et al. 1983).

Clinical studies

Ebselen is a lipid soluble seleno-organic compound that potently inhibits lipid peroxidation through a glutathione peroxidase-like action. Because it is active against membrane hydroperoxides, such as phospholipid hydroperoxide glutathione peroxidase, this agent effectively inhibits both nonenzymatic and enzymatic lipid peroxidation including the lipoxygenase pathway of the arachidonate cascade. In a recent clinical study ebselen reduced brain damage and extend of low-density areas in patients with delayed neurological deficits after SAH (Saito et al. 1998).

Plasmin and plasminogen activating factor and vasospasm

Experimental studies

In experimental SAH in the pig, intracisternal plasmin resulted in a markedly less initial proliferation and medial necrosis of the vessels (Alksne et al. 1986). Experimental studies have demonstrated that intrathecal administration of tissue-type plasminogen activator (tPA) is effective in removing the remaining hematoma and preventing vasospasm. (Findley et al. 1988, Seifert et al. 1989).

Clinical studies

Also clinical studies have demonstrated that intrathecal administration of tissue-type plasminogen activator (tPA) is effective in removing the remaining hematoma and preventing vasospasm (Konishi et al. 1990, Mizoi et al. 1991, Öhman et al. 1991c, Zabramski et al. 1991). Nevertheless, failure in tPA in the prevention of vasospasm has been described (Steinberg et al. 1994). In comparison with urokinase only tPA is effective in prevention of vasospasm (Usui et al. 1994). In one study injection of 2 mg tPA daily for 5 days (a total of 10 mg) is effective in preventing the development of vasospasm (Mizoi et al. 1993). In another study even repeated doses of 0.1 mg were useful for preventing vasospasm (Sasaki et al. 1994). In a randomised trial of 100 patients with SAH recombinant tPA was administrated into the opened basal subarachnoid cistern immediately following aneurysm clipping. The overall incidence of angiographic vasospasm measured between the 7th and 11th day following SAH was similar for the two groups. However, there was a trend towards lesser degree of vasospasm in the tPA-treated patients. Thus, the efficacy of tPA in preventing clinical vasospasm and its clinical consequence require examination in larger randomised trials (Findlay et al. 1995).

In a review Seifert (1994) concluded that the risks inherent with this aggressive form of pharmacological blood removal seem to be acceptable in the light of the devastating effects of the so far untreatable development of cerebral vasospasm.

Nitric oxide (NO)

Experimental studies

Vasodilation is normally maintained by NO and/or other dilators. The NO binds to hem moity of the enzyme guanyl cyclase, which catalyzes the conversion of guanosine triphosphate to cyclic guanosine-5'.phosphate in smooth-muscle cells and thereby decreases intracellular free calcium levels, causing vascular smooth-muscle cells to relax. The hem moity of guanyl cyclase is ferrous. Because NO preferentially reacts with Fe^{++}, the ferrous component of oxyhaemoglobin competitively binds NO in SAH, limiting the availability of NO for vasodilation. In a primate model of SAH prevention of cerebral vasospasm was demonstrated by treatment with a chelator of Fe^{++} (2,2′-dipyridyl) (Horky et al. 1998).

Inhibition of K^+ channel function also contributes to the pathophysiology of cerebral vasospasm. It has been suggested that NO liberated from nitrovasodilators can produce relaxation by activating K^+ channels in cerebral arteries. In cerebral arteries exposed to SAH, smooth muscle cells are depolarised because of decreased membrane conductance to K^+. Zuccarello et al. (1996b) demonstrated that smooth muscle cells from spastic basilar arteries are depolarised and that this depolarisation can be overcome by a K^+ channel activator cromakalim. The same authors reported that vascular narrowing after experimental SAH can be reversed by topical application of cromakalin. Other studies in experimental SAH in the rabbit support this concept, indicating that cromakalin attenuates the development of vasospasm in a dose-dependent manner with effect achieving significance at doses of 0,1 and 0,3 mg/kg (Kwan et al. 1998).

NO has a modest influence of CBF under basal conditions and inhibits constriction of large cerebral arteries to serotonin, but not to hypocapnia (Faraci and Heistad 1992). Furthermore, studies in rats suggest that inhibition of NO synthesis affects the relation between cerebral artery diameter and CBF, and can lead to subtle cerebral vascular pathological changes consistent with focal brain ischaemia (Prado et al. 1992). In the canine basilar artery subjected to chronic vasospasm after SAH this relaxing factor is abolished (Kim et al. 1988). Another study in rabbits suggests that impairment of NO-derived vasodilation following SAH may be involved in the pathogenesis of cerebral vasospasm (Nakagomi et al. 1987). Intra-carotid infusion of a NO-donating compound reverses angiographic confirmed vasospasm, increases CBF, and decreases flow velocity. However, only NO-donation compounds with a short half-life avoided a concomitant decrease in blood pressure (Pluta et al. 1997). In monkeys subjected to vasospasm by placement of blood clots around the middle cerebral artery, intra-carotid infusion of NO increased CBF, decreased cerebral vascular resistance, reversed arteriographic vasospasm, and decreased CBF velocities in the vasospastic artery. The effects of NO on CBF and velocity, however, disappeared shortly after terminating NO infusion (Afshar et al. 1995). In a rabbit SAH-model tape containing nitroglycerin was applied onto the skin. An improvement of cerebral vasospasm after SAH without any significant changes in the systemic circulation was found (Ito et al. 2000). In monkeys brief intra-carotid and continuous intravenous infusion of L-arginine, the substance of the NO-producing enzyme nitric oxide synthase, did not influence the incidence or degree of cerebral vasospasm. After SAH, intra-carotid infusion of L-arginine markedly increased rCBF in this primate model of SAH. Thus, discordance between degree of vasospasm and rCBF was found (Pluta et al. 2000).

In a canine study it was found that the release of NO is not impaired during chronic vasospasm. Thus, the loss of relaxation could be due to a decreased transfer of endothelial-derived relaxing factor or a reduced responsiveness of the smooth muscle (Kim et al. 1989). In another study it was found that segments of cerebral arteries from rabbits subjected to SAH contract to uridine triphosphate, serotonin, and noradrenalin, and this reaction is not related to impaired NO relaxation (Debdi et al. 1992).

In intact dogs, intracisternal injections of L-arginine produce a dose-dependent increase in basilar artery diameter; conversely L-NMMA reduced the diameter. Intracisternal injection of superoxide dismutase (SOD), which caused no effect on vascular diameter per se, enhances the duration of the vasodilatory effect of L-arginine, suggesting that inactivation of NO by superoxide anion contributes to the development of vasospasm (Kajita et al. 1994).

Clinical studies

The experimental findings are in accordance with studies of human basilar arteries indicating that the endothelium-dependent relaxation responses to thrombin, bradykinin and calcium ionophore were less for vessels subjected to SAH than for control (Hatake et al. 1992). In another study NO metabolites were analysed after cisternal drainage in patients with SAH. The concentrations of nitrite and nitrate were significantly elevated in the CSF, and the concentrations correlated with the amount of bleeding as evaluated by Fishers graduation. Steroids, which are known to prevent the formation of inducible NO synthase mediated by inflammatory cytokines, did not influence the concentration of NO metabolites (Suzuki et al. 1997).

Sodium nitroprusside

Intrathecal administration of sodium nitroprusside, a NO donor, has recently been introduced in the treatment of vasospasm after SAH (Thomas et al. 1999a). Angiography demonstrated reversal or amelioration of vasoconstriction in 83% of established vasospasm treated by intrathecal sodium nitroprusside alone. Among patients treated prophylactically, none developed clinical vasospasm (Thomas et al. 1999b)

Neuropeptides

Patients with cognitive impairments after aneurysmal SAH exhibited higher cerebrospinal fluid concentrations of -endorphins, corticotropin-releasing factor, and delta sleep-inducing peptide than did those patients with normal cognitive capacity (Uski et al. 2000).

Vasoactive intestinal polypeptide (VIP)

Experimental studies

Vasoactive intestinal polypeptide (VIP) induces a dose-dependent relaxation of the cerebral arteries in animals (Lee et al. 1975, Larsson et al. 1976, Tods 1982). VIP acts directly on vascular smooth muscle, rather than indirectly through endothelial cells (Duckles and Said 1982), Edvinsson and Ekman 1984). In cat cerebral arteries VIP may be released from nerve terminals to induce vasodilation by transmural stimulation (Lee et al. 1984, Bryden and Bevan 1986). The dilatory effect of VIP is exerted via an increase in the cAMP level in the smooth muscle (Huang and Rorstad 1984, Iton et al. 1985, Ganz et al. 1986). Uemura et al. (1987) found that VIP immunoreactivity in the cerebral arteries was decreased after experimental SAH. In vitro studies of rabbit cerebral artery indicate that in normal arteries the content was increased by VIP, whereas the increase in cAMP was less in arteries evaluated 2 days after SAH (Tsukahara et al. 1989).

Clinical studies

Vasoactive intestinal polypeptide (VIP) induces a dose-dependent relaxation of the cerebral arteries in human (Edvinsson and Ekman 1984).

Neuropeptide Y

Experimental studies

In a primate model a relationship between neuropeptide Y levels in the CSF or peripheral plasma and delayed cerebral vasospasm was not confirmed (Pluta et al. 1992).

Clinical studies

Neuropeptide Y-like immunoreactivity levels are increased in patients with SAH, and in some patients correlated to Doppler sonographic changes (Edvinsson et al. 1990). Calcitonin gene-related peptide levels were also increased in connection with vasospasm (Edvinsson et al. 1990).

Heat shock protein

Experimental studies

Induction heat shock protein, HSP70, in the brain is an indicator of cellular injury. Focal and global ischaemia, heat shock, status epilepticus, and neural toxins induce HSP70 in neurones outside the region of infarction. Following focal ischaemia HSP70-induction is a more sensitive indicator of cellular injury than histological staining. HSAP70 induction in neurones and glia cells have been demonstrated following injection of lysed blood in the cisterna magna in rats (Matz et al. 1996a). Using the endovascular model of SAH in rats, HSAP70 was induced in the basal forebrain, thalamus, neocortex, striatum and hippocampus. Immunostaining with HSP70 occurred primarily in neurones, but was also observed in glia and the endothelium (Matz et al. 1996b).

Antithrombin III

Experimental studies

In rabbits subjected to SAH antithrombin III, injected intracisternally, reverses delayed narrowing of the basilar artery (Vollmer et al. 1989b). In dogs White and Robertson (1985) found that antithrombin III relaxed isolated canine basilar arteries that were precontracted with plasmin, thrombin and uridine triphosphate.

Clinical studies

Studies of isolated human basilar arteries indicate that antithrombin III is a potent and non-specific vasodilator (White 1987). Other studies suggest that antithrombin III, if present in the CSF during SAH, protects patients from vasospasm (White and Robertson 1987).

The plasma thrombin-antithrombin III complex and the plasma-$_2$-plasmin inhibitor complex were investigated in patients with SAH. It was found that both factors may reflect the severity of brain damage induced by SAH, but there was no significant difference in the levels between patients who experienced arterial vasospasm and those who did not (Itoyama et al. 1994).

Platelet-activating factor (PAF) and antagonist

Experimental studies

The role of inflammatory processes in causing cerebral vasospasm following SAH has been studied (Kasell et al. 1985, Peterson et al. 1990). Intrathecal administration of PAF alone or together with autologous blood produced basilar artery constriction and neurological deterioration in rabbits (Hirashima et al. 1993). In addition, the intrathecal administration of anti-PAF immunoglobulin and PAF antagonists prevented vasoconstriction of the main trunk arteries and/or neurological deterioration in the rabbit model of SAH (Hirashima et al. 1994b, Hirashima et al. 1996).

Clinical studies

The involvement of platelet activating factor, a potent mediator of inflammation has been studied. In patients with SAH the concentration of PAF in the CSF (Hirashima et al. 1994a) and plasma (Hirashima et al. 1994b) peaked 7 days after SAH. In the same studies the concentration of CSF-PAF was higher in those patients with cerebral infarction after vasospasm.

Heparin

Clinical studies

Rapp et al. (1982) in a study of patients with SAH where the carotid artery was ligated compared the effect of heparin with the result of carotid ligation without heparin from another clinical trial (Perret and Nibbelink 1981). The incidence of ischaemic complications in patients receiving heparin was 6%, compared with 23% in the control study. The mortality was reduced from 16 to 10%. In a later study including 104 patients treated prophylactically with heparin during gradual carotid ligation neurological deficit was 19% compared with 39% in the control group (Kapp et al. 1987). Chimowitz and Pessin (1987), in a review, concluded that data concerning a role for heparin in the management of vasospasm are promising, but further controlled studies are needed prior to clinical application.

Papaverine

Experimental studies

Papaverine, a potent vasodilator, has been used for treatment of experimental vasospasm by intravenous or intrathecal administration (Kapp et al. 1970, Kuwayama et al. 1972, Nagai et al. 1975, Ogata et al. 1975). However, these preliminary studies have not shown significant therapeutic effect. Dogs subjected to SAH were studied angiographically at 4, 7, 10 and 14 days after intercisternal blood injection. The papaverine insensitive component of vasospasm increased with increasing time after SAH, and with increasing severity of vasospasm (MacDonald et al. 1995). In dogs subjected to subarachnoid haemorrhage, a prolonged-release preparation of papaverine that could be implanted intracranially prevented vasospasm (Shiokawa et al. 1998).

Clinical studies

Papaverine has been used for treatment of vasospasm by intravenous or intrathecal administration (Kapp et al. 1970, Kuwayama et al. 1972, Nagai et al. 1975, Ogata et al. 1975, Segawa et al. 1988, Tsukahara et al. 1990). However, these preliminary studies have not shown significant therapeutic effect.

In a recent study 8 of 12 patients had marked angiographic reversal of arterial narrowing following intra-arterial papaverine infusion, four of whom showed reversal of neurological deficits (Kassell et al. 1992). In patients with vasospasm intra-arterial papaverine increases the arterial diameter significantly (Milbrun et al. 1998). Selective intra-arterial papaverine infusion in connection with transluminal angioplasty successfully dilated 34 of 37 vascular territories in 10 patients, and in eight patients improvement in neurological function was found (Kaku et al. 1992). Sawada et al. (1997) found that a 0.4% intra-arterially infused solution at the top of the internal carotid artery was a safe and adequate concentration for treating cerebral vasospasm. Other authors using intra-arterially papaverine, however, conclude that papaverine as it is currently used does not provide added benefits, compared with medical treatment of vasospasm alone (Polin et al. 1998).

Significant elevations of ICP, blood pressure and pulse rate have been demonstrated during papaverine infusion. Failure to perform adequate monitoring during papaverine infusion might potentially produce an uncontrolled ICP-increase (McAuliffe et al. 1995). Case report of severe thrombopenia after papaverine administration to patients with SAH has been published (Miller et al. 1995).

Methylprednisolone

Experimental studies

In a rat model adventitial hyperpermeability of the basilar artery was successfully prevented by intrathecal steroid (Ogane et al. 1982). A massive dose of methylprednisolone markedly reduces experimental posthemorrhagic chronic vasospasm in dogs, and also reduces the histological vasculopathy associated with vasospasm (Chyatte et al. 1983). In a canine model intrathecal steroid prevented arterial contraction elicited by vasoactive substances (Sohma et al. 1991).

Clinical studies

In a clinical study of 21 patients judged to be at high risk of vasospasm because of either poor admitting grade or large amount of subarachnoid blood, methylprednisolone reduced the incidence of delayed cerebral ischaemia (Chyatte et al. 1987). In a retrospective study the incidence of postoperative vasospasm was significantly low compared with a historic control group (Suzuki et al. 1994).

α_2 adrenoreceptor agonist

Tizanidine is a selective $_2$ adrenoreceptor agonist which inbibits aspartic acid and glutamic acid release. Tizanidine is an effective agent in the prevention of focal cerebral ischaemia in rats (Berkman et al. 1998). Berkman et al. (2000) analysed the effects of tizanidine using a femoral artery vasospasm model described by Okada et al. (1990). The study showed that tizanidine administration before the vasospasm reduced ultrastructural and morphometric vasospastic insult significantly.

Endothelin blockade

Experimental studies

Endothelin is produced by endothelial cells, and has been shown to produce vasoconstriction of cerebral arteries both *in vivo* and *in vitro* (Ide et al. 1989, Mima et al. 1989, Asano et al. 1989, Saito et al. 1989, Sokolovsky 1992, Cosentino and Katusic 1994). In a study of perfused rabbit arteries the effect of endothelin on the basilar arteries was greater than on the femoral or mesenteric arteries. The effect of intraluminal endothelin was enhanced by extraluminal oxyhaemoglobin and L-NAME, but not by extraluminal indomethacin (Kazuki et al. 1997). Domindo et al. (2000) performed diffusion weighted MRI spectroscopy in rats following application of endothelin-1 to the middle cerebral artery. In endothelin-1 treated animals a 10% loss of phosphocreatine and ATP was observed, and the area of the hemisphere with a low apparent diffusion coefficient was 27% after 30 min.

Endothelin acts on at least two receptor subtypes (ET_A and ET_B). Oxyhaemoglobine increases the release of endothelin-1 from endothelial and smooth cells (Kasuya et al. 1993). In dogs an increase of immunoreactive endothelin-1 has been demonstrated. Application of monoclonal antibody against endothelin-1 reverses cerebral spasm in the early phase after SAH, but the maintenance of cerebral vasospasm at later stages was independent on endothelin-1 (Yamaura et al. 1992).

Cisternal injection of endothelin causes severe vasoconstriction of the canine basilar artery (Kobayashi et al. 1991). This constriction is prevented by pre-treatment with the calcium blocker nicardipine (Kobayshashi et al. 1990), and by endothelin receptor antagonist in the rabbit (Foley et al. 1994, Wanebo et al. 1998, Zuccarello et al. 1998). Other studies indicate that drugs that antagonise the action of endothelin reverse experimental vasospasm (Itoh et al. 1994, Zuccarelli et al. 1994a, Hino et al. 1995). In a rat SAH-model administration of endothelin-1 receptor antagonist BQ-123 in the late phase (48 hrs. after SAH) caused dilatation of the basilar artery (Josko et al. 2000). In rabbits attenuation of vasospasm is also prevented by CGS 26303, an endothelin-converting enzyme inhibitor (Kwan et al. 1997, Kwan et al. 1998). Studies in a two haemorrhage canine model indicate that endothelin-1 initiates the development of vasospasm through protein kinase C activation, but does not contribute to prolonged vasospasm (Nishizawa et al. 2000).

Bosentan is a competitive and elective antagonist of endothelin-1 on endothelin_A and endothelin_B receptors. In the double-haemorrhage model in rabbits oral bosantan administrated after the initial SAH decreased the magnitude of angiographic arterial constriction by 9% of control (Zuccarello et al. 1996). Bosentan has shown efficacy in *in vitro* experiments (Clozel et al. 1994, Roux et al. 1990). In the two-haemorrhage dog model bosentan effectively relaxed cerebral arteries (Shigeno et al. 1995, Zimmermann et al. 1996).

In a study of monkeys subjected to SAH the levels of mRNA for the two endothelin precursors (pre-pro ET_1 and prepro ET_3) were determined. Specific agonist binding to endothelin_A and endothelin_B in cerebral arteries was also measured. The study did not support the hypothesis that overexpression of endothelin_1 is the principle cause of vasospasm, but rather suggests that SAH causes complex changes in the endothelin system that are responsible for the cellular response to SAH (Hino et al. 1996). This opinion is in concert with Pluta et al. (1997). They demonstrated that endothelin-1 is released from astrocytes, but not endothelial cells, during hypoxia and is released from the brain after transient ischaemia. They did not find correlation between CSF-endothelin_1 and vasospasm *in vivo*, or between CSF-endothelin_1 and oxyhaemoglobin *in vitro*. Thus, they emphasize that the increase in CSF-endothelin_1 after SAH appears to be the result of cerebral ischaemia, rather than reflecting the cause of cerebral vasospasm. In contrast, Ohkuma et al. (1999) found that antisera preproendothelin-oligoDNA therapy combined with clot lysis by recombinant tissue plasminogen activator reduced vasospasm in a canine model of SAH, and this effect appeared to be related to reduced endothelin-1 synthesis. Furthermore, Fassbender et al. (2000) found that activated mononuclear leukocytes in the CSF of SAH patients synthesise and release endothelin-1, and subsequent haemolysis of blood is sufficient to induce endothelin-1 production.

Clinical studies

The CSF-endothelin concentration is increased in patients with SAH, and during symptomatic vasospasms the endothelin level in CSF increases even more (Shirakami et al. 1994). The time course of the occurrence of vasospasms and that of the increase in cerebrospinal fluid endothelin-1 like immunoactivity coincides precisely (Suzuki et al. 1992). Even plasma endothelin concentrations seem to correlate with delayed cerebral ischaemia and vasospasm after SAH. The highest levels of endothelin are predictive of the symptoms of cerebral ischaemia and vasospasms, and endothelin may also worsen ischaemia with a history of hypertension (Juvela 2000). In another study, however, it was found that increased endothelin-1 in CSF was found when cerebral vasospasms were already clinically evident suggesting that endothelin-1 expression is associated with severe vasospasms responsible for clinical evident ischaemia but does not play a role in the pathogenesis of vasospasm (Mascia et al. 2000). Fassbender et al. (2000) found that endothelin-1 is produced by activated CSF mononuclear leukocytes. This finding suggests that subarachnoid inflammation may represent a therapeutic target to prevent vasospasm.

An inverse relationship between atrial natriuretic peptide and endothelin has been suggested. In a recent clinical study, however, plasma atrial natriuretic peptide and brain natriuretic peptide were differentially regulated in the presence of SAH, but not by the level of plasma endothelin (Wijdicks et al. 1997).

In a review Zimmermann and Seifert (1998) conclude that the results of current clinical and experimental investigations support the hypothesis that endothelin-1 is a major cause of cerebral vasospasms after SAH. Other studies indicate that SAH causes complex changes in the endothelin system and increased ET_1 levels after SAH, which are mot solely responsible for the development of vasospasm but may occur after cerebral ischaemia. In a recent phase II trial an endothelin (A/B) receptor antagonist (TAK-044) was examined. Three months after SAH there were no significant differences in clinical outcome in the placebo-treated and TAK-044-treated groups. A lower incidence of delayed ischaemic events in the TAK-044-treated group was found (Shaw et al. 2000).

Monitoring

Grading system

Hunt and Hess (1968) analysed surgical risks as related to time of intervention in the repair of intracranial aneurysm. Since then this grading system has been world-wide accepted. The clinical grading system is as follows:

Grade	Clinical condition
0	Unruptured
I	Asymptomatic or minimal headache, nuchal rigidity
II	Moderate to severe headache, nuchal rigidity, no neurological deficit other than cranial nerve palsy
III	Drowsiness, confusion, mild focal deficit
IV	Stupor, moderate to severe hemiparesis, possible early decerebrate rigidity and vegetative disturbances
V	Deep coma, decerebrate rigidity, moribund appearance
+ 1 grade	For vasospasm or systemic disease

The World Federation of Neurological Surgeons (WFNS) Committee has modified the original Glasgow Coma Scale (Drake 1988)

WFNS Grade	GCS Score	Motor deficit
I	15	absent
II	14–13	absent
III	14–13	present
IV	12–7	present or absent
V	6–3	present or absent

A grading system based upon CT findings was constructed by Fisher et al. (1980). The graduation is based upon density of subarachnoid haemorrhage as revealed during CT examination. In a recent study it was found that the severity of SAH evaluated by Fishers graduation correlates with cognitive deficits (Hütter et al. 1998).

Score	Description
0	Unruptured
0	No blood detected
1	Diffuse or vertical layers < 1 mm thick
2	Localised clot and/or vertical layers ≥ 1 mm
3	Intracerebral or intraventricular clot with diffuse or no subarachnoid haemorrhage

For evaluation of outcome Glasgow Outcome Scale (GOS) has been used for most current studies. A modification of GOS was defined by Ogilvy and Carter (1998) as follows:

Points	Definition	
4	excellent	= no neurological deficit; patient able to return to previous level or lifestyle
4	Good	= mild deficit; patient able to return to premorbid work or lifestyle
3	Fair	= neurological deficit; patient unable to return to previous work or lifestyle but able to live at home with minimal or no assistance
2	Poor	= significant deficit; patient requiring full-time nursing care in an institution or at home
1	Death	

Common for the two grading scales and for the outcome scale is the dichotomised nature of the scales, making classification difficult. Furthermore, the U-shaped nature of the scales when used for population studies is a drawback in studies of comparison.

CT scanning

Preoperative CT scan findings are of prognostic value, and may even be superior to clinical grading by Hunt and Hess in predicting outcome. Thus, among patients with SAH as the only neuroradiological finding, the rate of good outcome was 93% when the preoperative neurological grade according to Hunt and Hess was 1 or 2; but even with grade 3 and 4, good outcome was accounted for in 84% of the patients. By contrast, in patients with additional intracerebral and/or intraventricular haemorrhage, the good outcome rate was only 44% (Auer et al. 1986).

In other studies CT findings proved to be a simple, yet accurate, prognostic indicator of ischaemic neurological dysfunction (Gurusingle and Richardson 1984). The extend and location of blood in the subarachnoid space determine the severity and location of vasospasm (Kistler et al. 1983). In one study low density areas were always detected when vasospasm occurred in the ascending branches of the middle cerebral artery (Saito et al. 1979).

Comparison of transcranial Doppler with digital subtraction angiography has been studied in patients with vasospasm. Mean flow velocity is inadequate for estimation of the severity of vasospasm in vessels more peripheral than the M1 segment. Furthermore, severe vasospasms extending to more peripheral regions can produce more serious ischaemic insults, compared with vasospasms localised to basal vessels. In patients with negative transcranial Doppler results and clinical features suggesting the development of vasospasm quantitative studies of cerebral circulation transit time, using intra-arterial digital subtraction angiography are of value (Okada et al. 1999).

The ventriculocranial ratio (VCR), defined as the ratio of the width of the ventricles behind the frontal horns between the caudate nucleus, where the walls are almost parallel, to the width of the brain at the same level, has been used as an outcome index in SAH. No patients with a VCR of more than 0.25, as calculated from the initial CT scan, survived (Mohr et al. 1983). On the other hand, an increase in ventricular size owing to hydrocephalus is accompanied by clinical deterioration and by a reduced CBF (Menon et al. 1981).

Transcranial Doppler (TCD)

Experimental studies

In studies in rabbit SAH, the time course of changes in flow velocity following SAH has been demonstrated. Differences in the flow velocity and the CBF responses to hypercapnia, hypocapnia and trimethaphan-induced hypotension were found, indicating that TCD cannot be considered a simple alternative to CBF measurement for studies of cerebrovascular reactivity and cerebral autoregulation (Nelson et al. 1990). Also experimental studies in normally autoregulating rabbits indicate that pulsative index cannot be interpreted simply as an index of cerebrovascular resistance (CVR). Thus, during hypercapnic challenge a positive correlation was found between pulsative index and cortical resistance.

Clinical studies

In studies where cerebral perfusion pressure was reduced a negative correlation between pulsative index and CVR was disclosed (Czosnyka et al. 1996).

Vasospasm, clinical studies

Blood velocity studies have been used in diagnosis of vasospasms. When angiographic spasms were present in the middle cerebral artery, the blood velocity was higher in this territory in contrast to low blood velocity found in the distal internal carotid artery (Lindegaard et al. 1989). Serial TCD studies in the early period after SAH are of value in identifying patients who can be selected for prophylactic therapy for delayed ischaemic deficits (Grosset et al. 1993).

Jacobsen et al. (1990c) defined a spasm index as the ratio between flow velocity in the middle cerebral artery and the rCBF. This index seems stable in spite of day-to-day fluctuations in CBF, and seems to enable estimation of the progress in the development of vasospasm, even in cases with great day to day fluctuation in CBF.

In SAH patients with disturbed cerebral autoregulation induced hypertension by phenylephrine might alter flow velocity. Thus, the level of cerebral autoregulation needs to be considered when interpreting studies where transcranial velocity are implicated (Manno et al. 1998).

Recently transcranial color-coded sonography was compared with TCD in patients with SAH. The sensitivity and specificity of color-coded sonography were higher than for TCD for both the middle cerebral artery and the internal corotid artery (Proust et al. 1999).

ICP, clinical studies

In patients with SAH the correlation between ICP and mean flow velocity and the index of cerebral circulatory resistance were studied. In patients with a resistance index of less than 0.5, changes in the mean flow velocity reflect the actual severity and time course of vasospasm. During the time course of vasospasm, an increase in the resistance index above values of 0.6, with a simultaneously decreased mean flow velocity indicates a rise in ICP rather than a reduction in vasospasm (Klingelhöfer et al. 1991).

Critics

As blood velocity is related to flow, but inversely related to the area of the vessel, the use of transcranial Doppler has been criticised in studies of vasospasm. Thus, Laumer et al. (1993) found that in patients admitted within 48 hours after SAH or with a poor grade SAH, transcranial Doppler sonography seems to be of dubious value. Even in patients admitted later than 72 hours, the indication for TCD depends on the management. If surgery is performed in cases of asymptomatic vasospasm, the clinical value of TCD also is questionable.

In a retrospective study of 50 patients Xe-CT flow was correlated to TCD sonography. The result suggests that increased blood velocity revealed by TCD correlates with increased rCBF, and not with ischaemia. No difference in rCBF was found in territories with and without rapid increase in blood velocity in the middle cerebral artery. Furthermore, although focal neurological deficits corresponded with decreased contralateral rCBF in the middle cerebral artery, increased velocity did not correlate with neurological findings. Therefore, therapeutic decisions based only on blood flow velocity might be inappropriate and potential harmful (Clyde et al. 1996).

In another study correlations between flow velocity, CBF, and delayed ischaemia were analysed. Vasospasm and hypoperfusion were present in patients with delayed ischaemia and lateralizing neurological deficits; discordant results seem to reflect inherent limitations by to two methods (Davis et al. 1992).

In contrast to these negative attitudes Wardlaw et al. (1998) concluded that TCD service provided by neuroradiographers is accurate and useful in diagnosing and managing elevated blood velocities and ischaemic neurological deficit following SAH. They postulate that if the information gleaned from TCD findings was used more often in patient management outcome might be improved.

Jugular venous saturation

In a recent study jugular venous saturation was performed in 26 patients with SAH. The incidence of normal (56–74%) and pathological saturation values was evaluated. On serial measurements 37 og 354 (10%) samples indicated desaturation episodes. ICP was significantly higher during desaturation episodes, and during desaturation episodes lower values of $PaCO_2$ and CPP were more frequently observed (Citerio et al. 1998).

Microdialysis

Intracerebral microdialysis has been used for routine monitoring of patients with SAH. In a study including 10 patients microdialysis was performed for periods ranging from 6 to 11 days after the bleeding.

Concentration of energy-related substances including lactate, pyruvate, glucose and hypoxanthine was measured, and supplemented with the excitatory amino acids, glutamate and aspartate. Microdialysis was found to be a promising tool for chemical monitoring of the brain and generated a working hypothesis, that the pattern of lactate, lactate/pyruvate ratio, hypoxanthine, and glutamate changes can be used to detect disturbances in brain metabolism. Furthermore, a correlation between glutamate and outcome supports the importance of overactivation of excitatory amino acids (Persson et al. 1996). Simultaneous samplings from two vascular territories (middle and anterior cerebral arteries) indicate that a rise in glutamate and aspartate in one territory is not necessarily parallel with a rise in the other (Säveland et al. 1996). By combining PET with microdialysis (lactate, lactate/pyruvate ratio, hypoxanthine, glutamate and aspartate) it has been demonstrated that the presence of whole-brain ischaemia and/or regional ischaemia within the region of the microdialysis probe was associated with increased levels of energy-related metabolites and excitatory amino acids (Enblad et al. 1996). In a recent study two patterns related to clinical outcome were found. Patients with good outcome were characterised by decreasing glucose levels parallel to an increase of both lactate and pyruvate, suggesting hyperglycolysis. In severely disabled patients or patients who died, another pattern with no decrease of glucose levels and no increase of pyruvate was observed (Cesarini et al. 2000).

Brain tissue oxygen tension

Probes used for brain tissue oxygenation have been developed. In one study hyoxic values of brain oxygen tension (<10 mm Hg) occurred more frequently in patients developing infarction. It was concluded that monitoring brain tissue oxygen tension provides an additional independent parameter to detect hypoxic events and to guide triple-H therapy (Veath et al. 2000).

During surgery a clear correlation was found between brain oxygen tension and MABP below a threshold of 80 mm Hg (KettWhite et al. 2000).

Multimodal monitoring

Multimodal monitoring including laser flowmetry, ICP, and MABP gives the opportunity to evaluate cerebral autoregulation and CO_2 reactivity. By combining the use of multimodal monitoring (brain tissue oxygen tension, brain carbon dioxide, pH and temperature) with microdialysis, a potential to assist in the perioperative management of SAH patients has been documented (Hutchinson et al. 2000). Combined with transcranial Doppler flowmetry and CT-scanning it gives valuable information. Concerning the early development of ischaemia, evidence has been presented indicating that the presence of angiographic vasospasm and increased flow velocities not always correlate with ischaemia in the microcirculation as determined with Laser flowmetry (Johnson et al. 1996).

Perioperative management

Delayed and early operation

Risk of rebleeding

Delayed operation for SAH has been routine in many neurosurgical units. On one hand, a clear correlation has been demonstrated between an improvement in neurological status and operative conditions and neurological status and postoperative outcome. On the other hand, with a delayed regime the incidence of rebleeding is increased.

Within the first two weeks of acute SAH a daily rebleeding rate from 0.2 to 2.1% has been observed (Rosenørn et al. 1987). The mortality in rebleeding is about 50%, and the risk of further rebleeding is increased in survivors of the first rebleeding to 47% (Hijdra et al. 1987). In a retrospective study the incidence of rebleeding in early- and late surgery groups was 2.7 and 9.5% respectively (Miyaoka et al. 1993). On the other hand, the mortality rate during "ultra early" rebleeding during transportation and preparation for surgery was only 7%, compared with 9% combined mortality rate from complications and late ischaemia (Hillman et al. 1988).

In a series of 179 patients with spontaneous SAH 17.3% had ultra-early rebleeding. A particular high risk of ultra-early rebleeding was observed in those patients who had platelet hypoaggregation, patients who were admitted shortly after their SAH, and in those whose thrombin-antithrombin complex levels were extremely high (Fuji et al. 1996).

Studies with Doppler sonography also favour early surgery. Thus, postoperative flow velocities are lower in patients operated within 48 hours of SAH (Romner et al. 1990). In the co-operative North American study, early operation improved the rate of good recovery (71 versus 62%) (Haley et al. 1992). In an international co-operative study including 3521 patients it was concluded, however, that early surgery was neither more hazardous nor beneficial, than delayed surgery. Thus the postoperative risk following early surgery is equivalent to the risk of rebleeding and vasospasm in patients waiting for surgery (Kassell et al. 1990a, Kassell et al. 1990b).

Mortality

With delayed operation a mortality rate of 36% was found. 18% of the patients survived with seriously neurological sequelae and 46% with a favourable outcome was found (Adams et al. 1981).

Timing of operation

The timing of surgery does not affect the development of vasospasm. Thus any increased risk of cerebral ischaemia associated with surgery performed between 4 and 12 days after SAH is due to factors other than aggravation of vasospasm (MacDonald et al. 1994).

Timing of surgery in clinical grade I and II is not a major factor (Miyaoka et al. 1993). In poor grade patients the attitude concerning early clipping is controversial. Hunt and Hess scale graduation is not a sufficient basis for decision. If space-occupying hematoma is present urgent removal even in grade V patients should be performed. (Arnold et al. 1994, Steudel et al. 1994). Patients in grade IV and V are improved by external ventricular drainage. It also appears recommendable to operate patients who persist for several days in a condition no better than grade IV, rather than to assume an expectative attitude because re-rupture mostly terminates the life, whereas clipping gives a chance of recovery (Arnold et al. 1994).

Haematoma

In the moribund patients with intracerebral hematoma, angiographic verification, although preferable, is not necessary. In these patients CT angiography provides sufficient information concerning vascular anatomy to allow emergency craniotomy and clipping (le Roux et al. 1993).

Clot removal

Experimental studies

Theoretically, early clot removal reduces the occurrence of delayed vasospasm. Studies in monkeys indicate that clot removal at early operation is likely to reduce the incidence of vasospasm, if performed within 48 hours of SAH (Handa et al. 1987). In a study by Nosko et al. (1987), clot removal 24 hours after experimental SAH in primate, completely prevented chronic cerebral vasospasm.

Clinical studies

Clinical studies support these observation. Thus, vasospasm was only observed in moderate degree when blood clot was successfully removed by operation (Mizukami et al. 1982). In consequence, early removal of significant intracerebral hematoma with simultaneous clipping of the aneurysm is recommended (Whelock et al. 1983). On the other hand, another study indicates that the arterial territories involved in infarction are not reflected by the distribution of subarachnoid blood, and even the side of the infarct corresponds only weekly with the side on which most extravasated blood was observed. In the same study infarction was not related to the clearance rate of extravasated blood. These findings argue against a direct role of extravasated blood and in favour of systemic factors, dependent on the severity of the initial haemorrhage (Brouwers et al. 1992).

Ventricular and spinal drainage

The safety of spinal drainage has been studied consecutively in 432 patients. Unless contraindicated by mass effect of associated pathology in all grade I-III patients (n = 314) referred within 14 days were treated with spinal drainage at surgery. There were no cases of meningitis or nerve root injury. Only one case of rebleeding was associated with spinal drainage. In grade IV-V patients 47% required preoperative ventriculostomy, and 11% were unfit for spinal drainage due to mass effect (Connolly et al. 1997).

Unruptured intracranial aneurysm

Using evidence-based criteria Brennan and Schwartz (2000) reviewed the literature on unruptured aneurysms. As a therapeutic guideline, conservative treatment was recommended for small aneurysms (< 10 mm) and asymptomatic nongiant aneurysms in older people, wheras surgery is recommended for larger aneurysms in younger people and symptomatic aneurysms in fit patients.

Aneurysm rupture

Intraoperative rupture of cerebral aneurysm occurs in 19%. Rupture occurs early or predisectionally in 7%, during dissection in 48%, and during clip application in 45%. Outcome after rupture during predissection was poor with only 1 of 4 patients surviving. Rupture during clip application was attributed to incomplete dissection in 65%, poor clip application in 31%, and a mechanical clip failure in one of 58 ruptures (Batjer and Samson 1986a). Thiopental protection (5–15 mg/kg) has been used successfully during temporary vessel occlusion, even when the aneurysm ruptured (McDermott et al. 1989).

Hunt and Hess grade IV and V

Even in moribund patients with middle cerebral artery aneurysm, presenting with deep coma, dilated and fixed pupils and decerebrate rigidity, operative closure of the aneurysm has been performed, and the patients have still regained full consciousness within a few days (Brandt et al. 1987).

Temporary occlusion

Many neurosurgeons avoid the use of induced hypotension when there is angiographic evidence of vasospasm (Ruta et al. 1991). In fact, routine use of temporary proximal occlusion of the parent vessel, rather than induced hypotension is preferred by many neurosurgeons (Charbel et al. 1991). In a retrospective analysis Giannotta et al. (1991) concluded that controlled hypotension may not be necessary in the management of aneurysm surgery. On the other hand, the use of induced hypotension and hypervolemia as part of the anaesthetic management have been recommended in patients with symptomatic vasospasm (Buckland et al. 1988).

In a consecutive study Samson et al. (1994) analysed the effects of temporary arterial occlusion, and found that several parameters were related to postoperative development of ischaemic injury. Thus, patients more than 61 years of age and those in poor neurological condition (Hunt and Hess III and IV) did not tolerate temporary occlusion as well as patients who were younger and in better condition. Patients occluded for less than 14 minutes tolerated temporary occlusion, while all patients occluded for more than 31 minutes had evidence of cerebral infarction. In a consecutive study of 132 patients it was found that the following factors were associated with a stroke outcome: patients age, intraoperative aneurysm rupture, temporary clipping lasting more than 20 min, clipping between the 4th and the 10th day after SAH, and multiple clipping episodes. All patients were subjected to mild hypothermic hypotension and mannitol treatment. Overall 5.2% of the patients had postoperative stroke (Ogilvy et al. 1996). In another study, including 49 patients subjected to temporary middle cerebral artery occlusion MCAO, intravenous agents like propofol, etomidate and pentobarbital were used for cerebral protection. The authors concluded that patients in whom focal iatrogenic MCAO is induced have an advantage when pentobarbital was given, compared with those receiving isoflurane, propofol and etomidate titrated to achieve EEG burst suppression, particularly if more than 10 min of occlusion time is required. Furthermore, it was concluded that 10 min is a general guideline for safe temporary MCAO (Lavine et al. 1997) For review Taylor et al. 1996.

Intravascular balloon occlusion

Intravascular technique for treatment of aneurysm of the internal carotid artery in and around the cavernous sinus reserves special attention. Coil treatment is an attractive choice, but intravascular balloon occlusion has also been practised. Test for tolerance of occlusion is performed. Temporary occlusion of the internal carotid artery is performed for 10 min combined with a 30% decrease in baseline blood pressure. For permanent occlusion the balloon catheter is navigated into the internal carotid artery, and inflated at or just proximal to the aneurysm neck. In a report including 58 patients a morbidity rate of 10% caused by transient cerebral ischaemia, a permanent ischaemic morbidity of 5%, and a mortality rate of 5% were found (Larson et al. 1995).

Treatment of giant aneurysm

Rebleeding from giant aneurysm occurs at a rate comparable with that associated with smaller aneurysms (Khurana et al. 1998). In another study temporary occlusion of the parent vessel was necessary in 67% of direct procedures, with an average occlusion time of 15.5 min. Among surgically treated patients, a favourable outcome was achieved in 72% of patients with aneurysm of the anterior cerebral circulation, and 78% of the patients with rupture of the posterior lesions (Piepgras et al. 1998).

Cardiopulmonary by-pass

Cardiopulmonary by-pass has been used successfully in the operative treatment of giant anterior aneurysm, and basilar aneurysm. At 20°C the circulation is stopped for up to 45 minutes (Silverberg et al. 1981, Richards et al. 1987). In a recent study deep hypothermic circulatory arrest was used in 14 patients. All aneurysms were successfully treated, but two patients developed stroke (Solomon et al. 1991).

Intraoperative angiography

Intraoperative angiography has been proposed by Payner et al. (1998). They studied 151 patients with SAH and found that selective use of intraoperative angiography led to successful treatment as shown by postoperative angiography with a low incidence of unexpected residual aneurysm (3.2%), distal branch occlusion (1.9%), and parent vessel stenosis (0%). Intraoperative angiography led to immediate repositioning of the aneurysm clip in 27% of these cases.

Endovascular treatment of cerebral aneurysm (Coil treatment)

Aneurysm occlusion with coils was first reported by Hilal in 1988, and has since been refined. In a study of 71 patients with intracranial aneurysms endovascular technique with the placement of minicoils inside the aneurysmal sac was used. At 1-year follow-up examination the outcome was good in 85% of the cases, the morbidity and mortality were 4.2% and 11.3% respectively. It was found that aneurysms in the posterior circulation were particularly well suited for endovascular treatment (Casasco et al. 1993). In another study of 42 patients with posterior fossa aneurysms, the overall morbidity and mortality rates related to this treatment were 4.8% and 2.4% respectively. Excellent results with low morbidity and mortality were also demonstrated in posterior circulation aneurysms (Nichols et al. 1997). In a study of 327 patients the interval between Coil treatment and SAH did not affect morbidity rates or 6-month outcomes (Baltsavias et al. 2000). Close postoperative angiography and clinical monitoring of patients with wide-necked subtotally occluded aneurysms, however, are mandatory to check for potential aneurysmal recanalization, regrowth, and rupture (Guglielmi et al. 1992). The balloon-assisted Guglielmi detachable coil technology is a promising adjunct to the treatment of wide necked aneurysms (Lefkowitz et al. 1999). However, temporary increase of pressure within the aneurysm while occluding the aneurysm may potentially be the cause of aneurysm rupture (Akiba et al. 1999). If long-term effectiveness of treatment with endovascular coils can be established, it is apparent that this treatment will play a major role in the treatment of intracranial aneurysms. It is emphasised that prospective studies comparing surgical versus endovascular treatment of ruptured aneurysms are important (Nichols 1993).

Although endovascular treatment of aneurysms has gained some popularity, a conservative attitude still is appropriate. In a retrospective study Sturaitis et al. (2000) did not demonstrate any significant impact of integration of the detachable coil modality on clinical outcome, mortality, morbidity or effectiveness of treatment. Baskin et al. (1998) in their discussion summarised as follows: The role of endovascular occlusion for the treatment of aneurysms remains controversial. Data do not exist to substantiate this therapy as more than a temporising adjunctive intervention for patients with SAH, and its application is most appropriately reserved for lesions for which the anticipated morbidity accompanying open treatment is prohibitive. Until proven otherwise through the appropriate class-I studies, direct clip obliteration remains the definitive treatment for aneurysms, at both the basilar bifurcation and other locations.

Angioplasty of vasospasm

Experimental studies

In vitro studies in the canine double-haemorrhage model indicate that vasospastic vessels dilated with balloon angioplasty immediately after, have a significant reduction of responses to vasoconstrictors and vasorelaxants. Both normal and vasospastic vessels showed flattening and patchy denudation of the endothelium, and straightening and occasional rupturing of the internal elastic lamina (Chan et al. 1995).

Clinical studies

Cerebral angioplasty involves physical dilation of cerebral arteries which are affected by vasospasms. The technique was described by Zubkov et al. (1984), and has since been introduced in the treatment of vasospasm.

In selected studies intravascular balloon dilation of the spastic cerebral arteries is promising (Higashida et al. 1992). In a recent clinical study of 89 patients with vasospasm after SAH it was concluded that for best results, angioplasty should be performed before angiopathic features became florid. This helps to preserve flow through the short arteries to the brain stem and deep brain nuclei, which may be involved indirectly in the vasospastic process (Zubkov et al. 1994). Firlik et al. (1997) found a significant improvement of CBF after angioplasty in areas of brain at risk of infarction.

In another study of unclipped but ruptured aneurysm, urgent clipping of the aneurysm followed by immediate postoperative angioplasty was performed. Following angioplasty transcranial Doppler and SPECT studies indicated improved cerebral perfusion compared with preoperative determinations (leRoux et al. 1994).

In a retrospective uncontrolled study of 50 consecutive patients, where 46 had objective clinical deterioration despite maximal medical therapy, a total of 170 vessel segments were dilated. 61% of the patients showed sustained neurological improvement. 6% deteriorated within 72 hours after angioplasty, with 4% (two patients) dying as a result of vessel rupture. The authors concluded that timely balloon angioplasty can reverse delayed ischaemic deficit caused by vasospasm in patients for whom medical therapy failed (Eskrige et al. 1998). In another retrospective study of 31 patients angioplasty was found to be a safe and effective treatment for vasospasm that is refractory to hyperdynamic hypervolemic therapy, and when used early (< 24 hours), it led to significant clinical improvement (Bejjani et al. 1998). These results are in concert with another study including 51 patients unresponsive to traditional treatment. A 2-hour window exists for restoration of blood flow to ultimately improvement of the patients outcome (Rosenwasser et al. 1999). Prophylactic use of angioplasty in patients with Fisher Grade 3 SAH was investigated by Muizelaar et al. (1999). In 13 patients they found extremely low incidence of vasospasm and delayed ischaemic neurological deficit after treatment.

Cerebral vasospasm after early surgical versus early angioplastic treatment was compared in a nonrandomised series of 156 patients. The infarction rate was higher with endovascular treatment versus surgery (37,7 versus 21,6%), but this significant difference was found to be a result of a skewed Fisher grade 4 infarction pattern in the endovascular treatment group versus the surgery treatment group (Gruber et al. 1998).

In a recent study comparison of balloon angioplasty and papaverine infusion for the treatment of proximal anterior circulation vasospasm was performed. Papaverine treated patients demonstrated a 20% mean decrease in blood velocity on post-treatment day 1, but velocities were not significantly lower than pre-treatment levels by post-treatment day 2. In comparison balloon angioplasty resulted in a 45% mean decrease in velocity to a normal level, and this decrease was sustained (Elliott et al. 1998).

Extracranial-intracranial by-pass

In a clinical study of 11 patients extracranial-intracranial by-pass for symptomatic vasospasm was successful i 8 patients who responded neurologically within 24 hours (Batjer and Samson 1986b).

Laser surgery

Laser energy, at a wavelength of 480 nm, applied in 1 sec pulses has been studied experimentally. Prophylactic Laser application seems to attenuate the development of vasospasm. Morphological examination demonstrates focal loss of endothelial cells immediately after Laser application, followed approximately 7 days later by the development of intimal hyperplasia (Macfarlane et al. 1991).

Thrombotic treatment

Direct thrombosis of aneurysms with cellulose acetate polymer has been introduced. In aneurysms considered inoperable because of their size or location, or because of the patient's neurological condition this technique has been used (Kinugasa et al. 1992).

Anaesthetic Management

Morphine

In experimental studies in rats with SAH morphine partially restores CBF autoregulation, but attenuates CO_2 reactivity (Ma et al. 1999).

Nimodipine

During anaesthesia for cerebral aneurysm pre-treatment with nimodipine reduces systemic arterial pressure (Stullken et al. 1985).

Mannitol

Mannitol is used in the control of peroperative ICP-hypertension. However, mannitol treatment increases the risk of aneurysmal rupture during surgery. An increased pressure gradient across the aneurysm wall is supposed to be the reason (Rosenørn et al. 1983).

Controlled hypotension

During profound peroperative controlled hypotension to MABP 30–40 mm Hg, severe CBF disturbances have been observed postoperatively, at the site of cerebral retractors. However, no correlation between intraoperative reduction of CBF, and immediate postoperative neurological deficits was found (Farrar et al. 1981). It has been argued that many patients with SAH have impaired cerebral autoregulation. Controlled hypotension under this circumstance increases the incidence of cerebral ischaemia, infarction, and postoperative neurologic deficits (Kelly et al. 1977). In a recent retrospective study intraoperative hypotension had a significantly adverse effect on the outcome of patients with SAH, and hypotension was also related to more frequent and severe manifestations of vasospasm (Chang et al. 2000). In another study a clear correlation between prain tissue oxygenation and mean arterial blood pressure below a threshold of 80 mm Hg was found (KettWhite et al. 2000). Studies with isoflurane are reviewed in chapter 4 and 8. Barbiturate is reviewed in chapter 5 and 8.

Hypothermia

In a recent study patients with ruptured internal carotid or middle cerebral artery aneurysms were randomized to mild hypothermia (33.5°C) or normothermia (37°C). The cerebral aneurysms were clipped via the pterional approach through a unilateral frontotemporal craniotomy, and were subjected to temporary vessel occlusion. Studies with SPECT were performed on Days 4,7, and 14 after subarachnoid haemorrhage. CBF in the frontal cortex ipselateral to the aneurysm was higher in the hypothermia group than in the normothermic group on Day 4 but not Day 7 and 14. No differences in rCBF in the ipselateral cingulate cortex or basal ganglia or in any contralateral region were detected. The authors argue that mild hypothermia may reduce the severity of ischaemia induced by intraoperative temporary vessel occlusion and brain retraction, thus ameliorating postoperative CBF impairment (Karibe et al. 2000). A randomized prospective pilot study of mild hypothermia used during clipping of aneurysm was promising (Hindman et al. 1999), and a multicentre study is in progress.

Propofol anaesthesia

During propofol anaesthesia the threshold of ICP above which cerebral swelling occurs after opening of dura is 10 mm Hg (Bundgaard et al. 1998). The CO_2 reactivity is reduced during propofol/fentanyl anaesthesia, but the relaxation of the brain is better than during sevoflurane and isoflurane anaesthesia (Petersen et al. 2000). A fairly good correlation between preoperative Hunt and Hess and ICP measured during propofol/fentanyl anaesthesia, has been observed (Cold and Landsfeldt 1999).

Desflurane anaesthesia

During 4–6% desflurane anaesthesia tissue oxygen tension and tissue pH are low in patients with SAH compared with patients without SAH. Low pH was correlated to Fisher grade. Increasing the desflurane concentration to 9% increased brain tissue oxygen tension and pH (Hoffman et al. 2000).

References

Abe K, Fujino Y, Demizu A, et al. The effect of prostaglandin E_1 on local cerebral blood flow during cerebral aneurysm clip ligation. Europ J Anaesthesiol 1991: 8: 359–363.

Adams HP, Kassell NF, Torner CJ, et al. Early management of aneurysmal subarachnoid haemorrhage. J Neurosurg 1981: 54: 141–145.

Afshar JKB, Pluta RM, Boock RJ et al. Effect of intracarotid nitric oxide on primate cerebral vasospasm after subarachnoid haemorrhage. J Neurosurg 1995: 83: 118–122.

Akiba Y, Murayama Y, Vinuela F, et al. Balloon-assisted Guglielmi detachable coiling of wide-necked aneurysms. Part I - Experimental evaluation. Neurosurgery 1999: 45: 519–530.

Alcock JM, Drake CG. Ruptured intracranial aneurysms. The role of arterial spasm. J Neurosurg 1965: 22: 21–29.

Allen GS, Ahn HS, Preziosi TJ. et al. Cerebral arterial spasm – A controlled trial of nimodipine in patients with subarachnoid henorrhage. N Engl J Med 1983: 308: 619–624.

Allen JM, Schon F, Todd N, et al. Presence of neuropeptide Y in human circle of Willis and its possible role in cerebral vasospasm. Lancet 1984: 2: 550–552.

Alksne JF, Greenhoot JH. Experimental catecholamine-induced chronic vasospasm: myonecrosis in vessel wall. J Neurosurg 1974: 41: 440–445.

Alksne JF, Branston PJ, Bailey M. Modification of experimental post-subarachnoid haemorrhage vasculopathy with intercisternal plasmin. Neurosurgery 1986: 19: 20–25.

Ameriso S, Wong VLY, Ishii H, et al. Hematogenous factors and prediction of delayed ischaemic deficit after subarachnoid haemorrhage. Stroke 1992. 23: 1404–1409.

Amin-Hanjani B, Schwartz RB, et al. Hypertensive encephalopathy as a complication of hyperdynamic therapy for vasospasm: Report of two cases. Neurosurgery 1999: 44: 1113–1116.

Andreoli A, di Pasquale G, Pinelli G, et al. Subarachnoid haemorrhage: Frequency and severity of cardiac arrhytmia. A survey of 70 cases studied in the acute phase. Stroke 1987: 18: 558–564.

Andrews RJ, Spiegel PK. Intercranial aneurysms. Age, sex, blood pressure and multiplicity in an unselected series of patients. J Neurosurg 1979: 51: 27–32.
Antiplatelet trialists collaboration: Collaboration overview of randomized trials of antiplatelet therapy. Br Med J 1994: 308: 81–106.
Arnold H, Schwachenwald R, Nowak G, Schwachenwald D. Aneurysm surgery in poor grade patients. Results, and value of external ventricular drainage. Neurol Res 1994: 16: 45–48.
Asano T, Sasaki T, Koide T, et al. Experimental evaluation of the beneficial effect of an antioxidant on cerebral vasospasm. Neurol Res 1984: 6: 49–53.
Asano T, Koide T, Gotoh O, et al. The role of free radical and eicosanoids in the pathogenesic mechanism underlying ischaemic brain edema. Mol Chem Neuropath 1989: 10: 101–103.
Asano T, Ikegaki I, Sazuki Y et al. Endothelin and the production of cerebral vasospasm in dogs. Biochem Biophys Res Commun 1989: 159: 1245–1451.
Asano T, Takakura K, Sano K, et al. Effects of hydroxyl radical scavenger on delayed ischaemic neurological deficits following aneurysmal subarachnoid haemorrhage: Results of a multicenter, placebo-controlled-double-blind trial. J Neurosurg 1996: 84: 792–803.
Auer LM, Preventive nimodipine and acute aneurysm surgery: Heading for control of complications after aneurysmal subarachnoid haemorrhage. Neurochirurgica (Stuttg) 1985: 28: 87–92.
Auer LM, Schneider GH, Auer T. Computerized tomography and prognosis in early aneurysm surgery. J Neurosurg 1986: 65: 217–221.
Austin GM, Schievink W, Williams R. Controlled pressure volume factors in the enlargment of intracranial aneurysms. Neurosurgery 1989: 24: 722–730.
Awad IA, Carter LP, Spetzer RF, et al. Clinical vasospasm after subarachnoid haemorrhage: Response to hypervolemic hemodilution and arterial hypertension. Stroke 1987: 18: 365–372.
Balsavias GS, Byrne JV, Halsey J, et al. Effects of timing of Coil embolization after aneurysmal subarachnoid hemorrhage on procedural morbidity and outcomes. Neurosurgery 2000: 47: 1320–1331.
Barker FG, Ogilvy C. Efficacy of prophylactic nimodipine for delayed ischaemic deficit after subarachnoid haemorrhage: A metaanalysis. J Neurosurg 1996: 84: 405–414.
Baskin JJ; Vishteh AG, Theodore N, et al. Endovascular treatment of basilar artery aneurysms. Crit Rev Neurosurg 1998: 8: 50–60.
Batjer H, Samson D. Intraoperative aneurysmal rupture: Incidence, outcome and suggestions for surgical management. Neurosurgery 1986a: 18: 701–707.
Batjer H, Samson D. Use of extracranial-intracranial bypass in the management of symptomatic vasospasm. Neurosurgery 1986b: 19: 235–246.
Bederson JB, Levy AL, Ding WH, et al. Acute vasoconstriction after subarachnoid haemorrhage. Neurosurgery 1998: 42: 352–362.
Bejjani GK, Bank WO, Olan WJ, Sekhar LN. The efficacy and safety of angioplasty for cerebral vasospasm after subarachnoid haemorrhage. Neurosurgery 1998: 42: 979–987.
Bergvall U, Steiner L, Forster DMC, Early pattern of cerebral circulatory disturbances following subarachnoid haemorrhage. Neuroradiology 1973: 5: 24–32.
Berkman MZ, Zirh TA, Berkman K, Pamir N. Tizanidine is an effective agent in the prevention of focal cerebral ischaemia in rats: an experimental study. Surg Neurol 1998: 50: 264–271.
Berkman MZ, Iplikcioglu AC, Berkman MK, et al. The effect of tizanidine on chronic vasospasm in rats. Acta Neurochir 2000: 142: 1047–1054.
Bevan JA, Bevan RD, Frazee JG. Functional arterial changes in chronic cerebral vasospasm in monkeys: An in vitro assessment of contribution to arterial narrowing. Stroke 1987: 18: 472–481.
Bornstein RA, Weir BKA, Petruk KC, Disney LB, Neurophyschological function in patients after subarachnoid haemorrhage. Neurosurgery 1987: 21: 651–654.
Boullin DJ, Bunting S, Blaso WP, et al. Responses of human and baboon arteries to prostaglandin endoperoxides and biologically generated and synthetic prostacyclin: Their relevance to cerebral arterial spasm in man. Br J Clin Pharmacol 1979: 7: 139–147.
Boullin DJ, Brandt L, Lundgren B, Tagari P. Vasoconstrictor activity in cerebrospinal fluid from patients subjected to early surgery for ruptured intracranial aneurysms. J Neurosurg 1981: 55: 237–245.
Brandt L, Sonesson B, Ljunggren B, Säveland H. Ruptured middle cerebral artery aneurysm with intracerebral haemorrhage in younger patients appearing moribund: Emergency operation? Neurosurgery 1987: 20: 925–929.
Brawley BW, Sttrandness DE, Kelly WA. The biphasic response of cerebral vasospasm in experimental subarachnoid haemorrhage. J Neurosurg 1968: 22: 1–8
Brennan JW, Schwartz ML. Unruptured intracranial aneurysms: appraisal of the literature and suggested recommendations for surgery, using evidence-based medicine criteria. Neurosurgery 2000: 47: 1359–1372.
Brinker T, Seifert V, Stolke D. Acute changes in the dynamics of the cerebrospinal fluid system during experimental subarachnoid haemorrhage. Neurosurgery 1990: 27: 369–372.
Brinker T, Seifert V, Stolke D. Effect of intrathecal fibronolysis on cerebralspinal fluid absorption after experimental subarachnoid haemorrhage. J Neurosurg 1991: 74: 789–793.
Brinker T, Sefert V, Dietz H. Cerebral blood flow and intracranial pressure during experimental subarachnoid haemorrhage. Acta Neurochir (Wien) 1992: 115: 47–52.
Brouwers PJAM, Wijdicks EFM, van Gijn J. Infarction after aneurysm rupture does not depend on distribution of clearance rate of blood. Stroke 1992: 23: 274–279.
Bryden JE, Bevan JA. Evidence that vasoactive intestinal polypeptide (VIP) mediates neurogenic vasodilation of feline cerebral arteries. Stroke 1986: 17: 1189–1192.
Buckland MR, Batjar HH, Giesecke AH. Anesthesia for cerebral aneurysm surgery: Use of induced hypertension in patients with symptomatic vasospasm. Anesthesiology 1988: 69: 116–119.
Bundgaard H, Landsfeldt U, Cold GE. Subdural monitoring of ICP during craniotomy. Thresholds of cerebral swelling/herniation. Acta Neurochir 1998 (suppl) 71: 276–278.
Caner H, Kwan AL, Bavbek M, et al. Systemic administration of mexiletine for attenuation of cerebral vasospasm fol-

lowing experimental subarachnoidal haemorrhage. Acta Neurochir (Wien) 2000: 142: 455–461.
Casasco AE, Aymard A, Gobin P, et al. Selective endovascular treatment of 71 intracranial aneurysms with platinum coils. J Neurosrug 1993: 79: 3–10.
Cesarini KG, Enblad P, et al. Cerebral hyperglycolysis, a favourable metabolic response after severe SAH. Proceeding XI ICP symposium, Cambridge 2000: O10-3, page 83.
Chan PDS, Findley JM, Vollrath B, et al. Pharmacological and morphological effects of *in vitro* transluminal balloon angioplasty on normal and vasospastic canine basilar arteries. J Neurosurg 1995: 83: 522–530.
Chang HS, Hongo K, Nakagawa H. Adverse effects of limited hypotensive anaesthesia on the outcome of patients with subarachnoid hemorrhage. J Neurosurg 2000: 92: 971–975.
Chapleau CE, White RP. Effects of prostacyclin on the isolated canine basilar artery. Prostaglandins 1979: 17: 573–580.
Charbel FT, Ausman JI, Diaz FG, et al. Temporary clipping in aneurysm surgery: Technique and results. Surg Neurol 1991: 36: 83–90.
Chiang VLS, Claus EB, Awad IA. Toward more rational prediction of outcome in patients with high-grade subarachnoid hemorrhage. Neurosurgery 2000: 46: 28–36.
Chimowitz MI, Pessin MS. Is there a role of heparin in the management of complications of subarachnoid haemorrhage? Stroke 1987: 18: 1169–1172.
Chung RY, Carter BS, Norbash A, et al. Management outcomes for ruptured and unruptured aneurysms in the elderly. Neurosurgery 2000: 47: 827–833.
Chyatte D, Rusch N, Sundt TM Jr. Prevention of chronic experimental cerebral vasospasm with ibuprofen and high-dose methylprednisolone. J Neurosurg 1983: 59: 925–932.
Chyatte D, Fode NC, Nichols DA, Sundt TM Jr. Preliminary report: Effects of high dose methylprednisolone on delayed cerebral ischemia in patients at high risk for vasospasm after aneurysmal subarachnoid haemorrhage. Neurosurgery 1987: 21: 157–160.
Citerio G, Cormio M, Portella G, et al. Jugular saturation ($SjvO_2$) monitoring in subarachnoid hemorrhage (SAH). J Neurosurg 1998 (suppl) 71: 316–319.
Clozel M, Breu V, Gray GA, et al. Pharmacological characterisation of bosantan, a new potent orally active non-peptidic endothelin receptor antagonist. J Pharmacol Exp Ther 1994: 270: 228–235.
Clyde BL, Resnick DK, Yonas H, et al. The relationship of blood velocity as measured by transcranial Doppler ultrasonography to cerebral blood flow as determined by stable Xenon computed tomographic studies after aneurysmal subarachnoid haemorrhage. Neurosurgery 1996: 38: 896–905.
Cold GE, Landsfeldt U. Studies of ICP during craniotomy for cerebral aneurysm. Correlation to Hunt and Hess graduation and other perioperative data. Acta Anaesthesiol Scand (suppl) 1999: 43: 115
Cole DJ, Nary JC, Reynolds LW, et al. Experimental subarachnoid haemorrhage in rats. Anesthesiology 1997: 87: 1486–1493.
Connolly ES, Kader AA, Frazzini VI, et al. The safety of intraoperative lumbar subarachnoid drainage for acutely ruptured aneurysm: Technical note:. Surg Neurol 1997: 48: 338–344.
Consentino T, Katusic Z. Does endothelin-1 play a role in the pathogenesis of cerebral vasospasm? Stroke 1994: 25: 904–908.
Conway LW, McDonald LW. Structural changes of the intradural arteries following subarachnoid haemorrhage. J Neurosurg 1972: 37: 715–723.
Critchley GR, Bell BA. Intracranial pressure, cerebral blood flow and tissue oxygenation changes following experimental subarachnoid haemorrhage. Proceeding XI ICP symposium, Cambridge 2000, O7-4, page 68.
Crompton MR. The pathogenesis of cerebral infarction following the rupture of cerebral berry aneurysms. Brain 1964: 87: 491–510.
Cropp GJ, Manning GW. Electrocardiographic changes simulating myocardial ischemia and infarction associated with spontaneous intracranial haemorrhage. Circulation 1960: 22: 25–38.
Cruickshank JM, Neil-Dwyer G, Scott AW. Possible role of catecholamines, corticosteroids, and potassium in production of electrocardiographic abnormalities associated with subarachnoid hemorrhage. Br Heart J 1974: 36: 697–706.
Cummins BH, Lothian D. Amine levels in the cerebrospinal fluid after subarachnoid haemorrhage (abstract). Br J Surg 1973: 60: 910.
Cummins BH, Griffith HB. Intracarotid phenoxybenzamine for cerebral arterial spasm. Br Med J 1971: 1: 382–383.
Czosnyka M, Richards HK, Whitehouse HE, Pickard JD. Relationship between transcranial Doppler-determined pulsative index and cerebrovascular resistance: an experimental study. J Neurosurg 1996: 84: 79–84.
Dahlström A. Fuxe K. Evidence for the existence of monoamine-containing neurons in the central system. 1. Demonstration of monoamines in the cell bodies of brain stem neurons. Acta Phsyiol Scand 1964: 62 (suppl 232): 1–55.
Davis SM, Andrews J, Lichtenstein M, et al. A single-photon emission computed tomography study of hypoperfusion after subarachnoid haemorrhage. Stroke 1990: 21: 252–259.
Davis SM, Andrews JT, Lichtenstein M, et al. Correlations between cerebral arterial velocities, blood flow, and delayed ischemia after subarachnoid haemorrhage. Stroke 1992: 23: 492–497.
Debdi M, Seylas J, Sercombe R. Early changes in rabbit cerebral artery reactivity after subarachnoid haemorrhage. Stroke 1992: 23: 1154–1162.
Delgado RJ, Arbab Ma-R, Diemer NH, Scendgaard N-Aa. Subarachnoid haemorrhage in the rat: Cerebral blood flow and glucose metabolism during the late phase of cerebral vasospasm. J Cereb Blood Flow Metab 1986a: 6: 590–599.
Delgado RJ, Diemer NH, Svendgaard N-Aa. Subarachnoid haemorrhage in the rat: Cerebral blood flow and glucose metabolism after selective lession of the catecholamine systems in the brainstem. J Cereb Blood Flow Metab 1986b: 6: 600–606.
Delgado RJ, Arbab Ma-R, Rosengren E, Svendgaard N-Aa. Effect of neonatal 6-hydroxydopamine treatment on experimental vasospasm following a subarachnoid haemorrhage in the rat. J Cereb Blood Flow Metab 1987: 7: 289–294.
Delgado TJ, Arbab A-R, Edvinsson L, et al. Prevention of cerebral vasospasm in the rat by depletion or inhibition of substance P in conducting vessels. J Neurosurg 1990: 72: 917–925.
Dernbach PD, Little JR, Jones SC, Ebrahim ZY. Altered cerebral autoregulation and CO_2 reactivity after aneurysmal subarachnoid haemorrhage. Neurosurgery 1988: 22: 822–826.

Dillon PF, Aksoy MO, Driska SP, et al. Myosin phsophorylation and the cross-bridge cycle in arterial smooth muscle. Science 1981: 211: 495–497.

Dilray A, Botha JH, Rambiritch V, et al. Levels of catecholamine in plasma and cerebrospinal fluid in aneurysmal subarachnoid haemorrhage. Neurosurgery 1992: 31: 42–51.

Dinh YRT, Lot G, Benrabah R, et al. Abnormal cerebral vasodilation in aneurysmal subarachnoid haemorrhage: Use of serial 133-Xe cerebral blood flow measurement plus acetazolamide to assess cerebral vasospasm. J Neurosurg 1993: 79: 490–493.

Diringer MN, Kirsch JR, Hanley DF, Traystman RJ. Altered cerebrovascular CO_2 reactivity following subarachnoid haemorrhage in cats. J Neurosurg 1993: 78: 915–921.

Diringer MN, Kirsch JR, Traystman RJ. Reduced cerebral blood flow but intact reactivity to hypercapnia and hypoxia following subarachnoid haemorrhage in rabbits. J Cereb Blood Flow Metab 1994: 14: 59–63.

Dóczi T. The patogenetic and prognostic significance of blood-brain barrier damage at the acute stage of aneurysmal subarachnoid haemorrhage. Clinical and experimental studies. Acta Neuchir (Wien) 1985: 77: 110–132.

Dóczi T, Joó F, Adám G, Bozóky B, Szerdahelyi P. Blood-brain barrier damage during the acute stage of subarachnoid haemorrhage, as exemplified by a new animal model. Neurosurgery 1986: 18: 733–739.

Domingo Z, Bradley JK, Blamire AM. et al. Diffusion weighted imaging and magnetic resonance spectroscopy in a low flow ischaemic model due to endothelin induced vasospasm. NMR Bioned 2000: 13: 154–162.

Doshi R, Neil-Dwyer G. A clinicopathological study of patients following a subarachnoid haemorrhage. J Neurosurg 1980: 52. 295–301.

Drake CG. Intracranial aneurysms. Proc R Soc Med 1971: 64: 477–481.

Drake CG Report of World Federation of Neurological Surgery Committee on a universal subarachnoid hemorrhage grading scale. J Neurosurg 1988: 68: 985–986.

Dreier JP, Ebert N, Priller J, et al. Products of hemolysis in the subarachnoid space inducing spreading ischemia in the cortex and focal necrosis in rats: A model for delayed ischemic neurological deficits after subarachnoid hemorrhage? J Neurosurg 2000: 93: 658–666.

Duckles SP, Said SI. Vasoactive intestinal peptides as a neurotransmitter in the cerebral circulation. Eur J Pharmacol 1982: 78: 371–374.

Duff TA, Feilbach JA, Scott G. Does cerebral vasospasm result from denervation supersensitivity? Stroke 1987: 18: 85–91.

Dutton J. Acrylic investment of intracranial aneurysms. A report of 12 years experience. J Neurosurg 1969: 31: 652–657.

Edner G, Kågström E, Wallstedt L. Total overall management and surgical outcome after aneurysmal subarachnoid haemorrhage in a defined population. Br J Neurosurgery 1992: 6: 409–420.

Edvinsson L, Ekman R. Distrubution and dilatory effect of vasoactive intestinal polypeptide (VIP) in human cerebral arteries. Peptide 1984: 329–331.

Edvinsson L, Emson P, McCulloch J et al. Neuropeptide Y: Immunocytochemical localization and effect upon feline pial arteries and veins *in vitro* and *in situ*. Acta Physiol Scand 1984: 122: 155–163.

Edvinsson L, Uddman R, Juul R. Peptidergic innervation of the cerebral circulation. Role in subarachnoid haemorrhage in man. Neurosurg Rev 1990: 13: 265–272.

Elderik OP, Kristiansen K, Torvik A. Subarachnoid haemorrhage and cerebrovascular spasm. Morphological study in intracranial arteries based on animal experiments and human autopsies. J Neurosurg 1981: 55: 869–876.

Elliott JP, Newell DW, Lam DJ. Et al. Comparison of balloon angioplasty and papaverine infusion for the treatment of vasospasm following aneurysmal subarachnoid haemorrhage. J Neurosurg 1998: 88: 277–284.

Enblad P, Valtysson J, Andersson J, et al. Simultaneous intracerebral microdialysis and positron emission tomography in the detection of ischaemia in patients with subarachnoid haemorrhage. J Cereb Blood Flow Metab 1996: 16: 637–644.

Eskesen V, Sørensen EB, Rosenørn J, Schmidt K. The prognosis in subarachnoid haemorrhage of unknown etiology. J Neurosurg 1984: 61: 1029–1031.

Eskesen V, Rosenørn J, Schmidt K, et al. Clinical features and outcome in 48 patients with unruptured intracranial saccular aneurysms. A prospective consecutive study. Br J Neurosurg 1987: 1: 47–52.

Eskrige JM, Mcauliffe W, Song JK, et al. Balloon angioplasty for the treatment of vasospasm. Results of the first 50 cases. Neurosrugery 1998: 42: 510–517.

Espinosa F, Weir B, Overton T, et al. A randomized placebo-controlled double-blind trial of nimodipine after SAH in monkeys. J Neurosurg 1984: 60: 1167–1175.

Faleiro LCM, Machado CRS, Gripp A et al. Cerebral vasospam: Presence of mast cells in human cerebral arteries after aneurysm rupture. Preliminary note. J Neurosurg 1981: 54: 733–735.

Faraci FM, Heistad DD. Endothelium-derived relaxing factor inhibits constrictor responses of large cerebral arteries to serotonin. J Cereb Blood Flow Metab 1992: 12: 500–506.

Farrar JK, Gamache FW, Ferguson GG et al. Effects of profound hypotension on cerebral blood flow during surgery for intracranial aneurysm. J Neurosurg 1981: 55: 857–864.

Fassbender K, Hodapp B, Rossol S, et al. Endothelin-1 in subarachnoid hemorrhage: An acute-phase reactant produced by cerebrospinal fluid leukocytes. Stroke 2000: 31: 2971–2975.

Fein JM, Flor WJ, Cohen SL. Sequential changes of vascular ultrastructure in experimental cerebral vasospasm: Myonecrosis of subarachnoid arteries. J Neurosurg 1974: 41: 49–58.

Fein JM. Cerebral energy metabolism after subarachnoid hemorrhage. Stroke 1975: 6: 1–8.

Ferguson GG, Harper AM, Fitch W, et al. Cerebral blood flow measurements after spontaneous subarachnoid haemorrhage Europ Neurol 1972: 8: 15–22.

Findley JM, Weir BKA, Steinke D et al. Effect of intrathecal thrombolytic therapy on subarachnoid clot and chronic vasospasm in a primate model of SAH. J Neurosurg 1988: 69: 723–735.

Findlay JM, Kassell NF, Weir KBA, et al. A randomized trial on intraoperative, intracisternal tissue plasminogen activator for the prevention of vasospasm. Neurosurgery 1995: 37: 168–178.

Finn SS, Stephensen SA, Miller CA, et al. Observations on the peroperative management of aneurysmal subarachnoid haemorrhage. J Neurosurg 1986: 65: 48–62.

Firlik AD, Kaufmann AM, Jungries CA, Yonas H. Effect of transluminal angioplasty on cerebral blood flow in the management of symptomatic vasospasm following aneu-

rysmal subarachnoid haemorrhage. J Neurosurg 1997: 86: 830–839.
Fisher CM, Kistler JP, Davis JM. Relation of cerebral vasospasm to subarachnoid haemorrhage visualized by CT scanning. Neurosurgery 1980: 6: 1–9.
Flamm ES, Yasargil G, Ransohoff J. Control of cerebral vasospasm by parenteral phenoxybenzamine. Stroke 1972a: 3: 421–426.
Flamm ES, Yasargil G, Ransohoff J. Alteration of experimental cerebral vasospasm by adrenergic blockade. J Neurosurg 1972b: 37: 294–301.
Flamm ES, Adams HP, Beck DW et al. Dose-escalation study of intravenous nicardipine in patients with aneurysmal subarachnoid haemorrhage. J Neurosurg 1988: 68: 393–400.
Foley PL, Caner HH, Kassell NF, Lee KS. Reversal of subarachnoid haemorrhage-induced vasoconstriction with an endothelin receptor antagonist. Neurosurgery 1994: 34: 108–113.
Fortuny LA, Prieto-Valiente L. Long term prognosis in surgically treated intracranial aneurysms. Part 1: Mortality. J Neurosurg 1981: 54: 26–54.
Frazer RAR, Stein BM, Barrett RE, Pool JL. Noradrenergic mediation of experimental cerebrovascular spasm. Stroke 1970: 1: 356–362.
Froman C, Smith AC. Metabolic acidosis of the cerebrospinal fluid associated with subarachnoid haemorrhage. Lancet 1967: 1: 965–967.
Fuji Y, Takeuchi S, Sasaki O, et al. Ultra-early rebleeding in spontaneous subarachnoid haemorrhage. J Neurosurg 1996: 84: 35–42.
Fujishima M, Sugi T,Choki J, et al. Cerebrospinal fluid and arterial lactate, pyruvate and acid-base balance in patients with intracranial haemorrhage. Stroke 1975: 6: 707–714.
Fukomori T, Tani E, Maeda Y, Sukenaga A. Effects of prostacyclin and indomethacin on experimental delayed cerebral vasospasm. J Neurosurg 1983: 59: 829–834.
Gade A. Amnesia after operations on aneurysms of the anterior communicating artery. Surg Neurol 1982: 18: 46–49.
Galloon S, Rees GAD, Briscoe CE, et al. Prospective study of electrocardiography changes associated with subarachnoid haemorrhage. Br J Anesth 1972: 44: 511–514.
Ganz P, Sandrock AW, Landis SC, et al. Vasoactive intestinal peptide: Vasodilation and cyclic AMP generation. Am J Physiol 1986: 250: H755–H760.
Gelmers HJ, Beks JWF, et al. Regional cerebral blood flow in patients with subarachnoid haemorrhage. Acta Neurochir 1979: 47: 245–251.
Géraud G, Tremoulet M, Guell A. Bes A. The prognostic value of noninvasive CBF measurement in subarachnoid haemorrhage. Stroke 1984: 15: 301–305.
Germann P, Aloy A, Zabloudil B, et al. Treatment of subarachnoid haemorrhage with the calcium entry blocker nimodipine affects pulmonary gas exchange in patients requiring controlled mechanical ventilation. Anesthesiology 1987: A115.
Germano A, d'Aella D, Cicciarello R, et al. Blood-brain barrier permeability changes after experimental subarachnoid haemorrhage. Neurosurgery 1992: 30: 882–886.
Germano A, dAvella D, Imperatore C, et al. Time-course of blood-brain barrier permeability changes after experimental subarachnoid haemorrhage. Acta Neurochir (Wien) 2000: 142: 575–581.
Gianotta SL, McGillicuddy JE, Kindt GW. Diagnosis and treatment of postoperative cerebral vasospasm. Surg Neurol 1978: 8: 286–290.
Gianotta SL, Oppenheimer JH, Levy ML, Zelman V. Management of intraoperative rupture of aneurysm without hypotension. Neurosurgery 1991: 28: 531–536.
Giller CA. The frequency-dependent behavior of cerebral autoregulation. Neurosurg 1990: 27: 362–368.
Gilsbach JM, Reulen HJ, Ljunggren B. et al. Early aneurysm surgery and prevention therapy with intravenously administered nimodipine: A multicenter, double-blind, dose-comparison study. Neurosurgery 1990: 26: 458–464.
Gioia AE, White RP, Bakhitial R, Robertson JT. Evaluation of the efficacy of intrathecal nimodipine in canine models of chronic cerebral vasospasm. J Neurosurg 1985: 62: 721–728.
Greenblatt SH. Cerebrospinal fluid creatinine phosphokinase in acute subarachnoid haemorrhage. J Neurosurg 1976: 44: 50–54.
Grosset DG, Straiton J, McDonald I, et al. Use of transcranial Doppler sonography to predict development of a delayed ischaemic deficit after subarachnoid haemorrhage. J Neurosurg 1993: 78: 183–187.
Grote E, Hassler W. The critical first minutes after subarachnoid haemorrhage. Neurosurgery 1988: 22: 654–661.
Grotenhuis JA, Bettag W, Fiebach BJO, Dabir K. Intracarotid slow bolus injection of nimodipine during angiography for treatment of cerebral vasospasm after SAH. J Neurosurg 1984: 61: 231–240.
Grubb RL, Raichle ME, Eichling JO, Gado MH. Effects of subarachnoid haemorrhage on cerebral blood volume, blood flow, and oxygen utilization in humans. J Neurosurg 1977: 46: 466–453.
Gruber A, Ungersböck K, Reinprecht A, et al. Evaluation of cerebral vasospasm after early surgical and endovascular treatment of ruptured intracranial aneurysms. Neurosurgery 1998: 42: 258–268.
Guglielmi G, Vinuela F, Duckwiler G, et al. Endovascular treatment of posterior circulation aneurysms by electrothrombosis using electrically detachable coils. J Neurosurg 1992: 77: 515–524.
Gurusinghe NT, Richardson AE. The value of computerized tomography in aneurysmal subarachnoid haemorrhage. J Neurosurg 1984: 60: 763–770.
Haley EC, Kassell NF, Torner CJ, et al. The international cooperative study on the timing of aneurysm surgery. The North Americal Experience. Stroke 1992: 23: 205–214.
Haley EC, Kassell NF, Torner JC, et al. A randomized controlled trial of high-dose intravenous nicardipine in aneurysmal subarachnoid haemorrhage. J Neurosurg 1993a: 78: 537–547.
Haley EC, Kassell NF, Torner JC, et al. A randomized trial of nicardipine in subarachnoid haemorrhage: Angiographic and transcranial Doppler ultrasonic results. J Neurosurg 1993b: 78: 548–553.
Haley EC, Kassell NF, Torner JC, et al. A randomized trial of two doses of nicardipine in aneurysmal subarachnoid haemorrhage. J Neurosurg 1994: 80: 788–796
Haley EC, Kassell NF, Alves WM, et al. Phase II trial of tirilazad in aneurysmal subarachnoid haemorrhage. J Neurosurg 1995: 82: 786–790.
Haley EC, Kassell NF, Apperson-Hansen C, et al.A randomized, double-blind, vehicle-controlled trial of tirilazad mesylate in patients with aneurysmal subarachnoid hemorrhage. A

cooperative study in North America. J Neurosurg 1997: 86: 467–474.
Handa Y, Weir BKA, Nosko M, Mosewich R, Tsuji T, Grace M. The effect of timing of clot removal on chronic vasospasm in a primate model. J Neurosurg 1987: 67: 558-564.
Handa Y, Hayashi M, Takeuchi H, et al. Time course of the impairment of cerebral autoregulation during chronic cerebral vasospasm after subarachnoid haemorrhage in primates. J Neurosurg 1992: 76: 493-501.
Handa Y, Kubota T, Tsuchida A, et al. Effect of systemic hypotension on cerebral energy metabolism during chronic cerebral vasospasm in primates. J Neurosurg 1993: 78: 112–119.
Hartmann A. Continuous monitoring of CSF pressure in acute subarachnoid haemorrhage. In Intracranial Pressure IV, Shulman K, Marmarou Am Miller JD, Becker DP, Hochwald GM, Brock M (eds). Springer Verlag 1980: 220-228.
Hasan D, Vermeulen M, Wijdicks EFM et al. Effect of fluid intake and antihypertensive treatment on cerebral ischemia after subarachnoid haemorrhage. Stroke 1989: 20: 1511-1515.
Hase U, Reulen H-J, Fenske A, Schürmann K. Intracranial pressure and pressure volume relation in patients with subarachnoid haemorrhage. Acta Neurochir 1978: 44: 69–80.
Hashi K, Meyer JS, Shinmaru S, et al. Cerebral hemodynamic and metabolic changes after experimental subarachnoid haemorrhage. J Neurol Sci 1972: 17: 1–14.
Hatake K, Wakabayashi I, Kakishita E, Hishida S. Impairment of endothelium-dependent relaxation in human basilar artery after subarachnoid haemorrhage. Stroke 1992: 23: 1111–1117.
Hauerberg J, Juhler M, Rasmussen G. Cerebral blood flow autoregulation after experimental subarachnoid hemorrhage during hyperventilaiton in rats. J Neurosurg Anesthesiol 1993: 5: 258-263.
Hayashi M, Marukawa H, Fujii H, et al. Intracranial hypertension in acute stage of ruptured intracranial aneurysm. In: Keks JWF, Bosch DA, Brock M (eds). Intracranial Pressure III. Springer Verlag, Berlin. 1976: 162-167.
Hayashi M, Marukawa S, Fujii H et al. Intracranial pressure in patients with diffuse cerebral arterial spasm following ruptured intracranial aneurysms. Acta Neurochir 1978: 44: 81–95.
Hayashi M, Kobayashi H, Kawano H et al. Cerebral blood flow and ICP patterns in patients with communicating hydrocephalus after aneurysm rupture. J Neurosurg 1984: 61: 30–36.
Heilbrun MP, Olesen J, Lassen NA. Regional cerebral blood flow studies in subarachnoid haemorrhage. J Neurosurg 1972: 37: 36–44.
Heinsoo M, Eelmäe J, Kuklane M, et al. The posible role of CSF hydrodynamic parameters following in management of SAH patients. Acta Neurochir 1998 (suppl) 71: 13-15.
Higashida RT, Halbach VV, Dowd CF et al. Intravascular balloon dilatation therapy for intracranial arterial vasospasm: Patient selection, technique, and clinical results. Neurosurg Rev 1992: 15: 89–95.
Hijdra A, Vermeulen M, van Gijn J et al. Rerupture of intracranial aneurysms. A Clinicoanantomical study. J Neurosurg 1987a: 67: 29–33.
Hijdra A, Braakman R, van Gijn J, et al. Aneurysmal subarachnoid haemorrhage complications and outcome in a hospital population. Stroke 1987: 18: 1061-1067.
Hilal SK. Synthetic fibre coated platinum coils successfully used for the endovascular treatment of arteriovenous malformations, aneurysms and direct arteriovenous fistulae of the central nervous system. Radiology 1988 [suppl] (abstract) 28–29.
Hillman J, von Essen C, et al. Significance of "ultra early" rebleeding in subarachnoid haemorrhage. J Neurosurg 1988: 68: 901–907.
Hindman BJ, Todd MM, Gelb AW et al. Mild hypothermia as a protective therapy during intracranial aneurysm surgery: a randomized prospective trial. Neurosurgery 1999:44:23–33
Hino A, Mizukawa N, Tenjin H, et al. Postoperative hemodynamic and metabolic changes in patients with subarachnoid haemorrhage. Stroke 1989: 20: 1504–1510.
Hino A, Weir B, MacDonald RL, et al. Prospective randomized, double-blind trial of BQ-123 and bosentan for prevention of vasospasm following subarachnoid haemorrhage in monkeys. J Neurosurg 1995: 83: 503-509.
Hino A, Tokuyama Y, Kobayashi M, et al. Increased expression of endothelin-B receptor MRNA following subarachnoid haemorrhage in monkeys. J Cereb Blood Flow Metab 1996: 16: 688–697.
Hirashima Y, Endo S, Otsuji T, et al. Platelet-activating factor and cerebral vasospasm following subarachnoid haemorrhage. J Neurosurg 1993: 78: 592–597.
Hirashima Y, Endo S, Kurimot M, et al. Platelet-activating factor and antiphospholipid antibodies in subarachnoid haemorrhage. Acta Neruochir 1994a: 128: 144–149.
Hirashima Y, Endo S, Ohmori T, et al. Platelet-activating factor (PAF) concentration and PAF acetylhydrolase activity in cerebrospinal fluid of patients with subarachnoid haemorrhage. J Neurosurg 1994b: 80: 31–36.
Hirashima Y, Endo S, Kato R. Prevention of cerebral vasospasm following subarachnoid haemorrhage in rabbits by platelet-activating factor antagonist E5880. J Neurosurg 1996: 84: 826-830.
Hoffman WE, Wheeler P, Edelman G, et al. Hypoxic brain tissue following subarachnoid haemorrhage. Anesthesiology 2000: 92: 442–446.
Hollin SA, Decker RE. Microsurgery treatment of internal carotid artery aneurysms. J Neurosurg 1977: 47: 142–149.
Horky LL, Pluta RM, Boock RJ, Oldfield EH. Role of ferrous iron chelator 2,2'-dipyridyl in preventing delayed vasospasm in a primate model of subarachnoid haemorrhage. J Neurosurg 1998: 88: 298-303.
Huang M, Rorstad OP. Cerebral vascular adenylate cyclase: Evidence for coupling to receptors for vasoactive intestinal peptide and parathyroid hormone. J Neurochem 1984: 43: 894-896.
Hughes JFM, Schianchi PM. Cerebral artery spasm: A histological study at necropsy of the blood vessels in the cases of subarachnoid haemorrhage. J Neurosurg 1978: 48: 515–525.
Hunt WE, Hess RM. Surgical risks as related to time of intervention in the repair of intracranial aneurysms. J Neurosurg 1968: 28: 14–20.
Hutchinson PJ, Al-Rawi PG, OConnell MT, et al. Biochemical changes related to hypoxia during cerebral aneurysm surgery: Combined microdialysis and tissue oxygen monitoring: Case report. Neurosurgery 2000: 46: 201–206.
Hütter BO, Kreitschmann.Andermahr I, Gilsbach JM. Cognitive deficits in the acute stage after subarachnoid hemorrhage 1998: 43: 1054–1065.

Ide K, Yamakawa K, Nakagomi T et al. The role of endothelin in the pathogenesis of vasospasm following subarachnoid haemorrhage. Neurol Res 1989: 11: 101–104.

Inagawa T. Cerebral vasospasm in elderly patients treated by early operation for ruptured intracranial aneurysms. Acta Neurochir 1992: 115: 79–85.

Ishii R. Regional cerebral blood flow in patients with ruptured intracranial aneurysms. J Neurosurg 1979: 50: 587–594.

Ito Y, Isotani E, Mizuno Y, et al. Effective improvement of the cerebral vasospasm after subarachnoid hemorrhage with low-dose nitroglycerin. J Cardiovasc Pharmacol 2000: 35: 45–50.

Itoh S, Sasaki T, Asai A, et al. Prevention of delayed vasospasm by an endothelin ET-a receptor antagonist BQ-123: change of ET-a receptor MRNA expression in a canine subarachnoid haemorrhage model. J Neurosurg 1994: 81: 759–764.

Itoh T, Sasaguri T, Makita Y et al. Mechanisms of vasodilation induced by vasoactive intestinal polypeptide in rabbit mesenteric artery. Am J Physiol 1985: 249: H231–H240.

Itoyama Y, Fujioka S, Takaki S, et al. Significance of elevated thrombin-antithrombin complex and plasminogen-$_2$-plasmin inhibitor complex in the acute stage of non-traumatic subarachnoid haemorrhage. Neurosurgery 1994: 35: 1055–1060.

Jakobsson KE, Säveland H, Hillman J, et al. Warning leak and management outcome in aneurysmal subarachnoid haemorrhage. J Neurosurg 1996: 85: 995–999.

Jakobsen M. Overgaard J, Marcussen E, Enevoldsen EM. Relation between angiographic cerebral vasospasm and regional CBF in patients with SAH. Acta Neurol Scand 1990a: 82: 109–115.

Jakobsen M, Enevoldsen E, Bjerre P. Cerebral blood flow and metabolism following subarachnoid haemorrhage: Cerebral oxygen uptake and global blood flow during the acute period in patients with SAH. Acta Neurol Scand 1990b: 82: 174–182.

Jakobsen M, Enevoldsen E, Dalager T. Spasm index in subarachnoid hemorrhage: Consequences of vasospasm upon cerebral blood flow and oxygen extraction. Acta Neurol Scand 1990c: 82: 311–320.

Jakobsen M, Skjødt T, Enevoldsen E. Cerebral blood flow and metabolism following subarachnoid haemorrhage: Effect of subarachnoid blood. Acta Neurol Scand 1991: 83: 226–233.

Jakubowski J, McCleery WNC, Todd JH, Smart RC. Cerebral blood flow changes in acute experimental hemorrhagíc vasospasm. Acta Neurochirurgica 1976: 34: 265–268.

James IM. Changes in cerebral blood flow and in systemic arterial pressure following spontaneous subarachnoid haemorrhage. Clin Sci 1968: 35: 11–22.

Jarman DA, du Boulay GH, Kendall B. et al. Responses of baboon cerebral and extracerebral arteries to prostacyclin and prostaglandin endoperoxide *in vitro* and *in vivo*. J Neurol Neurosurg Phsychiatr 1979: 42: 677–686.

Johnson WD, Bolognese P, Miller JI, et al. Continuous postoperative lCBF monitoring in aneurysmal SAH patients using a combined ICP-Laser, Doppler, fiberoptic probe. J Neurosurg Anesthesiol 1996: 8: 199–207.

Josko J, Hendryk S, Jedrzejowska-Szypulka H, Slowinski J, et al. Effect of endothelin-1 receptor antagonist BQ-123 on basilar artery diameter after subarachnoid hemorrhage (SAH) in rats. J Physiol Pharmacol 2000: 51: 241–249.

Juul R, Hara H, Gisvold SE, et al. Alterations in perivascular dilatory neuropeptides (CGRP, SP, VIP) in the external jugular vein and in the cerebrospinal fluid following subarachnoid haemorrhage in man. Acta Neurochir 1995: 132: 32–41.

Juvela S. Aspirine and delayed ischemia after aneurysmal subarachnoid haemorrhage. J Neurosurg 1995: 82: 945–952.

Juvela S. Plasma endothelin concentrations after aneurysmal subarachnoid hemorrhage. J Neurosurg 2000: 92: 390–400.

Kajita Y, Suzuki Y, Oyama H, et al. Combined effect of L-arginine and superoxide dismutase on the spastic basilar artery after subarachnoid haemorrhage in dogs. J Neurosurg 1994: 80: 476–483.

Kak VK, Taylor AR. Cerebral blood flow in subarachnoid haemorrhage. Lancet 1967: 1: 875–877.

Kaku Y, Yonekawa Y, Tsukahara T, Kazekawa K. Superselective intra-arterial infusion of papaverine for the treatment of cerebral vasospasm after subarachnoid haemorrhage. J Neurosurg 1992: 77: 842–847.

Kanamaru K, Weir BKA, Findley JM, et al. A dosage study of the effect of 21-aminosteroid U-74006F on chronic cerebral vasospasm in a primate model. Neurosurgery 1990: 27: 29–38.

Kanamary K, Weir BKA, Simpson I, et al. Effect of 21-aminosteroid U-74006F on lipid peroxidation in subarachnoid clot. J. Neurosurg 1991: 74: 454–459.

Kaplan BJ, Gravenstein N, Friedman WA, et al. Effects of induced hypotension during experimental vasospasm: A neurological electrophysiological, and pathological analysis. Neurosurgery 1986: 19: 41–48.

Kapp J Mahaley MS, Odom GI. Cerebral arterial spasm Part 2: Experimental evaluation of mechanical and humoral factors in pathogenesis. J Neurosurg 1968a: 29: 339–349.

Kapp J Mahaley MS, Odom GI. Cerebral arterial spasm Part 1: Evaluation of experimental variables affecting the diameter of the exposed basilar artery. J Neurosurg 1968b: 29: 331–338.

Kapp J, Mahaley MS Jr, Odom GL. Experimental evaluation of potential spasmolytic drugs. J Neurosurg 1970: 32: 468–472.

Kapp JP, Neill WR, Neill CL, et al. The three phases of vasospasm. Surg Neurol 1982: 18: 40–45.

Kapp J, Neill WR, Salter JE, Barnes TY. Systemic heparin in early management of ruptured intracranial aneurysms: Review of 104 consecutive cases and comparison with concurrent controls. Neurosurgery 1987: 20: 564–570.

Karibe H, Sato K, Shimizu H, et al. Intraoperative mild hypothermia ameliorates postoperative cerebral blood flow impairment in patients with aneurysmal subarachnoid hemorrhage. Neurosurgery 2000: 47: 594–601.

Kassell NK, Peerless SJ, Reilly PL. ICP, aneurysms, and subarachnoid haemorrhage. In: Beks JWF, Bosch DA, Brock M (eds). Intracranial Pressure III, Springer Verlag, Berlin, Heidelberg, New York, 1976: pp 147–150.

Kassell NK, Torner JC. Epidemiology of intracranial aneurysms. Int. Anaestesiol Clin 1982: 20: 13–17.

Kassell NF, Sasaki T, Colohan ART, et al. Cerebral vasospasm following subarachnoid haemorrhage. Stroke 1985: 16: 562–572.

Kassell NK, Torner CJ, Haley C et al. The international cooperative study on the timing of aneurysm surgery. Part 1: Overall management results. J Neurosurg 1990a: 73: 18–36.

Kassell NK, Torner CJ, Jane JA et al. The international cooperative study on the timing of aneurysm surgery. Part 2: Surgical results. J Neurosurg 1990b: 73: 37–47.

Kassell NF, Helm G, Simmons N, et al. Treatment of cerebral vasospasm with intra-arterial papaverine. J Neurosurg 1992: 77: 848–852.

Kassell NF, Haley C, Apperson-Hansen C, et al. Randomized double-blind, vehicle-controlled trial of tirilazad mesylate in patients with aneurysmal subarachnoid haemorrhage: A cooperative study in Europe, Australia, and New Zealand. J Neurosurg 1996: 84: 221–228.

Kasuya H, Weir BKA, White DM, et al. Mechanism of oxy-hemoglobin-induced release of endothelin from cultured vascular endothelial cells and smooth-muscle cells. J Neurosurg 1993: 79: 892–898.

Kaye AH, Brownbill D. Postoperative intracranial pressure in patients operated for cerebral aneurysms following subarachnoid haemorrhage. J Neurosurg 1981: 54: 726–732.

Kazuki S, Ohta T, Ogawa R, et al. Effects of intraluminal or extraluminal endothelin on perfused rabbit basilar arteries. J Neurosurg 1997: 86: 859–865.

Kelly PJ, Gorten RJ, Grossman RG et al. Cerebral perfusion, vascular spasm, and outcome in patients with ruptured intracranial aneurysms. J Neurosurg 1977: 47: 44–49

KettWhite R, Hutchinson PJ, et al. Effects of variation in cerebral haemodynamics during aneurysm surgery on tissue oxygenation and metabolisme.Proceeding XI ICP symposium, Cambridge 2000, O10-1, page 81.

Khurana VG, Piepgras DG, Whisnant JP. Ruptured giant intracranial aneurysms. Part I. A study of rebleeding. J Neurosurg 1998: 88: 425–429.

Kim P, Yakch TL, Romero SD, Sundt TM Jr. Production of uric acid in cerebrospinal fluid after subarachnoid haemorrhage in dogs. Investigation of the possible role of Xanthine oxidase in chronic vasospasm. Neurosurgery 1987: 21: 39–44.

Kim P, Sundt TM Jr, Vanhoutte PM. Loss of endothelium-dependent relaxations and maintenance of endothelium-dependent contractions in chronic vasospasm following subarachnoid haemorrhage. In Wilkins RH (ed) Cerebral Vasospasm, New York, Raven Press, 1988: pp 145–150.

Kim P, Lorenz RR, Sundt TM Jr, Vanhoutte PM. Release of endothelium-derived relaxing factor after subarachnoid haemorrhage. J Neurosurg 1989: 70: 108–114.

Kim P, Jones JD, Sundt TM. High-energy phosphate levels in the cerebral artery during chronic vasospasm after subarachnoid haemorrhage. J Neurosurg 1992: 76: 991–996.

Kinugasa K, Mandai S, Terai Y et al. Direct thrombosis of aneurysms with cellulose acetate polymer Part II: Preliminary clinical experience. J Neurosurg 1992: 77: 501–507.

Kistler JP, Crowell RM, Davis KR et al. The relation of cerebral vasospasm to the extent and location of subarachnoid blood visualized by CT scan: A prospective study. Neurology 1983: 33: 424–436.

Klingelhöfer J, Sander D, Holzgraefe M, et al. Cerebral vasospasm evaluated by transcranial Doppler ultrasonography at different intracranial pressures. J Neurosurg 1991: 75: 752–758.

Kobayashi H, Hayashi M, Kobayashi S, et al. Effect of endothelin on the canine basilar artery. Neurosurgery 1990: 27: 357–361.

Kobayashi H, Hayashi M, Kobayashi S, et al. Cerebral vasospasm and vasoconstriction caused by endothelin. Neurosurgery 1991: 28: 672–679.

Kobayashi H, Ide H, Handa Y, et al. Effect of leukotrine antagonist on experimental delayed cerebral vasospasm. Neurosurgery 1992: 31: 550–556.

Konichi Y, Maemura E, Sato E et al. A therapy against vasospasm after subarachnoid haemorrhage: Clinical experience of balloon angioplasty. Neurol Res 1990: 12: 103–105.

Kosnik EJ, Hunt WE. Postoperative hypertension in the management of patients with intracranial arterial aneurysms. J Neurosurg 1976: 45: 148–154.

Kosteljanetz M. CSF dynamics in patients with subarachnoid and/or intraventricular haemorrhage. J Neurosurg 1984: 60: 940–946.

Krasznai L, Grote EH. Acute vasoparalysis after subarachnoid haemorrhage and cerebral trauma: General reflex phenomenon? Neurol Res 1994: 16: 40–44.

Krayenbühl HA, Yasargil MG, Glamm ES et al. Microsurgical treatment of intracranial saccular aneurysms. J Neurosurg 1972: 37: 678–686.

Kudo T, Suzuki S, Iwabuchi T. Importance of monitoring the circulation blood volume in patients with cerebral vasospasm after subarachnoid haemorrhage. Neurosurgery 1981: 9: 514–520.

Kuwamura Sh, Sayama I, Yasui N, Uemura K. Sequential changes in cerebral blood flow and metabolism in patients with subarachnoid haemorrhage. Acta Neurochir (Wien) 1992: 114: 12–15.

Kuwayama A, Zervas NT, Shintani A, et al. Papaverine hydrochoride and experimental haemorrhagic cerebral arterial spasm. Stroke 1972: 3: 27–33.

Kwan A-L, Bavbek M, Jeng AY, et al. Prevention and reversal of cerebral vasospasm by an endothelin-converting enzyme inhibitor, CGS 26303, in an experimental model of subarachnoid haemorrhage. J Neurosurg 1997: 87: 281–286.

Kwan A-L, Lin C-H, Yanamoto H, et al. Systemic administration of the potassium channel activator cromakalim attenuates cerebral vasospasm after experimental subarachnoid haemorrhage. Neurosurgery 1998: 42: 347–351.

Kwan AL, Bavlek M, Jeng AY, et al. Attenuation of experimental subarachnoid hemorrhage-induced cerebral vasospasm by CGS 26303, an endothelin-converting enzyme inhibitor. J Cardiovasc Pharmacol 1998: 31 (suppl 1): S320–322.

Lam JMK, Smielewski P, Czosnyka M, et al. Predicting delayed ischemic deficits after aneurysmal subarachnoid hemorrhage using a transient hyperemic response test of cerebral autoregulation. Neurosurgery 2000: 47: 819–826.

Lang EW, Diehl RR, Mehdorn HM. Cerebral autoregulation testing after aneurysmal subarachnoid hemorrhage. The phase relationship between arterial blood pressure and cerebral blood flow velocity. Crit Care med 2001: 29: 158–163.

Lanzino G, Kassell NF, Germanson T, et al. Plasma glucose levels and outcome after aneurysmal subarachnoid haemorrhage. J Neurosurg 1993: 79: 885–891.

Lanzino G, Kongable GL, Kassell NF. Electrocardiographic abnormalities after non-traumatic subarachnoid haemorrhage. J Neurosurg Anesthesiol 1994: 6: 156–162.

Lanzino G, Kassell NF, Dorsch NW, et al. Double-blind, randomized, vehicle-controlled study of high-dose tirilazad mesylate in women with aneurysmal subarachnoid hemorrhage. Part I. A cooperative study in Europe, Australia, New Zealand, and South Africa. J Neurosurg 1999: 90: 1011–1017.

Lanzine G, Kassell NF. Double-blind, randomized, vehicle-controlled study of high-dose tirilazad mesylate in women with aneurysmal subarachnoid hemorrhage. Part 2. A cooperative study in North America, J Neurosurg 1999: 90: 1018–1024.
Larson JL, Tew JM, Tomsick TA, et al. Treatment of aneurysms of the internal carotid artery by intravascular balloon occlusion. Long-term follow-up of 58 patients. Neurosurgery 1995: 36: 23–30.
Larsson LI, Edvinsson L, Fahrenkrug J, et al. Immunohistochemical localization of a vasodilatory polypeptide (VIP) in cerebrovascular nerves. Brain Res 1976: 113: 400–404.
Laumer R, Steinmeier R, Gönner F, et al. Cerebral hemodynamics in subarachnoid haemorrhage evaluated by transcranial Doppler sonography. Part 1. Reliability of flow velocities in clinical management. Neurosurgery 1993: 33: 1–9.
Lavine SD, Masri LS, Levy ML, et al. Temporary occlusion of the middle cerebral artery in intracranial aneurysm surgery: time limitation and advantage of brain protection. J Neurosurg 1997: 87: 817–824.
Lee TJF, Su C, Bevan JA. Nonsympathetic dilator innervation of cat cerebral arteries. Experientia 1975: 31: 1424–1426.
Lee TJF, Saito A, Berezin I. Vasoactive intestinal polypeptide-like substance: The potential transmitter for cerebral vasodilation. Science 224: 1984: 898–901.
Lefkowitz MA, Gobin P, Akiba Y, et al. Balloon-assisted Guglielmi detachable coiling of wide-necked aneurysms. Part II - Clinical results. Neurosurgery 1999: 45: 531–538.
Le Roux PD, Dailey AT, Newell DW, et al. Emergent aneurysm clipping without angiography in the moribund patient with intracerebral haemorrhage: The use of infusion computed tomography. Neurosurgery 1993: 33: 189–197.
Le Roux PD, Newell DW, Eskridge J, et al. Severe symptomatic vasospasm: The role of immediate postoperative angioplasty. J Neurosurg 1994: 80: 224–229.
Le Roux PD, Elliott JP, Newell DW, et al. Predicting outcome in poor-grade patients with subarachnoid haemorrhage: A retrospective review of 159 aggressively managed cases. J Neurosurg 1996: 85: 39–49.
Le Veen RF, Wolf GL, Biery D. Angioplasty-induced vasospasm in rabbit model: Mechanisms and treatment. Invest Radiol 1985: 20: 938–944.
Levy ML, Giannotta SL. Induced hypertension and hypervolemia for treatment of cerebral vasospasm. Neurosurg Clin N Am 1990: 1: 357–365.
Levy ML, Rabb CH, Zelman V, Gianotta SL. Cardiac performance enhancement from dobutamine in patients refractory to hypervolemic therapy for cerebral vasospasm. J Neurosurg 1993: 79: 494–499.
Lewis PJ, Weir BKA, Nosko MG, et al. Intrathecal nimodipine therapy in a primate model of chronic cerebral vasospasm. Neurosurgery 1988: 22: 492–500.
Lindegaard K-F, Nornes H, Bakke SJ, et al. Cerebral vasospasm diagnosis by means of angiography and blood velocity measurements. Acta Neurochir (Wien) 1989: 100: 12–24.
Liszczak TM, Varsos VG, Black PM, et al. Cerebral arterial constriction after experimental subarachnoid haemorrhage is associated with blood components within the arterial wall. J Neurosurg 1983: 58: 18–26.
Loach AB, Benedict CR. Plasma catecholamine concentration associated with cerebral vasospasm. J Neurol Sci 1980: 45: 261–271.
Lobato RD, Marin J, Salaices M, et al. Cerebrovascular reactivity to noradrenaline and serotonin following experimental subarachnoid haemorrhage. J Neurosurg 1980: 53: 480–485.
Loch Macdonald R, Weir BKA, Runzer TD, et al. Effect of intrathecal superoxide dismutase and catalase on oxyhemoglobin-induced vasospasm in monkeys. Neurosurgery 1992: 30: 529 - 539.
Luer MS, Slavin KV, Hernandez-Avila G, et al. Regional cerebral oxygen saturation during intra-arterial papaverine therapy for vasospasm. Case report. Neurosurg 1995: 36: 1033–1036.
Ma X-D, Hauerberg J, Pedersen DB, Juhler M. Effects of morphine on cerebral blood flow autoregulation and CO_2-reactivity in experimental subarachnoid hemorrhage. J Neurosurg Anesthesiol 1999: 11: 264–272.
Ma X-D, Willumsen L, Hauerberg J, et al. Effects of graded hyperventilation on cerebral blood flow autoregulation in experimental subarachnoid hemorrhage. J Cereb Blood Flow Metab 2000: 20: 718–725.
MacDonald RL, Wallace MC, Coyne TJ. The effect of surgery on the severity of vasospasm. J Neurosurg 1994: 80: 433–439.
MacDonald RL, Cerebral vasospasm. Neurosurg Quarterly 1995: 5: 73–97.
MacDonald RL, Zhang J, Sima B, et al. Papaverine-sensitive vasospasm and arterial contractility and compliance after subarachnoid haemorrhage in dogs. Neurosurgery 1995: 37: 962–968.
Macfarlane R, Teramura A, Owen CJ et al. Treatment of vasospasm with a 480-nm pulsed-dye laser. J Neurosurg 1991: 75: 613–622.
Maeda Y, Tani E, Iyamoto T. Prostaglandin metabolism in experimental cerebral vasospasm. J Neurosurg 1981: 55: 779–785.
Manninen PH, Belb AW, et al. Perioperative electrocardiographic monitoring of patients with cerebral aneurysms. Can J Anaesth. P 107.
Manno EM, Gress DR, Schwamm LH, et al. Effects of induced hypertension on transcranial Doppler untrasound velocities in patients with subarachnoid hemorrhage. Stroke 1998: 29: 422–428.
Marion DW, Segal R, Thompson ME. Subarachnoid haemorrhage and the heart. Neurosurgery 1986: 18: 101–106.
Maroon JC, Nelson PB. Hypovolemia in patients with subarachnoid haemorrhage. Therapeutic implications. Neurosurgery 1979: 4: 223–226.
Marston SB. The regulation of smooth muscle contractile proteins. Prog Biophys Molec Biol 1982: 41: 1–41.
Martins AN, Wiley JK. Side effects of spasmolytic agents in the monkey. Intracisternal phenoxybenzamine and phentolamine. J Neurosurg 1973: 39: 629–635.
Masaoka H, Suziki R, Hirata Y et al. Raised plasma endothelin in aneurysmal subarachnoid haemorrhage. Lancet (letter) 1989: 2: 1402.
Mascia L, Ranieri VM, Zhang H, et al. The role of pro-inflammatory and anti-inflammatory cytokines in the development of vasospasm after subarachnoid hemorrhage. Proceeding XI ICP symposium, Cambridge 2000: P6-1, page 175.
Mascia L, Stewart DJ, Fedorko L. et al. The role of endothelin-1 in the pathogenesis of cerebral vasospasm in patients with aneurysmal subarachnoid hemorrhage. Proceeding XI ICP symposium, Cambridge 2000: P6-2, page 176.

Massicotte EM, del Bigio MR. Human arachnoid villi response to subarachnoid haemorrhage: Possible relationship to chronic hydrocephalus. J Neurosurg 1999: 91: 80–84.
Mathiesen T, Andersson B, Loftenius A, von Holst H. Increased interleukin-6 levels in cerebrospinal fluid following subarachnoid haemorrhage. J Neurosurg 1993: 78: 562–567.
Mathiesen T, Edner G, Ulfarson E, Andersson B. Cerebrospinal fluid interleukin-1 receptor antagonist and tumor necrosis factor- following subarachnoid haemorrhage. J Neurosurg 1997: 87: 215–220.
Matsui T, Kaizu H, Itoh S, Asano T. The role of active smooth-muscle contraction in the occurrence of chronic vasospasm in the canine two-haemorrhage model. J Neurosurg 1994. 80: 276–282.
Matsui T, Asano T. Effects of new 21-aminosteroid tirilazad mesylate (U74006F) on chronic cerebral vasospasm in a "two-haemorrhage" model of beagle dogs. Neurosurgery 1994: 34: 1035–1039.
Matz PG, Weinstein P, States B, et al. Subarachnoid injections of lysed blood induce the hsp70 stress gene and produce DNA fragmentation in focal areas of the rat brain. Stroke 1996a: 27: 504–512.
Matz PG, Sundaresan S, Sharp FR, et al. Induction of HSP70 in rat brain following subarachnoid haemorrhage produced by endovascular perforation. J Neurosurg 19956b: 85: 138–145.
Mayer SA, LiMandri G, Sherman D. Electrocardiographic markers of abnormal left ventricular wall motion in acute subarachnoid haemorrhage. J Neurosurg 1995: 83: 889–896.
McAuliffe W, Townsend M, Eskrige JM, et al. Intracranial pressure changes induced during papaverine infusion for treatment of vasospasm. J Neurosurg 1995: 83: 430–434.
McDermott MW, Durity FA, Borozny M, et al. Temporary vessel occlusion and barbiturate protection in cerebral aneurysm surgery. Neurosurgery 1989: 25: 54–62.
McGillicuddy J, Kindt G, Gianotta S, Ostrowski P. Focal cerebral blood flow in cerebral vasospasm: The effect of intravascular volume expansion. Acta Neurol Scand 1979: 60 (suppl 72): 490–491.
McKissock W, Richardson A, Walch L. Middle cerebral aneurysms. Further results in the controlled trial of conservative and surgical treatment of ruptured intracranial aneurysms. Lancet 1962: 2: 417–421.
McKissock W, Richarson A, Walch L. Anterior communicating aneurysms. A trial of conservative and surgical treatment. Lancet 1965: 1: 873–876.
Medlock MD, Dulebohm SC, Elwood PW. Prophyllactic hypervolemia without calcium channel blockers in early aneurysm surgery. Neurosurgery 1992: 30: 12–16.
Mee E, Dorrance D, Lowe D, Neil-Dwyer G. Controlled study of nimodipine in aneurysm patients treated early after subarachnoid haemorrhage. Neurosurgery 1988: 22: 484–491.
Mendelow AD, McCalden TA, Hattingh J, et al. Cerebrovascular reactivity and metabolism after subarachnoid haemorrhage in baboons. Stroke 1981: 12: 58–65.
Mercier P, Alhayek G, Rizk T, et al. Are the calcium antagonists really useful in cerebral aneurysmal surgery? A retrospective study. Neurosurgery 1994: 34: 30–37.
Merory J, Thomas DJ, Humprey PRD et al. Cerebral blood flow after surgery for recent subarachnoid haemorrhage. J Neurol Neurosurg Psychiat 1980: 43: 214–221.
Messeter K, Brandt L, Ljunggren B, et al. Prediction and prevention of delayed ischaemic dysfunction after aneurysmal subarachnoid haemorrhage and early operation. Neurosurgery 1987: 20: 548–553.
Meyer CHA, Lowe D, Meyer M, et al. Subarachnoid haemorrhage: Older patients have low cerebral blood flow. Br Med J 1982: 285: 1149–1153.
Meyer CHA, Lowe D, Meyer M, et al. Progressive change in cerebral blood flow during the first three weeks after subarachnoid haemorrhage. Neurosurgery 1983: 12: 58–76.
Mickey B, Vorstrup S, Voldby B, et al. Serial measurement of regional cerebral blood flow in patients with SAH using 133 Xe inhalation and emission computerized tomography. J Neurosurg 1984: 60: 916–922.
Milbrun JM, Moran CJ, Cross DT, et al. Increase in diameter of vasospastic intracranial arteries by intraarterial papaverine administration. J Neurosurg 1998: 88: 38–42.
Miller JA, Cross DT, Moran CJ, et al. Severe thrombocytopenia following intraarterial papaverine administration for treatment of vasospasm. J Neurosurg 1995: 83: 435–437.
Millikan CH. Cerebral vasospasm and ruptured intracranial aneurysm. Arch Neurol 1975: 32: 433–449.
Mima T, Yanagisawa M, Shigeno T, et al. Endothelin acts in feline and canine cerebral arteries from adventitial side. Stroke 1989: 20: 1553–1556.
Minami N, Tani E, Maeda Y, et al. Effects of inhibitors of protein kinase C and calpain in experimental delayed cerebral vasospasm. J Neurosurg 1992: 76: 111–118.
Miyaoka M, Sato K, Ishii S. A clinical study of the relationship of timing to outcome of surgery for ruptured cerebral aneurysms. J Neurosurg 1993: 79: 373–378.
Mizoi K, Yoshimoto T, Fujiwara S et al. Prevention of vasospasm by clot removal and intrathecal bolus injection of tissue-type plasminogen activator: Preliminary report. Neurosurgery 1991: 28: 807–813.
Mizoi K, Yoshimoto T, Takahashi A, et al. Prospective study on the prevention of cerebral vasospasm by intrathecal fibrinolytic therapy with tissue-type plasminogen activator. J Neurosurg 1993: 78: 430–437.
Mizukami M, Kawase T, Usami T, Tazawa T. Prevention of vasospasm by early operation with removal of subarachnoid blood. Neurosurgery 1982: 10: 301–307.
Mohr G, Ferguson G, Khan M, et al. Intraventricular hemorrhage from ruptured aneurysm. J Neurosurg 1983: 58: 482–487.
Morgan MK, Day MJ, Little N, et al. The use of intraarterial papaverine in the management of vasospasm complicating arteriovenous malformation resection. J Neurosurg 1995: 82: 296–299.
Moskowitz MA, Kiwak KJ, Hekimian K, Levine L. Synthesis of compounds with properties of leucotrienes C4 and D4 in gerbil brains after ischemia and reperfusion. Science 1984: 224: 886–889.
Mountz JM, McGillicuddy JE, Wilson MW, et al. Pre- and post-operative cerebral blood flow changes in subarachnoid hemorrhage. Acta Neurochir (Wien) 1991: 109: 30–33.
Muizelaar JP, Becker DP. Induced hypertension for the treatment of cerebral ischemia after subarachnoid hemorrhage. Surg Neurol 1986: 25: 317–325.
Muizellar JP, Zwienenberg M, Rudisill NA, Hecht ST. The prophylactic use of transluminal balloon angioplasty in patients with Fisher grade 3 subarachnoid hemorrhage: a pilot study. J Neurosurg 1999: 91: 51–58.

Murayama Y, Malisch T, Guglielmi G, et al. Incidence of cerebral vasospasm after endovascular treatment of acutely ruptured aneurysms: report of 69 cases. J Neurosurg 1997: 87: 830–835.

Naderi S, Ozgüven A, Bayhan H, et al. Evaluation of cerebral vasospasm in patients with subarachnoid hemorrhage using single photon emission computed tomography. Neurosurg Rev 1994: 17: 261–265.

Nagai H, Noda S, Mabe H. Experimental cerebral vasospasm. Part 2: Effects of vasoactive drugs and sympathectomy on early and late spasm. J Neurosurg 1975: 42: 420–428.

Nakagomi T, Kassell NF, Sasiki T, et al. Impairment of endothelium-dependent vasodilation induced by acetylcholine and adenosine triphosphate following experimental subarachnoid hemorrhage. Stroke 1987: 18: 482–489.

Nakashima T, Takenaka K, Nishinura Y et al. Phospholipase C activity in cerebrospinal fluid following subarachnoid hemorrhage related to brain damage. J Cereb Blood Flow Metab 1993: 13: 255–259.

Näveri L, Strömberg C, Saavedra JM. Angiotensin IV reverses the acute cerebral blood flow reduction after experimental subarachnoid hemorrhage in the rat. J Cereb Blood Flow Metab 1994: 14: 1096–1099.

Neil-Dwyer G, Walter P, Cruickchank JM, et al. Effect of propranolol and phentolamine on myocardial necrosis after subarachnoid hemorrhage. Br Med J 1978: 2: 990–992.

Nelson RJ, Perry S, Hames TK, Pickard JD. Transcranial Doppler ultrasound studies of cerebral autoregulation and subarachnoid hemorrhage in the rabbit. J Neurosurg 1990: 73: 601–610.

Nichols DA. Endovascular treatment of the acutely ruptured intracranial aneurysm [guest editorial] J Neurosurg 1993: 79: 1–2.

Nichols DA, Brown RD, Thielen KR, et al. Endovascular treatment of ruptured posterior circulation aneurysms using electrolytically detachable coils. J Neurosurg 1997: 87: 374–380.

Nishizawa S, Peterson JW, Shimoyama I, Uemura K. Relation between protein kinase C and calmodulin systems in cerebrovascular contraction: Investigation of the pathogenesis of vasospasm after subarachnoid hemorrhage. Neurosurgery 1992: 31: 711–716.

Nishizawa S, Nezu N, Uemura K. Direct evidence for a key role of protein kinase C in the development of vasospasm after subarachnoid hemorrhage. J Neurosurg 1992: 76: 635–639.

Nishizawa S, Chen D, Yokoyama T, et al. Endothein-1 initiates the development of vasospasm after subarachnoid haemorrhage through protein kinase C activation, but does not contribute to prolonged vasospasm. Acta Neurochir (Wien) 2000: 142: 1409–1415.

Nornes H, Magnæs B. Intracranial pressure in patients with ruptured saccular aneurysm. J Neurosurg 1972: 36: 537–548.

Nosko M, Weir BKA, Lunt A, et al. Effect of clot removal at 24 hours on chronic vasospasm after SAH in the primate model. J Neurosurg 1987: 66: 416–422.

Nosko M, Schultz R, Weir B, et al. Effects of vasospasm on level of prostacyclin and thromboxane A2 in cerebral arteries of the monkey. Neurosurgery 1988: 22: 45–50.

Ogata M, Marshall BM, Lougheed WM. Observations on the effects on intrathecal papaverine in experimental vasospasm. J Neurosurg 1975: 38: 20–25.

Ogilvy CS, Carter BS, Kaplan S, et al. Temporary vessel occlusion for aneurysm surgery. Risk factors for stroke in patients pretreated by induced hypothermia and hypertension and intravenous mannitol administration. J Neurosurg 1996: 84: 785–791.

Ogilvy CS, Carter BS. A proposed comprehensive grading system to predict outcome for surgical management of intracranial aneurysms. Neurosurgery 1998: 42: 959–970.

Ogane K, Suzuki S, Ohkuma H, et al. Adventitial hyperpermeability after subarachnoid hemorrhage, and its prevention with intrathecal steroid administration in rats. Proceeding of the 8-th symposium of Cerebral Vasospam, Tokyo 1982: 8: 245–251.

Ohkuma H, Parney I, Megyesi J, et al. Antisera preproendothelin-oligoDNA therapy for vasospasm in a canine model of subarachnoid hemorrhage. J Neurosurg 1999: 90: 1105–1114.

Öhman J, Heiskanen O. Effect of nimodipine on the outcome of patients after aneurysmal subarachnoid hemorrhage and surgery. J Neurosurg 1988: 69: 683–686.

Öhman J, Servo Am Heiskanen O. Risks factors for cerebral infarction in good-grade patients after aneurysmal subarachnoid hemorrhage and surgery: A prospective study. J Neurosurg 1991a: 74: 14–20.

Öhman J, Servo A, Heiskanen O. Long-term effects of nimodipine on cerebral infarcts and outcome after aneurysmal subarachnoid hemorrhage and surgery. J Neurosurg 1991b: 74: 8–13.

Öhman J, Servo A, Heiskanen O. Effect of intrathecal fibrinolytic therapy on clot lysis and vasospasm in patients with aneurysmal subarachnoid hemorrhage. J Neurosurg 1991c: 75: 197–201.

Ohta H, Yasui N, Suzuki A. et al. [Hemorrhagic infarction following vasospasm due to a ruptured intracranial aneurysm] (Jpn) Neurol Med Chir 1982: 22: 716–724.

Okada T, Harada T, Bark DH, et al. A rat femoral artery model for vasospasm. Neurosurgery 1990: 27: 349–356.

Okada Y, Shima T, Nishida M, et al. Comparison of transcranial Doppler investigation of aneurysmal vasospasm with digital subtraction angiographic and clinical findings. Neurosurgery 1999: 45: 443–450.

O'Laoire SA. Intracranial aneurysms: An analysis of the results of microneurosurgery and the causes of operative mortality and morbidity. University of Cork (Ireland), Thesis 1978.

O`Neill P, Walton S, Foy PM, Shaw MDM. Role of prostaglandins in delayed cerebral ischemia after subarachnoid hemorrhage. Neurosurgery 1991: 30: 17–22.

Onoue H, Katusic ZS. Subarachnoid hemorrhage and the role of potassium channels in relaxations of canine basilar artery to nitrovasodilators. J Cereb Blood Flow Metab 1998: 18: 186–195.

Pakarinen S. Incidence, aetiology, and prognosis of primary subarachnoid hemorrhage: A study based on 589 cases diagnosed in a defined urban population during a defined period. Acta Neurol Scand 1967: 43 (suppl 29): 1–128.

Pasqualin A, Tsukahara T, Kassell NF, Torner JC. Effect of nicardipine on basilar artery vasoactive responses after subarachnoid hemorrhage. Neurosurgery 1992: 31: 697–704.

Park CC, Shin ML, Simard JM. The complement membrane attack complex and the bystand effect in cerebral vasospasm. J Neurosurg 1997: 87: 294–300.

Park S, Rasmussen H. Carcachol-induced protein phosphorylation changes in bovine tracheal smooth muscle. J Biol Chem 1986: 261: 15734–15739.

Paul KS, WhalleY ET, Forster C, et al. Prostacyclin and cerebral vessel relaxation. J Neurosurg 1982: 57: 344–350.

Payner TD, Horner TG, Leipzig TJ, et al. Role of intraoperative angiography in the surgical treatment of cerebral aneurysm. J Neurosurg 1998: 88: 441–448.

Peerless S, Yasargil M. Adrenergic innervation of the cerebral blood vessels in the rabbit. J Neurosurg 1971: 35: 148–154.

Pellettieri L, Carlsson C-A, Lindholm L. Is the vasospasm following subarachnoid hemorrhage an immunoreactive disease? Experientia 1981: 37: 1170.

Pellettieri L, Nilsson B, Carlsson C-A, Nilsson U. Serum immunocomplexes in patients with subarachnoid hemorrhage. Neurosurgery 1986: 19: 767–771.

Pelofsky S, Jacobson DW. Effects of prostaglandin E1 on experimental cerebral vasospasm. J Neurosurg 1972: 36: 634–639.

Perret GE, Nibbelink DW. Randomized treatment study. Carotid ligation. In: Sahs AL, Nibbelink DW, Torner CJ (eds). Aneurysmal subarachnoid hemorrhage. Baltimore, Urban and Schwarzenberg 1981: 121–143.

Persson L, Valtysson J, Enblad P, et al. Neurochemical monitoring using intracerebral microdialysis in patients with subarachnoid hemorrhage. J Neurosurg 1996: 84: 606–616.

Petersen KD, Landsfeldt U, Cold GE, et al. ICP during three anaesthetics for elective craniotomy. J Neurosurg Anesthesiol 2000: 12: A-15: 167.

Peterson EW, Cardoso ER. The blood-brain barrier following experimental subarachnoid hemorrhage. Part I: Response to insult caused by arterial hypertension. J Neurosurg 1983: 58: 388–394.

Peterson JW, Kwun BD, Hackett JD, et al. The role of inflammation in experimental vasospasm. J Neurosurg 1990: 72: 767–774.

Petruk KC, West GR, Marriott MR, et al. Cerebral blood flow following induced subarachnoid hemorrhage in the monkey. J Neurosurg 1972: 37: 316–324.

Petruk KC, West M. Mohr G et al. Nimodipine treatment in poor-grade aneurysm patients. J Neurosurg 1988: 68: 505–517.

Pickard JD, MacDonell LA, MacKenzie ET et al. Prostaglandin-induced effects on the primate cerebral circulation. Eur J Pharmacol 1977: 43: 343–351.

Pickard JD, Matheson M, Patterson J, Wyper D. Prediction of late ischemic complications after cerebral aneurysm surgery by the intraoperative measurement of cerebral blood flow. J Neurosurg 1980: 53: 305–308.

Pickard JD, Murray GD, Illingwoth R, et al. Effect of nimodipine on cerebral infarction and outcome after subarachnoid hemorrhage: British Aneurysm Nimodipine Trial. Br Med J 1989: 298: 636–642.

Pickard JD, Walker V, Brandt L, et al. Effect of intraventricular haemorrhage and rebleeding following subarachnoid haemorrhage on CSF eicosanoids. Acta Neurochir (Wien) 1994: 129: 152–157.

Piepgras DG, Khurana VG, Whisnant JP. Ruptured giant intracranial aneurysms. Part II. A retrospective analysis of timing and outcome of surgical treatment. J Neurosurg 1998: 88: 430–435.

Pluta RM, Zauner A, Morgan JK, et al. Is vasospasm related to proliferative arteriopathy? J Neurosurg 1992: 77: 740–748.

Pluta RM, Deka-Starosta A, Zauner A. et al. Neuropeptide Y in the primate model of subarachnoid hemorrhage. J Neurosurg 1992: 77: 417–423.

Pluta RM, Oldfield EH, Boock RJ. Reversal and prevention of cerebral vasospasm by intracarotid infusions of nitric oxide doners in a primate model of subarachnoid hemorrhage. J Neurosurg 1997: 87: 746–751.

Pluta RM, Boock RJ, Afshar JK, et al. Source and cause of endothelin-1 release into cerebrospinal fluid after subarachnoid hemorrhage. J Neurosurg 1997: 87: 287–293.

Pluta RM, Afshar JKB, Thompson BG, et al. Increased cerebral blood flow but no reversal or prevention of vasospasm in response to L-arginine infusion after subarachnoid hemorrhage. J Neurosurg 2000: 92: 121–126.

Polin RS, Hansen CA, German P, et al. Intra-arterially administered papaverine for the treatment of symptomatic cerebral vasospasm. Neurosurgery 1998: 42: 1256–1267.

Prado R, Watson BD, Kuluz J, Dietrich WD. Endothelium-derived nitric oxide synthase inhibition. Effects on cerebral blood flow, pial artery diameter, and vascular morphology in rats. Stroke 1992: 23: 1118–1124.

Pritz MB, Giannotti SL, Kindt GW, et al. Treatment of patients with neurological deficits associated with cerebral vasospasm by intravascular volume expansion. Neurosurgery 1978: 3: 364–368.

Proust F, Callonec F, Clavier E, et al. Usefulness of transcranial color-coded sonography in the diagnosis of cerebral vasospasm. Stroke 1999. 30: 1091–1098.

Quintana L, Konda R, Ishibashi Y et al. The effect of prostacyclin on cerebral vasospasm. An experimental study. Acta Neurochir 1982: 62: 187–193.

Qureshi AI, Sung GY, Asad M, et al. Prognostic value and determinants of ultraearly angiographic vasospasm after aneurysmal subarachnoid hemorrhage. Neurosurgery 1999: 44: 967–974.

Rabow L, Algers G, Elfversson J, et al. Does a routine operation for intracranial aneurysm incur brain damage? Acta Neurochir 1995: 133: 13–16.

Rasmussen G, Bergholt B, Dahl B, et al. Effect of nimodipine on cerebral blood flow and cerebrovascular reactivity after subarachnoid hemorrhage. Acta Neurol Scand 1999: 99: 182–186.

Rasmussen H, Haller H, Takuwa Y, et al. Messenger Ca++, protein kinase C, and smooth muscle contraction. Prog Clin Biol Res 1990: 327: 89–106.

Richards PG, Marath A, Edwards JMR, Lincoln C. Management of difficult intracranial aneurysms by deep hypothermia and elective cardiac arrest using cardiopulmonary bapass. Br J Neurosurg 1987: 1: 261–269.

Romner B, Ljunggren B, Brandt L, Säveland H. Correlation of transcranial Doppler sonography findings with timing of aneurysm surgery. J Neurosurg 1990: 73: 72–76.

Rosenblum WI, Guilianti D. Participation of cerebrovascular nerves in generalized sympathetic discharge. Arch Neurol 1973: 25: 51–54.

Rosenblum WI. Contricting effect of leucotrienens on cerebral arterioles of mice. Stroke 1985: 16: 262–263.

Rosenstein J, Wang AD-J, Symon L, Suzuki M. Relationship between hemispheric cerebral blood flow, cerebral conduction time, and clinical grade in aneurysmal subarachnoid hemorrhage. J Neurosurg 1985: 62: 25–30.

Rosenwasser RH, Delgado TE, Buchheit WA, Freed MH. Control of hypertention and prophylaxis against vasospasm in cases of subarachnoid hemorrhage. A preliminary report. Neurosurgery 1983: 12: 658–661.

Rosenwasser RH, Jallo JI, Getch CC, et al. Complications of Swan-Ganz catheterization for hemodynamic monitoring in patients with subarachnoid hemorrhage. Neurosurgery 1995: 37: 872–876.

Rosenwasser RH, Armomda RA, Thomas JE, et al. Therapeutic modalities for the management of cerebral vasospasm: Timing of endovascular options. Neurosurgery 1999: 44: 975–980.

Rosenørn J, Westergaard L, Hansen PH. Mannitol-induced rebleeding from intracranial aneurysm. J Neurosurg 1983: 59: 529–530.

Rosenørn J, Eskesen V, Schmidt K, et al. Clinical features and outcome in 1076 patients with ruptured intracranial saccular aneurysms. A prospective consecutive study. Br J Neurosurgery 1987: 1: 33–46.

Rouesseaux M, Huglo D, Steinling M. Cerebral blood flow in frontal lesions of aneurysms of the anterior communicating artery. Stroke 1994: 25: 135–140.

Roux S, Löffler B-M, Gray GA, et al. The role of endothelin in experimental cerebral vasospasm. Neurosurgery 1995: 37: 78–86.

Roux S, Breu V, Giller T, et al. Ro 61-1760, a new hydrosoluble endothelin antagonist: general pharmacology and effects on experimental cerebral vasospasm. J Pharmacol Exp Ther 1997: 283: 1110–1118.

Ruta TS, Mutch WAC. Controlled hypotension for cerebral aneurysm surgery: Are the risks worth the benefit?. J Neurosurg Anesthesiol 1991: 3: 153–156.

Saito A, Shiba R, Kimura S, et al. Vasoconstrictor response of large arteries of cats to endothelin, an endothelin-derived vasoactive peptide. Eur J Pharmacol 1989: 162: 353–358.

Saito I, Ueda Y, Sano K. Significance of vasospasm in the treatment of ruptured intracranial aneurysms. J Neurosurg 1977: 47: 412–429.

Saito I, Shigeno T, Aritake K, et al. Vasospasm assessed by angiography and computerized tomography. J Neurosurg 1979: 51: 466–475.

Saito I, Asano T, Sano K, et al. Neuroprotective effect of an antioxidant, ebselene, in patients with delayed neurological deficitis after aneurysmal subarachnoid hemorrhage. Neurosurgery 1998: 42: 269–278.

Sakai T, Tanikake T, Kyoi K. Pathological study of the late arterial spasm. Neurol Med Chir (Tokyo) 1979: 19: 1085–1093.

Sako M, Nishihara J, Ohta S, et al. Role of protein kinase C in the pathogenesis of cerebral vasospasm after subarachnoid hemorrhage. J Cereb Blood Flow Metab 1993: 13: 247–254.

Samson D, Batjar HH, Bowman G. A clinical study of the parameters and effects of temporary arterial occlusion in the management of intracranial aneurysms. Neurosurgery 1994: 34: 22–29.

Sano K, Asano T, Tanishima T, Sasaki T. Lipid peroxidation as a cause of cerebral vasospasm. Neurol Res 1980: 2: 253–272.

Sano K. Acute ischemic and delayed ischemic neurological deficits as the cause of bad grading in aneurysmal subarachmoid hemorrhage. Neurol Res 1994: 16: 35–39.

Sasaki T, Murota S, Wakai S, et al. Evaluation of prostaglandin, biosynthetic activity in canine basilar artery following subarachnoid injection of blood. J Neurosurg 1981: 55: 771–778.

Sasaki T, Ohta T, Kikuchi H, et al. A Phase II clinical trial of recombinant human tissue-type plasminogen activator against cerebral vasospasm after aneurysmal subarachnoid hemorrhage. Neurosurgery 1994: 35: 597–605.

Säveland H, Nilsson OG, Boris Møller F, et al. Intracerebral microdialysis of glutamate and aspartate in two vascular territories after subarachnoid hemorrhage. Neurosurgery 1996: 38: 12–20.

Sawada M, Hashimote N, Tsukahara T, et al. Effectiveness of intra-arterially infused papaverine solutions of various concentrations for the treatment of cerebral vasospasm. Acta Neurochir 1997: 139: 706–711.

Schievink WI, Hageman LM, Velis DNV, et al. Relationship between blood viscocity and cerebral ischemia after surgical treatment of ruptured intracranial aneurysms. Surg Neurol 1987: 27: 537–542.

Segawa H, Saito I Okada T, et al. Efficacy of intracisternal papaverine on symptomatic vasospasm. In Wilkins RH (ed) Cerebral Vasospasm, Raven Press, New York 1988, 433–441.

Seifert V, Eisert WG, Stolke D, et al. Efficacy of single intracisternal bolus injection of recombinant plasminogen activator to prevent delayed cerebral vasospasm after experimental subarachnoid hemorrhage. Neurosurgery 1989: 25: 590–598.

Seifert V. Intrathecal fibrinolysis using recombinant tissue plasminogen activator (rTPA) for prevention of cerebral vasospasm and delayed ischaemic deficits after aneurysmal subarachnoid haemorrhage. Experimental and clinical data. Neurol Res. 1994: 16: 54–58.

Sekhar LN, Heros RC. Origin, growth, and rupture of saccular aneurysms. A review. Neurosurgery 1981: 8: 248–260.

Shapiro SA, Campbell RL, Scully T. Hemorrhagic dilation of the fourth ventricle: An ominous predictor. J Neurosurg 1994: 80: 805–809.

Shaw MD, Vermeulen M, Murray GD, et al. Efficacy and safety of the endothelin receptor antagonist AK-044 in treating subarachnoid hemorrhage: a report by the Steering Committee on behalf of the UK/Netherlands/Eire TAK-044 Subarachnoid Haemorrhage Study Group. J Neurosurg 2000: 93: 992–997.

Sheehan JP, Polin RS; Sheehan JM, et al. Factors associated with hydrocephalus after aneurysmal subarachnoid hemorrhage. Neurosurgery 1999: 45: 1120–1128.

Shibuya M, Suzuki Y, Sugita K et al. Effect of AT877 on cerebral vasospasm after aneurysmal subarachnoid hemorrhage. J Neurosurg 1992: 76: 571–577.

Shigeno T. Norepinephrine in cerebrospinal fluid of patients with cerebral vasospasm. J Neurosurg 1982: 56: 344–349.

Shigeno T, Fritschka E, Schramm J Brock M. Cerebral oedema following experimental subarachnoid hemorrhage. In: Brock M (ed). Modern Neurosurgery, Springer Verlag, Berlin 1982: 396–399.

Shigeno T, Clozel M, Sakai S, et al. The effect of bosentan, a new potent endothelin receptor antagonist, on the pathogenesis of cerebral vasospasm. Neurosurgery 1995: 37: 87–91.

Shimoda M, Oda S, Tsugane R, Sato O. Intracranial complications of hypervolemic therapy in patients with a delayed ischemic deficit attributed to vasospasm. J Neurosurg 1993: 78: 423–429.

Shiokawa K, Kasuya H, Miyajima M, et al. Prophylactic effect of papaverine prolonged-release pellets on cerebral vasospasm in dogs. Neurosurgery 1998: 42: 109–116.

Shiokawa Y, Delgado-Zygmunt TJ, Arbab MA-R, Svendgaard NAa. Effect of unilateral pre- and postganglionic lesioning of the trigeminal nerve on the development of cerebral va-

sospasm in the squirrel monkey: Angiographic findings. Br J Neurosurg 1992: 6: 445–455.
Shirakami G, Magaribuchi T, Shingu K, et al. Changes of endothelin concentration in cerebrospinal fluid and plasma of patients with aneurysmal subarachnoid hemorrhage. Acta Anaesthesiol Scand 1994: 38: 457–461.
Simeone FA, Trepper PJ, Brown DJ. Cerebral blood flow evaluation of prolonged experimental vasospasm. J Neurosurg 1972: 37: 302–311.
Silverberg GD, Reitz BA, Ream AK. Hypothermia and cardiac arrest in the treatment of giant aneurysms of the cerebral circulation and hemangioblastoma of the medulla. J Neurosurg 1981: 55: 337–346.
Smigiel MR, Sundt TM. Comparative effectiveness of alpha blockade and beta-stimulation in modifying experimental basilar arterial spasm. J Neurosurg 1974: 41: 300–305.
Smith SL, Scherch HM, Hall ED. Protective effects of tirilazad mesylate and metabolite U-89678 against blood-brain barrier damage after subarachnoid hemorrhage and lipid peroxidative neuronal injury. J Neurosurg 1996: 84: 229–233.
Sohma M, Suzuki S, Kimura S, et al. Adventitial hyperpermeability of cerebral artery in pathophysiology of cerebral vasospasm. Cerebrovasc Disease Tohoku 1991: 13: 83–87.
Sokolovsky M. Endothelins and sarafotoxins: Physiological regulation, receptor subtypes and transmembrane signaling. Pharmacol Ther 1992: 54: 129–149.
Solomon RA, McCormack BM, Lovitz RN, et al. Elevation of brain norepinephrine concentration after experimental subarachnoid hemorrhage. Neurosurgery 1986: 19: 363–366.
Solomon RA, Lovitz RL, Hegemann MT, et al. Regional cerebral metabolic activity in the rat following experimental subarachnoid hemorrhage. J Cereb Blood Flow Metab 1987: 7: 193–198.
Solomon RA, Smith CR, Raps EC, et al. Deep hypothermic circulatory arrest for the management of complex anterior and posterior circulation aneurysms. Neurosurgery 1991: 29: 732–738.
Steinberg GK, Vanefsky MA, Marks MP, et al. Failure of intracisternal tissue plasminogen activator to prevent vasospasm in certain patients with aneurysmal subarachnoid hemorrhage. Neurosurgery 1994: 34: 809–814.
Steiner L, Löfgren J, Zwetnow N. Cerebral blood flow and metabolism in the acute phase of experimental subarachnoid bleed. Zbl Neurochirurgie 1978: 39. 223–230.
Steinke DE, Weir BKA, Findley JM, et al. A trial of the 21-aminosteroid U-74006F in a primate model of chronic cerebral vasospasm. Neurosurgery 1989: 24: 179–186.
Steudel W-I, Reif J, Voges M. Modulated surgery in the management of ruptured intracranial aneurysm in poor grade patients. Neurol Res 1994: 16: 49–53.
Stornelli SA, French JD. Subarachnoid hemorrhage factors in prognosis and management. J Neurosurg 1964: 21: 769–780.
Stullken EH, Johnston WE, Prough DS, et al. Implications of nimodipine prophylaxis of cerebral vasospasm in anaesthetic management during intracranial aneurysm clipping. J Neurosurg 1985: 62: 200–205.
Sturaitis MK, Rinne J, Chaloupka JC, et al. Impact of Guglielmi detachable coils on outcomes of patients with intracranial aneurysms treated by a multidisciplinary team at a single instittition. J Neurosurg 2000: 93: 569–580.
Sundberg G, Pontén U. ICP and CSF absorption impairment after subarachnoid hemorrhage. In: Beks JWA, Bosch DA, Brock M (eds) Intracranial Pressure III, Springer Verlag, Berlin, Heidelberg, New York 1976: 139–146.
Sutter B, Suzuki S, Arthur AS, et al. Effects of subarachnoid hemorrhage on vascular responses to calcitonin gene-related peptide and its related second messengers. J Neurosurg 1995: 83: 516–521.
Suzuki R, Masaoka H, Hirata Y, et al. The role of endothelin-1 in the origin of cerebral vasospasm in patients with aneurysmal subarachnoid hemorrhage. J Neurosurg 1992: 77: 96–100.
Suzuki S, Ogane K, Souma M, et al. Efficacy of steroid hormone in solution for intracranial irrigation during aneurysmal surgery for prevention of the vasospasm syndrome. Acta Neurochir 1994: 131: 184–188.
Suzuki Y, Sato S, Suzuki H et al. Increased neuropeptide Y concentrations in cerebrospinal fluid from patients with aneurysmal subarachnoid hemorrhage. Stroke 1989: 20: 1680–1684.
Suzuki Y, Osuka K, Noda A, et al. Nitric oxide metabolites in the cisternal cerebral spinal fluid of patients with subarachnoid hemorrhage. Neurosurgery 1997: 41: 807–812.
Symon L. Vasospasm in aneurysm. In: Moossy J, Janeway R (eds) Cerebral Vascular diseases. Grune and Stratton, New York 1971: 232–240.
Svendgaard N-Aa, Brismar J, Delgado TJ, Rosengren E. Subarachnoid hemorrhage in the rat: Effect on the development of vasospasm of selective lesions of the catecholamine systems in the lower brain stem. Stroke 1985: 16: 602–608.
Svendgaard N-Aa, Delgado TJ, Brun A. Effect of selective lesions in the hypothalamus-pituitary region on the development of cerebral vasospasm following an experimental subarachnoid hemorrhage in the rat. J Cereb Blood Flow Metab 1986: 6: 650–657.
Svendgaard NAa, Arbab MA-R, Delgado TJ, Rosengren E. Effect of selective lesions of medullary catetholamine nuclei on experimental cerebral vasospasm in the rat. J Cereb Blood Flow Metab 1987: 7: 21–28.
Tagari P, du Boulay GH, Aitken V, Bouillin DJ. Leucotriene D4 and the cerebral vasculature *in vivo* and in *vitro*. Prostaglandin Leurotrienes Med 1983: 11: 281–297.
Takuwa Y, Matsui T, Abe Y, et al. Alterations in protein kinase C activity and membrane lipid metabolism in cerebral vasospasm after subarachnoid hemorrhage. J Cereb Blood Flow Metab 1993: 13: 409–415.
Tanabe Y, Sakata K, Yamada H. Cerebral vasospasm and ultrastructural changes in cerebral arterial wall. An experimental study. J Neurosurg 1978: 49: 229–238.
Taylor CL, Selman WR, Kiefer SP, et al. Temporary vessel occlusion during intracranial aneurysm repair. Neurosurgery 1996: 39: 893–906.
Terada T, Hyoutani G, Uematsu Y et al. [Hemorrhagic infarction following vasospasm due to ruptured cerebral aneurysms] (Jpn) Neurol Med Chir 1987: 27: 83–89.
Thomas JE, Rosenwasser RH. Reversal of severe cerebral vasospasm in three patients after aneurysmal subarachnoid hemorrhage: Initial observations regarding the use of intraventricular sodium nitroprusside in humans. Neurosurgery 1999a: 44: 48–58.
Thomas JE, Rosenwasser RH, Armonda RA, et al. Safety of intrathecal sodium nitroprusside for the treatment and prevention of refractory cerebral vasospasm and ischaemia in humans. Stroke 1999b: 30: 1409–1416.

Toda N. Relaxant responses to transmural stimulation and nicotine of dog and monkey cerebral arteries. Am J Physiol 1982: 243: H145–H153.

Toda N, Kowakami M, Yoshida K. Constrictor action of oxy-haemoglobin in monkey and dog basilar arteries *in vivo* and *in vitro*. Am J Physiol 1991: 260: 420–425.

Toshima M, Kassell NF, Sasaki T, et al. The effect of hemoglobin on vasodilatory effect of calcium antagonists in the isolated rabbit basilar artery. J Neurosurg 1992: 76: 670–678.

Trojanowski T. Blood-brain barrier changes after experimental subarachnoid hemorrhage. Acta Neurochir (Wien) 1982: 60: 45–54.

Tsukahara T, Hongo K, Kassell NF, Ogawa H. The influence of experimental subarachnoid hemorrhage in the relaxation induced by vasoactive intestinal polypeptide in the cerebral arteries of the rabbit. Neurosurgery 1989: 24: 731–735.

Tsukahara T, Yonekawa Y, Yamamoto M, et al. The endothelium-dependent response of human cerebral arteries and its changes after subarachnoid hemorrhage. In: Sano K, Takakura K, Kassell NF et al. (eds) Cerebral Vasospasm, University of Tokyo Press 1990: 227–230.

Uemura U, Sugimoto T, Okamoto S, et al. Changes of neuropeptide immunoreactivity in cerebrovascular nerve fibers after experimentally produced SAH: Immunohistochemical study in the dog. J Neurosurg 1987: 66: 741–747.

Umansky F, Kaspi T, Shalit MN. Regional cerebral blood flow in the acute stage of experimentally induced subarachnoid hemorrhage. J Neurosurg 1983: 58: 210–216.

Uski T, Andersson K-E, Brandt L, et al. Responses of isolated feline and human cerebral arteries to prostacyclin and some metabolites. J Cereb Blood Flow Metab 1983: 3: 238–245.

Uski TK, Lilja Å, Säveland H. et al. Cognitive functioning and cerebrospinal fluid concentrations of neuropeptides for patients with good neurological outcomes after aneurysmal subarachnoid hemorrhage. Neurosurgery 2000: 47: 812–818.

Usui M, Saito N, Hoya K, Todo T. Vasospasm prevention with postoperative intrathecal thrombolytic therapy: A retrospective comparison of urokinase, tissue plasminogen activator, and cisternal drainage alone. Neurosurgery 1994: 34: 235–245.

Vaeth A, Kunze E, Roosen K, Meixenberger J. Therapeutic aspects of brain tissue PO_2 monitoring after subarachnoid hemorrhage. Proceeding XI ICP symposium, Cambridge 2000: O10-2, page 82.

Veelken JA, Laing RJ, Jakubowski J. The Sheffield model of subarachnoid hemorrhage in rats. Stroke 1995: 26: 1279–1284.

Voldby B, Enevoldsen EM. Intracranial pressure changes following aneurysm rupture. Part 1: Clinical and angiographic correlations. J Neurosurg 1982a: 56: 186–196.

Voldby B, Enevoldsen EM. Intracranial pressure changes following aneurysm rupture. Part 2: Associated cerebrospinal fluid lactacidosis. J Neurosurg 1982b: 56: 197–204.

Voldby B, Enevoldsen EM. Intracranial pressure changes following aneurysm rupture. Part 3: Recurrent hemorrhage. J Neurosurg 1982c: 56: 784–789.

Voldby B, Enevoldsen EM, Jensen FT. Cerebrovascular reactivity in patients with ruptured intracranial aneurysms. J Neurosurg 1985a: 62: 59–67.

Voldby B, Enevoldsen EM, Jensen FT. Regional CBF, intraventricular pressure, and cerebral metabolism in patients with ruptured intracranial aneurysms. J Neurosurg 1985b: 62: 48–58.

Vollmer DG, Kassell NF, Honga K. et al. Effect of the nonglucocorticoid 21-aminosteroid U74006F on experimental cerebral vasospasm. Surg Neurol 1989a: 31: 190–194.

Vollmer DG, Honga K, Kassell NF, et al. Effect of intracisternal antithrombin III on subarachnoid hemorrhage-induced arterial narrowing. J Neurosurg 1989b: 70: 599–604.

Vollrath BAM, Weir BKA, MacDonald RL, Cook DA. Intracellular mechanisms involved in the responses of cerebrovascular smooth-muscle cells to hemoglobin. J Neurosurg 1994: 80: 261–268.

von Horst H, Granström E, Hammarström S, et al. Effect of leucotriens C4, D4, prostacyclin, and thromboxane A2 on isolated human cerebral arteries. Acta Neurochir 1982: 62: 177–185.

Walker V, Pickard JD, Smythe P, et al. Effects of subarachnoid hemorrhage in intracranial prostaglandins. J Neurol Neurosurg Psychiatr 1983: 46: 119–125.

Wanebo JE, Arthur AS, Louis HG, et al. Systemic administration of the endothelin-A receptor antagonist TBC 11251 attenuates cerebral vasospasm after experimental subarachnoid hemorrhage: dose study and review of endothelin-based therapies in the literature on cerebral vasospasm. Neurosurgery 1998: 43: 1409–1417.

Wang J, Ohta S, Sakaki S, et al. Changes in Ca++-ATPase activity in smooth-muscle cell membranes of the canine basilar artery with experimental subarachnoid hemorrhage. J Neurosurg 1994: 80: 269–275.

Wardlaw JM, Offin R, Teasdale GM, Teasdale EM. Is routine transcranial Doppler ultrasound monitoring useful in the management of subarachnoid hemorrhage. J Neurosurg 1998: 88: 272–276.

Wheelock B, Weir B, Watts R, et al. Timing of surgery for intracerebral hematomas due to aneurysm rupture. J Neurosurg 1983: 58: 476–481.

Weir B, Menon D, Overton T. Regional cerebral blood flow in patients with aneurysms. Estimation by Xenon 133 inhalation. Can J Neurol Sci 1978: 5: 301–305.

Weir B, Disney L, Grace M, Roberts P. Daily trends in white blood cell count and temperature after subarachnoid hemorrhage from aneurysm. Neurosurgery 1989: 25: 161–165.

White RP, Hagen A, Robertson JT. Experimental evaluation of the spasmogenicity of dopamine on the basilar artery. J Neurosurg 1976: 44: 45–49.

White RP, Huang S-P, Hagen AA, Robertson JT. Experimental assessment of phenoxybenzamine in cerebral vasospasm. J Neurosurg 1979: 50: 158–163.

White RP, Robertson JT. Role of plasmin, thrombin and antithrombin III as etiological factors in delayed cerebral vasospasm. Neurosurgery 1985: 16: 27–35.

White RP. Comparison of the inhibitory effects of antithrombin III, alpha-2-macroglobulin, and thrombin in human basilar arteries: Relevance to cerebral vasospasm. J Cereb Blood Flow Metab 1987: 7: 68–73.

White RP, Robertson JT. Pharmacodynamic evaluation of human cerebral arteries in the genesis of vasospasm. Neurosurgery 1987: 21. 523–531.

Wiebers DO, Whisnant JP, 0`Fallon WM Jr. The natural history of unruptured intracranial aneurysms. N Eng J Med 1981: 304: 696–698.

Wiebers DO, Whisnant JP, Sundt TM, 0'Fallon WM Jr. The significance of unruptured saccular aneurysms. J Neurosurg 1987: 66: 23–29.

Wijdicks EFM, Schievink WI, Burnett JC. Natriuretic peptide system and endothelin in aneurysmal subarachnoid hemorrhage. J Neurosurg 1997: 87: 275-280.

Winkling M, Müller HW, Deinsberger W, et al. Levels of immunoreactive cysteinyl-leukotrienes in CSF after subarachnoid haemorrhage correlate with blood flow-velocity in TCD. Acta Neurochir 1997: 139: 764-769.

Wurtman RJ, Zervas NT. Monoamine neurotransmitters and the pathophysiology of stroke and central nervous system trauma. J Neurosurg 1974: 40: 34-36.

Yamakama I, Isobe K, Yamaura A. Effects of intravascular volume expansion of cerebral blood flow in patients with ruptured cerebral aneurysms. Neurosurgery 1987: 21: 303-309.

Yamamoto M. Meyer J, Naritomi H, et al. Noninvasive measurement of cerebral vasospasm in patients with subarachnoid hemorrhage. J Neurol Sci 1979: 43. 301-311.

Yamamoto S, Teng W, Nishizawa S, et al. Improvement in cerebral blood flow and metabolism following subarachnoid hemorrhage in response to pryphyllactic administration of the hydroxyl radical scavenger, AVS, ()-N,N-propylenedinicotinamide: A positron emission tomography study in rats. J Neurosurg 2000: 92: 1009-1015.

Yamaura I, Tani E, Maeda Y, et al. Endothelin-1 of canine basilar artery in vasospasm. J Neurosurg 1992: 76: 99-105.

Yokota M, Tani E, Maeda Y, Kokubu K. Effect of 5-lipoxygenase inhibitor on experimental delayed cerebral vasospasm. Stroke 1987: 18: 512-518.

Yokota M, Peterson JW, Kaooutzanis MC, et al. Protein kinase C and diacylglycerol content in basilar arteries during experimental cerebral vasospasm in the dog. J Neurosurg 1995: 82: 834-840.

Yonas H, Sekhar L, Johnson DW, Gur D. Determination of irreversible ischemia by xenon-enhanced computed tomographic monitoring of cerebral blood flow in patients with symptomatic vasospasm. Neurosurgery 1989: 24: 369-372.

Zabramski LH, Spetzler RF, Bonstelle C. Chronic cerebral vasospasm: Effect of calcium antagonists. Neurosurgery 1986: 18: 129-135.

Zabramski JM, Spetzler RF, Lee KS, et al. Phase I trial of tissue plasminogen activator for the prevention of vasospasm in patients with aneurysmal subarachnoid hemorrhage. J Neurosurg 1991: 75: 189-196.

Zea Longa E, Weinstein RP, Calson S. et al. Reversible middle cerebral artery occlusion without craniectomy in rats. Stroke 20: 84-91.

Zimmermann M, Seifert V, Löffler B-M, et al. Prevention of cerebral vasospasm after experimental subarachnoid hemorrhage by RO 47-0203, a newly developed orally active endothelin receptor antagonist. Neurosurgery 1996: 38: 115-120.

Zimmermann M, Seifert V. Endothelin and subarachnoid hemorrhage: an overview. Neurosurgery 1998: 43: 863-876.

Zingesser LH, Schechter MM, Dexter J, et al. On the significance of spasm associated with rupture of a cerebral aneurysm. Arch Neurol 1968: 18: 520-528.

Zubkov YN, Nikiforov BM, Shustin VA. Balloon-catheter technique for dilatation of constricted cerebral arteries after aneurysmal SAH. Acta Neurochir 1984: 70: 65-79.

Zubkov YN, Alexander LF, Smith RR et al. Angioplasty of vasospasm: Is it reasonable?. Neurol Res 1994: 16: 9-11.

Zuccarello M, March JT, Schmidt G, et al. Effect of 21-aminosteroid U-74006F on cerebral vasospasm following subarachnoid hemorrhage. J Neurosurg 1989: 71: 98-104.

Zuccarello M, Lewis AI, Rapoport RM, et al. Endothelin ET_a and ET_b receptors in subarachnoid hemorrhage-induced cerebral vasospasm. Eur J Pharmacol 1994: 259: 1-2

Zuccarello M, Soattin GB, Lewis AI, et al. Prevention of subarachnoid hemorrhage-induced cerebral vasospasm by oral administration of endothelin receptor antagonists. J Neurosurg 1996a: 84: 503-507.

Zuccarello M, Bonasso CL, Sperelakis N, Rapoport RM. Relaxation of subarachnoid hemorrhage-induced spasm of rabbit basilar artery by the K^+ channel activator cromakalim. Stroke 1996b: 27: 311-316.

Zuccarello M, Boccaletti R, Romano A, Rapoport RM. Endothelin B receptor antagonists attenuate subarachnoid hemorrhage-induced cerebral vasospasm. Stroke 1998: 29: 1924-1929.

Østergaard JR, Kristensen BO, Svehag S-E, et al. Immune complees and complement activation following rupture of intracranial saccular aneurysms. J Neurosurg 1987: 66. 891-897.

CHAPTER 12

Ischaemia

Experimental ischaemia can be global of focal. In experimental studies forebrain ischaemia is of the global type, and in many respects, it mimics cardiovascular arrest. Focal ischaemia, on the other hand, is typically performed by middle cerebral artery occlusion (MAC), which simulates stroke. Ischaemia can be incomplete or complete, depending on the preservation of blood flow to the ischaemic area. Other ischaemic models of traumatic cerebral injury and retractor ischaemia are of interest. Moreover, ischaemic injury is elicited by changes in the relationship between oxygen/substrate supply and cerebral metabolism. Typical examples are anoxia/hypoxia, hypoglycaemic, excitatory insult and epilepsy.

In this review focus has been paid upon experimental studies, and to lesser degree clinical studies. Clinical studies of ischaemia secondary to traumatic lesion and subarachnoid haemorrhage are only mentioned superficially, but are reviewed in Chapter 9 and 10. Clinical studies of stroke are not reviewed, as patients within this category are not admitted to neurosurgical intensive units.

Ischaemic threshold

Experimental studies

Neurological deficits

In experiments of reversible middle cerebral artery occlusion (MCAO) in cats and monkeys, reversible paralysis occurs when CBF is reduced to 23 ml/100g/min and irreversible paralysis supervenes when CBF is permanently reduced to about 17–18 ml (Heiss et al. 1976, Jones et al. 1981).

EEG

In analogy with these findings isoelectric EEG is observed at controlled hypotension to MABP 10–30 mm Hg and disappearance of evoked potentials occurs at MABP 15–20 mm Hg. Studies in rats have demonstrated that the EEG suppression and anoxic depolarisation do not occur as a simple function of progressive oxygen decline during cerebral ischaemia. Thus, EEG suppression spares oxygen stores while anoxic depolarisation accelerates the decline in oxygen stores (Raffin et al. 1991).

Threshold

In gerbils, subjected to acute cerebral ischaemia by carotid ligation, an ischaemia CBF threshold of 20 CBF ml/100g/min has been defined. Below this threshold MR spectroscopy shows metabolic failure with phosphocreatine and ATP decline. These changes combined with lactate accumulation and a fall in intracellular pH indicate that failure of synaptic function is a direct consequence of energy failure (Crockard et al. 1987). In experiments with primates subjected to MCAO, pH in the extracellular space remains stable until CBF levels of 20 ml/100g/min; below this value, pH fell rapidly (Harris et al. 1987), and an increase in brain water was observed (Symon et al. 1979). In baboons direct cortical electrical response is lost at the same level of CBF (Farman et al. 1994).

If CBF falls to about 10 ml/100g/min, cytotoxic oedema occurs as a result of sodium passage into the cells. Unless the cells have been severely damaged, the formation of oedema is reversible (Hossmann 1976). Studies in baboons indicate that if the duration of ischaemia is too long, reperfusion will increase cerebral oedema (Bell et al. 1985).

In animal experiments the ischaemia threshold of evoked potential suppression is reached at CBF values of 15–17 ml/100g/min (Branston et al. 1974, Heiss et al. 1976, Astrup et al. 1977).

A difference in vulnerability has been observed with a lower threshold in the basal ganglia and the medial lemniscus in the brain-stem (Okada et al. 1983, Branston et al. 1984). Furthermore, studies of spontaneous firing of nerve cells in the cat suggest differences in flow thresholds ranging from 6 to 20 ml/100g/min (Heiss and Rosner 1983). If CBF is reduced below the level of 6–8 ml influx of Ca^{2+}, efflux of K^+ and depletion of ATP occur (Astrup et al. 1977, Branston et al. 1977, Astrup et al. 1979) and calcium homeostasis is exhausted (Harris et al. 1981). At this low values cellular integrity and viability are severely impaired and cellular death and infarction are threatening (Symon and Brierley 1976, Astrup 1982). Using MR spectroscopy these findings are in accordance with studies in gerbils indicating a decrease in intracellular pH at CBF levels of 18–23 ml, a decrease in ATP at CBF levels of 12–14 ml followed by disappearance of ATP and phosphocreatine and a decrease in ^{23}Na signal (Naritomi et al. 1988). In small animals cats, rats and gerbils with a higher oxygen consumption, the threshold of membrane failure has been found to be higher (Hossman and Schuier 1980, Strong et al. 1983, Mies et al. 1984, Harris and Symon 1984).

In rats subjected to MCAO the ischaemic threshold approached 50 ml/100g/min. This threshold is about 3 times higher than in primates. The authors argue that since neuronal density is also threefold greater in rats than in primates, the higher ischaemic threshold in the rat may reflect a neuronal primacy in determining the brains susceptibility to ischaemia (Jacewicz et al. 1992). In another study in rats subjected to forebrain ischaemia, ischaemic changes in the deepest layers in the cortex were correlated to CBF values of 50 ml (Mendelow et al. 1984). Furthermore, in the same animal it was observed that at CBF averaging this value, changes in protein synthesis (Mies et al. 1991), the expression of heat shock proteins (Jacewicz et al. 1986) and cerebral acidosis occur (Nakai et al. 1988).

In rats subjected to MCAO and ipselateral common carotid occlusion it was found that the ultimate extent of infarction in a region does not seem to be predictable from a knowledge of the early postischaemic CBF. Thus, postischaemic CBF may determine whether a particular region will show infarction, but it is not possible to use CBF as a reliable index of an infarcts topography (Hakim et al. 1992).

As indicated species influence ischaemic threshold. According to Byron (2001) the threshold of CBF below which neuronal function is impaired and the tissue is at risk of infarction is around 22 ml/100g/min in awake or lightly anaesthetised monkey, and around 30–35 ml/100g/min in the cat and the rat. The threshold of CBF below which the tissue becomes irreversibly damaged and will progress to infarction depends on the duration of ischaemia, and is around 10 ml/100g/min for 1–2 hrs., and around 18 ml/100g/min for permanent ischaemia in the monkey.

Penumbra

In regions where CBF levels range from 8 to 23 ml synaptic transmission failure threshold has been partly or completely exceeded, but membrane failure has not occurred. This state, called an ischaemic penumbra (Symon et al. 1974, Branston et al. 1974, Astrup et al. 1977, Symon 1980, Astrup et al. 1981), has gained considerable interest, because therapeutic measures aiming at an increase in CBF theoretically may re-establish synaptic transmission and reduce neurological deficits. The results obtained demonstrated that there are separate thresholds for cessation of electrical activity and for loss of ion homeostasis due to overt energy failure. Such findings led to the definition of penumbra as tissues containing electrically inexcitable but essentially viable cells. Studies in cats subjected to electrical cortical stimulation have shown, that even in the penumbra after MCAO some degree of flow reactivity persists suggesting that the microcirculation in the penumbra is not maximally vasodilated (Strong et al. 1988). In experimental studies high-speed MR imaging of ischaemia brain injury following MCAO is diagnostically useful in differentiating severely hypoperfused permanently injured tissue from the mildly hypoperfused ischaemic penumbra (Roberts et al. 1993).

By sequential multitracer PET, including studies of penumbra CBF, $CMRO_2$, oxygen extraction fraction, CBV and CMR-glucose, viable tissue can be detected up to several hours after MCAO in cats. The transition of misery-perfused regions into necrosis or preserved tissue can be followed over time. This observation supports the concept of a dynamic penumbra, in which, for up to 24 hours, tissue damage spreads progressively from the centre to the periphery of the ischaemia zone (Heiss et al. 1994).

Infarct

If ischaemic threshold is exceeded, cellular necrosis takes place and an infarct develops. During complete cerebral ischaemia, a selective vulnerability has been observed, involving the CA1 subfield of the hippocampus, the caudo-putamen, the layers III-V in the cerebral neocortex, the cerebellar Purkinje cells, and the lateral reticular nucleus of the thalamus (Ito et al. 1975, Ginsberg et al. 1979, Diemer and Siemkowicz 1981, Pulsinelli et al. 1982a, Blomquist and Wieloch 1985). In animal studies of focal ischaemia after MCAO, a demarcated area of ischaemia develops in the occluded territory of the artery (Brierley and Graham 1984). With ^{31}P-nuclear magnetic resonance it is possible to follow changes in the ratio creatine phosphate (PCr) to inorganic phosphate (P_i), depletion of ATP and intracellular pH in cats subjected to

MCAO. The results suggest that in severe stroke, in comparison with mild stroke, the depletion in ATP, the decrease in intracellular pH and the decrease in the ratio PCr/P_i are more pronounced (Komatsumoto et al. 1987). In the periinfarct zone a mantle with reduced CBF and increased glucose consumption has been observed (Nedergaard et al. 1986).

Apoptosis or programmed cell death

Some proliferating cells are eliminated under physiological and pathological conditions by a process called programmed cell death, whose morphological counterpart is apoptosis. Apoptosis differs from necrosis in several important ways. Morphologically, apoptosis shows typical chromatin condensation and DNA fragmentation, and in later stages cell shrinkage. Biochemically, the nuclear changes indicate a characteristic laddering, reflecting breakage of DNA at internucleosomal bridges. In a review Graham and Chen (2001) conclude that there is convincing evidence for the induction of programmed cell death after ischaemia including altered expression and activity in the ischaemic brain of deduced key death-regulating genes.

Duration of ischaemia

The duration of flow deprivation influences ischaemic threshold; hence a CBF reduction to 8 ml is only tolerated for about one hour (Morawetz et al. 1979, Marcoux et al. 1982). However, neuronal transmission can be re-established at flow of 10–12 ml for less than 2-3 hours. With permanent MCAO neuronal necrosis occurs at CBF in the range of 15–17 ml, and flows ranging from 18 to 23 ml are tolerated for more than two weeks. On the other hand, in studies of complete cerebral ischaemia of 30 min duration, restoration of phosphocreatine and lactate concentration and recovery of the adenylate energy charge were complete after a recirculation period of 90 min (Nordström et al. 1976). In another study of temporary MCAO in the rat it was found that 15 min of occlusion produced a small, deep infarction, and progressively longer periods of occlusion caused a larger infarction with cortical necrosis. 120–180 minutes of occlusion produced an infarction comparable in size to permanent occlusion (Memezawa et al. 1992). This is also in accordance with another study, where the shortest occlusion time to produce a maximal infarct was 3 to 4 hours (Kaplan et al. 1991, Degraba et al. 1993).

In contrast to these studies Hossmann et al. (1987) described functional and metabolic recovery in a cat following 1 hour of complete global ischaemia. However, the animal had complete atrophy of the dorsal hippocampus and striatum and enlargement of the ventricular system.

Blood pressure

Studies of graded hypotension in MCAO rats have demonstrated that blood pressure plays a greater role in determining infarct size than did MCAO duration. At a blood pressure of 40 mm Hg, 60 min of MCAO produced 25% damage, accelerating every 20 min during a two hour period. At blood pressure 80 mm Hg, 120 min of MCAO produced the same damage as only 80 min of MCAO at blood pressure 60 mm Hg, and at 60-, 80-, 100-, and 120-min duration of MCAO, infarct size was significantly reduced with increasing blood pressure (Zhu and Auer 1995).

Rheology and haemodilution

One theoretically approach towards brain protection is to improve the rheological properties of blood by lowering the viscosity. Haemodilution increases CBF and generally there is an inverse relationship between CBF and haematocrit. Several studies have pointed on the fact that haemodilution is an effective way to increase perfusion in the ischaemic brain. However haemodilution also decreases the oxygen-carrying capacity. In a recent study a haematocrit of 30% was found to be optimum for protecting the brain (Lee et al. 1994).

In rabbits subjected to MCAO marked haemodilution induced with 6% hydroxyethyl strach exacerbated neurologic injury at haemoglobin concentration at 6g/100 ml (Reasoner et al. 1996).

Clinical studies

Hyperventilation to $PaCO_2$ level of 2.7 kPa in man is accompanied by EEG changes compatible with cerebral hypoxia. These changes are normalised by hyperbaric oxygen. Furthermore, a moderate increase in CMR-glucose, indicating anaerobic metabolism, has been observed at extreme hyperventilation with CBF levels ranging from 10 to 20 ml, which corresponds to jugular venous oxygen tensions of 2.7 kPa (Alexander et al. 1968). Clinical studies in patients with stroke indicate that penumbra flow ranges from 7 to 17 ml/100g/min. (Furlan et al. 1996) and 10 to 22 ml/100g/min. (Marchal et al. 1996). It is therefore thought that ischaemic threshold for synaptic transmission in humans is CBF levels of 17–22 ml/100g/min.

Critical levels of brain tissue oxygen tension range from 5 to 23 mm Hg, dependent upon technology (Santbrink et al. 1996, Kiening et al.1 1996, Doppenberg et al 1998).

In a series of PET studies performed 5–18 hrs. after stroke onset the threshold for penumbra was around 20 ml/100g/min, and the thresholds for irreversible damage were around 8 ml/100g/min for CBF and around 0,9 ml O_2/100g/min for $CMRO_2$ (Byron 2001).

In view of more recent studies it is justified to redefine the "penumbra" to denote tissue containing neurones that are at risk but are potentially salvageable even when MCAO is permanently occluded. The penumbra, thus defined, is that part of the ischaemic tissue that is recruited in the infarction process if no treatment is instituted, but may be salvaged by appropriate treatment, for example, pharmacological intervention (Kuroda and Siesjö 1997). For reveiw see Heiss (2000).

Anaesthesia

Anaesthetic agents seem to influence ischaemic threshold. During endarterectomy in patients anaesthetized with less than 1% halothane, EEG changes with flattening and isoelectric recordings were observed during clamping when CBF fell to levels ranging between 18–23 ml (Tr¢jaborg and Boysen 1973, Sharbrough et al. 1973). An identical threshold of CBF was found during carotid ligation in patients operated for cerebral aneurysm (Leech et al. 1974). During neurolept anaesthesia, however, a higher stump pressure and lower CBF was observed (McKay et al. 1976), and during isoflurane anaesthesia the ischaemic EEG changes were observed, when CBF was reduced to values below 10 ml (Messick et al. 1987).

MR and PET studies

In stroke patients, studies with MR spectroscopy suggest that irreversible neuronal damage occurs within 6 hours (Gideon et al. 1992).

In patients with chronic cerebral infarcts studies with ^{123}I Isopropyl Iodo-Amphetamine have demonstrated that a central area of infarct is surrounded by a peripheral area with moderate CBF decrease. It is supposed that this periinfarct area is caused by deafferentation of areas not directly affected by the ischaemic insult and/or selective neuronal loss (Raynaud et al. 1987). Studies of cortical evoked potential in cats subjected to MCAO suggest that restoration of blood supply to regions with cortical deafferentation normalises somatosensory evoked potentials (Kataoka et al. 1987).

In patients with acute ischaemic stroke diffusion-weighted MR image lesions have been identified as early as 39 minutes after the stroke (Yoneda et al. 1999) Quantitative data, including the diffusion-weighted imaging, indicated lower apparent diffusion coefficients in tissue 105 minutes after onset of stroke (Warach et al. 1992). Also perfusion-weighted MR image demonstrates haemodynamic abnormalities (Sorensen et al. 1996). Combined perfusion- and diffusion weighted MR images have been used to deliniate regions at risk for eventual infarction (Sorensen et al. 1997).

Brain retraction ischaemia

During craniotomy retractors produce a pressure on the brain surface. This pressure, measured by transducers fixed at the retractor, is transmitted to the adjacent brain tissue. A decrease in regional CPP below the transducer with risk of developing ischaemic brain damage has been demonstrated (Albin et al. 1975, Albin et al. 1977). In normotensive patients the threshold of brain retractor pressure in developing cerebral ischaemia is 30–40 mm Hg. In hypotensive patients it is lower (Rosen¢rn 1989). This threshold corresponds to thresholds of rCBF of 10–13 ml/100g/min. If the brain retractor pressure after 6–8 minutes remains above 30 mm Hg, intermittent placement of retractor is recommended.

In a mongrel dog model evoked potential and Laser-Doppler flow measurements were undertaken during brain retraction. Loss of evoked potential was associated with low blood pressure, low CBF, hypocapnia and older age (Andrews and Muto 1992). In the same model mannitol plus nimodipine is superior to either agent alone in maintaining both CBF and evoked potential (Andrews and Muto 1992).

Spreading depression (SD)

Neuronal damage

Spreading depression (SD) seems to be a stereotyped response of brain cortical tissues to noxious stimuli. SD has been detected in low perfused areas and is supposed to play a role in the development of selective neuronal damage (Nedergaard 1988). During SD a period of 2–3 min duration with increased CBF is followed by a prolonged cortical oligaemia. The early phase of increased CBF is not observed in conscious restrained rats, but a long lasting (3 hours) reduction in CBF is still observed (Duckrow 1991). During this period the CO_2 reactivity is abolished, autoregulation to hypotension preserved and the spontaneous vasomotor activity in the cortical microcirculation is decreased (Piper et al. 1991).

Excitatory amino acids

SD is blocked by N-methyl-D-aspartate (NMDA)-receptor blockage (Gill et al. 1992) while 2,3-dihydroxy-6-nitro-7-sulfamoyl-benzo(F)-quinoxaline (NBQX) blockade is without influence in one study (Lauritzen and Hansen 1992). Suppression of SD, however, has been found in another study (Mies et al. 1994).

Nitric oxide (NO)

Studies in rats indicate that rCBF during SD is not regulated by nitric oxide (Zhang et al. 1994).

pH

In normal cerebral tissue SD is accompanied by triphasic changes in extracellular pH and an increase in lactate concentration (Mutch and Hansen 1984). Accumulation of arachidonic acid occurs, whilst energy charge is preserved (Lauritzen et al. 1990). In ischaemic tissue SD is associated with a pronounced acidic shift (Mutch and Hansen 1984).

It is suggested that the majority of the spontaneous depolarisations evoked by focal ischaemia are SD-like phenomenon probably evoked by a high values of K^+_e or glutamate in the ischaemic focus, while other SD phenomenons are elicited by independent foci of low CBF within the ischaemia border areas (Nedergaard and Hansen 1993)

Promotion and inhibition of SD

Hypoglycaemia prolongs the calcium transient associated with depolarisation of the SD type. This result supports the contention that repeated depolarisations, occurring in the penumbra-zone of a focal ischaemic lesion, could lead to calcium-related damage (Gidö et al. 1993). Other studies, in rats subjected to photothrombotic infarction and focal cerebral ischaemia, indicate that ischaemia under this circumstance provokes SD, which was triggered either within the infarct core or in the infarct rim and spread to more distant sites (Dietrich et al. 1994, Nedergaard and Hansen 1993).

Spreading depression is promoted by hypoglycaemia and inhibited by hyperglycaemia, chlorpromazine and ganglioside (Somjen et al. 1990).

SD and tolerance to cerebral injury

It has been demonstrated that certain minor cortical injury makes neurones more tolerant to subsequent ischaemic injury. This tolerance-inducing effect is long-lasting. Cortical spreading depression is one way to accomplish this tolerance (Abe et al. 1995). Recent experimental studies indicate that SD-induced neuronal depolarisation, when induced 1 day before cerebral ischaemia, induces tolerance to neuronal damage (Kawahara et al. 1994, Kawahara et al. 1995, Kobayashi et al. 1995). In rats subjected to forebrain ischaemia preinschaemic SD induced by KCl application to the cerebral cortex, and applied from 1 day to 7 days before cerebral ischaemia, decreased the number of injured neurones. Ketamine blocked this effect (Taga et al. 1997).

The mechanism by which SD produces ischaemia preconditioning is not clear. One possibility is that SD causes the synthesis of substances that can reduce the vulnerability of neurones to ischaemia injury. SD has been shown to lead to synthesis of mRNA for nerve growth factor (NGF) (Herrera et al. 1993) and brain derived neurotrophic factor (BDNF) (Kokaia et al. 1994). In addition, cortical synthesis of basic fibroblast growth factor mRNA, that occur after cortical ablation injury, has been attributed to SD (Yuguchi et al. 1994). It is also possible that SD reduces the rate at which energy depletion occurs during ischaemia. Data by Kawahara et al. (1994) indicate that SD reduces CMR glucose as long as 3 days after SD is elicited.

Reperfusion after ischaemia

It has repeatedly been observed that ischaemia is followed by a reactive hyperaemic period (Hossmann et al 1973, Steen et al. 1978, Hossmann 1988) and later on by a period with postischaemic hypoperfusion. Reperfusion as such has both positive and negative elements as regards restitution of cerebral tissue and salvage of brain cells.

CBF and $CMRO_2$

In the postischaemic period commensurate changes in CBF and cerebral blood volume (CBV) have been demonstrated in rats (Todd et al. 1986, Crumrine and LaManna 1991). $CMRO_2$ during this phase is initially low, but an increase in time is generally observed. In incomplete ischaemia the same authors found that hyperaemia is a consequence of reperfusion into the maximally vasodilated vessel bed, and this hyperaemia is reduced following longer periods of ischaemia. The hyperaemic period is accompanied by glucose hypermetabolism (Diemer and Siemkowicz 1980, Choki et al. 1983).

Experimental studies show that during the evolving stage of focal ischaemia, the ischaemic centre is surrounded by a band of increased 2-deoxyglucose uptake, that indicates the border zone of ischaemic neuronal damage (Hasegawa et al. 1990, Nedergaard et al. 1986). These findings have been determined in stroke models using normotensive animals. Normotensive rats usually do not have infarction after occlusion of the distal MCA alone (Coyle 1987). Collateral supply from the anterior cerebral artery is thought to protect against infarction in these animals. In contrast stroke-phrone spontaneously hypertensive rats develop infarction after occlusion of the distal MCA (Coyle and Jokelainen 1983).

Increased glucose utilisation related to postischaemic neuronal damage was observed 7 days after transient ischaemia in normotensive animals (Komatsumoto et al. 1989, Rischke and Kriegstein 1991). In spontaneously hypertensive rats studies of local CBF and glucose utilisation on the seventh day after infarction, unveiled a narrow band of increased glucose uptake in the border zone at the periphery of the infarcted area. The local CBF in the ischaemic cortex revealed a graded reduction from the ischaemic centre to surrounding tissue. The ischaemic areas had a significant increase in water content (Shima et al. 1994).

During focal ischaemia the reduction of CBF is not equally dense in all affected regions. Although the actual CBF values vary with species and with technique of MCAO, typical values are 5–15% of control in the focus and 15–35% in the penumbra areas (Nedergaard et al. 1988, Takagi et al. 1995, Tsuchidate et al. 1996). The ischaemic areas receive blood from leptomeningeal anastomoses from the anterior and posterior cerebral arteries. The reduction in flow in affected areas are relatively stable for up to 6 hr of MCAO, with small additional alterations after the initial reduction.

In the core of ischaemia CBF is too low to sustain normal ATP values, and to prevent anaerobic production of lactate and H^+. Values typical for 2 hrs. of MCAO in the neocortical focus, were a decrease in ATP from 2.9 to 0.5 mM, and an increase in lactate from 2.0 to 14.1 mM. In the penumbra ATP decreased from 2.8 to 1.5 mM, and lactate increased from 1.0 to 10 mM. An extensive deterioration of the bioenergetic state of the focus was observed, while the changes in the penumbra were less pronounced. Studies with diffusion-weighted MR technique suggest, that the area of lactic acidosis extends beyond that of ATP depletion (Hoehn-Berlage et al. 1995, Kohno et al. 1995).

Release of K^+ and uptake of Ca^{2+} are permanent in the focus. Penumbra areas show repeated depolarisation waves of the spreading depression or ischaemia type, accompanied by transient efflux of K^+ and uptake of Ca^{2+}. The rise in Na^+ and the depolarisation of the cell membrane are supposed to be responsible for presynaptic release of glutamate and the associated increase of extracellular glutamate concentrations. Microdialysis studies indicate sustained extracellular elevation of glutamate in the ischaemic core (Margaill et al. 1996, Matsumoto et al. 1996, Yang et al. 1996), but only a transient increase in the penumbra area (Morimoto et al. 1996). In the penumbra zone it is supposed that repeated spreading depression or ischaemic depolarisations create calcium "overload" in the penumbral cells, and that the gradual extension of the infarct into the penumbra zone represents calcium-mediated cell damage. Several studies indicate that the NMDA antagonist, MK-801, reduces the depolarisation waves in the penumbra and the infarct volume (Gill et al. 1992, Idiom et al. 1992, Back et al. 1996). MK-801, however, can only reduce the infarct volume when given before or just after the induction of focal ischaemia (Disci et al. 1994, Yang et al. 1994, Martial et al. 1996).

Restoration of CBF occurs within 15 min following 1–3 hrs. of focal ischaemia (Shogun et al. 1985, Kurita et al. 1988, Memezawa et al. 1992, Tsuchidate et al. 1996). CBF is then maintained close to the normal in both the ischaemic core and the penumbral areas (Buchan et al. 1992, Tsuchidate et al. 1966).

Hyperaemia has been attributed to vasoparalysis due to accumulation of lactic acidosis or the accumulation of vasoactive substances (ADP, AMP, potassium) during ischaemia. The mechanisms underlying delayed hypoperfusion remain obscure. The imbalance between oxygen demand and oxygen availability during hypoperfusion may lead to secondary postischaemic hypoxia as a potential damaging consequence of transient ischaemia. This relationship, however, remains an issue of controversy. In contrast to the substantial amount of data describing absolute postischaemic CBF levels in different brain regions at distinct time points, not much is known about the dynamics of postischaemic flow derangements. The transition period from hyperaemia to hypoperfusion after transient global ischaemia has been considered to be a gradual process. A variety of mechanisms could be involved, including rheological changes and microvascular obstruction due to aggregation of blood elements and hemoconcentration, capillary obstruction by endothelial microvilli formation or by neuronal, glial and endothelial swelling. Vasomotion due to the accumulation of vasoconstrictive substances such as arachidonic acid could also be involved. Studies in rats also indicate that cortical hypoperfusion can be triggered by a neuronal mechanism (Frerichs et al. 1992)

In contrast to forebrain ischaemia, focal ischaemia is not followed by delayed postischaemic hypoperfusion. Changes in bioenergetic state during reperfusion are rather complicated. ATP concentration recovers partially at 1 hour of reperfusion, but decreases again after 4 hours (Folbergrová et al. 1995). The decrease in ATP is followed by an increase in lactate. These changes suggest mitochondrial dysfunction, either because of deficient oxygen supply or damage of the respiratory chain. Studies of Garcia et al. (1994) suggest that the patience of capillaries is compromised by "sticking" of polymorphonuclear leukocytes to the endothelial walls. The secondary bioenergetic failure during reperfusion correlates well with changes in mitochondrial function, which recovered at 1 hr, but progressively deteriorated at 2–4 hrs. (Kuroda et al. 1996). This reduction of mitochondrial function affects ADP-stimulated respiration, with glutamate and malate as substrates.

Oedema

Reperfusion after an occlusion of MCA may be followed by massive brain oedema, especially the vasogenic component. This damage is triggered by resupply of water and osmotic agents and by oxygen, which triggers the formation of free radicals.

PET studies

Clinical studies of PET scanning have given some insight into the metabolic and haemodynamic events which characterise the evolution of ischaemia tissue (Hakim et al. 1989, Baron 1991, Heiss et al. 1992). These reports describe the occurrence of a marked decrease in CBF, $CMRO_2$ and oxygen extraction fraction (OEF) in the ischaemic core within 6–48 hours following the onset of stroke. At follow-up PET studies a few days later, $CMRO_2$ and OEF did not change in the core of ischaemia. Only CBF increased slightly. In the border zone of ischaemia $CMRO_2$ was reduced and deteriorated, and OEF initially close to the contralateral side progressively decreased. The progressive metabolic derangement was without concomitant change in flow, but was reflected in a decrease in $CMR_{glucose}$. In the border zone of ischaemia with increased OEF $CMRO_2$ was only slightly affected, while CBF was reduced. Within 2 weeks $CMRO_2$, $CMR_{glucose}$ and OER deteriorated, indicating progressive derangement of metabolism. This evoluation, however, has not been found in baboons subjected to MCAO and followed up to four hours after ischaemia (Pappata et al. 1993).

Blood pressure

During reperfusion, after MCAO, a short interval of phenylephrine-induced hypertension effectively augments local CBF (Cole et al. 1992). In chronically hypertensive rats subjected to focal ischaemia, cerebrovascular adaptation enables the microregional oxygen balance to be maintained at a level similar to that of normotensive animals. However, in normotensive animals with focal ischaemia, an acute increase in blood pressure improved regional oxygen balance (Chi et al. 1996)

No reflow

The reactive hyperaemic period can be absent because of erythrostasis (Hekmatpanah 1973), increased blood viscosity and swelling of perivascular glia cells, all of which prevent cerebral circulation. Ames et al. in (1968) described this "no reflow" phenomenon. In another study of unilateral carotid occlusion in the gerbil, a reduction of number of perfused capillaries was found during the ischaemia period, and during the early reperfusion period a mismatch between capillary perfusion and CBF was found (Ennis et al. 1990).

According to Ito et al. (1980) and Kågstr¢m et al. (1983) low or no perfused vessels require a high opening pressure to establish a vascular "flush" otherwise observed after complete ischaemia. It has since been demonstrated that early reflow in selected vulnerable areas, i.e. hippocampal CA1, is higher than controls (Pulsinelli et al. 1982) indicating that the selective vulnerability is not related to the "no-reflow" phenomenon as described by Ames. Recently de la Torre et al. (1992) have questioned the existence of no-reflow. Their data indicate that "no-reflow" is a post-mortem phenomenon. They injected carbon black intravenously instead of originally intra-arterially and found normal cerebrovascular filling whether global brain ischaemia was present or not.

Neuronal function

Postischaemic hypometabolism is correlated to outcome and the duration of the ischaemic period (Michenfelder and Milde 1990). During this period intracellular alkalosis is present, the degree of which is associated to neurological outcome (Chopp et al. 1990).

After complete ischaemia the hypoperfusion period lasts 4-8 hours (Nordström and Rhencrona

1977). During the hypoperfusion period the CO_2 reactivity is low or absent, but CBF response to hypoxia is preserved (Kågstr¢m 1982). The level of CBF is higher in fasting animals (Kågstr¢m et al. 1983). Postischaemic hypoperfusion is attenuated by Calcium blocking agents (Steen et al. 1984) which also improve neurologic damage and outcome (Steen et al. 1984, Gisvold et al. 1984). Nimodipine abolishes cerebral autoregulation, impair CO_2 reactivity (Schmidt et al. 1991) and increases the critical level of CBF at which cytotoxic oedema formation occurs (Harris 1982).

A pronounced cumulative effect on the development of oedema formation and tissue injury has been observed, when the ischaemic periods were carried out during the period of marked postischaemic hypoperfusion (Tomida et al. 1987).

Autoregulation and CO_2 reactivity

Todd et al. 1986 found that the hypoperfusion period started earlier after shorter periods of ischaemia. In established hypoperfusion CBF is independent by the duration of ischaemia, and the CO_2 reactivity is abolished (Schmidt-Kastner et al. 1987). Other studies indicate that following complete global ischaemia, autoregulation is better preserved than CO_2 reactivity (Nemoto et al. 1975, Hossmann et al. 1973). These observations have recently been re-evaluated in dogs subjected to complete ischaemia. The results indicated that after 12 and 18 min, autoregulation and CO_2 reactivity were both present, but attenuated (Christopherson et al. 1993).

Recovery from severe prolonged hypoxia, combined with carotid ligation has been studied in newborn lambs. One hour after severe hypoxia CBF was increased by 110%, whereas oxygen consumption was unchanged. Cerebral autoregulation was disrupted during the recovery phase (Short et al. 1994).

Deafferentiation

When the excitatory afferents from CA3 to CAI are removed, the postischaemic metabolism in the vulnerable CA1 is reduced to the same low level as in other ischaemia-resistant regions (J¢rgensen et al. 1990).

Calcium

Energy failure gives rise to Ca^{2+} influx into the cells (Deshpande et al. 1987). CBF threshold for Ca^{2+} entry into the cell is close to 10 ml/100g/min. Together with impaired intracellular calcium sequestration, activation of catabolic enzymes occurs. These processes ultimately cause neuronal death. A therapeutic window for reperfusion damage has been defined for three types of substances: Pre- and postsynaptically acting blockers of Na^+, Ca^{2+}, and K^+ channels, glutamate antagonists acting on postsynaptic AMPA receptors, and Cyclosporin, which blocks the megapore of the inner mitochondrial membrane.

Brain oedema

Water and ion balances

Cerebral ischaemia is followed by accumulation of water, cations and albumin in brain tissue. In experimental studies of MCAO the increase in cations and water accounts for nearly all brain oedema, while the increase in albumin plays no role in oedema development (Menzies et al. 1993). Chloride accumulates with sodium in brain during the early stages of ischaemia. The BBB permeability to ^{22}Na is high relative to that of other cations, indicating a specific transport mechanism for sodium (Betz et al. 1994).

Ischaemia

The water accumulation during ischaemia is dependent on the level of CBF during ischaemia (Crockard et al. 1980). Thus, in baboons, ischaemic oedema develops when CBF is reduced below a threshold of 20 ml/100g/min (Symon et al. 1979). Furthermore, it is dependent on the duration of the ischaemia period (Ito et al. 1979, Klatzo et al. 1981) and whether ischaemia is complete or incomplete (Schuier et al. 1980, Todd et al. 1986). In the gerbil repeated ischaemic insults result in pronounced oedema formation (Tomida et al. 1987).

Hydrostatic pressure gradients

Increases in hydrostatic pressure gradients between arterial- and tissue pressure are important stimulus for oedema formation (Hatashita and Hoff 1986). Studies of pial arterial pressure in cats subjected to MCAO have shown that brain water content correlates inversely with pial pressure in the core of ischaemia, and correlates positively with pial pressure in the periphery of the ischaemic core (Yamaguchi et al. 1989). However, in another study CBF and CBV were found to be normal during the time of severe oedema formation, suggesting that changes in CBF and CBV reflect the status of larger vessels and that values in the normal range may be observed even under conditions of severe oedema and impaired perfusion at the capillary level (Pluta et al 1989).

Reperfusion

Other studies indicate that during recirculation after cerebral ischaemia the formation of brain oedema is increased (Hossmann 1976, Todd et al. 1986). Resolution of oedema also occurs in this period (Crockard et al. 1980, Ianotti and Hoff 1983). An increase in oedema formation has been related to the degree of postischaemic hyperaemia (Kogure et al. 1981, Auer 1977, Mchedlishvili et al. 1984). In gerbils, a threshold of ischaemia CBF at 10 ml/100g/min below which resolution of brain oedema does not occur, has been described (Ianotti and Hoff 1983).

Blood-brain barrier (BBB)

During complete global ischaemia the BBB remains intact for several hours (Ito et al. 1979, Schuier and Hossmann 1980, Katzman et al. 1977). On the other hand, during recirculation BBB damage is accelerated (Ito et al. 1979, Nishimoto et al. 1979), and brain oedema rapidly occurs (Ianotti and Hoff 1983, Avery et al. 1984). The degree of BBB damage is dependent on the duration of the ischaemia period (Todd et al. 1986, Nishimoto et al. 1979). In focal cerebral ischaemia blood flow restoration may exacerbate brain oedema as well (Ito et al. 1979, Iannotti and Hoff 1983). Thus, reperfusion presents a dilemma as it may reduce the infarct area and attenuate oedema formation, but it may also disrupt the BBB and enhance oedema formation. In a recent study of MAC in rats it was demonstrated that brain infarct and BBB disruption was exacerbated after reperfusion, and that BBB disruption was related to the degree of CBF recovery (Yang and Betz 1994).

Vasogenic oedema

Vasogenic oedema results from increased permeability of brain capillaries, and is characterized by an increase in extracellular volume. Several biochemical agents seem to be involved in the formation of vasogenic oedema. Prostaglandins seem to play a role in experimental brain trauma (Shohami et al. 1987), phospholipase C is elevated (Wei et al. 1982), release of glutamate and of free fatty acids in brain tissue is increased (Baethmann et al. 1989) and the concentration of bradykinin as well (Unterberg and Baethmann 1984). Bradykinin is responsible for disruption of the blood-brain barrier (Unterberg et al. 1984) and global loss of CO_2 reactivity (White et al. 1992).

Arachidonic acid

Release of free arachidonic acid from membrane phospholipids may play an important role in the pathogenesis of vasogenic brain oedema (Agardh et al. 1980, Bazan et al. 1980, Rehncrona et al. 1982, Siesjö et al. 1982). The level of free arachidonic acid is normally maintained at a very low level in extra- and intracellular spaces (Kuwashima et al. 1976, Rodrigues et al. 1983). It has been demonstrated that intracerebral injection of arachidonic acid induces vasogenic oedema as well as cytotoxic oedema (Chan et al. 1983). Arachidonic acid produces opening of the BBB and affects the vasomotor response of cerebral vessels (Unterberg et al. 1985). It has been suggested that arachidonic acid increases the capillary permeability of the brain at least in two different ways. One is an action of the acid itself, which stimulates perturbation of the membrane of the capillary endothelial cells, thus promoting an increase in capillary permeability. The other action includes an activation of the cascade reaction. This reaction may be initiated by activation of membrane-bound enzymes such as phospholipase A2 and phospholipase C (Ohnishi et al. 1992).

Cytotoxic or ischaemic oedema

The principal reason for the formation of ischaemic or cytotoxic oedema appears to be a disturbance of the energy-dependent sodium-potassium pump on the cell membrane. Unlike vasogenic oedema ischaemic oedema forms primarily in the cerebral cortex and not in the white matter. Initially the blood-brain barrier is intact. However, a continuing decrease in CBF leads to cellular damage, damage to the capillary endothelium and disruption of the blood-brain barrier.

It is proposed that failure of oxidative metabolism during ischaemia increases the concentration of H^+, lactate, pyruvate (Hossmann and Matsuoka 1982). Experimental studies indicate that lactacidosis contributes to formation of cytotoxic oedema (Kraig et al. 1987, Kimelberg 1995). *In vitro* adminsitration of lactic acid causes glial swelling in a dose-dependent manner together with intracellular acidification (Staub et al. 1990). Another study indicates that lactacidose-induced glial swelling depends on the presence of extracellular Ca^{2+} ions (Plesnila et al. 1998).

Initially, the accumulation of water is intracellular owing to the increase in intracellular Na^+ resulting from membrane failure (Hossmann et al. 1977, Harris et al. 1981) or a reduction of sodium and water clearance from the tissue (Lo et al. 1987). Other studies demonstrate that blood to brain sodium transport is increased in ischaemic tissue at early times before the BBB is disrupted. It is supposed that stimulation of the Na^+, K^+ pumps in the capillary endothelium by elevated interstitial fluid K^+ concentration may mediate this effect (Schielke et al. 1991). During complete ischaemia, in comparison with incomplete, less oedema is formed, because oedema formation presumes a functional vascular bed (Crockard et al. 1980, Ianotti and Hoff 1983). In incomplete ischaemia substrate supply and the generation of ideogenic osmoles are continued (Siesjö 1981, Myers 1979).

Glucose

In rats subjected to forebrain ischaemia normoglycaemic animals are capable of resolving postischaemic oedema, whilst hyperglycaemia results in a delayed secondary increase in oedema followed by the onset of seizure activity (Warner et al. 1987).

Excitatory amino acids

Following opening of the blood-brain barrier, NBQX (2,3-dihydroxy-6-nitro-7-sulfamoyl-benzo(F)-quin oxaline) and AMPA (amino-3-hydroxy-5-methyl-4-isozole propionic acid) receptor antagonists reduce the development of oedema, indicating that these antagonists may play a role in brain oedema formation (Westergren and Johansson 1993).

Arachidonic acid, leukotrienes and lipooxygenase

Arachidonic acid (AA) plays an important role in cytotoxic swelling. Glial swelling from AA or linoleic acid is completely inhibited by U-74389F, an antagonist of lipid peroxidation (Staub et al. 1994).

Leucotrienes with their strong vasoconstrictor activity and ability to increase vascular permeability, may contribute to the development of ischaemic oedema (Minamisawa et al. 1988). The efficacy of lipoxygenase inhibitors in modifying oedema formation has been studied in several models of brain injury. The studies of Unterberg et al. (1991) indicated that BW755C, a non-specific inhibitor of lipoxygenases, did not attenuate oedema formation after freezing cortical injury in the cat. However, the BW755C that was used in those studies, inhibits 5-, 12-, and 15-lipoxygenases as well as cyclooxygenase. In another study nordihydroguaiaretic acid, a non-specific inhibitor of lipoxgenases, reduces oedema formation after transient ischaemia in gerbils (Dempsey et al. 1986). Unlike non-specific lipoxygenase inhibitors, specific 5-lipoxygenase inhibitors appear to be more consistent in reducing oedema formation in models of cerebral ischaemia. Thus, after transient forebrain ischaemia in spontaneously hypertensive rats, decreased oedema formation was observed with specific inhibitors (Minamisawa et al. 1988, Mabe et al. 1990). During transient forebrain ischaemia in the gerbil, production of leucotriene C_4 was prohibited by pre-treatment with AA-861, a specific 5-lipoxygenase inhibitor, and in the same animals oedema formation was reduced (Baskaya et al. 1996).

Biochemical changes in ischaemic cells

Calcium

Intracellular Calcium

A rise in intracellular Ca^{2+} ($Ca^{2+}{}_i$) is one of the keys in the development of ischaemic brain damage (Siesjö 1992). The intrusion of Ca^{2+} is through voltage-sensitive channels and more importantly, via agonist-operated calcium channels, notable those gated by glutamine and related excitatory amino acids.

Ca^{2+} stores

The uptake of Ca^{2+} in intracellular stores requires energy as ATP. If intracellular Ca^{2+} increases markedly, mitochondria accumulates large amounts of Ca^{2+}. The necessary energy for this sequestration is the potential across the inner mitochondrial membrane, upheld in the presence of oxygen or ATP.

Siesjö and Bengtsson (1989) and Siesjö (1992) have suggested that calcium fluxes is a unifying pathological event, which is liberated by ischaemia, excitotoxins, hypoglycaemia and spreading depression.

Mitochondrial function

Membrane lipids are essential to mitocondrial function. Degradation of the lipid skeleton occurs during ischaemia/reperfusion. Several factors are involved in this process. Mitochondrial phospholipids such as cardiolipin decreases progressively, or shows no resynthesis (Nakahara et al. 1992, Sun and Gilboe 1994), probably because of Ca^{2+}-dependent activation of mitochondiral phsopholipase A_2 (Rordorf et al. 1991). Cardiolipin is a mitochondria-specific phospholipid, synthesised in the inner membrane of mitochondria, which synthesis is inhibited by an increase in $[Ca^{2+}]_i$ (Daum 1985). Cardiolipin is sensitive to oxidative stress (Soussi et al. 1990). Many enzymes localised to the inner mitochondrial membrane, such as respiratory chain enzymes (Complex I-V), and adenine nucleotide translocase, bind cardiolipin and require the complete composition of the mitochondrial membrane for full activity.

Oxidation stress leads to the inhibition of mitochondrial respiratory chain in other ways. Both ·OH and O_2^- inactivate respiratory chain enzymes, and such inactivation does not depend on only lipid peroxydation (Zhang et al. 1990). NO binds and inhibit complex IV (Cytochrom c oxidase), which induces the inhibition of complex 1 (NADH-Q-reductase), and complex II (Succinate-Q reductase) by further formation of free radical species (Cleeter et al. 1994). NO also affects mitochondria via an effect upon membrane potential and mitochondrial calcium homeostasis (Richter et al. 1994), Sweitzer and Richter 1994). Other studies have demonstrated that the peroxynitrite anion is a potent inhibitor of NADH dehydrogenase, succinate dehydrogenase, and ATPase, but not cytochrom c oxidase (Radi et al. 1994).

Pyruvate dehydrogenase activity is also reduced just after the start of reperfusion, probably because of free radical-mediated, site-specific protein oxidation (Katayama and Welch 1989, Bogaert et al. 1994). During transient forebrain ischaemia, followed by (3-6 hours) reperfusion, a reduction of pyruvate dehydrogenase has also been demonstrated, probably due to an increase in Ca^{2+} (Zaiden and Sims 1994).

Further targets of secondary mitochondrial damage exist. Adenine nucleotide translocase is localised on the inner mitochondrial membrane and exchanges matrix ATP for outside ADP. Its functions are coupled with those of oxidative phosphorylation in mitochondria (Aliev and Saks 1993). Elevation of free fatty acids and their CoA esters inhibits ANT activity during ischaemia/reperfusion in the brain (Kurup et al. 1990). ANT may also play an important role in mitochondrial permeability transition (Griffith and Halestrap 1991).

It was originally hypothesised that, once Ca^{2+}_i reached the set point for net mitochondrial calcium accumulation, the result is mitochondrial dysfunction, and cell death (Deshpande et al. 1987, Kristían and Siesjö 1996). A new concept, however, has recently been advanced. This involves the activation of a permeability transition (PT) pore in the inner mitochondrial membrane, which opens the membrane to H^+, and allows calcium to leave the mitochondria (Bernardi et al. 1994, Zoratti and Szabo 1995). The opening of these megapore is caused by oxidative stress and mitochondiral Calcium accumulation (Crompton et al. 1988, Duchen et al. 1993, Richter et al. 1995). Formation of megapore has been considered the most important event in the cascade causing cell death, and is thought as a trigger of apoptosis (Zamzami et al. 1996). The formation of megapore could be secondary to the production of reactive oxygen species, or to the release of protein which acts as a transcription factor. For review (Siesjö and Siesjö 1996, Kristián and Siesjö 1996, Kuroda and Siesjö 1997).

The immunosuppressant cyclosporin A is a blocker of the permeability transition. Cyclosporin ameliorates CA1 damage after transient forebrain ischaemia in rats (Uchino et al. 1995).

Phospholipase and DAG

In response to stimuli neurones also release Ca^{2+} from intracellular stores, Acetylcholine and some peptides activate a surface receptor coupled to phospholipase C, which catalyses the formation of diacylglyceride (DAG) and isositol from phosphatidylinositol. Glutamate, acting on metabotropic receptors, also initiates Ca^{2+}_i increase. Ca^{2+}_i increase as such also triggers releasing mechanisms from intracellular stores. This amplification mechanism is duplicated by caffeine. Ryanodine and Dantrolene reduce intracellular Ca^{2+} release.

Proteases and endonuchleasis

A rise in Ca^{2+}_i causes activation of lipases, proteases and endonuchleases which may alter the functions of receptors, membrane channels and give rise to break down of the cytoskeleton.

Calmodulin

Intracellular calcium is buffered to calmodulin and by other proteins such as calcibindin (McBurney and Neering 1987). The Ca^{2+}-calmodulin complex is in part responsible for the activation of phospholipases, proteases and kinases. Regional differences in Ca^{2+}-calmodulin binding after ischaemia correlate with subsequent delayed neuronal damage (Grotta et al. 1990).

Calcium/calmodulin-dependent kinase II (CaM kinase II) is a multifunctional protein kinase critical to multiple signal transduction pathways responsive to changes in intracellular Ca^{2+} concentrations. CaM kinase II and its substrates, which include enzymes and proteins involved in neurotransmitter synthesis and release, carbohydrate metabolism, and formation of cytoskeleton, are found in multiple cellular compartments in neuronal tissue. CaM kinase II also phosphorylates the cytoskeletal components, tubulin, MAP-2 and (Steiner et al. 1990), affecting the dynamic structure of the neuronal cytoskeleton. In the nucleus, activation of CaM kinase II can affect gene transcription by phosphorylation of transcription factors such as cAMP response element-binding protein (Kapiloff et al. 1991). Cerebral ischaemia causes a rapid loss of CaM kinase II activity (Schackelford et al. 1995), but does not affect all protein kinases similarly. In ischaemic models protein kinase A is not reduced in the rabbit, rat and gerbil (Aronowski et al. 1992, Yamamoto et al. 1992).

Calpain

One potential pathogenic event that has generated considerable interest is the activation of calpain, an intracellular protease, that has been implicated in a number of neuropathologic conditions. Calpain is activated by intracellular Ca^{2+}, causing proteolysis of neuronal cytoskeletal and regulatory proteins. It has thus been argued that the accumulation of numerous, irreversible changes to these multiple substrate proteins must eventually be lethal to the cell. Independent support for an important role of calpain in focal ischaemia has come from studies reporting significant reductions in neocortical infarct volume when selective calpain inhibitors were administrated (Bartus et al. 1994, Hong et al. 1994, Bartus et al. 1995). In a study of focal cerebral ischaemia (MCAO) in the rat, administration of AK275, a calpain inhibitor, demonstrated a reliable and robust neuroprotective effect over the concentration rage of 10 to 200 M, perfused supracortically for 21 hr. Moreover, a 75% reduction in infarct volume was observed when initiation of drug treatment was delayed for 3 hr postocclusion (Bartus et al. 1994).

Calcium antagonists

Calcium antagonists are potent dilator of vascular smooth vessels. Although studies in rats (Mohamed et al. 1984), and primates (Harper et al. 1981, Haws et al.1983) have shown a marked increase in CBF after administration of calcium antagonists, other studies in rats (Edvinsson et al. 1983, primate (Harris et al. 1982) and human (Forsman et al. 1986) have not been able to confirm this finding. It is supposed that differences in methodology, species, and dose of nimodipine may explain these differences.

Nimodipine

Nimodipine has been shown to increase CBF in the reperfusion period after complete ischaemia in the rat (Young et al. 1987) dog (Steen et al. 1983, Steen et al. 1984) and in primate (Steen et al. 1985). This effect is even seen when given after complete ischaemia (Steen et al. 1985, Milde et al. 1986). In the rat nimodipine does not affect post-ischaemic regional hypometabolism (Young et al. 1987). Experimental studies have demonstrated that nimodipine does not increase ICP, even during compromised intracranial compliance (Hadley et al. 1987). Nevertheless, verapamil, another calcium blocker, increases ICP in patients with brain tumour (Bedford et al. 1983).). On the other hand, nimodipine abolishes cerebral autoregulation, impairs CO_2 reactivity (Schmidt et al. 1991)

Nimodipine has a favourable influence on histopathology and neurological outcome in both complete cerebral ischaemia (Steen et al. 1985, Mohamed et al. 1985, Mabe et al. 1986, Jacewicz et al. 1990), and after focal cerebral ischaemia (Germano et al. 1987).

The promotion of recovery by nimodipine treated animals is predominantly due to improvement of postischaemic hypoperfusion by means of increasing CBF in the peripheral or penumbra regions of the ischaemia focus (Scriabine et al. 1985). Although Michenfelder and Milde (1987) found that nimodipine does not affect cerebral lactate levels following complete ischaemia in dogs, other studies indicate that post-treatment with nimodipine in rats subjected to MCAO normalises cerebral acidosis (Hakim 1986), and that pre-treatment with nimodipine reduces brain oedema in conscious rats subjected to focal cerebral ischaemia (Jacewicz et al. 1990).

Although nimodipine increases plasma-glucose concentration (Mohamed et al. 1984), it also prevents the enhancement of cerebral tissue acidosis produced by hyperglycaemia before incomplete focal ischaemia (Berger and Hakim 1989).

In primates (Harris et al. 1982), cats (Haws and Heistad 1984) and baboons (McCalden et al. 1984) the CO_2 reactivity is severely impaired. However, nimodipine does not increase CBF during hypocapnia in rats (Young et al. 1990). In the same animal nimodipine pre-treatment did not interfere with the ability to use hyperventilation for CBF manipulation (Young and Chien 1989).

In spite of the general statement that nimodipine improves recovery, failure of nimodipine to improve recovery has been demonstrated in other studies of cerebral ischaemia (Barnett et al. 1986, Vibulsresth et al. 1987). Moreover, in normal dogs (Forsman et al. 1986) and in focal ischaemia, nimodipine fails to augment CBF regardless of whether the cortex was severely or mildly ischaemic (Dirnagl. et al. 1990). One reason to these discrepancies could be failure in maintenance of blood pressure during nimodipine treatment. In studies by Marinov et al. (1991) it was demonstrated that neuronal damage was reduced when blood pressure was maintained. However, studies in cats with MCAO indicate that nimodipine together with dopamine-induced hypertension, might provoke BBB damage and increase oedema formation (Sakabi et al. 1991).

Preischaemic, in comparison with postischaemic drug administration, has convincingly demonstrated to have neuroprotective effect. According to Gotoh et al. (1986) the timing of nimodipine administration relative to the production of the ischaemia insult, is a very important factor. Thus, therapeutical attempts to reduce the ischaemia damage should be started earlier than 4-6 hours after the ischaemia insult.

In vivo binding studies in rats have demonstrated that nimodipine binding increases earlier in the more severely ischaemic structures than in those with more moderate reductions in perfusion, and that when the binding declines in a region where it was previously increased, infarction is likely (Hakim and Hogan 1991)

Other calcium blockers

Other calcium blockers with better penetration through the BBB improves CBF, brain-pH and EEG recovery in focal ischaemia (Meyer et al. 1990). Cerebral protective effects have been demonstrated with lidoflazin (Rosenthal et al. 1987) and emopamil (Bielenberg et al. 1987a,b). Flunarizine improves survival after prolonged global ischaemia Cohan et al. 1989), improves functional recovery after focal ischaemia, even when the agent is administrated after termination of the ischaemia (de Ryck et al. 1989). This effect is not a result of altered brain temperature (Cohan et al. 1992).

Nicardipine was administrated 10 min following focal cerebral ischaemia in rats. It was found that this Calcium blocker attenuates focal ischaemia brain injury by exerting direct neuroprotective and antioedematous effects that did not depend on CBF, which was unaffected both during the ischaemia and the reperfusion period (Kittala et al. 1997).

SB 201823A a novel blocker, is selective for calcium channels. This blocker is neuroprotective in both gerbil bilateral carotid artery occlusion and in the rat photothrombotic lesions model (Benham et al. 1993). In the rat middle artery occlusion model a reduced lesion volume was found, but the drug also caused a decrease in heart rate at a neuroprotective dose (Barone et al. 1995). Another study confirms the neuroprotective effect in MCAO model, and in the rat photochemical model even when treatment was delayed until 4 hrs after occlusion (Wood et al. 1997).

Conopeptides are potent inhibitors of Ca^{2+} entry sides through N-type Ca^{2+} channels. These channels are widely distributed in the central nervous system, primarily localised presynaptically. Initial studies indicate, that the conopeptide (SNX-111) has protective effect also when delaying the start of therapy 6 hours following ischaemia (Valentino et al. 1993). A study demonstrated that conopeptide prevents CA1 injury 24 hours following severe forebrain ischaemia and reduces infarction following focal ischaemia (Buchan et al. 1994).

Another N-type calcium channel antagonist (SNX-111) was studied in focal ischaemia in rats. SNX-111 reduced total amount of extracellular glutamate after occlusion, and reduced the cortical infarct size (Takizawa et al. 1995).

A novel series of compounds have been developed which inhibit lipid peroxidation and block calcium entry. U92032 is one of these "dual function compounds" which is more potent than flunarizine or nicardipine for inhibiting calcium influx induced by hypoxia or glutamate (Takashima et al. 1993). U92032 has protective effects against hypoxia, ischaemia neuronal damage and transient focal ischaemia (Goto et al. 1994). It inhibits delayed neuronal death in the hippocampus after transient global ischaemia (Takahashi et al. 1993).

Clinical studies

The number of ischaemia strokes complicating aneurysmal subarachnoid haemorrhage has been consistently reduced by nizofenone (Ohta et al. 1986) or nimodipine pre-treatment (Allen et al. 1983, Auer 1984, Philippon et al. 1986, Brandt et al. 1988, Jan et al. 1988, Ohman and Heiskanen 1988, Petruk et al. 1988, Pickard et al. 1989). Other experimental and clinical studies have shown that intracisternal administration of nimodipine (Auer et al. 1982, Zabramski et al. 1986) or other calcium blockers (Takayasu et al. 1986) increase the arterial diameter. However, systemic treatment with nimodipine does not reduce the incidence and severity of cerebral vasospasm detected by arteriography (Petruk et al. 1988).

Clinical controlled studies of the effect of nimodipine in stroke (Gelmers et al. 1988) and acute head injury (Harders et al. 1996) have been equivocal. In cardiac arrest, nimodipine antagonises postischaemic hypoperfusion, and it enhances the rate at which recovery occur (Forsman et al. 1989)

Excitatory amino acids

The predominant mechanism for excitation in the brain encompasses ion channels gated by amino acids. Glutamate, the most important excitatory amino acid, is a mixed agonist. When released form presynaptic endings, glutamate will activate both AMPA and NMDA receptors. By allowing Na+ to enter, the opening of AMPA channels leads to depolarisation. By causing depolarisation, Na+ influx via the AMPA receptor-linked channels result in Calcium influx via NMDA channels. Additionally Na^+ and Ca^{++} influx allow further Ca^{++} influx through calcium channels.

In experimental studies of cerebral ischaemia the excitatory amino acids (EAA), glutamate, aspartate and glycine seem to play an important role. Certain neurones in discrete brain regions are destroyed. This selective neuronal death is supposed to be caused by release of excitatory amino acids. It is generally believed that ATP depletion and consequently rise in intracellular Ca^{2+} are the main reason of failure of uptake of excitatory amino acids. However, Astrocytes in culture can maintain glutamate uptake during hypoxia if glucose is available (Swanson 1992), and in studies of global cerebral ischaemia in rats, it has been demonstrated that oxygen is not required to maintain efficient uptake of extracellular glutamate during hyperglycaemia (Swanson et al. 1994).

Ischaemia

In cats subjected to global ischaemia, the concentration of glutamate in cortical tissue, measured by microdialysis, increases at CBF levels below 20 ml/100g/min (Shimada et al. 1989). An increase in glutamate has been observed in the ovine fetal brain during maternal haemorrhage (Penning et al. 1995). In global ischaemia the concentrations of glutamate and glycine in dialysate are correlated to the duration of ischaemia. In cerebral ischaemia it has been demonstrated that extracellular glutamate in the CA1 region of hippocampus reaches toxic concentrations. A clear correlation between ischaemia-induced glutamate accumulation and a decrease in extracellular calcium has been found (Benveniste 1991).

During short periods of penumbral ischaemia an increase of glutamate occurs in the rat, but the concentration does not reach critical levels (Ueda et al. 1992). In other studies of MCAO the threshold for glutamate release was a CBF reduction to 48%. Mean CBF during ischaemia exhibited an inverse relationship with infarct volume, and the magnitude of glutamate release during ischaemia was positively related with infarct volume (Takagi et al. 1993).

Marked astrocyte swelling is a prominent occurrence during and after ischaemia. In models of astrocytic swelling cultures of astrocytes exposed to hypotonic or high K^+ solutions have been used. Swelling in these cultures is accompanied by release of taurine, glutamate and aspartate. Uptake of glutamate and aspartate by astrocytes is predominantly Na^+ -dependent, the process being coupled to influx of Na^+ and efflux of K^+ (Kimelberg et al. 1995). In rat astrocyte cultures, hypoxia reduced glutamate uptake by 40%. Reduction in pH from 7.4 to 5.8 also reduced the glutamate uptake. However, the combination of hypoxia and acidosis reduced glutamate uptake to below 10% of controls (Swanson et al. 1995).

Glutamate transporters

Normal functioning of glutamate transporters clear the synaptically released glutamate to prevent excitatory neuronal death. In rats subjected to MCAO blockage of the glial glutamate transporter GLT-1 led to increased infarct volume. In contrast, blockade of the neuronal EAAC1 transporter did not influence the infarct volume (Rao et al. 2001).

Blockers of glutamate receptors

Inhibitors of excitatory receptors, especially the N-Methyl-D-Aspartate (NMDA) groups, have been studied in the CAl region of hippocampus. Bezomorphan ((+)SKF 10.047), acting on of the NMDA receptor, is effective in gerbil global ischaemia (Lysko et al. 1992). Other NMDA antagonists have no effect in complete global ischaemia but are to some degree effective in preventing neuronal damage in incomplete ischaemia, repeated normothermic global ischaemic insults, hypoglycaemia (Choi et al. 1990, Papagapiou and Auer 1990, Lin et al. 1993) and in focal ischaemia (Ozyurt et al. 1988, Steinberg et al. 1991, Sauer et al. 1995). In the penumbra the energy depletion is sufficient to release glutamine, and pH is sufficiently high to maintain NMDA receptor function, which otherwise is eliminated at pH 6.0. In experimental studies NMDA receptor antagonists reduce the volume of ischaemia even in respiratory acidosis (Park et al. 1993) which otherwise seems to attenuate the protective effect of NMDA antagonists (Park et al. 1991b). In rats subjected to subdural hematoma, NMDA antagonists attenuate the ICP increase otherwise found (Kurudo et al. 1991). NMDA also exhibits protection against redistribution of calmodulin and thus changes the activity of protein kinases (Aronowski et al. 1993).

Both NMDA receptor agonists and antagonists produce cerebral vasodilation *in vitro* and *in vivo.* It is unclear whether this action is due to direct effects on the cerebral vasculature or other indirect mechanisms. In isolated bovine cerebral arteries NMDA receptors mediating vasomotion are not present. Competitive NMDA agonists and antagonists have negligible effects on cerebral arterial tone. Non-competitive NMDA antagonists dilate preconstricted arteries, but by mechanisms which were not stereospecific (Wendling et al. 1996).

Diemer (1990) stresses the importance of other antagonists to excitatory amino acids, especially the alpha-amino-3-hydroxy-5-methyl-4-isovasole proprionic acid (AMPA) receptor blockers. AMPA receptors especially should be present in the hippocampus. In this region denervation of ischaemia-vulnerable pyramidal cells has a protective effect, and most synapses are glutaminergic. The vulnerability during ischaemia seems to be best correlated to the occurrence of AMPA receptors. Thus, a therapeutic window has been defined for AMPA-blockers. According to this Nellgård and Wieloch (1992), in rats, found that AMPA, but not NMDA receptor antagonists, decreased neuronal damage following transient severe cerebral ischaemia. Pretreatment with a new AMPA receptor antagonist, LY-293558, reduced significantly infarct size in focal cerebral ischaemia in cats (Bullock et al. 1994).

In forebrain ischaemia NBQX is effective in reducing degeneration of CA1 cells even after 12 hours (Li and Buchan 1993). In experimental studies the occurrence of repeated spreading depression (SD) in the periinfarct surrounding has been documented (Nedergaard and Astrup 1986). These electrophysiological disturbances are associated with increased energy demand which is not matched with an adequate supply of oxygen. In rats subjected to MCAO prevention of periinfarct SD with NBQX has been shown. It is suggested that suppression of SD and the decreased metabolic workload is one factor improving neuronal survival (Mies et al. 1994).

Methionine sulfoximine (MS)

Methionine sulfoximine irreversibly inhibits brain glutamine synthase, which is localised to glia cells (Norenberg et al.1979). This enzyme is essential to the astrocyte-neuronal shuttle by which glutamine is provided to neurones (Waniewski and Martin 1986). In rats subjected to MACO, pre-treatment with methionine sulfoximine, reduces neuronal damage, and an increase in brain glycogen stores has been found, which is supposed to benefit penumbra tissue metabolism (Swanson et al. 1990). Limiting ischaemic injury by inhibition of excitatory amino acid release has recently been demonstrated (Graham et al. 1993).

Riluzole

Riluzole reduces the degree of neuronal injury after exposure to anoxia or to excitatory amino acids (Dessi et al. 1993, Estevez et al. 1995). Its neuroprotective effect has been demonstrated in models of cerebral ischaemia (Pratt et al. 1992, Malgouris et al. 1989). Riluzole prevents seizures induced by a variety of stimuli (Romettino et al. 1991). The mechanism by which riluzole is able to reduce neuronal injury and possible prevent cell death is not fully understood. It has been demonstrated that it reduces potassium-induced glutamate release *in vitro*, and spontaneous glutamate release *in vivo* (Martin et al. 1993, Cheramy et al, 1992). These effects can in part be attributed to the capability of riluzole to block neuronal ion channels, including Na^+, K^+ and Ca^{2+} channels (Dessi et al. 1993, Hebert et al. 1994). In Rabbits subjected to transient global cerebral ischaemia riluzole was not able to attenuate glutamate release (Kwon et al. 1998),

Glycine antagonists

Glycine is required to coactivate the NMDA receptor before the associated ionophore becomes permeable to calcium (Lester et al. 1993). Glycine has been demonstrated to be required in cell culture medium to allow glutamate toxicity in cultured neurones (Johnson and Ascher 1987). Furthermore, interstitial glycine concentrations become substantially increased during an ischaemic insult and remain elevated for prolonged intervals after reperfusion (Baker et al. 1991, Globus et al. 1991). Rats subjected to glycine receptor antagonists demonstrated reduced cerebral infarct volumes after MCAO, and were associated with a reduced incidence of hemiparesis resulting from MCAO. In the forebrain ischaemia model, glycine receptor antagonism had no effect on delayed neuronal necrosis in the CA1 region, neocortex, or caudoputamen (Warner et al. 1995). Another glycine antagonist (L-687,414) was effective in producing neuroprotection in focal cerebral ischaemia at doses that did not affect MABP or had any other of the adverse effects associated with the administration of NMDA receptor blockers (Gill et al. 1995)

Adenosine

CBF regulation

Adenosine is a potent vasodilator and plays a role in the normal regulation of CBF (Berne et al.1974, Winn et al. 1981), and the regulation under pathophysiologic conditions (Van Wylen et al. 1986, Hagberg et al. 1987, Phillis et al. 1987, Meno et al. 1991). During hypoxia an increase in interstitial fluid adenosine concentration has been observed in piglet (Park et al. 1987).

Ca^{2+} uptake and excitatory amino acids

It has been shown that adenosine and its agonist inhibit intracellular calcium uptake (Dragunow and Faull 1988) and the release of excitotoxic compounds (Coradetti et al. 1984, Fastbom and Fredholm 1985). Interstitiel fluid concentrations of glutamate and aspartate are increased in the presence of adenosine receptor blockade (Sciotti et al. 1992). With some exceptions adenosine A_1 receptors and NMDA binding sites have similar distributions in the brain (Goodman and Snyder, Young and Fagg 1990).

Leukocyte function

Neutrophil generation by superoxide anions (Cronstein et al. 1986), and leukocyte-endothelial cell interactions are attenuated (Cronstein et al. 1986).

Protection

Adenosine suppresses neuronal activity (Phillis et al. 1975). Rudolphi et al. (1987) and Phillis et al. (1989) proposed adenosine to be an endogenous neuroprotector. Adenosine agonist limits the neuronal loss following ischaemia (Block and Pulsinelli 1987, Evans et al. 1987, von Lubitz et al. 1988, Bielenberg 1989, Roucher et al. 1991), and attenuates traumatic cell death in rat hippocampal cells (Mitchell et al. 1995). Studies in rats indicate a protective effect of adenosine on both normo- and hyperglycaemic ischaemia-reperfusion injury (Zhou et al. 1994).

Antagonists

Adenosine antagonists exacerbate the consequences of ischaemia (Rudolphi et al. 1987, Sturm et al. 1993, Perés-Pinzón et al. 1993, Wieloch et al. 1986). A worsening of brain ischaemia with the adenosine antagonist, theophylline, has been found (Wieloch et al. 1986, Zhou et al. 1994).

Propentofylline, an adenosine uptake blocker increases GABA (Vukadinovic et al. 1986) and adenosine levels in the brain, and reduces glutamate release under ischaemic conditions (Andiné et al. 1990, Miyashita et al. 1992). A neuroprotective effect against brain damage in gerbils has been demonstrated (DeLeo et al. 1988). In clinical studies of stroke pentofylline increased glucose utilisation in the infarct zone (Huber et al. 1993).

Nitric oxide (NO)

EDRF and NO

In 1980 an endothelium-derived relaxing factor (EDRF), which exerts an influence on vascular tone was described (Furchgott and Zawadzki 1980). Later on EDRF was identified as nitric oxide or closely related compounds produced by the amino acid L-arginine by NO synthetase (Myers et al. 1990, Moncada et al. 1991). Other studies indicated that NO influences tone in the cerebral vessels (Moncata et al. 1991, Faraci 1992). NO stimulates soluble guanylate cyclase, resulting in an increase in cGMP and dilation of cerebral vessels. Whether NO is involved in the increase in CBF elicited by neuronal activation remains controversial.

There is evidence suggesting that certain nitric oxide-containing compounds such as nitrosothiols resemble the EDRF generated by acetylcholine more closely than does NO itself. One of these compounds is S-Nitroso-L-cysteine (Kukreja et al. 1993). Nitroglycerine and nitroprusside stimulate the formation of cGMP, while methylene attenuates relaxation by inhibiting guanylate cyclase (Watanabe et al. 1988, Kim et al. 1992).

Although some of the discrepancy in recent studies may be related to the degree of NO synthase inhibition in the different studies, NO is unlikely to be the universal mediator of "metabolic vasodilation" in the brain as originally proposed (Iadecola et al. 1994).

NO synthesis

In the brain NO synthase (NOS) is localised to the endothelium (eNOS), parenchymal neurones and perivascular neurones (nNOS). The enzyme is separated into a constitutive and inducible form. A third form (iNOS) is normally absent in the brain, but becomes an important source after infiltration of inflammatory cells. Concerning the gene expression of NOS (see page 41).

The constitutive form is present in brain tissue and endothelium and is active under basal conditions. This enzyme is stimulated by an increase in intracellular Ca^{2+}, acetylcholine, serotonin, substance P, histamine, bradykinin, vasopressin, ATP and prostaglandin. Besides, endothelium-dependent responses can be elicited by platelets by ADP liberation (Shimokawa et al. 1988, Oyama et al. 1993, Kurkeja et al. 1993), and from astrocytes by lipoxygenase products (Murphy et al. 1994). The activity of NO synthase can be regulated in a negative feedback manner by NO (Rogers and Ignarro 1992, Rengassamy and Johns 1993).

Inducible NO synthase activity is of minor importance during normal basal conditions. Expression of this form happens as a response to immunologic stimuli which liberates lipopolysaccharide and cytokines, interferon gamma, tumour necrosis factor and interleukin-1. The NO production by the inducible form is much higher than the constitutive form (Marletta 1993, Schmidt et al. 1993). This is critical because NO can be toxic to cells. The induction of NO synthetase can be inhibited by glucocorticoids and some cytokines (Moncada et al. 1991).

Localisation

Within the brain tissue NO production has been localised to neurones and perivascular fibres. However, neurones that contain NO synthase represent only 1% of cortical neurones (Dawson et al. 1992). Increased neuronal activity from the fastigial nucleus of the cerebellum and cholinergic fibres that project to the cerebral cortex is attenuated by inhibitors of NO synthetase (Adachi et al. 1992, Iadecola 1992).

Two types of reactive neurones have been found in neural parenchyma. Type I neurones, medium-sized, bipolar or multipolar, were distributed in the cerebral cortex and white matter. Type II, lightly stained, small oval neurones, were distributed in the cerebral cortex. Endothelial cells were intensively reactive in the arteries, arterioles, and capillaries, but weakly in the veins (Tomimoto et al. 1994).

Excitatory amino acids

Activation of glutamate receptors stimulates NO formation (Garthwaite 1991), and dilation of cerebral vessels in response to NMDA is dependent on NO formation (Faraci and Breese 1993). Also cerebral vasodilation during penthylenetetrazole- and harmaline-induced seizures (Faraci et al. 1993), and the dilation occurring during spreading depression (Northington et al. 1992, Duckrow 1993) are induced by increased NO formation.

Cerebral vessels

Perivascular neurones are innervated by NO-synthase-containing nerves. The source of these nerves seems to be the sphenopalatine ganglion (Toda et al. 1993). Activation of these fibres within the vessel wall produces NO-dependent relaxation *in vitro* (Toda and Okamura 1992). Also electrical stimulation of the parasympathetic fibres from the sphenopalatine ganglion produces NO-mediated increased in CBF (Morita-Tsuzuki et al. 1993).

Glia cells

Glia cells function as cellular stores for the substrate for NO formation (Aoki et al. 1991). The constitutional NO synthase in astrocytes responds to stimuli including Ca^{2+}, bradykinin, glutamate and norepinephrine (Agullo and Garcia 1992, Murphy et al. 1991). In response to lipopolysaccharide and cytokines induction of inducible NOS in astrocytes, microglia and glioma cells occurs (Simmons and Murphy 1992, Lee et al. 1993, Merrill et al. 1993, Colasanti et al. 1993). However, relatively little is known regarding the regulation of induction of NO synthase in glia. Induction can be inhibited by dexamethasone, norepinephrine, interleukin-10 and some cytokines (Simmons and Murhpy 1993, Galea et al. 1993, Mollace et al. 1993, Feinstein et al. 1993).

NO-synthase inhibitors

Many studies of NO are based on the activity of NOS and especially the use of analogous of L-arginine, which act as specific enzyme inhibitors. These inhibitors include N-monomethyl L-arginine (L-NMMA), N-nitro-L-arginine (L-NNA) and N-nitro-L-arginine-methyl ester (L-NAME). Inhibitors of NO synthase all decrease CBF while glucose utilisation is not influenced. Consequently, the normal ratio of CBF to glucose consumption is reduced (Macrae et al. 1993). In a recent study the CO_2 sensitivity of CBF was completely abolished by L-NAME (Bonvento et al. 1994). However, reversal of CO_2 sensitivity was observed after L-arginine administration (Sandor et al. 1994). Cerebral vasodilation during hypercapnia is dependent in large part on production of NO (Faraci et al. 1994). L-NAME does not influence α_2-adrenergic-mediated decrease in CBF by dexmedetomidine (McPherson et al. 1994).

Ischaemia

Using NO sensitive electrodes an increased local concentration of NO has been demonstrated in cerebral ischaemia. With electron paramagnetic resonance NO-trapping technique, it was found that the amount of trapped NO during forebrain ischaemia increased seven times that of control (Tominaga et al. 1994). This increase occurs rapidly within minutes. However, as ischaemia continues, the NO-level falls slowly with a half-life of approximately 30 min, but increases again during reperfusion (Malinska et al. 1993). After focal cerebral ischaemia, biochemical and immunocytochemical evidence of expression of the inducible isoform of NO-synthase has been demonstrated (Iadecola et al. 1995).

In the periphery of the area of necrosis the expression of NO synthase is delayed, but remains constant throughout the duration of ischaemia (Zhang et al. 1993).

Protection

An increase in nitrite, nitrate and cGMP and citrulline production has been observed in MCAO (Kader et al. 1993, Kumura et al. 1994). Beneficial effects of NO during ischaemia include maintenance of CBF and inhibition of aggregation and adherence of platelets and leukocytes (Nishimura et al. 1991). In spontaneously hypertensive rats subjected to MCAO the concentration in cerebral tissue of NO was lower, the release of oxygen radicals higher, and the infarst size larger than in normotensive rats (Dobrucki et al. 2000). Moreover, an increase in NO blocks NMDA receptors (Manzoni et al. 1992), and neurones that contain NO synthase are resistant to damage caused by excitatory amino acids (Dawson et al. 1992).

One explanation for the neuroprotection is that NO improves perfusion in the ischaemic penumbra. Theoretically there are several actions of NO that are relevant in this respect. First, NO can increase cGMP synthesis in vascular smooth muscle of arteries and arterioles and promote vasodilation. Second, NO, by preventing platelet aggregation and neutrophile adhesion may limit additional vascular occlusion. However, excessive concentration of NO may be cytotoxic due to the formation of superoxide (Beckman et al. 1990, Radomski et al. 1991). Third, studies of transient focal ischemia in rats indicate that early NO production exerts a neuroprotective effect by modulating neutrophil infiltration (Batteur-Parmentier et al. (2000). As a consequence of these effects some studies with repeated administration of low doses of NO synthase demonstrate a reduction of infarct size and cerebral oedema together with a decrease in CBF (Buisson et al.1992, Nagafuji et al. 1992, Nowicki et al. 1991). In other studies acute administration of NO synthase inhibitors has a protective effect during focal cerebral ischaemia in rats (Trifiletti 1992, Buisson et al. 1993, Achwal et al. 1993) and cats (Nishikawa et al. 1993). In one study co-administration of L-arginine reversed this effect (Yoshida et al. 1994).

A recent study indicated that in spite of the decrease in CBF, inhibition of NO synthase mildly improved the oxygen supply and consumption balance in ischaemia cortex (Wei et al. 1994). In other studies, however, NO synthase inhibitors have enhanced brain damage (Weismann et al. 1992, Yanamoto et al. 1992, Zhang and Iadecola 1993, Kuluz et al. 1993), and in *in vivo* studies no effect of NO synthase on brain damage after ischaemia has been demonstrated (Dawson et al. 1992, Moncada et al. 1992). In a recent study it was demonstrated that inhibition of endothelial and neuronal NO synthase activity does not modify resistance of NO-producing neurones to transient ischaemia (Sancesario et al. 1994). Other studies have shown that administration of L-arginine, the substrate of NO production, before and after MCAO in hypertensive rats, increases CBF and reduces infarct size (Morikawa et al. 1992), suggesting that L-arginine becomes a limiting factor for production of NO during ischaemia. The effect of L-arginine on CBF is sustained throughout the observation period of 70–105 min (Morikawa et al. 1994).

The administration of NO donors like nitroprusside and 3-morholino-sydnonimin after MCAO reduces infarct volume and increases CBF (Zhang et al. 1993, Zhang et al. 1994). However, in other studies L-arginine did not have these effects (Buisson et al. blood 1993). In this context it shall be emphasized that some NOS inhibitors increase blood pressure in a dose-dependant manner, and consequently an increase in blood flow in regions dependent on collateral circulation has been observed (Muhonen et al. 1994). In one study of spinal cord ischaemia development of spinal cord infarct during long-term inhibition of nitric oxide synthase in rats was found (Blot et al. 1994).

One reason to discrepancy in results could be that NO only improves cerebral damage when given early in the reperfusion stage. Thus, NO-producing agents do not increase CBF or reduce infarct size when they are administrated 2 hrs. after induction of ischaemia (Zhang and Iadecola 1994), suggesting that the beneficial effects of NO occur only in the early phase of cerebral ischaemia. In another study of rats subjected to MCAO inhibition of NO synthesis worsened ischaemia damage when instituted shortly after induction of ischaemia, but did not affect or reduce the ischaemic damage at later times (Zhang et al. 1995).

Free radicals

It has been proposed that the oxidation/reduction state of NO may be of importance. Reduction of NO by superoxide generates peroxynitrite ion, which is cytotoxic. On the other hand, oxidation of NO also generates nitrosonium, which can nitrosylate NMDA receptors, and thus prevent excessive stimulation (Lipton et al. 1993). Other path-ways are possible. Production of messenger RNA for interleukin-lb occurs in ischaemia tissue and may induce NO synthase activation (Liu et al. 1993). If L-arginine becomes a limiting factor in production of NO after ischaemia, then increased activity of NOS may lead to production of superoxide and hydrogen peroxide which are both cytotoxic (Schmidt et al. 1993, Heinzel et al. 1992, Pou et al. 1992).

Subarachnoid haemorrhage

In subarachnoid haemorrhage NO relaxation of large arteries is impaired (Hatake 1992, Vollmer et al. 1992). Some studies indicate that this impairment is caused by reduced formation of cGMP. Other studies suggest that the production of cGMP is normal (Kanamura et al. 1989, Katusic et al. 1993).

Radical oxygen species (ROS)

Free radicals are formed in all cells. As they are toxic, the cell possesses a defence mechanism. If oxygen accepts one electron superoxide radicals including H_2O_2 and O_2^- are formed. This reduction is coupled to the enzymatic process catalysed by xanthine oxidase in which hypoxanthine and zanthine are oxidised to uric acid. By the so called "Haber-Weiss reaction" O_2^-, ·OH and H_2O_2 react to form the extremely toxic .OH radical. This process is catalysed by Iron, which is normally tightly bound to ferritin and transferrin, but released from ferritin by O_2^- and reduced flavins, and from transferrin by acidosis.

Radical oxygen species play an important role in ischaemic damage in the reperfusion period (Hall and Braughler 1989, Floyd 1990, Carney and Floyd 1991, Siesjö 1992, Chan 2001). Following ischaemia reperfusion leads to formation of radical oxygen species (ROS), and scavengers of ROS ameliorate damage. Overexpression of CuZn-SOD or knockout of neuronal nitric oxide synthase (nNOS) reduce the infarct size after transient focal ischaemia in transgenic mice (Huang et al. 1994, Yang et al. 1994). Dirnagl et al. (1995) demonstrated a burst-like formation of $O2^{\cdot-}$ during the first 10–12 min. of reperfusion after forebrain ischaemia, suggesting that if the aim of therapeutic intervention is to prevent ROS formation and accumulation, scavengers of free radicals are to be given before ischaemia, or at the time of reperfusion.

Inflammatory cells represent one of the major sources of ROS. Reperfusion up-regulates cell adhesion molecules such as ICAM-1 and P-selectin on endothelial cells, and β2-integrins on leukocytes. Leukocytes exhibit in turn rolling, firm adherence to the endothelial cells, and migration. Activated PMN leukocytes can produce ROS, leading to reperfusion damage (Winn et al. 1995). In support P-selectin can be detected continuously during reperfusion following focal ischaemia (Okada et al. 1994). ICAM-1 is up-regulated from 163 hrs. up to 1 week after reperfusion (Matsuo et al. 1994, Okada et al. 1994). PMN leukocytes begin to infiltrate into the ischaemia tissue between 6 and 12 hrs. after reperfusion (Garcia et al. 1994, Marsuo et al. 1994). It has been shown that extracellular ROS generation is biphasic, with an increase within one hr, and after 24 hrs. after reperfusion, and that circulating and infiltrating PMN leukocytes are involved in both the first and second phase of ROS production (Matsuo et al. 1995). NO is produced in endothelial cells, macrophages, and leukocytes. Endothelial (eNOS) and /or inducible NOS (iNOS) are activated during reperfusion. Their activities increase in the period 1–12 hrs. and peak at 1–2 days after the start of reperfusion (Iadecola et al. 1995, Nakashima et al. 1995). In the reperfusion period platelets are also supposed to play a role (Bazan and Allan 1996). Furthermore, it has also been proposed that microglia produces cytotoxic mediators, such as ROS and inflammatory cytokines (IL-1, Il-6, TNF-α), which may accelerate tissue damage (Gehrmann et al. 1995). This contention is supported by studies indicating that intracerebral or systemic administration of IL-1 receptor antagonist reduces the infarct volume after permanent focal ischaemia (Relton and Rothwell 1992, Garcia et al. 1995).

Another source of ROS is the neuronal cell. Experiments have demonstrated that activation of NMDA receptors and the associated increase in intracellular Ca^{2+} concentration lead to the formation of ROS in neurones (Dawson et al. 1991, Bondy and LeBel 1993, Coyle and Puttfarcken 1993, McNamara and Fridovich 1993, Yang et al. 1996). Some of the generation of ROS must emanate from mitochondria, another source being arachidonic acid oxidation via cyclo-oxygenase and lipoxygenase (Bazan et al. 1991, Bazan and Allan 1996). Furthermore, Ca^{2+}-dependent activation of phospholipase A_2 and of peptidases, such as calpain I, yields $O_2^{\cdot-}$. Neuronal nitric oxide synthase is also activated by an increase in $[Ca^{2+}]_i$, generating NO. More recently, *in vitro* and *in vivo* experiments have provided information on mitochondria as a major source of oxygen free radicals (Ambrosio et al. 1993, Dugan et al. 1995, Reynolds and Hastings 1995, Piantadosi and Zhang 1996). Mitochondria generates $O_2^{\cdot-}$ when reducing O_2 to H_2O in the respiratory chain, at the site of NADH dehydrogenase and ubiquinone. Under pathological conditions, such as ischaemia-reperfusion and hypoxia-re-oxygenation, the imbalance between restoration of oxygen supply and mitochondrial respiratory function results in a massive generation of ROS in mitochondria. Under these conditions, defensive mechanisms, such as manganese superoxide dismutase (Mn-SOD) and glutathione peroxidase, are not able to prevent the efflux of ROS from mitochondria.

NO

NO, derived from endothelial cells, can elicit toxic peroxynitrate ion (NO_3^-), which is decomposed rapidly at acid pH yielding ·OH and NO_2. This process is initiated by NO synthase, which is activated by an increase in $Ca^{2+}{}_i$

Iron

There is increasing interest in brain iron metabolism, because abnormal iron deposition in various brain regions has been reported in many neurodegenerative disorders such as Alzheimer disease, Parkinson disease, amyotrophic lateral sclerosis, and multiple sclerosis. Iron in various organs is involved in the formation of free radicals, thus contributing to lipid peroxidation (Mead 1976). It has been argued that re-circulation of blood after transient cerebral ischaemia causes an increase in low molecular weight species of iron (Krause et al. 1987), and that free radical formation initiated by iron ions leads to brain damage by lipid peroxidation (Siesjö 1988). In spite of many studies concerned with a role of iron in neuronal damage during early phases of cerebral ischaemia, abnormal iron deposition at a late stage after cerebral ischaemia has only sparsely been reported. In rats subjected to transient forebrain ischaemia, it was demonstrated that iron deposits in the CA1 region occurred after four weeks. The depositions gradually increased and formed clusters by week 24.

An increase in astroglia reaction, and the appearance of ferritin-immunopositive microglia paralleling the accumulation in the CA1 regions, indicate that iron deposition probably is produced in the process of gliosis. At least three different types of iron deposition in the chronic phase after transient ischaemia have been disclosed, suggesting that late-onset iron deposition may be relevant to the pathogenesis of chronic brain dysfunction seen at a late stage after cerebral ischaemia (Kondo et al. 1995).

Low iron diet for 8 weeks decreases brain and serum iron levels, and in the gerbil fewer neurological deficits and decreased brain oedema after temporary unilateral carotid ligation have been observed (Patt et al. 1990).

In clinical practice high serum ferritin levels within the first 24 hours of hospitalisation for an acute ischaemia stroke are related to a poor prognosis, independent of the stress response (Dávalos et al. 1994).

Free radical scavengers

In some studies of cerebral ischaemia radical scavengers have been demonstrated to have a beneficial effect (Lim et al. 1986, Cerchiari et al. 1987, Abe et al. 1988, Liu et al. 1989). In other studies a lack of effect has been found (Forsman et al. 1988). Vitamine E, a non-toxic free radical scavenger, protects against anoxic brain damage in hippocampal slice (Acosta et al. 1986).

Oxygen free radicals are decomposed by superoxide dismutase and glutathione peroxidase but also react with ferritin giving rise to reduction of Fe^{3+} to Fe^{2+} which again may create oxygen radicals with their effect on lipid peroxidase (Pulsinelli et al. 1985). Studies in cats subjected to MCAO suggest that the histoprotective action of superoxide dismutase is due to its ability to attenuate increases in intracellular Ca^{2+} during the re-circulation period (Araki et al. 1992). Superoxide dismutase concentration in the CSF is a marker of acute brain lesion. The enzyme leaks rapidly from ischaemically injured brain cells, and determination of the concentration in CSF is supposed to have some prognostic value (Strand and Marklund 1992). Superoxide dismutase reduces permeability and oedema induced by hypertension in rats (Zhang and Ellis 1990).

Lazaroids

Lazaroids are 21-aminosteroids which act as free-radical scanvengers and, at as iron chelators. In temporary focal ischaemia lazaroid improves survival rate (Hall et al. 1988) and reduces infarct size (Silvia et al. 1987, Xue et al. 1990). In complete focal ischaemia (MCAO) lazaroid reduces oedema formation (Young et al. 1988) and infarct size (Hall et al. 1990). In global cerebral ischaemia in gerbil Hall et al. (1990) found preservation of the CA1 structure. In the rat, however, no effect was found (Lesink et al. 1990, Xue et al. 1990). In dogs subjected to cardiac arrest Natale et al. (1988) found improved survival rate and better neuronal function. In the same animal, subjected to ICP-hypertension, Perkins et al. (1988) found improved neurologic function and better recovery.

In rabbits tiralazad pre-treatment reduced neurologic deficits from multiple cerebral emboli (Clark et al. 1994).

Mice subjected to a concussive injury showed improved neurologic score (Hall et al. 1988) and cats subjected to another concussion model demonstrated reduced posttraumatic brain lactate acidosis (Dimlich et al. 1990).

In cats subjected to spinal cord trauma prevention of posttraumatic hypoperfusion was found

(Hall 1988). In cats subjected to experimental subarachnoid haemorrhage, prevention of hypoperfusion and ICP-hypertension were observed (Hall and Travis 1988). In primates lazaroids reduced severe spasms and improved neurological outcome (Steinke et al. 1989).

Other studies have shown that lazaroids prevent secondary collapse in cats subjected to haemorrhage shock (Hall et al. 1988). Furthermore, lazaroids, in experimental studies enhance the recovery of evoked potential, improve postischaemic blood pressure and block spreading depression-induced hypoperfusion. (For Review see Hall and Braughler 1989ab).

In cats subjected to MCAO (Myers et al. 1990), and in rats subjected to forebrain ischaemia (Buchan et al. 1992) no effects on ischaemia injury were found. Helfaer et al. (1992) in mongrel dogs subjected to 12 min ventricular fluid infusion to raise ICP above systolic pressure, did not find any improvement of metabolic recovery. In cats subjected to transient focal ischaemia, administration of tirilazad at the onset of either ischaemia or reperfusion does not ameliorate infarct volume assessed during early reperfusion (Takeshima et al. 1994). However, it cannot be excluded that higher dose, different timing of administration, and a longer recovery period would be beneficial in a less severely injured model of focal ischaemia. Differences of aminosteroids in efficacy may also be due to species, difference in incomplete and complete ischaemia models and administration dose.

In clinical studies tirilazad treatment have been disappointing in acute stroke (The RANTTAS investigators 1996, The RANTTAS II investigators 1998), in acute head injury (Marshall et al. 1998), and in spinal cord injury (Bracken et al. 1997). In subarachnoid haemorrhage patients doses of 6 mg/kg/day seems to improve recovery in men (Kassell et al. 1996). In woman 15 mg/kg decreased the incidence of vasospasm, but did not improve recovery (Lanzino et al. 1999), and the same dose given daily reduced the mortality among patients who were neurological grade IV or V on admission (Lanzino and Kassell 1999).

Superoxide dismutase (SOD) and catalase

Superoxide dismutase and catalase, both free radical scavengers, inhibit arachidonic acid metabolites and normalise CO_2 reactivity in experimental cerebral ischaemia and traumatic brain injury (Kontos et al. 1981, Wei et al. 1981). In transgenic mice that overexpress human copper/zinc superoxide dismutase, an attenuated activation of the transcription factor (NF-kappaB) occurs. This attenuation is supposed to block expression of deleterious genes like c-myc, thereby reducing ischaemic damage (Huang et al. 2001). However, these enzymes do not pass the blood-brain barrier (Chan et al. 1987) and both enzymes have very short half-life.

In anaesthetised piglets subjected to fluid percussion injury, it has been demonstrated that pial artery vasoconstriction associated with elevated CSF opioids level. Furthermore, opioid-induced vasodilation and cyclic GMP production are attenuated. Superoxide dismutase/catalase partially restore these effects (Thoregood and Armstead 1996).

Preconditioning with the endotoxin analog diphsophoryl lipid A indices tolerance against ischaemic/reperfusion injury in the rat. An enhancement of basal superoxide dismutase activity was observed before ischaemia, and a further enhancement was seen in the ischaemic penumbra 24 hours after reperfusion (Toyoda et al. 2000).

N-acetylcystein

N-acetylcystein, another free radical scavenger, passes the blood-brain barrier. In experimental studies this drug normalises the CO_2 reactivity after traumatic brain injury (Ellis et al. 1991).

Dihydrolipoat

Dihydrolipoat, a drug with antioxidant activity against lipid peroxidation, protects neurones against ischaemia damage by diminishing the accumulation of free radicals within the cerebral tissue (Prehn et al. 1992).

Spin trapping agents

Spin trapping agents are compounds which react with unstable free radicals to form relatively stable adducts with a typical electron spin resonance signal. The free radical trapping agent N-*TERT.*-butyl-α-phenylnitrone has been studied in gerbils subjected to forebrain ischaemia. When the agent is administrered 30 min. before carotid occlusion, prevention of the increased locomotor activity documented in saline-injected ischaemic animals was observed, and a significant reduced damage of the CA1 pyramidal cell layer was found 5 days post-ischaemia (Phillis and Clough Helfman 1990). When the agent was administrated 2 hrs. post-ischaemia protection failed against cerebral ischaemia (Clough-Helfman and Phillis 1991).

In experimental studies the spin trapping agents, possess free radical scavenger effect, reduce infarct size and prevent a secondary mitochondrial dysfunction due to reperfusion. Probably they scavenge free radicals at the blood-endothelial cell interface.

These drugs attenuate ·OH formation during reperfusion following transient forebrain ischaemia in rats (Sen and Phillis 1993), and one of the agents, S-PBN, reduces the formation and related brain damage due to stereotactic injection of malonate into the striatum (Schulz et al. 1995a,b).The effect of spin trapping agents was first demonstrated in gerbils, when the agent was administrated 30 min before ischaemia.(Cao et al. 1988, Floyd 1990, Oliver et al. 1990, Phillis and Claugh-Helfman 1990). Subsequently, the effect also has been demonstrated when given up to 12 hrs. following middle cerebral artery occlusion (Cao and Phillis 1994). An amelioration has also been demonstrated, when the drug is administrated 1 or 3 hrs. after the start of recirculation (Zhao et al. 1994). Other studies indicate that when given 1 hr. after recirculation, prevention of mitochondrial dysfunction and bioenergetic failure after 4 hrs. of recirculation are found (Folbergrová et al. 1995, Kuroda et al. 1996a, Kuroda et al. 1996b).

Eicosanoids

Metabolites arising from the result of cyclooxygenase and lipoxygenase activity include prostaglandins, leucotriens and thromboxane. Another pathway, via phospholipase A_2 activity, gives rise to the formation of prostaglandins, leucotriens, thromboxane and platelet-activating factor (PAF). The latter is proinflammatory and leads to activation of platelets as well as activation and adherence of leukocytes to endothelial cells. For review see (Siesjö 1992).

Studies by *ex vivo* incubation of tissue slices demonstrate that ischaemia and subsequently re-circulation cause site- and time specific changes of tissue eicosanoids production (Kempski et al. 1987). However, regional heterogeneity in the postischaemic eicosanoid production in the brain has also been demonstrated (Patel et al. 1992).

Lipid peroxidase

Lipid peroxidases are catabolic enzymes which catalyse the formation of free fatty acids, which are synthesised to prostaglandins and thromboxanes by cyclooxygenase and leucotrienes by lipooxygenase. After forebrain ischaemia in the rat a delayed and long-lasting increase in lipid peroxidation has been found (Bromont et al. 1989). Phenothiazines are inhibitors of iron- dependent lipid peroxidation (Yu et al 1992a). In a transient rat focal stroke model phenothiazine reduced cortical infarct volume (Yu et al. 1992b).

Thromboxane

Thromboxane A_2 has vasoconstrictor properties and may worsen postischaemic hypoperfusion. However in a rat microdialysis study thromboxane did not increase following MCAO (Cole et al. 1993). During forebrain ischaemia, microdialysis technique has shown a relationship between the duration of ischaemia and thromboxane production. During the reperfusion period both thromboxane and 6-keto-PGF-1_α are present in increased concentrations.

Epoxygenase pathway

Recently another pathway of arachidonic metabolism has been demonstrated referred to as the epoxygenase pathway (Fitzpatrick and Murphy 1989). The epoxygenase metabolites are called epoxyeicotrienoic acids (EET). Two EETs have been demonstrated in brain tissue (Amruthesh and Ellis 1990) of which 5.6-EET is the most abundant. This agent produces cerebral vasodilation, an effect prevented by indomethacin (Ellis et al. 1990).

Cyclooxygenase inhibitors

Indomethacin

Indomethacin is a blocker of cyclooxygenase and thereby prostaglandin synthesis. Indomethacin acts as a cerebral vasoconstrictor and reduces CBF, while $CMRO_2$ remains unchanged (Pichard and MacKenzie 1973, Sakabe and Siesjö 1979, Dahlgren et al. 1981, Wennmalm et al. 1981).

Experimental studies of canine basilar arteries indicate that prostaglandins mediate cerebral oedema (Shohami et al. 1987). In cats subjected to focal ischaemia (Dempsey et al. 1985) and rats subjected to freezing lesions (Yen and Lee 1987), indomethacin reduces cerebral oedema. Also the rapid accumulation of eicosanoids during reperfusion is blocked by indomethacin (Gaudet et al. 1980). In other experimental studies of focal ischaemia (Harris et al. 1982; Awad et al. 1983, Sutherland et al. 1988, Suzuka et al. 1989) and traumatic head injury (Shapira et al. 1988) indomethacin administration was not followed by a decrease in cerebral oedema. Other experimental studies suggest that the infarct size in focal cerebral ischaemia was not influenced by indomethacin (Harris et al. 1982, Koide et al. 1986).

Indomethacin reduces cerebral infarct size in focal ischaemia (Sasaki et al. 1988), enhances post-ischaemia re-perfusion after MCAO (Shigeno et al. 1985) and reduces the detrimental effect of cerebral fluid compression (Hallenbeck and Furlow 1979).

Furthermore, in rats subjected to fluid percussion trauma pre-treatment with indomethacin an improved recovery has been observed (Kim et al. 1989).

The vasoconstrictor effect of indomethacin has been used in the treatment of ICP-hypertension in patients with head injury. In one study, indomethacin 30 mg was followed by an immediate decrease in ICP of about one hour duration. The fall in ICP was accompanied by a decrease in CBF, an increase in $AVDO_2$ and $AVD\text{-}_{lactate}$, whilst $CMRO_2$ was unchanged (Jensen et al. 1991). In another study the effect of a bolus doses (30 mg) of indomethacin on ICP was comparable with the effect of a 1.5 kPa decrease in $PaCO_2$ (Dahl et al. 1996).

Zometirac

The cyclooxygenase inhibitor zomepirac has been studied in cats after global ischaemia. Zomepirac-treated animals displayed higher flow during the hypoperfusion phase, the CO_2 reactivity was intact and the EEG showed prominent recovery (Stevens et al. 1986).

Ibuprofen

In dogs subjected to global cerebral ischaemia, another cyclooxygenase inhibitor, ibuprofen, has been found to improve postischaemic hypoperfusion and decrease cerebral venous levels of thromboxane A2 (Grice et al. 1986).

Combined therapy with cyclooxygenase and lipoxygenase

In a rat model of temporary focal ischaemia the mixed cyclooxygenase-lipoxygenase inhibitor BW755C was administrated near the rime of reperfusion. A significant attenuation of postischaemic hypoperfusion combined with a reduced extravasation of Evans blue were demonstrated. Hemispheric swelling as well as total infarct volume were reduced in treated animals (Chen et al. 1995).

Phospholipase C

Phospholipase C, an enzyme that catalyses the phosphodiesteratic cleavage of phosphatidylinositol, is activated by a receptor-mediated mechanism coupled to a guanosine triphosphate-binding protein (G-protein). By this enzymatic process 1,4,5-inositol triphosphate (IP3) is formed. In the endoplasmatic reticulum IP3 releases Ca^{2+}. Another enzymatic product is 1,2-diacylglycerol an activator of proteinkinase C (Nahorski 1988).

In rats subjected to forebrain ischaemia phenylmethylsulfonyl fluoride, a Phospholipase C inhibitor, ameliorates delayed neuronal damage in the hippocampal CA1 subfield (Umemura et al. 1992).

Protein synthesis and proteolysis

Delayed neuronal death in selectively vulnerable areas has been demonstrated (Bodsch et al. 1985, Thilmann et al.1986, Widmann et al. 1991). Repeated episodes of global ischaemia have been attributed to the irreversible suppression of protein synthesis. It is, therefore, conceivable that synthesis of protective macromolecules such as calcium-binding proteins or neuropeptides may become a limiting factor for cell survival. Persisting inhibition of protein synthesis following cerebral ischaemia is an early manifestation of neuronal injury (Widmann et al. 1992).

It has been suggested that metal-catalysed oxidation of proteins is a site-specific process involving the interaction of free radicals and Fe^{2+} at metal binding sites on the protein. Protein oxidation increases during reperfusion following 10 min ischaemia in gerbils (Olivier et al. 1990). However, in another study of ischaemia of one or three hours duration oxidative damage of proteins was not documented (Folbergrová et al. 1993).

In the ischaemic core local cytoskeletal proteolysis, assessed regionally by an immunoblotting procedure to detect spectrin breakdown products, begin within 2 hrs. of MCAO (Yao et al. 1995)

Tau protein

Tau proteins belong to the microtubule-associated protein family, and are localised in neurones. Tau proteins bind to microtubules through repetitive regions in their carboxy-terminal part. This binding is regulated by the degree of Ser/Thr phosphorylation of the tau proteins. Recent studies indicate that tau dephosphorylation is an early event that occurs during ischaemia, but does not persist during reperfusion regardless of the neurological outcome (Burkhart et al. 1998, Shackelford and Yeh 1998). It is suggested that phosphorylation of particular sites on tau proteins may reflect microtubule dynamics and activation of different transduction signals. Mailliot et al. (2000) found that the sequential and differential recovery of tau phosphorylation after ischaemia followed by reperfusion, is a useful marker with which to monitor integrity after cerebral ischaemia.

Ornithine decarboxylase

Following ischaemia, activation of ornithine decarboxylase (ODC) has been noticed. Induction of ODC and accumulation of putrescine are hypothesised to be responsible for vasogenic oedema and neuronal death (Dempsey et al. 1991). Inhibition of ODC with α-difluoromethylornithine (DFMO) significantly reduced infarct size after transient focal ischaemia (Muszynski et al. 1993), and delayed neuronal death in the hippocampus (Kindy et al. 1994).

Gene expression

The temporal profile of gene expression after MCAO in the rat comprises immediate early genes, which are expressed within minutes *(Fos, jun and zif)*, heat shock protein, eNOS, growth factors, expressed within hours, and cytokines, adhesion molecules, bcl-2, and p53 expressed within days.

The molecular regulation of apoptosis has been studied from different perspectives, with emphasis on the conserved phylogenetic nature of cell death mechanisms, and its interlocking with the control of cell proliferation in conjunction with influence of extracellular factors such as cytokines.

At least two families of gene expressed mechanisms are of interest: The BCL-2 family which represent both apoptosis inhibitors and inducers, and the Caspases, which represent a family of executioners. For review: Kristian and Siesjö (1996), MacManus and Linnik (1997), Papadopoulos et al. (2000).

There are reports of increases in neurotrophins and various excitatory amino acid receptors following an ischaemia insult. This issue has been reviewed by Akins et al. (1996). The link between cell proliferation and apoptosis has been touched by many (Desbarats et al. 1996, McConkey and Orrenius 1996) and extended to neurogenesis and neuronal apoptosis as well (Ross 1996). After Kainic acid treatment, an increase of the cell-cycle proteincyclin D1 was reported in astrocytes (Liu et al. 1996). Ischaemia-induced increases in gene expression in astrocytes was described for β-amyloid precursor proteins (Kositonabo et al. 1996), clusterin (Walton et al. 1996), and the neurofibromatosis gene product NF1 (Giordano et al. 1996).

Immediate early genes (Fos and Jun)

Reams of data have been accumulated on the rapid but transient induction of immediate early genes (IEG) after various stimuli including either a focal or global ischaemic insult. These transcription factors, exemplified by the leucine-zipper protein *Fos* and *Jun*, are considered to be nuclear third messengers that link extracellular signals to longer term alterations in effector gene expression, and to be a paradigm for transcription-dependent i.e. programmed cell death (apoptosis) even in a situation of overall defective protein synthesis such as ischaemia (Wiessner et al. 1996). In the normal CNS these proteins are present at relatively low levels but correlations have been made between increased expression of *fos* and *jun* and subsequent delayed neuronal death induced by ischaemia or a variety of disease states as epilepsy. A causal link between IEG expression to subsequent death was made in cultured neurones, using antibodies or dominant-negative *Jun* that prevented the ultimate demise of treated cells (Herzog and Morgan 1996).

Despite apparently irrefutable evidence for a role in cell death for the IEG, a disconcerting alternate view suggests that *fos* and *jun* may be components of an adaptive or repair/regeneration process, because many cells that have increased expression actually survive insults such as excitotoxicity (Akins et al. 1996, Herzog and Morgan 1996, Hughes and Dragunow 1995). Such an idea comes from the finding of normal cell death in *fos*-null mice, and the lack of effect in neuronal cell death in the spinal cord after sciatic nerve resection in knockout animals (Roffler-Tarlov et al. 1996). This is in concert with findings indicating an increase in *fos* and *jun*DmRNA in the resistant hippocampal dentate area in a model of transient cerebral ischaemia (Tseng et al. 1997), and after transient global ischaemia with postischaemic hypothermia (Kamme and Wieloch 1996).

The Bcl-2 gene family

This family includes several members, that are structurally, but not functionally homogenous. Some members of the family protect from cell death (Bcl-2, Bcl-x_l, whilst others (Bax, Bad, Bid and Bcl-x_s) promote cell death. *In vitro* studies indicate that Bcl-2 protected against a wide variety of insults, including excitatoxicity, elevated Calcium, lipid peroxidation, and free radical damage. A neuroprotective effect of Bcl-2 has been shown in transgenic animals that overexpressed Bcl-2, or when viral vectors are used to overexpress Bcl-2 in focal, or global ischaemia (Choi 1966, Chopp and Li 1996, Linnik 1996, Lawrence et al. 1996).

Several studies have analysed the expression of the proapoptotic and antiapoptotic members of the Bcl-2 family after focal and global cerebral ischaemia. These studies have concentrated on the protective proteins Bcl-2 and Bcl-x_L and the death enhancing Bax protein, as these proteins have been shown to be important determinants of neuronal apoptosis in the developing brain (Deckwerth et al. 1996, Shindler et al. 1997). In general, the result from stroke studies have been consistent with the known functions of these proteins. Thus, the proapoptotic Bax protein is upregulated in neurones that are destined to die in both global ischaemia (Chen et al, 1996, Hara et al. 1996) and focal ischaemia (Gillardon et al. 1996), while its expression remains constant in neurones that survive the ischaemia insult.

Bcl-2 inhibits both apoptosis and necrosis. Bcl-2 expression has little effect on metabolic function in normal cells. Several lines are suggest as to the way Bcl-2 prevent cell death:

Regulation by dimerization

The cumulative response to the Bcl-2 family members in a cell is in part regulated by dimerization domains within the family. The ability of Bcl-2 to inhibit apothosis is blocked by the formation of a heterodimer with Bax (Yang and Korsmeyer 1996). The binding of these proteins is dependent on three conserved regions, BH1, BH2, and BH3. Deletion studies indicate that the BH1 and BH2 domains are responsible for the formation of Bcl-2 homodimers, whereas the BH3 domain has an important functional role in the death promoting family members, including Bax, Bak and Bip (Zha et al. 1996, Sattler et al. 1997). At present the majority of dimerization data can be fit to two potential models. In the first model, the formation of toxic Bax homodimers is dominant, and Bcl-2/Bcl-x_L dimers may be dominant repressors of cell death, and heterodimerization with Bax and Bad inhibits the ability of these molecules to prevent apoptosis (Gajewski and Thompson 1996).

Phosphorylation-dependent regulation.

Bcl-2 family members can be phosphorylated in a manner that modifies function and intracellular localisation. Phosphorylation attenuates the protective effect of Bcl-2 while deleting the target serine residue enhances the activity of Bcl-2 (Gajewski and Thompson 1996). Phosphorylation of proapoptotic Bad alters its normal affinity for Bcl-x_L (Zha et al. 1996). Thus, different phosphorylation states of the Bcl-2 family members alter the activities of these proteins, possibly by altering their affinity for Bcl-2 family members and other protein in the cell.

Local inhibition of free radical production.

Bcl-2 inhibits the accumulation of lipid peroxides (Yang and Korsmeyer 1996). This antioxidant effect, however, was not observed in all models, and subsequently this hypothesis has attracted less interest.

Formation of a ionic conductance channel in membranes

The Bcl-x_L protein contains two central hydrophobic α helices, surrounded by five anphipathic helices (Muchmore et al. 1996). Minn et al. (1997) demonstrated that Bcl-x_L can insert into membranes and form a ionic conductance channel that is cation selective at physiological pH. The implications for ischaemia include the possibility that Bcl-x_L regulates the sequestration of intracellular calcium, which is an important component of the excitotoxic cell death mechanism.

Regulation of permeability transition in mitochondria

When Bcl-2 is expressed in the outer mitochondrial membrane, it inhibits the permeability transition to several apoptosis inducers (Zamzami et al. 1996, Marchetti et al. 1996). Bcl-2 also enhances the calcium uptake capacity of the mitochondria and provides mitochondria with a greater resistance to Ca^{2+} induced respiratory injury (Murphy et al. 1966).

Prevention of cytochrom c release from mitochondria

Cytochrom c released from the mitochondria can activate CPP32-like caspases and drive apoptotic cell death (Kluck et al. 1997). Bcl-2 expression prevents the release of cytochrom c from the mitochondria, and prevents the activation of caspases (Yang et al. 1997).

Interactions with Ced-4 and Ced-5.

The nematode C elegans has two important genes for cell killing. Ced-3 is the parent gene of the caspase family. Intensive investigation has still not revealed a mammalian homolog of Ced-4. Ced-4 interacts with Bcl-2, which inhibits the cell killing effect of Ced-4 (Chinnaiyan et al. 1997, Wu et al. 1997).

The Caspases family

The Ced-3/ICE family of cysteine proteinases, called caspases, have received a great deal of attention because of their key role as a final common excecutioner of apoptosis. The caspases are expressed as proenzymes that undergo proteolytic processing and subunit rearrangement to yield active enzymes. The caspase family contains several members with unique tissue distribution, substrate specificity, and activation criteria..

Several important nuclear proteins have been identified as caspase substrates, and the degradation of these proteins may contribute to chromatin condensation and/or DNA fragmentation. Some of the caspase substrates localised in the nucleus are identified below:

In the Mongolian gerbil treatment with caspase inhibitor ameliorates brain injury after transient cerebral ischaemia, probably by inhibiting the activity of interleukin-1beta (Hayashi et al. 2001).

Poly (ADP-ribose)polymerase (PARP)

This is a repair enzyme, which functions upstream of p53 to identify DNA strand breaks. Caspase mediates cleavage of PARP, blocks DNA repair, and prevents the reduction in the cellular pool of NAD associated with PARP activity (Schwartz and Milligan 1996, Ashkens and Werb 1996).

DNA-PKcs (DNA-dependent protein kinase)

DNA-PKcs is a DNA repair enzyme. DNA-PKcs may be involved in the repair of double stranded DNA breaks. A caspase-mediated loss of DNA-PKcs activity would also inhibit the ability of the cell to repair DNA damage (Casciola-Rosen et al. 1966, Song et al. 1996).

Actin

Actin is an important cytoskeletal protein. Its degradation by caspases could compromise cellular and nuclear structure. Actin is an effective inhibitor of Dnase I, an enzyme capable of double-stranded DNA cleavage. Caspase-mediated cleavage of actin could contribute to cellular and nuclear collapse and lead to activation of Dnase I (Kayalar et al. 1996).

Lamin

The nuclear lamins are structural proteins that contribute to the nuclear cytoskeleton. Specifically inhibiting caspase-mediated cleavage of lamin did not prevent chromatin condensation, but it did prevent the progression to nuclear shrinkage and fragmentation into apoptotic bodies (Rao et al. 1996, Takahashi et al. 1996).

HnRNP (heteronuclear ribonucleo proteins)

The hnRNP are a family of proteins that are involved in RNA splicing and processing. Caspase-mediated degradation of hnRNP could compromise the ability of the cells to recover from an apoptotic-initiating event by altering the processing of newly transcribed proteins (Waterhouse et al. 1996).

Transcription factors

Many of the stroke-induced changes in gene expression result from changes in the relative distribution of the transcription factor that transactivates these genes. Some changes in transcription factor expression can be directly linked to cell death, such as the induction of the transcription factor p53 transactivating the proapoptotic protein Bax (Smith and Fornace 1996, Levine 1997). However, interpreting the consequences of changes in the expression of transcription factors requires careful analysis, because these factors are highly context dependent. A good example of this context dependency is NF-KB, a factor that is sequestrated in the cytoplasm by the inhibitory protein IKB (Lipton 1997, Baichwal and Baeurele 1997). When IKB is phosphorylated and/or cleaved, NF-KB is free to translocate to the nucleus, where it influences the expression of a wide variety of genes, including many stress activated genes. The levels of NF-KB are elevated in several degenerative diseases, including stroke (Terai et al. 1996) and Alzheimer's disease (Kaltschmidt et al. 1997, Terai et al. 1996. Grilli et al. (1996) showed that blocking NF-KB activation by aspirin or sodium salicylate could protect neurones against an excitatoxic insult. While these data suggest that NF-KB is detrimental, several studies have shown that NF-KB activation blocks apoptosis to a variety of insults (Beg and Baltimore 1996, Liu et al. 1996), and can be neuroprotective (Goodman and Mattson 1996). Thus, this transcription factor can be both protective and detrimental, depending on the context in which it is expressed and the nature of the insult.

P53

This transcription factor sits at a crossroad between surveillance of the genome for DNA damage, recruitment of the repair machinery, or alternatively tipping of the cell into an apoptosic cell death pathway, as a final solution in maintenance of tissue integrity. Experiments with p53-knockout-mice indicate a less severe outcome in neurones after kainic acid treatment (Morrison et al. 1996) adrenalectomy (Sakhi et al. 1996). These observations add to those which have shown attenuation of ischaemia damage (Choi 1996, Chopp and Li 1996, Linnik 1996).

Cultured neurones from p53-deficient animals, however, have a decreased sensitivity to either glutamate excitotoxicity or genotoxins (Enokido et al. 1996, Xiang et al. 1996). In addition, overexpression of p53 in either cultured cortical, hippocampal, or superior cervical ganglion leads to apoptosis (Jordan et al. 1996, Slack et al. 1996, Xiang et al. 1996). Increased expression of p53 has been reported after cerebral ischaemia insult (Chopp and Li 1996, Tomasevic et al. 1996).

c-Myc

Research has led to the recognition of the importance of another transcription factor c-Myc, in regulating apoptosis (Zorning and Evans 1996). The nuclear phosphoprotein c-Myc is involved in cell cycle regulation and is not generally expressed in non-proliferating or quiescent cells. Few genes have actually been identified as targets for c-Myc transactivation, but one is p53. Overexpression of c-Myc primes cells for apoptosis and facilitates the adverse effects of lack of nutrients or oxygen (Alarcon et al. 1966, Graeber et al. 1996). Such conditions exist in the ischaemia brain, and it is therefore of interest that an up-regulation of c-myc expression has been reported after focal occlusion (Nakagomi et al. 1996). Another target gene of c-Myc is ornithine decarboxylase (Henriksson and Luscher 1996), which has been seen to increase after cerebral ischaemia, although its overexpression in transgenic rats was unsuccessful in influencing infarct volume (Lukkarinen et al. 1997).

Leukocyte activation and adhesion molecules

Activation of leukocytes is important in the complex pathophysiological cascade leading to vasomotor reactions in cerebral arteries. Activated polymorphonuclear leukocytes have been shown to produce vasospastic reactions in arteries from different vascular beds, indicating that these vasoactive substances may contribute to cerebral ischaemia (Faraci et al. 1991, Akopov et al. 1992). In a study of rabbits intravascular leukocyte activation induced an acute disturbance of the endothelium-dependent relaxation, and under this circumstance, platelet activation might result in marked angiospastic reactions of large cerebral arteries (Akopov et al. 1994). This reaction is independent of NO synthesis from L-arginine (Akopov et al. 1994).

The leukocyte adhesion molecules are supposed to be important control factors in the pathophysiology of secondary brain injury. There are three families of adhesion molecules (Foresee et al. 1994). The first includes the glycoproteins L-selectin, E-selectin and P-selectin. L-selectin is present on the surface of leukocytes while E- and P-selectins are expressed on the endothelial surface after injury. P-selectin is also expressed on platelets. The glycoproteins mediate the initial tethering of leukocytes to the vessel wall by binding to counter-receptors within moments of tissue injury (Spertini et al. 1991). Deficiency of either the selectins or their ligands causes failure of the migration process and recurrent infection (Etzioni et al. 1992). In a recent study inhibition of L-selectin did not alter ischaemic injury in a rabbit stroke model (Yenari et al. 2001).

The two other families mediate strong adhesion and migration across the endothelium into tissues. The immunoglobulin consists of ICAM-1, ICAM-2 and vascular cell adhesion molecule (VCAM-1), which are present on the endothelial surface, and ICAM-3 which is present on the leukocyte cell surface. Their counter-receptors form the third family, the integrins (e.g. CD11b, CD18, Mac-1). The blood of healthy humans contains soluble, active forms of the selectins and immunoglobulins, termed sL-selectin and sICAM-1.

Experimental studies suggest that IL-1β, IL-6 and TNFα up-regulate the activity of the adhesion molecules. Thus treatment of endothelial cell cultures with IL-1β caused increased leukocyte adhesion by acting on endothelial cells (Bevilacqua et al. 1985). IL-1β increases ICAM-1 expression in fibroblasts, and IL-1β and TNFα increase ICAM-1 expression in other cell cultures. TNFα and interferon-gamma cause induction of ICAM-1 expression in microglia (Zielasek et al. 1993), and administration of TNFα to cultured CNS endothelial cells causes increased expression of VCAM-1 and E-selectin (DoreDuffy et al. 1994). Similarly IL-1β, TNFMα, interferon-gamma and lipopolysaccharide increase ICAM-1 expression (Wong et al. 1992).

Leukocytes accumulate in damaged brain tissue and there is significant correlation between the degree of leukocyte accumulation and the extent of cerebral oedema in rats. (Schoettle et al. 1990), In a rat stroke model an increase in cortical E-selectin expression by 6 hrs. after injury, which peaked at 12 hrs. and returned to basal concentrations by day 5 was found. ICAM-1 expression 3 hr after injury was also found (Wang and Feurstein 1995). In the reperfusion period after MCAO in rats an increase in cortical ICAM-1 expression from 1 h after injury was found. This correlated with moderate infiltration of leukocytes in the areas of ICAM-1 expression (Clark et al. 1995). An up-regulation of cortical E-selectin during reperfusion has been demonstrated in primates (Haring et al. 1996). Another recent study showed that ICAM-1 deficient mice were less susceptible of cerebral ischaemia/reperfusion injury (Soriano et al. 1996).

There are only a small number of studies which have investigated adhesion molecules in neurological disease and non-traumatic brain injury. ICAM-1 expression is increased in the cerebral vessels of patients with multiple sclerosis, viral encephalitis and cerebral infarct (Sobel et al. 1990), and there is a high concentration of sICAM-1 in the CSF and blood of patients with bacterial meningitis, which correlates with measures of blood-brain barrier dysfunction (Rieckmann et al. 1993). In patients with stroke or transient cerebral ischaemia increased expression of CD11a and CD18 were found (Kim et al. 1995), and in brain sections from patients dying from stroke an increased expression of endothelial ICAM-1 was found (Lindsberg et al. 1995).

Anti-adhesion molecule therapy

Antibodies to the intercellular adhesion molecule-1 (ICAM-1) reduce infarct size volume when given at 1 hr. of reperfusion following 2 hrs. of MCAO, and that antibodies to adhesion molecules on the surface of leukocytes, also ameliorate the infarct volume, even when administrated after 4 hrs. of reperfusion (Chopp et al. 1994, Zhang et al. 1995). In addition, an anti-neutrophil monoclonal antibody attenuates reactive oxygen species formation during reperfusion and reduces infarct size (Matsuo et al. 1995). These findings are in good agreement with other studies showing that leukocytes and cell adhesion molecules such as ICAM-1 play an important role in reperfusion damage following focal ischaemia (Zoppe et al. 1991, Barone et al. 1992, Zhang et al. 1995). More recently it was demonstrated that homozygous null ICAM-1 mice show a marked reduction of the infarct size due to transient focal ischaemia (Connolly et al. 1996). Adhesion molecule antibodies in CNS ischaemia have been studied in spinal cord ischaemia. Antibody to the integrin CD 18 and to the immunoglobulin ICAM-1 produced a reduction in neurological deficits (Clark et al. 1991, Clark et al. 1991). Pretreatment with anti-CD18 decreased the extent of neurologic damage in a reperfusion spinal cord ischaemia model (Clark et al. 1991), and improved microvascular patience when administrated before reperfusion in a baboon transient MCAO model (Mori et al. 1992). Other studies in rat stroke models indicate that antibodies to various adhesion molecules reduce infarct size and leukocyte infiltration (Chen et al. 1994, Jiang et al. 1994, Zhang et al. 1994). Treatment with anti-integrin or anti-ICAM-1 antibodies several hours after the onset of ischaemia also results in reduced infarct size (Chopp et al. 1996, Zhang et al. 1995).

However, in other studies leukocyte antibodies did not improve cerebral injury (Takeshima et al. 1992).

Glia cell activation

Effect

Transformations of postischaemic glia cells appear 15 min. after cerebral ischaemia. These transformations include swelling of cisterns of Golgi apparatus, endoplasmatic reticulum and microtubule (Pepito 1986). Cerebral ischaemia changes astrocyte and other glia cells into reactive species. In gerbil subjected to MCAO, reactive astrocytes were detected in the cerebral cortex and caudo-putamen as early as 24 hours after reperfusion (Yamamoto et al. 1987). Kraig and Jaeger (1990) suggested that the reactive glioses is triggered by elevation of interstitial K^+ and intracellular pH.

Hypoxia-regulated genes

The expression of a novel oxygen regulated stress protein ORP150 was described in ischaemic mouse brain (Kuwabara et al. 1996). Another helix-loop-helix transcription factor first described in 1993, the hypoxic-inducible factor, has been shown to influence the expression of many oxygen-regulated genes (Dachs and Stratford 1996). The recognised target repertoire of hypoxic-inducible factor-1 includes genes such as erythropoitin, vascular endothelial growth factor, aldolase, enolase, lactate dehydrogenase, and heme-oxygenase-1 (Lee et al. 1997, Semenza et al. 1996). Hypoxia-inducible factor-1 is present in the brain, and its expression increases after exposure to hypoxia (Wiener et al. 1996). Therefore increased gene expression for heme-oxygenase after either global or focal ischaemia may come to no surprise (Takeda et al. 1996).

Cytokines

The cytokines are low-molecular weight polypeptides, which are synthesised and released by multiple cell types throughout the body. Their actions are numerous but they act primarily as mediators of the inflammatory process and as growth factors. Many of the clinical signs which are seen after an acute brain injury (pyrexia, neutrophilia and cerebral oedema, secondary to disruption of the blood-brain barrier) are influenced by cytokine activity (Ott et al. 1994). Cytokines also stimulate the formation or release of many types of secondary mediators such as the oxygen-derived free radicals, neuropeptides and arachidonic acid derivates, and up-regulate the activity of the adhesion molecules.

Interleukin 1_β (IL-1_β) and tumour necrosis factor$_\alpha$ (TNF$_\alpha$)

Cerebral IL-1β and TNF8Ma are increased acutely after cerebral ischaemia in animal stroke models, particularly in the first hours after injury (Liu et al. 1993, Liu et al. 1994, Szaflarski et al. 1995). These findings suggest that IL-1β and TNFα55M are released very early after injury, and explain partly why these two cytokines are often not detected in serum in clinical studies of brain injury.

Several studies have demonstrated the toxic effect of IL-1β and TNFα (Okusawa et al. 1988, Waage et al. 1993). IL-1β acts to stimulate production of other cytokines, including TNFα, and in particular IL-6, by both astrocytes and microglia (Shalaby et al. 1989). Similarly TNFα causes the release of other cytokines, particularly IL-6 (McIntoch 1993, Shalaby et al. 1989). IL-1β is increased in the CSF of patients who have sustained a stroke (Tarkowski et al. 1995).

In a rat MCAO model, administration of an IL-1 blocker reduced cerebral oedema (Yamasaki et al. 1992).

Interleukin-6 (IL-6)

IL-6 differs from IL-1β and TNFα, as it both causes and inhibits inflammation. IL-1β and TNFα together with many other mediators, including platelet activating factor, interferon and the bradykinins, promote IL-6 production. The part played by IL-6 in the regulation of the intracranial inflammatory process is complex, because it has pro- and anti-inflammatory actions, and has negative feedback effect on the production of IL-1β and TNFα (Schindler et al. 1990).

Clinical studies in non-traumatic brain injury implicate IL-6 as a mediator in the secondary inflammatory response. IL-6 concentrations in CSF are increased after SAH, peaking day 6 (Mathiesen et al. 1993). The concentration of IL-6 in plasma increases at the time of diagnosis of brain death (Amado et al. 1995).

Heat shock protein (HSP)

Another aspect of adaptive/regeneration response in the brain to ischaemic insults concerns heat shock protein, the expression of which is increased in both neurones and glia cells (Akins et al. 1996, Kirino 1996, Massa et al. 1996). HSP prevents initiation of inflammatory gene expression via inhibition of the transcription factor NFκB activation. It also inhibits nitric oxide synathase type 2 expression and macrophage/microglial activation in the brain (Heneka et al. 2000).

Production

Exposure of cultured cells to a mild heat stress has been found to enhance cell survival after a subsequent lethal elevation in body temperature (Gerner and Schneider 1975). This protective effect has been reported to correlate with the production of heat shock protein (HSP) (Li and Werb 1982).

Global ischaemia induces heat shock protein expression throughout the hippocampal area before any degeneration of the CA1 layer (Wiessner et al. 1996). Also during brief focal ischaemia in the rat expression of the heat shock protein was found in the territory of the insult (Galzier et al. 1994). After focal ischaemia, cells that had increased expression of heat shock protein did not show DNA fragmentation (States et al. 1996).

Localisation

Immunoreactive HSP is localised in neurones, most strikingly in hippocampus. Its accumulation, however, is minimal in the CA1 pyramid cells, which are extremely vulnerable to ischaemia injury (Vass et al. 1988, Nowak 1989).

Protection

There is a hierarchy of cell types and anatomic sites that express HSP. This hierarchy seams to reflect cellular and anatomic vulnerability to ischaemia cell damage (Li et al. 1992). It has been suggested that HSP induction in neurones bordering a necrotic ischaemia core, may be the morphological equivalent of the ischaemic penumbra. Studies in rats subjected to focal ischaemia indicate that expression of HSP is prolonged in regions of undergoing injury, but is transient in surrounding regions that recover (Welsh et al. 1992). Chopp et al. (1989) demonstrated that transient hyperthermia, before a period of cerebral ischaemia, had a neuroprotective effect against ischaemic cell damage. Kitagawa et al. (1991) demonstrated that an optimal neuroprotective effect was achieved by a single hyperthermic episode applied 18 hours before forebrain ischaemia. There is now growing evidence concerning the critical role of HSP in enhancing survival during thermo stress (Li and

Laszlo 1985, Riabowol et al. 1988). Studies with localisation of HSP protein mRNA induction in gerbil brain after ischaemia have demonstrated a prolonged postischaemic stress response in vulnerable hippocampal neurones (Nowak 1991).

Nitric Oxide synthase

During cerebral ischaemia three isoforms of nitric oxide synthase (NOS) are of interest. They include neuronal (nNOS), endothelial (eNOS) and inflammatory (iNOS). In focal ischaemia all three types of NOS are expressed. nNOS and eNOS increase within few hours, while iNOS is induced after one day. eNOS may be beneficial to the ischaemic tissue, whereas excessive NO formation synthesised by nNOS and iNOS may be detrimental. The effects of NO in cerebral ischaemia are considered in chapter 2 and page 352.

Serine proteases

Tissue-type plasminogen activator (t-PA), one of the serine protease, has been used in the acute treatment of thromboembolic stroke (Hacke et al. 1995). When administered within three hours after the onset of stroke an improvement in neurological recovery was observed (Adams et al. 1995).

Serine proteases have been identified to occur in neurones and glial cells. Their enzymatic activity regulates the balance between the accumulation and the degradation of the extracellular matrix. The balance between the degradation and accumulation of the extracellular matrix is the integral to pathological processes involved in cerebral ischaemia. Serpins, including type 1 plasminogen activator inhibitor, neuroserpin and protease nexin-1, are compounds that modulate the activity of serine proteases, and exhibit neuroprotective activity (For review Vivien and Buisson 2000).

Peptide growth factor

Peptide growth factor is increasingly being linked to the neurodegenerative effects of cerebral ischaemia. In animal models, increased expression of basic fibroblast growth factor has been documented during both focal (Kumon et al. 1993) and global (Takami et al. 1992) models of cerebral ischaemia. Fibroblast growth factor and epidermal growth factor are of interest because they are present throughout the brain and are protective during ischaemia (Yamada et al. 1991, Freese et al. 1992). Fibroblast growth factor has been shown to activate protein kinase C, but is also dependent on protein kinase C for cell proliferation (Presta et al. 1991). The mechanism of protection by epidermal- and fibroblast growth factors during hypoxia and NO toxicity appears to be dependent on a minimum degree of protein kinase C activity. Other signal transduction pathways independent of protein kinase C also may mediate protection by these growth factors (Meiese and Boccone 1995).

Brain-derived neurotrophic factor (BDNF)

BDNF is one of the best characterised neurotrophic factors in the nerve growth family. It plays a critical role in the maintenance and repair of specific neural groups in the central nervous system. It is especially important in the degenerative change that occurs in the hippocampal cells after seizures and forebrain ischaemia. Hippocampus has the highest BDNF messenger ribonucleic acid (mRNA) content (Hofer et al. 1990). A marked increase of BDNFmRNA expression has been reported during brief hippocampal seizures (Isackson et al. 1991). In transient forebrain ischaemia a marked increase in BDNF in dentate gyrus has been demonstrated after two hours (Lindvall et al. 1992), and intraventricular infusion of BDNF prevented the neurodegeneration of hippocampal CA1 neurones after transient forebrain ischaemia (Tsukahara et al. 1994).

Neuronal apoptosis inhibitory protein (NAIP)

Recently, a gene for spinal muscular atrophy was found. This gene is encoding neuronal apoptosis inhibitory protein (NAIP). An overexpression of NAIP protects several different cell lines form apoptotic death induced by a variety of triggers. A close correspondence between the regional distribution of NAIP-like immunoreactivity in the CNS and the reported neurodegenerative alterations in spinal muscular atrophy has been found. Transient forebrain ischaemia selectively elevates levels of NAIP in rat neurones that are resistant to the injurious effects of ischaemia, suggesting that increasing levels of NAIP may confer protection against ischaemia cell death (Xu et al. 1997).

β-Amyloid precursor protein

The β-amyloid precursor protein (APP) harbours the βA4 fragment, which is a major component of the amyloid plaques found in aged brains, Alzheimer disease and other neurodegenerative diseases. The majority of APP immunoprecipitated from total brain is derived from neurones. Under pathological conditions, however, non-neuronal APP isoforms are up-regulated. APP has been detected directly in different glia cell types *in vivo* and *in vitro* (Haass et al. 1991, Banati et al. 1994), suggesting a glia origin of APP in the lesioned brain. In the four-vessel occlusion model of rats it was found that APP is expressed in reactive glia cells with spatial differences in the distribution pattern of APP induction in astrocytes and microglia (Banati et al. 1995).

Cerebral Acidosis and Glucose

Cerebral acidosis

Neuronal damage

Using H^+ selective electrode it has been shown by Thorn and Heitmann (1954) that the brain becomes acidotic during ischaemia. Furthermore, studies with H^+ selective microelectrodes indicate that the acidosis occurs in the interstitial tissue (Siemkowicz and Hansen 1981). Other experimental studies indicate that the degree of intracellular and interstitial acidosis contributes to neurological damage (Myers and Yamaguchi 1977, Nordström et al. 1978, Siemkowicz and Hansen 1981, Rehncrona et al. 1981, Pepito et al. 1987).

Lactate

Lactic acidosis as such is detrimental to brain tissue (Rehncrona et al. 1981). The lactic acidosis may increase to high levels because of suppression of the activity of pyruvate dehydrogenase (Katayama et al. 1989). Activation of pyruvate dehydrogenase by dichloroacetate results in a decrease in lactate concentration in the rat brain (Kuroda et al. 1984). However, in another study it was shown that the mechanism by which dichloroacetate decreases brain lactate does not involve stimulation of pyruvate dehydrogenase (Dimlich and Nielsen 1992).

In hippocampal slice preparation it has been shown that lactate can fuel synaptic function (Schurr et al. 1988). In another study in rats it was demonstrated that blockade of lactate transport into neurones prevented its utilisation and, consequently, exacerbated delayed ischaemic neuronal damage (Schurr et al. 2001). These observations indicate that lactate accumulated during ischaemia is not only a harmful waste product. Other studies of isolated perfused rat brain indicate that during complete ischaemia the brain is able to recover some cellular ion transport and electrical activity without supply of glucose, but preferentially by combustion of lactate accumulated in brain tissue. However, this mechanism is only useful during a limited time period (Bock et al. 1993).

Glia cells

Recent studies indicate that glia cells become more acidotic than other brain cells (Kraig and Chesler 1987, Kraig and Nicolson 1987), and that an ischaemia infarction occurs when pH is less than 5.30 for more than 20 min (Kraig et al. 1987). The same group has hypothesised that astroglia cells act as a zinc for protons and that astroglia proliferation is stimulated by extracellular K+ increase (Kraig et al. 1990). Siesjö et al. (1990), however, in experimental studies have rejected this theory, and Katsura et al. (1992) in studies of normo- and hypercapnic rats demonstrated a linear relationship between lactate and tissue PCO_2 over the lactate range 2–40 mmol/kg; a finding which weakens any argument for gross compartmentation of H^+.

Hypercapnia

The detrimental effect of preischaemic hyperglycaemia has been explained as an exaggeration of intra- and extracellular acidosis. Data are conflicting. Several studies have demonstrated that acidosis associated with extreme hypercapnia does not interfere with cellular energy production (Litt et al. 1985, Xu et al. 1991). Extreme hypercapnia of 75 min duration fails to cause histologic damage (Cohen et al. 1990, Xu et al. 1991). On the other hand, it has been shown that hypercapnia (PaCO2 level 300 mm Hg) clearly enhanced ischaemic brain damage, as assessed histologically after 7 days of recovery (Katsura et al. 1994).

Pyruvate and carnitine

When neurones are cultured in serum free medium, they depend mainly on energy supplied by pyruvate, because these neurones are immature and possess little capability to gain energy from glycolysis. Under these circumstances, astrocytes may protect neurones from pyruvate deprivation by providing pyruvate (Matsumoto et al. 1994).

Carnitine as well as acetyl-l-carnitine can increase the metabolic rate of mitochondria, thus improving oxygen utilisation (Siliprandi et al. 1965, Bellei et al. 1989). These drugs also stimulate aerobic pyruvate metabolism, thereby inhibiting flux of pyruvate to lactic acid (Hutson et al. 1989). Postischaemic administration of acetyl-l-carnitine potentiates normalisation of the brain energy metabolism and improves neurological outcome in global cerebral ischaemia (Rosenthal et al. 1992).

Fructose-1,6,-biphosphate

In vivo and *in vitro* animal studies indicate that pre-treatment with fructose-1,6,-biphosphate (FBP) provides protection of haemodynamic and vital organs during shock, hypoxia, and ischaemia. Subsequent studies that focused on cerebral hypoxia and ischaemia demonstrated that pre-treatment with FBP reduced central nervous system injury (Gregory et al. 1989, Sola et al. 1996, Kuluz et al. 1993, Kellcher et al. 1994). When FBP is cerebroprotective during oxygen deprivation, ATP is preserved and levels of extracellular glutamate are reduced (Bickler and Buck 1996). In neonatal rat brain slices subjected to severe hypoxia, pre-treatment with FBP completely preserved ATP, and almost completely preserved cell morphology, but did not alter hypoxia-induced decrease in intracellular pH. Furthermore, pre-treatment substantially augments the flux of glucose into the pentose-phosphate pathway (Espanol et al. 1998). Other studies, however, indicate that FBP fails to provide protection during cerebral ischaemia. Some authors have explained that there is a lack of protection if FBP is given after ischaemia, if ischaemia is "too severe," or if the administration of FBP dose is lower than threshold value. Exceptions to these points are studies by Kuluz et al. (1993) who found that postischaemic administration of FBP reduced infarct size in a rat MCAO model, and studies by Sola et al. (1996) which demonstrated that FBP reduced CNS injury in neonatal rats after hypoxia.

Glucose

Ischaemia

The level of plasma-glucose influences the development of ischaemia. As demonstrated by Myers and Yamaguchi (1977), non-fasting monkeys subjected to global ischaemia develop more brain damage than fasting animals, and hyperglycaemic rats made a poorer recovery than did normoglycaemic and hypoglycaemic rats after 10 min of complete ischaemia (Siemkowicz and Hansen 1978). These observations have been extended by Rehncrona et al. (1981) who demonstrated that hyperglycaemic rats subjected to complete, in contrast to incomplete ischaemia, showed improved recovery, that tissue lactic-acid accumulation especially developed during incomplete ischaemia, and that a lactate concentration exceeding 20 mol/g was associated with impaired recovery. Evidence suggests that recovery in hyperglycaemic animals subjected to incomplete ischaemia is poorer than it is with complete ischaemia, and if hyperglycaemia develops prior to the insult, tissue lactic-acidosis has a detrimental effect on recovery (Siesjö 1984).

There was a marked difference in the amount of lactate accumulated between hypo- and hyperglycaemic rats. In hypoglycaemic animals massive depolarisation occurred at a tissue lactate content of about 4 mM, corresponding to a decrease in intracellular pH to 6.9. In the hyperglycaemic rats depolarisation occurred at a lactate content of about 12 mM, corresponding to a pH_i of 6.4. The time to depolarisation varied between 30 s. (hypoglycaemia) and 90 s. (hyperglycaemia) (Ekholm et al. 1993).

Recently it was demonstrated that hyperglycaemia decreases blood-brain barrier transport measured by permeability surface area product for glutamate during focal ischaemia in rats (Kawai et al. 1998).

Acute and chronic hyperglycaemia

Some experimental studies suggest that the duration of hyperglycaemia may influence outcome. Wagner and Lanier (1994), in rats subjected to complete cerebral ischaemia, found that high-energy phosphate depletion was similar in acute and chronic hyperglycaemic animals, suggesting that energy failure is not the origin of difference in postischaemic neurologic injury.

CBF thresholds

In rats subjected to MCAO, triple-hold tracer autoradiography has demonstrated that the threshold of local CBF for cerebral tissue pH reduction was lower in normoglycaemic compared with hyperglycaemic animals. In the same study the threshold of local CBF for local glucose hypermetabolism was found to be 20 and 30 ml/100g/min in normoglycaemic and hyperglycaemic rats respectively (Nakai et al. 1988).

Mechanism

The mechanism of the detrimental effects of hyperglycaemia is still unclear. Thus, in contrast to lactic-acid accumulation, MR studies in rats indicate that hypercapnic-induced intracellular acidosis is tolerated well (Litt et al. 1985). Furthermore, the effect of pre-existing hypoglycaemia on ischaemic brain damage is inconclusive (Diemer and Siemkowicz 1981, Pulsinelli et al. 1982). In focal ischaemic of

MCAO in rats (Nedergaard and Diemer 1987) and cats (Zasslow et al. 1987), and in rats subjected to photochemically induced cortical lesion (Ginsberg et al. 1987), hyperglycaemia diminishes the selective neuronal injury in the periinfarct zone (infarct rim) and the infarct size. Nedergaard and Astrup (1986) demonstrated that metabolism in the cortical infarct rim is stimulated by spontaneous changes in extracellular potassium and that the metabolism remained normal in hyperglycaemic rats owing to an inhibition of transient increases of extracellular potassium.

Calcium

From experimental studies in rats it has been suggested that accumulation of intracellular calcium is not an early event in ischaemia-hyperglycaemic brain damage (Macmillan 1989).

Collateral circulation

Studies in rats subjected to MCAO with or without common carotid artery occlusion suggest that infarcted regions having collateral circulation are vulnerable to the deleterious effects of hyperglycaemia, whereas regions with end-arterial vascular supply are more resistant (Prado et al. 1988). Other studies in rats suggest that blood flow alterations after MCAO are not influenced by the plasma glucose utilisation. In contrast, glucose utilisation depends on the combination of plasma glucose concentration and blood flow (Nedergaard et al. 1988).

Hypoglycaemia

In hypoglycaemic coma restoration of oxidative phosphorylation occurs within few min and with a rapid restoration of K^+_e levels. However free fatty acid remained elevated for longer time. Tissue lactate content increased only moderately and production of metabolic acids did not lead to intracellular acidosis (Katsura et al. 1993).

Clinical studies

In cardiac arrest survivors, elevated blood glucose levels on admission were predictive for unfavourable neurologic recovery (Longstreth and Inui 1984). This finding was explained by prolonged cardiopulmonary resuscitation, leading to both a greater increase in blood glucose level and a worsening in neurological outcome. In a recent study including 145 nondiabetic cardiac arrest patients, a high admission blood glucose level was associated with a poor neurological outcome (Müllner et al. 1997). In another study this correlation was not found, and the authors argue that the correlation found in other studies is a epiphenomenon (Steingrub and Mundt 1996).

Temperature

Protection

Hypothermia exerts a protective effect on the brain in global ischaemia (Chopp et al. 1989), incomplete ischaemia (Hoffman et al. 1991) and in experimental head injury (Clifton et al. 1991). Even a temperature decrease of 3°C has a protective effect in experimental brain ischaemia (Busto et al. 1989). In rats with permanent MCAO hypothermia, even when its induction is delayed for up to 1 hour after the unset of ischaemia, decreases brain injury (Baker et al. 1992). In global ischaemia in the rat, studies with NMR spectroscopy indicate that mild hypo- and hyperthermia affect intracellular acidosis during ischaemia and reperfusion period in a stepwise manner with more profound acidosis during ischaemia and a slower rate of recovery in reperfusion with increasing temperature (Haraldseth et al. 1992). In rats subjected to transient MCAO during hypo- and normothermia, studies by diffusion- and perfusion-weighted NMR imaging indicate, that the protective effect of hypothermia on ischaemia cell damage is reflected in an early return of apparent diffusion coefficient of water during reperfusion, and that the reduction of ischaemic cell damage by hypothermia is mediated by an improved CBF during acute recovery (Jiang et al. 1994). Prolonged hypothermia during later reperfusion improves neurologic outcome after global ischaemia in the rat, and attenuated the increase in HSP70 expression in the hippocampus, but did not affect the Hsp70 induction in the cerebellum (Hicks et al. 2000).

Also in studies of spinal ischaemia a slight decrease in the temperature in the peri-ischaemic period provides protection as measured by histopathological and neurological function (Marsala et al. 1994).

Chronic protection of brain ischaemia by hypothermia has been studied. The results indicated that intraischaemic, but not postischaemic, hypothermia provides chronic protection to the hippocampus after transient brain ischaemia. The inability of postischaemic hypothermia to protect chronically after 3 days indicates, that postischaemic hypothermia merely delays ischaemia cell death and/or the postischaemic undergoes a secondary insult (Dietrich et al. 1993).

Excitatory amino acids

The mechanism by which hypothermia confers neural protection is poorly understood. The concept that hypothermia protects by preserving cellular energy stores and aerobic metabolism is based on the observation that $CMRO_2$ is an inverse exponential function of temperature (Michenfelder and Milde 1991). During transient global ischaemia in rabbits brain oxygen tension is unaltered during mild and moderate hypothermia (Bacher et al. 1998). This finding suggests that other mechanisms are important for hypothermic neuroprotection.

Studies of the brain by microdialysis have documented an attenuation of postischaemic glutamate spike during intraischaemic hypothermia (Busto et al. 1989, Mitani and Katoka 1991, Illievich et al. 1994). Mild hypothermia also reduces penumbra glutamate levels in the rat permanent focal cerebral ischaemia model (Winfree et al. 1996). Both transient mild hypothermia and single-dose MK-801, a glutamate receptor antagonist, produce similar but not additive cerebroprotective effects, suggesting that transient alteration of NMDA-gated calcium influx produces a reduction in infarct size (Frazzini et al. 1994). In hippocampal slices the death of neurones from simulated ischaemia was predominantly due to activation of glutamate receptors. Isoflurane, sodium pentothal, NMDA antagonist and mild hypothermia prevented cell death to similar degrees (Popovoc et al. 2000).

Triple-therapy (hypothermia, hypertension, and mannitol)

In a rabbit model of temporary four-vessel occlusion mild hypothermia was combined with induced hypertension and mannitol treatment. In the control group the infarct volume was 193 mm^3 against 32- for the hypertensive animals, 41 -for the hypothermic- and 58 mm^3 for the mannitol treated animals. After triple treatment the infarct volume was reduced to 1 mm^3 (Ogilvy et al. 1996).

In another study rats were subjected to MACO. Both mild intraischaemic hypothermia and mannitol reduced infarct size and neurological deficit. However, hypothermia reduced infarct size more effectively than mannitol, and mannitol adds no significant protection to hypothermia, whereas hypothermia adds significant protection beyond that afforded by mannitol after brief focal ischaemia followed by reperfusion (Karibe et al. 1995).

Head injury

Two randomised studies of patients with severe head injury indicated that mild hypothermia (32–34° C) reduced ICP, CBF and $CMRO_2$. A trend to improved outcome was demonstrated in both studies, supporting the initiation of multicenter trial of therapeutic moderate hypothermia for the treatment of severe closed head injury (Marion et al. 1993, Shiozaki et al. 1993). Although the possibility of a hypothermia-induced coagulopathy is present, short-term use of hypothermia does not increase the risk for intracranial haemorrhagic complications in head injury (Resnick et al. 1994).

Meningitis

In experimental studies of pneumococcal meningitis moderate hypothermia the increase in CBF was blocked by hypothermia and the reduction of ICP correlated with the decrease in temperature (Angstwurm et al. 2000).

Different receptors

γ-aminobutyric acid (GABA)receptors

Localisation

GABA is ubiquitous in the brain, with very high concentration in cortex and striatum. GABA application to cells completely blocks the effects of glutamate, EAA including depolarisation and voltage-gated calcium influx (Riveros and Orrego 1986, Saji and Reis 1987, Calabresi et al. 1990). GABAergic neurones are particularly resistant to ischaemia in culture and in tissue slices (Tecoma et al. 1989).

Seizures

Susceptibility to audiogenic seizures was investigated in rats subjected to complete cerebral ischaemia. Glutamic acid decarboxylase revealed a 50% loss of this activity in the inferior colliculi. A conspicuous sprouting of GABA-ergic terminals in the ventral thalamic nuclei, which peaked about 1 month after the insult was found. Loss of $GABA_A$ inhibition coincided with the onset of audiogenic seizures (Kawai et al. 1995).

Muscinol

A new GABA agonist, muscinol, was found to be an effective neuroprotector during ischaemia. Other authors have found similar results with other GABA-mimetic agents (Brailowsky et al. 1986, Lyden and

Hedges 1992, Sternau et al. 1989). Combination therapy with muscinol and NMDA receptor blocker in embolic cerebral ischaemia in rats appeared to be more effective than either agent used alone (Lyden and Lonzo 1994).

Another $GABA_A$ receptor partial agonist, PNU-101017, that has a high affinity for the receptor subtypes containing α_1 and α_2 subunits was studied in the gerbil forebrain ischaemia model. Administration of this drug during reperfusion resulted in a decrease in CA1 damage at 5 days. Even with delay of the initial dosing until 4 hrs. after reperfusion PNU-101017 reduced Ca1 neuronal loss (Hall et al. 1997).

Endothelin (ET) receptors

Three endothelins (ET-1, ET-2 and ET-3) have been implicated in cerebrovascular pathological conditions. All three isoforms of ET are present in the brain (Sakurai et al. 1992). The effects are mediated via two receptors subtypes, endothelin type A (ET_A) and endothelin type B (ET_B). The predominant effect of ET_A receptor activity is cerebral vasoconstriction, whereas ET_B receptors mediate vasodilation (Masaki et al. 1994).

Topical or intraparenchymal application of ET-1 are associated with reduction in cerebral blood flow, and development of irreversible ischaemic damage (Robinson et al. 1990, Fuxe et al. 1992, Sharkey et al. 1993). Blockade of ET_A receptor prevents ET-1-induced vasoconstriction in isolated pial vessels (Patel et al. 1996). Endogenous endothelins have been implicated in the pathophysiology of cerebral ischaemia (Patel et al.1996). Combined ET_A/ET_B antagonists, however, do not improve hypoperfusion after global cerebral ischaemia (Patel and McCulloch 1996). Neither does administration of a selective endothelin receptor type A antagonist improve outcome in focal cerebral ischaemia in the cat (Bhardwaj et al. 2000).

Serotonergic receptors

Localisation

Anatomical studies have disclosed serotonin 5-HT_2 receptors in cerebral cortex and striatum of rat. 5-HT_2 receptors are also recognised on cerebral vessels, and immunohistochemical studies show that pial arteries are innervated by serotonergic fibres (Adell et al. 1991, Itakura et al. 1985, Wiersperger 1990, Leysen et al. 1981).

Ischaemia

Serotonergic denervation partially protects the striatum from kainic acid-mediated damage (Berger et al. 1982). Involvement of serotonin in ischaemic neuronal damage of transient forebrain ischaemia has been documented (Globus et al. 1992). Freezing lesion in the rat induces an increase in serotonin metabolism in the cortex, as well as a depression in cortical norepinephrine content, but no changes in dopamine and its metabolites (Pappius and Dadoun 1986, 1987).

Antagonists

Serotonin inhibitors reduce neurologic deficits in a rabbit spinal cord ischaemia model (Zivin and Venditto 1984, Zivin 1985). In later studies, by the same group, significant changes of biogenetic amines after treatment with serotonin inhibitors were not documented (Zivin and DeGirolami 1986), and blockade of serotonin receptors had no effect on outcome in patients with acute cerebral infarction (Ramirez-Lessepas et al. 1986). Ritanserin, a 5-HT_2 receptor antagonist did not have any protective effect in permanent focal ischaemia (Takagi et al. 1994).

Pappius et al (1988) showed that the depressed state of the lesioned brain, as assessed by glucose utilisation, could be ameliorated by inhibition of serotonin synthesis with p-chlorophenylalanine.

Adrenergic receptors

Nucleus ceruleus

In rats cerebral cortex is widely innervated by noradrenergic fibres arising from the nucleus ceruleus. Electrical activity of nucleus ceruleus neurones appears to be regulated by both positive and negative feedback mechanisms mediated by α_1- and α_2-adrenergic receptors (Nakamura et al. 1988).

Prazosin

Prazosin, a specific norepinephrine antagonist at the postsynaptic α_1 receptor, increases glucose utilisation after a focal freezing lesion and decreases the cortical accumulation of serotonin (Inoue et al. 1991).

Idazoxan

Idazoxan, an α_2 adrenergic antagonist, also reduces the magnitude of the delayed neuronal degeneration elicited by cerebral ischaemia (Yasuda et al. 1978).

Imidazole receptors

Recently another class of receptors, termed imidazole receptor has been classified. IM receptors differ from the α_2-adrenergic receptors with respect to anatomical distribution in the brain (Ernsberger et al. 1987, Bricca et al. 1989, Wickberg and Uhlen 1990), and they bind substituted imidazolines such as clonidine and its congeners (Michel et al. 1989). Blockers of IM receptors including rilmemidine and the before mentioned idazoxan protect against neuronal damage in global ischaemia (Gustafson et al. 1989, Gustafson et al. 1990) and in focal cerebral ischaemia Maiese et al. 1992). It is unknown whether the effects of these drugs are due to direct actions on ischaemic neurones or indirect activation of neural networks that transneuronally modify cerebral ischaemic injury (Maiese et al. 1992). Binding studies have demonstrated that IM receptors are sparse in the human cortex (Ernsberger et al. 1987, Bricca et al. 1988, Bricca et al. 1989). Consequently, a protective effect of these agents is supposed to be an unlikely mechanism.

Histamine receptors

Blood-brain barrier

There is some evidence that brain histamine may play an important role in the regulation of blood-brain barrier permeability (Dux and Joó 1982, Gross et al. 1982, Oichi et al. 1989).

Oedema

Pretreatment with H_2 receptor antagonists attenuates brain oedema elicited by systemic kainic acid injection (Sztriha et al. 1987). During MCAO a gradual increase in the level of brain histamine has been documented (Adachi et al. 1991). Treatment with H_2 antagonist prevents this increase (Adachi et al. 1992).

Insulin receptors

Blood-brain barrier

Insulin crosses the blood-brain barrier (Margolis and Altszuler1967, Wallum et al. 1987). Insulin receptors are distributed throughout the brain (Havrankova and Roth 1978, Pacold and Blakard 1979, Zahniser et al. 1984) on astrocyte (Albrecht et al. 1982) and cerebral capillaries (Frank and Pardridge 1981).

Effect

Insulin causes neurophysiologic inhibition (Palovcik et al. 1984) except in specific regions such as area postrema (Carpenter and Briggs 1986). In a recent study glucose-induced hyperinsulinemia under normoglycaemic condition, increased glucose utilisation in the ventromedial, dorsomedial, and anterior hypothalamic nuclei (Lucigmani et al. 1987). The protein kinase Akt/PKB, which is implicated in antiapoptosis and neuronal survival is activated by insulin (Burgering and Coffer 1995, Franke et al. 1995).

Protection

Insulin reduces ischaemic damage in both the brain (LeMay et al. 1988, Voll and Auer 1988) and the spinal cord (Robertson and Grossman 1987). In Global ischaemia, a substantial portion of the beneficial effect of insulin appears related to a direct central nervous system effect of insulin (Voll and Auer 1991). In focal ischaemia, the effects of insulin have been studied by Hamilton et al. (1995), who found that insulin benefits transient focal ischaemia. A decrease in glucose concentration was explained as a potential causal factor.

Insulin protects against ischaemia-initiated excitatory damage, reduces glucose utilisation and thereby reduces lactic acidosis. Insulin acts centrally by promoting neuronal survival through neural growth-like factors (Hill et al. 1988, Araujo et al. 1989). Other studies indicate that during ischaemia insulin acts directly on the brain independent of hypoglycaemia, to reduce ischaemia brain necrosis (Voll and Auer 1991). In a recent study metabolism of glucose, glycogen and high-energy phosphate during transient forebrain ischaemia in diabetic and non-diabetic rats were studied during insulin treatment. Pre-ischaemic brain glycogen was similar in all groups. At the completion of ischaemia, brain lactate in diabetic animals was higher than in non-diabetic animals, reflecting a higher intra-ischaemic consumption of glucose plus glycogen in diabetic animals. High-energy phosphates were better preserved in diabetic animals. Thus, a greater intra-ischaemic carcohydrate consumption and lactate production were found. The results suggest that primary energy failure during ischaemia is not the origin of greater injury in hyperglycaemic animals, nor is energy enhancement the origin of improved outcome after acute insulin treatment (Lanier et al. 1996).

Insulin treatment of corticosteroid-associated hyperglycaemia was studied in rats subjected to forebrain ischaemia. Dexamethasone administration before brain ischaemia resulted in a worsening of outcome that was related to drug-induced hyperglycaemia. Restoration of normoglycaemia, by insulin, resulted in a functional outcome similar to normoglycaemic animals, and an attenuation of steroid-associated histologic injury (Wass et al. 1996).

Chatecholamine release

Insulin modulates catecholamine release and uptake in CNS. The net result is an elevation of norepinephrine levels in the extracellular space. Early postischaemic administration of catecholamine was found to reduce neuronal necrosis in the rat (Koide et al. 1986). Insulin also inhibits glial uptake of GABA (Bouhaddi et al. 1988).

Magnesium receptors

Blood-brain barrier

Magnesium crosses the blood-brain barrier poorly. The concentration in the CNS is dependent on the plasma concentration. In human a bolus of 60 mg/kg of $MgSO_4$ leads after 90 min to a significant increase in CSF Magnesium concentration (Fuchs-Buder et al. 1997).

Cerebral spasm

Mg^{2+} causes a dose-dependent vasodilation of pial arterioles. This effect is probably due to a reduction in the influx of Ca^{2+} into vascular smooth muscle cells (Seelig et al. 1983, Altura and Altura 1984). Magnesium also induces dilation of the basilar artery in cats with arterial spasms (Kapp et al. 1970) and improves blood flow in the cortical territory of the occluded middle cerebral artery (Chi et al. 1990).

Calcium and NMDA receptors

Magnesium competes with Ca^{2+} to prevent entry into brain cells and might thereby prevent cell death. The rise in intracellular Ca^{2+} produced by ischaemia is reduced by Mg^{2+}, and Mg^{2+} binds to the NMDA-gated ionophore (Novak et al. 1984, Goldman and Kinkbeiner 1988).

Protection

Systemic injection of Mg^{2+} induces protection of the brain in experimental head trauma (McIntoch et al. 1989), spinal cord ischaemia (Vacanti and Ames 1984. Robertson et al. 1986, Simpson et al. 1994), and ischaemia after MCAO (Izumi et al. 1991). High levels of magnesium protect cultured hippocampal cells from anoxia (Rothman 1983, Kass et al. 1988). Moreover, in cultured hippocampal cells magnesium has been shown to have protective effect against applied glutamate (Finkbeiner and Stevens 1988). In rats subjected to traumatic injury by a weight drop device postinjury treatment with Magnium attenuates brain oedema formation and improves neurological outcome (Feldman et al. 1996). In rats subjected to MCAO, intra-arterially $MgSO_4$ administered before the ischaemia period, is neuroprotective indicated by a 40–60% reduction of infarct volume. This effect was dependent on dose and period of administration (Marinov et al. 1996). In the study of MCAO by Izumi et al. (1991) it was found that Mg^{2+} induced hyperglycaemia. Insulin further reduced the infarct volume. Intrathecal magnesium sulphate protects the spinal cord from ischaemia injury during thoracic aortic cross-clamping (Simpson et al. 1994).

Opioid receptors

Ischaemia

It has been postulated that endogenous opioids might play an important role in the pathophysiology of cerebral ischaemia (Hosobuchi et al. 1982a. Faden et al. (1981) found an elevation of β-endorphin-like immunoreactivity following spinal injury. This increase is associated with a decrease in systemic blood pressure and reduction of flow in both grey and white matter in the spinal cord, particularly at the injury site (Balentine 1978). Traumatic spinal cord injury causes enhanced binding to the kappa-opioid receptor (Krumins and Faden 1984, Faden et al. 1985). Naloxone improved the spinal cord blood flow and facilitated subsequent neurological recovery.

Protection

Only few endogenous opioids have been studied during cerebral ischaemia. Hosobuchi et al.(1982b) found no effect, while Sándor et al. (1983) found that one of the stable long-acting enkephalins led to a dose-dependent decrease of tissue blood flow and oxygen tension in awake cats. In a later study the same group with the same drug, injected intracarotically, found an increase in CVR and a decrease in CBF in focal ischaemia after MCAO (Sándor et al. 1986).

Antagonist

Baskin and Hosobuchi (1981) reported that naloxone reversed ischaemic neurological deficits in man. Several studies have confirmed that naloxone has a protective effect upon experimental cerebral ischaemia (Baskin et al. 1982, Faden et al. 1982, Levy et al. 1982, Pietronigro et al. 1983, Zambramski et al. 1983). However, other studies failed to confirm this beneficial effect (Holoday and D'Amato 1982, Kastin et al. 1982, Hubbard and Sundt 1983, Claperon et al. 1983, Fallis et al. 1983, Nehls et al. 1983). Generally naloxone improves neurological outcome in gerbils, but not in cats or primates.

Rats treated with the σ_1 -receptor ligand, (+)-pentazocine during cerebral ischaemia using the filament occlusion technique for 2 hrs., followed by 22 hrs. Reperfusion, showed reduced infarct volume. (-)-pentazocine had no effect (Takahashi et al. 1997).

Other drugs

Steroids

Effect

Methylprednisolone inhibits oxygen free radical-induced lipid peroxidation (Braughler et al. 1982, Hall and Braughler 1981). In rats the drug inhibits peroxydation in brain synaptosomal membranes when present in a 100M concentration, while lower and higher concentration produced less effect (Braughler 1985). A bolus dose of 30 mg/kg should be sufficient to attain this level. Methylprednisolone prevents progression of posttraumatic ischaemia (Hall et al. 1984, Young and Flamm 1982), reverses accumulation of intracellular calcium (Young and Flamm 1982), prevents neurofilament degradation (Braughler and Hall 1984) and inhibits membrane lipid hydrolysis (Anderson et al. 1985). As a consequence methylprednisolone augments recovery of evoked potential (Young and Flamm 1982).

Protection

Methylprednisolone enhances recovery of mice subjected to cerebral concussion (Hall 1985) and in clinical setting it seems to increase survival (Giannotta et al. 1984). On the other hand, pre-treatment with mega doses of methylprednisolone did not improve striatal lesions caused by NMDA receptor agonist in the rat (Uhler et al. 1994).

Head injury

Steroid has been shown to enhance the early recovery of mice subjected to moderate severe concussive head trauma when administrated at 5 min. postinjury. The dose-response curve for this effect is similar to that found in spinal injury, a dose of 30 mg/kg being optimal (Hall 1982). Consistent with this result one controlled trial has demonstrated that high-dose regimen within 6 hrs. of severe head injury in Glasgow Scale score 3–8 patients significantly increase survival and the recovery of speech (Giannotta et al. 1984). However, flaws in the study prevent it from being a definite result. Other clinical studies with conventional steroid dosing regimens showed no apparent effect (Braakman et al. 1983, Hall 1982)

Subarachnoid haemorrhage

Studies in dogs subjected to experimental subarachnoid haemorrhage indicate that methylprednisolone delayed cerebral spasms (Chyatta et al. 1983, Chyatta and Sundt 1984) and acute spasms in cats (Hall and Travis 1988). Other studies in rats with experimental subarachnoid haemorrhage have shown that formation of brain eicosanoid is attenuated (Gaetani et al. 1990). Clinical studies in subarachnoid haemorrhage indicate a reduction of angiographically vasospasms (Chyatta et al. 1987), but clinical controlled outcome studies are still not available.

Spinal injury

Pre-treatment of cats with an intravenous dose of methylprednisolone served to protect homogenates of uninjured spinal cord, removed 1 hour after steroid administration from *in vitro* lipid peroxidation (Braughler and Hall 1984, Hall and Braugler 1981). Most striking was the demonstrated need for a very large dose of 30 mg/kg because pre-treatment with lower doses was ineffective. On the other hand, the dose response curve for this antioxidant effect was biphasic. Doubling the dose to 60 mg/kg caused a loss of effect, and tripling the dose actually promoted subsequent in vitro lipid peroxidation. In other words, the steroid had to be present in the spinal tissue in a critical concentration in order to protect against lipid peroxidation. Other studies indicated that a 30 mg/kg dose of methylprednisolone given to cats subjected to blunt spinal cord injury could attenuate posttraumatic lipid peroxidation (Anderson et al. 1985, Hall and Brauhler 1982)

In spinal cord injury methylprednisolone, when administrated within 8 hours after trauma, improves motor function. The dose of methylprednisolone in this study was an initial bolus dose of 30 mg/kg, followed by 5.4 mg/kg/hour for 23 hours (Bracken et al. 1992).

Progesterone and oestrogen

In experimental studies less susceptibility to postischaemic and posttraumatic brain injury in female animals has been demonstrated. This finding is likely due to the effects of circulating estrogens and progesterone.

In transient MCAO in the rats and in global ischaemia in cats progesterone provides neuroprotection (Jiang et al. 1996, Gonzales-Vidal et al. 1998). Administration of progesterone to male rats 2 hours after MCAO reduces ischaemic brain damage and improves neurological deficit even seven days after ischaemia (Kumon et al. 2000).

The mechanism by which progesterone provides neuroprotection is supposed to be its potentiating effect upon GABA inhibition and attenuation of excitatory amino acid responsiveness. Other effects include an amplification of adenosines inhibitory action on neuronal activity, a reduction of brain oedema and action as a free-radical scavenger.

In rats subjected to MAC oestrogen therapy during reperfusion improves tissue outcome. Oestrogen rapidly promotes CBF recovery, and reduces hemispheric no-reflow zones (McCullough et al. 2001). In female rats subjected to subarachnoid haemorrhage 17-beta oestradiol reduced the mortality and secondary ischaemic damage without affecting the clot volume (Yang et al. 2001). Oestrogens putative effects include preservation of autoregulatory function, free-radical scavenger function, reduction of β amyloid production, reduced excitotoxicity, increased expression of the antiapoptotic factor bcl-2 and activation of mitogen activated protein kinase pathways (for reveiw Roof and Hall 2000).

Erythropoietin

According to Siren et al. (2001) systemic administration of erythropoietin after MAC in rats reduces the volume of infarction 24 hrs. later, and in neuronal cultures erythropoietin inhibits apoptosis induced by serum deprivation or kainic acid exposure.

Fibroblast growth factor

Fibroblast growth factor reduces infarct volume when infused intravenously in animal models of focal cerebral ischaemia. Intravenous basic fibroblast growth factor decreases DNA fragmentation and prevents down-regulation of Bcl-2 expression in the ischaemic brain following MAC in rats (Ay I, et al. 2001). Another growth factor, keratinocyte growth factor prevents ischaemic-induced delayed neuronal death in the hippocampal CA1 field of the gerbil brain (Sadohara et al. 2001).

Gangliosides

Localisation

Gangliosides are glycosphingolipids with hydrophilic and lipophilic biochemical groups. They are constituents of cell-surface membranes and intracellular structures (golgi membranes, endoplasmatic reticulum, lysosome).

Effect

Gangliosides promote functional recovery after traumatic and ischaemia lesions; the mechanisms being increased collateral sprouting, protection against Wallerian degeneration, increased axonal sprouting from proximal end of injured nerves and reduction of oedema.

Protection

Gangliosides reduce histopathologic damage in cats subjected to MCAO (Tanaka et al. 1986) and improves recovery of the EEG (Komatsumoto et al. 1988). However, in other studies of focal ischaemia in rats these findings have not been confirmed (Mayer and Pulsinelli 1992). In gerbil a reduction in mortality after cerebral ischaemia has been found (Karpiak et al. 1987). In rats ganglioside prevented accumulation of eicosanoids, thromboxane and 6-keto prostaglandins (Petroni et al. 1989), and in monkeys subjected to global ischaemia an improved neurological outcome of survived animals has been found (Cahn et al. 1989).

Clinical application

Favourable results have been found in clinical studies of peripheral radiculopathy after lumbar disc operation (Cubells et al. 1980) and in other peripheral neuropathies (Gai et al. 1980).

GM-1

A new ganglioside, monosialoganglioside (GM-1) has been developed. This ganglioside inhibits glutamate-mediated proteinkinase C translocation in cultures of cerebellar neurones (Vaccarino et al. 1987). Clinical trials with GM-1 suggest a therapeutic efficacy in acute stroke (Argentino et al. 1989, Angeleri et al. 1992, Lenzi et al. 1994) and in subarachnoid haemorrhage (Papo et al. 1991).

Cronassial

Cronassial was suspended from clinical use due to the possibility that this drug was involved in the development of Guillain-Barré polyradiculitis in several patients (Roemmer 1989). For review see Rodden et al. 1991).

Heparin

Administration of massive doses of heparin reduces brain injury after ischaemia and reperfusion (Smith et al. 1969). In rats subjected to transient forebrain ischaemia heparin resulted in reduced leukocyte accumulation, infarct size and neurological dysfunction 48 hrs. after reperfusion when compared to untreated animals (Yanaka et al. 1996a). Also animals receiving heparin 3 hrs. after reperfusion showed significant better results than untreated animals (Yankee et al. 1996b).

References

Abe H, Xu ZC, Nowak TS (1995): Threshold depolarization intervals for ischemic tolerance vs. Expression of hsp 72 and other ischemia-induced mRNAs. J Cereb Blood Flow Metab 15 (suppl 1): S67.

Abe K, Yuki S, Kogure K (1988) Strong attenuation of ischemic and postischemic brain edema in rats by a novel free radical scavenger. Stroke 19: 480–485.

Acosta D, Kass I, Cottrell JE (1986) Vitamin E protects against anoxic brain damage in the hippocampal slice. Anesthesiology 65: A317.

Adachi N, Oishi R, Saeki K (1991) Changes in the metabolism of histamine and monoamines after occlusion of the middle cerebral artery in rats. J Neurochem 57: 61–66.

Adachi N. Itoh Y, Oichi R, Saeki K (1992) Direct evidence for increased continuous histamine release in the striatum of conscious freely moving rats produced by middle cerebral artery occlusion. J Cereb Blood Flow Metab 12: 477–483.

Adachi T, Inanami O Sato A (1992) Nitric oxide (NO) is involved in increased cerebral cortical blood flow following stimulation of the nucleus basilis of Meynert in anesthetized rats. Neurosci Lett 139: 201–204.

Adams RJ, Fisher M, Furlan AJ, del Zopepe G (1995) Acute stroke treatment trials in the United States. Rethinking strategies for success. Stroke 26: 2216–2218.

Adell A, Carceller A, Artigas F (1991) Regional desitribution of extracellular 5-hydroytryptamine and 5-hydroxyindoleacetic acid in the brain of freely moving rats. J Neurochem 56: 709–712.

Agardh CD, Westergerg E, Siesjö BK (1980) Severe hypoglycemia leads to accumulation of arachidonic acid in brain tissue. Acta Physiol Scand 109: 115–116.

Akins PT, Liu PK, Hsu CY (1996) Immediate early gene expression in response to cerebral ischemia: Friend or foe? Stroke 27: 1982–1687.

Akopov SE, Grygorian MR, Gabrielian ES, Balayan BH (1992) Investigation of the dependence of human middle artery contractile activity on the presence of an atherosclerotic patch. Heart Vessels 7: 196–199.

Akopov SE, Sercombe R, Seylas J (1994) Leukocyte-induced acute endothelial dysfunction in middle cerebral artery in rabbits. Response to aggregating platelets. Stroke 25: 2246–2252.

Akopov SE, Sercombe R, Seylas J (1994) Endothelial dysfunction in cerebral vessels following carotid artery infusion of phorbol ester in rabbits: The role of polymorhonuclear leukocytes. J Cereb Blood Flow Metab 14: 1078–1087.

Alarcon RM, Rupnow BA, Graeber TG et al. (1996) Modulation of c-Myc activity and apoptosis in vivo. Cancer Res 56: 4315–4319.

Albin MS, Bunegin L, Dujovny M, et al. (1975) Brain retraction pressure during intracranial procedures. Surg Forum 26: 199–200.

Albin MS, Bunegin L, Bennett MH et al. (1977) Clinical and experimental brain retraction pressure monitoring. Acta Neurol Scand 56: (suppl 64): 522–573.

Albrecht J, Wróblewska B, Mossakowski M (1982) The binding of insulin to cerebral capillaries and astrocyte of the rat. Neurochem Res 7: 489–494.

Alexander SC, Smith TC, Strobel G, Stephen GW, Wollman H (1968) Cerebral carcohydrate metabolism of man during respiratory and metabolic alkalosis. J Appl Physiol 24: 66–72.

Aliev M, Saks V (1993): Quantitative analysis of the "phosphocreatine shuttle": I. A probability approach to the description of phosphocreatine production in the coupled creatine kinase-ATP/ADP translocase-oxidative phosphorylation reactions in heart mitochondria. Biochim Biophysic Acta 1143: 291–300.

Allen GS, Ahn HS, Preziosi TJ, Battye MB, Boone SC, Chou SN, Kelly DL, Weir BK (1983) Cerebral arterial spasms - a controlled trial of nimodipine in patients with subarachnoid hemorrhage N Eng J Med 308: 619–624.

Altura BT, Altura BM (1984) Interactions of Mg and K on cerebral vessels. Aspects in view of stroke, review of present status and new findings. Magnesium 3: 195–211.

Amado JA, LopezEspadas F, VazquezBarquero A, et al. (1995) Blood levels of cytokines in brain-death patients: relationship with circulating hormones and acute-phase reactants. Metabolism Clinical and Experimental 44: 812–816.

Ambrosio G, Zweier J, Duilio C, et al. (1993): Evidence that mitochondrial respiration is a source of potentially toxic oxygen free radicals in intact rabbit heart subjected to ischemia and reflow. J Biol Chem 25: 18532–18541.

Ames A III, Wright RL, Kowada M, Thurston JM, Majno G (1968) Cerebral ischemia. II. The no-reflow phenomenon. Am J Pathol 52: 437–453.

Amruthesh SC, Ellis EF (1990) Formation and identification of novel, vasodilator metabolites of arachidonate in mouse brain. FASEB J 4: A993.

An G, Lin TN, Liu JS, et al. (1993) Expression of c-fos and c-jun family genes after focal cerebral ischemia. Ann Neurol 33: 457–464.

Anderson DK, Saunders RD, Demediuk P, et al. (1985) Lipid hydrolysis and peroxidation in injured spinal cord: partial protection with methylprednisolone of vitamin E and silenium. Cent Nerv Syst Trauma 2: 257–267.

Andiné P, Rudolphi KA, Fredholm BB; Hagberg H (1990) Effect of pentofylline /HWA 285) on extracellular purines and excitatory amino acids in CA1 of rat hippocampus during transient inschemia. Br J Pharmacol 1000: 814–818.

Andrews RJ, Muto RP (1992) Retraction brain ischemia: cerebral blood flow, evoked potentials, hypotension and hyperventilation in a new animal model. Neurological Research 14: 12–18.

Andrews RJ, Muto RP (1992) Retraction brain ischemia: Mannitol plus nimodipine preserves both cerebral blood flow and evoked potentials during normoventilation and hyperventilation. Neurological Reserach 14: 19–25.

Angstwurm K, Reuss S, Freyer D, et al. (2000) Induced hypothermia in experimental pneumococcal meningitis. J Cereb Blood Flow Metab 20: 834–838.

Aoki E, Semba R, Mikoshita K, Kashiwamata S (1991) Predominant localization in glial cells of free L-arginine: immunocytochemical evidence. Brain Res 547: 190–192.

Araki N, Greenberg JH, Uematsu D, et al. (1992) Effect of superoxide dismutase on intracellular calcium in stroke. J Cereb Blood FLow Metab 12: 43–52.

Araujo DM, Lapchak PA, Collier B, et al. (1989) Insuline-like growth factor-I (somatomedin-C) receptors in the rat brain: distribution and interaction with the hippocampal cholinergic system. Brain Res 484: 130–138.

Angeleri F, Scarpino O, Martinazzo C, et al. (1992) GM1 ganglioside therapy in acute ischemic stroke. Cerebrovasc Dis. 2: 163–168.

Argentino C, Sacchetti ML, Toni D, et al. (1989) GM1 ganglioside therapy in acute ischemic stroke. Stroke 20: 1143–1149.

Aronowski J, Waham MN, Grotta JC (1993) Neuronal protection and preservation of calcium/clamodulin-dependent protein kinase II and protein kinase C activity by dextrorphan treatment in global ischemia. J Cereb Blood Flow Metab 13: 550–557.

Ashkenas J, Werb Z (1996) Proteolysis and the biochemistry of life-or-death decisions. J Exp Med 183: 1947–1951.

Ashwal S, Cole DJ, OSborne TN, Pearce WJ (1993) Low dose L-NAME reduces infarct volume in the rat MCAO/reperfusion model. J Neurosurg Anestheiol. 5: 241–249.

Astrup J, Symon L, Branston NM, Lassen NA (1977) Cortical evoked potential and extracellular K^+ and H^+ at critical levels of brain ischaemia. Stroke 8: 51–57.

Astrup J, Blennow G, Nilsson B (1979) Effects of reduced cerebral blood flow upon EEG pattern, cerebral extracellular potassium, and energy metabolism in the rat cortex during bicuculline-induced seizures. Brain Res 177: 115–126.

Astrup J, Skovsted P, Gjerris F, S¢rensen HR (1981a) Increase in extracellular potassium in the brain during circulatory arrest: Effects of hypothermia, lidocaine, and thiopental. Anesthesiology 55: 256–262.

Astrup J, M¢ller S¢rensen P, S¢rensen HR (1981b) Inhibition of cerebral oxygen and glucose consumption in the dog by hypothermia, pentobarbital, and lidocaine. Anesthesiology 55: 263–268.

Astrup J (1982) Energy-requiring cell functions in the ischemic brain. Their critical supply and possible inhibition in protective therapy. J Neurosurg 56: 482–497.

Auer L (1977) The role of cerebral perfusion pressure as origin of brain edema in acute arterial hypertension. Eur Neurol 15: 153–156.

Auer LM, Ito Z, Suzuki A, Ohta H (1982) Prevention of symptomatic vasospasm by topically applied nimodipine. Acta Neurochir (Wien) 63: 297–302.

Auer LM (1984) Acute operation and preventive nimodipine outcome in patients with ruptured cerebral aneurysms. Neurosyrgery 15: 57–66.

Avery S, Crockard HA, Ross Russell RW (1984) Evolution and resolution of edema following severe temporary cerebral ischemia in the gerbil. J Neurol Neurosurg Psychiat 47: 604–610.

Awad I, Little JR, Lucas F, et al. (1983) Modification of focal cerebral ischemia by prostacyclin and indomethacin. J Neurosurg 58: 714–719.

Ay I I, Sugimori H, Finklestein SP (2001) Intravenous basic fibroblast growth factor (bFGF) decreases DNA fragmentation and prevents downregulation of Bcl-2 expression in the ischemic brain following middle cerebral artery occlusion in rats. Brain Res Mol Brain Res 87: 71–80.

Back T, Ginsberg M, Dietrich W, Watson B (1996): Induction of spreading depression in the ischemic hemisphere following experimental middle cerebral artery occlusion: effect on infarct morphology. J Cereb Blood Flow Metab 16: 202–213.

Backer A, Kwon JY, Zornow MH (1998) Effects of temperature on cerebral tissue oxygen tension, carbon dioxide tension, and pH during transient global ischemia in rabbits. Anesthesiology 88: 403–409.

Baethmann A, Maier-Hauff K, Schürer L, et al. (1989) Release of glutamate and of free acids in vasogenic brain edema. J Neurosurg 70: 578–591.

Baker A, Zornow M, Scheller M, et al. (1991) Changes in extracellular concentrations of glutamate, aspartate, glycine, dopamine, serotonin, and dopamine metabolites after transient global ischemia in the rabbit brain. J Neurochem 57: 1370–1379.

Baker CJ, Onesti ST, Solomon RA (1992) Reduction by delayed hypothermia of cerebral infarction following middle cerebral artery occlusion in the rat: a time-course study. J Neurosurg 77: 438–444.

Balentine JD (1978) Pathology of experimental spinal cord trauma. I. The necrotic lesion as a function of vascular injury. Lab Invest 39: 236–253.

Banati RB, Gehrmann J, Kreutzberg GW (1994) Glial β-amyloid precurser protein: expression in the dentate gyrus after entorhinal cortex lesion. Neurol Report 5: 1359–1361.

Banati RB, Gehrmann J, Wiessner C, et al. (1995) Glial expression of the β-amyloid precurser protein (APP) in global ischemia. J Cereb Blood Flow Metab 15: 647–654.

Barnett GH, Bose B, Little JR, Jones SC, Friel HT (1986) Effects of nimodipine on acute focal cerebral ischemia. Stroke 17: 884.

Baron JC, Bousser MG, Comar D, Castaigne O (1980) "Crossed cerebellar diaschisis" in human supratentorial brain infarction. Trans Amer Neurol Ass 8: 128.

Baron JC (1985) Positron tomography in cerebral ischemia: a review. Neuroradiology 27: 509–516.

Baron JC, Bousser MG, Comar D, Castaigne P (1980) "Crossed cerebellar diaschisis" in human supratentorial brain infarction. Ann Neurol (abstract) 8: 128.

Baron JC (1991) Pathophysiology of acute cerebral ischemia: PET studies in humans. Cerebrovasc Dis 1 (suppl): 22–31.

Barone F, Schmidt B, Hillegass L, et al. (1992) Reperfusion increases neutrophils and leukotrien B4 receptor binding in rat focal ischemia. Stroke 23: 1337–1348.

Barone FC, Lysko PG, Price WJ, et al. (1995) Sb201823-A antagonizes calcium currents in central neurones and reduces the effects of focal ischemia in rats and mice. Stroke 26: 1083–1690.

Bartus RT, Baker KL, Heiser AD, et al. Postischemic administration of AK275, a calpain inhibitor provides substantial protection against focal ischemic brain damage. J Cereb Blood Flow Metab 1994: 14: 537–544.

Bartus RT, Dean RL, Cavanaugh K, et al. Time-related neuronal changes following middle cerebral artery occlusion: Implications for therapeutic intervention and the role of calpain. J Cereb Blood Flow Metab 1995: 15: 969–979.

Baskaya MK, Hu Y, Donaldson D, et al. (1996) Protection effect of the 5-lipoxygenase inhibitor AA-861 on cerebral edema after transient ischemia. J Neurosurg 85: 112–116.

Baskin DS, Hosohuchi Y (1981) Naloxone reversal of ischemic neurological deficits in man. Lancet 2: 272–275.

Baskin DS, Kieck CF, Hosobuchi Y (1982) Naloxone reversal of ischemic neurological deficits in baboons is not mediated by systemic effect. Life Sci 31: 2201–2204.

Batteur-parmentier S, Margaill I, Plotkine M (2000) Modulation by nitric oxide of cerebral neutrophil accumulation after transient focal ischemia in rats. J Cereb Blood Flow Metab 20: 812–819.

Bazan NG, Rodriguez de Turco EB (1980) Membrane lipids in the pathogenesis of brain edema: Phospholipids and arachidonic acid, the earliest membrane components changed at the onset of ischemia. Adv Neurol 28: 197–205.

Bazan NG, Squinto SP, Braquet P et al. (1991): Platelet-activation factor and polyunsaturated fatty acids in cerebral ischemia or convulsions: Intracellular PAF-binding sites and activation of FOS/JUN/AP-1 transscriptional signaling system. Lipids 26: 1236–1242.

Bazan NG, Allan G (1996): Platelet-activating factor is both a modulator of synaptic function and a mediator of cerebral injury and inflammation. In: Siesjö BK, Wieloch T (eds): Advances in Neurology 71. Philadelphia: Lippincott-Raven, pp 475-484.

Beckman JS, Beckman TW, Chen J, et al. (1990) Apparent hydroxyl radical production by peroxynitrite: implications for endothelial injury from nitric oxide and superoxide. Proc Natl Acad Sci USA 87: 1620–1624.

Bedford RF, Dacey R, Winn R, Lynch C (1983) Adverse impact of a calcium entry-blocker (verapamil) on intracranial pressure in patients with brain tumors. J Neurosurg 59: 800–802.

Beg AA, Baltimore D (1996) An essential role for NF-kappaB in preventing TNF-alpha-induced cell death. Science 274: 782–784.

Bell BA, Symon L, Branston NM (1985) CBF and time thresholds for the formation of ischemic cerebral edema, and effect of reperfusion in baboons. J Neurosurg 62: 31–41.

Bellei M, Batteli D, Guarriero DM, Muscatello U, et al. (1989) Changes in mitochondrial activity caused by ammonium salts and protective effect of carnitine. Biochem Biophys Res Commun 158: 181–188.

Benham CD, Brown TH, Cooper DG, et al. (1993) SB201823-A, a neuronal calcium channel antagonist is neuroprotective in two models of cerebral ischemia. Neuropharmacology 32: 1249–1257.

Benveniste H (1991) The excitotoxin hypothesis in relation to cerebral ischemia. Cerebrovascular and Brain Metabolism Reviews 3: 213–245.

Berger L, Hakim AM (1989) Nimodipine prevents hyperglycemia-induced cerebral acidosis in middle cerebral artery occluded rats. J Cereb Blood Flow Metab 9: 58–64.

Berger M, Sperk G, Hornykiewicz O (1982) Serotonergic denervation partially protects rat striatum from kainic acid toxity. Nature 299: 254–256.

Bernardi P, Broekemeier KM, Pfeiffer DR (1994) Recent progress on regulation of the mitochodrial permeability transient pore: a cyclosporin-sensitive pore in the inner mitochondrial membrane. J Bioenerg Biomemb 26: 509–517.

Berne RM, Rubio R, Curnish RR (1974) Release of adenosine from ischemic brain. Effect on cerebral vascular resistance and incorporation into cerebral adenine nucleotides. Circ Res 35: 262–271.

Betz AL, Keep RF, Beer ME, Ren (1994) Blood-brain barrier permeability and brain concentration of sodium, potassium, and cloride during focal ischemia. J Cereb blood flow Metab 14: 29–37.

Bickler PE, Buck LF, (1996) Effects of fructose-1,6,-biphosphate on glutamate release and ATP loss from rat brain slices during hypoxia. J Neurochem 67: 1463–1468.

Bevilacqua MP, Pobers JS, Wheeler ME, et al. (1985) Interleukin 1 acts on cultured human vascular endothelium to increase the adhesion of polymorphonuclear leukocytes, monocytes, and related leukocyte cell lines. J Clin Invest 76: 2003–2011.

Bhardwaj A, Wu Y, Hurn PD, et al. (2000) Administration of selective endothelin receptor type A antagonist RO 61–1790 does not improve outcome in focal cerebral eschemia in cat. J Cereb Blood Flow Metab 20: 499–504.

Bielenberg GW, Haubruck H, Krieglstein J (1987a) Effects of calcium entry blocker emopamil on postischemic energy metabolism of the isolated perfused rat brain. J Cereb Blood Flow Metab 7: 489–496.

Bielenberg GW, Beck T, Sauer D, et al. (1987b) Effects of cerebroprotective agents on cerebral blood flow and on postischemic energy metabolism in the rat brain. J Cereb Blood Flow Metab 7: 480–488.

Bielenberg GW (1989) R-PIA protects cortical tissue in permanent MCA occlusion in the rat. J Cereb Blood Flow Metab 9 (suppl 1): S645.

Block GA, Pulsinelli WA (1987) The adenosine agonist R-Phenylisopropyladenosine, attenuates ischemic neuronal damage. J Cereb Blood Flow Metab 7 (suppl 1): S258.

Blomqvist P, Wieloch T (1985) Ischemic brain damage in rats following cardiac arrest using a long-term recovery model. J Cereb Blood Flow Metab 5: 420–431.

Blot S, Arnal J-F, Xu Y, Gray F, Michel J-B (1994) Spinal cord infarcts during long-term inhibition of nitric oxide synthase in rats. Stroke 25: 1666–1673.

Bock A, Tegtmeier F, Hansen AJ, Höller M (1993) Lactate and postischemic recovery of energy metabolism and electrical activity in the isolated perfused rat brain. J Neurosurg Anesthesiology 5: 94–013.

Bodsch W, Takahashi K, Barbier A, et al. (1985) Cerebral protein synthesis and ischemia. Prog Brain Res 63: 197–210.

Bogaret Y, Ronsenthal R, Fiskum G (1994): Postischemic inhibition of cerebral cortex pyruvate dehydrogenase. Free Radical Biol Med 6: 811–820.

Bondy S, LeBel C (1993): The relationship between excitatoxicity and oxidative stress in the central nervous system. Free Radical Biol Med 14: 633:–642.

Bonvento G, Seylas J, Lacombe P (1994) Widespread attenuation of the cerebrovascular reactivity to hypercapnia following inhibition of nitric oxide synthase in the conscious rat. J Cereb Blood Flow Metab 14: 699–703.

Braakman R, Schouten HJA, et al. (1983) Megadose steroids in severe head injury. Results of a prospective double-blind clinical trial. J Neurosurg 58: 326–330.

Bracken MB, Shepard MJ, Collins WF et al. (1992) Methylprednisolone or naloxone treatment after acute spinal cord injury: 1-year follow-up data. J Neurosurg 76: 23–31.

Bracken MB, Shephard MJ, Holford TR, et al. (1997) Administration of methylprednisolone for 24 or 48 h or tirilazad mesylate for 48 h in the treatment of acute spinal cord injury; results of the third national acute spinal cord injury randomized controlled trial. JAMA 277: 1597–1604.

Brailowsky S, Knight RT, Blood K, Scabini D (1986) GABA-induced potentiation of cortical hemiplegia. Brain Res 362: 322–330.

Brandt L, Ljunggren B, Saveland H, Andersson K-E (1988) Use of a calcium antagonist in aneurysmal subarachnoid hemorrhage. Ann NY Acad Sci 522: 667–675.

Branston NM, Symon L, Crockard HA, Pasztor E (1974) Relationship between the cortical evoked potential and local cortical blood flow following acute middle cerebral artery occlusion in the baboon. Exp Neurol 45: 195–208.

Branston NM, Strong AJ, Symon L (1977) Extracellular potassium activity, evoked potential and tissue blood flow. Relationships during progressive ischaemia in baboon cerebral cortex. J Neurol Sci 32: 305–321.

Branston NM, Hope DT, Symon L (1979) Barbiturates in focal ischaemia of primate cortex: effects on blood flow distribution, evoked potential and extracellular potassium. Stroke 10: 647–653.

Branston NM, Ladds A, Symon L, Wang AD (1984) Comparison of the effects of ischaemia on early components of the somatosensory evoked potential in the brainstem, thalamus and cerebral cortex. J Cereb Blood Flow Metab 4: 68–81.

Braughler JM, Hall ED (1982) Correlation of methylprednisolone levels in cat spinal cord with its effect on (Na^+/ K^+) - ATPase, lipid peroxidation, and alpha motor neuron function. J Neurosurg 56: 838–844.

Braughler JM, Hall ED (1984) Effects of multi-dose methylprednisolone sodium succinate administration on injured cat spinal cord neurofilament degradation and energy metabolism. J Neurosurg 61: 290–295.

Braughler JM (1985) Lipid peroxidation-induced inhibition of gamma-aminobutyric acid uptake in rat brain synaptosomes: protection by glucocorticoids. J Neurochem 44: 1282–1288.

Bricca G, Dontenwill M, Molines A, et al. (1988) Evidence of the existence of a homogeneous population of imidazoline receptors in the human brainstem. Eur J Pharmacol 150: 401–402.

Bricca G, Dontenwill M, Molines A, et al. (1989a) Rilmenidine selectivity for imidazoline receptors in human brain. Eur J Pharmacol 163: 373–377.

Bricca G, Dontenwill M, Molines A, et al. (1989b) The imidazoline preferring receptor: binding studies in bovine, rat and human brainstem. Eur J Pharmacol 162: 1–9.

Brierley JB, Graham DI (1984) Hypoxia and vascular disorders of the central nervous system. In: Adams H, Corsellis JAN, Duchen LW (Eds). Greenfields Neuropathology. London: Edwards Arnold 125–207.

Bromont C, Marie C, Bralet J (1989) Increased lipid peroxidation in vulnerable brain regions after transient forebrain ischemia in rats. Stroke 20: 918–924.

Buchan A, Xue D, Slivka A (1992): A new model of temporary focal neocortical ischemia in the rat. Stroke 23: 273–279.

Buchan AM, Bruederlin B, Heinicke E, Li H (1992) Failure of the lipid peroxidation inhibitor, U74006F, to prevent postischemic selective neuronal injury. J Cereb Blood Flow Metab 12: 250–256.

Buchan A, Xue D, Slivka A, (1992): A new model of temporary focal neocortical ischemia in the rat. Stroke 23: 273–279.

Buchan AM, Gertler SZ, Li H, et al. (1994) A selective N-type Ca^{2+}-channel blocker prevents CA1 injury 24h following severe forebrain ischemia and reduces infarction following focal ischemia. J Cereb Blood Flow Metab 14: 903–910.

Buisson A, Plotkine M, Boulu RG (1992) The neuropretective effect of a nitric oxide inhibitor in a rat model of focal cerebral ischemia. Br J Pharmacol 106-766-767.

Buisson A, Margaill I, Callebert J, et al. (1993) Mechanisms involved in the neuroprotevtive activity of nitric oxide synthase inhibitor during focal cerebral ischemia. J Neurochem 61: 690–696.

Bullock R, Graham DI, Swanson S, McCulloch J (1994) Neuroprotective effect of the AMPA receptor antagonist LY-293558 in focal cerebral ischemia in the cat. J Cereb Blood Flow Metab 14: 466–471.

Burda J, Marsala M, Radonak J, Marsala J (1991) Graded postischemic reoxygenation ameliorates inhibition of cerebral cortical protein symthesis in dogs. J Cereb Blood Flow Metab 11: 1001–1004.

Burgering BMT, Coffer PJ (1995) Protein kinase B (c-Akt) in phosphatidylinositol-3-OH kinase signal transduction. Nature 376: 599–602.

Burkhart KK, Beard DC, Lehman RA, Billingsley ML (1998) Alterations in tau phosphorylation in rat and human neocortical slices following hypoxia and glucose deprivation. Exp Neurol 154: 464–472.

Busto R, Globus MYT, Dietrich WD, et al. (1989) Effect of mild hypothermia on ischemic-induced release of neurotransmitters and free fatty acids in the rat brain. Stroke 20: 904–910.

Busto R, Dietrich WD, Globus MY-T, Ginsberg MD (1989) Postischemic moderate hypothermia inhibits CA1 hippocampal ischemia neuronal injury. Neurosci Lett 101: 299–304.

Byron C (2001) Perfusion thresholds in human cerebral ischemia: historical perspective and therapeutic implications. Cerebrovasc Dis 11: 2–8.

Cahn R, Borziex MG, Aldino C, et al. (1989) Influence of monosialoganglioside inner ester on neurologic recovery after global cerebral ischemia in monkeys. Stroke 20: 652–656.

Calabresi P, Mercuri NB, De Murtas M, Bernardi B (1990) Endogenous GABA mediates presynaptic inhibition of spontaneous and evoked excitatory synaptic potentials in the rat neostriatum. Neurosci Lett 118: 99–102.

Cao W, Carney J, Duchon A, et al (1988) Oxygen free radical involvment in ischemia and reperfusion injury to brain. Neurosci lett 88: 233–238.

Cao X, Phillis J (1994) α-phenyl-tert-butyl-nitrone reduced cortical infarct and edema in rats subjected to focal ischemia. Brain Res 644: 267–272.

Carney J, Floyd R, (1991): Protection against oxidative damage to CNS by α-phenyl-tret-bytyl nitrone (PBN) and other

spin trapping agents: A novel series of non-lipid free radical scavengers. J Mol Neurosci 3: 47–57.
Carperter DO, Briggs DB (1986) Insulin excites neurons of the area postrema and causes emesis. Neurosci Lett 68: 85–89.
Casciola-Rosen L, Nicholson DW, Chong T, et al. (1996) Apocain/CPP32 cleaves proteins that are essential for cellular repair: a fundamental principle of apoptotic death J Exp Med 183: 1957–1964.
Cerchiari EL, Hoel TM, Safar P, Sclabassi RJ (1987) Protective effects of combined superoxide dismutase and deforeoxamine on recovery of cerebral blood flow and function after cardiac arrest in dogs. Stroke 18: 869–878.
Chan PH, Fishman RA, Caronna J; et al. (1983) Induction of brain edema following intracerebral injection of arachidonic acid. Ann Neurol 13: 625–632.
Chan PH, Longar S, Fishman RA (1987) Protective effects of liposome-entrapped superoxide dismutase on posttraumatic brain edema. Ann Neuro 21: 540–547.
Chan PH. Reactive oxygen radicals in signaling and damage in the ischemic brain. J Cereb Blood Flow Metab 2001: 21: 2–14.
Chen H, Chopp M, Zhang RL et al. (1994) Anti-CD11b monoclonal antibody reduces ischemic cell damage after transient focal cerebral ischemia in rat. Ann Neurol 35: 458–463.
Chen J, Weinstein PR, Graham SH. Attenuation of postischemic brain hypoperfusion and reperfusion injury by the cyclooxygenase-lipoxygenase inhibitor BW755C. J Neurosurg 1995: 83: 99–104.
Chen J, Graham SH, Nakayama M, et al. (1997) Apoptosis repressor genes Bcl-2 and Bcl-x-long are expressed in the rat brain following global ischemia. J Cereb Blood Flow Metab 17: 2–10.
Cheramy A, Barbeito L, Godeheu G, Glowinski J (1992): Riluzole inhibits the release og glutamate in the caudate nucleus of the cat in vivo. Neurosci Lett 147: 209–212.
Chi OZ, Pollak P, Weiss HR (1990) Effects of magnesium sulfate and nifedipine on regional cerebral blood flow during middle cerebral artery ligation in the rat. Arch Int Pharmanodyn Ther 304: 196–205.
Chi OZ, Wei HM, Tse J, et al. Cerebral microregional oxygen balance during chronic versus acute hypertension in middle cerebral artery occluded rats. Anest Analg 1996: 82: 587–592.
Chinnaiyan AM, O'Rourke K, Lane RB, Dixit VM (1997) Interaction of CED-4 with CED-3 and CED-9: A molecular framework for cell death. Science 275: 1122–1126.
Choi DW (1990) Possible mechanisms limiting N-methyl-D-aspartate receptor overactivation and the therapeutic efficacy of N-Methyl-D-Aspartate antagonists. Stroke 21 (suppl III) III-20-III-22.
Choi DW, Li Y (1996) Ischemia-induced neuronal apoptosis. Curr Opinion Neurobiol 8: 667–672.
Choki J, Greenberg J, Reivich M (1983) Regional cerebral glucose metabolism during and after bilateral cerebral ischemia in the gerbil. Stroke 14: 568–574.
Chopp M, Chen H, Ho KL, et al. (1989) Transient hyperthermia protects against subsequent forebrain ischemic cell damage in the rat. Neurology 39: 1396–1398.
Chopp M, Knight R, Tidwell CD, et al. (1989) The metabolic effects of mild hypothermia on global cerebral ischemia and recirculation in the cat: Comparison to normothermia and hyperthermia. J Cereb Blood Flow Metab 9: 141–148.
Chopp M, Chen H, Van de Linde AMQ, et al. (1990) Time course of postischemic intracellular alkalosis reflects the duration of ischemia J Cereb Blood Flow Metab 10: 860–865.
Chopp M, Zhang R, Chen H, et al. (1994): Postischemic administration of an anti-Mac-1 antibody reduces ischemic cell damage after transient middle cerebral artery occlusion in rats. Stroke 25: 869–876.
Chopp M, Li Y (1996) Apoptosis in focal cerebral ischemia. Acta Neurochir Suppl 66: 21–26.
Chopp M, Li Y, Jiang N, et al. (1996) Antibodies against adhesion molecules reduce apoptosis after transient middle cerebral artery occlusion in rat brain. J Cereb Blood Flow Metab 16: 578–584.
Christopherson TJ, Milde JH, Michenfelder JD (1993) Cerebral vascular autoregulation and CO_2 reactivity following onset of the dalayed postischemic hypoperfusion state in dogs. J Cereb Blood Flow Metab 13: 260–268.
Chyatta D, Rusch N, Sundt TM Jr (1983) Prevention of chronic experimental cerebral vasospasm with ibuprofen and high-dose methylprednisolone. J Neurosurg 59: 925–932.
Chyatta D, Sundt TM Jr (1984) Response of chronic experimental cerebral vasospasm to methylprednisolone and dexamethasone. J Neurosurg 60: 923–926.
Chyatta D, Fole NC, Nichols DA et al. (1987) Preliminary report: effect of high dose methylprednisolone on delayed cerebral ischemia in patients at high risk for vasospasm after aneurysmal subarachnoid hemorrhage. Neurosurgery 21: 157–160.
Claperon N, Durussel JJ, Rossignol P (1983) Effect of naloxone on rat brain hypoxia. J Pharm Pharmacol 35: 681–682.
Clark WM, Madden KP, Rothlein R, et al. (1991) Reduction of central nervous system ischemic injury in rabbits using leukocyte adhesion antibody treatment. Stroke 22: 877–883.
Clark WM, Madden KP, Rothlein R, et al. (1991) Reduction of central nervous system ischemic injury by monoclonal antibody to intercellular adhesion molecule. J Neurosurg 75: 623–627.
Clark WM, Hotan T, Lauten JD, Coull BM. (1994) Therapeutic efficacy of tirilazad in experimental multiple cerebral emboli: A randomized, controlled trial. Crit Care Med 22: 1161–1166.
Clark WM, Lauten JD, Lessov N, et al. (1995) Time course of ICAM-1 expression and leukocyte subset infiltration in rat forebrain ischemia. Mol Chem Neuropathol 26: 213–230.
Cleeter M, Cooper J, Darley-Usmar V, et al. (1994) Reversible inhibition of cytochrom c oxidase, the terminal enzyme of the mitochondrial respiratory chain, by nitric oxide. FEBS Lett 345: 50–54.
Clifton GL, Jiang JY, Lyeth BG, et al. (1991) Marked protection by moderate hypothermia after experimental traumatic brain injury. J Cereb Blood Flow Metab 11: 114–121.
Clough-Helfman C, Phillis JW (1991) The free radical trapping agent N-tret.-butyl-α-phenylnitrone (PBN) attenuates cerebral ischemic injury in gerbils. Free Rad Res Comms 15: 177–186.
Cohan SL, von Lubitz D, Redmond D, et al. (1989) The effects of flunarizine on survival following prolonged cerebral ischemia in the gerbil. In: Hartmann A, Kuschinsky W (eds): Cerebral Inschemia and Calcium. Berlin/Heidelberg, Springer-Verlag, pp 483–493.

Cohan SL, Redmond D, Chen M (1992) Effect of flunarizine on electroencephalogram recovery and brain temperature in-gerbils after brain ischemia. Stroke 23: 229–233.
Cohen Y, Chang L-H, Litt L, et al. (1990) Stability of brain intracellular lactate and 31P-metabolite levels at reduced intracellular pH during prolonged hypercapnia in rats. J Cereb Blood Flow Metab 10: 277–284.
Colasanti M, Mollace V, Cundari E, et al. (1993) The generation of nitric oxide participates in IFN-induced MHC class II antigen expression by cultured astrocytoma cells. Int J Immunopharmacol 15: 763–771.
Cole DJ, Matsumura JS, Drummond JC, Schell RM (1992) Focal cerebral ischemia in rats: Effects of induced hypertension, during reperfusion, on CBF. J Cereb Blood Flow Metab 12: 64–69.
Cole DJ, Patel PM, Schell RM, et al. (1993) Train eicosanoid levels during temporal focal cerebral ischemia in rats: A microdialysis study. J Neurosurg Anesthesiology 5: 41–47.
Connolly EJ, Winfree C, Springer T, et al. (1996): Cerebral protection in homozygous null ICAM-1 mice after middle cerebral artery occlusion. Role of neutrophil adhesion in the pathogenesis of stroke. J Clin Invest 97: 209–216.
Coradetti R, LoConte G, Moroni F, et al. (1984) Adenosine decreases aspartate and glutamate release from rat hippocampal slices. Eur J Pharmacol 104: 19–26.
Coyle J, Puttfarcken P (1993): Oxidative stress, glutamate, and neurogenerative disorders. Science 262: 689–695.
Coyle P, Jokelainen PT (1983) Differential outcome to middle cerebral artery occlusion in spontaneously hypertensive stroke-phrone rats. Stroke 14: 605–611.
Crockard A, Ianotti F, Hunstock AT, et al. (1980) Cerebral blood flow and edema following carotid occlusion in the gerbil. Stroke 11: 494–498.
Crockard HA, Gadian DG, Frackowiak RSJ, et al. (1987) Acute cerebral ischaemia: Concurrent changes in cerebral blood flow, energy metabolites, pH and lactate measured with hydrogen clearance and 31P and 1H nuclear magnetic resonance spectroscopy. II. Changes during ischaemia. J Cereb Blood Flow Metab 7: 394–402.
Crompton M, Ellinger Hm Costi A (1988): Inhibition of cyclosporin A of a Ca++ dependent pore in heart mitochondria activated by inorganic phosphate and oxidative stress. Biochem J 255: 357–360.
Cronstein BN, Levin RI, Belanoff J, et al. (1986) Adenosine an endogenous inhibitor of neutrophil-mediated injury to endothelial cells. J Clin Invest 78: 760–770.
Crumrine RC, LaManna JC (1991) Regional cerebral metabolites, blood flow, plasma volume, and mean transit time in total cerebral ischemia in the rat. J Cereb Blood Flow Metab 11: 272–282.
Cubells JM, de Blas A, Rodriquez H, et al. (1980) Los gangliosidos de corteza cerebral bovine en el tratamiento de las lesiones radiculares. Med Cmil 75: 156–180.
Dachs GU, Stratford IJ (1996) The molecular response to mammalian cells to hypoxia and the potential for exploitation in cancer therapy Br J Can 74 (suppl 27): S126–S132.
Dahl B, Bergholt B, Kjærgaard JO, et al. (1996) The correlation between CO_2- and indomethacin reactivity in severe head injury. Acta Neurochir 1996: 138: 265–273.
Dahlgren N, Nilsson B, Sakabe T, Siesjö BK (1981) The effect of indomethacin on cerebral blood flow and oxygen consumption in the rat at normal and increased carbon dioxide tensions. Acta physiol Scand 111: 475–485.
Dávalos A, Fernandez-Real J, Ricart W, et al. (1994) Iron-related damage in acute stroke. Stroke 25. 1543–1546.
Dawson DA, Kusumoto K, Graham DI, et al. (1992) Inhibition of nitric oxide synthase does not reduce infarct volume in a rat model of focal cerebral ischemia. Neurosci Lett 142: 151–154.
Dawson TM, Dawson VL, Snyder SH (1992) A novel neuronal messenger molecule in brain: The free radical, nitric oxide. Ann Neurol 32: 297–311.
Dawson V, Dawson T, London E (1991) Nitric oxide mediates glutamate neurotoxicity in primary cortical cultures. Proc Natl Acad Sci USA 88: 6368–6371.
Daum G. (1985): Lipids of mitochondria. Biochim Biophys Acta 822: 1–42.
Deckweth TL, Elliot JL, Knudson CM, et al. (1996) BAX in required for neuronal death after trophic factor deprivation and during development. Neuron 17: 401–411.
DeGraba TJ, Ostrow PT, Grotta JC (1993) Threshold of calcium disturbances after focal cerebral ischemia in rats. Implications of the window of therapeutic opportunity. Stroke 24: 1212–1217.
de la Torre JC, Fortin T, Saunders JK, et al. (1992) The no-reflow phenomenon is a post-mortem artefact. Acta Neuchir (Wien) 115: 37–42.
De Leo J, Toth L, Schubert P, et al. (1987) Ischemic-induced neuronal cell death, calcium accululation, and glial response in the hippocampus of the mongolian gerbil and protection by pentofylline (HWA 285). J Cereb Blod Flow Metab 7: 745–751.
de Ryck M, van Reempts J, Borgers M, et al. (1989) Photochemical stroke model: Flunarizine prevents sensorimotor deficits after neocortical infarcts in rat. Stroke 20: 1383–1390.
Dempsey RJ, Roy MW, Meyer KL, Donaldson DL (1985) Indomethacin-mediated improvement following middle cerebral artery occlusion in cats. Effects of anesthesia. J Neurosurg 62: 874–881.
Dempsey RJ, Roy MW, Cowen DE, et al. (1986) Lipoxygenase metabolites of arachidonic acid and the development of ischemic cerebral oedema. Neurol Res 8: 53–56.
Dempsey RJ, Carney JM, Kindy MS (1991) Modulation of ornithine decarboxylase mRNA following trasient ischemia in the gerbil brain. J Cereb Blood Flow Metab 11: 979–985.
Desbarats L, Schneider A, Muller D, et al. (1996) Myc: a single gene controls both proliferation and apoptosis in mammalian cells Experientia 52: 1123–1129.
Deshpande JK, Siesjö BK, Wieloch T (1987) Calcium accumulation and neuronal damage in the rat hippocampus following cerebral ischemia. J Cereb Blood Flow Metab 7: 89–95.
Dessi F, Ben-Ari Y, Charriaut-Marlanque C (1993) Riluzole prevents anoxic injury in cultured cerebellar granule neurons. Eur J Pharmacol 250: 325–328.
Dezsi L, Greenberg J, Sladky J, et al (1994): Prolonged effects of MK-801 in the cat during focal cerebral ischemia and recovery: Survival, EEG activity and histopathology. J Neurol Sci 121: 110–120.
Diemer NH, Siemkowicz E (1980) Regional glucose metabolism and nerve cell damage after cerebral ischemia in normo- and hypoglycemic rats. In: Circulatory and Developmental Aspects of Brain Metabolism (Spatz M, Mrsulja BB, Rakie LJ, Lust WD, eds), New York, Plenum, pp 23–32.

Diemer NH, Siemkowicz E (1981) Regional neurone damage after cerebral ischaemia in the normo- and hypoglycemic rat. J Neuropath Exp Neurol 7: 217–227.

Diemer NH, Johansen FF, J¢rgensen MB (1990) N-Methyl-D-Aspartate and non-N-Methyl-D-Aspartate antagonists in global cerebral ischemia. Stroke 21 (suupl III): III-39-III-42.

Dietrich WD, Busto R, Alonso O, et al. (1993). Intraichemic but not postischemic brain hyperthermia protects chronically following global forebrain ischemia in ras. J Cereb Blood Flow Metab 13: 541–549.

Dietrich WD, Feng Z, Leistra H, et al. (1994) Photothrombotic infarction triggers multiple episodes of cortical spreading depression in distant brain regions. J Cereb Blood Flow Metab 14: 20–28.

Dimlich RV, Tornheim PA, Kindel RH, et al. (1990) Effects of a 21-aminostroid (U 74006F) on cerebral metabolites and edema after severe experimental head trauma. Adv Neurol 52: 365–375.

Dimlich RVW, Nielsen MM (1992) Facilitating postischemic reduction of cerebral lactate in rats. Stroke 23: 1145–1153.

Dirnagl U, Jacewicz M, Pulsinelli W (1990) Nimodipine post-treatment does not increase blood flow in rats with focal cortical ischemia. Stroke 21: 1357–1261.

Dirnagl U, Lindauer U, Them A, et al. (1995): Global cerebral ischemia in the rat: Online monitoring of oxygen free radical production using chemiluminescense in vivo. J Cereb Blood Flow Metab 15: 929–940.

Dobrucki LW, Kalinowski L, Uracz W, Malinski T (2000) The protective role of nitric oxide in the brain ischemia. J Physiol Pharmacol 51: 695–703.

Doppenberg EMR, Zauner A; Watson JC, Bullock R (1998) Determination of ischemic threshold for brain oxygen tension. Acta Neurochir (suppl) 71: 166–169.

DoreDuffy P, Washington RA, Balabanov R, (1994) Cytokine mediated activation of cultured CNS microvessels: a system for examining antigenic modulations of CNS endothelial cells, and evidence for long-term expression of the adhesion protein E-selectin. J Cereb Blood Flow Metab 14: 837–844.

Dragunow M, Faull RLM (1988) Neuroprotective effects of adenosine. Trends Pharmacol Sci 9: 193–194.

Duchen M, McGuinness O, Brown L, Crompton M (1993): On the involvement of a cyclosporin A sensitive mitochondrial pore in myocardial reperfusion injury. Cardiovasc Res 27: 1790–1794.

Duckrow RB (1991) Regional cerebral blood flow during spreading cortical depression in conscious rats. J Cereb Blood Flow Metab 11: 150–154.

Duckrow RB (1993) A brief hypoperfusion precedes spreading depression if nitric oxide synthesis is inhibited. Brain Res 618: 190–195.

Dugan l, Sensi S, Canzoniero L, et al. (1995): Mitochondrial production of reactive oxygen species in cortical neurons following exposure to N-Methyl-D-aspartate. J Neurosci 15: 6377–6388.

Dux E, Joó F (1982) Effects of histamine on brain capillaries. Exp Brain Res 47: 252–258.

Edvinsson L, Johansson BB, Larsson B, et al. (1983) Calcium antagonists: Effect on cerebral blood flow and blood-brain larrier permeability in the rat. Br J Pharmacol 79: 141–148.

Ekholm A, Katsura K, Siesjö BK (1993) Coupling of energy failure and dissipative K^+ flux during ischemia: Role of preischemic plasma glucose concentration. J Cereb Blood Flow Metab 13: 193–200.

Ellis EF, Police RJ, Yancey L, et al. (1990) Dilation of cerebral arterioles by cytochrome P-450 metabolites of arachidonic acid. Am J Physiol 259: H1171–H1177.

Ellis EF, Dodson LY, Police RJ (1991) Restoration of cerebrovascular responsiveness to hyperventilation by the oxygen free radical scavenger n-acetylcysteine following experimental traumatic brain injury. J Neurosurg 75: 774–779.

Ennis SR, Keep RF, Schielke GP, Betz AL (1990) Decrease in perfusion of cerebral capillaries during incomplete ischemia and reperfusion. J Cereb Blood Flow Metab 10: 213–220.

Ernsberger PR, Meeley MP, Mann JJ, Reis DJ (1987) Clonidine binds to imdazole binding sites as well as α_2-adrenoceptors in the ventrolateral medulla. Eur J Pharmacol 134: 1–14.

Enokido Y, Araki, Tanaka K, et al. (1996) Involvement of p53 in DNA strand break-induced apoptosis in postmitotic CNS neurons. Eur J Neurosci 8: 1812–1821.

Espanol MT, Litt L, Hasegawa K, et al. (1998) Fructose-1,6,-biphosphate preserves adenosine triphosphate but not intracellular pH during hypoxia in respiring neonatal rat brain slices. Anesthesiology 88: 461–472.

Esteve AG, Stutzmann JM, Barteibo L. (1995): Protective effect of riluzole on excitatory amino acid-mediated neurotoxicity in motoneuron-enriched cultures. Eur J Pharmacol 280: 47–53.

Etzioni A, Frydman M, Pollack S, et al. (1992) Brief report: Recurrent severe infections caused by a novel leukocyte adhesion deficiency. New Engl J Med 327: 1789–1792.

Evans MC, Swan JH, Meldrum BS (1987) An adenosine analoque, 2-chloroadenosine, protects against long term development of ischemic cell loss in the rat hippocampus Neurosci Lett 83: 287–292.

Faden AI, Jacobs TP, Mougey E, Holoday JW (1981) Endorphins in experimental spinal injury: therapeutic effect of naloxone. Ann Neurol 10: 326–332.

Faden AI, Molineaux CJ, Rosenberger JG, et al. (1985) Endogenous opioid immunoactivity in rat spinal cord following traumatic injury. Ann Neurol 17: 386–390.

Faden AI, Hallenbeck JM, Brown CQ (1982) Treatment of experimental stroke: comparison of naloxone and thyrotropin releasing hormone. Neurology (NY) 32: 1084–1087.

Fallis R, Fisher M, Lobo R (1983) A double-blind trial of naloxone in acute stroke. Stroke 14: 124.

Faraci FM, Lopez AG, Breese K, et al. (1991) Effect of atherosclerosis on cerebral vascular responses to activation of leukocytes and platelets in monkeys. Stroke 22: 790–796.

Faraci FM (1992) Regulation of the cerebral circulation by endothelium. Pharmacol Ther 56: 1–22.

Faraci FM, Breese KR, Heistad DD (1993) Nitric oxide contributies to dilation of cerebral arterioles during seizures Am J Physiol 265: H2209–H2212.

Faraci FM, Breese K (1993) Nitric oxide mediates vasodilation in response to activation of N-methyl-D-aspartate receptors in brain. Cric res 72: 476–480.

Faraci FM, Breese KR, Heistad DD (1994) Cerebral vasodilation during hypercapnia. Role of glibenclamide-sensitive potassium channels and nitric oxide. Stroke 25: 1679–1683.

Farman C, Chen ZP, Branston N, Symon L (1994) The effect of haemodilution and hypercapnia on the recovery of cerebral function from experimental focal ischemia. Acta Neurochir (Wien) 127: 210–214.

Fastbom J, Fredholm BB (1985) Inhibition of [^{3}H]-glutamate release from rat hippocampal slices by L-isopropyladenosine. Acta Physiol Scand 125: 121–123.

Feinstein DL, Galea E, Reis DJ (1993) Norepinephrine suppresses inducible nitric oide synthase activity in rat astroglial cultures. J Neurochem 60: 1945–1948.

Feldman Z, Gurevitch B, Artru AA, et al. (1996) Effect of magnesium given 1 hour after trauma on brain edema and neurological outcome. J Neurosurg 85: 131–137.

Finkbeiner SM, Stevens CF. (1988) Application of quantitative measurements for assessing neurotoxicity. Proc Natl Acad Sci USA 85: 4071–4074.

Fitzpatrick FA, Murphy RC (1989) Cytochrom P-450 metabolism of arachidonic acid: formation and biological actions of "epoxygenase"-derived eicosanoids. Pharmacol Rev 40: 229–241.

Floyd RA (1990) Role of oxygen free radicals in carcinogenesis and brain ischemia. FASEB J 4: 2587–2597.

Folbergrová J, Kiyota Y, Pahlmark K, et al. (1993) Does ischemia with reperfusion lead to oxidative damage to proteins in the brain. J Cereb Blood Flow Metab 13: 145–152.

Folbergrová J, Zhao Q, Katsura K, Siesjö BK (1995) N-tret-butyl-α-phenylnitrone improves recovery of brain energy state in rats following transient focal ischemia. Proc Natl Acad Sci USA 92: 5057–5061.

Forsman M, Fleischer JE, Milde JH, et al. (1986) The effect of nimodipine on cerebral blood flow and metabolism. J Cereb Blood Flow Metab 6: 763–767.

Forsman M, Fleischer JE, Milde PA, et al. (1988) Superoxide dismutase and catalase failed to improve neurologic outcome after complete cerebral ischemia in the dog. Acta Anaesthesiol Scand 32: 152–155.

Forsman M, Aarseth HP, Nordby HK, et al. (1989) Effects of nimodipine on cerebral blood flow and cerebrospinal fluid pressure after cardiac arrest: Correlation with neurologic outcome. Anesth Analg 68: 436–443.

Frank HJL, Pardridge WM (1981) A direct in vitro demonstration of insulin binding to isolated brain microvessels. Diabetes 30: 757–761.

Franke TF, Yang SI, Chan TO et al. (1995) The protein kinase encoded by the Akt proto-oncogene is a target of the PDGF-activated phosphatidylinositol 3-kinase. Cell 81: 727–736.

Frazzini VI, Winfree CJ, Choudhri HF, et al. (1994) Mild hypothermia and MK-801 have similar but not additive degrees of cerebroprotection in the rat permanent focal ischemia model. Stroke 34: 1040–1046.

Freese A, Finklestein SP, Figlia M (1992) Basic fibroblast growth factor protects striatal neurons in vitro from NMDA-receptor mediated excitotoxicity. Brain Res 575: 351–355.

Frerichs KU, Sirén A-L, Feurstein GZ, Hallenbeck JM. The onset of postischemic hypoperfusion in rats is precipitous and may be controlled by local neurons. Stroke 1992: 23: 399–406.

Froese S, Shephard E, Adams S, et al. (1994) Integrins, selectins and CAMs- The glue of life. South African Med J 84: 759–764.

Fuchs-Buder T, Tramèr MR, Tassonyi E. (1997) Cerebrospinal fluid passage of intravenous magnesium sulfate in neurosurgical patients. J Neurosurg Anesthesiol 9: 324–328.

Furchgott RF, Zawadzki JV (1980) The obligatory role of endothelial cells in the relaxation of arterial smooth muscle by acetylcholine. Nature 288: 373–376.

Furlan M, Marchal G, Viader F, et al. (1996) Spontaneous neurological recovery after stroke and the fate of the ischemic penumbra. Ann Neurol 40: 216–226.

Fuxe K, Kurasawa N, Cintra A, et al. (1992) Involvement of local ischemia in endothelin-1 induced lesions of the neostriatum of the anesthetized rat. Exp Brain Res 88: 131–139.

Gaetani P, Marzatico F, Renault B et al. (1990) High-dose methylprednisolone and ex vivo release of eicosanoids after experimental subarachnoid haemorrhage. Neurol Res 12: 111–116.

Gai AM, Sessa MB, Angeli S (1980) Valutazioni prognostiche in funzione di nuovi protocolli farmacologici in alcune lesioni del sistema nervosa periferico. Eur Medicophys 16: 221–232.

Gajewski TF, Thompson CB (1996) Apoptosis meets signal transduction: elimination of a BAD influence. Cell 87: 589–592.

Galea E, Reis DJ, Feinstein DL (1993) Cloning and expression of rat astroglial inducible nitric oxide synthase. Sos Neurosci Abstracts 19: 1121.

Garcia JH, Liu K-F, Yoshida Y, et al. (1994): Influx of leukocytes and platelets in an evolving brain infarct. Am J Pathol 144: 188–199.

Garcia JH, Liu K-F, Relton JK. (1995): Interleukin-1 receptor antagonist decreases the number of necrotic neurons in rats with middle cerebral artery occlusion. Am J Pathol 147: 1477–1486.

Garthwaite J (1991) Glutamate, nitric oxide and cell-cell signaling in the nervous system. Trends Neurosci 14: 60–67.

Gaudet RJ, Alam I, Levine L (1980) Accumulation of cyclooxygenase products of arachidonic acid metabolism in gerbil brain during reperfusion after bilateral common carotid artery occlusion. J Neurochem 35: 653–658.

Gehrmann J, Banati R, Wiessnert C, et al. (1995): Reactive microglia in cerebral ischemia: an early mediator of tissue damage: Neuropathol Appl Neurobiol 21: 277–289.

Germano IM, Bartkowski HM, Cassel ME, Pitts LH (1987) The therapeutic value of nimodipine in experimental focal cerebral ischemia: Neurological outcome and histopathological findings. J Neurosurg 67: 81–87.

Gerner EW, Schneider MJ (1975) Induced thermal resistance in Hela cells. Nature 256: 500–502.

Giannotta SL, Weiss MH, Apuzzo MLJ, et al. (1984) High dose glucocorticoids in the management of severe head injury. Neurosurgery 15: 497–501.

Gideon P, Henriksen O, Sperling B, et al. (1992) Early time course of N-acetylaspartate, creatinine and phosphocreatinine, and compounds containing choline in the brain after acute stroke. A proton magnetic resonance spectroscopy study. Stroke 23: 1566–1572.

Gidö G, Katsura K, Kristian T, Siesjö BK (1993) Influence of plasma glucose concentration on rat brain extracellular calcium transients during spreading depression. J Cereb Blood Flow Metab 13: 179–182.

Gill R, Andine O, Hillered L, et al. (1992): The effect of MK-801 on cortical streading depression in the penumbra zone following focal ischemia in the rat. J Cereb Blood Flow Metab 12: 371–379.

Gill R, Hargreaves RJ, Kemp JA (1995) The neuroprotective effect of the glycine site antagonist 3-R-(+)-cis-4methyl-

HA966 (L-687,414) in rat model of focal ischemia. J Cereb Blood Flow Metab 15: 197-204.

Ginsberg MD, Graham DI, Path MRC, et al. (1979) Diffuse cerebral ischaemia in the cat: III. Neuropathological sequelae of severe ischaemia. Ann Neurol 5: 350–358.

Ginsberg MD, Prado R, Dietrich WD, et al. (1987) Hyperglycemia reduces the extend of cerebral infarction in rats. Stroke 18: 570–574.

Girodano JM, Mahadeo DK, He YY, et al. (1996) Increased expression of the neurofibromatosis 1 (NF1) gene product, neurofibromin, in astrocytes in response to cerebral ischemia. J Neurosci Res 43: 246-253.

Gisvold SE, Safar P, Hendricks HHL, Rao G, Moossy G., Alexander H (1984) Thiopental treatment after global ischaemia in pigtailed monkeys. Anesthesiology 1984: 60: 88–96.

Glazier SS, O'Rourke DM, Graham DI, Welsh FA (1994) Induction of ischemic tolerance following brief focal ischemia in rat brain. J Cereb Blood Flow Metab 14: 545–553.

Globus M, Ginsberg M, Busto R (1991) Excitotoxic index - a biochemical marker of selective vulnerability. Neurosci Lett 127: 39–42.

Globus MY-T, Wester P, Busto R, Dietrich WD (1992). Ischemic-induced extracellular release of serotonin plays a role in CA1 neuronal cell death. Stroke 23: 1595–1601.

Goldman RS, Finkbeiner SM. (1988) Therapeutic use of magnesium sulfate in selected vases of cerebral ischemia and seizures. N Eng J Med 319: 1224-1225.

Gonzales-Vidal MD, Cervera-Gaviria M, Ruelas R et al. (1998) Progesterone: Protective effects on the cat hippocampal neuronal damage due to acute global cerebral ischemia. Arch Med Res 29: 117–124.

Goodman RR, Snyder SH (1982) Autoradiographic localization of adenosine receptors in rat brain using [^{3}H] cyclohexyladenosine. J Neurosci 9: 1230–1241.

Goodman Y, Mattson MP (1996) Ceramide protects hippocampal neurons against excitotoxic and oxidation insults, and amyloid betapeptide toxicity. J Neurochem 66: 869–872.

Goto Y, Kassell NF, Hiramatsu K, et al. (1994) Effect of two dual-function compounds, U92798 and U92032, on transient focal ischemia in rats. Neurosurgery 34: 332–338.

Graeber TG, Osmanian C, Jacks T, et al. (1996) Hypoxia-mediated selection of cells with deminished apoptotic potential in solid tumours. Nature 379: 88–91.

Graham SH, Chen J, Sharp FR, Simon RP (1993) Limiting ischemic injury by inhibition of excitatory amino acid release. J Cereb Blood Flow metab 13: 88–97.

Graham SH, Chen J. Programmed cell death in cerebral ischemia. J Cereb Blood Flow Metab 2001: 21: 99–109.

Gregory GA, Yu AC, Chan PH (1989) Fructose-1,6,-biphosphate protects astrocytes from hypoxic damage. J Cereb Blood Flow Metab 9: 29–34.

Grice SC, Chappell ET, Prough DS, et al. (1986) Ibuprofen improves cerebral blood flow after global cerebral ischemia in dogs. Anesthesiology 65: A312.

Griffiths E, Halestrap A (1991): Further evidence that cyclosporin A protects mitochondral from calcium overload by inhibiting a matrix peptidyl-propyl *cis-trans* isomerase. Implication for the immunosuppressive and toxic effects of cyclosporin. Biochem J 274: 611–614.

Grilli M, Pizzi M, Memo M, et al. (1996) Neuroprotection by aspirin and sodium salicylate through blockade of NF-kappaB activation. Science 274: 1383–1385.

Gross PM, Teasdale GM, Graham DI, et al. (1982) Intra-arterial histamine increases blood-brain transport in rats. Am J Phys 243: H307–H317.

Grotta JC, Dedman JR, Rhoades HM, et al. (1990) Neuronal protection correlates with prevention of calcium-calmodulin binding in rats. Stroke 21: (suppl III): III28–III31.

Gustafson I, Yoshitoyo M, Wieloch TW (1989) Postischemic administration of idazoxan, an α_2-adrenergic receptor antagonist, decreases neuronal damage in the rat brain. J Cereb Blood Flow Metab 9: 171–174.

Gustafson I, Westerberg E, Wieloch T (1990) Protection against ischemia-induced neuronal damage by the α_2-adrenoceptor antagonist idazoxan: influence of time of administration and possible mechanisms of action. J Cereb Blood Flow Metab 10: 885–894.

Haass C, Hung AY, Selkoe DJ (1991) Processing of β-amyloid precurser protein in microglia and astrocytes favors an internal localization over constitutive secretion. J Neurosci 11: 3783–3793.

Hacke W, Zeumer H, Ferbert A, et al. (1988) Intra-arterial thrombolytic therapy improves outcome in patients with acute vertebrobasilar occlusive desease. Stroke 19: 1216–1222.

Hacke W, Kaste M, Fieschi C, et al. (1995) Intravenous thrombolysis with recombinant tissue plasminogen activator for acute hemispheric stroke. The European Cooperative Acute Stoke Study. JAMA 274: 1017–1025.

Hadley MN, Spetzler RF, Fifield MS, et al. (1987) The effect of nimodipine on intracranial pressure. Volume-pressure studies in a primate model. J Neurosurg 66: 387–393.

Hagberg H, Andersson P, Lacarewicz J, et al. (1987) Extracellular adenosine, inosine, hypoxanthine adn xanthine in relation to tissue nucleotides and purines in rat striatum during transient ischemia. J Neurochem 49: 227–231.

Hakim AM (1986) Cerebral acidosis in focal ischemia: II. Nimodipine and verapamil normalize cerebral pH following middle cerebral artery occlusion in the rat. J Cereb Blood Flow Metab 6: 676–683.

Hakim AM, Evans AC, Berger L, et al. (1989) The effect of nimodipine on the evolution of human cerebral infarction studied by PET. J Cereb Blood Flow Metab 9: 523–534.

Hakim AM, Hogan MJ (1991) In vivo binding of nimodipine in the brain: I. The effect of focal cerebral ischemia. J Cereb Blood Flow Metab 11: 762–770.

Hakim AM, Hogan MJ, Carpenter S (1992) Time course of cerebral blood flow and histological outcome after focal cerebral ischemia. Stroke 23: 1138–1144.

Hall ED, Braughler JM (1981) Acute effect of intravenous glucocorticoid pretreatment on the in vitro peroxidation of cat spinal cord tissue. Exp Neurol 73: 321–324.

Hall ED, Braughler JM (1982) Effects of intravenous methylprednisolone on spinal cord lipid peroxidation and (Na^+ +K^+)-ATPase activity. Dose response analysis during 1st hour after contusion injury in the cat. J Neurosurg 57: 247–253.

Hall ED (1982) Glucocorticoid effect on central nervous excitability and synaptic transmission. Int Rev Neurobiol 23: 165–195.

Hall ED, Wolf DL (1984) Effects of single large dose of methylprednisolone sodium succinate on experimental posttraumatic spinal cord ischemia. Dose-reponse and time-action analysis. J Neurosurg 61: 124–130.

Hall ED (1985) High-dose glucocorticoid treatment improves neurological recovery in head-injured mice. J Neurosurg 62: 882–887.

Hall ED, Yonkers PA, McCall JM (1988) Attenuation of hemorrhagic shock by the non-glucocorticoid 21-aminosteroid U 74006F. Eur J Pharmacol 147: 299–303.

Hall ED Pazara KE, Braughler JM (1988) The 21-aminosteroid lipid peroxidation inhibitor U 74006F protects against cerebral ischemia in gerbils. Stroke 19: 997–1002.

Hall ED, Travis MA (1988) Inhibition of arachidonic acid-induced vasogenic brain edema by the non-glucocorticoid 21-aminosteroid U 74006F. Brain Res 451: 350–352.

Hall ED, Travis MA (1988) Attenuation of progressive brain hypoperfusion following experimental subarachnoid hemorrhage by large intravenous doses of methylprednisolone. Exp Neurol 99: 594–606.

Hall ED, Yonkers PA, McCall JM, Braughler JM (1988) Effects of a 21-aminosteroid U74006F on experimental head injury in mice. J Neurosurg 68: 456–461.

Hall ED (1988) Effect of a 21-aminosteroid U74007F on post-traumatic spinal cord ischemia in cats. J Neurosurg 68: 462–465.

Hall ED, Travis MA (1988) Effects of the non-glucocorticoid 21-aminosteroid U74006F on progressive brain hypoperfusion following experimental subarachnoid hemorrhage. Exp Neurol 1988: 102: 244–248.

Hall ED, Braughler JM (1989) Central nervous system trauma and stroke. I. Biochemical considerations for oxygen radical formation and lipid peroxidation. Free Radical Biology Medicine 6: 289–301.

Hall ED, Braughler JM (1989) Central nervous system trauma and stroke. II. Physiological and pharmacological evidence for involvement of oxygen radicals and lipid peroxidation. Free Radical Biology Medicine 6: 303–313.

Hall ED, Pazara KE, Tang AH, et al. (1990) 21 aminosteroids-limiting the extent of damage after ischemia. In Rose FC (ed) New Drug Strategies in the prevention and treatment of stroke. Smith-Gordon Publischer. London, in press.

Hall ED, Andrus PK, Fleck TJ, et al. (1997) Neuroprotective properties of the benzodiazepine receptor partial agonist PNU-101017 in the gerbil forebrain ischemia model. J Cereb Blood Flow Metab 17: 875–883.

Hallenbeck JM, Furlow TW (1979) Prostaglandin I2 and indomethacin prevent impairment of post-ischemic brain reperfusion in the dog. Stroke 10: 629–637.

Halsey JH, Conger KA, Garcia JH, Sarvary E (1991) The contribution or reoxygenation to ischemic brain damage. J Cereb Blood FLow Metab 11: 994–1000.

Hamilton MG, Tranner BI, Auer RN.(1995) Insulin reduction of cerebral infarction due to transient focal ischemia. J Neurosurg 82: 262–268.

Hara H, Iwai T, Niwa M, et al. (1996) Immunohistochemical detection of Bax and Bcl-2 proteins in gerbil hippocampus following transient forebrain ischemia. Brain Res 711: 249–253.

Haraldseth O, Gr¢nås T, Soutnon T, et al. (1992) The effects of brain temperature on temporary global ischemia in rat brain. A ^{31}phosphorous NMR spectroscopy study. Acta Anaesthesiol Scand 36: 393–399.

Harders A, Kakarieka A, Braakman R, et al. (1996) Traumatic subarachnoid hemorrhage and its treatment with nimodipine. J Neurosurg 85: 82–89.

Haring H, Berg EL, Tsurushita N et al. (1996) E-selectin appears in nonischemic tissue during experimental focal cerebral ischemia. Stroke 27: 1386–1391.

Harper AM, Craigen L, Kazda S (1981) Effect of the calcium antagonist, nimodipine, on cerebral blood flow and metabolism in primates. J Cereb Blood Flow Metab 1: 349–356.

Harris RJ, Symon L, Branston NM, Bayhan M (1981) Changes in extracellular cation activity in cerebral ischemia. J Cereb Blood Flow Metab 1: 203–209.

Harris RJ, Branston NM, Symon L, et al. (1982) The effect of a calcium antagonist, nimodipine, upon physiological responses of the cerebral vasculature and its possible influence upon focal cerebral ischemia. Stroke 13: 759–766.

Harris RJ, Bayhan M, Branston NM, et al. (1982) Modulation of the pathophysiology of primate focal cerebral ischaemia by indomethacin. Stroke 13: 17–24.

Harris RJ, Symon L (1984) Extracellular pH, potassium, and calcium activities in progressive ischaemia of rat cortex. J Cereb Blood Flow Metab 4: 178–186.

Harris RJ, Richards PG, Symon L, et al. (1987) pH, K^+, and PO_2 of the extracellular space during ischaemia of primate cerebral cortex. J Cereb Blood Flow Metab 7: 599–604.

Hasegawa Y, Choki J, Yamaguchi T. (1990) Cerebral blood flow, glucose utilization, and electrocorticograms following common caritd artery occlusion in gerbil. Stroke 21: 112–118.

Hatake K, Wakabayashi I, Kakishita E, Hishida S (1992) Impairment of endothelium-dependent relaxation in human basilar artery after sybarachnoidal hemorrhage. Stroke 23: 1111–1117.

Hatashita S, Hoff JT (1986) Role of a hydrostatic pressure gradient in the formation of early ischemic brain edema. J Cereb Blood Flow Metab 6: 546–522.

Havrankova J, Roth J (1978) Insulin receptors are widely distributed in the central nervous system of the rat. Nature 272: 827–829.

Haws VW, Heistad DD (1984) Effects of nimodipine on cerebral vasoconstrictor responses. Am J Physiol 247: H170–H176.

Hayashi Y, Jikihara I I, Yagi T, et al. (2001) Immunohistochemical investigation of caspase-1 and effect of caspase-1 inhibitor in delayed neuronal death after transient cerebral ischemia. Brain Res 893: 113–120.

Heinzel B, John M, Klatt P, Bohme E, Mayer (1992) Ca^{2+}/calmodulin-dependent formation of hydrogen peroxide by brain nitric oxide synthase. Biochem J 281: 627–630.

Heiss WD, Hayakawa T, Waltz AG (1976) Cortical neuronal function during ischaemia. Effects on occlusion of one middle cerebral artery on single unit activity in cats. Arch Neurol 33: 813–820.

Heiss WD, Rosner G (1983) Functional recovery of cortical neurons as related to degree and duration of ischaemia. Ann Neurol 14: 294–301.

Heiss WD, Huber M, Fink GR, et al. (1992) Progressive derangement of periinfarct viable tissue in ischemic stroke. J Cereb Blood FLow Metab 12: 193–203.

Heiss WD, Wienhard RGK, Löttgen J, et al. (1994) Dynamic penumbra demonstrated by sequential multitracer PET after middle cerebral artery occlusion in cats. J Cereb Blood Flow Metab 14: 892–902.

Heiss WD (2000) Ischemic penumbra: Evidence from fuctional imaging in man. J Cereb Blood Flow Metab 20: 1276–1293.

Hekmatpanah J (1973) Cerebral blood flow dynamics in hypotension and cardiac arrest. Neurology 23: 174–180.

Helfaer MA, Kirsch JR, Hurn PD, et al. (1992) Tiralazad mesylate does not improve early cerebral metabolic recovery following compression ischemia in dogs. Stroke 23: 1479–1486.

Heneka MT, Sharp A, Klockgether T, et al. (2000) The heat shock response inhibits NF-κB activation, nitric oxide synthase type 2 expression, and macrophage/microglial activation in brain. J Cereb Blood Flow Metab 20: 800–811.

Henriksson M, Lusher B (1996) Proteins of the Myc network: essential regulators of cell growth and differentiation. Adv Cancer Res 68: 115–182.

Herbert T, Drapeau P, Pradier L, Dunn RJ (1994): Block of the rat brain IIA sodium channel alpha subunit by the neuroprotective drug roluzole. Mol Pharmacol 45: 1055–1060.

Herrera DG, Maysinger D, Gadient R, et al. (1993): Spreading depression induces c-*fos*-like immunoreactivity and NGF mRNA in the rat cerebral cortex. Brain Res 602: 99–103.

Herzog KH, Morgan JL (1996) Cellular immediate-early genes and cell death in the nervous system. Neuropath Applied Neurobiol 22: 484–488.

Hicks SD, DeFranco DB, Callaway CW (2000) Hypothermia during reperfusion after asphyxial cardiac arrest improves functional recovery and selective alters stress-induced proteim expression. J Cereb Blood Flow Metab 20: 520–530.

Hill JM, Lesniak MA, Pert CB (1988) Co-localization of IGF-II receptors, IL-1 receptors and Thy 1.1 in the rat brain. Peptides 9 (suppl 1): 91–96.

Hoehn-Berlage M, Norris D, Kohne K, et al. (1995): Evolution of regional changes in apparent diffusion coefficent during focal iscehmia of rat brain. J Cereb Blood Flow Metab 15: 1002–1011.

Hofer M, Pagliusi SR, Hohn A, et al. (1990) Regional distribution of brain-derived neurotrophic factor mRNA in the adult mouse brain. EMBO J. 9: 2459–2464.

Hoffman WE, Werner C, Baugman VL, et al. (1991) Postischemic treatment with hypothermia improves outcome from incomplete cerebral ischemia in rats. J Neurosurg Anesthesiology 3: 34–38.

Holaday JW, D'Amato RJ (1982a) Naloxone and ischemic neurologic deficits in the gerbil: is there an effect? Science 218: 292–294.

Holaday JW, D'Amato RJ (1982b) Naloxone or TRH fails to improve neurologic deficits in gerbil models of "stroke". Life Sci 31: 385–392.

Hong S-C, Goto Y, Lanzino G, et al. Neuroprotection with a calpain inhibitor in a model of focal cerebral ischemia. Stroke 1994: 25: 663–669.

Hosobuchi Y, Baskin DS, Woo SK (1982a) Reversal of induced ischemic neurologic deficit in gerbils by the opiate antagonist naloxone. Science 215: 69–71.

Hosobuchi Y, Baskin DS, Woo SK (1982b) Reversal of neurological deficits by opiate antagonist naloxone after cerebral ischemia in animals and humans. J Cereb Blood Flow Metab 2 (suppl 1): S98–100.

Hossmann K-A, Lechtabe-Gruter H, Hossmann V (1973) The role of cerebral blood flow for the recovery of the brain after prolonged ischemia. Z Neurol 204: 281.

Hossmann K-A (1976) Development and resolution of ischemic brain swelling. In: Pappius HM, Feindel W (eds): Dynamics of Brain Edema, Springer Verlag, pp 219–277.

Hossmann K-A, Sakaki S, Zimmerman V (1977) Cation activities in reversible ischemia of the cat brain. Stroke 8: 77–81.

Hossmann K-A, Schuier FJ (1980) Experimental brain infarction in cats. Stroke 11: 583–592.

Hossmann K-A, Matsuoka Y (1982) Brain tissue osmolality following middle cerebral artery occlusion in cats. J Cereb Blood Flow Metab 2: 262–263.

Hossmann K-A, Schmidt-Kastner R, Grosse Ophoff B (1987) Recovery of integrative central nervous function after one hour global cerebro-circulatory arrest in normothermic cat. J Neurological Sciences 77: 305–320.

Hossmann K-A (1988) Resuscitation potentials after prolonged global cerebral ischemia in cats. Critical Care Medicine 16: 964–971.

Huang CY, Fujimura M, Noshita N, et al. (2001) SOD1 down-regulates NF-kappaB and c-Myc expression in mice after transient focal cerebral ischemia. J Cereb Blood Flow Metab 21: 163–173.

Huang Z, Huang P, Panahian N, e tal. (1994): Effects of cerebral ischemia in mice deficient in neuronal nitric oxide synthase. Science 265: 1883–1885.

Hubbard JL, Sundt TM Jr (1983) Failure of naloxone to affect focal incomplete cerebral ischemia and collateral blood flow in cats. J Neurosurg 59: 237–244.

Huber M, Kittner B, Hojer C, et al. (1993) Effect of propentofylline on regional cerebral glucose metabolism in acute stroke. J Cereb Blood Flow Metab 13: 526–530.

Hudges P Dragunow M (1995) Induction of immediate-early genes and the control of neurotransmitter-regulated gene expression within the nervous system. Pharmacol Rev 47: 133–178.

Hutson SM, van Dop C, Lardy HA (1977) Mitichondrial metabolism of pyruvate in bovine spermatozoa. J Biol Chem 252: 1309–1315.

Iadecola C (1992) Nitric oide participates in the cerebrovasodilation elicited from cerebellar fastigial nuchleus. Am J Physiol 263: R1156–R1161.

Iadecola C, Pelligrino DA, Moskowitz MA, Lassen NA (1994) Nitric oxide synthase inhibition and cerebrovascular regulation. J Cereb Blood Flow Metab 14: 175–192.

Iadecola C, Zhang F, Xu S, et al. (1995) Inducible nitric oxide synthase gene expression in brain following cerebral ischemia. J Cereb Blood Flow Metab 15: 378–384.

Iannotti F, Hoff JT (1983) Ischemic brain edema with and without reperfusion: An experimental study in gerbils. Stroke 14: 562–567.

Illievich UM, Zornow MH, Choi KT, Scheller MS, Strnat MAP (1994) Effect of hypothermic metabolic suppression on hippocampal glutamate concentrations after transient global cerebral ischemia. Anesth Analg 78: 905–911.

Inoue M, McHugh M, Pappius HM (1991) The effect of α-adrenergic receptor blockers prazosin and yohimbine on cerebral metabolism and biogenic amine content of traumatized brain. J Cereb Blod Flow Metab 11: 242–252.

Isackson P, Huntsman MM, Murray KD, Gall CM (1991) BDNFmRNA expression is increased in adult rat forebrain after limbic seizures. Temporal patterns of induction distinct from NGF. Neuron 6: 937–948.

Itakura T, Yokota H, Kimura H, et al. (1985) 5-hydroxytryptamine innervation of vessels in the rat cerebral cortex. J Neurosurg 62: 42–47.

Ito U, Spatz M, Walker JT, Klatzo I (1975) Experimental cerebral ischaemia in mongolian gerbils. I. Light microscopic observations. Acta Neuropathol (Berl.) 32: 209–223.

Ito U, Ohno K, Nakamura R, Saganuma F, Inada Y (1979) Brain edema during ischemia and after restoration of blood flow.

Measurement of water, sodium, potassium content and plasma protein permeability. Stroke 10: 542–547.

Ito U, Ohno K, Yamaguchi T, Tomita H, Inaba Y, Kashima M (1980) Transient appearance of "no-reflow" phenomenon in mongolian gerbils. Stroke 11: 517–521.

Izumi Y, Roussel S, Pinard E, Seylaz J (1991) Reduction of infarct volume by magnesium after middle cerebral artery occlusion in rats. J Cereb Blood Flow Metab 11: 1025–1030.

Jacewicz M, Kiessling M, Pulsinelli WA (1986) Selective gene expression in focal cerebral ischemia. J Cereb Blood Flow Metab 6: 263–272.

Jacewicz M, Brint S, Tanabe J, et al. (1990) Nimodipine pretreatment improves cerebral blood flow and reduces brain edema in conscious rats subjected to focal cerebral ischemia. J Cereb Blood Flow Metab 10: 903–913.

Jacewicz M, Brint S, Tanabe J, Pulsinelli WA (1990) Continuous nimodipine treatment attenuates cortical infarction in rats subjected to 24 hours of focal cerebral ischemia. J Cereb Blood Flow Metab 10: 89–96.

Jacewicz M, Tanabe J, Pulsinelli WA (1992) The CBF threshold and dynamics for focal cerebral infarction in spontaneously hypertensive rats. J Cereb Blood Flow Metab 12: 359–370.

Jan M, Buchheit F, Tremoulet M (1988) Therapeutic trial of intravenous nimodipine in patients with established cerebral vasospasms after rupture of intracranial aneurysms. Neurosurgery 23: 154–157.

Jensen K, Öhrström J, Cold GE, Astrup J (1991) The effects of indomethacin on intracranial pressure, cerebral blood flow, and cerebral metabolism in patients with severe head injury and intracranial hypertension. Acta Neurochir (Wien) 108: 116–121.

Jiang Q, Chopp M, Zhang ZG, et al. (1994) The effect of hypothermia on transient focal ischemia in rat brain evaluated by diffusion- and perfusion-weighted NMR imaging. Journal CBF and Metabolism 14: 732–741.

Jiang N, Zhang RL, Chen H, et al. (1994) Anti-CD11b monocloncal antibody reduces ischemic cell damage after transient (2h) but not after permanent MCA occlusion in the rat. Neurosci Res Comm 15: 85–93.

Jiang N, Chopp M, Stein D, et al. (1996) Progesterone is neuroprotective after transient middle cerebral artery occlusion in male rats. Brain Res 735: 101–107.

Johnson J, Ascher P (1987) Glycine potentiates the NMDA response in cultured mouse brain neurons. Nature 325: 529–531.

Jones TH, Morawetz RB, Crowell RM, et al. (1981) Thresholds of focal cerebral ischaemia in awake monkeys. J Neurosurg 54: 773–782.

Jordan J, Galindo MF, Prehn JHM, et al. (1996) p53 expression induces apoptosis in hippocampal pyramidal neuron cultures J Neurosci 17: 1397–1405.

J¢rgensen MB, Whright DC, Diemer NH (1990) Postischemic glucose metabolism is modified in the hippocampal CA1 region depleted of excitatory input or pyramidal cells. J Cereb Blood Flow Metab 10: 243–251.

Kabayashi S, Harris VA, Welsk FA (1995): Spreading depression induces tolerance of cortical neurons to ischemia in rat brain. J Cereb Blood Flow Metab 15: 721–727.

Kader A, Frazzini VI, Solomon RA, Trifiletti RR (1993) Nitric oxide production during focal cerebral ischemia in rats. Stroke 24: 1709–1716.

Kaltschmidt B, Uherek M, Volk B, et al. (1997) Transcription factor NF-kappaB is activated in primary neurons by amyloid beta peptides and in neurons surrounding early plaques from patients with Alzheimer deisease. Proc Natl Acad Sci USA 94: 2642–2647.

Kamatsumoto S, Greeberg JH, Hickey WF, et al. (1989) Local glucose utilization in chronic middle cerebral artery occlusion in the cat. J Cereb Blood Flow Metab 9: 535–547.

Kamme F, Wieloch T (1996) Induction of junDmRNA after transient forebrain ischemia in the rat. Effect of hypothermia. Mol Brain Res 43: 51–56.

Kanamaru K, Waga S, Kojima T, et al. (1987) Endothelium-dependent relaxation of canine basilar arteries. Stroke 18: 932–937.

Kanamura K, Weir BKA, Findlay JM, et al. (1989) Pharmacologiclal studies on relaxation of spastic primate cerebral arteries in subarachnoidal hemorrhage. J Neurosurg 71: 909–915.

Kapiloff MS, Mathis JM, Nelson SA, et al. (1991) Calcium/calmodulin-dependent protein kinase mediates a pathway for transscriptional regulation. Rpoc Natl Acad Sci USA 88: 3710–3714.

Kaplan B, Brint S, Tanabe J, et al. (1991) Temporal thresholds for neocortical infarction in rats subjected to reversible focal cerebral ischemia. Stroke 22: 1032–1039.

Kapp J, Mahaley MS Jr, Odom GI (1970) Experimental evaluation of potential spasmolytic drugs. J Neurosurg 32: 468–472.

Karibe H, Zarow GJ, Weinstein PR. Use of mild intraischemic hypothermia versus mannitol to reduce infarct size after temporary middle cerebral artery occlusion in rats. J Neurosurg 1995: 83: 93–98.

Karpiak SE, Li YS, Mahadik SP (1987) Ganglioside (GM1 and AGF2) reduce mortality due to ischemia: protection of membrane function. Stroke 18: 184–187.

Kass IS, Cottrell JE, Chambers G. (1988): Magnesium and cobalt, not nimodipine, protect neurons against anoxic damage in the rat hippocampal slice. Anesthesiology 69: 710–715.

Kastin AJ, Nissen C, Olson RD (1982) Failure of MIF-1 or naloxone to reverse inschemic-induced neurologic deficits in gerbils. Pharmacol Biochem Behav 17: 1083–1085.

Kataoka K, Graf R, Rosner G, Heiss W-D (1987) Experimental focal ischemia in cats: Changes in multimodality evoked potentials as related to local cerebral blood flow and ischemic brain edema. Stroke 18: 188–194.

Katayama Y, Welch F (1989): Effect of dichloroacetate on regional energy metabolites and pyruvate dehydrogenase activity during ischemia and reperfusion in gerbil brain. J Neurochem 52: 1817–1822.

Katsura K, Ekholm A, Siesjö BH (1992) Tissue PCO_2 in brain ischemia related to lactate content in normo- and hypercapnic rats. J Cereb Blood Flow Metab 12: 270–280.

Katsura K, Folbergrová J, Bengtsson F, et al. (1993) Recovery of mitochondrial and plasma membrane function following hypoglycemic coma: Coupling of ATP synthesis, K^+ transport, and changes in extra- and intracellular pH. J Cereb Blood Flow Metab 13: 820–826.

Katsura K, Kristián T, Smith M-L, Siesjö BK (1994) Acidosis induced by hypercapnia exaggerates ischemic brain damage. J Cereb Blood Flow Metab 14: 243–250.

Katusic ZS, Milde JH, Cosentino F, Mitrovis BS (1993) Subarachnoid hemorrhage and endothelial L-arginine pathway in small brain stem arteries. Stroke 24: 392–399.

Katzman R, Clasen R, Klatzo I, et al. (1977) Report of Joint Commitee for Stroke Resources IV Brain Edema in Stroke. Stroke 8: 512–54o.

Kawahara N, Reutzler CA, Wiegand SJ, et al. (1994): Induction of protective mechanisms in cerebral ischemia. Soc Neurosci (abstract) 20: 1480.

Kawahara N, Ruetzler CA, Klatzo I (1995): Protective effect of spreading depression against neuronal damage in cerebral ischemia. Neurol Res 17: 9–16.

Kawai K, Penix LP, Kawahara N, et al. (1995) Developement of susceptibility to audiogenic seizures following cardiac arrest cerebral ischemia in rats. J Cereb Blood Flow Metab 15: 248–258.

Kawai N, Keep RF, Betz AL, Nagao S (1998) Hyperglycemia induces progressive changes in the cerebral microvasculature and blood-brain barrier transport during focal cerebral ischemia. Acta Neurochir (suppl) 71: 219–221.

Kayalar C, Ord T, Testa MP, et al. (1996) Cleavage of actin by interleukin 1 beta-converting enzyme to reverse DNase 1 inhibition. Proc Natl Acad Sci USA 93: 2234–2238.

Kellcher JA, Gregory GA, Chan PH (1994) Effect of FBP on glutamate uptake and glutamate synthetase activity in hypoxic astrocyte cultures. Neurochem Res 19: 209–215.

Kempski O, Shohami E, von Lubitz D, et al. (1987) Postischemic production of eicosanoids in gerbil brain. Stroke 18: 111–119.

Kiening KL, Unterberg AW, Bardt TF et al. (1996) Monitoring of cerebral oxygenation in patients with severe head injuries: Brain tissue pO_2 versus jugular vein saturation. J Neurosurg 85: 751–757.

Kim HJ, Levasseur JE, Patterson JL, et al. (1989) Effect of indomethacin prestreatment on acute mortality in experimental brain injury. J Neurosurg 71: 565–572.

Kim JS, Chopp M, Chen H, et al. (1995) Adhesive glycoproteins CD11a and CD18 are upregulated in the leukocytes from patients with ischemic stroke and transient ischemic attacks. J Neurol Science 128: 45–50.

Kim P, Schini VB, Sundt TM, Vanhoutte PM (1992) Reduced production of cGMP underlies the loss of endothelium-dependent relaxations in the canine basilar artery after subarachnoidal hemorrhage. Circ Res 70: 248–256.

Kimelberg HK, Rutledge E, Goderie S, Charniga C, (1995) Astrocytic swelling due to hypotonic or high K+ medium causes inhibition of glutamate and aspartate uptake and increases their release. J Cereb Blood Flow Metab 15: 409–416.

Kimelberg HK (1995) Current concepts of brain edema. Review of laboratory investigations. J Neurosurg 83: 1051–1059.

Kindy MS, Hu Y, Dempsey RJ (1994) Blockade of ornithine decarboxylase enzyme protects against ischemic brain damage. J Cereb Blood FLow Metab 14: 1041–1045.

Kirino T (1996) Ischemic cell death in the hippocampus. Int Acad Biomed Drug Res 11: 62–75.

Kitagawa K, Matsumoto M, Tagaya M, et al. (1991) Hyperthermia-induced neuronal protection against ischemic injury in gerbils. J Cereb Blood Flow Metab 11: 449–452.

Kittaka M, Giannotta SL, Zelman V, et al. (1997) Attenuation of brain injury and reduction of neuron-specific enolase by nicardipine in systemic circulation following focal ischemia and reperfusion in a rat model. J Neurosurg 87: 731–737.

Klatt P, Schmidt K, Uray G, Mayer B (1993) Multiple catalytic fluctuations of brain nitric oxide synthase. J Biol Chem 268: 12781–14787.

Klatzo I, Schuier F, Orzi F, Wilmes F, et al. (1981) Inter-relationships between cerebral blood flow (CBF) and brain edema (BE). In: Minderhond JM (ed): Cerebral Blood Flow: Basic Knowledge and Clinical Implications. Excerpta Medica Amsterdam, Oxford, Princeton, pp 160–173.

Kluck RM, Bossy-Wetzel E, Green DG, Newmeyer DD (1997) The release of cytochrom C from mitochondria: a primary site for Bcl-2 regulation of apoptosis. Science 275: 1132–1136.

Kogure K, Busto R, Scheinberg P (1981) The role of hydrostatic pressure in ischemic brain edema. Ann Neurol 9: 273–282.

Kohno K, Hoehn-Berlage M, Mies G, et al. (1995) Relationship between diffusion-weighted MR images, cerebral blood flow, and energy state in experimental brain infarction. Magn Reson Imaging 13: 73–80.

Koide T, Wieloch TW, Siesjö BK (1986) Circulating catecholamine modulate ischemic brain damage. J Cereb Blood FLow Metab 6: 559–565.

Koide T, Wieloch TW, Siesjö BK (1986) Chronic dexamethasone pretreatment aggravates ischemic neuronal necrosis. J Cereb Blood Flow Metab 6: 395–404.

Koistinaho J, Pyykonen I, Keinanen R, Hokfelt T (1996) Expression of β-amyloid precursor protein mRNAs following transient focal ischemia. Neuroreport 7: 2727–2731.

Kokaia Z, Othberg A, Kokaia M, et al. (1994) BDNF makes cultured dentate granule cells more resistant to hyherglycaemic damage. Neuroreport 5: 1241–1244.

Komatsumoto S, Nioka S, Greenberg JH, et al. (1987) Cerebral energy metabolism measured in vivo by ^{31}P-NMR in middle cerebral artery occlusion in the cat. Relation to severity of stroke 7: 557–562.

Komatsumoto S, Greenberg J, Hickey W et al. (1988) Effect of ganglioside GM1 on neurologic function, electroencephalogram amplitude and histology in chronic middle cerebral artery occlusion in cats. Stroke 19: 1027–1035.

Kondo Y, Ogawa N, Asanuma M, et al. (1995) Regional differences in late-onset iron deposition, ferritin, transferrin, astrocyte proliferation, and microglial activation after transeient forebrain ischemia in rat brain. J Cereb Blood Flow Metab 15: 216–226.

Kontos HA, Wei EP, Dietrich WD et al. (1981) Mechanism of cerebral arteriolar abnormalities after acute hypertension. Am J Physiol 240: H511–H527.

Kraig RP, Chesler M (1987) Glial acid-base behaviour in brain ischaemia (abstract). J Cereb Blood Flow Metab 7: suppl 1: S 126.

Kraig RP, Nicolson C (1987) Profound acidosis in presumed glia during ischaemia. In: Cerebrovascular diseases, 15th Priceton-Williamberg Conference (Raichle ME, Powers WJ eds), New York, Raven Press, pp 97–102.

Kraig RP, Pepito CK, Plum F, Pulsinelli WA (1987) Hydrogen ions kill brain at concentrations reached in ischaemia. J Cereb Blood Flow Metab 7: 379–386.

Kraig RP, Jaeger CB (1990) Ionic concomitants of astroglial transformation to reactive species. Stroke 21 (suupl III): III-184-III-187.

Krause GS, Nayini NR, White BC et al. (1987) Natural course of iron delocalization and lipid peroxidation during the first eight hours following a 15-minute cardiac arrest in dags. Ann Emerg Med 16: 1200-1205.

Kristían T, Siesjö BK (1995): Temporal profile of extracellular ion concentrations after transient middle cerebral artery occlusion in the rats. In Abstracts of 25th Annual meeting of Soc of Neuroscience Part 1, pp 216.

Kristián T, Siesjö BK (1996): Calcium related damage in ischemia. Life Science 59: 357–367.

Krumins SA, Faden AI (1984) Traumatic injury alters opiate receptor binding in rat spinal cord. Ann Neurol 19: 498–501.

Kwon J-Y, Bacher A, Zornow MH (1998): Riluzole does not attenuate increases in hippocampal glutamate concentrations in a rabbit model of repeated transient global ischemia. Anesth Analg 86: 128–133.

Kuluz JW, Prado RJ, Dietrich WD, et al. (1993) The effect of nitric oxide synthase inhibition on infarct volume after reversible focal cerebral ischemia in conscious rats. Stroke 24: 2023–2029.

Kuluz JW, Gregory GA, Han Y, et al. (1993) Fructose-1,6,-diphosphate reduces infarct volume after reversible middle cerebral artery occlusion in rats. Stroke 24: 1576–1583.

Kumon Y, Sakaki S, Kadota O, et al. (1993) Transient increase in endogenous basic fibroblast growth factor in neurons of ischemic rat brains. Brain Res 605: 169–174.

Kumon Y, Kim SC, Tompkins P, et al. (2000) Neuroprotective effect of postischemic adminsitration of progesterone in spontaneously hypertensive rats with focal cerebral ischemia. J Neurosurg 92: 848–852.

Kumura E, Kosaka H, Shiga T, et al. (1994) Elevation of plasma nitric oxide end products during focal cerebral ischemia and reperfusion in the rat. J Cereb Blood Flow Metab 14: 487–491.

Kurkeja RC, Wei EP, Kontos HA, Bates JN (1993) Nitric oxide and S-nitroso-L-cysteine as endothelium-derived relaxing factors from acetylcholine in cerebral vessels in cat. Stroke 24: 2010–2015.

Kuroda S, Katsura K, Tsuchidate R, Siesjö BK (1996a) Secondary bioenergetic failure after transient focal ischemia is due to mitochondrial injury. Acta Physiol Scand 156: 149–150.

Kuroda S. Katsura K, Hillered L, et al (1996b) Delayed treatment with α-phenyl-N-tert-butyl nitrone (PBN) attenuates secondary mitochondrial dysfunction after transient focal cerebral ischemia in the rat. Neurobiol Dis 3: 149–157.

Kuroda S, Siesjö BK (1997). Reperfusion damage following focal ischemia: Pathophysiology and therapeutic windows. Clin Neurosci 4: 199–212.

Kuroda Y, Toshima K, Watanabe T, et al. (1984) Effects of dichloroacetate on pyruvate metabolism in rat brain in vivo. Pediatr Res 18: 936–938.

Kuroiwa T, Shibutani M, Okeda R (1988): Blood-brain barrier disruption and exaxerbation of ischemic brain edema after restoration of blood flow in experimental focal cerebral ischemia. Acta Neuropathol 76: 62–70.

Kurup C, Kumaroo K, Dutka A (1990): Influence of cerebral ischemia and postischemic reperfusion on mitochondrial oxidative phosphorylation. J Bioenerget Biomembr 22: 61–78.

Kuwabara K, Matsumoto M, Ikeda J, et al. (1996) Purification and characterization of a novel stress protein the 150-kDa oxygen-regulated protein (ORP150), from cultured rat astrocytes and its expression in ischemic mouse brain. J Biol Chem 271: 5025–5032.

Kuwashima J, Fujitani B, Nakamuru K e t al (1976) Biochemical changes in unilateral brain injury in the rat: a possible role of free fatty acid accumulation. Brain Res 110: 547–557.

Kågström E, Smith M-L, Siesjö BK (1983) Recirculation in the rat brain following incomplete ischemia. J Cereb Blood Flow Metab 3: 183–192.

Kågstr¢m E, Smith M-L, Siesjö BK (1983) Local cerebral blood flow in the recovery period following complete cerebral ischemia in the rat. J Cereb Blood Flow Metab 170–182.

Lanier WL, Hofer RE, Gallagher WJ (1996) Metabolism of glucose, glycogen, and high-energy phosphates during transient forebrain ischemia in diabetic rats. Anesthesiology 84: 917–925.

Lassen NA (1959) Cerebral blood flow and oxygen consumption in man. Physiol Rev 39: 183–238.

Lassen NA, Astrup J (1987) Ischemic penumbra. In Cerebral Blood Flow, Physiologic and Clinical Aspects. Wood JH (ed). McGraw-Hill Book Company. 458–466.

Lanzino G, Kassell NF, Dorsch NW, et al. (1999) Double-blind randomized vehicle-controlled study of high-dose tirilaxad mesylate in women with aneurysmal subarachnoid hemorrhage. Part I. A cooperative study in Europe, Australia, New Zealand and South Africa. J Neurosurg 90: 1011–1017.

Lanzino G, Kassell NF (1999) Double-blind, randomized, vehicle-controlled study of high-dose tirilasat mesylate in women with anerysmal subarachnoid hemorrhage. Part II. A cooperative study in North America. J Neurosurg 90: 1018–1024.

Lawrence MS, Ho DY, Sun GH, et al. (1996) Overexpression of Bcl-2 with herpes simplex vectors protects CNS neurons against neurological insult in vitro and in vivo. J Neurosci 16: 486–496.

Lauritzen M, Hansen AJ (1992) The effect of glutamate receptor blockade on anoxic depolarization and cortical spreading depression. J Cereb Blood Flow Metab 12: 223–229.

Lee PJ, Jiang BH, Chin BY, et al. (1997) Hypoxia-inducible factor-1 mediates transcriptional activation of heme oxygenase-1 gene in response to hypoxia. J Biol Chem 272: 5375–5381.

Lee SC, Dickson DW, Liu W, Brosnan CF (1993) Induction of nitric oxide synthase activity in human astrocytes by interleukin-lb and interferon-gamma. J Neuroimmunol 46: 19–24.

Lee SH, Heros RC, Mullan JC, Korosue K (1994) Optimum degree of hemodilution for brain protection in a canine model of cerebral ischemia. J Neurosurg 80: 469–475.

Leech PJ, Miller JD, Fitch W, Barker J (1974) Cerebral blood flow, internal carotid artery prssure, and EEG as a guide to the safety of carotid ligation. J Neurol Neurosurg Psychiat 37: 854–862.

LeMay DR, Gehua L, Zelenock GB, et al. (1998) Insulin administration protects neurologic function in cerebral ischemia in rats. Stroke 19: 1411–1419.

Lenzi GL, Grigoletto F, Gent M et al. (1994) Early treatment of stroke with monosialoganglioside GM-1 Efficacy and safety results of the early stroke trial. Stroke 25: 1552–1558.

Lesiuk HJ, Sutherland GR, Peeling J, et al. (1990) The effect of U74006F on forebrain ischemia evaluated with magnetic resonance imaging and histopathology. Can J Neurol Sci 17: 228.

Lester R, Tong G, Jahr C (1993) Interaction between the glycine and glutamate binding sites of the NMDA receptor. J Neurosci 13: 1088–1096.

Levy R, Fenstel P, Severinghaus J, Hosobuchi Y (1982) Effect of naloxone on neurologic deficit and cortical blood flow during focal cerebral ischemia in cats. Life Sci 31: 2205–2208.
Leysen JE, Awouters F, Kennis L et al (1981) Receptor binding profile of R 41468, a novel antagonist at 5-HT2 receptors Life Sci 28: 1015–1022.
Li GC, Werb Z (1982) Correlation between synthesis of heat shock proteins and development of thermotolerance in Chinese hamster fibroblasts. Proc Natl Acad Sci USA 79: 3218–3222.
Li GC, Laszlo A (1985) Thermotolerance in mammalian cells: a possible role for heat shock proteins. In: Changes in Eukaryotic Gene Expression in Response to Environmental Stress, (eds) Atkinson BG, Walden DB, New York, Academic Press, pp 227–256.
Li H, Buchan AM (1993) Treatment with AMPA antagonist 12 hours following severe normothermic forebrain ischemia presvents CA1 neuronal injury. J Cereb Blood Flow Metab 15: 933–939.
Li Y, Chopp M, Garcia JH, et al. (1992) Distribution of the 72-kd heat shock protein as a function of transient focal cerebral ischemia in rats. Stroke 23: 1292–1298.
Lim KH, Connolly M, Rose D, et al. (1986) Prevention of reperfusion injury of ischemic spinal cord: use of recombinant superoxide dismutase. Ann Thorac Surg 42: 282–286.
Lin B, Dietrich WD, Ginsberg MD, et al. (1993) MK-801 (dizocilpine) protects the brain from repeated normothermic global ischemic insults in the rat. J Cereb blood Flow Metab 13: 925–932.
Lindsberg PJ, Siren AL; Feuerstein GZ, et al. (1995) Antagonism of neutrophil adherence in the deteriorating stroke model in rabbits. J Neurosurg 82: 269–277.
Lindvall O, Ernfors P, Bengzon J, et al. (1992) Differential regulation of mRNAs for nerve growth factor, brain-derived neurotrophic factor, and neurotrophin 3 in the adult rat following cerebral ischemia and hypoglycemic coma. Proc Natl Acad Sci USA 89: 648–652.
Lipton SA, Choi Y-B, Pan Z-H, et al. (1993) A redox-based mechanism for the neuroprotective and neurodestructive effects of nitric oxide and related nitroso-compounds. Nature. 364: 626–632.
Lipton SA (1997) Janus faces of NF-kappa B: Neurodestruction versus neuroprotection. Nat Med 3: 20–22.
Litt L, Gonzales-Mendez R, Severinghaus JW, et al. (1985) Cerebral intracelluar changes during supercarbia: an in vivo 31P nuclear magnetic resonance study in rats. J Cereb Blood Flow Metab 5: 537–544.
Liu T, Bechman JS, Freeman BA, et al. (1989) Polyethylene glycol-concungated superoxide dismutase and catalase reduce ischemic brain injury Am J Physiol 256: H589–H593.
Liu T, McDonnell PC, Young PR, et al. (1993) Interleukin-lb mRNA expression in ischemic rat cortex. Stroke 24: 1746–1751.
Liu T, Clark RK, McDonnell PC, et al. (1994) Tumor necrosis factor-alpha expression in ischemic neurons. Stroke 25: 1481–1488.
Liu W, Bi X, Tocco G, et al. (1996) Increased expression of cyclin D1 in the adult rat brain following kainic acid treatment. Neuro Report 7: 2785–2789.
Liu ZG, Hsu H, Goeddel DV, Karin M (1996) Dissection of TNF receptor 1 effector functions: JNK activation is not linked to apoptosis while NF-kappaB activation prevents cell death. Cell 87: 565–576.
Lo WD, Betz L, Schielke GP, Hoff JT (1987) Transport of sodium from blood to brain in ischemic brain edema. Stroke 18: 150–157.
Longstreth WT Jr. Inui TS (1984) High blood glucose level on hospital admission and poor neurological recovery after cardiac arrest. Ann Neurol 15: 59–63.
Lucignani G, Namba H, Nehlig AM et al. (1987) Effects of insulin on local cerebral glucose utilization in the rat. J Cereb Blood Flow Metab 7: 309–314.
Lukkarinen J, Grohn OHJ, Sinevirta R, et al. (1997) Transgenic rats as models for studying the role of ornithine decarboxylase expression in permanent middle cerebral artery occlusion. Stroke 28: 639–645.
Lyden PD, Hedges B (1992) Protective effect of synaptic inhibition during cerebral ischemia. Stroke 23: 1463–1470.
Lyden PD, Lonzo L (1994) Combination therapy protects ischemic brain in rats. A glutamate antagonsit plus GABA acid agonist. Stroke 25: 189–196.
Lysko PG, Yue T-L, Gu J-L, Feurstein G (1992) Neuroprotective mechanism of (+) SKF 10.047 In vitro and in gerbil global ischemia. Stroke 23: 1319–1324.
Lythgoe DJ, Little RA, O'Shaughnessy CT, Steward MC (1990) Effect of U74006F on oedema and infarct volumes following permanent occlusion of the middle cerebral artery in the rat. Br J Pharmacol 100: 454P.
Mabe H, Nagai H, Takagi T, et al. (1986) Effect of nimodipine on cerebral functional and metabolic recovery following ischemia in the rat brain. Stroke 17: 501–505.
Mabe H, Nagai H, Suzuka T (1990) Role of brain leukotriene in brain oedema following cerebral ischemia: effect of 5-lipoxygenases inhibitor, AA-861. Neurol Res 12: 165–168.
MacManus JP, Linnil MD (1997) Gene expression induced by cerebral ischemia: An apoptotic perspective. J Cereb Blood Flow Metab 17: 815–832.
MacMillan V (1989) Influence of lactate accumulation on calcium content of ischemic and postischemic brain. J Cereb Blood Flow Metab 9: 640–645.
Macrae IM, Dawson DA; Norrie JD, McCulloch J (1993) Inhibition of nitric oxide synthesis: Effect on cerebral blood flow and glucose utilization in the rat. J Cereb Blood Flow Metab 13: 985–992.
Maiese K, Boccone L (1995) Neuroprotection by peptide growth factors against anoxia and nitric oxide toxicity requires modulation of protein kinase C. J Cereb Blood Flow Metab 15: 440–449.
Mailliot C, Podevin-Dimster V, Rosenthal RE, et al. (2000) Rapid tau protein dephosphorylation and differential rephosphorylation during cardiac arrest-induced cerebral ischemia and reperfusion. J Cereb Blood Flow Metab 20: 543–549.
Malanski T, Bailey F, Zhang ZG, Chopp M (1993) Nitric oxide measured by a prophyrinic nicrosensor in rat brain after transient middle cerebral artery occlusion. J Cereb Blood Flow Metab 13: 355–358.
Malgouris C, Bardot F, Daniel M, et al. (1989): Rilizole, a novel antiglutamate, prevents memory loss and hippocampal neuronal damage in ischemic gerbils. J Neurosci 9: 3720–3727.
Manzoni O, Prezeau L, Marin P, et al. (1992) Nitric oxide-induced blockade of NMDA receptors. Neuron 8: 654–662.
Marinov M, Harbaugh KS, Hoopes PJ, et al. (1996) Neuroprotective effects of preischemic intraarterial magnesium sulfate in reversible focal cerebral ischemia. J Neurosurg 85: 117–124.

Matsumoto K, Yamada K, Kohmura E, et al. (1994) Role of pyruvate in schemia-like conditions on cultured neurons. Neurol Res 16: 460–464.

McPherson RW, Kirsch JR, Traystman RJ (1994) Inhibition of nitric oide synthase does not affect α_2-adrenergic-mediated cerebral vasoconstriction. Anesth Analg 78: 67–72.

Marchal G, Beaudouin V, Rioux P, et al. (1996) Prolonged persistence of substantial volumes of potentially brain tissue after stroke. A correlation PET-CT study with voxel-based data analysis. Stroke 27: 599–606.

Marchetti P, Susin SA, Decaudin D, et al. (1996) Apoptosis-associated derangment of mitochondrial function in cells lacking mitochondrial DNA. Cancer Res 56: 2033–2038.

Marcoux FW, Morawetz RB, Crowell RM, et al. (1982) Differential regional vulnerability in transient focal cerebral ischaemia. Stroke 13: 339–346.

Margaill I, Parmentier S, Callebert J, et al. (1996): Short therapeutic window for MK-801 in transient focal cerebral ischemia in normotensive rats. J Cereb Blood Flow Metab 16: 107–113.

Margolis R, Altszuler N (1967) Insulin in the cerebrospinal fluid. Nature 215: 1275–1276.

Marinov M, Wassmann H, Natschev S (1991) Effect of nimodipine in treatment of experimental focal cerebral ischemia. Neurological Research 13: 77–83.

Marion DW, Obrist WD, Carlier PM, et al. (1993) The use of moderate therapeutic hypothermia for patients with severe head injuries: a preliminary report. J Neurosurg 79: 354–362.

Marletta MA (1993) Nitric oxide synthase structure and mechanism. J Biol Chem 268: 12231–12234.

Marsala M, Vanicky I, Yaksh TL (1994) Effect of graded hypothermia (27 to 34C) on behavioral function, histopathology, and spinal blood flow after spinal ischemia in rat. Stroke 25: 2038–2046.

Marshall LF, Maas AI, Marshall SB, et al. (1998) A multicentre trial on the efficacy of using tirilazad mesylate in cases of head injury. J Neurosurg 89: 519–525.

Martin D, Thompson MA, Nadler JV (1993): The neuroprotective agent riluzole inhibits the release og glutamate and aspartate from slices of hippocampus are CA1. Eur J Pharmacol 250: 473–476.

Masaki T, Vane J, Vanhoutte PM (1994) International Union of Pharmacology nomenclature of endothelin receptors. Pharmacol Rev 46: 137–142.

Massa SM, Swanson RA, Sharp FR (1996) The stress gene response in brain. Cerebrovasc Brain Metab Rev 8: 95–158.

Mathiesen T, Andersson B, Loftenius A, et al. (1993) Increased interleukin-6 levels in cerebrospinal fluid following subarachnoid hemorrhage. J Neurosurg 78: 562–567.

Matsumoto K, Lo, E, Pierce A, et al. (1996): Secondary elevation of extracellular neurotransmitter aminoacids in the reperfusion phase following focal cerebral ischemia. J Cereb Blood Flow Metab 16: 114–124.

Matsuo Y, Onodera H, Shiga Y et al. (1994): Correlation between myeloperoxidase-quantified neutrophil accumulation and ischemic brain injury in the rat. Effects of neutrophil depletion. Stroke 25: 1469–1475.

Matsuo Y, Onodera H, Shiga Y et al (1994): Role of cell afhesion molecules in brain injury after transient middle cerebral artery occlusion in the rat. Brain Res 656: 344–352.

Matsuo Y, Kihara T, Ikeda M, et al. (1995): Role of neutrophils in radical production during ischemia and reperfusion of the rat brain: Effect of neutrophil depletion on extracellular ascorbyl radical formation. J Cereb Blood Flow Metab 15: 941–947.

Mayer SA, Pulsinelli WA (1992) Failure of GM1 ganglioside to influence outcome in experimental focal ischemia. Stroke 23: 242–246.

McBurney RN, Neering IR (1987) Neuronal calcium homeostasis. Trends Neurosci 10: 164–169.

McCalden TA, Nath RG, Thiele K (1984) The effect of a calcium antagonist (nimodipine) on basal cerebral blood flow and reactivity to various agonist. Stroke 15: 527–530.

McConkey DJ, Orrenius S (1996) Signal transduction pathways in apoptosis. Stem Cells 14: 619–631.

McCullough LD, Alkayed NJ, Traystman RJ, et al. (2001) Postischemic estrogen reduces hypoperfusion and secondary ischemia after experimental stroke. Stroke 32: 796–802.

Mchedlishvili G, Mossakowski M, Itkis M, Januszewski SS (1984) Cerebral blood volume changes during the development of brain edema. In: Go KG, Baethmann A (eds): Recent Progress in the Study and Therapy of Brain Edema. Plenum Press, pp 137–150.

McIntosh TK, Vink R, Yanakami I Faden AI (1989) Magnesium protects against neurological deficit after brain injury. Brain Res 482: 252–260.

McIntosh TK (1993) Novel pharmacologic therapies in the treatment of experimental traumatic brain injury. Br J Anaesth 78: 520–523.

McKay RD, Sundt TM, Michenfelder JD, et la. (1976) Internal carotid artery stump pressure and cerebral blood flow during carotid endarterectomy: Modification by halothane, enflurane, and innovar. Anesthesiology 45: 390–399.

McNamara J, Fridovich I (1993): Did radicals strike Lou Gehrig? Nature 362: 20–21.

Memezawa H, Smith ML, Siesjö BK (1992) Penumbra tissue salvaged by reperfusion following middle cerebral artery occlusion in rats. Stroke 23: 552–559.

Memezawa H, Zhao Q, Smith M, Siesjö BK (1995): Hyperthermia nullifies the ameliorating effect of dizocilpine maleate (MK-801) in focal cerebral ischemia. Brain res 670: 48–52.

Mendelow AD, Graham DI, McCulloch J, Mohamed AA (1984) The distribution of ischemic damage and cerebral blood flow after unilateral carotid occlusion and hypotension in the rat. Stroke 15: 704–710.

Meno JR, Ngai AC, Ibayashi S, Winn HR (1991) Adenosine release and changes in pial arteriolar diameter during transient cerebral ischemia and reperfusion. J Cereb Blood Flow Metab 11: 986–993.

Merrill JE, Agnarro LJ, Sherman MP, Melinek J, Lane TE (1993) Microglial cell cytotoxicity of oligodendrocytes is mediated through nitric oxide. J Immunol 151: 2132–2141.

Messick JM, Casement B, Sharbrough FW, et al. (1987) Correlation of regional cerebral blood flow (rCBF) with EEG changes during isoflurane anesthesia for carotid endarterectomy: Critical rCBF. Anesthesiology 66: 344–349.

Meyer FB, Andersson RE, Sundt TM Jr (1990) The novel dihydronaphthyridine Ca^{2+} channel blocker CI-951 improves CBF, brain-pH_i, and EEG recovery in focal cerebral ischemia. J Cereb Blood Flow Metab 10: 97–103.

Mezies SA, Betz AL, Hoff JT (1993) Contribution of ions and albumin to the formation and resolution of ischemic brain edema. J Neurosurg 78: 257–266.

Michenfelder JD, Milde JH (1987) Nimodipine does not affect cerebral lactate levels following complete ischemia in dogs. J Cereb Blood Flow Metab 7: 619–624.

Michenfelder JD, Milde JA (1990) Postischemic canine cerebral blood flow appears to be determined by cerebral metabolic needs J Cereb Blood Flow Metab 10: 71–76.

Michenfelder JD, Milde JH (1991) The relationship among canine brain temperature, metabolism, and function during hypothermia. Anesthesiology 75: 130–136.

Mies G, Koiber O, Drewes LR, Hossmann K-A (1984) Cerebral blood flow and regional potassium distribution during focal ischaemia of gerbil brain. Ann Neurol 16: 232–237.

Mies G, Ishimaru S, Xie Y, Seo K, Hossmann K-A (1991) Ischemic thresholds of cerebral protein synthesis and energy state following middle cerebral artery occlusion in rat. J Cereb Blood Flow Metab 11: 753–761.

Mies G, Kohno K, Hossmann K-A (1994) Prevention of periinfarct direct current shifts with glutamate antagonist NBQX following occlusion of the middle cerebral artery in the rat. J Cereb Blood Flow Metab 14: 802–807.

Minamisawa H, Terashi A, Katayama Y, et al. (1988) Brain eicosanoid levels in spontaneously hypertensive rats after ischemia with reperfusion: leukotriene C_4 as a possible cause of cerebral edema. Stroke 19: 372–377.

Minn AJ, Velez P, Schendel SL, et al. (1997) Bcl-x(l) forms an ion channel in synthetic lipid membranes. Nature 385: 353–357.

Mitani A, Katoka K (1991) Critical levels of extracellular glutamate mediating gerbil hippocampal delayed neuronal death during hypothermia: Brain microdialysis study. Neuroscience 42: 661–670.

Mitchell H, Frisella WA, Brooker RW, Yoon K-W. (1995) Attenuation of traumatic cell death by an adenosine A_1 agonist in rat hippocampal cells. Neurosurgery 36: 1003–1008.

Miyashite K, Nakajima T, Ishikawa A, Miyatake T (1992) An adenosine uptake blocker, propentofylline, reduces glutamate release in gerbil hippocampus following transient forebrain ischemia. Neurochem Res 17: 147–150.

Milde LN, Milde JH, Michenfelder JD (1986) Delayed treatment with nimodipine improves cerebral blood flow after complete cerebral ischemia in the dog. J Cereb Blood Flow Metab 6: 332–337.

Miller RJ (1988) Ca^{2+} channels, excitatory amino acids and cerebral ischemia. In Pharmacology of Cerebral Ischemia (Krieglstein J, ed), Orlando, CRC Press, pp 139–149.

Mohamed AA, McCulloch J, Mendelow AD, et al. (1984) Effect of the calcium antagonist nimodipine on local cerebral blood flow: Relationship to arterial blood pressure. J Cereb Blood Flow Metab 4: 206–211.

Mohamed AA, Gotoh O, Graham DI, et al. (1985) Effect of pretreatment with the calcium antagonist nimodopine on local cerebral blood flow and histopathology after middle cerebral artery occlusion. Ann Neurol 18: 705–711.

Mollace V, Colasanti M, Persichine T, et al. (1993) HIV gp 120 glycoprotein stimulates the inducible isoform of NO synthase in human cultured astrocytoma cells. Biochem Biophys Res Commun 194: 439–445.

Moncada C, Lekieffre D, Arvin B, Meldrum B (1992) Effect of NO synthase inhibition on NMDA- and ischemic-induced hippocampal lesions. Neuroport 3: 530–532.

Moncada S, Palmer RMJ, Higgs EA (1991) Nitric Oxide: physiology, pathophysiology, and pharmacology. Pharmacol Rev 43: 109–142.

Morawetz RB, Marcoux FW, Crowell RM, et al. (1979) Identical thresholds for cerebral ischaemia in white and grey matter. Acta Neurol Scand 60: suppl 72: 282–283.

Mori E, del Zoppo GJ, Chambers JD, et al. (1992) Inhibition of polymorphonuclear leukocyte adherence suppresses noreflow after focal cerebral ischemia in baboons. Stroke 23: 712–718.

Mori E. (1993) Safety and efficacy of fibrinolytic agents in acute ischemic stroke. Cerebrovasc Dis 3: 264–268.

Morikawa E, Rosenblatt S, Moskowitz MA (1992) L-arginine dilates rat pial arterioles by nitric oxide-dependent mechanisms and increases blood flow during focal cerebral ischemia. Br J Pharmacol 107: 905–907.

Morikawa E, Moskowitz MA, Huang Z, Yoshida T, Irikura K, Dalkara T (1994) L-arginine infusion promotes nitric oxide-dependent vasodilation, increases regional cerebral blood flow, and reduces infarction volume in the rat. Stroke 25: 429–435.

Morimoto T, Globus M-T, Busto R, et al. (1996): Simultaneous measurement of salicylate hydroxylation and glutamate release in the penumbral cortex following transient middle cerebral artery occlusion in rats. J Cereb Blood Flow Metab 16: 92–99.

Morita-Tsuzuki Y, Hardebo JE, Bouskela E (1993) Inhibition of nitric oxide synthase attenuates the cerebral blood flow response to stimulation of postganglionic parasympathetic nerves in the rat. J Cereb Blood Flow Metab 13: 993–997.

Morrison RS, Wenzel HJ, Kinoshita Y, et al. (1996) Loss of the p53 tumor suppressor gene protects neurons from kainic-induced celle death. J Neurosci 16: 1337–1345.

Muchmore SW, Sattler M, Liang H, et al. (1996) X-ray and NMR structure of human Bcl-2-xL, an inhibitor of programmed cell. Nature 381: 335–341.

Muhonen MG, Heistad DD, Faraci FM, Loftus CM (1994) Augmentation of blood flow through cerebral collaterals by inhibition of nitric oxide synthase. J Cereb Blood Flow Metab. 14: 704–714.

Müllner M, Sterz F, Binder M, et al. (1997) Blood glucose concentration after cardiopulmonary resuscitation influences functional neurological recovery in human cardiac arrest survivors. J Cereb Blood Flow Metab 17: 430–436.

Murphy AN, Bredesen DE, Cortopassi G, et al. (1996) Bcl-2 potentiates the maximal calcium uptake capacity of neural cell mitochondria. Proc Natl Acad Sci USA 93: 9893–9898.

Murphy S, Rich G, Orgren KI, et al. (1994) Astrocyte-derived lipoxygenase product evokes endothelium-dependent relaxation of the basilar artery. J Neurosci Res 38: 314–318.

Muszynski CA, Robertson CS, Goodman JC, Henley CM (1993) DFMO reduces cortical infarct volume after middle cerebral artery occlusion in the rat. J Cereb Blood Flow Metab 13: 1033–1037.

Mutch WAC, Hansen AJ (1984) Extracellular pH changes during spreading depression and cerebral ischemia: Mechanisms of brain pH regulation. J Cereb Blood Flow Metab 4: 17–27.

Myers RE, Yamaguchi S (1977) Nervous system effects of cardiac arrest in monkeys. Arch Neurol 34: 65–74.

Myers RE (1979) Lactic acid accumulation as a cause of brain edema and cerebral necrosis resulting from oxygen deprivation. In: Korobkin R, Guilleliault (eds): Advances in Perinatal Neurology. Jamaica, N. Y. Spectrum 1, pp 85–114.

Myers RE, Kleinholz M, Wagner KR, de Couten-Myers GM (1990) Effects of experimental aminosteroid on outcome of cerebrovascular occlusion in cats. Stroke 21: 179.

Nagafuji T, Matsui T, Koide T, Asano T (1992) Blockade of nitric oxide formation by N-nitro-L-arginine mitigates is-

chemic brain edema, and subsequent cerebral infarction in rats. Neurosci Lett 147: 159–162.
Nahorski SR (1988) Inositol polyphosphates and neuronal calcium hemostasis. Trends Neurosci 11: 444–448.
Nakagomi T, Asai A, Kanemitsu H, et al. (1996) Up-regulation of c-myc gene expression following focal ischemia in the rat brain. Neurol Res 18: 599–563.
Nakahara I, Kikuchi H, Taki W, et al. (1992): Changes in major phospholipids of mitochondria during postischemic reperfusion in rat brain. J Neurosurg 76: 244–250.
Nakai H, Yamamoto YL, Diksic M, et al. (1988) Tripple-tracer autoradiography demonstrates effects of hyperglycemia on cerebral blood flow, pH, and glucose utilization in cerebral ischemia of rats. Stroke 19: 764–772.
Nakamura S, Sakaguchi T, Kimura F, Aoki F (1988) The rose of α-adrenoceptor-mediated collateral excitation in the regulation of the electrical activity of locus coeruleus neurons. Neuroscience 27: 921–929.
Nakashima M, Yamashita K, Kataoka Y, et al. (1995): Time course of nitric oxide synthase activity in neuronal, glial, and endothelial cells of rat striatum following focal cerebral ischemia. Cell Mol Neurobiol 15: 341–349.
Naritomi H, Sasaki M, Kanashiro M, et al. (1988) Flow thresholds for cerebral energy disturbance and Na^+ pump failure as studied by *in vivo* ^{31}P and ^{23}Na nuclear magnetic resonance spectroscopy. J Cereb Blood Flow Metab 8: 16–23.
Natale JE, Schott RJ, Hall ED, et al. (1988) The 21-aminosteroid U74006F reduces systemic lipid peroxidation, improves neurological function, and reduces mortality after cardiopulmonary arrest in dogs. Stroke 19: 1371–1378.
Nedergaard M, Astrup J (1986) Infarct rim: Effect of hyperglycemia on direct current potential and [^{14}C]2-deoxyglucose phosphorylation. J Cereb Blood Flow Metab 6: 607–615.
Nedergaard M, Gjedde A, Diemer NH (1986) Focal cerebral ischaemia of the rat brain: Autoradiographic determination of cerebral glucose utilization, glucose content and blood flow. J Cereb Blood Flow Metab 6: 414–424.
Nedergaard M, Diemer NH (1987) Focal ischaemia of the rat brain, with special reference to the influence of plasma glucose concentration. Acta Neuropath (Berl). 73: 131–137.
Nedergaard M (1988) Mechanisms of brain damage in focal cerebral ischaemia. Acta Neurol Scand 77: 1–24.
Nedergaard M, Jakobsen J, Diemer NH (1988) Autoradiographic determination of cerebral glucose content, blood flow, and glucose utilization in focal ischaemia of the rat brain: Influence of the plasma glucose concentration. J Cereb Blood Flow Metab 8: 100–108.
Nedergaard M, Hansen AJ (1993) Characterization of cortical depolarizations evoked in focal cerebral ischemia. J Cereb Blood Flow Metab 13: 568–574.
Nehls DG, Gaines C, Robert M (1983) Effect of naloxone in the treatment of experimental stroke in awake monkeys. Stroke 14: 123.
Nellgard B, Wieloch T (1992) Postischemic blockade of AMPA but not NMDA reseptors mitigates neuronal damage in the rat brain following transient severe cerebral ischemia. J Cereb Blood Flow Metab 12: 2–11.
Nemoto EM, Snyder JV, Carroll RG, Morita H (1975) Global ischemia in dogs: cerebrovascular CO_2 reactivity and autoregulation. Stroke 6: 425–431.
Nishikawa T, Kirsch JR, Koehler RC, et al. (1993) Effect of nitric oxide synthase inhibition on cerebral blood flow and injury volume during focal ischemia in cats. Stroke 24: 1717–1724.
Nishimoto K, Kakari S, Pappius HM, et al. (1979) Behavior of the blood-brain barrier (BBB) in cerebral ischemia. In: Mrsulja BB, Rokio LM, Klatzo I, Spatz M (eds): Pathophysiology of Cerebral Energy Metabolism. New York, Plenum Press, pp 99–108.
Nishimura H, Rosenblum WI, Nelson GH, Boynton S (1991) Agents that modify EDRF formation after antiplatelet properties of brain arteriolar endothelium *in vivo*. Am J Phys 261: H15-H21.
Nordström C-H, Rehncrona S, Siesjö BK (1976) Restitution of cerebral energy state after complete and incomplete ischemia of 30 min duration. Acta Physiol Scand 97: 270–272.
Nordström C-H, Rehncrona S (1977) Postischaemic cerebral blood flow and oxygen utilization rate in rats anaesthetized with nitrous oxide or phenobarbital. Acta Physiol Scand 101: 230–240.
Nordström C-H, Rehncrona S, Siesjö BK (1978) Effect of phenobarbitone in cerebral ischaemia. Part II: Restitution of cerebral energy state, as well as of glycolytic metabolites, citric acid cycle intermediates and associated aminoacids after pronounced incomplete ischemia. Stroke 9: 335–343.
Norenberg MD, Martinez-Hernandez A (1979) Fine structural localization of glutamine synthetase in astrocyte of rat brain. Brain Res 161: 303–310.
Northington FJ, Matherne GP, Berne RM (1992) Competitive inhibition of nitric oxide synthase prevents the cortical hyperemia associated with peripheral nerve stimulation. Proc Natl Acad Sci USA 89: 6649–6652.
Nowak L, Bregestovski P, Ascher P, et al. (1984) Magnesium gates glutamine-activated channels in mouse central neurons. Nature 307: 462–465.
Nowak TS Jr (1989) MK-801 prevents 70 kDa stress protein induction in gerbil brain after ischemia: The heat shock response as a marker for excitotoxic pathology. In Pharmacology of Cerebral Ischemia . Proceedings of the Second International Symposium on the Pharmacology of Cerebral Ischemia (Krieglstein J ed), Boca Raton, CRC Press, pp 229–234.
Nowak TS (1991) Localization of 70 kDa stress protein mRNA induction in gerbil brain after ischemia. J Cereb Blood Flow Metab 11: 432–439.
Ogilvy CS, Chu D, Kaplan S (1996) Mild hypothermia, hypertension, and mannitol are protective against infarction during experimental intracranial temporary vessel occlusion. Neurosurgery 38: 1202–1210.
Ohman J, Heiskanen O (1988) Effect of nimodipine on the outcome of patients after aneurysmal subarachnoid hemorrhage and surgery. J Neurosurg 69: 683–686.
Ohnishi T, Posner JB, Shapiro WR (1992) Vasogenic brain edema induced by arachidonic acid: Role of extracellular arachidonic acid in blood-brain barrier dysfunction. Neurosurgery 30: 545–551.
Ohta T, Kikuchi H, Hashi K (1986) Nizofenone administration in the acute stage following subarachnoid hemorrhage. J Neurosurg 64: 420–426.
Oishi R, Baba M, Nishibori M, et al. (1989) Involvement of central histaminergic and cholinergic systems in the morphine-induced increase in blood-brain barrier permeability to sodium fluorscein in mice. Naunyn Schmiedegergs Arch Pharmacol 339: 159–165.
Okada Y Shima T, Yamamoto M, Uozumi J (1983) Regional cerebral blood flow, sensory evoked potentials, and intrac-

ranial pressure in dogs with MCA occlusion by embolization or trapping. J Neurosurg 58: 500-507.
Okada Y, Copeland B, Mori E, et al. (1994): P-selectin and intracellular adhesion molecule-1 expression after focal brain ischemia and reperfusion. Stroke 25: 202-211.
Okusawa S, Gelfand JA, Ikejima T, et al. (1998) Interleukin 1 induces a shock-like state in rabbits. Synergism with tumor necrosis factor and the effect of cyclooxygenase inhibition. J Clin Invest 81: 1162-1172.
Oliver C, Starke-Reed P, Stadtman E, et al (1990) Oxidative damage to brain proteins, loss of glutamine synthetase activity, and production of free radicals during ischemia/reperfusion-induced injury to gerbil brain. Proc Natl Acad Sci USA 87: 5144-5147.
Ott L, McClain CJ, Gillespie M, et al. (1994) Cytokines and metabolic dysfunction after severe head injury. J Neurotrauma 11: 447-472.
Oyama H, Suzuki Y, Satoh S, et al. (1993) Role of nitric oxide in the cerebral vasodilatory responses to vasopressin and oxytocin in dogs. J Cereb Blood Flow Metab 13: 285-290.
Ozyurt E, Graham DI, Woodruff GN, McCulloch J (1988) Protective effect of the glutamate antagonist, MK-801 in focal cerebral ischemia in the cat. J Cereb Blood Flow Metab 8: 138-143.
Pacold ST, Blackard WG (1979) Central nervous system insulin receptors in normal and diabetic rats. Endocrinology 105: 1252-1457.
Palovcik RA, Phillips MI, Kappy MS, Raizada MK (1984) Insulin inhibits pyramidal neurons in hippocampal slices. Brain Res 309: 187-191.
Papadopoulos MC, Giffard RG, Bell BA (2000) An introduction on the changes in gene expression that occur after cerebral ischaemia. Br J Neurosurg 14: 305-313.
Papagapiou MP, Auer RN (1990) Regional neuroprotective effects of the NMDA receptor antagonist MK-801 (dizocilpine) in hypoglycemic brain damage. J Cereb Blood Flow Metab 10: 270-276.
Pappata S, Fiorelli M, Rommel T, et al. (1993) PET study of changes in local brain hemodynamics and oxygen metabolism after unilateral middle cerebral artery occlusion in baboons. J Cereb Blood Flow Metab 13: 416-424.
Pappius HM, Dadoun R (1986) Biogenic amines in injured brain. Trans Am Soc Neurochem 17: 298.
Pappius HM, Dadoun R (1987) Effect of injury on the indoleamines in cerebral cortex. J Neurochem 49: 321-325.
Pappius HM, Dadoun R, McHugh M (1988) The effect of p-chlorophenylalanine on cerebral metabolism and biogenic amine content of traumatized brain. J Cereb Blood Flow Metab 8: 324-344.
Park CK, McCullocj J, Lang JK, Choi CR (1993) Effect of respiratory depression on cytoprotective effect of the competitive NMDA antagonist D-CPPene. In Intracranial Pressure VIII (eds) Avezaat CJJ, van Eijndhoven JHM, Maas AIR, Tans JThJ, Springer Verlag 162-166.
Park TS, van Wylen DGL, Rubio R, Berne RM (1987) Increased brain interstitiel fluid adenosine concentration during hypoxia in newborn piglet, J Cereb Blood Flow Metab 7: 178-183.
Patt A, Horesh IR, Berger EM, et al. (1990) Iron depletion or chelation reduces ischemic/reperfusion-induced edema in gerbil brain. J Pediatr Surg 25: 224-228.
Patel PM, Drummond JC, Mitchell MD, et al. (1992) Eicosanoid production in the caudate nucleus and dorsal hippocampus after forebrain ischemia: A microdialysis study. J Cereb Blood Flow Metab 12: 88-95.
Patel TR, McCulloch J (1996) Failure of an endothelin antagonist to modify hypoperfusion after transient global ischaemia in the rat. Cereb Blood Flow Metab 16: 490-499.
Patel TR, Galbraith S, McAuley MA, McCulloch J (1996a) Endothelin-mediated vascular tone following cerebral sichemia in the cat. J Cereb Blood Flow Metab 16: 679-687.
Patel TR, Galbraith S, Graham DI, et al. (1996b) Endothelin receptor antagonist increases cerebral perfusion and reduces ischemic damage in feline focal cerebral ischemia. J Cereb Blood Flow Metab 16: 950-958.
Penning DH, Chestnut DH, Dexter F, et al. (1995) Glutamate release from the ovine fetal brain during maternal hemorrhage. Anesthesiology 82: 521-530.
Pepito CK (1986) Transformation of postischemic perineuronal glial cells. I. Electron microscopic studies. J Cereb Blood Flow Metab 6: 616-624.
Pepito CK, Kraig RP, Pulsinelli WA (1987) Light and electromicroscopy evaluation of hydrogen ion-induced brain necrosis. J Cereb Blood Flow Metab 7: 625-632.
Pérez-Pinzón MA, Lutz PL, Sick TJ, Rosenthal M (1993) Adenosine a retaliatory" metabolite, promotes anoxia tolerance in turtle brain. J Cereb Blood Flow Metab 13: 728-732.
Perkins WJ, Milde LN, Milde JH, Michenfelder JD (1989) Effect of a 21-aminosteroid oxygen radical scavenger on neurological outcome following complete cerebral ischemia in dogs. J Cereb Blood Flow Metab 9 (suppl 1): S562.
Petroni A, Bertazzo A, Sarti S et al. (1989) Accumulation of arachidonic acid cyclo- and lipoxygenase products in rat brain during ischemia and reperfusion: effect of treatment with GM1-lactone. J Neurochem 53: 747-752.
Petruk KC, Weir BKA, et al. (1988) Nimodipine treatment in poor-grade aneurysm patients. J Neurosurg 68: 505-517.
Philippon J, Grob R, Agreou F, et al. (1986) Prevention of vasospasm in subarachnoid hemorrhage. A controlled study with nimodipine. Acta Neurochir 82: 110-114.
Phillis JW, Kostopoulos GK, Limacher JJ (1975) A potent depressant action of adenine derivates on cerebral cortical neurones. Eur J Pharmacol 30: 125-129.
Phillis JW, Walter GA, O'Regan MH, Stair RE (1987) Increases in cerebral cortical perfusate adenosine and inosine concentrations during hypoxia and ischemia. J Cereb Blood Flow Metab 7: 679-686.
Phillis JW, Clough-Helfman (1990) Protection from cerebral ischemic injury in gerbils with the spin trap agent N-tret-bubyl-α-phenylnitrone (PBN). Neurosci Letters 116: 315-319.
Piantadosi C, Zhang J, (1996): Mitochondrial generation after brain ischemia in the rat. Stroke 27: 327-332.
Pichard JD, MacKenzie ET (1973) Inhibition of prostaglandin synthesis and the response of baboon cerebral circulation to carbon dioxide. Nature New Biol 245: 187-188.
Pickard JD, Murray GD, Illingworth R, et al. (1989) Effect of oral nimodipine on cerebral infarction and outcome after subarachnoid hemorrhage: British aneurysm nimodipine trial. Br Med J 298: 636-642.
Pietronigro DD, Hovsepian M, Demopoulos HB, Flamm ES (1983) Effect of naloxone on ascorbic acid loss from ischemic cerebral cortex. Stroke 14: 123.
Piper RD, Lambert GA, Duckworth JW (1991) Cortical blood flow changes during spreading depression in cats. Am J Physiol 261: H96-H102.

Plesnila N, Ringel F, Chang RCC et al. (1998) Relevance of Calcium homeostasis in glial cell swelling from acidosis. Acta Neurochir (suppl) 71: 203–205.

Pluta R, Tomida S, Ikeda J, et al. (1989) Cerebral vascular volume after repeated ischemic insults in the gerbil: Comparison with changes in CBF and brain edema. J Cereb Blood Flow Metab 9: 163–170.

Popovic R, Liniger R, Bickler PE, (2000) Anesthetic and mild hypothermia semilarly prevent hippocampal neuron death in an *in vitro* model of cerebral ischemia. Anesthesiology 92: 1343–1349.

Pou S, Pou WS, Bredt DS, et al. (1992) Generation of superoxide by purified brain nitric oxide synthase. J Biol Chem 267: 24173–14176.

Prado R, Ginsberg MD, Dietrich WD, et al. (1988) Hyperglycemia increases infarct size in collaterally perfused but not end-arterial vascular territories. J Cereb Blood Flow Metab 8: 186–192.

Pratt J, Rataud J, Bardot F, et al. (1992): Neuroprotective actions of rilizole in rodent models of global and focal cerebral ischemia. Neurosci Lett 140: 225–230.

Prehn JHM, Karkoutly C, Nuglisch J, et al. (1992) Dihydrolipoate reduces neuronal injury after cerebral ischemia. J Cereb Blood Flow Metab 12: 78–87.

Presta M, Tiberio L, Rusnati M, et al. (1991) Basic fibroblast growth factor requires a long-lasting activation of protein kinase C to induce cell proliferation in transformed fetal bovine aortic endothelial cells. Cell Regul 2: 719–726.

Pulsinelli Wa, Levy DE, Duffy TE (1982) Regional cerebral blood flow and glucose metabolism following transient forebrain ischaemia. Ann Neurol 11: 499–509.

Pulsinelli WA, Bierley IB, Plum F (1982) Temporal profile of neuronal danage in a model of transient forebrain ischaemia. Ann Neurol 11: 491–498.

Pulsinelli WA, French J, Rawlinson D, Plum F (1982) Cerebral ischaemia damages neurons despite lowered brain lactate levels. Ann Neurol 12: 86–92.

Pulsinelli WA, Kraig RP, Plum F (1985) Hyperglycemia, cerebral acidosis, and ischemic brain damage. In: Cerebrovascular Diseases (Plum F, Pulsinelli WA, eds). New York, Raven Press, pp 201–210.

Radi R, Rodriquez M, Castro L, Telleri R (1994): Inhibition of mitochondrial function in the rat after complete and incomplete cerebral ischemia. Stroke 10: 437–446.

Radomski NW, Palmer RM, Moncada S (1991) Modulation of platelet aggregation by an L-arginine-nitric oxide pathway. Trends Pharmacol Sci 12: 87–88.

Raffin CN, Harrison M, Sick TJ, Rosenthal M (1991) EEG suppression and anoxic depolarization: Influences on cerebral oxygenation during ischemia. J Cereb Blood Flow Metab 11: 407–415.

Ramirez-Lessepas M, Patrick BK, et al. (1986) Failure of central nervous system serotonin blockage to influence outcome in acute cerebral infarction. A double blind randomized trial. Stroke 17: 953–961.

The RANTTAS investigators (1996) A randomized trial of tirilazad mesylate in patients with acute stroke (RANTTAS). Stroke 27: 1453–1458.

The RANTTAS II investogators (1998) High dose tirilaxad for acute stroke (RANTTAS II). Stroke 29: 1256–1257.

Rao L, Perez D, White E, (1996) Lamin proteolysis facilitates nuclear events during apoptosis. J Cell Biol 135: 1441–1455.

Rao VL, Dogan A, Todd KG, et al. (2001) Antisense knockdown of the glial glutamate transporter GLT-1, but not the neuronal glutamate transporter EAAC1, exacerbates transient focal cerebral ischemia-induced neuronal damage in rat brain. J Neurosci 15: 1876–1883.

Raynaud C, Rancurel G, Samsom Y, et al. (1987) Pathophysiologic study of chronic infarcts with I-123 Isopropyl Iodo-Amphetamine (IMP): The importance of periinfarct area. Stroke 18: 21–29.

Reasoner DK, Ryu KH, Hindman BJ, et al. (1996) Marked hemodilution increases neurologic injury after focal cerebral ischemia in rabbits. Anesth Analg 82: 61–67.

Rehncrone S, Rosen I, Siesjö BK (1981) Brain lactic acidosis and ischemic cell damage: 1. Biochemistry and neurophysiology. J Cereb Blood Flow Metab 1: 297–311.

Rehncrona S, Westerberg E, Akesson B, Siesjö BK (1982) Brain cortical fatty acids and phospholipids during and following complete and severe incomplete ischemia. J Neurochem 38: 84–93.

Relton J, Rothwell N. (1992): Interleukin-1 receptor antagonist inhibits ischemic and excitatoxic neuronal damage in the rat. Brain Res Bull 29: 243–246.

Rengasamy A, Johns RA (1993) Regulation of nitric oxide synthase by nitric oxide. Mol Pharmacol 44: 124–128.

Resnick DK, Marion DW, Darby JM (1994) The effect of hypothermia on the incidence of delayed traumatic intracerebral hemorrhage. Neurosurgery 34: 252–256.

Reynolds J, Hastings T (1995): Glutamate induces the production of reactive oxygen species in cultured forebrain neurons following NMDA receptor activation. J Neurosci 15: 3318–3327.

Riabowol KL, Mizzen LA, Welch WJ (1988) Heat shock is lethal to fibroblasts microinjected with antibodies against hsp 70. Science 242: 433–436.

Richter C, Gogvadze V, Schlapbach R, et al. (1994): Nitric oxide kills hepatocytes by mobilizing mitochondrial Calcium. Biochem Biophys Res Commun 205: 1143–1150.

Richter C, Gogvadze V, Laffranchi R, et al. (1995): Oxidants in mitochondria: from physiology to diseases. Biochem Biophys Acta 1271: 67–74.

Rieckmann P, Nunke K, Burchhardt M et al. (1993) Soluble intercellular adhesion molecule-1 in cerebrospinal fluid: An indicator for the inflammatory impairment of the blood-cerebrospinal fluid barrier. J Neuroimmunology 47: 133–140.

Rischke R, Krieglstein J (1989) Postischemic neuronal damage causes astroglial activation and increase in local cerebral glucose utilization of rat hippocampus. J Cereb Blood Flow Metab 11: 106–113.

Riveros N, Orrogo F (1986) N-methylaspartate-activated calcium channels in rat brain cortex slices: effect of calcium channel blockers and of inhibition and depressant substances. Neuroscience 17: 541–546.

Roberts TPL, Vexler Z, Derugin N, et al. (1993) High-speed MR imaging of ischemic brain injury following stenosis of the middle cerebral artery. J Cereb Blood Flow Metab 13: 940–946.

Robertson CS, Foltz R, Grossman RG, et al. (1986) Protection against experimental ischemic spinal cord injury. J Neurosurg 64: 633–642.

Robertson CS, Grossman RG (1987) Protection against spinal cord ischemia with insulin-induced hypoglycemia. J Neurosurg 67: 739–744.

Robinson MJ, Macrae IM, Todd M, et al. (1990) Reduction of local cerebral blood flow to pathological levels by endothelin-1 applied to the middle cerebral artery of the rat. Neurosci Lett 118: 269–272.

Rodden FA, Wiegandt H, Bauer BL (1991) Ganglioside: the relevanve of current research to neurosurgery. J Neurosurg 74: 606–619.

Rodrigues de Turco EB, Morelli de Liberti S, Bazan NG (1983) Stimulation of free fatty acid and diacylglycerol accumulation in cerebrum and cerebellum during bicuculline-induced status epilepticus. J Neurochem 40: 252–259.

Roemmer E (1989) Arzneimitter-induziertes Guillain-Barré Syndrom. Dtsch Artzebl 86: 452.

Roffler-Tarlov S, Brown JJG, Tarlov E, et al. (1996) Programmed cell death in the absence of *c-Fos* and *c-Jun*. Development 122: 1–9.

Rogers NE, Ignarro LJ (1992) Constitutive nitric oxide synthase from cerebellum is reversibly inhibited by nitric oxide formed from L-arginine. Biochem Biophys Res Commun 189: 242–249.

Romettino S, Lazdunski M, Gottesmann C.(1991) Anticonvulsant and sleep-waking influences of riluzole in a rat model og absence epilepsy. Eur J Pharmacol 199: 371–373.

Roof RL, Hall ED (2000) Gender differences in acute CNS trauma and stroke: Neuroprotective effects of estrogen and progesterone. J Neurotrauma 17: 367–388.

Rordrof G, Uemura Y, Bonventre J (1991): Characterization of phospholipase A_2 activity in gerbil brain: Enhanced activities of cytosolic mitochondral, and microsomal forms after ischemia and reperfusion. J Neurosci 11: 1829–1836.

Rosenthal RE, Hamud F, Fiskum G, et al. (1987) Cerebral ischemia and reperfusion: Prevention of brain mitochondrial injury by lidoflazine. J Cereb Blood Flow Metab 7: 752–758.

Rosenthal RE, Williams R, Bogaert YE, et al. (1992) Prevention of postischemic canine neurological injury through potentiation of brain energy metabolism by acetyl-l-carnitine. Stroke 23: 1312–1318.

Ross ME (1996) Cell devision and the nervous system: regulating the cycle from neural differentiation to death. Trends Neurosci 19: 62–68.

Rothman SM, (1983) Synaptic activity mediates death of hypoxic neurons. Science 220: 536–537.

Simpson JI, Eide TR, Schiff GA, et al. (1994) Intrathecal magnesium sulfate protects the spinal cord from ischemic injury during thoracic aortic cross-clamping. Anesthesiology 81: 1493–1499.

Roucher O, Méric P, Corrèze JL, et al. (1991) Metabolic effects of R-phenylisopropyladenosine during reversible forebrain ischemia studied by vivo ^{31}P nuclear magnetic resonance spectroscopy. J Cereb Blood Flow Metab 11: 453–458.

Rudolphi KA, Keil M, Hinze H-J (1987) Effect of theophylline on ischemically induced hippocampal damage in Mongolian gerbils: a behavioral and histopathological study. J Cereb Blood Flow Metab 7: 74–81.

Sadohara T, Sugahara K, Urashima Y, et al. (2001) Keratinocyte growth factor prevents ischemic-induced delayed neuronal death in the hippocampal CA1 field of the gerbil brain. Neuroreport 12: 71–76.

Sagar SM (1993) The molecular biology of brain ischemia: Trendy genes in sick neurons. Ann Neurol 33: 437–438.

Saji M, Reis DJ (1987) Delayed transneuronal death of substantia nigra neurons prevented by GABA agonist. Science 2000: 66–69.

Sakabe T, Siesjö BK (1979) The effect of indomethacin on blood flow-metabolism couple in the brain under normal, hypercapnic and hypoxic conditions. Acta Physiol Scand 107: 283–284.

Sakaki T, Tsunoda S, Morimoto T (1991) The influence of the calcium antagonist nimodipine and induced hypertension on behavior of the cerebral pial arteries, the blood-brain barrier, cerebral edema, and cerebral infarction in cats with one-hour occlusion of the middle cerebral artery. Neurosurgery 28: 267–272.

Sakhi S, Gilmore W, Tran ND, Schreiber SS (1996) p53-deficient mice are protected against adrenalectomy-induced apoptosis. NeuroReport 8: 233–235.

Sakurai T, Yamagisawa M, Masaki T (1992) Molecular characteristics of endothelin receptors. Trend Pharmacol Sci 13: 103–108.

Sancesario G, Iannone M, Morello M, et al. (1994) Nitric oxide inhibition aggravates ischemic damage of hippocampal but not of NADPH neurons in gerbils. Stroke 25: 436–444.

Sándor P, Demchenko IT, Morgalyov YN, et al. (1983) Cerebral blood flow and tissue $p0_2$ changes following local Met-enkephalin administration in awake, freely moving cats. Acta Physiol Hung 61: 155–161.

Sándor P, Gotoh F, Tomita M, et al. (1986) Effects of stable enkephalin analoque, (D-Met-2,pro-5)-Enkephalinamide, and naloxone on cortical blood flow and cerebral blood volume in experimental brain ischemia in anesthetized cats. J Cereb Blood Flow Metab 6: 553–558.

Sándor P, Komjati K, Reivich M, Nyary I (1994) Major role of nitric oxide in the mediation of regional CO_2 responsiveness of the cerebral and spinal cord vessels of the cat. J Cereb Blood Flow Metab 14: 49–58.

Santbrink van H, Maas AIR, Avezaat CJ (1996) Continuous monitoring of partial pressure of brain tissue oxygen in patients with severe head injury. Neurosurgery 38: 21–31.

Sasaki K (1979) Cerebro-cerebellar interconnections in cats and monkeys. In: Massion J, Sasaki K, eds. Cerebro-cerebellar Interactions. Amsterdam, The Netherlands: Elsevier/Nort-Holland. 105–124.

Sasaki O, Takeuchi S, Koike T, et al. (1995) Fibrinolytic therapy for acute embolic stroke: Intravenous, intracarotid, and intra-arterial local approaches. Neurosurgery 36: 246–253.

Sasaki T, Nakagomi T, Kirino T, et al. (1988) Indomethacin ameliorates ischemic neuronal damage in the gerbil hippocampal CA1 sector. Stroke 19: 1399–1403.

Sattler M, Liang H, Nettesheim D, et al. (1997) Structure of Bcl-cL-Bak peptide complex: recognition between regulators of apoptosis. Science 275: 983–986.

Sauer D, Weber E, Lüönd G, et al. (1995) The competitive NMDA antagonist CGP 40116 permanently reduces brain damage after middle cerebral artery occlusion in rats. J Cereb Blood Flow Metab 15: 602–610.

Schielke GP, Moises HC, Betz L (1991) Blood to brain sodium transport and interstitial fluid potassium concentration during early focal ischemia in the rat. J Cereb Blood Flow Metab 11: 466–471.

Schindler KS, Latham CB, Roth KA (1997) Bax deficiency prevents the increased cell death of immature neurons in bcl-x-deficient mice. J Neurosci 17: 3112–3119.

Schindler R, Mancilla J, Endres S, et al. (1990) Correlations and interactions in the production of interleukin-6 (IL-6), IL-1, and tumor necrosis factor (TNF) in human blood mononuclear cells. Blood 75: 40–47.

Schmidt HHHW, Lohmann SM, Walter U (1993) The nitric oxide and cGMP signal transduction system: regulation and mechanism of action. Biochem Biophys Acta 1178: 153–175.

Schmidt JF, Waldemar G, Paulson OB (1991) The acute effect of nimodipine on cerebral blood flow, its CO_2 reactivity, and cerebral oxygen metabolism in human volunteers. Acta Neurochir (Wien) 111: 49–53.

Schmidt-Kastner R, Hossmann K-A, Ophoff BG (1987) Pial artery pressure after one hour of global ischemia. J Cereb Blood Flow Metab 7: 109–117.

Schwartz LM, Milligan CE (1996) Cold thoughts of death: the role of ICE proteases in neuronal death. Trends Neurosci 19: 555–562.

Schweitzer M, Richter C (1994): Nitric oxide potently and reversibly deenergizes mitochondria at low oxygen tehsion. Biochem Biophysic Res Commun 204: 169–175.

Schoettle RJ, Kochanek PM, Magargee MJ, et al. (1990) Early polymorphonuclear leukocyte accumulation correlates with the development of posttraumatic cerebral edema in rats. J Neurotrauma 7: 207–217.

Schuier FJ, Hossmann K-A (1980) Experimental brain infarct in cats II: Ischemic brain edema. Stroke 11: 593–601.

Schulz J, Henshaw D, Siwek D, et al (1995a) Involvement of free radicals in excitatoxicity *in vivo*. J Neurochem 64: 2239–2247.

Schulz J, Matthews R, Jenkins B, et al (1995b) Improved therapeutic window for treatment of histotoxic hypoxia with a free radical spin trap. J Cereb Blood Flow Metab 15: 948–952.

Schurr A, West CA, Rigor B (1988) Lactate-supported synaptic function in the rat hippocampal slice preparation. Science 240: 1326–1328.

Schurr A, Payne RS, Miller JJ, et al. (2001) Blockade of lactate transport exacerbates delayed neuronal damage in a rat model of cerebral ischemia. Brain Res 23: 895: 268–272.

Sciotto VM, Roche FM, Grabb MC, van Wylen DGL (1992) Adenosine receptor blockade augments interstitial fluid levels of excitatory amino acids during cerebral ischemia. J Cereb Blood Flow Metab 12: 646–655.

Scriabine A, Battye R, Hoffmeister F, et al. (1985) Nimodipine. New Drugs Ann 3: 197–218.

Seelig JM, Wei EP, Kontos HA, et al. (1983) Effect of changes in magnesium ion concentration on cat cerebral arterioles. Am J Physiol 43: H22–H26.

Semenza GL, Jiang BH, Leung SW, et al. (1996) Hypoxia response elements in the aldolase A, enolase 1, and lactate dehydrogenase A gene promotes contain essential binding sites for hypoxia-inducible factor-1. J Biol Chem 271: 32529–32537.

Sen S, Phillis J (1993) Alpha-phenyl-tret-butyl-nitrone (PBN) attenuates hydroxyradical production during ischemia-reperfusion injury of rat brain: a EPR study. Free Radic Res Comm 19: 255–265.

Shackelford DA, Xeh RY, Hsu M, et al. (1995) Effect of cerebral ischemia on calcium/calmodulin-dependent protein kinase II activity and phsophorylation. J Cereb Blood Flow Metab 15: 450–461.

Shackelford DA, Yeh RY (1998) Dephosphorylation of tau during transient forebrain ischemia in the rat. Mol Chem Neuropathol 34: 103–120.

Shalaby MR, Waage A, Aarden L, et al. (1989) Endotoxin, tumor necrosis factor-alpha and interleukin 1 induce interleukin-6 production *in vivo*. Clin Immunol Immunopath 53: 488–498.

Shapira Y, Davidson E, Weidenfeld Y, et al. (1988) Dexamethasone and indomethacin do not affect brain edema following head injury in rats. J Cereb Blood Flow Metab 8: 395–402.

Sharbrough FW, Messick JM, Sundt TM Jr (1973) Correlation of continuous electroencephalograms with cerebral blood flow measurements during carotid endarterectomy. Stroke 4: 674–683.

Shigeno S, Fritschka E, Shigeno T, Brock M (1985) Effects of indomethacin on rCBF during and after focal cerebral ischemia in the cat. Stroke 16: 235–240.

Shigeno T, Teasdale G, McCulloch J, Graham D (1985): Recirculation model following MCA occlusion in rats. Cerebral blood flow, cerebrovascular permeability, and brain edema. J Neurosurg 63: 272–277.

Shima K, Umezawa H, Chigaski H, et al. (1994) Local cerebral blood flow and glucose metabolism in chronic focal ischemia of stroke-phrone spontaneously hypertensive rats. Stroke 16: 289–296.

Shimada N, Graf R, Rosner G, Wakayama A, et la. (1989) Ischemic flow threshold for extracellular glutamate increase in cat cortex. J Cereb Blood Flow Metab 9: 603–606.

Shimokawa H, Kim P, Vanhoutte PM (1988) Endothelium-dependent relaxation of aggregating platelets in isolated basilar arteries of control and hypercholesterolemic pigs. Circ Res 63: 604–612.

Shiozaki T, Sugimoto H, Taneka M. et al. (1993) Effect of mild hypothermia on uncontrollable intracranial hypertension after severe head injury. J Neurosurg 79: 363–368.

Shizumi K (1988) Intra-arterial urokinase infusion in the very early stage of cerebral artery occlusion and stenosis at their main trunks. Jpn J Stroke 10: 83–93.

Shohami E, Shapira Y, Sidi A. Cotev S (1987) Head injury induces increased prostaglandin synthesis in rat brain. J Cereb Blood Flow Metab 7: 58–63.

Short BL, Walker LK, Traystman RJ. (1994) Impaired cerebral autoregulation in the newborn lamb during recovery from severe, prolonged hypoxia, combined with carotid artery and jugular vein ligation. Crit Care Med 22: 1262–1268.

Siemkowicz E, Hansen A (1978) Clinical restitution following cerebral ischaemia in hypo-, normo, and hyperglycemic rats. Acta Neurol Scand 58: 1–8.

Siemkowicz E, Hansen AJ (1981) Brain extracellular ion composition and EEG activity following 10 min ischaemia in normo- and hyperglycemic rats. Stroke 12: 236–240.

Siesjö BK (1981) Cell damage in the brain. A speculative synthesis. J Cereb Blood Flow Metab 1: 155–185.

Siesjö BK, Ingvar M, Westerberg E (1982) The influence of bicuculline-induced seizures on free fatty acid concentration in cerebral cortex, hippocampus, and cerebellum. J Neurochem 39: 796–802.

Siesjö BK. (1984) Cerebral circulation and metabolism. J Neurosurg 60: 883–908.

Siesjö BK (1988) Mechanisms of ischemic brain damage. Crit Care Med 16: 954–963.

Siesjö BK, Bengtsson F (1989) Calcium fluxes, calcium antagonists, and calcium-related pathology in brain ischemia, hypoglycemia, and spreading depression: A unifying hypothesis. J Cereb Blood Flow Metab 9: 127–140.

Siesjö BK, Ekholm A, Katsura K, Theander S (1990) Acid-base changes during complete brain ischemia. Stroke: 21 (suppl III): III-194–III-199.

Siesjö BH (1992) Pathophysiology and treatment pf focal cerebral ischemia. Part I: Pathophysiology. J Neurosurg 1992: 77: 169–184.
Siesjö BH (1992) Pathophysiology and treatment of focal cerebral ischemia. Part II: Mechanisms of damage and treatment. J Neurosurg 1992: 77: 337–354.
Siesjö BK, Siesjö P. Mechanisms of secondary brain injury. Europ J Anaesthesiol 1996: 13: 247–268.
Siliprandi N, Siliprandi D, Ciman M (1965) Stimulation of oxidation of mitochondrial fatty acids and of acetate by acetylcarnitine. Biochem J 96: 777–780.
Silvia RC, Piercey MF, Hoffmann WE, et al. (1987) U74006F, an inhibitor of lipid peroxidation protects against lesion development following experimental stroke in cat: Histological and metabolic analysis. Neurosci Abstr 13: 1499.
Simmons ML, Murphy S (1992) Induction of nitric oxide synthase in glial cells. J Neurochem 59: 897–905.
Simmons ML, Murphy S (1993) Cytokines regulate L-arginine-dependent cyclic GMP production in rat glial cells. Eur J Neurosci 5: 825–832.
Simpson JI, Eide TR, Schiff GA, et al. (1994) Intrathecal magnesium sulfat protects the spinal cord from ischemic injury during thoracic aortic cross-clamping. Anesthesiology 81: 1493–1499.
Siren AL, Fratelli M, Brines M, et al. (2001) Erythropoietin prevents neuronal apoptosis after cerebral ischemia and metabolic stress. Proc Natl Acad Sci USA. PMID 1125943.
Slack RS, Belliveau DJ, Rosenberg M, et al. (1996) Adenovirus-mediated gene transfer of the tumor suppressor p53 induces apothosis in postmitotic neurons. J Cell Biol 135: 1085–1096.
Sobel RA, Mitchell ME, Fondren G (1990) Intercellular adhesion moleculte-1 (ICAM-1) in cellular immune reactions in the human central nervous system. Am J Path 136: 1309–1316.
Sola A, Berrios M, Sheldon RA, et al. (1996) Fructose-1,6,-diphosphate after hypoxic ischemic injury is protective to neonatal rat brain. Brain Res 741: 294–299.
Somjen GG, Aitken PG, Balestrino M, et al. (1990) Spreading depression-like depolarization and selective vulnerability of neurons. Stroke 21 (suppl III): 179–183.
Song Q, Burrows SR, Smith G, et al. (1996) Interleukin-1 beta-converting emzyme-like protease cleaves DNA-dependent protein kinase in cytotoxic T cell killing. J Exp Med 184: 619–626.
Sorensen AG, Buonanno FS, Gonzales RG, et al. (1996) Hyperacute stroke: evaluation with combined multisection diffusion-weighted and hemodynamically weighted echoplanar MR imaging. Radiology 199: 391–401
Sorensen AG, Gonzales RG, Copen WA et al. (1997) Quantitation of diffusion/perfusion MRI mismatch in acute human cerebral infarction. Stroke 28: 252.
Soriano SG, Lipton SA, Wang YF, et al. (1996) Intercellular adhesion molecule-1-deficient mice are less susceptible to cerebral ischemia-reperfusion injury. Ann Neurol 39: 618–624.
Soussi B, Idstrom-JP, Schersten T, Bylund-Fellenius A (1990): Cytochrom c oxidase and cardiolipin alterations in response to skeletal muscle ischemia and reperfusion. Acta Physiol Scand 138: 107–114.
Spertini O, Luscinskas FW, Kansas GS et al. (1991) Leukocyte adhesion molecule-1 (LAM-1), L-selectin) interacts with an inducible endothelial cell ligand to support leukocyte adhesion. J Immunol 147: 2565–2573.
States BA, Honkaniemi J, Weinstein PR, et al. (1996) DNA fragmentation and HSP70 protein induction in hippocampus and cortex occurs in separate neurons following permanent middle cerebral artery occlusions. J Cereb Blood Flow Metab 16: 1165–1175.
Staub F, Baethmann A, Peters J, et al. (1990) Effects of lactacidosis on glial cell volume and viability. J Cereb Blood Flow Metab 10: 866–876.
Staub F, Winkler A, Peters J, et al. (1994) Swelling, acidosis, and irreversible damage of glial cells from exposure to arachidonic acid *in vivo*. J Cereb Blood Flow Metab 14: 1030–1039.
Steen PA, Milde JH, Michenfelder JS (1978) Cerebral metabolic and vascular effect of barbiturate therapy following complete global ischemia. J Neurochem 31: 1317–1324.
Steen PA, Newberg LA, Milde JH, Michenfelder JD (1983) Nimodopine improves cerebral blood flow and neurologic recovery after complete global ischemia in the dog. J Cereb Blood Flow Metab 3: 38–43.
Steen PA, Newberg LA, Milde JH, Michenfelder JD (1984) Cerebral blood flow and neurologic outcome when nimodipine is given after complete cerebral ischemia in the dog. J Cereb Blood Flow Metab 4: 82–87.
Steen PA, Gisvold SE, Milde JH, et al. (1985) Nimodipine improves outcome when given after complete cerebral ischemia in primates. Anesthesiology 62: 406–414.
Steinberg GK, Kunis D, Saleh J, DelaPaz R (1991) Protection after transient focal cerebral ischemia by the N-Methyl-D-Aspartate antagonist Dextrophan is dependent upon plasma and brain levels. J Cereb Blood FLow Metab 11: 1015–1024.
Steiner B, Mandelkow E-M, Biernat J, et al. (1990) Phosphorylation of microtubule-associated protein tau: identification of the site for Ca^{2+}-calmodulin dependent kinase and relationship with tau phosphorylation in Alzheimer tangles. EMBO J 9: 3539–3544.
Steingrub S, Mundt DJ (1996) Blood glucose and neurologic outcome with global brain ischemia. Crit Care Med 24: 802–805.
Steinke DE, Weif BKA, Findley JM, et al (1989) A trial of the 21-aminosteroid U 74006F in a primate model of chronic cerebral vasospasms. Neurosurgery 24: 179–186.
Sternau LL, Lust WD, Ricci AJ, Ratcheson R (1989) Role of GABA in selective vulnerability in gerbils. Stroke 20: 281–287.
Stevens MK, Yaksh TL, Hansen II RB, Anderson RE (1986) Effect of preischemia cyclooxygenase inhibition by zomepirac sodium on reflow, cerebral autoregulation, and EEG recovery in the cat after global ischemia. J Cereb Blood Flow Metab 6: 691–702.
Strand T, Marklund SL (1992) Release of superoxide dismutase into cerebrospinal fluid as a marker of brain lesion in acute cerebral infarction. Stroke 23: 515–518.
Strong AJ, Venables GS, Gibson G (1983) The cortical ischemic penumbra associated with occlusion of MCA in the cat. Topography of changes in blood flow, potassium ion activity, and EEG. J Cereb Blood Flow Metab 3: 86–96.
Strong AJ, Gibson G, Miller SA, Venables GS (1988) Changes in vascular and metabolic reactivity as indices of ischaemia in the penumbra. J Cereb Blood Flow Metab 8: 79–88.
Sturm CD, Frisella WA, Yoon K-W (1993) Attenuation of potassium cyanide-mediated neuronal cell death by adenosine. J Neurosurg 79: 111–115.

Sun D, Gilboe D. (1994): Ischemia-induced changes in cerebral mitochondrial free fatty acids, phospholipids, and respiration in the rat. J Neurochem 62: 1921–1928.

Sutherland G, Lesiuk H, Bose R, Sima A (1988) Effect of mannitol, nimodipine, and indomethacin singly or in combination on cerebral ischemia in rats. Stroke 19: 571–578.

Suzuka T, Mabe H, Nagai H (1989) Role of arachidonic acid metabolites on development of ischemic cerebral edema in rat middle cerebral artery occlusion. J Cereb Blood Flow Metab 9: suppl 1, S 89.

Swanson RA (1992) Astrocyte glutamate uptake during chemical hypoxia *in vitro*. Neursci Lett 147: 143–146.

Swanson RA, Chen J, Graham SH (1994) Glucose can fuel glutamate uptake in ischemic brain. J Cereb Blood Flow Metab 14: 1–6.

Swanson RA, Farrell K, Simon RP (1995) Acidosis causes failure of astrocyte glutamate uptake during hypoxia. J Cereb Blood Flow Metab 15: 417–424.

Symon L, Pasztor E, Branston N (1974): The distribution and density of reduced cerebral blood flow following acute middle cerebral artery occlusion: An experimental study by the technique of hydrogen clearance in baboons. Stroke 5: 355–346.

Symon L, Brierley J (1976) Morphological changes in cerebral blood vessels in chronic ischemic infarction: flow correlation obtained by the hydrogen clearance method. In: The Cerebral Vessel Wall, Cervos Navarro J, Matakas F (eds). New York, Raven Press, pp 165–174.

Symon L, Branston NM, Chikovani O (1979) Ischemic brain edema following middle cerebral artery occlusion in baboons: relationship between regional cerebral water content and blood flow at 1 and 2 hours. Stroke 10: 184–191.

Symon L (1980) The relationship between CBF, evoked potentials, and the clinical features in cerebral ischaemia. Acta Neurol Scand 62 (suppl 78): 175–190.

Swanson RA, Shiraishi K, orton MT, Sharp FR (1990) Methionine sulfoximine reduces cortical infarct size in rats after middle cerebral artery occlusion. Stroke 21: 322–327.

Szaflarski J, Burtrum D, Silverstein FS, et al. (1995) Cerebral hypoxia-ischemia stimulates cytokine gene expression in perinatal rats. Stroke 26: 1093–1100.

Sztriha L, Joó F, Szerdahelyi P (1987) Histamine H2-receptors participate in the formation of brain edema induced by kainic acid in rat thalamus. Neurcsi Lett 75: 334–338.

Taga K, Patel PM, Drummond JC, et al. (1997): Transient neuronal depolarization induces tolerance to subsequent forebrain ischemia in rats. Anesthesiology 87: 918–925.

Takagi K, Ginsberg MD, Globus MY, et al. (1993) Changes in amino acid neurotransmitters and cerebral blood flow in the ischemic penumbra region following middle cerebral artery occlusion in the rat: correlation with histopathology. J Cereb Blood Flow Metab 13: 575–585.

Takagi K, Ginsberg MD, Globus MY, et al. (1994) The effect of ritanserin, a $5\text{-}HT_2$ receptor antagonist, on ischemic cerebral blood flow and infarct volume in rat middle cerebral artery occlusion. Stroke 25: 481–486.

Takagi K, Zhao W, Busto R, Ginsberg MD (1995): Local hemodynamic changes during transient middle cerebral artery occlusion and recirculation in the rat: A [^{14}C]iodoantipyrine autoradiographic study. Brain Res 691: 160–168.

Takahashi A, Alnemri ES, Lazebnik YA, et al. (1996) Cleavage of lamin A by Mch2 alpha but not CPP32: multiple interleukin 1 beta-converting enzyme-related proteases with distinct substrate recognition properties are active in apoptosis. Proc Natl Acad Sci USA 93: 8395–8400.

Takahashi H, Traystman RJ, Hashimoto K, et al. (1997). Postischemic brain injury is affected steriospecifically by pentazocine in rats. Anest Analg 85: 353–357.

Takahashi M, Takagi H, Ito C. et al. (1993) Protective effect of U92032, a novel calcium blocker, with anti-peroxidative activity, on cerebral ischemic injury. Jpn J Pharmacol (abstract) 61: 289P.

Takami K, Iwane M, Kiyota Y et al. (1992) Increase of basic fibroblast growth factor immunoreactivity and its mRNA level in rat brain following transient forebrain ischemia. Exp Brain Res 90: 1–10.

Takashima M, Liou SY, Kunihara M (1993) Differential effect of U92032, a novel Ca^{2+} channel blocker, on Ca^{2+} influx evoked by high K^+, glutamate and hypoxia. Jpn J Pharmacol (abstract) 61: 166P.

Takayasu M, Suzuki Y, Shibuya M, et al. (1986) The effects of HA compound calcium antagonists on delayed cerebral vasospasm in dogs. J Neurosurg 65: 80–85.

Takeda A, Kimpara T, Onodera H, et al. (1996) Regional difference in induction of heme oxygenase-1 protein following rat transient forebrain ischemia. Neurosci Lett 205: 169–172.

Takeshima R, Kirsch JR, Koehler RC et al. (1992) Monoclonal leukocyte antibody does not decrease the injury of transient focal cerebral ischemia in cats. Stroke 23: 247–252.

Takeshima R, Kirsch JR, Koehler RC, Traystman RJ (1994) Tirilazad treatment does not decrease early brain injury after transient focal ischemia in cats. Stroke 25: 670–676.

Takizawa S, Matsushima K, Fujita H, et al. (1995) A selective N-type calcium channel antagonist reduces extracellular glutamate release and infarct volume in focal cerebral ischemia. J Cereb Blood Flow Metab 1995: 15: 611–618.

Tanaka K, Dora E, Urbanics R, et al. (1986) Effect of ganglioside GM1, on cerebral metabolism, microcirculation, recovery kinetics of ECoG and histology, during the recovery period following focal ischemia in cats. Stroke 17: 1170–1178.

Tarkowski E, Rosengren L, Blomstrand C, et al. (1995) Early intrathecal production of interleukin-6 predicts the size of brain lesion in stroke. Stroke 26: 1393–1398.

Tecoma ES, Choi DW (1989) GABAergic neocortical neurons are resistant to NMDA receptor-mediated injury. Neurology 39: 676–682.

Terai K, Matsuo A, McGeer EG, McGeer PL (1996) Enhancement of immunoreactivity for NF-kappaB in the hippocampal formation and cerebral cortex of Alzheimer's disease. Brain Res 735–159–168.

Thilmann R, Xie Y, Kleihues P, Kiesling M (1986) Persistent inhibition of protein synthesis precedes delayed neuronal death in psotischemic gerbil hippocampus. Acta Neuropathol (Berl) 71: 78–93.

Thorn W, Heitmann R (1954) pH der Gehirnrinde vom Kaninchen in Situ während perakuter, totaler Ischaemie, reiner Anoxie und in der Erholung. Phlügers Arch 258: 501–510.

Thorogood MC, Armstead WM. Influence of polyethylene glycol superoxide dismutase/catalase on altered opioid-induced pial artery dilation after brain injury. Anesthesiology 1996: 84: 614–625.

Toda N, Okamura t (1992) Regulation of nitroxinergic nerve of arterial tone. News Physiol Sci 7: 148–152.

Toda N, Ayajiki K, Yoshida K, et al. (1993) Impairment by damage for the pteryopalatine ganglion of nitroxinergic vasodilator nerve function in canine cerebral and retinal arteries. Circ Res 72: 206–213.

Todd NV, Picozzi P, Crockard A, Ross Russell RW (1986) Duration of ischemia influences the development and resolution of ischemic brain edema. Stroke 17: 466–471.

Todd NV, Picozzi P, Crockard HA (1986) Quantitative measurement of cerebral blood flow and cerebral blood volume after cerebral ischemia. J Cereb Blood Flow Metab 6: 338–341.

Todd NV, Picozzi P, Crockard A, Russell RR (1986) Reperfusion after cerebral ischemia: Influence of duration of ischemia. Stroke 17: 460–466.

Tomasevic G, Subberod P, Wieloch M, Wieloch T (1996) DNA damage and repair: changes in the tumor suppressor protein p53 and the proliferative nuclear antigen (PCNA) in the rat brain following transient cerebral ischemia. In Pharmacology of Cerebral Ischemia. (eds) Krieglestein J et al. Wissenschafliche Verlagsgesellschaft, Stuttgart, pp 1–5.

Tomida S, Nowak TS, Vass K, Lohr JM, Klatzo I (1987) Experimental model for repetive ischemic attacks in the gerbil: The cumulative effect of repeated ischemic insults. J Cereb Blood Flow Metab 7: 773–782.

Tomimoto H, Nishimura M, Suenaga T. et al. (1994) Distribution of nitric oxide synthase in the human cerebral blood vessels and brain tissues. J Cereb Blood Flow Metab 14: 930–938.

Tominaga T, Sato S, Ohnishi T, Ohnishi ST (1994) Electron paramagnetic resonance (ERP) detection of nitric oxide production during forebrain ischemia of the rat. J Cereb Blood Flow Metab 14: 715–722.

Toyoda T, Kassell NF, Lee KS (2000) Induction of tolerance against ischemia/reperfusion injury in the rat brain by preconditioning with the endotoxin analog diphosphoryl lipid A. J Neurosurg 92: 435–441.

Trifiletti RR (1992) Neuroprotective effects of N-nitro-L-arginine in focal stroke in 7-day old rat. Eur J Pharmacol 218: 197–198.

Tr¢jaborg W, Boysen G (1973) Relation between EEG, regional cerebral blood flow and internal carotid artery pressure during carotid endarterectomy. EEG Clin Neurophysiol 34: 61–69.

Tseng MT, Chan SA, Reid KH, Iyer VG (1997) Fos-like immunoreactivity in rat hippocampal neurons following transient global ischemia. Neurol Res 19: 89–91.

Tsuchidate R, He Q-P, Smith M-L, Siesjö BK (1997): Regional cerebral blood flow during and after 2 hours of middle cerebral artery occlusion in the rat. J Cereb Blood Flow Metab 17: 1066–1073.

Tsukahara T, Yonekawa Y, Tanaka K, et al. (1994) The role of brain-derived neurotrophic factor in transient forebrain ischemia in the rat. Neurosurgery 34: 323–331.

Uchino H, Elmer E, Uchino K, Siesjö BK (1995): Cyclosporin A dramatically ameliorates CA1 hippocampal damage following transient forebrain ischemia in the rat. Acta Phys Scand 155: 469–471.

Ueda Y, Obrenovitch TP, Lok SY, et al. (1992) Efflux of glutamate produced by short ischemia of varied severity in rat striatum. Stroke 23: 253–259.

Uhler TA, Frim DM, Pakzaban P, Isacson O (1994) The effect of megadose methylprednisolone and U-78517F on toxicity mediated by glutamate receptors in the rat neostriatum. Neurosurgery 34: 122–128.

Umemura A, Mabe H, Nagai H (1992) A Phospholipase C inhibitor ameliorates postischemic neuronal damage in rats. Stroke 23: 1163–1166.

Unterberg A, Baethmann AJ (1984) The kallikrein-kinin system as mediator in vasogenic brain edema. Part 1: Cerebral exposure to bradykinin and plasma. J Neurosurg 61: 87–96.

Unterberg A, Wahl M, Baethmann AJ (1984) Effects of bradykinin on permeability and diameter of pial vessels *in vivo*. J Cereb Blood Flow Metab 4: 574–585.

Unterberg A, Wahl M, Baethmann A (1985) Arachidonic acid induces opening of the blood-brain barrier. In: Brain Edema, eds.: Inaba Y, Klatzo I, Spatz M. Springer Verlag, pp 159–164.

Unterberg A, Schmidt W, Wahl M, et al. (1991) Evidence against leukotrienes as mediators of brain edema. J Neurosurg 74: 773–780.

Vacanti TX, Ames A III (1984) Mild hypothermia and Mg^{++} protect against irreversible damage during CNS ischemia. Stroke 15: 695–698.

Valentino K, Newcomb R, Gadbois T et al. (1993). A selective N-type calcium channel antagonist protects against neuronal loss after global cerebral ischemia. Proc Natl Acad Sci USA 90: 7894–7897.

Van Wylen DGL, Park TS, Rubio R, Berne RM (1986) Increases in interstitial fluid adenosine concentration during hypoxia, local potassium infusion, and ischemia. J Cereb Blood Flow Metab 6: 522–528.

Vass K, Welch WJ, Nowak TS Jr (1988) Localization of 70 kDa stress protein induction in gerbil brain after ischemia. Acta Neuropathol (Berl) 77: 128–135.

Vibulsresth S, Dietrich WD, Busto R, Ginsberg MD (1987) Failure of nimodipine to prevent ischemic neuronal damage in rats. Stroke 18: 210–216.

Vivien D, Buisson A (2000) Serine proteases inhibitors: Novel therapeutic targets for stroke? J Cereb Blood Flow metab 20: 755–764.

Voll CL, Auer RN (1988) The effect of postischemic blood glucose levels on ischemic brain damage in the rat. Ann Neurol 24: 638–646.

Voll CL, Auer RN (1991) Insulin attenuates ischemic brain damage independent of its hypoglycemic effect. J Cereb Blood Flow Metab 11: 1006–1014.

Vollmer DG, Takayasu M, Dacey RG (1992) An *in vitro* comparative study of conducting vessels and penetrating arterioles after experimental subarachnoidal hemorrhage in the rabbit. J Neurosurg 77: 113–119.

von Lubitz DKJE, Dambriosa JM, Kempski O, Redmond DJ (1988) Cyclohexyl adenosine protects against neuronal death following ischemia in the CA1 region of gerbil hippocampus. Stroke 19: 1133–1139.

Vukadinovic V, Stefanovich V, Rakic L (1986) Effect of profentofylline on GABA system of the rat brain. Drug Dev Res 7: 87–94.

Waage A, Halstensen A, Espevik T, et al. (1993) Compartmentalization of TNF and IL-6 in meningitis and septic shock Mediators of Inflammation 2: 23–25.

Wagner SR, Lanier WL (1994) Metabolism of glucose, glycogen, and high energy phosphates during complete cerebral ischemia. Anesthesiology 81: 1516–1526.

Wallum BJ, Taborsky GJ, Jr, Porte D Jr, et al. (1987) Cerebrospinal fluid insulin levels increase during intravenous insulin infusions in man. J Clin Endocrinol Metab 64: 190–194.

Walton M, Young D, Sirimane E, et al. (1996) Induction of clusterin in the immature brain following a hypoxic-ischemic injury. Mol Brain Res 39: 137-152.

Wang X, Feuerstein GZ (1995) Induced expression of adhesion molecules following focal brain ischemia. J Neurotrauma 12: 825-832.

Waniewski RA, Martin DL (1986) Exogenous glutamate is metabolized to glutamine and exported by rat primary astrocyte cultures. J Neurochem 47: 304-313.

Warach S, Chien D, Li W, et al. (1992) Fast magnetic resonance diffusion-weighted imaging of acute human stroke. Neurology 42: 1717-1723.

Warner DS, Smith -L, Siesjö BK (1987) Ischemia in normo- and hyperglycemic rats: Effects on brain water and electrolytes. Stroke 18: 464-471.

Warner DS, Martin H, Ludvig P, et al. (1995) *In vivo* models of cerebral ischemia: effects of parenterally administrated NMDA receptor glycine site antagonists. J Cereb Blood Flow Metab 15: 188-196.

Wass CT, Scheithauer BW, Bronk JT, et al. (1996). Insulin treatment of corticosteroid-associated hyperglycemia and its effect on outcome after forebrain ischemia in rats. Anesthesiology 84: 644-651.

Watanabe M, Rosenblum WI, Nelson GH (1988) *In vivo* effect of methylene blue on endothelium-dependent and endothelium-independent dilations of brain microvessels in mice. Circ Res 62: 86-90.

Waterhouse N, Kumar S, Song Q, et al. (1996) Heteronuclear ribonucleoproteins C1 and C2, components of the spliceosome, are specific targets of interleukin-1 beta-converting enzyme-like proteases in apoptosis. J Biol Chem 271: 29335-29341.

Wei EP, Kontos HA, Dietrich WD et al. (1981) Inhibition by free radical scavengers and by cyclooxygenase inhibitors of pial arteriolar abnormalities from concussive brain injury in cats. Circ Res 48: 95-103.

Wei EP, Lamp RG, Kontos HA (1982) Increased phospholipase C activity after experimental brain injury. J Neurosurg 56: 695-698.

Wei HM, Chi OZ, Liu X, et al. (1994) Nitric oxide synthase inhibition alters cerebral blood flow and oxygen balance in focal cerebral ischemia in rats. Stroke 25: 445-450.

Weissman BA, Kadar T, Brandeis R, Shapira S (1992) N-nitro-L-arginine enhances neuronal death following transient forebrain ischemia in gerbils. Neurosci Lett 146: 139-142.

Welsh FA, Moyer DJ, Harris VA (1992) Regional expression of heat shock protein-70 mRNA and c-fos mRNA following focal ischemia in rat brain. J Cereb Blood Flow Metab 12: 204-212.

Wendling WW, Chen D, Daniels FB, et al. (1996) The effect of N-methyl-D-aspartate agonists and antagonists on isolated bovine cerebral arteries. Anesth Analg 82: 264-268.

Wennmalm Å, Eriksson S, Wahren J (1981) Effect of indomethacin on basal and carbon dioxide stimulated cerebral blood flow in man. Clinical Physiol 1: 227-234.

Westergren I, Johansson BB (1993) Blockade of AMPA receptors reduces brain edema following opening of the blood-brain barrier. J Cereb Blood Flow Metab 13: 603-608.

White IR, Piper IR Miller JD (1992) The role of bradykinin in the etiology of vasogenic brain edema and perilesional brain dysfunction. Acta Neurochir (Wien) 115: 53-59.

Widdmann R, Kuroiwa T, Bonnekoh P, Hossmann K-A (1991) ^{14}C leucine incorporation into brain proteins in gerbils after transient inschemia: Relationship to selective vulnerability of hippocampus. J Neurochem 56: 789-796.

Widmann R, Weber C, Bonnekoh P, et al. (1992) Neuronal damage after repeated 5 minutes of ischemia in the gerbil is preceded by prolonged impairment of protein metabolism. J Cereb Blood Flow Metab 12: 425-433.

Wieloch T, Koide T, Westerberg E (1986) Inhibitory neurotransmitters and neuromodulators as protective agents against ischemic brain damage. In: Pharmacology of Cerebral Ischemia (Krieglstein J Ed), Amsterdam, Elsevier, pp 191-197.

Wiener CM, Booth G, Semenza GL, (1996) *In vivo* expression of mRNAs encoding hypoxia-inducible factor-1. Biochem Biophys Res Commun 225: 485-488.

Wiessner C, Vogel P, Neumann-Haefewlin T, Hossmann KA (1996) Molecular correlates of delayed neuronal death following transient forebrain ischemia in the rat. Acta Neurochir Suppl 66: 1-7.

Wikberg JES, Uhlen S (1990) Further characterization of the guinea pig cerebral cortex idazoxan receptor: solubilization, distinction from the imidazole site, and demonstration of cirazoline as an idazoxan receptor-selective drug. J Neurochem 55: 192-203.

Winn HR, Rubio R, Berne RM (1981) Brain adenosine concentration during hypoxia in the rat. Am J Physiol 241: H235-H242.

Winn RK, Sharar SR, Vedder NB, Harlan JM (1995): Leukocytes and endothelial adhesion molecules in ischemia/reperfusion injuries. In Wiley, Chichester Ciba Foundation. Symposium 189: Cell Adhesion and human disease, pp 63-76.

Wiernsperger N (1990) Serotonin $5\text{-}HT_2$ receptors and brain circulation. J Cardiovasc Pharmacol 16: (suppl): s20-s24.

Winfree CJ, Baker CJ, Connolly ES, et al. (1996) Mild hypothermia reduces penumbral glutamate levels in the rat permanent focal cerebral ischemia model. Neurosurgery 38: 1216-1222.

Wong D, Dorovinzis K, (1992) Upregulation of intercellular adhesion molecule-1 (ICAM-1) expression in primary cultures of human brain microvessel endothelial cells by cytokines and lipopolysaccharide. J Neuroimmunol 39: 11-22.

Wood NI, Barone FC, Benham CD, et al. (1997) The effect of SB 206284A, a novel neuronal calcium-channel antagonist, in models of cerebral ischemia. J Cereb Blood Flow Metab 17: 421-429.

Wu D, Wallen WD, Nunez G (1997) Interaction and regulation of subcellular localization of CED-4 by CED-9. Science 275: 1126-1129.

Xiang Hm Hochman DW, Saya H, et al. (1996) Evidence for p53-mediated modulation of neuronal viability. J Neurosci 16: 6753-6765.

Xu DG, Ckrocker SJ, Doucet J-P, et al. (1997) Elevation of neuronal expression of NAIP reduces ischemic damage in the rat hippocampus. Nature Medicine 3: 997-1004.

Xue D, Bruederlin B, Heinecke E, Li H, Slivka A, Buchan AM (1990) U74006F reduces neocortical infarction but does not attenuate selective hippocampal CA1 necrosis. Stroke 21: 178.

Yamada K, Kinishita A, Kohmura E, et al. (1991) Basic fibroblast growth factor prevents thalamic degeneration after cortical infarction. J Cereb Blood Flow Metab 11: 472-478.

Yamaguchi S, Kobayashi S, Yamashita K, Kitani M (1989) Pial arterial pressure contribution to early ischemic brain edema. J Cereb Blood Flow Metab 9: 597–602.

Yamamoto H, Fukunaga K, Lee K, et al. (1992) Ischemia-induced loss of brain calcium/calmodulin-dependent protein kinase II. J Neurochem 58: 1110–1117.

Yamamoto K, Akai F, Yoshimine T, Yanagihara T (1987) Immunohistochemical investigation of cerebral ischemia after middle cerebral artery occlusion in gerbils. J Neurosurg 67: 414–420.

Yamamoto S, Galonov EV, Berger SB, Reis DJ (1992) Inhibition of nitric oide synthesis increases focal ischemia infarction in rat. J Cereb Blood Flow Metab 12: 717–726.

Yamasaki Y, Suzuki T, Yamaya H, et al. (1992) Possible involvment of interleukin-1 in ischemic brain edema formation. Neurosci Lett 142: 45–47.

Yan HQ, Banos MA, Herregodts P, et al. (1992) Expression of interleukin (IL)-1beta, IL-6 and their respective receptors in the normal rat brain and after injury. Europ J Immunol 22: 2963–2971.

Yanaka K, Spellman SR, McCarthy JB, et al. (1996a) Reduction of brain injury using heparin to inhibit leukocyte accumulation in a rat model of transient focal cerebral ischemia. I. Protective mechanism. J Neurosurg 85: 1102–1107

Yanaka K, Spellman SR, McCarthy JB, et al. (1996b) Reduction of brain injury using heparin to inhibit leukocyte accumulation in a rat model of transient focal cerebral ischemia. II. Dose-response effect and the therapeutic window. J Neurosurg 85: 1108–1112.

Yang C-S, Lin N-N, Tsai P-J, et al. ((1996): *In vivo* evidence of hydroxyl radical formation induced by elevation of extracellular glutamate after cerebral ischemia in the cortex of anaesthetized rats. Free Radical Biol Med 20: 245–250.

Yang E, Korsmeyer SJ (1996) Molecular thanatopsis: a discource in the BCL-2 family and cell death. Blood 88: 386–401.

Yang G, Chan P, Chen S, et al. (1994): Reduction of vasogenic edema and infarction by MK-801 in rats after temporary focal cerebral ischemia. Neurosurgery 34: 339–345.

Yang G, Chan P, cen J, et al. (1994): Human copper-zinc superoxide dismutase transgenic mice are highly resistant to reperfusion injury after focal cerebral ischemia. Stroke 25: 165–170.

Yang G-Y, Betz AL (1994) Reperfusion-induced injury to the blood-brain barrier after middle cerebral artery occlusion in rats. Stroke 25: 1658–1665.

Yang J, Liu X, Bhalla K, et al. (1997) Prevention of apoptosis by BCL-2. Relase of cytochrome C from mitochondria blocked. Science 275: 1129–1132.

Yang SH, He Z, Wu SS, et al. (2001) 17-beta estradiol can reduce secondary ischemic damage and mortality of subarachnoid hemorrhage. J Cereb Blood Flow Metab 21: 174–181.

Yao H, Ginsberg MD, Eveleth DD, et al. (1995) Local cerebral glucose utilization and cytoskeletal proteolysis as indices of evolving focal ischemic injury in core and penumbra. J Cereb Blood Flow Metab 15: 398–408.

Yasuda H, Shuto S, Tsumagari T, Nakayima A (1978) Protective effect of a novel imidazole derivative against cerebral anoxia. Arch Int Pharmacodyn Ther 233: 136–144.

Yen MH, Lee SH (1987) Effects of cyclooxygenase and lipoxygenase inhibitors on cerebral edema induced by freezing lesions in rats. Europ J Pharmacol 144: 369–373.

Yenari MA, Sun GH, Kunis DM, et al. (2001) L-selectin inhibition does not reduce injury in a rabbit model of transient focal cerebral ischemia. Neurol Res 23: 72–78.

Yoneda Y, Tokui K, Hanihara T, et al. (1999) Diffusion-weighted magnetic resonance imaging: detection of ischemic injury 39 minutes after onset in a stroke pateint. Ann Neurol 45: 794–797.

Yoshida T, Limmroth V, Irikura K, Moskowitz MA (1994) The NOS inhibitor, 7-nitroindazole, decreases focal infarct volume but not the response to topical acetylcholine in pial vessels. J Cereb Blood Flow Metab 14: 924–929.

Young AB, Fagg GE (1990) Excitatory amino acid receptors in the brain: Membrane binding and receptor autoradiographic approaches. Trends Pharmacol Sci 11: 126–133.

Young W, Flamm ES (1982) Effect of high-dose corticoid therapy on blood flow, evoked potentials, and extracellular calcium in experimental spinal injury. J Neurosurg 57: 667–673.

Young W, Wojak JC, DeCrescito V (1988) Aminosteroid lipid peroxidation inhibitor reduces ion shifts and edema in the rat middle cerebral artery occlusion model of regional ischemia. Stroke 19: 1013–1019.

Young WL, Jsovitz K, Morales O, Chien S (1987) The effect of nimodipine on post-ischemic cerebral glucose utilization and blood flow in the rat. Anesthesiology 67: 54–59.

Young WL, Chien S (1989) Effect of nimodipine on cerebral blood flow and metabolism in rats during hyperventilation. Stroke 20: 275–280.

Young WL, Barkai A, Prohovnik I, et al. (1990) Nimodipine does not increase cerebral blood flow during hypocapnia in the rat. J Neurosurgical Anesthesiology 2: 284–289.

Yu MJ, McCowan JR, Thrasher KJ, et al. (1992a) Phenothiazines as lipid peroxidation inhibitors and cytoprotective agents. J Med Chem 35: 716–724.

Yu MJ, McCowan JR, Smalstig B, et al. A Phenothiazine derivate reduces rat brain damage after global or focal ischemia. Stroke 23: 1287–1291.

Yuguchi T, Kohmura E, Yamada K, et al. (1994): Messenger RNA and protein expression of basic fibroblast growth factor receptor after cortical ablation. Mol Brain Res 25: 50–56.

Zabramski JM, Spetzler RF, Selman WR, Hershey LA, Roessman U (1983) Naloxone improves neurologic function during, and outcome after, temporary focal cerebral ischemia. Stroke 14: 123.

Zabramski JM, Spetzler RF, Bonstelle C (1986) Chronic cerebral vasospasm: Effect of calcium antagonists. Neurosurgery 18: 129–135.

Zahniser NR, Goens MB, Hanaway PJ, Vinych JV (1984) Characterization and regulation of insulin receptors in rat brain. J Neurochem 42: 1254–1262.

Zaiden E, Sims N (1994): The calcium content of mitochondria from brain subregions following short-time forebrain ischemia and reperfusion in the rat. J Neurochem 63: 1812–1819.

Zamzami N, Susin SA, Manchetti P, et al (1996): Motochondrial control of nuclear apoptosis. J Exp Med 183: 1533–1544.

Zasslow MA, Pearl RG, Shuer LM, et al. Hyperglycemia decreases neuronal ischemic changes after middle cerebral artery occlusion in the cat. Anesthesiology 67: A 581.

Zha J, Harada H, Yang E, Ross ME, Iadecola C (1996) Serine phsophorylation of death agonist BAD in reponse to sur-

vival factor results in binding to 14-3-3 not BCL-X. Cell 87: 619–628.
Zhang F, Iadecola C (1992) Reduction of focal cerebral ischemic damage by delayed treratment with nitric oxide doners. J Cereb Blood Flow Metab 14: 574–580.
Zhang F, Iadecola C (1993) Nitroprusside improves blood flow and reduces brain damage after focal ischemia. Neuroreport 4: 559–562.
Zhang F. White JG, Iadecola C (1994) Nitric oxide doners increase blood flow and reduce brain damage in focal ischemia: evidence that nitric oide is benefial in the early stages of cerebral ischemia. J Cereb Blood Flow Metab 14: 217–226.
Zhang F, Xu S, Iadecola C, (1995) Time dependence of effect of nitric oxide synthase inhibition on cerebral ischemic damage. J Cereb Blood Flow Metab 15: 595–601.
Zhang Y, Marcillat O, Giulivi C, et al (1990). The oxidative inactivation of mitochondrial electron transport chain components and ATPase. J Biol Chem 265: 16330–16336.
Zhang ZG, Chopp M, Zaloga C, Pollock JS, Förstermann U (1993) Cerebral endothelial nitric oxide synthase expression after focal cerebral ischemia in rats. Stroke 24: 2016–2022.
Zhang ZG, Chopp M, Maynard KI, Moskowitz MA (1994) Cerebral blood flow changes during cortical spreading depression are not altered by inhibition of nitric oxide synthesis. J Cereb Blood Flow Metab 14: 939–943.
Zhang RL, Chopp M, Li Y, et al. (1994) Anti-ICAM-1 antibody reduces ischemic cell damage after transient middle cerebral artery occlusion in the rat. Neurology 44: 1747–1751.
Zhang Z, Chopp M, Tang W, et al. (1995): Postischemic treatment (2–4 hr) with the anti-CD11b and the anti-CD18 monoclonal antibodies are neuroprotective after transient (2h) focal cerebral ischemia in the rat. Brain Res 698: 79–85.
Zhang X-M, Ellis EF (1990) Superoxide dismutase reduces permeability and edema induced by hypertension in rats. Am J Physiol 259: H497–H503.
Zhao Q, Pahlmark K, Smith ML, Siesjö BK (1994) Delayed treatment with the spin trap α-phenyl-N-tret-butyl nitrone (PBN) reduced infarct size following transient middle cerebral artery occlusion in rats. Acta Physiol Scand 152: 349–450.
Zhou J, Meno JR, Hsu SSF, Winn HR (1994) Effects of theophylline and cyclohexyladenosine on brain injury follwoing normo- and hyperglycemic ischemia: A histopathologic study in the rat. J Cereb Blood Flow Metab 14: 166–173.
Zhu CZ, Auer RN (1995) Graded hypotension and MCA occlusion duration: Effect in transient focal ischemia. J Cereb Blood Flow Metab 15: 980-988.
Zielasek J, Archelos JJ, Toyka KV, et al. (1993) Expression of intercellular lesion adhesion moleculte-1 on rat microglial cells. Neurosci Lett 153: 136–139.
Zimmer R, Lanf R, Oberdörster G (1971) Post-ischemic reactive hyperemia of the isolated perfused brain of the dog. Pflügers Arch 328: 332–343.
Zivin JA, Venditto JA (1984) Experimental CNS ischemia: Serotonin antagonists reduce ro prevent damage. Neurology 34: 469–474.
Zivin JA (1985) Cyproheptadine reduces or prevents ischemia central nervous system damage. Neurology 35: 584–587.
Zivin JA, DeGirolami U (1986) Studies of the influence of biogenic amines on central nervous system ischemia. Stroke 17: 509–514.
Zoppo DGJ, Ferbert A, Otis S, et al. (1988) Local intra-arterial fibrinolytic therapy in acute carotid territory stroke: A pilot study. Stroke 19: 307–313.
Zoppo DGJ, Schmid-Schönbein GW, Mori E, et al. (1991): Polymorphonuclear leukocytes occlude capillaries following middle cerebral artery occlusion and reperfusion in baboons. Stroke 22: 1276–1283.
Zoratti M, Szabo I (1995): The mitochondrial permeability transient. Biochem Biophys Acta 1241: 139–176.
Zornig M, Evan GI (1996) Cell cycle: on target with myc. Current Biol 6: 1553–1556.
Zu Y, Cohen Y, Litt L, Change L-H, James TL (1991) Tolerance of low cerebral intracellular pH in rats during hyperbar hypercapnia. Stroke 22: 1303–1308.

Subject Index

A
Acetazolamide 26
Acetylcholine, 20,124,158
- Central ana lgetics 158
- Head injury 225
- Hypnotic agents 124
- Regulation of CBF 23
Acidosis (cerebral) 367
- Glia cell 367
- Head injury 221
- Hypercapnia 367
- Ischaemia 367
- Lactate 367
- Neuronal damage 367
- THAM 259
Actin 362
Adaptation
- CO2 (experimental) 23,54, 257
- CO2 (human) 25,54, 258
Adenosine 16, 189
- Autoregulation 190,191
- Blood-brain barrier 190
- Calcium uptake 352
- Cardiac arrythmia 191
- CBF 16, 189, 191, 351
- $CMRO_2$ 189, 191
- CO_2 reactivity 190
- CSF formation 190
- Excitatory amino acid 352
- Experimental studies 189
- Human studies 190
- Hyperaemia 242
- ICP 190
- Ischaemia 191
- Leukocyte function 352
- Protection 190, 352
- Rebound hypertension 189, 190
- Theophylline 352
Adrenergic receptors 371
Adrenogenic system
- Vasospasm (SAH) 300
Ageing
- CBF 12
- $CMRO_2$ 13
- Head injury 227
Air embolism 108, 212
Airway pressure 22
Alpha-agonists 20
Alfentanil 165
- Autoregulation 165
- CBF 165
- CO_2 reactivity 165
- Craniotomy 165
- CSF formation 165
- Experimental studies 165
- ICP 165
- Propofol 165
Althesin 132
- CBF 132
- $CMRO_2$ 132
- CO_2 reactivity 132
- Craniotomy 133
- EEG 133
- Experimental studies 132
- Head injury 133
- ICP 133
AMPA blockers 351
Aneurysmal SAH 15, 291
- Adrenogenic system 300
- Angiography 319
- Angioplasty of vasospasm 319
- Angiotensin IV 295
- Antithrombin III 310
- Aspirin 307
- Autoregulation 296, 300
- AVS 305
- Blood-brain barrier 296
- Bosentan 312
- Brain tissue oxygen tension 316
- Calcium (vasospasm) 298
- Cardiac arrhythmia 303
- Cardiopulmonary by-pass 318
- CBF 294, 295, 299, 301
- Cerebral blood volume 294
- Cerebral perfusion pressure 295
- Chatecholamine 301
- Clinical studies (CBF) 295
- Clinical studies ($CMRO_2$) 295
- Clot removal 316
- CMRO2 294, 295, 299
- Coagulation (vasospasm) 299
- Coil treatment 319
- Complement system (vasospasm) 299
- Controlled hypotension 98, 101, 183, 191, 321
- CO_2 reactivity 297, 300
- Creatine kinase (CSF) 302
- CSF dynamic 294
- CT scanning (Ficher) 314
- Cytokines (CSF) 302
- Denervation 301
- Desflurane 321
- Diamox 300
- Drainage 293, 317
- Ebselen 308
- ECG 303
- Eicosanoid 303, 307
- Endothelin 312
- Energy metabolism 298
- Epidemiology 291
- Experimental models 292
- Experimental studies 294, 297
- Extracranial/intracranial by-pass 320
- Fibrinolysis 294
- Free radical (vasospasm) 298
- Genetics 291
- Giant aneurysm 318
- Glasgow Outcome Scale 314
- Glucose utilisation 295
- Haemodilution 303
- Haemorrhagic infarct 304
- Heat shock protein 310
- Heparin 311
- Hunt and Hess 297, 313, 318
- Hydrocephalus 293
- Hyperaemia 295
- Hyperglycaemia 292
- Hypertensive encephalopathy 304
- Hyperventilation 297
- Hypervolaemia 304
- Hypothermia 321
- ICP 293
- Intraoperative angiography 319
- Intravascular balloon occlusion 318
- Jugular venous oxygen saturation 315
- Lactate (CSF) 302
- Laser surgery 320
- Lazaroid 305
- Leukotriens 307
- Lipid peroxidase 308
- Lipooxygenase 308
- Mannitol 320
- Median eminence 301
- Mexiletine 307
- Microdialysis 315
- Morphine 320
- Mortality 291, 317
- Multimodal monitoring 316
- Myocardial lesion 303

- Neuropeptides (vasospasm) 302, 309
- Neuropeptide Y 310
- Nicardipine 306
- Nimodipine 306, 320
- Nitric oxide 295, 308
- Operation 316
- Outcome 291
- Outflow resistance 294
- Papaverine 311
- Peak ICP pressure 293
- PET 296, 300
- pH (CSF) 302
- Phenoxybenzamine 301
- Phospholipase C 303
- Plasmin 308
- Plasmin activating factor 308
- Platelet function and activating factor 307, 310
- Prevalence and incidence 291
- Prognostic indices 291
- Propofol 321
- Prostacyclin 307
- Protein kinase C 298
- Pulmonary oedema 304
- Rebleeding 316
- Reduced CBF 295
- Rupture of aneurysm 318
- SPECT 296, 300
- Substance P 301
- Superoxide dismutase 305
- Swan-Ganz monitoring 304
- Temporal occlusion 318
- Tiralazad 305
- Tizanidine 312
- Transcranial Doppler 297, 314
- Traumatic SAH 236, 242
- Unruptured aneurysm 317
- Vasoactive intestinal polypeptide 310
- Vasospasm 293, 297
- Warning episodes 293
- Xenon CT scanning 300
- Zanthin oxidease 305

Aneurysm surgery 101,131
Angiography (SAH) 319
Angioplasty (SAH) 319
Angiotensin 200
- Aneurysmal SAH 295

Antithrombin III
- Aneurysmal SAH 310

Apoplexy
- Hyperventilation 258

Apoptosis 339
Arachidonic acid
- Oedema 345, 346

Aspartate, *see* also excitatory amino acid
- Head injury 232

Aspiration
- Risk 60

Aspirin
- Aneurysmal SAH 307

ATP *see* also Adenosine 189
- Head injury 224, 228

Atracurium 174
- CBF 174
- $CMRO_2$ 174
- ICP 175

Autoregulation 26,183
- Adenosine 190,191
- Alfentanil 165
- Anaesthetics 35
- Aneurysmal SAH 50, 296
- Blood-brain barrier 28
- Cardiac output 247
- Cerebral perfusion pressure 28
- CO_2 reactivity 30
- Dynamic studies 26
- Experimental studies 27
- False autoregulation 247
- Fentanyl 161
- Halothane 86, 88
- Head injury 30, 50, 223, 224, 246
- Hunt and Hess 297
- Hypertensive encephalopathy 29
- Hyperventilation 53
- Ischaemia 28, 344
- Isoflurane 34, 94
- Lower limit 27,29
- Ketamine 135
- Ketanserin 193
- Factors influencing CA 27
- Morphine 160
- Propofol 140,141
- Regional differences 28
- Reperfusion 344
- Sodium Nitroprusside 185
- Sevoflurane 102, 104
- Static studies 26
- Sufentanil 165
- Sympathetic innervation 29
- Time related changes 27, 29
- Transcranial Doppler 26, 297
- Transient hyperaemic response 248
- Vasoconstrictors 28
- Vasoparalysis 50
- Upper limit 29

Autoradiographic method 2
AVDO2
- Head injury 253

AVDO2 method 4
AVS (N,N-propylenedinedinicotinamide) 305

B

Barbiturate 18, 126
- Aneurysm 131
- A-V malformation 131
- Barbiturate reactivity 249
- Blood-brain barrier 127
- By pass operation 131
- Cardiac arrest 132
- Carotid surgery 131
- CBF 57, 126, 130
- Cerebral perfusion pressure 57
- Cerebral vasodilation 127
- Clinical studies 261
- $CMRO_2$ 57, 126, 130
- CO_2 reactivity 127
- Craniotomy 130
- EEG 58, 128, 130
- Energy metabolism 128
- Excitatory amino acid 18, 130
- Experimental studies 126, 261
- Free radical 129
- Glucose metabolism 128
- Guidelines (head injury) 268
- Halothane 89
- Head injury 131, 261
- Human studies 130
- Hypoxia 128
- ICP hypertension 129
- Inversesteal 128
- Ischaemia 129
- Metabolic regulation 18
- Nitric oxide 127
- Protection 18, 129
- Sedation 57
- Serotonin 130
- Tolerance 58, 127

Beta-Amyloid precurser protein 366
Bcl-2 gene family 360
Blood-brain barrier 32
- Adenosine 190
- Aneurysmal SAH 296
- Autoregulation 32
- Barbiturate 127
- Dopamine 199
- Head injury 222, 224
- Insulin 372
- Ischaemia 345
- Isoflurane 94
- Magnesium 373
- Mannitol 62
- Oedema 345
- Sodium Nitroprusside 185

Bohr effect 24, 52
Bold contrast 6
Bradykinin
- Bradykinin B_2 antagonist 262
- Cryogenic lesion 230
- Head injury 262

Brain-derived neurotrophic factor 366
Brain oedema *see* oedema
Brain retraction
- Ischaemia 340

Brain stem lesion
- CBF 243
- Head injury 226

Brain temperature
- Head injury 223

Brain tissue oxygen tension
- Aneurysmal SAH 316
- Cerebral perfusion pressure 255
- Head injury 255
- Head position 255
- Hyperventilation 255
- Ischaemia 339
- Jugular venous oxygen saturation 256

- Mannitol 256
- Outcome 255
- Oxygen fraction 256

C
Calcium 346
- Calmodulin 347
- Calpain 348
- Diacylglyceride 347
- Intracellular calcium 346
- Ischaemia 344, 346
- Magnesium 373
- Mitochondrial function 346
- Phospholipase 347
- Stores 346
- Vasospasm (SAH) 298
Calcium blockers (antagonists) 194, 306
- Conopeptide 349
- Emopamil 349
- Flunarizine 349
- Head injury 231, 232
- ICP 65
- Ischaemia 348
- Lidoflazin 349
- Mexiletine 307
- Nicardipine 194, 306, 349
- Nifidipine 194
- Nimodipine 262, 306, 348
- Vasospasm 306, 320
Calcitonin gene-related peptide
- Head injury 242
Calmodulin 347
Calpain 348
Captopril 197
Carbon dioxide *see* CO_2
Cardiac Arrhythmia
- Aneurysmal SAH 303
Cardiac output and CBF 16
- Autoregulation 247
Cardiolipin 346
Cardiopulmonary by-pass (SAH) 318
Carnitine 367
Caspase 361
Catalase 357
CBF methods 1
- $AVDO_2$ 4
- Autoradiographic method 2
- Doppler flowmetry 6
- Hydrogen clearance 1
- Inhalation method 4
- Intraarterial method 3
- Inhalation method 4
- Intravenous method 4
- Integral method 2
- Kety and Schmidt method 3
- Laser Doppler Flowmetry 7
- Microsphere technique 1
- MR imaging methods 6
- PET 5
- SPECT 4
- Stable Xenon method 5
- Venous outflow 2
CBF patterns
- Head injury 244
CBF regulation 12
- Adenosine 16
- CO_2 21
- Cardiacoutput 16
- Haemodilution 16
- Head injury 241
- Hypercapnia 21
- Hypocapnia 21
- Nitric oxide 16
- Oxygen tension 16, 17
- Viscosity 16
Central $\alpha 2$ agonists 194
Central venous pressure 48
Cerebral atrophy
- Head injury 226, 239
Cerebral autoregulation (CA) *see* autoregulation
Cerebral blood volume (CBV)
- Airway pressure 22
- Aneurysmal SAH 294
- Head injury 230, 241
- Hypocapnia 24
- ICP 47
Cerebral contusion
- Reduced CBF 242
Cerebral haemodynamics
- Aneurysmal SAH 294
Cerebral haemodynamic reserve 254
Cerebral perfusion pressure
- Aneurysmal SAH 295
- Cerebral perfusion targeted therapy 258
- Guidelines 267
- Head injury 244, 248, 258
- Mannitol 360
Cerebral oedema *see* oedema
Cerebral oligaemia, *see* reduced CBF
Cerebrospinal fluid
- Creatine kinase 251
- Lactate 251
- Nitric oxide 251
C-fos
- Head injury 226
- Ischaemia 360
Chatecholamine
- Insulin 373
- Vasospasm (SAH) 301
Chest injury, *see* lung injury
Children
- Head injury (outcome) 240
- Hyperaemia 241
Cholinergic receptors
- Head injury 233, 234
Cisatracurium 175
Clonidine 195
- Action 195
- Anaesthetic requierment 195
- CBF 195
- Central haemodynamics 195
- CO_2 reactivity 195
- Head injury 195, 264
- Protection 195
Clot removal (SAH) 317
CMRO2 14
- Ageing 14
- Aneurysmal SAH 15, 294, 299
- $CBF/CMRO_2$ coupling 14, 246
- CO_2 reactivity 249
- Dementia 15
- Diaschisis 15
- Endotoxaemia 15
- Epilepsy 15
- Free radical 249
- Head injury 15, 222, 245, 246
- Hypocapnia 22
- Infarction 246
- Mental performance 4
- Starvation 4
- Stress 4
c-Myc 363
Coagulopathy
- Head injury 240
Cognitive function
- Hyperaemia (head injury) 242
Coil treatment (SAH) 319
Collateral circulation 369
Consciousness (level)
- $CMRO_2$ 245
CO2 and CO2 reactivity 22, 25, 28, 52
- Adaptation 23,25
- Adenosine 190
- Althesin 132
- Alfentanil 165
- Aneurysmal SAH 297, 300
- Apoplexy 25, 258
- Autoregulation 30, 249
- Barbiturate 27
- Bohr effect 24, 52
- Brain tissue oxygen tension 255
- Clonidine 95
- Carotid surgery 25
- Cerebral blood volume 24
- $CMRO_2$ 249
- CSF formation 24
- Desflurane 105
- Experimental studies 25
- Fentanyl 161, 162
- Halothane 86, 88
- Head injury 25, 222, 224, 248
- Human studies 24
- Hypercapnia 21
- Impaired CO2 reactivity 23,24, 248
- Inverse steal 23,25
- Ischaemia 24, 344
- Isoflurane 94, 99
- Ketanserin 193
- Lactate 249
- Nitric oxide 24
- Outcome 248
- Propofol 140,141
- Protection 26
- Regional differences 248
- Reperfusion 344
- Sevoflurane 104
- Sodium Nitroprusside 185
- Steal phenomenon 22,24

- Sufentanil 164
- Time related changes 24
- Trimethaphan 188
Controlled hypotension 98, 183, 321
- Agents 184
- Baroreflex activity 184
- CBF 183
- Flow distribution 184
- Isoflurane 98, 101, 191
Corticosteroid 65
- Aneurysmal SAH 311, 374
- Head injury 374
- ICP hypertension 65
- Protection 374
- Spinal injury 374
COX2
- Head injury 231
CPAP
- ICP 49
Craniectomy (decompressive)
- Head injury 256
Craniotomy
- Alfentanil 165
- Althesin 133
- Barbiturate 130
- Droperidol 144
- Etomidate 134
- Halothane 89
- Isoflurane 99
- Propofol 142
- Remifentanil 167
Creatine kinase
- Aneurysmal SAH (CSF) 302
Cronassial 376
Cryogenic lesion 229
- Bradykinin 230
- Glucose utilisation 229
- ICP gradients 230
- Leukotriens 230
- Mannitol 230
- Vasopressin 230
CSF dynamic
- Aneurysmal SAH 294
CSF formation 27,64,68
- Adenosine 190
- Alfentanil 165
- CO_2 27
- Desflurane 105
- Enflurane 90
- Fentanyl 161
- Furosemide 64
- Halothane 87
- Head injury 238
- Midazolam 139
- Propofol 141
- Remifentanil 166
- Sevoflurane 102
CT scanning
- Aneurysmal SAH 313, 314
- Head injury 241, 250
Cyclooxygenase inhibitors 358
- Ibuprofen 359
- Indomethacin 358
- Ischaemia 358
- Zometirac 359
Cytokines
- Aneurysmal SAH 302
- Head injury 233
- Ischaemia 364

D
Dementia 15
Desflurane 104
- Aneurysmal SAH 321
- CBF 105
- $CMRO_2$ 105
- CO_2 reactivity 105
- Central haemodynamic 104
- CSF formation 105
- EEG 105
- Experimental studies 104
- Human studies 105
- ICP 105, 106
- Nitrous oxide 106
- Protection 105
Dexmedetomidine 196
- Action 196
- CBF 196
- $CMRO_2$ 196
- Cognition 197
- EEG 196
- Experimental studies 196
- Human studies 197
- ICP 196, 197
- Protection 196
Diamox
- Vasospasm (SAH) 300
Diaschisis 15
Diazepam 137
- CBF 137
- $CMRO_2$ 137
- Experimental studies 137
- GABA 137
- Glucose metabolism 138
- Human studies 138
- ICP 138
- Protection 138
Diffuse axonal injury 235
Diffuse swelling
- Head injury 243
Diffusion weighted MR imaging 6
Dihydroergotamine 49, 200, 264
- Clinical studies 264
- Experimental studies 264
- Head injury 264
- ICP 49
- Lund model 50, 264
Dihydrolipoat 357
Diltiazem 194
Dopamine 20, 199
- Experimental studies 199
- Head injury 259
- Human studies 200
Dipyridamole 191
Dopaminergic function
- Propofol 140
Doppler flowmetry 6
Dorsal raphe nucleus 19
Drainage (ventricular or spinal)
- Aneurysmal SAH 293, 317
- Head injury 256
Droperidol 143
- CBF 143,144
- $CMRO_2$ 143,144
- Craniotomy 144
- Experimental studies 143
- ICP 144
- Human studies 144
- Oedema 144
D-tubocuranine 174

E
ECG
- Aneurysmal SAH 303
EEG
- Althesin 133
- Barbiturate 58, 128, 130
- Desflurane 105
- Dexmedetomidine 196
- Enflurane 90, 91
- Etomidate 134
- Fentanyl 161,162
- Ischaemia 337
- Isoflurane 95, 100
- Ketamine 136, 137
- Mannitol 61
- Methohexitone 132
- Morphine 160
- Neurolept anaesthesia 163
- Nitrous oxide 108
- Propofol 141,143
- Remifentanil 166,
- Sevoflurane 102, 103
- Sufentanil 163, 164
Eicosanoid
- Aneurysmal SAH 303
- Clinical studies (SAH) 307
- Epoxygenase pathway 358
- Experimental studies (SAH) 307
- Ischaemia 358
- Lipid peroxidase 358
- Thromboxane 358
Emopamil
- Head injury 232
- Ischaemia 349
Enalaprilat 197
Endothelin and blockade
- Aneurysmal SAH 312
- Clinical studies (SAH) 313
- Experimental studies (SAH) 312
- Ischaemia 371
Endotoxaemia 15
Energy metabolism
- Vasospasm (SAH) 298
Enflurane 90
- CBF 90, 91
- Cerebral perfusion pressure 91
- $CMRO_2$ 90, 91
- CSF-formation 90
- EEG 90, 91

- Evoked potential 92
- Experimental studies 90
- Human studies 91
- ICP 90, 91
- Nitrous oxide 90

Epilepsy 15, 143, 176
- Guidelines for prophyllactic therapy 268

Epinephrine 199
Ergot alkaloids 200
Erythropoietin 375
Esmolol 192
Etanolone 145
- CBF 145
- $CMRO_2$ 145

Ethanol
- Head injury 225, 240

Etomidate 133
- Adrenocortical function 134
- CBF 133, 134
- Clinical studies 134
- $CMRO_2$ 133,134
- Craniotomy 134
- EEG 134
- Experimental studies 133
- Head injury 134
- ICP 133, 134
- Protection 133

Excitatory amino acid 125
- Adenosine 352
- AMPA blockers 351
- Barbiturate 125, 130
- Central analgetics 159
- Glycine antagonists 351
- Halothane 87
- Head injury 225, 231, 232
- Hypothermia 370
- Ischaemia 349
- Isoflurane 96
- Methionine sulfoximine 351
- NBQX blockers 351
- Nitric oxide 353
- NMDA blockers 350
- Oedema 346
- Propofol 140
- Riluzole 351
- Selfotel 262
- Spreading depression 341

Experimental models of aneurysmal SAH 292
- Femoral artery model 292
- Infusion model 292
- Pressure thresholds model 292
- Subarachnoid model 292

Experimental models of head injury 221
- Diffuse brain injury 227
- Fluid percussion model 223
- Impact model 222
- Mass expanding model 228
- Mock-CSF infusion model 228
- Non-impact acceleration model 221
- Piston model 223, 227
- Subdural haematoma 227
- Traumatic SAH 227
- Weight drop model 223

Extradural haematoma 235

F

"False" autoregulation
- CO_2 reactivity 249
- Head injury 247

Fentanyl 161
- Autoregulation 161
- CBF 161, 162
- Clinical application 163
- $CMRO_2$ 161, 162
- CO_2 reactivity 161, 162
- CSF formation 161
- EEG 161, 162
- Energy charge 161
- Experimental studies 161
- Head injury 262
- ICP 162
- Ischaemia 162
- Limbic system 161
- Protection 162
- Tolerance 161

Fibrinolysis
- Aneurysmal SAH 294

Fibroblast growth factor
- Head injury 226
- Ischaemia 375

Flumazenil 139
Flunarizine 349
Foramen ovale 213
Free radical and scavengers
- Aneurysmal SAH 298
- AVS 305
- Barbiturate 129
- Clinical studies 262
- CO_2 reactivity 249
- Dihydrolipoat 357
- Experimental studies 262, 304
- Head injury 231, 233
- Iron 356
- Lazaroid 231, 305
- N-acetylcystein 357
- Nitric oxide 354
- Propofol 140
- Spin trapping agents 357
- Superoxide dismutase 305
- Vasospasm (SAH) 298
- Zanthin oxidase 305

Fructose-1,6,-biphosphate 368
Furosemide 64
- CSF formation 64
- ICP 64

G

GABA 144, 370
- CBF 144
- $CMRO_2$ 144
- Diazepam 137
- Halothane 87
- Head injury 234
- Histamin 23
- Hypnotic agents 125
- Ischaemia 370
- Midazolam 138
- Muscinol 370
- Propofol 139

Gangliosides 375
- Cronassial 376
- GM-1 375
- Ischaemia 375
- Protection 375

Gender
- Head injury 240

Gene expression 360
Giant aneurysm 318
Glasgow Coma Scale 239, 249
Glasgow Outcome Scale 314
Glia cell
- Acidosis 367

Glia cell activation 364
Glucose
- Ischaemia 368

Glucose utilisation
- Aneurysmal SAH 295
- Cryogenic lesion 229
- Head injury 223

Glutamate, *see* also excitatory amino acid
- Head injury 232

Glycerol 63
GM-1 (monosialoganglioside) 375
Guidelines (head injury)
- Americal guidelines 266
- EBIC-guidelines 265

H

Haemodilution
- CBF regulation 16
- Clinical studies (SAK) 303
- Experimental studies (SAH) 303

Halothane 85
- Autoregulation 86, 88
- $AVDO_2$ 88
- Barbiturate 89
- Blood-brain barrier 86
- CBF 85, 88
- CBF/$CMRO_2$ 85, 88
- Cerebral oedema 86
- Cerebral perfusion pressure 86, 88
- $CMRO_2$ 85, 88, 245
- CO_2 reactivity 86, 88
- Craniotomy 89
- CSF formation 87
- CVR 85, 88
- Experimental studies 85
- Excitatory amino acids 87
- GABA 87
- Hyperventilation 89
- ICP 86, 88
- Nitric oxide 85
- Protection 86

Head injury 15, 221
- Age 227

- Althesin 133
- American Guidelines 266
- ATP 224
- Autoregulation 223, 224, 246, 247, 253
- AVDO2 253
- Barbiturate 131, 261
- Barbiturate reactivity 249
- Blood-brain barrier 222, 224
- Bradykinin B2 antagonist 262
- Brain stem 226
- Brain temperature 223, 226
- Brain tissue oxygen tension 255
- Calcium blocker 232
- Calcium homeostasis 231
- CBF patterns 244
- Cerebral atrophia 226, 239
- Cerebral blood volume 230, 241
- Cerebral contusion 235, 242
- Cerebral haemodynamic reserve 254
- Cerebral perfusion pressure 244, 248, 255, 258
- Cholinergic receptors 233
- Clonidine 195, 264
- $CMRO_2$ 245
- CO_2 reactivity 222, 224, 253
- Contre coup 235
- COX2 231
- CPP targeted therapy 258
- Craniectomy (decompressive) 256
- Creatine kinase 251
- CSF formation 238
- CT scanning 241, 250
- Cytokines 233
- Dextromethorphan 232
- Dihydroergotamine 264
- Diffuse axonal injury 235
- Diffuse swelling 237
- Dopamine 259
- Emopamil 232
- EBIC-guidelines 265
- Ethanol 225, 240
- Excitatory amino acid 225, 231, 232
- Experimental studies 221
- Extradural haematoma 235
- Fentanyl 161, 262
- Fibroblast growth factor 226
- Free radical 231
- Free radical scavenger 233, 263
- GABA 234
- Genetic aspect 227
- Glasgow Coma Scale 239, 249
- Glucose utilisation 223, 246
- Heat shock protein 226, 231, 234
- Hyperaemia 237, 241, 242
- Hyperbar oxygen therapy 262
- Hyperglycaemia 240, 252
- Hypertonic saline 263
- Hyperventilation 51,52, 247, 257
- Hypothermia 260, 370
- ICP 237, 244
- ICP-targeted therapy 259
- Indomethacin 55, 264
- Intracellular pH 229
- Intracerebral haematoma 235
- Inverse steal 249
- Ischaemia 228, 237, 238, 243
- Jugular venous oxygen saturation 253, 254, 256
- Ketamine 232
- Lactate 224, 251
- Lactate/oxygen index 253
- Leukocyte function 226, 233
- Lund model 50, 264
- Lung injury 236, 240
- Magnesium 234
- Mannitol 256, 263
- Microdialysis 252
- Mitochondiral function 224
- Morphine 262
- Neurogenic pulmonary oedema 236
- Neurological assessment 249
- Neuroworsening 250
- Nicardipine 262
- Nimodipine 262
- Near infrared spectroscopy (NIRS) 254
- Nitric oxide 225, 251
- Nociceptin orphanin 225
- Norepinephrine 259
- Nutritional support (guidelines) 268
- Oedema 223, 229, 235, 238
- Outcome assessment 239, 255
- PET scanning 246
- Phosphocreatinine 224
- Platelet function 226, 231
- Pressure volume relation 238
- Primary damage 235
- Prognostic indicators 239
- Propofol 143, 262
- Prostaglandin 231
- Reduced CBF 242
- Secondary damage 236
- S-100B 252
- Selfotel 262
- Spasm of arteries 224, 245
- Spinal drainage 256
- Stable Xenon-CT 245
- Subdural haematoma 235, 242
- Thalamic lesion 239
- THAM 259
- Therapy 256
- Tissue peaks 247
- Transcranial Doppler 250
- Transneuronal degeneration 226, 239
- Traumatic SAH 236
- Vasoreactivity cascade 248
- Ventricular drainage 256
- Ventricular volume 237
- Water shed ischaemia 238

Head position and ICP 48
- Brain tissue oxygen tension 255

Heat shock protein
- Aneurysmal SAH 310
- Head injury 226, 231, 234
- Ischaemia 365

Heparin
- Aneurysmal SAH 311
- Ischaemia 376

Hibernation 13

Histamine
- CBF 21
- Ischaemia 372

Histopathology
- Vasospasm (SAH) 299

Human studies of CBF 13

Human studies of $CMRO_2$ 14

Hunt and Hess 313, 318

Hydrocephalus 47, 293
- Aneurysmal SAH 293

Hydrogen clearance and CBF 1

Hyperaemia
- Aneurysmal SAH 295
- Calcitonin gene-related peptide 242
- Cognitive function 242
- Head injury 241, 242
- Transcranial Doppler 242

Hyperbar oxygen therapy 262

Hypercapnia 367

Hyperglycaemia
- Aneurysmal SAH 292
- Head injury 240, 252
- Ischaemia 368
- Oedema 346

Hypertensive drugs 198

Hypertensive encephalopathy
- Autoregulation 29
- Aneurysmal SAH 304

Hyperthermia
- Aneurysmal SAH 321
- Head injury 226

Hypertonic saline 63
- Clinical studies 263
- Experimental studies 263
- Head injury 263

Hyperventilation 21, 51
- Adaptation 257
- Aneurysmal SAH 297
- Autoregulation 53, 247
- Beneficial effects 55
- Bohr effect 52
- Brain tissue oxygen tension 255
- Detrimental effects 55
- Diaschisis 24
- Guidelines 267
- Halothane 66
- Head injury 257
- ICP 24, 51-54
- Inverse steal 23, 28 ,51, 53
- Ischaemia 52, 255, 339
- Mechanism 21
- Nitric oxide 22
- Pediatric patients 52
- Prolonged continuous hyperventilation 25

Hypervolaemia
- Clinical studies (SAH) 304
- Haemorrhagiv infarct 304
- Hypertensive encephalopathy 304
- Pulmonary oedema 304

Hypocapnia *see* hyperventilation
Hypoglycaemia 369
Hypothermia 17, 56
- Aneurysmal SAH 321
- Brain temperature 77
- Clinical studies 19, 57, 260
- Excitatory amino acid 370
- Experimental studies 260
- Head injury 260, 370
- Ischaemia 369
- Isoflurane 97
- Mechanism 18
- Meningitis 370
- Protection 17
- Q-10 17
Hypoxia-inducible factor 364
Hypoxia *see* oxygen tension

I

Ibubrofen 359
ICAM
- Head injury 233
ICP 43
- Adenosine 190
- Alfentanil 165
- Althesin 133
- Aneurysmal SAH 293
- Atracurium 175
- Barbiturate 129, 130
- Critical levels of ICP 45, 237
- Desflurane 105, 106
- Dexmedetomidine 196, 197
- Diazepam 138
- Droperidol 144
- Enflurane 90, 91
- Etomidate 133, 134
- Fentanyl 162
- Furosemide 64
- Gradients 230
- Guidelines 267
- Halothane 86, 88
- Head injury 237
- Hypocapnia 24
- Indication for ICP monitoring 46, 238, 267
- Isoflurane 95, 100
- Ketamine 136,
- Ketanserin 193
- Labetalol 192
- Lidocaine 177
- Mannitol 61
- Methodology 43
- Midazolam 139
- Monitoring technology 46
- Morphine160
- Neurolept anaesthesia 163
- Nitroglycerin 186, 187
- Nitrous oxide 108
- Normal values of ICP 44
- Phenoperidine 160
- Pressure gradients 228
- Pressure volume relationship 46, 228
- Pressure waves 44,
- Propofol 140
- Regional difference in ICP 45
- Remifentanil 166
- Sodium Nitroprusside 185, 186
- Sevoflurane 102, 104
- Succinylcholine 174
- Sufentanil 164
- Threshold for ICP treatment (guidelines) 267
- Trimethaphan 188
- Vasospasm (SAH) 315
- Xenon 109
ICP-hypertension 47
- Analgetics 59
- Aneurysmal SAH 65
- Body position 48
- Calcium blockers 65
- Central venous pressure 48
- Cerebral perfusion pressure 258
- Control of CBV 47
- Corticosteroid 65
- CPAP
- CPP-targeted therapy 258
- CSF formation 48
- Dihydroergotamine 49
- Furosemide 64
- Glycerol 63
- Guidelines 267, 268
- Head injury 65, 237
- Head position 48
- Hypertonic saline 63, 263
- Hyperventilation 51-55
- Hypnotic agents 57
- Hypothermia 56
- ICP-targeted therapy 259
- Indomethacin 55
- Kappa-opioid 65
- Lidocaine 59
- Mannitol 60
- Medical approach 47
- Muscular relaxation 60
- PEEP 49
- Sodium 60
- Strategies in the control of ICP 66–69
- Suction procedure 49
- Surgical approach 47
- THAM 66
- Theophyllamine 56
Idaxoxan 371
Imidazole receptors 372
Immediate early genes 360
Immunoreactivity
- Vasospasm (SAH) 299
Indomethacin 55
- Experimental studies 55, 264
- Head injury 55, 264
- Human studies 55, 264
- Ischaemia 358
Infarction
- CMRO2 (head injury) 246
- Ischaemia 338
Inflammatory response
- Head injury 233
Inhalation anaesthetics 83
- Ca^{2+} -ATPase 84
- Cellular enzyme systems 83
- Excitatory amino acids 84
- GABA 84
- K^+ channels 84
- Nitric oxide 84
Inhalation method of CBF 4
Insulin 372
- Blood-brain barrier 372
- CBF regulation 21
- Chatecholamine 373
- Ischaemia 372
- Protection 372
Integral method of CBF measurement 2
Interleukins
- Ischaemia 365
Intraarterial method of CBF 3
Intracellular pH
- Ischaemia 228
Intracerebral haematoma 235
Intraoperative angiography (SAH) 319
Intravascular balloon occlusion (SAH) 318
Intravenous method of CBF 4
Inverse steal
- Head injury 249
- Hyperventilation 23, 28, 51, 53, 249
- Barbiturate 128
Iron 356
Ischaemia 337
- Acidosis (cerebral) 367
- Actin 362
- Adenosine 351
- Adrenergic receptors 371
- AMPA blockers 351
- Anaesthesia 340
- Apoptosis 339
- Arachidonic acid 345
- Autoregulation 344
- Bcl-2 gene family 360
- Beta-amyloid precurser protein 366
- Brain-derived neurotrophic factor 366
- Brain retractor 340
- Calcium 344, 346
- Calcium blockers 348
- Calmodulin 347
- Calpain 348
- Carnitine 367
- Caspase family 361
- Catalase 357
- CBF 337, 341
- $CMRO_2$ 341
- c-Myc 363
- Conopeptide 349
- Complete ischaemia
- CO_2 reactivity 344
- Corticosteroid 374
- Cyclooxygenase inhibitors 358
- Cytokines 364
- Cytotoxic oedema 345

- Diacylglyceride 347
- Diffuse weighted MR imaging 6
- Dihydrolipoat 357
- Eicosanoids 358
- Emopamil 349
- Endonuchleasis 347
- Endothelin 371
- Erythropoietin 375
- Excitatory amino acid 349
- Fibroblast growth factor 375
- Flunarizine 349
- Free radical 354
- Free radical scavengers 356
- Fructose-1,6,-biphosphate 368
- GABA 370
- Gangliosides 375
- Gene expression 360
- Glia cell activation 364, 367
- Glucose 368
- Glycine antagonist 351
- Head injury 238, 243
- Heat shock protein 365
- Heparin 376
- Histamine 372
- Hyperglycaemia 368
- Hyperventilation 52
- Hypoglycaemia 369
- Hypothermia 369
- Hypoxia-inducible factor 364
- ICP 244
- Idazoxan 371
- Imidazole receptors 372
- Immediate early gene 360
- Incomplete ischaemia 228
- Indomethacin 358
- Infarct 338
- Interleukins 365
- Iron 356
- Jugular venous oxygen saturation 254
- Lactate 367
- Lamin 362
- Lazaroid 356
- Leukocyte activation 363
- Lidoflazin 349
- Lipid peroxidase 358
- Magnesium 373
- Mannitol 61
- Methionin sulfoximine 351
- Mitochondrial function 346
- MR studies 6, 340
- Muscinol 370
- N-acetylcystein 357
- NBQX blockers 351
- Neuronal apoptosis inhibitory factor 366
- Nicardipine 349
- Nimodipine 348, 349
- Nitric oxide 352
- Nitric oxide synthase 366
- NMDA blockers 350
- No reflow 343
- Nucleus ceruleus 371
- Oedema 343, 344
- Oestrogen 375
- Opioid receptors 373
- Ornithine decarboxylase 360
- Penumbra 338
- Peptide growth factor 366
- PET studies 340, 343
- Phospholipase 347, 359
- Prazosin 371
- Progesterone 375
- Programmed cell death 339
- Protease 347
- Protein synthesis 359
- Pyruvate 367
- Reperfusion 341
- Riluzole 351
- Serine proteases 366
- Serotonin 371
- Spin trapping agents 357
- Spreading depression 340
- Subdural haematoma 227
- Superoxide dismutase 357
- Tau protein 359
- Theophylline 352
- Transcription factor
- Threshold 254, 337
- Thromboxane 358
- Tirilazad 357
- Tumour necrosis factor 365
- Vasogenic oedema 345
- Water shed areas 238

Isoflurane 92, 191
- Aneurysm surgery 101
- Autoregulation 94, 99
- Blood-brain barrier 94
- Brain temperature 97
- CBF 92, 99
- Cerebral perfusion pressure 100
- Cerebrovascular resistance 92
- $CMRO_2$ 92, 99
- Controlled hypotension 98, 101, 191
- CO_2 reactivity 94, 99
- Coronary by-pass 100
- Craniotomy 99, 100
- EEG 95, 100
- Evoked potential 101
- Excitatory amino acid 96
- Experimental studies 92
- Glucose metabolism 94
- ICP 95, 100
- Labetalol
- Nitrous oxide 97, 99
- Nitric oxide 93
- Oedema 98
- Pial vessels 93
- Protection 95, 101
- Spreading depression 97

J

Jugular venous saturation 4
- Aneurysmal SAH 315
- Brain tissue oxygen tension 256
- Near infrared spectroscopy 254

K

Kappa-opioid 65
Ketamine 135
- Autoregulation 135
- CBF 135,136
- Clinical application 137
- $CMRO_2$ 135,136
- EEG 136, 137
- Experimental studies 135
- Glucose metabolism 136
- Head injury 232
- Human studies 136
- ICP 136
- Protection 136
- Receptor action 135

Ketanserin 193
- Autoregulation 193
- CBF 193
- $CMRO_2$ 193
- CO_2 reactivity 193
- Experimental studies 193
- Human studies 193
- ICP 193

Kety and Schmidt method 3

L

Labetalol 192
- CBF 192
- ICP 192
- Isoflurane 192

Lactate
- Aneurysmal SAH 302
- CO_2 reactivity 249
- False" autoregulation 247
- Head injury 221, 224
- Hyperaemia 242
- Ischaemia 367

Lamin 362
Laser Doppler flowmetry 7
Laser surgery (SAH) 320
Laxaroid 356
Leukocyte adhesion molecules 363
Leukocyte function
- Adenosine 352
- Head injury 226
- Ischaemia 363

Leukotriens 307
- Clinical studies (SAH) 307
- Cryogenic lesion 230
- Experimental studies (SAH) 307

Lidocaine 59, 175
- Air embolism 216
- CBF 176
- Clinical studies 59, 177
- $CMRO_2$ 176
- Endotracheal intubation 177
- Epilepsy 176
- Experimental studies 59, 175
- Human studies 59, 177
- ICP 59, 177
- Oedema 346
- Protection 59, 176

Lidoflazin 349
Limbic system 161
Lipid peroxidase 358
Locus ceruleus 21
Lung injury
- Head injury 236, 240

M

Magnesium 373
- Blood-brain barrier 373
- Head injury 234
- Ischaemia 373
- Protection 373
Mannitol 60
- Aneurysmal SAH 320
- Blood-brain barrier 62
- Brain tissue oxygen tension 256
- CBF 61, 263
- Cerebral perfusion pressure 62
- $CMRO_2$ 61, 263
- Cryogenic lesion 230
- EEG 61
- Experimental studies 61
- Guidelines 268
- Head injury 263
- ICP 61
- Ischaemia 61
- Oedema 61
- Osmotic gradient 60
- Rebound phenomenon 62
Mass lesion 47
Median eminence
- Vasospasm (SAH) 301
Medical approach to ICP control 47
Meningitis
- Hypothermia 370
Methionin sulfoximine 351
Methohexitone 132
- CBF 132
- $CMRO_2$ 132
- EEG 132
- Experimental studies 132
- Human studies 132
Mexiletine 307
Microdialysis
- Aneurysmal SAH 315
- Head injury 252
- Propofol 142
Microglia
- Head injury
Microsphere method of CBF 1
Midazolam 138
- CBF 138, 139
- $CMRO_2$ 138, 139
- CSF formation 139
- Experimental studies 138
- Flumazenil 139
- GABA 138
- Human studies 139
- ICP 139
- Nitrous oxide 138, 139
- Protection 138
Mitochondrial function
- Ischaemia 346
MR imaging techniques 6
MR scanning
- Ischaemia 340
Morphine 159
- Aneurysmal SAH 320
- Autoregulation 160
- CBF 159, 160
- $CMRO_2$ 159, 160
- EEG 160
- Experimental studies 159
- Head injury 262
- ICP 160
- Human studies 160
Moyamoya disease 102
Muscinol 370
Myeoloperoxidase
- Head injury 240
Myocardial lesion
- Aneurysmal SAH 303

N

N-acetylcystein 357
Nalaxone 168
- CBF 168
- $CMRO_2$ 168
- Ischaemia 373
- Neurolept anaesthesia 163
- Protection 168
Near infrared spectroscopy (NIRS)
- Jugular oxygen saturation 254
- Head injury 254
Nephrotoxicity (sevoflurane) 103
Neurogenic pulmonary oedema
- Head injury 236
Neurogenic regulation of CBF 19
- Acetylcholine 19
- Alpha-agonist 20
- Dopamine 20
- Dorsal raphe nucleus 19
- Locus ceruleus 19
- Neuropeptides 20
- Sympathectomy 20
- Trigeminal system 19
- Vasopressin 20
Neurolept anaesthesia 163
- CBF 163
- $CMRO_2$ 163
- EEG 163
- ICP 163
- Nalaxone 163
- Oedema 163
- Physiostigmin 163
Neuronal apoptosis inhibitory protein 366
Neuropeptides 22
- Vasospasm (SAH) 302, 309
Neuropeptide Y
- Aneurysmal SAH 310
Neuroworsening 250
Nicardipine 194
- Clinical studies (SAH) 306
- Cryogenic lesion 232
- Experimental studies (SAH) 306
- Head injury 262
- Ischaemia 348, 349
Nifidipine 194
Nimodipine
- Experimental studies (SAH) 306
- Clinical studies (SAH) 306, 320
- Head injury 262
- Intrathecal 306
- Vasospasm (SAH) 306
Nitric oxide
- Aneurysmal SAH 295, 308
- Barbiturate 127
- Blood-brain barrier 185
- Cerebrospinal fluid 251
- Clinical studies (SAH) 309
- CO_2 21
- Glia cell 353
- Excitatory amino acid 353
- Experimental studies (SAH) 308
- Free radical 354, 355
- Head injury 225
- Ischaemia 352
- NMMA 21
- NO-synthase inhibitors 353
- NO synthesis 352
- Protection 354
- Regulation of CBF 16, 20
- Spreading depression 341
Nitric oxide synthase 366
Nitroglycerin 186
- Action 196
- CBF 196
- $CMRO_2$ 186
- Experimental studies 196
- Human studies 187
- ICP 186, 187
- Pulmonary function 187
Nitrous oxide 106
- Air embolism 213
- CBF 106, 107
- $CMRO_2$ 106
- EEG 108
- Experimental studies 106
- ICP 108
- Midazolam 138, 139
- Propofol 142
- Sitting position 108
- Stress 107
- Supplement to anaesthesia 107
- Protection 107
NBQX blockers 351
NMDA blockers
- Ischaemia 350
Norepinephrine 126, 199
- CBF 199
- $CMRO_2$ 199
- Head injury 259
- Hypnotic agents 126
- Receptor 199
NO synthase inhibitors 353
NO-synthesis 352
Nuclei A1 and A2, *see* adrenogenic system

Nucleus ceruleus 371

O

Oedema 98 ,144,183, 229, 344
- Arachidomic acid 345
- Blood-brain barrier 345
- Cryogenic lesion 229
- Cytotoxic oedema 345
- Droperidol 144
- Excitatory amino acid 346
- Glucose 346
- Glucose utilization 229
- Head injury 223
- Hydrostatic pressure gradient 344
- Isoflurane 98
- Leukotriens 346
- Mannitol 61
- Head injury 223, 229, 233, 238
- Ischaemia 229, 343, 344
- Reperfusion 343, 345
- Vasogenic oedema 345

Oestrogen 375
Opioid receptors 373
Ornithine decarboxylase 360
Outcome
- Aneurysmal SAH 291
- $CMRO_2$ (head injury) 246
- CO_2 reactivity (head injury) 248
- Head injury (children) 240

Outflow resistance
- Aneurysmal SAH 294

Oxygen tension and CBF 17
- Adenosine 16
- Barbiturate 128
- CBF 16
- Head injury 17, 223
- Hyperbar oxygen therapy 262
- Nitric oxide 16

P

Pancuronium 174
Papaverine
- Clinical studies (SAH) 311
- Experimental studies (SAH) 311

PEEP
- Air embolism 214
- ICP-hypertension 49

Penumbra 338
Peptide growth factor 366
Perfusion weighted MR imaging 6
PET 5
- Aneurysmal SAH 296
- Head injury 246
- Ischaemia 340
- Vasospasm (SAH) 300

Pethidin 160
- CBF 160
- $CMRO_2$ 160
- Shivering 160

Phenoperidine 160
- CBF 160
- ICP 160

Phenoxybenzamine
- Vasospasm (SAH) 301

Phosphocreatine
- Head injury 224, 228

Phospholipase C 347
- Aneurysmal SAH 303
- Ischaemia 359

Physiostigmin 163
Pipecuronium 175
Plasmin and Plasmin activating factor
- Aneurysmal SAH 308

Platelet function and activating factor
- Aneurysmal SAH 307, 310
- Head injury 226, 231

Postoperative period 193
Prazosin 371
Pressure reactivity index 248
Pressure volume relation 46
- Head injury 228, 238

Pressure waves
- Aneurysmal SAH 293

Primary damage (head injury) 235
Procaine 178
Progesterone 375
Prognostic indicators
- Aneurysmal SAH 291
- Head injury 239

Propofol 139
- Aneurysmal SAH 321
- Autoregulation 140,141
- CBF 140,141
- Clinical application 143
- $CMRO_2$ 140,141
- CO_2 reactivity 140, 141
- Craniotomy 142
- CSF formation 141
- Dopaminergic system 140
- EEG 141,143
- Epilepsy 143
- Experimental studies 139
- Excitatory amino acid 140
- Free radical 140
- GABA 139
- Glucose metabolism 141
- Head injury 143, 262
- Human studies 141
- ICP 140
- Microdialysis 142
- Nitrous oxide 142
- Protection 141, 143
- Total intravenous anaesthesia 142

Propranolol 192
Prostacyclin
- Aneurymal SAH 307

Prostaglandin 197
- Head injury 231

Protease 347
Protection
- Adenosine 190, 352
- Barbiturate 18, 129
- Clonidine 195
- Desflurane 105
- Dexmedetomidine 196
- Diazepam 138
- Etomidate 133
- Fentanyl 162
- Gangliosides 375
- Halothane 86
- Heat shock protein 365
- Hypothermia 369
- Insulin 372
- Isoflurane 95, 101
- Ketamine 136
- Lidocaine 59, 176
- Magnesium 373-
- Midazolam 138
- Naloxone 168
- Nitric oxide 354
- Nitrous oxide 107
- Opioid receptors 373
- Propofol 141,143

Protein kinase C
- Vasospasm (SAH) 298

Protein synthesis
- Ischaemia 359

Pulmonary oedema
- Aneurysmal SAH 304

Purkince cell
- Head injury 226

Pyruvate 367

R

Rebleeding (SAH) 316
Rebound phenomenon (hypertension) 184
- Adenosine 189
- Sodium nitroprusside 184, 186

Rebound phenomenon (ICP hypertension)
- Mannitol 62

Reduced CBF
- Aneurysmal SAH 295
- Brain stem lesion 243
- Diffuse swelling 243
- Head injury 242, 243
- Oedema 243
- Water shed areas 243

Regulation of CBF
Remifentanil 166
- CBF 166
- CO_2 reactivity 166
- Craniotomy 167
- CSF formation 166
- EEG 166, 167
- Experimental studies 166
- Human studies 166
- ICP 166, 167

Reperfusion (ischaemia) 341
- Autoregulation 344
- Calcium 344
- CBF 341
- $CMRO_2$ 31
- CO_2 reactivity 344
- Hyperaemia 342
- No reflow 343
- Oedema 343
- PET studies 343

Ropivacaine 178
Rupture of aneurysm 318

S

SAH *see* Subarachnoid haemorrhage
Secondary damage (head injury) 236
Selfotel 262
Septicaemia
- Head injury 240
Serine proteases 366
Serotonin 371
- Barbiturate 130
Sevoflurane 102
- Autoregulation 102, 103
- CBF 102, 103
- Central haemodynamic 103
- $CMRO_2$ 102, 103
- CO_2 reactivity 104
- CSF formation 102
- EEG 102, 103
- Experimental studies 102
- ICP 102, 104
- Human studies 103
- Nephrotoxicity 103
S-100B
- Head injury 252
Sitting position 211
- Air embolism 212
- Anaesthesia 211
- CBF 212
- Deoxycycline 216
- Diagnosis 214
- Durant 216
- ECG 211
- Foramen ovale 213
- Hypotension 216
- Lidocaine 216
- Morbidity 215
- Nitrous oxide 258
- PEEP 214
- Pneumocephalon 212
- Surgical procedure 213
- Treatment 215
- Venous pressure 214
Sodium Nitroprusside 184
- Action 184
- Aneurysmal SAH 309
- Autoregulation 185
- Baroreflex activity 186
- Blood-brain barrier 185
- CBF 185, 186
- $CMRO_2$ 185, 186
- CO_2 reactivity 185
- Experimental studies 184
- Human studies 186
- Hypoxia 186
- ICP 185, 186
- Pulmonary shunt 186
- Rebound phenomenon 184, 186
- Tissue oxygen tension 185
- Toxicity 184
SPECT 4
- Aneurysmal SAH 296
- Vasospasm (SAH) 300
Spinal CSF drainage 47
Spin trapping agents 357
Spreading depression 340
- Excitatory amino acid 341
- Nitric oxide 341
- Neuronal damage 340
- Tolerance 341
Stable Xenon method 5
- Head injury 245
Starvation 14
Steal phenomenen 22, 51
Steroid *see* corticosteroid
Stress 14
Subarachnoid haemorrhage (SAH) *see* aneurysmal SAH
Subdural Haematoma 235
- CBF 242
Substance P
- Vasospasm (SAH) 301
Succinylcholine 60, 174
- CBF 174
- ICP 60, 174
Sufentanil 163
- Autoregulation 164
- CBF 163, 164
- $CMRO_2$ 163, 164
- CO_2 reactivity 164
- EEG 163, 164
- Experimental studies 163
- Humans studies 164
- ICP 164, 167
Superoxide dismutase
- Aneursmal SAH
- Head injury 233, 263
- Ischaemia 357
Surgical approach to ICP control 47
- Craniectomy 256
Sympathectomy 20
Swan-Ganz monitoring
- Aneurysmal SAH 304

T

Tau protein 359
Temporal occlusion (SAH) 318
Tetracaine 178
Thalamic lesion
- Head injury 239
THAM 66
- Experimental studies 259
- Clinical studies 260
- Head injury 259
- ICP Hypertension 66
Theophylline 56, 191
- Adenosine 351
- Apoplexy 56
- Inverse steal 56
- Ischaemia 56, 352
Therapy
- Air embolism 215
- Aneurysmal SAH 303
- Head injury 256
Threshold of ischaemia 337
Thromboxane 358
Tiralazad
- Experimental studies (SAH) 305
- Clinical studies (SAH) 305
- Ischaemia 356
Tissue peaks 247
Tizanidine 312
Total intravenous anaesthesia
- Propofol 142
Torasemide
- Cryogenic lesion 230
Toxaemia 15
Transcranial Doppler
- Aneurysmal SAH 297, 314
- Clinical studies (SAH) 315
- Experimental studies (SAH) 314
- Head injury 250
- Transient hyperaemic response 248
Transcription factors 362
Transient hyperaemic response 248
Transneuronal degeneration
- Head injury 226, 239
Traumatic SAH 236, 242
Trigeminal system 19
Trimethaphan 187
- Action 187
- CBF 188
- Clinical application 189
- CO_2 reactivity 188
- Experimental studies 187
- Human studies 188
- ICP 188–
- Renin 188
Tumour necrosis factor 365

U

Urapidil 193

V

Vasogenic oedema 345
Vasoparalysis
- Aneurysmal SAH 293
Vasopressin 20
- Cryogenic lesion 230
Vasoreactivity cascade
- Head injury 248
Vasoactive intestinal polypeptide
- Clinical studies (SAH) 310
- Experimental studies (SAH) 310
Vasospasm
- Adrenogenic system 300
- Aneurysmal SAH 297
- Angioplasty 319
- Autoregulation 300
- Brain tissue oxygen tension 316
- Calcium (SAH) 298
- CBF 299, 300
- Cerebrospinal fluid 302
- Chatecholamine 301
- $CMRO_2$ 299, 300
- Coagulation 299
- Complement system 299

- CO_2 reactivity 300
- Diamox 300
- Endothelin 312
- Energy metabolism 298
- Experimental studies (SAH) 297
- Extra/intracranial by pass 320
- Free radical 298
- Head injury 224, 245
- Histopathology 299
- ICP 315
- Jugular venous oxygen saturation 315
- Median eminence 301
- Microdialysis 315
- Multimodal monitoring 316
- Neuropeptides 302
- PET 300
- Phenoxybenzamine 301
- Protein kinase C 298
- SPECT 300
- Substance P 301
- Transcranial Doppler 314
- Xenon CT scanning 300

Vecuronium 175
Venous outflow technique 2
Ventricular drainage 47
Ventricular volume
- Head injury 237

Viscosity and CBF 16
Vitamin E
- Head injury 240

W

Warning episode (ICP) 293

X

Xenon 108
- Action109
- CBF 109
- ICP 109

Xenon-CT scanning
- Vasospasm (SAH) 300

Z

Zanthin oxidase 305
Zometirac 359

MIX
Papier aus verantwortungsvollen Quellen
Paper from responsible sources
FSC® C105338

If you have any concerns about our products,
you can contact us on
ProductSafety@springernature.com

In case Publisher is established outside the EU,
the EU authorized representative is:
Springer Nature Customer Service Center GmbH
Europaplatz 3, 69115 Heidelberg, Germany

Printed by Libri Plureos GmbH
in Hamburg, Germany